S0-DXO-641

Assistant Editors

MICHAEL E. MATLAK, M.D.

Associate Professor of Surgery and Pediatrics
Department of Surgery and Pediatrics
University of Utah College of Medicine
Full-time Staff Pediatric Surgeon
Primary Children's Medical Center
University of Utah Medical Center
Salt Lake City, Utah

GEORGE W. NIXON, M.D.

Associate Professor of Radiology
University of Utah College of Medicine
Pediatric Radiologist
Primary Children's Medical Center
Salt Lake City, Utah

MARION L. WALKER, M.D.

Assistant Professor of Neurosurgery
University of Utah College of Medicine
Chairman, Division of Pediatric Neurosurgery
Primary Children's Medical Center
Salt Lake City, Utah

EMERGENCY MANAGEMENT OF PEDIATRIC TRAUMA

THOM A. MAYER, M.D.

Clinical Assistant Professor of Pediatrics
and Emergency Medicine
Georgetown University School of Medicine
Washington, D.C.
Director of Emergency Medicine
North Broward Hospital District
Ft. Lauderdale, Florida

1985

W. B. SAUNDERS COMPANY

Philadelphia London Toronto
Mexico City Rio de Janeiro Sydney Tokyo

W. B. Saunders Company: West Washington Square
Philadelphia, PA 19105

1 St. Anne's Road
Eastbourne, East Sussex BN21 3UN, England

1 Goldthorne Avenue
Toronto, Ontario M8Z 5T9, Canada

Apartado 26370—Cedro 512
Mexico 4, D.F., Mexico

Rua Coronel Cabrita, 8
Sao Cristovao Caixa Postal 21176
Rio de Janeiro, Brazil

9 Waltham Street
Artarmon, N.S.W. 2064, Australia

Ichibancho, Central Bldg., 22-1 Ichibancho
Chiyoda-Ku, Tokyo 102, Japan

Library of Congress Cataloging in Publication Data

Mayer, Thom A.
Emergency management of pediatric trauma.

1. Pediatric emergencies. 2. Children—Wounds and injuries. 3. Chronic diseases in children. I. Title. [DNLM: 1. Chronic Disease—in infancy & childhood. 2. Emergencies—in infancy & childhood. 3. Wounds and Injuries—complications. 4. Wounds and Injuries—in infancy & childhood. WS 200 M468e]

RJ370.M39 1985 618.92′0025 84–14039

ISBN 0–7216–6189–0

Emergency Management of Pediatric Trauma ISBN 0–7216–6189–0

Last digit is the print number: 9 8 7 6 5 4 3 2 1

To my wife, Maureen,
my son, Josh,
and my parents, Jim and Bette

Their love has sustained me in all endeavors

CONTRIBUTORS

JEROME E. ADAMSON, M.D.

Professor and Residency Program Director, Department of Surgery and Plastic Surgery, Eastern Virginia Medical School, Norfolk, Virginia

Hand Injuries

JOANN ATER, M.D.

Assistant Clinical Professor of Pediatrics, University of Colorado School of Medicine; Attending Oncologist, Children's Hospital of Denver, Denver, Colorado

Injuries to Children with Hematologic Disorders

CHARLES L. BRORING, D.D.S., F.A.C.D., F.I.C.D.

Associate Professor and Chairman, Department of Pedodontics, Georgetown University School of Dentistry; Chief of Dentistry, Children's Hospital National Medical Center; Attending Staff, Georgetown University Hospital, Washington, D.C.

Dental Injuries

BRUCE A. BUEHLER, M.D.

Director, Meyer Children's Rehabilitation Institute; Director, Center for Human Genetics; Associate Professor of Pediatrics and Pathology, University of Nebraska Medical Center, Omaha, Nebraska

Injuries to Children with Endocrine and Metabolic Disease

JUDITH G. CHEEK, M.D.

Clinical Faculty, Georgetown University Hospital; Associate Faculty, Sibley Memorial Hospital; Courtesy Faculty, Columbia Hospital for Women, Washington, D.C.

Sexual Abuse of Children

JOHN L. COLOMBO, M.D.

Assistant Professor of Pediatrics, Director of Pediatric Pulmonology, Active Staff, University of Nebraska Medical Center; Consulting Staff, Medical Director, Respiratory Therapy, Children's Memorial Hospital, Omaha, Nebraska

Injuries to Children with Chronic Lung Disease

T. PETER DOWNING, M.D.

Chief Resident Associate, Department of Cardiothoracic Surgery, Mayo Clinic, Rochester, Minnesota

Vascular Injuries

GREGORY S. GEORGIADE, M.D.

Assistant Professor of Surgery, Duke University School of Medicine; Director, Burn Unit, Assistant Director, Trauma Services, Duke University Medical Center, Durham, North Carolina

Burns

J. ALEX HALLER, Jr., M.D., F.A.C.S., F.A.A.P.

Robert Garrett Professor of Pediatric Surgery, The Johns Hopkins University School of Medicine; Children's Surgery-in-Charge, Johns Hopkins Hospital, Baltimore, Maryland

Organization of a Regional Pediatric Trauma and Emergency Center

RICHARD B. JAFFE, M.D.

Associate Professor of Radiology, University of Utah College of Medicine; Pediatric Radiologist, Primary Children's Medical Center, Salt Lake City, Utah

Radiographic Evaluation of the Injured Child

KENT W. JONES, M.D.

Clinical Associate Professor of Surgery, University of Utah College of Medicine; Clinical Staff, Latter-Day Saints Hospital; Clinical Staff, Primary Children's Medical Center; Clinical Associate Professor of Surgery, University of Utah Medical Center; Consultant, Veterans Administration Hospital, Salt Lake City, Utah

Thoracic Trauma

DAVID L. KERNS, M.D.

Medical Director for Ambulatory Services, Children's Hospital Medical Center of Northern California, Oakland, California

Child Abuse

MICHAEL E. MATLAK, M.D., F.A.C.S., F.A.A.P.

Associate Professor of Surgery and Pediatrics, Department of Surgery and Pediatrics, University of Utah College of Medicine; Full-time Staff, Pediatric Surgery, Primary Children's Medical Center and University of Utah Medical Center, Salt Lake City, Utah

Abdominal Injuries; Genitourinary Injuries in Children; Foreign Bodies

THOM A. MAYER, M.D.

Clinical Assistant Professor of Pediatrics and Emergency Medicine, Georgetown University School of Medicine, Washington, D.C.; Director of Emergency Medicine, North Broward Hospital District; Chief Medical Officer and Executive Vice President, The Coastal Group, Inc., Ft. Lauderdale, Florida

Initial Evaluation and Management of the Injured Child; Management of Hypovolemic Shock; Intensive Care Monitoring; Head Injuries; Genitourinary Injuries in Children; Animal, Snake, and Insect Bites; Transportation of the Injured Child; Care of the Injured Child in the General Emergency Department

RICHARD G. MIDDLETON, M.D.

Professor of Surgery, Chairman, Division of Urology, University of Utah College of Medicine; Chief of Urology, University of Utah Medical Center, Salt Lake City, Utah

Genitourinary Injuries in Children

JOSEPH MOYLAN, M.D.

Professor of Surgery, Duke University School of Medicine; Chief of Trauma Services, Duke University Medical Center, Durham, North Carolina

Burns

LEONARD B. NELSON, M.D.

Associate Professor of Ophthalmology and Pediatrics, Jefferson Medical College of Thomas Jefferson University; Assistant Surgeon, Pediatric Ophthalmology, Wills Eye Hospital, Philadelphia, Pennsylvania

Eye Injuries

GEORGE W. NIXON, M.D.

Associate Professor of Radiology, University of Utah College of Medicine; Pediatric Radiologist, Primary Children's Medical Center, Salt Lake City, Utah

Radiographic Evaluation of the Injured Child; Genitourinary Injuries in Children

RICHARD T. O'BRIEN, M.D.

Professor of Pediatrics, University of Utah College of Medicine; Attending Pediatric Hematologist, Primary Children's Medical Center and University of Utah Medical Center, Salt Lake City, Utah

Injuries to Children with Hematologic Disorders

GARTH ORSMOND, M.B., B.Ch., F.C.P.

Associate Professor of Pediatrics, University of Utah College of Medicine; Director of Echocardiography, Primary Children's Medical Center, Salt Lake City, Utah

Injuries to Children with Chronic Cardiac Disease

ROBERT L. RAYBURN, M.D.

Assistant Clinical Professor of Anesthesiology and Pediatrics, University of Utah College of Medicine; Staff Anesthesiologist and Pediatrician, Primary Children's Medical Center, Salt Lake City, Utah

Ventilatory Therapy, Anesthesia, and Respiratory Support

ROBERT B. SALTER, O.C., M.D., M.S., F.R.C.S.C.

Professor and Head of Orthopedic Surgery, University of Toronto Faculty of Medicine; Senior Orthopedic Surgeon, Hospital for Sick Children, Toronto, Ontario, Canada

Musculoskeletal Injuries

ITZHAK I. SHASHA, M.D.

Attending Surgeon, Department of Surgery, Good Samaritan Hospital, West Palm Beach, Florida

Intensive Care Monitoring

RICHARD L. SIEGLER, M.D.

Associate Professor of Pediatrics, Director, Division of Nephrology and Hypertension, University of Utah College of Medicine; Director, Intermountain Pediatric-Adolescent Renal Disease Program, University Hospital; Attending Physician, University Hospital and Primary Children's Medical Center, Salt Lake City, Utah

Fluid and Electrolyte Management; Nutritional Support; Post-Traumatic Renal Failure; Injuries to Children with Chronic Renal Disease

CLIFFORD C. SNYDER, M.D.

Professor and Chairman, Division of Plastic Surgery, University of Utah College of Medicine; Chief of Plastic Surgery, Shriners Hospital for Crippled Children, Salt Lake City, Utah

Animal, Snake, and Insect Bites

THOMAS E. SPICER, M.D., F.A.C.S.

Assistant Professor, University of Texas Health Science Center at Dallas; Attending Physician, Parkland Memorial Hospital, Children's Medical Center, Baylor University Medical Center, Dallas, Texas

Facial and Soft Tissue Trauma in Childhood

BRUCE B. STORRS, M.D.

Assistant Professor of Neurosurgery, University of Utah College of Medicine; Attending Neurosurgeon, Primary Children's Medical Center, Salt Lake City, Utah

Spinal Cord Injury; Head Injuries

ANTHONY R. TEMPLE, M.D.

Adjunct Associate Professor, Department of Pediatrics, University of Pennsylvania; Clinical Staff, Children's Hospital of Philadelphia, Philadelphia, Pennsylvania; Medical Director, McNeil Consumer Products Co., Fort Washington, Pennsylvania

Poisoning

JOEL THOMPSON, M.D.

Associate Professor of Pediatrics and Neurology, Division of Pediatric Neurology, University of Utah College of Medicine and Primary Children's Medical Center, Salt Lake City, Utah

Near Drowning

MARION L. WALKER, M.D.

Assistant Professor of Neurosurgery, University of Utah College of Medicine; Chairman, Division of Pediatric Neurosurgery, Primary Children's Medical Center, Salt Lake City, Utah

Spinal Cord Injury; Head Injuries

PREFACE

Caring for a seriously injured child presents an ambiguous challenge to the physician, as well as to all other members of the health care team. Successfully evaluating and treating pediatric trauma patients can be extremely rewarding both professionally and personally. However, provision of such care is also extremely demanding for several reasons. In many cases, the physician responsible for the initial diagnosis and treatment may not have had extensive experience and training in pediatric trauma. Although trauma is responsible for over half of all deaths in children between ages one and fifteen years and causes nearly one third of deaths in children less than one year of age, these injuries are spread over so large a population base and geographic area that it is uncommon for any single physician or treatment facility to have extensive experience in caring for pediatric trauma victims.

There are numerous and significant differences between adult and pediatric trauma patients that preclude a totally unified approach to diagnosis and treatment in these two groups of patients. A working familiarity of these differences is frequently necessary if optimal care is to be provided to the pediatric patient. Furthermore, although the care of all seriously ill or injured patients can be emotionally taxing, there are few experiences more demanding than caring for a mortally wounded child. Finally, there is a precariously thin margin for error in caring for injured children, which requires that the physician be familiar with the appropriate elements of evaluation and resuscitation. Thus, although providing emergency care to injured children can be among the most satisfying of personal, professional, and emotional experiences, it is also among the most challenging.

The major causes of pediatric trauma include motor vehicle accidents, auto–pedestrian collisions, fires, falls, poisonings, and child abuse. It should therefore not be surprising that the majority of pediatric trauma victims present to local hospitals in the community in which these injuries occur. For this reason, the initial evaluation and therapy of these patients are usually provided by emergency physicians, pediatricians, family practitioners, general surgeons, and surgical subspecialists in the community. Although some patients are transferred to regional centers with specialists in pediatric emergency medicine, pediatric critical care, and pediatric surgery, the vast majority of care is necessarily provided in the local setting. More importantly, the initial resuscitation and evaluation of these patients are critical aspects of their care and are provided most commonly by emergency physicians and pediatricians. Thus, any physician who cares for pediatric trauma victims should be readily familiar with the principles of pediatric trauma resuscitation, evaluation, and diagnosis.

This textbook is intended to be a resource for all physicians caring for injured children, regardless of whether their training has been in pediatrics, emergency medicine, family practice, surgery, or surgical subspecialties (including pediatric surgery). The specific goals of this textbook include the following:

1. Provide a comprehensive, yet accessible, source of information on the evaluation, resuscitation, and therapy of major pediatric trauma.

2. Provide specific details on evaluation and management of minor pediatric trauma.

3. Provide an approach to evaluation and therapy of injuries to specific areas of the body, as well as specific types of injuries.

4. In conjunction with the preceding, provide the physician with sufficient knowledge of definitive care of the injury. Such details of definitive care are not intended to be exhaustive in nature but are included to ensure that the physician responsible for initial evaluation and treatment is aware of the need for specific consultation and therapy. Addressing this goal also assists the physician in communicating clearly, appropriately, and concisely with the family regarding the need for definitive therapy.

5. Provide appropriate references on the organization and management of pediatric trauma care within the emergency department. Thus, in addition to familiarizing the physician with the principles of pediatric trauma care, the textbook is intended to provide information on equipment needs, transportation systems, logistics of care, drug dosages, and so forth.

In order to meet these goals, the editor has asked over thirty physician authors to contribute to this textbook, each of whom is an extremely experienced and well-trained provider of emergency care to children. Most of the authors are either clinical or basic science researchers who have published extensively on various aspects of pediatric or pediatric surgical care. The authors were specifically informed of the goals of this text and were asked to address the practical needs of the physician responsible for the initial evaluation, diagnosis, and treatment of these patients.

As with any multiauthored text, it was necessary to accommodate a broad range of styles and of personal communication. In addition, because this textbook will likely be consulted as a reference on specific areas of interest, as opposed to being read from "front to back," there are a number of necessary repetitions in it. For example, because certain aspects of initial evaluation and treatment are critical to understanding the pathophysiology and care of a number of different types of injuries, there are references to these subjects in a number of chapters, including those on anesthesia, shock, head injury, thoracic injury, poisonings, and so on. However, the first chapter provides a detailed approach to overall systems management of initial evaluation, resuscitation, and therapy. Furthermore, when repetition has been necessary, the editor has striven for consistency among the chapters. Because a number of areas in pediatric trauma are the subjects of continuing controversy, the authors have addressed such controversy directly, with appropriate references for each side of the question. However, in most cases, the authors have also indicated a preferred method of diagnosis and/or treatment.

The textbook is divided into four sections, the first of which provides a comprehensive approach to the evaluation and management of the injured child. This includes a chapter detailing a protocol approach to resuscitation, evaluation, and initial therapy. For the most part, this chapter includes most of the information on technical procedures, such as cardiac resuscitation, endotracheal intubation, venous access, surgical control of the airway, tube thoracostomy, and so on. Additional chapters address the topics of pediatric shock, anesthesia and respiratory support, fluid and electrolyte management, intensive care unit monitoring, nutritional therapy, and post-traumatic renal failure. The final chapter of the initial section eloquently describes the radiologic evaluation of the child; it includes a discussion of specific differences between pediatric and adult patients.

Because of numerous diagnostic and therapeutic advances over the past several years, many children with severe chronic diseases are now able to lead more active lives, which has led to their exposure to a variety of forms of pediatric trauma. It is not uncommon to see patients with such chronic diseases present to the emergency department with major or minor injuries. In many cases, this represents a significant challenge in addressing both the acute injury and the implications for the chronic disease process. For this reason, the second section addresses the care of children with injuries and chronic diseases, including cardiac, hematologic, endocrine/metabolic, renal, and pulmonary disorders.

The third section of the textbook contains chapters on injuries to specific body areas (spinal cord, thorax, head, abdomen, etc.), as well as on specific types of injury (burns, child abuse, sexual abuse, poisonings, near drowning, etc.). Each of these chapters is carefully cross-referenced, both to chapters within the same section and to those in the section on initial evaluation and management. Most importantly, each author has specifically focused on practical details of interest to the emergency physicians, pediatricians, and surgeons who are responsible for the initial care of the injured patient. Specific attention has been focused on identifying injuries of sufficient severity to require consultation with specialists.

The fourth section of the book covers elements of organization and management of pediatric trauma care, including concepts of regional trauma centers, transportation of the injured child, and specific elements of caring for the injured child in the general emergency department.

Finally, to the extent that the textbook is successful in attaining its goals, the authors and assistant editors deserve full credit. I accept full responsibility for any errors of commission or omission and enthusiastically welcome comments or criticisms concerning the textbook.

THOM A. MAYER, M.D.

ACKNOWLEDGMENTS

Preparation and compilation of a textbook such as this requires the combined efforts of a large number of people with a broad range of talents. It is with great pleasure and a deep sense of personal satisfaction that I acknowledge the efforts of the Assistant Editors, Michael E. Matlak, M.D., George W. Nixon, M.D., and Marion L. Walker, M.D. Their patience with the long hours of consultation necessary to integrate the efforts of the authors was exceeded only by their enthusiasm and warm support of this project.

To the contributing authors goes the credit for any success the textbook might achieve. Each author is an extremely well respected and busy clinician caring for pediatric patients; most are also active in teaching and research. Their willingness to spend the long hours necessary for preparation of their chapters could only have come at the expense of their personal time and that of their families. In addition, each contributor kindly and graciously accepted editorial suggestions and, in some cases, revisions. Of particular note were the numerous contributions of Richard L. Siegler, M.D., who contributed four chapters to the textbook, during which time he also served as Acting Chairman of the Department of Pediatrics at the University of Utah. Despite the burden of numerous clinical and administrative responsibilities, he contributed eloquent and insightful chapters that greatly enhance the textbook.

In keeping with Hippocrates' dictum to "honor him who teaches you the art," a profound debt of gratitude is owed to the mentors who gave me a deep respect for scholarly pursuits. These include Harry McGoon, Enos Pray, Ph.D., Madison Spach, M.D., David C. Sabiston, Jr., M.D., the late Lowell A. Glasgow, M.D., and Dale G. Johnson, M.D.

I am particularly grateful to John Bernard Henry, M.D., an exemplary scientist, physician, educator, editor, and father-in-law. I relied on him regularly and heavily for advice on the multiple details involved in editing a medical textbook.

The majority of the medical illustrations were produced by Dwight D. Collman, M.D., my friend, colleague, and medical illustrator for many years. His illustrations are an important and significant part of the book.

I am grateful to Paul Laughlin, M.D., Raymond L. Cohen, M.D., Edward Cestaric, M.D., and Owen Chadwick, M.D., and others for reviewing several chapters and offering their insightful suggestions.

For her sustained loyalty, meticulous attention to detail, and patience in accepting numerous revisions, I express my deepest appreciation to Therese Bottiglieri. Her dedication and hard work have made this project much more enjoyable. In addition, Mrs. Jerry Powell was kind enough to lend her gracious support in preparing a number of the original manuscripts.

To my partner, Steven M. Scott, M.D., goes my deepest appreciation for his kind understanding and support of my long preoccupation with this textbook.

During the course of the preparation of this book, I was fortunate in having the expert assistance of three highly professional, gracious, and competent medical editors of the W. B. Saunders Company. Mary Cowell was instrumental in the development and initial stages of this project. It could not have been developed without her assistance. Linda Belfus was responsible for overseeing the majority of the manuscript preparation and submission, as well as numerous other details pertaining to the preparation of this work. It is difficult to overstate the role she played in bringing the book to print, as well as in making the entire process much more enjoyable. Finally, Carroll Cann was responsible for ably handling the final stages of textbook preparation. Finally, my sincere thanks to my wife, Maureen, who patiently accepted the long hours required for the editorial process. In addition, she offered numerous suggestions, which greatly clarified the text.

THOM A. MAYER, M.D.

CONTENTS

SECTION I
Evaluation and General Management of the Injured Child 1

CHAPTER 1
Initial Evaluation and Management of the Injured Child 1
Thom A. Mayer

CHAPTER 2
Management of Hypovolemic Shock 39
Thom A. Mayer

CHAPTER 3
Ventilatory Therapy, Anesthesia, and Respiratory Support 52
Robert L. Rayburn

CHAPTER 4
Fluid and Electrolyte Management 98
Richard L. Siegler

CHAPTER 5
Intensive Care Monitoring 113
Thom A Mayer and Itzhak I. Shasha

CHAPTER 6
Nutritional Support 125
Richard L. Siegler

CHAPTER 7
Post-Traumatic Renal Failure 139
Richard L. Siegler

CHAPTER 8
Radiographic Evaluation of the Injured Child 160
George W. Nixon and Richard B. Jaffe

SECTION II
Trauma to Children with Chronic Disease 205

CHAPTER 9
Injuries to Children with Chronic Cardiac Disease 205
Garth Orsmond

CHAPTER 10
Injuries to Children with Hematologic Disorders 216
Richard T. O'Brien and Joann Ater

CHAPTER 11
Injuries to Children with Endocrine and Metabolic Disease 226
Bruce A. Buehler

CHAPTER 12
Injuries to Children with Chronic Renal Disease 233
Richard L. Siegler

CHAPTER 13
Injuries to Children with Chronic Lung Diseases 241
John L. Colombo

SECTION III
Specific Types of Trauma 249

CHAPTER 14
Spinal Cord Injury 249
Bruce B. Storrs and Marion L. Walker

CHAPTER 15
Thoracic Trauma 254
Kent W. Jones

CHAPTER 16
Head Injuries 272
Marion L. Walker, Bruce B. Storrs, and Thom A. Mayer

CHAPTER 17
Facial and Soft Tissue Trauma in Childhood 287
T. E. Spicer

CHAPTER 18
Eye Injuries 301
Leonard B. Nelson

CHAPTER 19
Dental Injuries 317
Charles L. Broring

CHAPTER 20
Abdominal Injuries 328
Michael E. Matlak

CHAPTER 21
Genitourinary Injuries in Children 341
Richard G. Middleton, Michael E. Matlak, George W. Nixon, and Thom A. Mayer

CHAPTER 22
Musculoskeletal Injuries 353
Robert B. Salter

CHAPTER 23
Hand Injuries 390
Jerome E. Adamson

CHAPTER 24
Vascular Injuries 406
T. Peter Downing

CHAPTER 25
Burns 413
Gregory S. Georgiade and Joseph Moylan

CHAPTER 26
Child Abuse 421
David L. Kerns

CHAPTER 27
Sexual Abuse of Children 435
Judith G. Cheek

CHAPTER 28
Poisoning 444
A. R. Temple

CHAPTER 29
Near Drowning 459
Joel Thompson

CHAPTER 30
Animal, Snake, and Insect Bites 466
Clifford C. Snyder and Thom A. Mayer

CHAPTER 31
Foreign Bodies 484
Michael Matlak

SECTION IV
Organization and Management of Pediatric Emergency Care 501

CHAPTER 32
Organization of a Regional Pediatric Trauma and Emergency Center 501
J. Alex Haller, Jr.

CHAPTER 33
Transportation of the Injured Child 508
Thom A. Mayer

CHAPTER 34
Care of the Injured Child in the General Emergency Department 524
Thom A. Mayer

Index 534

SECTION

I Evaluation and General Management of the Injured Child

CHAPTER

1 Initial Evaluation and Management of the Injured Child

THOM A. MAYER

Unlike many other medical problems, the care of children with serious injuries does not afford the luxury of casual contemplation or a search for appropriate references for assistance. Children with serious injuries require rapid assessment and treatment in order to preserve life and limb. Perhaps no other emergency creates as much anxiety as that of a critically injured child. The notoriously thin margin for error in caring for critically ill children; the smaller total blood volumes of children; the fact that pulse and respiratory rates, blood pressure, and drug dosages vary with age; and the relative inexperience of most physicians in caring for children with trauma account in part for this uneasiness. It is precisely for these reasons that preparation is vital if the disability and death so often associated with trauma are to be circumvented.

This chapter presents a protocol approach to the care of injured children, the central aim of which is to provide concise and practical information on the initial evaluation, resuscitation, and stabilization of the injured child. It is divided into sections that correspond to the priorities of evaluation and treatment. The *primary survey* assesses the following: *A*irway (with cervical spine protection), *B*reathing, *C*irculation, and *D*iagnosis and treatment of shock. Appropriate resuscitative measures must be instituted when indicated, concurrently with the primary survey. Thus, the primary survey and resuscitative phase occur simultaneously. Resuscitation includes provision of a patent airway with adequate ventilation, control of hemorrhage, and detection and treatment of shock. Regional evaluation in the *secondary survey* provides systematic assessment of each body area: thorax, head and neck, abdomen, genitourinary tract, skin, and extremities. As in the primary survey, the regional evaluation of the secondary survey may need to be interrupted in order to provide emergency treatment. For example, a child in an auto-pedestrian collision requires assessment of the airway, breathing, and circulation and consideration of the possibility of the presence of shock. During this initial phase, the patient may need to be intubated or even have external cardiac massage applied. During the survey of the chest, a tension pneumothorax may be diagnosed, requiring immediate treatment. Whenever either the primary or secondary survey is interrupted to provide treatment, the physician must return to the same point in the systematic assessment of the patient following such treatment. This assures that no body area will fail to be evaluated and that evaluation and treatment occur according to the potential threat to life.

Although no systematic national pediatric trauma registry currently exists, several studies estimate that approximately 80 per cent of pediatric trauma are due to blunt injuries.[1, 2] Motor vehicle accidents, auto-pedestrian collisions, burns, and falls constitute the majority of these injuries.[3, 4] Penetrating trauma constitutes 20 per cent or less of total childhood injuries and is much more common in urban areas and among older children.[4] Thus blunt trauma is emphasized in the following discussion.

PRIMARY SURVEY—RESUSCITATIVE MEASURES

Airway and Breathing

The first priority in caring for the injured child is establishing a patent airway with adequate ventilation. This begins with careful positioning of the head and neck. Every seriously injured child should be assumed to

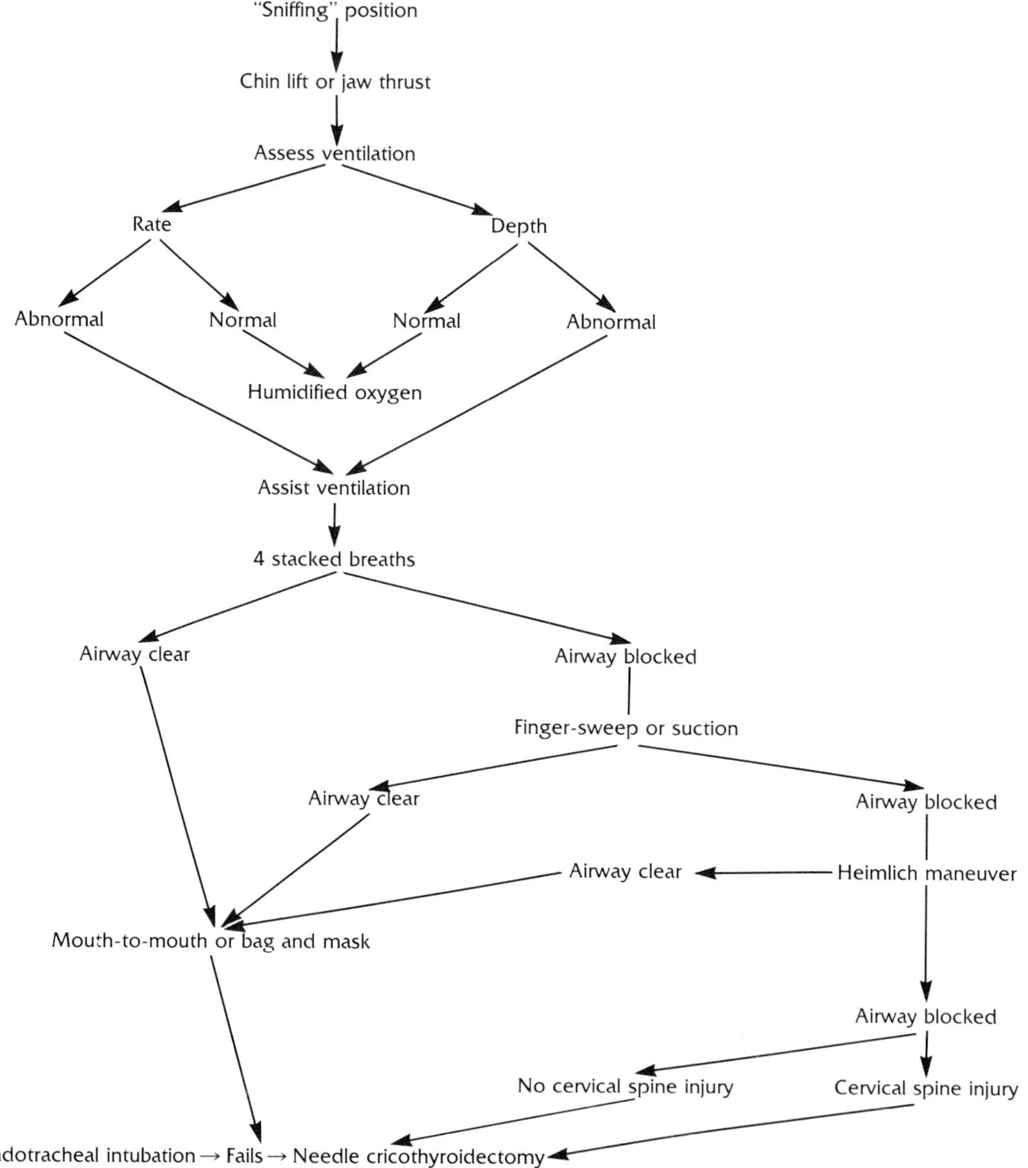

Figure 1–1. Flow sheet for airway management in pediatric patients.

have a cervical spine injury until proved otherwise. Although cervical spine injuries are much less common in children than in adults, precautions should nonetheless be taken to protect the cervical spine by means of "sandbags and tape," a back board, a rigid cervical collar, or Gardner-Wells tongs. Clearly, establishment of an airway is the highest priority, but consideration should simultaneously be given to cervical spine injury. The emphasis should not be on definitive treatment of the injury at this time, but rather on providing stability to the cervical spine while providing an airway. Gentle longitudinal traction on the head during airway manipulation is necessary to prevent the devastating sequelae that may result from cervical spine fracture. Immobilization of the neck with sandbags or rigid cervical collars may also be necessary.

Steps of Emergency Airway Control

Airway Positioning

A flow sheet for airway management is presented in Figure 1–1. The child should be placed in the "sniffing" position, which is classically described as that with the neck slightly flexed on the chest and the head slightly extended on the neck (Fig. 1–2). In practical terms, the occiput of the head should first be slightly raised above the level of the shoulders. This is easily accomplished by placing a folded towel or the rescuer's hand under the victim's head. Second, one hand should be placed at the angle of the mandible, with gentle forward pressure exerted (jaw thrust), since in the unconscious patient the mandible is relaxed and posterior displacement of the tongue may produce airway obstruction. Foreign matter should be quickly removed with a finger-sweep or gentle suction.

Ventilation Assessment

The rescuer's cheek should be placed near the child's mouth to feel if sufficient air movement is occurring. Further, looking at the thorax assists in determining if there is adequate chest wall expansion. Lightly moistening the rescuer's cheek may assist in detecting the small tidal volumes of infants and small children. Simultaneously, the carotid, femoral, or radial pulse should be palpated to assess the general circulatory status (see section on circulation).

This early stage in the assessment and treatment of the child is absolutely critical and is often either neglected or performed inadequately. Maintenance of a patent airway is the cornerstone of efficient resuscitation, since both ventilation and oxygenation depend on it. For this reason, proper airway positioning and assessment should be practiced either on mannikins or on volunteers.

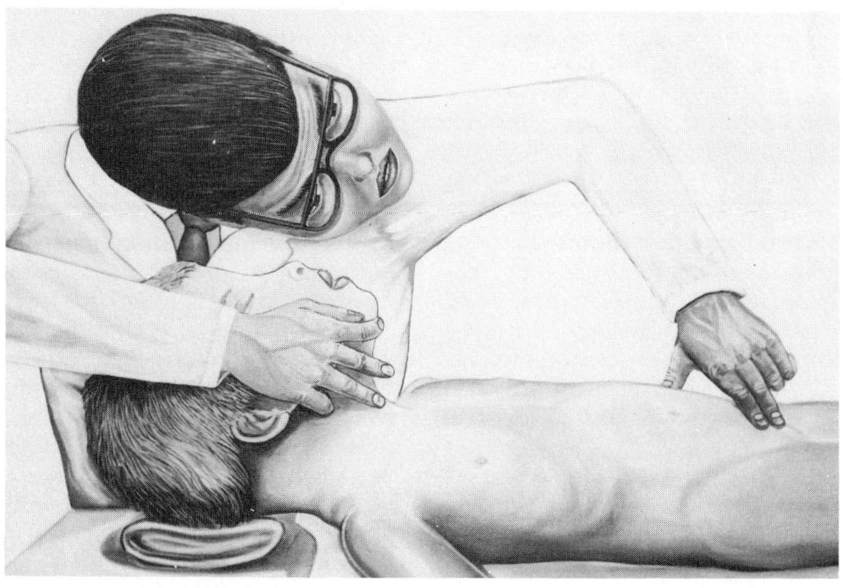

Figure 1–2. In the initial approach to the patient, an airway should be provided and ventilation and circulation should be assessed. A towel is placed under the patient's head and the right hand performs a jaw-thrust maneuver, which places the patient in the "sniffing" position. Ventilation is assessed by placing the cheek near the mouth (to assess air movement) and observing chest wall expansion. The left hand palpates the pulse to determine its strength, rate, and regularity.

Table 1–1. BASELINE CARDIORESPIRATORY VALUES IN CHILDREN

	Infants	Preschoolers	School-age
Normal respiratory rate	20–30	16–20	12–15
Maximum pulse rate	≤140	≤120	≤100

At this early stage, the rescuer is able to provide important resuscitative efforts (airway maintenance) as well as to assess critical aspects of the patient's status (ventilation and circulation.

Normal ventilation rates vary with age, as shown in Table 1–1. If the child's respiratory rate is inadequate for his age, or if spontaneous respiratory effort does not produce chest wall expansion, the child's ventilation should be supported by the most readily available means.

Mouth-to-Mouth and Bag and Mask Ventilation

Breathing support is usually provided first by mouth-to-mouth or bag and mask ventilation. Four rapid breaths, each sufficient to produce chest wall expansion, should be provided. If the chest wall does not rise with these breaths, the patient should be assumed to have airway obstruction. Reposition the patient in the sniffing position and recheck for foreign matter in the pharynx with a finger-sweep or suction. Repeat the four rapid breaths.

Blows and Thrusts

If chest wall expansion still does not occur, either four sharp back blows or four abdominal thrusts (Heimlich maneuver) should be used to clear the airway.[5] Unless cervical spine injuries can be clearly excluded, the abdominal thrust is the preferred method. The rescuer should take care to place the rescuer's hand below the xiphoid before the abdomen is compressed.

Oral and Nasal Tube Insertion

If the airway clears and spontaneous ventilation at adequate rates occurs, a plastic oral airway may be inserted if needed and if the child will accept it. Insertion of oral airways can produce vomiting or laryngospasm and the rescuer should be aware of this possibility.

Esophageal Obturator Airway. Esophageal obturator airways are available for children and may assume a role in the initial management of the airway at the scene of the accident for children over 120 cm in length. However, bag and mask ventilation is almost always the preferred alternative and nearly all children can be ventilated by the bag and mask method.

Endotracheal Tube. Indications for endotracheal intubation are the inability to adequately ventilate the child by mouth-to-mouth or bag and mask method and the need for prolonged control of the airway, including prevention of aspiration. When intubation is necessary, *preparation* is an absolute requirement. The proper-size endotracheal tube is easily selected by choosing a tube that fits comfortably in the child's nostril. An alternate method consists of choosing a tube that is approximately the same diameter as the child's little finger. Memorization of charts or formulas for proper sizing of endotracheal tubes is unnecessary and time-consuming and may be inaccurate. A stylet placed in the lumen of the tube facilitates placement and can be easily removed when the tube is in the trachea. The oropharynx should be cleared of secretions and foreign matter by a suction catheter. Prior to interrupting ventilation for an attempt at intubation, the laryngoscope should be checked to assure that it functions properly. In-line traction of the cervical spine should be maintained, and the head and neck should remain in the sniffing position.

Several rapid breaths should be given prior to the intubation attempt. Assisted ventilation should *never* be interrupted for more than 30 seconds for any reason. If an endotracheal tube cannot be placed within 30 seconds, ventilation should be resumed for several minutes prior to a second attempt at intubation. After the tube has been placed, the rescuer should auscultate both lung fields and observe for symmetric chest expansion to insure placement of the tube in the trachea. In infants and children it is extremely easy for the endotracheal tube to slide into the right mainstem bronchus, producing atelectasis and further decreasing ventilation. After assessment by auscultation and observation of chest expansion, the tube should be secured to the upper lip with tincture of benzoin and adhesive tape until tube position is verified by chest roentgenogram.

Ventilation should be continued by means of a pediatric anesthesia bag through the endotracheal tube at appropriate rates (see Table 1–2) and with sufficient tidal volume to produce chest wall expansion. Humidified oxygen should also be delivered. However, oxygen is not the cure for any traumatic disease. It is vital to find and appropriately treat the cause of inadequate ventilation immediately after providing a patent airway. Further information on pediatric airway maintenance is presented in Chapter 3.

Gastric Tube. In any child undergoing assisted ventilation, a gastric tube should be placed and gastric air and secretions should be evacuated by suction, since gastric distention routinely follows artificial ventilation. Owing to differences between chest wall compliance and diaphragmatic excursion in children, gastric distention may greatly impair ventilation, even when endotracheal intubation has been performed. An otherwise efficient resuscitation may be unsuccessful because the effects of gastric distention have not been prevented. Further, emptying the stomach contents may prevent aspiration and bradycardia produced by vagal stimulation.

A nasogastric tube is usually placed, unless there has been sufficient head or facial trauma to raise the question of cribriform plate fracture, in which case the tube should be passed through the mouth. A double-lumen tube* is preferred inasmuch as it can be easily cleared of particulate matter and thick secretions. Function of the gastric tube is best assured by injecting 10 to 15 cc of normal saline through the tube and verifying that a similar quantity can be aspirated.

Surgical Opening of the Airway

If the airway is still obstructed after the preceding measures, direct injury to the larynx or trachea may be the cause. However, these injuries are extremely unusual in children, rendering cricothyroidotomy or tracheostomy a rare necessity. The dictum "ventilate—don't operate" applies best to children. Almost all children can be adequately ventilated and oxygenated without surgical intervention. When necessary, the preferred surgical method in children is needle cricothyroidotomy, which can provide up to 30 minutes of airway control when used with jet ventilation.

Needle Cricothyroidotomy. Needle cricothyroidotomy should be performed with the patient's head in a neutral position, unless cervical spine injury has been clearly excluded, in which case slight extension may be used. After preparing the neck with antiseptic solution, one finger should be used to palpate the cricothyroid membrane in the midline, between the thyroid and cricoid cartilages (Fig. 1–3). It is imperative to stay precisely in the midline during this procedure; an assistant should always be present to hold the child's head and neck to facilitate this. Once the cricothyroid membrane has been clearly identified, a 5- to 10-cc syringe should be attached to a large (14 gauge) catheter. While palpating the cricothyroid cartilage in the midline, the rescuer should insert a catheter just below the midpoint of the cricothyroid membrane, with the needle angled 45 degrees caudally. Rapid aspiration of air into the syringe indicates entry into the tracheal lumen. The stylet should be carefully withdrawn while advancing the catheter caudally into the trachea, taking care not to perforate the posterior tracheal wall. Recheck the position of the catheter by again aspirating on the syringe. The hub of the catheter should be attached to a 3.5-mm pediatric endotracheal tube adapter. Bag ventilation can be delivered by this means or by connecting a high-flow oxygen source with a Y-connector between the oxygen source and cannula. Intermittent ventilation can be delivered by occluding the open port of the Y-connector with the thumb. This technique allows 30 to 45 minutes of ventilation and is thus a temporizing measure. Great care should be taken to ensure that the catheter remains patent, and arterial blood gases should be measured to ensure that oxygenation and ventilation are being provided.

*Andersen #11, Andersen Company, Cincinnati, Ohio.

Circulation

Determining circulatory status occurs simultaneously with assessment of the airway and breathing. Palpation of the carotid, femoral, or radial pulse may be accomplished during proper airway positioning. Although maintenance of a patent airway with adequate ventilation is the first priority, effective circulation is also a critical consideration. Circulatory assessment should include palpation of the pulse for quality (weak or strong), rate, and regularity and assessment of skin color and capillary refill. The last-named test is easily performed by pressing on the hypothenar eminence, nail beds, or mucous membranes and observing the time required for return of skin color. Under normal circumstances, the color should return

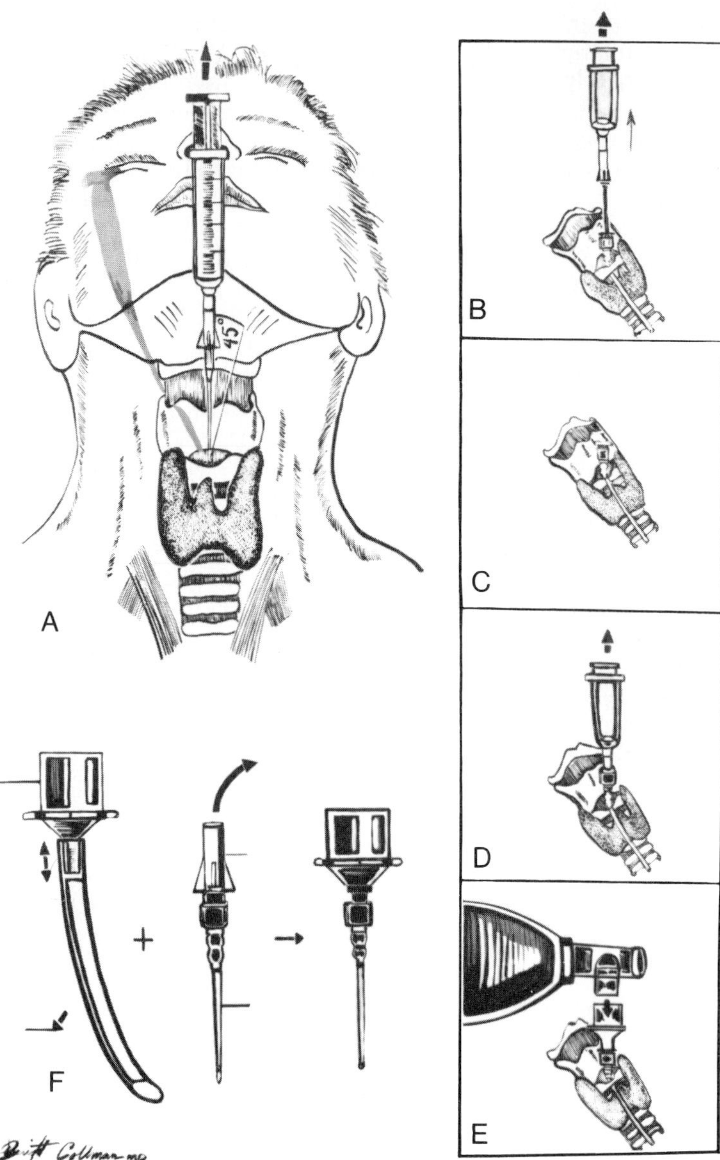

Figure 1–3. Needle cricothyroidotomy. *A,* The cricothyroid cartilage is palpated *in the midline,* between the thyroid and cricoid cartilage, and is punctured at a 45-degree angle with a 5- or 10-cc syringe attached to a 14-gauge catheter. *B,* As the catheter is advanced, the syringe should be aspirated, with free and rapid entry of air into the syringe indicating position in the trachea. *C,* After initial entry into the trachea, the catheter is carefully advanced distally. *D,* After the catheter is advanced, tracheal position should be carefully rechecked by again aspirating the syringe. *E,* Ventilation is provided either by bag and mask (as shown) or by jet ventilation. *F,* A 3.5-mm pediatric endotracheal tube adapter fits easily into the hub of the catheter, allowing ventilation.

within 2 seconds. If the child has been in a cold environment, refill on the extremities may be prolonged, in which case it should be assessed on the mucous membranes.

Cardiac Arrest

The traumatized child with an adequate airway but no pulse should be assumed to be in cardiac arrest. Cardiac arrest in injured children is usually due to a combination of hypoxia and blood loss, both of which must be aggressively treated. Principles of airway management are outlined above, and a detailed discussion of blood loss and shock follows. Any injured child in cardiac arrest must have a patent airway provided, and all children with evidence of internal or external hemorrhage should receive a bolus of 20 to 40 ml/kg body weight of lactated Ringer's solution (see pages 14–16). Blood loss may not be a contributing factor to cardiac arrest in some cases, such as in a child who aspirates a foreign body. However, most cases of pediatric trauma will have both hypoxia and hemorrhage as contributing factors.

During the initial phase of care, injured children in cardiac arrest may be assumed to have the electrocardiographic findings of either asystole or ventricular fibrillation. Asystole is a much more common arrhythmia in children, largely because the mechanism

Table 1–2. CARDIOPULMONARY ARREST: BASIC SUPPORT

Resuscitative Measure	Infants	Preschoolers	School-age
Sternal compressions	100/min	80/min	60/min
Depth of compressions	½–¾ in.	¾–1½ in.	1½–2 in.
Breaths	20/min	16/min	12/min
DC countershock	25–50 w-sec	50–100 w-sec	100–300 w-sec

of arrest is usually a combination of hypoxia and blood loss. In adults, ventricular fibrillation is a more common arrhythmia, largely because of the prevalence of heart disease in that age group. When electrocardiogram monitoring is available, it should be used to guide therapy. Cardiac arrest is treated by applying 60 to 100 sternal compressions per minute (Table 1–2) while maintaining adequate ventilation. Because the ventricles of infants and small children lie slightly higher in the chest and because the left lobe of the liver lies just underneath the xiphoid process, compressions should be applied to the mid sternum and should be ½ to ¾ in. in depth. Older children require ¾ to 1 in. of sternal compression to the lower sternum. Compressions should occupy one half of the cardiac cycle time. This is accomplished by a slight pause at the end of each compression. Pulses should be palpable with each compression in the neck, groin, or antecubital fossa.[6]

A dependable intravenous (IV) line should be established (see section on venous access, pages 9–12). Every child in cardiac arrest should receive 2 mEq/kg of IV sodium bicarbonate. The IV line should be flushed with saline prior to injecting 0.1 ml/kg of epinephrine (1:10,000 solution). Catecholamines are inactivated in alkaline solutions, so the precaution of flushing IV lines prior to epinephrine administration should be closely followed.

In patients with asystole, epinephrine stimulates myocardial contractility and enhances cardiac output. In addition, fine ventricular fibrillation is often converted to coarse fibrillation by epinephrine. This latter rhythm is much more amenable to electric cardioversion. The presence of cardiac arrest indicates that at least some degree of acidosis is present; therefore, bicarbonate is usually indicated. Thus, the initial medications for treatment of cardiac arrest in injured children are bicarbonate and epinephrine (Table 1–3).

However, the presence of either alkalosis or acidosis renders the myocardium markedly less sensitive to conversion to effective function.[7] Because excessive alkali infusion may result in alkalosis, potassium imbalance, hypercarbia, and hyperosmolality, further bicarbonate should be given only at a rate of 1

Table 1–3. EMERGENCY MEDICATIONS FOR CARDIAC ARREST IN CHILDREN

Drug	Dose	Indication
Sodium bicarbonate	2 cc/kg	Asystole Ventricular fibrillation Prolonged arrest
Epinephrine (1:10,000)	0.1 cc/kg	Asystole Ventricular fibrillation
Calcium chloride (10%)	20 mg/kg (dilute to 1%)	Asystole Electromechanical dissociation
Atropine	0.01 mg/kg	Asystole Bradycardia with hypotension
Isoproterenol*	0.1 μg/kg/min	Asystole Low cardiac output
Dopamine*	5–20 μg/kg	Asystole Low cardiac output
Lidocaine	1 mg/kg (bolus) 30 μg/kg/min (infusion)	Ventricular fibrillation Ventricular tachycardia
Bretylium	5–30 mg/kg	Refractory ventricular arrhythmia

*Use *only* after vascular volume is restored.

to 2 mEq/kg for each 10 minutes the child is in cardiac arrest or as arterial blood gases indicate.

If it is impossible to administer the emergency medications intravenously, epinephrine can be given either through intramuscular injection into the base of the tongue or through the endotracheal tube. Intratracheal epinephrine should be diluted with water (not saline) prior to instillation.[8]

Medications may be given by the intracardiac route but *only* if no other route is available. Complications from intracardiac injection include hemopericardium, cardiac tamponade, coronary artery laceration, pneumothorax, delay of cardiac massage, and inadvertent injection into the myocardium.[9] Because the parasternal approach to intracardiac injection involves a higher risk of left main coronary artery laceration, the subxiphoid approach is preferred. The cardiac needle should be inserted through the skin just below and to the patient's left of the xiphoid process and aimed posteriorly toward the left scapula. Gentle aspiration on the barrel of the syringe will produce return of blood when the needle enters the right ventricle. When this occurs, the needle advance should be stopped, the syringe should be gently aspirated again to ensure position in the ventricle, and *only* then should the drug be injected.

Asystole

If the EKG shows asystole or severe bradycardia, ventilation and massage should be continued. Atropine (0.01 to 0.02 mg/kg) should be given intravenously. Bicarbonate and epinephrine doses are repeated and if asystole persists, 10 per cent calcium chloride should be diluted to 1 per cent in a syringe and be given *slowly* in a dose of 2 cc/kg (20 mg/kg). If cardiac standstill continues, an isoproterenol infusion is begun at 0.1 to 0.5 mg/kg/minute. Both isoproterenol and dopamine require a microgram per kilogram per minute dose, which may be difficult to calculate. Although charts are available to assist in providing the proper dose, these may be difficult to use in an emergency situation.

A much easier method of preparing vasopressor infusions is by using the rule of six (Fig. 1–4). Isoproterenol concentrations are calculated in the following manner: 0.6 mg/kg should be placed in a metriset and enough 5 per cent dextrose and water added to make 100 ml. When this concentration is infused through an infusion pump with a microdrip set, the number of milliliters per hour on the pump equals the numbers of tenths of micrograms per kilogram per minute of isoproterenol infused into the patient. Similarly, dopamine concentrations can be easily calculated by adding 6 mg/kg to enough 5 per cent dextrose in water to equal 100 ml. Infusions through an infusion pump and microdrip set result in milliliters per hour on the pump equaling micrograms per kilogram per minute of dopamine infused into the patient.

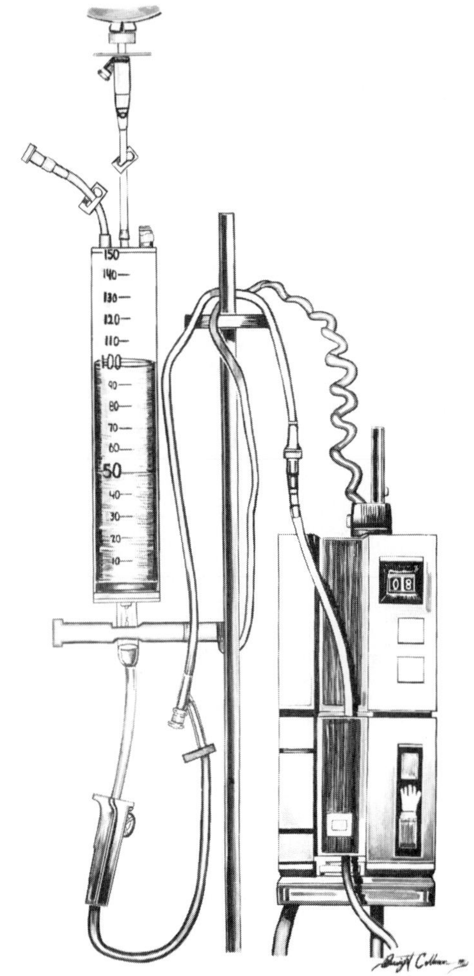

Figure 1–4. The rule of six method for dopamine and isoproterenol infusions. See text below for explanation.

If the preceding measures have not been successful, transvenous or transthoracic pacemaker insertion may be attempted, but the use of either method is rarely successful in asystole. Patients whose cardiac rhythm converts to bradycardia with hypotension may require atropine (0.01 mg/kg).

Ventricular Fibrillation

Ventricular fibrillation is rarer than asystole in pediatric trauma patients but may be present as either fine or coarse fibrillation. It is treated by immediate direct current (DC) countershock with 2 to 5 watt/seconds/kg, followed by bicarbonate and epinephrine administration. If the weight is not known or cannot be easily estimated, the current should be applied at 25 to 50 watt/seconds in infants, 50 to 100 watt/seconds in young children, and 100 to 300 watt/seconds in older children (see Table 1–2). If defibrillation is not affected with these doses, the current should be increased.

If fibrillation persists for 10 seconds after defibrillation is attempted, cardiac massage is resumed. Defibrillation should then be attempted again at the higher current level. After 2 minutes, administration of bicarbonate and epinephrine is repeated, again remembering to flush the line prior to epinephrine infusion.

Paddle placement in infants and small children may be difficult, particularly when using paddles made for adults. Infant and child attachments or adapters should be available for all defibrillators. If the paddles cannot be easily placed on the chest, an alternative method is to place one paddle over the precordium anteriorly, with the second paddle over the patient's back, behind the heart. This allows an effective vector to be transmitted to the myocardium and may effect cardioversion when chest placement of the paddles is unsuccessful.[10]

Although in some patients there is conversion from fibrillation to normal sinus rhythm, in many others there is conversion to asystole or other abnormal rhythms. The physician should be aware of this and should be prepared to treat any abnormal cardiac rhythm aggressively. When fibrillation recurs, lidocaine or bretylium tosylate infusion may be necessary (see Table 1–3).

Venous Access

The simplest, safest, and most rapid means of obtaining venous access is by percutaneous peripheral vein cannulation. Sites usually chosen for cannulation include the dorsum of the hand, the antecubital fossa, the saphenous vein at the ankle, and the external jugular vein in the neck. Because of the smaller size of veins in children and the fact that veins often collapse when a child is in shock, percutaneous peripheral cannulation may be difficult to perform and time-consuming. However, in most injured children, experienced physicians are able to successfully insert peripheral venous lines even in patients in profound shock.

Cannulation in small children can be facilitated by several simple steps. First, the extremity should be firmly secured to an arm or foot board, and the child should be restrained to prevent movement and inadvertent dislodgment of the catheter. Second, warm, moist compresses should be placed over the vein and a tourniquet placed proximal to the site of cannulation, whenever possible. This allows for venous dilation. Third, the catheter should be flushed with normal saline with 1 unit heparin per ml prior to the attempt at cannulation. This enables more rapid return of blood into the clear portion of the catheter when the vein is entered and may prevent puncture of the back wall of the vein. Fourth, puncturing the skin with a needle larger than the size of the catheter (e.g., a 20-gauge needle if a 22-gauge catheter will be used) may prevent both plugging of the catheter tip and shearing of the catheter as it enters the skin. Fifth, the bevel of the needle should initially be placed upward. When the vein is entered, as evidenced by the return of blood into the proximal portion of the catheter, the needle bevel should be rotated 180 degrees. This allows slightly more room for the advance of the catheter, which may be critical in preventing penetration of the back wall of the vein. Sixth, transillumination with a high intensity light is often helpful in locating veins on the extremities. Finally, application of military anti-shock trousers (MAST) may assist in increasing the filling of upper extremity veins, allowing easier cannulation. A particularly accessible vein for cannulation is the fifth interdigital vein, the position of which on the dorsum of the hand between the fourth and fifth metacarpals is quite constant in children. If percutaneous peripheral vein cannulation cannot be performed easily and rapidly, proceed to an alternative means immediately.

Alternatives to percutaneous peripheral cannulation include percutaneous central venous catheterization, peripheral venous cutdown, and intraosseous fluid infusion. Central venous lines via the subclavian, internal jugular, or femoral route are often used in adult patients when rapid venous access is needed. However, this procedure may involve significant complications, particularly when used in an emergency. Pneumothorax, tension pneumothorax, hemothorax, cardiac arrhythmias, and expanding hematoma at the puncture site are all possible complications of central venous catheterization.[11] More importantly, even large central veins may be much smaller in the patient in shock, making cannulation even more hazardous and difficult. Add to this the child's much smaller size, and the task becomes formidable. Subclavian vein catheterization in the young child may be particularly hazardous, since the risk of creating a pneumothorax is significant, particularly when the procedure is done under emergency conditions. Because the mediastinum is much more pliable and less firmly fixed to surrounding structures in infants and children, a pneumothorax may rapidly progress to a tension pneumothorax, especially when positive pressure ventilation is being applied.

A number of authorities advocate percutaneous cannulation of the femoral vein for emergency venous access in children.[11] Although this vein can be easily cannulated in the majority of cases, no studies have carefully assessed the complications from this procedure. However, avascular necrosis of the femoral head, femoral vein thrombosis, and femoral artery thrombosis (any one of which may result in shortening of the limb) have all been reported as complications of femoral vein cannulation.

For these reasons, in children under 5 years of age, percutaneous central venous cannulation should rarely be used for trauma resuscitation, except in the controlled circumstances of the operating room. Even in children over the age of 5, the procedure should be used with great caution, if at all.

Two reasons for avoiding central venous cannulation are the hazards associated with it and the fact that there are two safe, rapid, alternate methods for venous access—peripheral venous cutdown and intraosseous infusion. Several sites are available for cutdown, including the saphenous, brachial, cephalic, and external jugular veins, all of which can be easily cannulated within several minutes. The greater saphenous vein at the ankle is located 1 to 2 cm anterior and superior to the medial malleolus. This vein continues cephalad and can also be cannulated in the groin 2 to 3 cm caudal to the femoral pulse at the inguinal ligament. If the femoral pulse is not easily palpable, a line should be drawn between the anterior superior iliac spine and the pubic tubercle. The saphenous vein is located 2 to 3 cm inferior to the juncture of the medial and middle thirds of this line. The brachial vein lies 2 to 3 cm medial and superior to the medial epicondyle of the elbow. The cephalic vein is within the deltopectoral groove, or 1 to 2 cm inferior to the lateral-most aspect of the clavicle. The external jugular vein is usually visible in the neck, particularly when the child is in the Trendelenburg position. This vein runs from the angle of the jaw, crosses the midportion of the sternocleidomastoid muscle, and proceeds toward the middle of the clavicle. Most clinicians prefer to use the saphenous or brachial vein for peripheral cutdown, with the external jugular and cephalic veins less commonly used.

Regardless of the site chosen for cannulation, the technique is the same (Fig. 1–5). After preparing the skin with antiseptic and anesthetic, the physician makes a 1 to 2 cm skin incision, taking care to incise only the skin. A small curved hemostat is placed in the wound to gently probe for the vein. After the hemostat is placed underneath the vein, the instrument is gently opened to gradually free the vein from the surrounding tissue. The vein should be cleared from this surrounding tissue as well as possible because this tissue may impair cannulation. Once the vein has been dissected free for a distance of 1 to 2 cm, two strands of 4-0 absorbable suture are passed under the vein. The distal suture is tied around the most distal aspect of the vein. The proximal suture is not tied but simply provides countertraction while the vein is cannulated. A venotomy may be performed with a No. 11 scalpel blade by inserting the blade with the cutting edge up in the midportion of the vein (Fig. 1–5*F*). The tip of a hemostat may then be used to dilate the vein. However, this may result in creation of false tracts around the vein and unsuccessful cannulation. A simpler approach is to puncture the vein directly with an angiocatheter (Fig. 1–5G), advancing the catheter into the vein after puncture. When the catheter is in the vein, fluid should flow freely into the lumen. The catheter should be secured to the skin with nonabsorbable suture, and the IV tubing should be taped securely. Every physician caring for injured children must become adept at gaining access by venous cutdown. This simple and rapid method allows vascular access in many children in whom percutaneous cannulation is impossible.

As early as 1922, several reports demon-

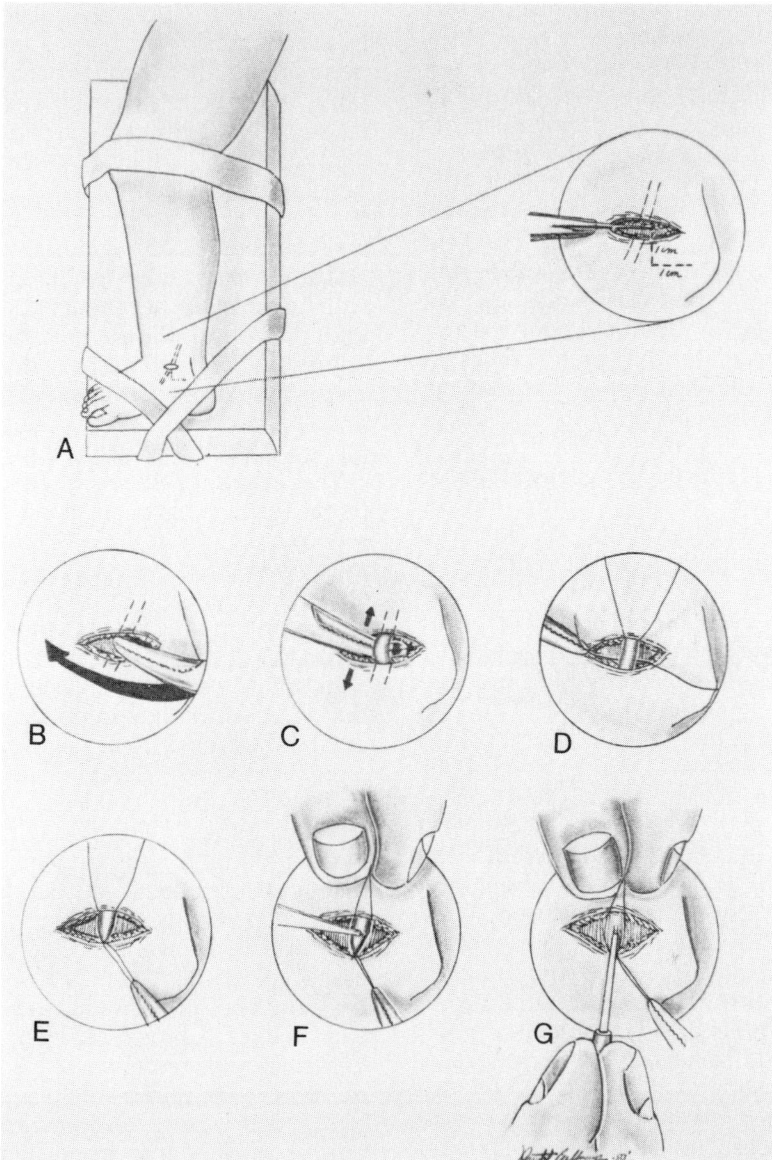

Figure 1–5. Saphenous vein cutdown. *A*, The leg is securely fastened to a foot board, and the area is prepped with antiseptic solution. A 1- to 2-cm incision is made through the skin 1 cm anterior and superior to the medial malleolus. *B*, A small curved hemostat is placed in the anterior aspect of the wound and swept toward the medial malleolus. *C*, The hemostat is used to gently dissect the vein free of fat and connective tissue. *D*, Two strands of absorbable suture are passed under the vein. *E*, The distal suture is tied around the most distal aspect of the vein, while the proximal suture simply provides counter traction while the vein is cannulated. *F*, A venotomy may be performed with a No. 11 scalpel blade by inserting the blade with the cutting edge up in the midportion. Once the vein has been entered, the tip of a hemostat may be used to dilate the vein. *G*, As an alternative, the vein may be punctured directly with an angiocatheter.

strated that bone marrow could be utilized as a route for fluid infusion.[11a] During the 1940s, numerous articles in the pediatric, anesthetic, and military literature demonstrated that crystalloids, colloids, blood, antibiotics, digitalis, heparin, insulin, anesthetic agents, epinephrine, and other sympathomimetic amines could be easily and safely infused into the marrow of the long bones.[11b–k] Bone marrow sinusoids communicate with large medullary venous channels that drain via nutrient and emissary veins into the systemic circulation.[11l] In this manner, the bone marrow functions as a noncollapsible route for venous access in the patient in shock. Furthermore, Papper[11m] demonstrated in 1942 that circulation times for IV and intraosseous injections were identical.[11m]

The advantages of intraosseous infusion are threefold. First, it is an extremely accessible route of vascular access, since the sternum, ileum, femur, or tibia may be utilized. Second, very little skill is necessary to perform the procedure. The easiest site for intraosseous infusion is the anterior tibia, just below the tibial tuberosity. After preparing the skin antiseptically and securing the leg adequately, a site is chosen on the flat, anterior portion of the tibia, 1 to 2 cm distal and slightly lateral to the tibial tuberosity. Several different types of needles may be utilized. Although a traditional bone marrow needle functions quite well, such needles are rarely kept in the emergency department. Other excellent needles are 16- to 20-gauge spinal needles, since these have a trocar to prevent the needle from being obstructed as it passes through the bony cortex into the marrow. However, any 14- to 20-gauge needle can be utilized in an emergency situation. The needle should be placed at a 90-degree angle to the bone and advanced firmly through the cortex into the marrow. Evidence that the needle is adequately within the marrow includes (1) a soft "pop" and lack of resistance after the needle has passed through the cortex, (2) aspiration of bone marrow into the needle, and (3) free flow of fluid into the marrow without evidence of subcutaneous infiltration. The needle can then be attached to standard IV tubing, and fluid, blood, or drugs may be infused.

The third advantage of intraosseous infusion is the remarkable lack of complications with the procedure. The most common complications are minimal subcutaneous infiltration of fluid and leakage from the puncture site after the needle has been removed. Although osteomyelitis and subcutaneous infections have been noted, these occur only when the intraosseous infusion is maintained for extended periods or when hypertonic fluids are infused.[11c–d]

Because intraosseous infusion is readily accessible, requires little skill, and has a low rate of complications, it should be considered for infusion of fluid, blood, and drugs during the initial minutes of resuscitation when percutaneous venous cannulation has failed to provide vascular access. This allows time for careful placement of a peripheral venous cutdown for more long-term vascular access.

Shock

Every physician who cares for injured patients must be trained to recognize the early development of shock in pediatric patients and to institute appropriate therapy.

In essence, shock, regardless of its cause, is a generalized state of inadequate tissue perfusion, which results in impaired respiration at the cellular level.[12] The development of shock is a dynamic process, involving many systems, which produce progressively developing clinical signs and symptoms of the disease. Although shock may be caused by a number of clinical entities, in the injured child, shock usually results from hypovolemia (most often secondary to hemorrhage), with or without the complication of hypoxia.

Although Chapter 2 provides a more complete discussion of the management of hypovolemic shock, recognition and initial management are addressed in this section.

The extent of shock is generally proportional to the degree of blood loss, which is reflected in physical signs and simple laboratory tests. However, if even mild shock is allowed to persist for a prolonged period, significant morbidity and mortality may result.[13]

In order to understand the classification of the degree of shock in children, a clear understanding of normal blood volume, pulse rates, and blood pressure is necessary. Compared with adults, children have larger total blood volumes.[14] For example, the average blood volume for an adult male is approximately 7 per cent of his body weight, whereas in children, a larger percentage of the total body weight is accounted for by blood volume.[15] A child's blood volume can be estimated as 85 ml/kg, regardless of the child's age. Anyone caring for injured patients should remember this figure, since transfusion requirements are dependent on total blood volume and amount and type of fluid loss. Similarly, upper limits of normal for pulse rates are dependent upon the child's age: 140 for infants, 120 for preschoolers, and 100 for school-age children. Although a large number of charts are available for determining normal blood pressure, a general estimate of normal systolic arterial pressure can be made by adding 80 to twice the child's age in years. Thus, a normal systolic blood pressure for a 5-year-old child is 90 mm Hg ($80 + [2 \times 5]$). Normal diastolic blood pressure is calculated by taking two thirds of the normal systolic pressure. These parameters should be kept in mind in the following discussion of hypovolemic shock in children.

Recognition of Shock

Physicians must be able to recognize the sometimes subtle signs and symptoms of developing shock. With a relatively small amount of blood loss (≤ 15 per cent), the only sign of shock may be a slight increase in the pulse rate. However, most children who have been injured are frightened and anxious, states which elevate the pulse. Tachycardia may be the only finding early in the course of the development of shock, and this may be due to either shock or anxiety. Thus, patients need to be carefully assessed and reassessed if there is evidence of even small amounts of blood loss.

When 15 to 25 per cent of blood volume has been lost, the effects of increased vasomotor tone and adrenergic stimulation result in the clinical findings of increased diastolic blood pressure (or decreased pulse pressure), prolonged capillary refill, and further increases in heart rate. In addition, increased respiratory rate, anxiety, and thirst may also be present. When blood loss reaches or exceeds 25 per cent, the above findings plus hypotension, confusion, decreased urine output and acidosis may be present.

Thus, valuable clinical indicators of progressing shock include the following: vital signs; skin temperature and color; capillary refill time; central nervous system status; and urine output. However, if the child has been in a cold environment or has a spinal cord injury, skin changes may be inaccurate in reflecting shock. Furthermore, in patients with head injuries, assessment of mental status may be more indicative of the degree of neurologic injury than it is of shock. Urine output is a classic indicator of blood flow to vital organs, since it generally reflects renal blood flow (in the absence of chronic renal disease or urinary obstruction). In this sense, it is an effective means of following the dynamic progression of shock and its resuscitation. A urine output of 1 ml/kg/hour in children or 2 ml/kg/hour in infants is indirectly indicative of restoration of adequate circulatory volume.[16]

However, this is a dynamic, not a static, measurement and requires observation over a period of time, usually at least 1 to 2 hours. Thus, urinary output is of little value in determining the immediate response to resuscitation in the injured child. Therefore changes in vital signs (pulse pressure, pulse rate, blood pressure) and simple laboratory tests (see the following section) may be the physician's sole aids in the early detection of shock.

Although the measurement of urine output is of little value in the *initial* phases of shock recognition and therapy, urinary output is nonetheless a critical parameter to follow in the *ongoing* care of the injured child. Following urine output usually requires the use of an indwelling bladder catheter, unless urethral injury is suspected (blood at the urethral meatus, perineal swelling, or scrotal hematoma). It is important to record the volume of urine initially drained via the bladder catheter and place the urine in separate container, since it usually has been produced prior to the traumatic event and should not be considered a part of the urine output following trauma.

Estimating the Degree of Blood Loss

Physicians caring for pediatric trauma victims must be able to estimate the degree of blood loss from the physical findings. For example, a mildly elevated diastolic blood pressure, mild tachycardia, and an otherwise normal examination indicates approximately 15 to 20 per cent blood loss. In a 50 kg, 10-year-old child, this represents approximately 850 ml of blood loss.

50	Weight (kg)
× 85	Blood (ml/kg)
4250	Blood volume (ml)
× 20	Blood loss (%)
850	Amount of blood loss (ml)

As a further example, if the child's blood pressure was 90/70, even more severe blood loss would be implied. The minimum systolic blood pressure in a 10-year-old child should be 100 mm Hg (80 + 2 × 10 years = 100), and the fact that the systolic pressure is below this indicates the presence of hypotension in this child. *Any child who presents with hypotension secondary to hypovolemia has usually lost at least 25 percent, and sometimes as much as 50 per cent, of the total blood volume.* Thus, the presence of hypotension in any injured child represents major blood loss until proved otherwise. Patients in whom over 25 per cent of the total blood volume has been lost may also present with hypotension, but often have acidosis as well and are more resistant to resuscitation. As mentioned previously, an additional clinical indicator of shock is the development of decreased urine output. Urine output of less than 1 ml/kg/hour in a child or 2 ml/kg/hour in an infant indicates the continued presence of shock.

Because the degree of blood loss dictates the blood replacement requirements, all physicians should have a working knowledge of the signs and symptoms that correlate with percentage of blood loss.

Simple laboratory indicators of shock reflect the presence of acidosis (arterial pH < 7.3, P_{CO_2} < 25 mm Hg, base deficit > 8 mEq/l, serum bicarbonate < 18 mEq/l) or *hemorrhage* (hematocrit < 35 ml/100 ml). Hematocrit and hemoglobin determinations are usually misleading in the initial phase of trauma, since they require 4 to 6 hours to equilibrate with extracellular fluid mobilization.[17] Thus, hematocrit values are often falsely high in the first hours following hemorrhage. However, a hematocrit of less than 35 ml/100 ml early in the course of shock is nonetheless significant and indicates either severe hemorrhage or pre-existing anemia.

In virtually every child with traumatic shock without heart or renal disease, there is some element of hypovolemia. Central venous pressure (CVP) catheters or pulmonary artery catheters are of little or no value in the initial stages of therapy for shock. CVP catheters may be of benefit in the ongoing resuscitation of severe shock, during operations in which continued fluid replacement is needed, or in the intensive care unit following the initial phase of therapy. Pulmonary artery catheters may also be of value when either operative or intensive care unit monitoring is required. They are of particular value when measurements of cardiac output are necessary to monitor therapy.

Treatment

Following recognition of the presence of shock and the determination of the degree of blood loss that caused it, the physician must rapidly and aggressively treat the shock state. The goals of therapy are to restore the effective circulatory volume, maximize oxygen delivery to the tissues, and decrease ongoing blood loss.

Restoring Circulatory Volume

The most critical aspect of therapy for shock is re-establishment of effective circulatory volume. Numerous studies document that early restoration of circulatory volume clearly decreases the morbidity and mortality from shock, even when blood cannot be transfused.[18-21] Virtually any patient with clinical signs or symptoms of shock requires rapid IV replacement of blood loss.

Fluid Therapy. Considerable controversy continues concerning the most appropriate fluid for infusion in shock resuscitation (see Chapter 2 for details).[22] For practical purposes, because whole blood or packed red blood cells require at least 45 minutes to type and crossmatch, an alternative fluid must be available for immediate resuscitation of shock. Type O negative blood and type specific blood require only a few minutes to prepare but may result in hemolytic reactions and may interfere with further crossmatching in the ongoing management of the traumatized patient. However, in children with *exsanguinating hemorrhage*, either type O or type specific blood should be immediately transfused. Otherwise, use of type O or type specific blood should be unnecessary.

The two general categories of therapeutic fluids for use as an alternative to blood in the initial phase of shock resuscitation are colloid and crystalloid solutions. The general types of colloid solutions are albumin, dextran, and, more recently, hetastarch. Disadvantages of albumin are that it causes an increase in salt and water retention,[23] altered pulmonary function,[24] compromised immunologic status,[25] and a tendency to coagulopathy.[26, 27] Dextran has been reported to cause anaphylactic reactions, coagulopathy, renal failure, and interference with blood typing and crossmatching.[28] Hetastarch has not been associated with as many complications and may be an effective alternative in initial shock resuscitation.[29] However, clinical experience with this agent has been limited in children. In addition to the use of colloids and crystalloids, perfluorochemicals and stroma-free hemoglobin have each shown some promise as oxygen-carrying blood substitutes. However, neither of these agents is widely used clinically at this time.

The majority of trauma surgeons, including the American College of Surgeons Committee on Trauma, recommend that crystalloid or balanced salt solutions be used for the initial resuscitation of the trauma victim.[30-33] Lactated Ringer's solution is the balanced salt solution that is used most often for resuscitation of the trauma victim. It should be infused at the rate 3 ml per ml of blood loss.[33]

For practical purposes, a child with any signs of shock should receive an initial bolus of fluid equal to one fourth of the total blood volume, or 20 ml/kg (Fig. 1–6). If hypotension or acidosis are present, the child should receive 40 ml/kg or one half of the total blood volume. This fluid should be infused rapidly, over the course of 5 to 10 minutes. In cases of exsanguinating hemorrhage, red blood cells (type specific or type O) and lactated Ringer's solution should be infused rapidly.

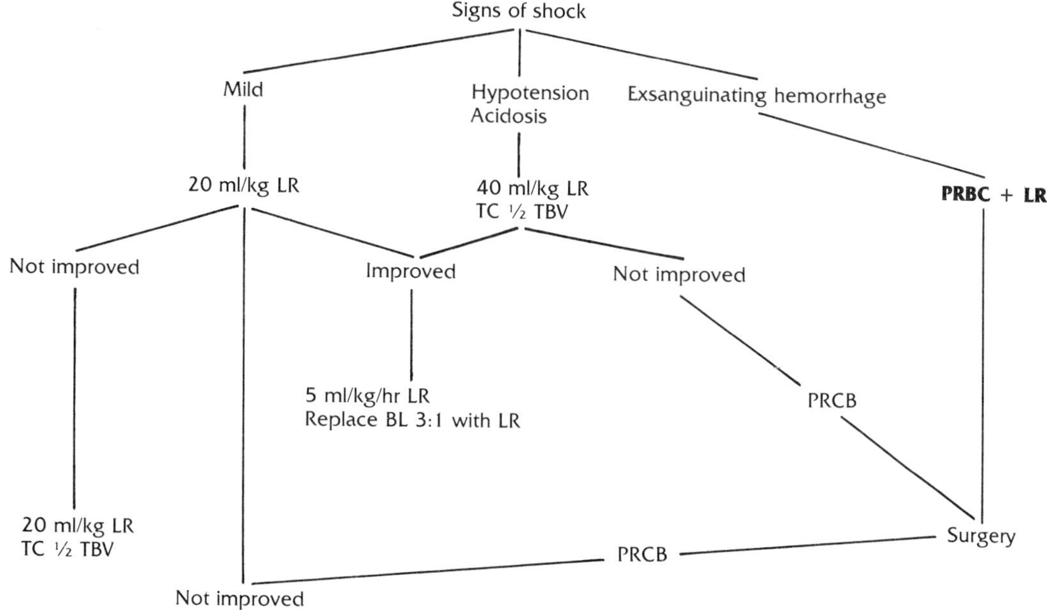

Figure 1–6. Fluid therapy in the pediatric trauma patient. In all patients with multiple trauma and mild symptoms of shock (tachycardia, tachypnea, decreased pulse pressure), 20 ml/kg of lactated Ringer's solution should be infused. If hypotension or acidosis is present, 40 ml/kg of lactated Ringer's solution (or one half of the total blood volume) should be given immediately. In cases of exsanguinating hemorrhage, red blood cells and lactated Ringer's solution should be given as soon as possible. Additional fluid therapy is guided by (1) the patient's response to initial fluid infusion; (2) replacement of blood loss up to 25 per cent of total blood volume with lactated Ringer's solution on the basis of 3 ml of crystalloid per ml of blood loss; and (3) replacement of blood loss in excess of 25 per cent of total blood volume, with one half of the volume replaced with red blood cells on a ml per ml basis and with the remainder 25 per cent blood loss replaced with 3 ml of lactated Ringer's solution per ml of blood loss. LR = lactated Ringer's solution; TC = type and crossmatch; TBV = total blood volume; PRBC = packed red blood cells; BL = blood loss.

Following the initial fluid bolus, additional fluid therapy is guided by three factors, the first and most important of which is the response to initial fluid infusion. *Careful attention must be paid to pre- and post-infusion parameters* (vital signs and physical examination), since these will often indicate whether a child has continued fluid losses. For example, if a patient with early signs of shock receives a bolus of 20 ml/kg of lactated Ringer's solution and responds with slight increase of the pulse and an increase in diastolic blood pressure and capillary refill time, he is probably suffering continuing losses and will require significant fluid replacement in addition to the original fluid bolus.

The second factor influencing fluid therapy is that blood loss up to 25 per cent of total blood volume may be replaced with crystalloid on the basis of 3 ml of lactated Ringer's solution per ml of blood loss. For example, in a 50 kg child with 20 per cent, or 850-ml, blood loss, a total of 2550 ml of crystalloid (3 ml per ml of blood loss × 850 ml blood loss) should be infused over the total course of the resuscitation. The third factor guiding fluid therapy is that patients with over 25 per cent blood loss require both crystalloid and blood transfusion. In general, half the fluid replacement for such patients is with red blood cells and half is with lactated Ringer's solution. For example, in a 50 kg patient with 1200-ml blood loss, one half of the replacement fluid (600 ml) should be in the form of packed red blood cells. The remaining blood loss should be replaced with lactated Ringer's solution based on the formula of 3 ml of lactated Ringer's solution per ml of blood loss. In this example, the child would thus receive one half of his blood loss replacement in the form of packed red blood cells and an additional 1800 ml of lactated Ringer's solution (3 ml lactated Ringer's solution per ml of blood loss × 600 ml of blood loss).

Because patients whose blood pressure falls below normal limits have lost at least 25 per cent of their total blood volume and usually require blood transfusion, routine typing and crossmatching of enough units to equal one half the child's blood volume should be undertaken if hypotension is present.

If the child's pulse systolic and diastolic blood pressures do not improve within 5 to 10 minutes of receiving the initial bolus of 20 ml/kg for mild shock or 40 ml/kg for patients with hypotension or acidosis, a second bolus of fluid equal in volume to the first is indicated. When this infusion is completed, the child has received at least one half of the total blood volume by bolus infusion. Virtually all children whose clinical findings do not improve following this infusion will require blood transfusion, and most will require surgery to control bleeding. In patients whose blood has been controlled and in whom the bolus infusion has improved the clinical findings, the infusion rate should be slowed to 5 ml/kg/hour for several hours of close observation, until the child has received the calculated amount of fluid required to replace blood loss. If the clinical status declines, additional bolus therapy may be indicated. If vital functions and urine output are normal, reduction of fluid infusion to maintenance levels (1500 ml per square meter body surface area) is acceptable.

In the past, platelets and clotting factors were often routinely transfused when patients received large volumes of blood products. At the present time, most traumatologists recommend that platelets and fresh frozen plasma be given only when the clinical status of the patient and appropriate laboratory studies indicate they are necessary.[31]

Although definitive therapy of the acidosis of shock requires aggressive fluid replacement, sodium bicarbonate may be of value in controlling the systemic effects of acidosis. Therefore, 2 ml/kg of bicarbonate should be given to patients whose arterial pH is less than 7.2, assuming the acidosis is not respiratory in nature.

Military Anti-Shock Trousers (MAST). An additional means of increasing the effective circulatory volume is through the use of military anti-shock trousers. These trousers have three separate air bladders, which wrap around the lower abdomen and each leg and are inflated with a foot pump, resulting in external counterpressure of up to 100 mm Hg. MAST can clearly be of benefit to the patient in shock, but the amount of "auto transfusion" that is provided to the circulatory volume is probably limited to from 5 to 10 per cent of the total blood volume.[34, 35] The primary benefit of MAST is probably secondary to its role in increasing total peripheral resistance, by stimulating vasocontriction in the lower extremity to diminish the size of the vascular bed being perfused.[36] In addition MAST may tamponade external and internal bleeding sites, stabilize leg and pelvic fractures, and increase the size of the veins in the upper extremity, facilitating venous cannulation.

Any child with a systolic blood pressure that is less than two thirds of normal and signs and symptoms of shock should have MAST applied. Patients with leg or pelvic fractures and those with major abdominal or lower extremity bleeding may also benefit from these trousers. The only absolute contraindication to the use of MAST trousers is the presence of pulmonary edema.[37]

Although MAST are of clear utility, they should be deflated slowly and with caution, since sudden removal may produce profound and refractory hypotension. Deflation should begin only after adequate fluid replacement has brought the vital signs toward normal limits. Deflation should be gradual, one segment at a time, beginning with the abdominal section. If blood pressure drops more than 5 mm Hg, the deflation process should be stopped and IV fluid replacement increased until blood pressure normalizes. At this point, deflation may be carefully resumed. In many patients, examination of the abdomen or lower extremities must be carried out during the phase of fluid replacement. When this is necessary, great caution should be exercised and the blood pressure should be followed closely. After a rapid examination, the MAST should be reinflated. Often MAST must remain on the patient until the patient has been taken to the operating room for exploratory laparotomy. Complications from MAST are infrequent but include the development of compartmental syndromes in the lower extremity.[38, 39]

Maximizing Oxygen Delivery

Providing tissue oxygenation is in many respects the central goal of shock therapy. However, restoration of circulatory volume is necessary to obtain this goal. In addition, several other aspects of therapy are specifically designed to maximize oxygen delivery. In general, the goal of therapy is to increase tissue oxygen supply while reducing oxygen demands.

Although oxygen is not the cure for any traumatic disease, hypoxia is often a factor in trauma patients, and increased oxygen delivery to the tissues is a critical goal.[40] Therefore, all injured children with signs of shock should have oxygen administered by the most readily available means. Principles of airway management outlined previously should be closely followed. Levels of arterial blood gases should guide the continuing rate and method of oxygen delivery.

An additional means of increasing the arterial oxygen content is through the provision of adequate quantities of oxygen-carrying capacity in the form of hemoglobin. Packed red blood cells will often need to be infused into injured patients. This should be done at the earliest appropriate time. In patients with 25 per cent or less blood loss, infusion of crystalloid may be sufficient to restore normal vital signs, and transfusion may not be required. However, in patients with 25 per cent or more blood loss or those in whom crystalloid does not immediately improve the clinical condition, transfusion is usually indicated. In some cases, tissue oxygen supply may need to be augmented by increasing cardiac output through the use of cardioactive drugs, such as dopamine.

Optimal oxygen delivery may also be assisted by decreasing oxygen demand or consumption. Control of temperature, physical activity, sepsis, and additional ongoing trauma may all be of assistance in this regard.

Decreasing Blood Loss

One of the key steps in the management of injured patients is to arrest the bleeding. Virtually any traumatic condition is worsened by ongoing blood loss. In addition, continuation of blood loss may result in devastating consequences. Bleeding may be external or internal; either may result in profound shock.

External Bleeding. External hemorrhage is generally easily recognized, since the manifestations of external bleeding are discernible to even the untrained eye. However, the magnitude of bleeding may not be obvious unless the patient is undressed; dressings that have been placed on wounds must also be removed. If a bulky dressing is placed over a site of bleeding, a significant amount of blood may be lost before it appears on the outer layer of dressing.

Systematic assessment of the entire body surface is necessary to insure that all areas of external hemorrhage are evaluated and treated. The magnitude of blood loss at the scene of the injury should be elicited from family, companions, or paramedical personnel. Any laceration may result in a great deal of bleeding, but scalp and facial wounds are particularly prone to profuse hemorrhage, owing to the inherent vascularity of these areas.

Measures to decrease external bleeding should begin with direct pressure over bleeding sites with sterile dressing.[41] Once pressure has been applied, it should be maintained, either with manual pressure or pressure dressings. If pressure dressings are used, they should be assessed frequently to quantify blood loss and to insure that they are not so tight that they occlude distal pulses. This assures that the pressure dressing is not acting as a tourniquet. Tourniquets should rarely be used, except in cases of exsanguinating hemorrhage, and even then, they should be used for only 15 to 20 minutes at a time.

The bleeding area should be elevated, as this often markedly decreases the amount of blood loss. In most cases, the combination of direct pressure and elevation will arrest external hemorrhage.

Hemostats to clamp spurting vessels should never be used except on the scalp. In virtually every area of the body except the scalp, major nerves are in proximity to major blood vessels, and clamping these vessels may result in peripheral nerve damage. This is of particular importance in the face and neck regions.

Internal Bleeding. Recognition of internal bleeding requires critical judgment, a thorough physical examination, and attention to the sometimes subtle changes present with major internal hemorrhage. A loudly crying child with a scalp laceration but no other serious injury may present to the emergency room "covered with blood." Often, such children have lost only 50 to 100 ml of blood, but the graphic manner in which it is lost may create a sense of urgency. Conversely, a child with a fractured femur and a ruptured spleen may be very quiet, with no obvious bleeding. Clearly, the latter child is more seriously injured and requires prompt therapy. However, unless the physician carefully examines each body area, significant blood loss may be missed (see following section).

Occult internal hemorrhage of a significant degree occurs in five body areas: chest, abdomen, retroperitoneum, pelvis, and femurs. Pain or swelling in any of these areas should alert the physician to the possibility of inter-

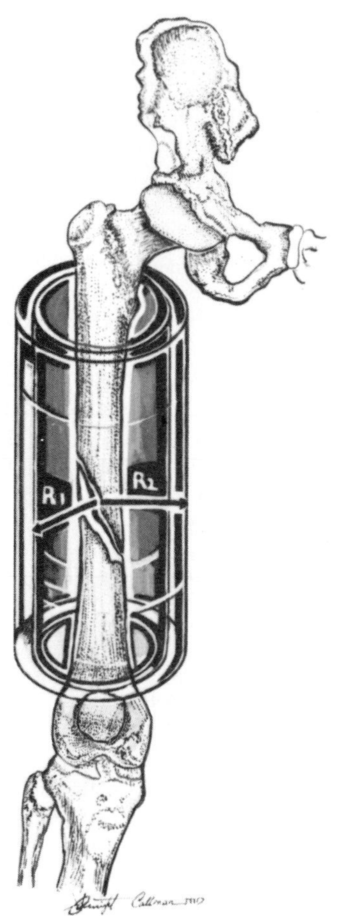

Figure 1–7. This diagram illustrates the magnitude of blood loss that may result from extremity fractures. In this diagram of the femur, R1 represents the radius of the thigh under normal circumstances. R2 represents the radius of the thigh after blood loss from a femoral fracture. Up to two units of blood may be lost from femoral fractures in older children, which may result in relatively small changes in the circumference of the thigh.

nal hemorrhage. Figure 1–7 illustrates the magnitude of blood loss that can be concealed in the thigh with a fractured femur. Even small changes in the circumference of the thigh or abdomen may be indicative of loss of a large percentage of the total blood volume.

Although restoration of vascular volume and treatment of specific injuries causing internal hemorrhage are two goals of treatment, external counterpressure devices have been useful in temporarily stabilizing internal hemorrhage (see page 16).

SECONDARY SURVEY—REGIONAL EVALUATION

Following the primary survey, initial stabilization of the cardiorespiratory system, and aggressive treatment of shock, each child should undergo a secondary survey, which consists of a timely, directed evaluation of every body region for trauma. The examination should be timely in that diagnostic evaluation should not delay treatment of life-threatening injuries. But it should also be a directed examination because even serious injuries can often be overlooked in children. As many as 25 per cent of patients with serious injuries admitted to major trauma centers have at least one injury missed at the time of initial evaluation.[42, 43] Thus, *every* child with either shock or injury to one body area must be carefully and systematically evaluated for injury to the remainder of the body.

History

The history of the injury may be crucial to the child's treatment, and must often be taken at the scene of the accident. The history should include events leading to the accident, the mechanism and time of injury, clinical course following the injury, contamination of wound sites, previous history of chronic illness (see Section Three) or injury, allergies, medication, and the time of the last meal eaten before injury. The American College of Surgeons recommends use of the mnemonic "Take an AMPLE history." The letters in the acronym stand for *a*llergies, *m*edications, *p*ast medical history, *l*ast meal, and *e*vents leading to the accident.[30]

Physical Examination

The order of physical examination of body regions may vary, but children's injuries should be evaluated in descending order of urgency. In most instances, highest priority is given to the cardiorespiratory and central nervous systems. Therefore, a logical plan is to evaluate the (1) thorax, (2) head and neck, (3) abdomen, (4) genitourinary tract, and (5) skin and extremities. Some clinicians prefer to do a "head-to-toes" examination, which is also acceptable, provided the cardiorespiratory system is not neglected for significant periods. Regardless of the order of examination, several principles are of vital importance. First, children should be assessed through a protocol in which *all body areas* are evaluated and each body area undergoes systematic assessment. Second, finding one severe injury should not cause the physician to cease the evaluation (except to treat life-threatening injuries). Assuming that a single injury is the sole cause of the patient's problem may have devastating consequences. Rather, any child with an injury to one body area should be assumed to have additional injuries until proved otherwise. Third, patients with head injuries who are in shock should always be evaluated with caution, since isolated head injuries rarely cause shock until late in the clinical course. Fourth, evaluation should always be gentle, particularly with regard to manipulation of the spinal axis. Further, any conscious child should be reassured, and every part of the physical examination or diagnostic work-up should be explained. Finally, the vital signs and, in most cases, the physical examination should be repeated frequently on patients with serious injuries. Continuous monitoring and careful reassessment are necessary, since children who arrive at the emergency room with normal vital signs may progress rapidly to shock.

The reader will notice that there is very little mention of radiography in this section on regional evaluation of trauma. This has been done purposefully for two reasons. First, the radiology chapter provides an excellent overview of the approach to ordering and interpreting radiographs in injured children, as well as specific indications for work-up of problems in given body areas. Second, and more importantly, the role of radiography in the first minutes of trauma care is limited. The physical examination is the clinician's first resource in caring for the patient. Indeed, a physician can hardly order appropriate x-rays if the patient has not been properly examined. Furthermore, determining which radiographs should be taken first is related to evaluation of the most life-threatening injuries. Therefore, chest and cervical spine films have the highest priority, whereas skull, abdominal, and extremity films are less urgently needed. This should not imply that radiologic evaluation of the injured child should not be undertaken but simply that the history and physical examination should guide timely and appropriate radiographs.

THORAX

Thoracic injuries frequently affect ventilation and circulation and may pose a serious threat to life. Any physician caring for injured children must be able to assess injuries to the thorax and institute appropriate therapeutic measures rapidly and efficiently. The principle of continual monitoring and reassessment is particularly important in thoracic injuries, since clinical deterioration frequently occurs.

The majority of thoracic injuries can be detected by carefully assessing airway position and patency, respiratory rate, chest wall movement, neck vein distention, tracheal position, and breath sounds and by palpation and percussion of the thorax. Concurrently, the circulation should be evaluated by checking carotid, femoral, or radial pulse for rate and intensity, as well as checking blood pressure, capillary refill, and heart sounds. A great deal of information can be gathered quickly by positioning the airway, palpating the pulse, and assessing chest wall movement, as shown in Figure 1–1. Neck vein distention is less commonly seen in children, but it should alert the physician to the possibility of pericardial tamponade or tension pneumothorax.

The chest wall should move symmetrically with each inspiration or assisted breath. Children with upper airway obstruction may have marked inspiratory effort but little or no chest wall movement. Symmetrically poor chest movement suggests airway obstruction or hypoventilation. Appropriate treatment measures consist of placing the airway in proper position, assessing airway patency, and assisting ventilation as necessary. When the chest wall rises asymmetrically, pneumothorax, tension pneumothorax, flail chest, and foreign body aspiration are possibilities.

The trachea should be in a midline position and is easily palpable in children. Tracheal deviation suggests tension pneumothorax. Auscultation of the left and right hemithoraces, including anterior and posterior aspects, should reveal equal breath sounds. Decreased breath sounds may accompany pneumothorax, hemothorax, or foreign body aspiration. Percussion of the thorax may show hyper-resonance (associated with tension pneumothorax) or dullness (noted with hemothorax). Palpation of the chest wall for tenderness or subcutaneous emphysema is important, inasmuch as these may be clues to underlying injury. Rib fractures are relatively less common in children than in adults, owing to children's more pliable rib cages. However, because considerable force is required to fracture a child's rib, this injury may indicate that additional injuries are present. Therefore rib fractures can be important findings, and virtually all children with rib fractures should be observed closely to insure that there are no additional injuries.

The majority of children with *severe* cardiorespiratory compromise secondary to thoracic injury have one of the following diagnoses: airway obstruction, tension pneumothorax, large hemo- or hemopneumothorax, flail chest, open pneumothorax (sucking chest wound), or pericardial tamponade. The last two injuries are less common in children than in adults, owing to the relative rarity of penetrating trauma in children. Other more rare causes of cardiorespiratory embarrassment are injuries to the heart and great vessels, rupture of the tracheobronchial tree, rupture of the esophagus, and pulmonary crush injuries. The following discussion is designed to acquaint the physician in a general sense with the clinical presentation of these entities and the appropriate emergency treatment measures. For a complete discussion of the pathophysiology and definitive treatment of thoracic injuries, please refer to Chapter 15.

Airway Obstruction

Any child with stridor, suprasternal or intercostal retractions, and bilateral or unilateral decrease in breath sounds and chest wall movement should be suspected of having partial or complete airway obstruction. If the airway is obstructed at a lower level, wheezing may be the only sign of obstruction.[44] Proper airway positioning and finger-sweep or suctioning of the oropharynx may clear the airway if the obstruction is in the superior oropharynx. Obstruction due to foreign bodies at a lower level may require back blows or the Heimlich maneuver, both of which should be applied firmly but judiciously.[4] Assisted ventilation may be necessary to adequately ventilate and oxygenate the child, but efforts to find and treat the cause of obstruction should not be neglected. Bronchial foreign bodies usually require bronchoscopic removal (see Chapter 31).

As noted previously, direct injuries to the larynx and trachea are uncommon in pediatrics, and almost all children can be ventilated without surgical intervention. In rare cases, cricothyroidotomy or tracheostomy may be necessary, but these methods should be considered last resorts. The cricoid area is the narrowest portion of the pediatric airway, and insertion of an airway at this level is fraught with complications.[45] When cricothyroidotomy is necessary, needle puncture with jet ventilation affords 30 to 45 minutes of ventilation if carefully applied and often allows time for more definitive control of the airway in the operating room (see pp. 5–6).

Tension Pneumothorax

Unilateral decrease in chest wall movement, decreased or absent breath sounds, hyper-resonance, cyanosis, neck vein distention, tracheal deviation, and corresponding deterioration of cardiorespiratory status all suggest tension pneumothorax. In this syndrome, the affected hemithorax becomes overdistended with air, resulting in mediastinal shift, compression of the heart and great veins, impedance of venous return, a fall in cardiac output, and decreased ventilation of the opposite lung. This is particularly devastating in children, in whom mediastinal fixation is less firm than in adults. Unless this problem is relieved immediately, death may be imminent. *Never wait for x-ray documentation when tension pneumothorax is suspected and the patient is in extremis.* Although tube thoracostomy is the definitive treatment, this should be instituted after needle aspiration has relieved the life-threatening problem.

A scalp-vein needle (for neonates and small infants) or IV catheter should be attached to a three-way stopcock and a 30- or 50-cc syringe. The stopcock is necessary because large quantities of air can frequently be aspirated from the hemithorax, and use of the stopcock prevents a pleural leak and redevelopment of tension while the syringe is being emptied of air. Needle aspiration is employed in the second or third intercostal space, taking care to avoid the internal mammary and intercostal arteries by placing the needle just lateral to the mid clavicular line and over the *top* of the rib at a 90-degree angle to the chest wall. Aspiration should continue until negative pressure has been reestablished in the hemithorax, as evidenced by inability to withdraw additional air into the aspirating syringe.

Following this, a chest tube should be placed in the fourth intercostal space in the mid or anterior axillary line. Many traumatologists place chest tubes somewhat lower in adults, but the child's wide diaphragmatic excursion predisposes to misplacement of the tube in the abdominal cavity when the lower interspaces are chosen. If possible, a nasogastric tube should be placed and the stomach emptied of air, since this may help lower the diaphragm and prevent inadvertent intra-abdominal placement of the tube.

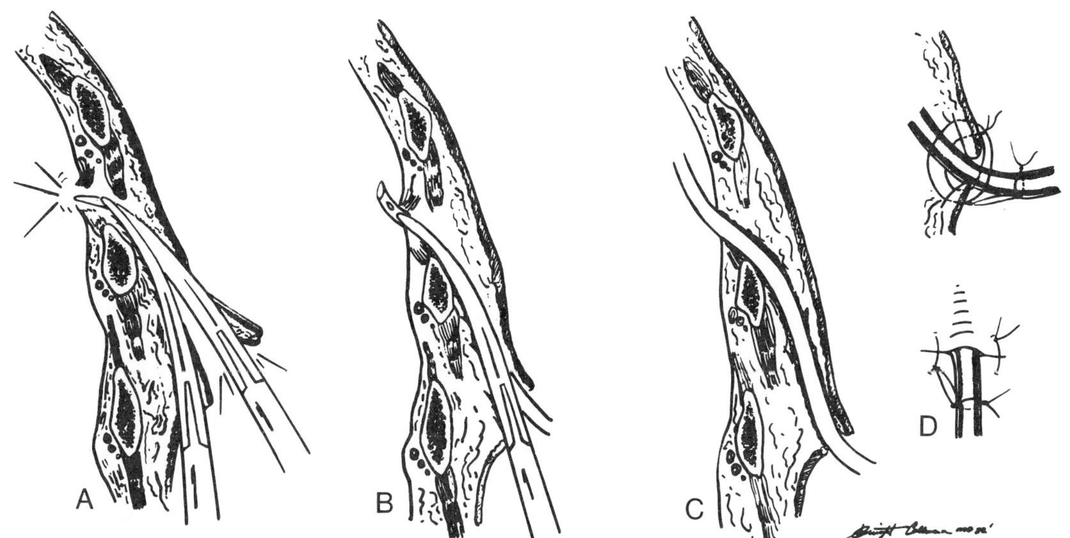

Figure 1–8. Chest tube placement in the pediatric patient. The patient is positioned rolled slightly on the side with the arm raised. The skin is anesthetized for a distance of 2 to 3 cm over the body of the sixth rib at the mid or anterior axillary line. *A*, After making a 1.5 cm skin incision over the middle of the sixth rib in the mid or anterior axillary line, a subcutaneous tunnel is created bluntly with a curved hemostat; it extends slightly posteriorly and over the top of the fifth rib, into the fourth intercostal space. The pleura is entered by firmly advancing the hemostat. *B*, The chest tube is then advanced into the pleural space with the hemostat. *C*, This creates a subcutaneous tunnel tract, which serves to anchor the chest tube. *D*, The chest tube is sutured to the skin, with the sutures then tied around the chest tube to help secure it.

The chest tube is placed as shown in Figure 1-8. Although trocar catheters are available, their use is contraindicated for *initial* entry into the pleural space, since significant pleural or mediastinal injuries may result. Instead, the curved hemostat should be used to enter the pleural space. Once entry into the pleural space has been effected (as evidence by a sharp "pop" and a rush of air), the tube should be placed with a hemostat (or *gently* with a trocar) into the hole originally created in the pleura. The chest tube should immediately be connected to a water seal and suction, and the skin incision should be closed snugly around the tube to avoid air leaks. The tube should be anchored to the skin securely and a chest roentgenogram obtained to verify resolution of the pneumothorax and chest tube position.

Pneumothorax and Hemothorax

Dullness to percussion, diminished or absent breath sounds, decreased chest wall movement, dyspnea, tachypnea, and subcutaneous emphysema are all possible signs of pneumothorax and hemothorax. In penetrating wounds, hemoptysis may also be present. A wide range of symptoms and physical findings may be present in children with pneumothorax and hemothorax, depending on the degree of injury.[46] Generally, most of these children will require tube thoracostomy, but this can usually be delayed, until the diagnosis is confirmed by x-ray, unless the child has tension pneumothorax. Most cases of pneumothorax due to blunt trauma and virtually all those associated with penetrating injury have at least some minor element of hemothorax as well. Thus, children with pneumothorax due to blunt trauma should be assumed to have some blood in the thorax, however minimal.

With more significant hemothorax, bleeding may progress until the hemorrhage is arrested by either a local tamponade effect or the development of shock. All children with physical signs or x-ray confirmation of pneumothorax should have an IV line placed in the upper extremity prior to tube thoracostomy, unless tension pneumothorax has developed. When hypovolemic shock is present, aggressive volume replacement should be undertaken. In cases of massive hemothorax, use of autotransfusion may be necessary.

Blood loss from the hemithorax must be carefully quantified. If blood loss exceeds 30 ml/kg in the initial 8 hours following injury or if bleeding into the chest cavity is the main cause of hemorrhagic shock, surgical intervention is generally undertaken. For a more detailed explanation of the indications for early thoracotomy, see Chapter 15.

Flail Chest

Although extremely uncommon in children, flail chest is an entity in which early recognition and treatment may be life-saving.[47] As noted, children have more pliable ribs, which are more resistant to fracture. Since the development of the flail segment requires several ribs fractured on both sides of the impact injury, this condition occurs in children only in cases of extremely severe trauma. High-speed motor vehicle accidents, auto-pedestrian collisions, or falls from a significant height account for most pediatric cases of flail chest. The anterior and lateral portions of the chest wall are most often affected, since the posterior thoracic cage is protected by the paraspinous muscles and the shoulder girdle.

Although x-ray confirms the diagnosis, physical findings include tenderness over the fracture sites, subcutaneous emphysema, dyspnea, cyanosis (in severe cases), and paradoxical motion of the flail segment with respiration. Treatment at the scene of injury includes placing the affected hemithorax down ("bad side down") and stabilization of the flail segment, preferably in the "out" position, as well as provision of appropriate respiratory support. Increasing evidence indicates that early internal pneumatic stabilization (intubation and positive pressure ventilation) should be applied to patients with significant flail segments.[47]

Open Pneumothorax

The classic "sucking chest wound" is produced by penetrating trauma, which is less common in children than in adults. Occasionally, severely fractured ribs may protrude through the skin, producing an open pneumothorax, but this is rare. The diagnosis is usually made by noting a penetrating chest wound through which air or blood moves with respiration. Subcutaneous emphysema, decreased breath sounds, decreased chest wall excursion, and dullness to percussion on the affected side may also be noted. The open wound should be covered with an airtight occlusive dressing as early as possible, usually with a petrolatum gauze dressing, after which tube thoracostomy and antibiotic therapy should be carried out.

Pericardial Tamponade

Pericardial tamponade is a rare cause of shock in a child and is nearly always due to penetrating trauma. Rents in the heart produce brisk bleeding into the pericardium, with resultant rise in pericardial pressure. This rise in pressure impairs cardiac filling and may produce profound hypotension. The classic findings of hypotension, distended neck veins, and muffled heart sounds are known as Beck's triad.[48] Additionally, pulsus paradoxus and an enlarged cardiac silhouette on chest radiogram may also be present.

Experience has shown that these "classic" findings are highly variable, and hypotension is perhaps the only feature that is invariably present.[49] Conversely, hypotension may be the *only* finding in a child with cardiac tamponade. Distended neck veins are an additional indicator of tamponade but they do not occur if significant hypovolemia is present. Heart sounds are often subjectively normal in children with tamponade, probably owing to the thinner chest wall. Pulsus paradoxus is an early, transient finding and is very difficult to elicit in a critically ill child. In adolescents, as much as 300 ml of blood may be necessary to appreciably increase the size of the cardiac silhouette, whereas as little as 200 ml may cause fatal tamponade. Thus hypotension is often the sole indicator of this life-threatening problem.

If persistent hypotension is present in a child with chest trauma who is ventilated adequately and in whom volume replacement has been instituted, either cardiac tamponade or occult exsanguinating hemorrhage should be considered. In patients in whom tamponade is suspected, a central venous catheter may be placed if the child is not in extremis. If the central venous pressure (CVP) is high (over 10), the diagnosis of cardiac tamponade is likely. If the CVP is normal or low, the diagnosis of tamponade is not necessarily excluded, since marked volume depletion and tamponade may be present simultaneously. Rapid volume infusion should be undertaken and the CVP response monitored. A rapid rise in the CVP with no improvement in the child's clinical course suggests tamponade.

Once cardiac tamponade has been diagnosed, or in those cases in which it is suspected and the patient is in profound shock, emergency treatment consists of needle pericardiocentesis (Fig. 1–9). A large-bore IV line must be in place whenever possible so that vascular volume can be rapidly expanded if necessary.

Aspiration of as little as 30 cc of blood from the pericardium may result in dramatic clinical improvement, although in some cases up to 250 to 500 cc may be withdrawn (thus the need for the three-way stopcock). If blood

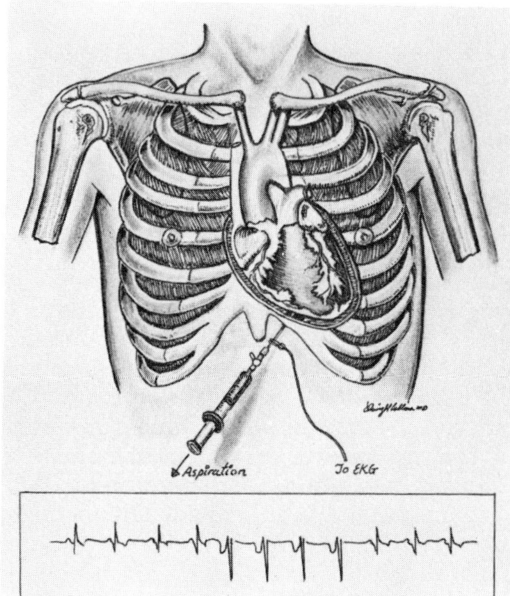

Figure 1–9. Needle pericardiocentesis. An 18-gauge needle with a three-way stopcock attached is inserted below and slightly to the patient's left of the xiphoid and is directed toward the left scapula. The needle should be aspirated as it is advanced, with blood entering the syringe when the pericardium has been entered. Defibrinated blood in the pericardium usually will not clot, whereas blood from the right ventricle does. The precordial (V) lead of an electrocardiogram (EKG) can be attached to the needle with a sterile alligator clip. When the pericardium has been entered, the EKG shows an increase in QRS voltage. Entry into the myocardium will produce ST segment elevation and/or premature ventricular contractions.

reaccumulates in the pericardium, hypotension may reoccur and reaspiration or thoracotomy may be necessary.

HEAD

Neurologic injuries are a significant cause of morbidity and mortality in pediatrics; greater than 75 per cent of children with multiple trauma suffer some degree of neurologic injury.[50, 51] In two thirds of these patients, the head is the most severely injured body area. The high incidence of head injuries, as well as the devastating problems that often follow them, requires that every physician treating emergency patients be thoroughly trained in the evaluation and the initial treatment of these injuries. Appropriate diagnostic and therapeutic intervention may be life-saving and an increasing number of reports indicate that aggressive treatment improves outcome in brain-injured patients.[52-54]

There is rarely a need for heroic speed in *surgical* intervention for head injury except in cases of massive hemorrhage or in which a rapidly expanding intracranial hematoma is producing tentorial or tonsillar herniation. Fortunately, these circumstances are less common in children than in adults. Other indications for surgical intervention include more slowly expanding hematomas and closed depressed skull fractures in which the fragment is depressed greater than the thickness of the skull. However, these latter cases usually do not require urgent surgery, although immediate neurosurgical consultation is necessary.

Although immediate neurosurgery is infrequently necessary, it is nonetheless critical that all children with neurologic injuries be evaluated and resuscitated rapidly and referred for appropriate neurosurgical care when indicated. Children with head injuries should be reassessed frequently in case neurologic deterioration occurs. To assure that appropriate care is immediately provided, assessment and simple therapeutic measures should begin at the scene of the accident. For example, documentation of deterioration of consciousness, arrest of scalp bleeding, and maintenance of a patent airway are three measures by which paramedical personnel at the scene of an accident may significantly improve the patient's care. In this sense, the ultimate outcome for patients with head injuries depends on cooperation and planning to assure timely, appropriate care. The following protocol is designed to facilitate such care.

History

In no other body area is the history as important as in neurologic injury. A clear history of neurologic deterioration following trauma may be critical in the decision for neurosurgical intervention. If a child is simply rushed from the scene of injury to the nearest hospital, the physician must rely solely on the patient's neurologic findings at the time of initial examination. In cases in which the child has a lucid interval following a period of unconsciousness, that initial unconsciousness is a vital piece of information. Paramedics and emergency medical teams must be instructed and trained carefully in this area, both to document the time and mechanism of injury and the initial course following the injury and to assure the performance of a brief early neurologic examination (see Mini-Neurologic Examination, pages 24–25). Witnesses to the accident, parents, and playmates may all need to be questioned with regard to the injury and the patient's level of consciousness following it. This can always be done quickly and seldom delays transporting the patient to emergency facilities. This information should be relayed to the physician as early as possible, since the urgency for surgical decompression may depend on the patient's clinical course following injury.

Oxygenation, Ventilation, and Perfusion

The highest priority in head-injured patients is maintenance of adequate oxygenation, ventilation, and perfusion.[55, 56] Hypoxia, hypercapnia, and hypotension all have devestating effects on the outcome of children with neurologic injury and should be treated aggressively to diminish secondary systemic brain injury as much as possible. Attention to optimizing function of the cardiorespiratory system is therefore central to the care of neurologic injuries. Appropriate measures that assure an adequate airway and effective circulation and prevent the development of shock are outlined in the preceding pages.

Hemorrhage

Following establishment of appropriate support for the cardiorespiratory system, the physician should control obvious bleeding from the head. The two most common sites causing massive external bleeding are the scalp vessels and the dural sinuses (in cases of open skull fracture). The vast majority of external hemorrhage from the head will be from scalp vessels, which may result in profound blood loss. However, profuse, uncontrolled bleeding should raise the suspicion of dural sinus tears, which require neurosurgical intervention.

Steps to control hemorrhage include placement of pressure dressings, elevation of the head (taking caution to maintain neutral cervical spine position), and the application of hemostats to spurting vessels in the scalp. Pressure dressings should be applied prior to elevating the head, since this prevents air embolism in cases of dural sinus tears.

Absence of Respiratory Effort

In children with no respiratory effort following massive neurologic injury, maximum resuscitative efforts should still be instituted. A significant number of patients with apnea survive their injuries and may return to a normal level of function.[57] The other consideration in patients with no respiratory effort is the possibility of high cervical spine injury; therefore, the spine should be appropriately stabilized.

Fixed, Dilated Pupils

Pupillary position and response are indicators of prognosis in patients with neurologic injury (see Mini-Neurologic Examination below). However, resuscitative efforts should never be withheld from a child with fixed, dilated pupils. A widely dilated, unreactive pupil may be caused by traumatic iridoplegia, direct third nerve damage, pressure on the third nerve secondary to increased intracranial pressure, profound shock, or cerebral anoxia. It is important to distinguish between these causes, since only the last three have significant prognostic significance. Three important questions assist in making the distinction of the cause of pupillary dilatation and unreactivity. First, Was the pupil dilated immediately following the injury? If so, this suggests either traumatic iridoplegia or direct third nerve injury. Second, What is the patient's level of consciousness? If the patient is awake and alert, a fixed, dilated pupil is unlikely to be secondary to shock, increased intracranial pressure, or cerebral anoxia. Third, What are the vital signs? Slowing of the pulse, increase in blood pressure, and a change in respirations all suggest increasing intracranial pressure.

Finally, even when a patient has bilaterally fixed and dilated pupils, aggressive therapeutic measures should be undertaken. Many children whose pupils are fixed and dilated on initial examination respond quickly to cardiorespiratory and neurologic resuscitation.[57]

Mini-Neurologic Examination

Although a detailed neurologic examination should be performed on every patient suffering significant trauma, this should be deferred during the initial survey. Instead, a mini-neurologic examination is the initial approach to the head-injured patient, since it provides a significant amount of information regarding the patient's neurologic state within the first few minutes of evaluation. The mini-neurologic examination consists of seven parts: history; level of consciousness; pupillary size, shape, and reactivity; movement of extremities; plantar responses; cerebrospinal fluid (CSF) otorrhea, rhinorrhea, or hemotympanum; and vital signs. Highlights are noted here—a more detailed discussion appears in Chapter 16.

As noted previously, the history of the injury, time to medical evaluation, and clinical course following the injury are critical pieces of information. The vital signs should be assessed and recorded, since they may reflect the development of compromised cardiorespiratory function, shock, or increased intracranial pressure. The respiratory pattern should be described as normal, shallow, or apneic, or requiring assisted ventilation (with both assisted and spontaneous respiratory rates recorded).

A general statement of the patient's overall level of consciousness is the most important part of the examination. This need not be a detailed statement and should always be written clearly. As Humphrey and associates noted, "Such phrases as 'comatose,' 'semi-comatose,' or 'semi-conscious' should be used only by poets." Describing the level of consciousness as "alert and oriented," "arousable to voice and touch," or "unresponsive to deep pain" imparts a great deal more information than "lethargic," "semi-comatose," and so on.

The Glasgow Coma Scale (GCS) (Table 1–4) tests the patient's best response in eye opening and best verbal and motor responses.[58] It should be used by all emergency medical personnel, since it clearly categorizes degree of neurologic injury.[59, 60] Use of the GCS is important for at least three reasons. First, GCS parameters are objective and easily assessed and give reproducible data concerning the level of consciousness. Second, use of the scale allows classification of head injuries. In general, patients with GCS scores of 10 or less are considered to have severe head injuries. Third, the GCS clearly documents neurologic deterioration. Decreases of 2 points are considered highly significant, whereas decreases of 3 points or more represent urgent neurosurgical emergencies.[61] (In evaluating motor response, the best response on either side is recorded, but notation should also be made separately of the response on the "worst side.") The most significant limitation of the GCS score relates to its use in children under 2 years of age. In children in this age group, verbal skills are developed to highly variable degrees. At the present time, pediatric neurosurgeons are testing several modifications of the scale for children in this pre-verbal age group. However, at the present time, we simply score all children who are able to cry with a full verbal score, since unconscious children cannot cry.

Table 1–4. GLASGOW COMA SCALE

Eye opening	Never	1
	To pain	2
	To speech	3
	Spontaneously	4
Best verbal response*	None	1
	Garbled	2
	Inappropriate	3
	Confused	4
	Oriented	5
Best motor response	None	1
	Extension	2
	Abnormal flexion	3
	Withdrawal	4
	Localizes pain	5
	Obeys commands	6

*Children 2 years of age or younger who cry are given a verbal score of 5.

Pupillary size and response should be assessed and the corneal reflex tested simultaneously. Detailed funduscopic examination can be delayed until the primary mini-neurologic exam has been completed. Oculocephalic reflexes (doll's eye movements) are a valuable sign, both of the severity of injury and of prognosis. However, the patient's neck should not be moved until the spine has been thoroughly evaluated. For this reason, oculocephalic reflexes are not routinely assessed until the diagnosis of cervical spine injury has been excluded. However, oculovestibular reflexes may be safely assessed.

Spontaneous and induced movements should be observed and the presence of hemiparesis, monoparesis, paraplegia, or quadriplegia assessed. Plantar reflexes should be elicited and recorded as upward, downward, or equivocal.

Assessment of the patient through history, level of consciousness (GCS score), pupillary position and reactivity, movements or lateralizing signs, plantar reflexes, presence of CSF otorrhea, rhinorrhea, or hemotympanum, and vital signs identifies virtually all patients with serious neurologic injuries. Following the mini-neurologic examination, a more detailed neurologic examination, including assessment of cranial nerves, oculocephalic or oculovestibular reflexes, extraocular movements, deep tendon reflexes, and motor or sensory function, should be performed.

Treatment

Outcome from head injuries is determined to a certain degree by the primary impact injury, but it is clearly affected to a significant degree by the secondary response to trauma, whether neurologic or systemic in nature. The therapy outlined below decreases the secondary injury to whatever degree possible. Following adequate attention to the airway and circulation and evaluation of the patient's neurologic status, basic therapy for

Table 1–5. THERAPY FOR HEAD INJURY

1. Maintain airway and circulation
2. Protect cervical spine
3. Position
   - Elevate head 30–45 degrees
   - Head in midline
4. Maintain systemic arterial pressure
5. Hyperventilation (PA_{CO_2} = 25–28 torr)
6. Antibiotics (for penetrating injuries or open fractures)
   - Ampicillin
   - Methicillin
7. Dilantin (for persistent seizures 10 mg/kg)
8. Diuretics (for documented deterioration)
   - Mannitol (1 g/kg)
   - Furosemide (1–2 mg/kg)
9. Burr holes

head injury should be undertaken (Table 1–5).

Any sudden documented decrease in the level of consciousness is a neurosurgical emergency. When accompanied by focal neurologic findings (a fixed, dilated pupil, eye deviated down and outward, and contralateral or ipsilateral hemiparesis or hemiplegia), the cause in the immediate period after injury is usually increased intracranial pressure from an expanding hematoma. Diffuse brain injury may also result in significant intracranial pressure elevation, but this usually takes longer to develop.[62]

All patients with documented neurologic deterioration must be treated rapidly. If neurosurgical consultation is immediately available, it should be sought. However, if this is not possible, the physician caring for the patient has two therapeutic options available to "buy time" until the child can be referred for neurosurgical care. First, the use of diuretics may decrease brain water sufficiently to decrease the development of increasing intracranial pressure.[63]

The cranial vault has a fixed volume, the contents of which are brain, CSF, water, and blood. Intracranial hematomas, vascular engorgement, or brain edema may result in increases in intracranial pressure if the brain's compensatory mechanisms are exceeded. If pressure continues unabated, tentorial herniation ensues. Diuretics such as furosemide and mannitol cause a temporary decrease in the intracranial pressure by decreasing the amount of brain water. Both act rapidly in producing diuresis and should never be used without an indwelling bladder catheter. However, these drugs should not be used routinely and are seldom indicated unless prior neurosurgical consultation has been obtained. Mannitol (1 g/kg intravenously) may cause increased bleeding of intracranial hematomas and increases cerebral hyperemia (which may cause increased intracranial pressure). Furosemide (1 to 2 mg/kg IV) has fewer side effects, but both diuretics provide only short-term benefit. Even when diuretic use slows the progression of tentorial herniation, it is a transient effect, and the patient should be referred to a neurosurgeon immediately.

Second, in the rare cases in which diuretic therapy does not reverse neurologic deterioration or in which neurosurgical care is many hours away, the use of burr holes should be considered. Burr holes may be placed with a twist drill or cranial perforator in the emergency room or operating room. The first burr hole should be placed on the side of the dilated pupil, just anterior to the ear and 1 to 2 cm above the zygomatic process, in the temporal bone. If blood is not present in the epidural space, the dura mater should be carefully incised. If blood is not found here, the procedure should be performed in the posterior frontal and parietal areas, or on the opposite side, until either a collection of blood is found or the patient's neurologic status improves.[64] Although placement of burr holes by non-neurosurgeons is rarely necessary, it can be life-saving.

Proper head positioning may greatly decrease intracranial pressure by assuring that venous drainage of the head is optimized. Elevating the head 30 to 45 degrees and maintaining it in a midline position are appropriate measures and may be instituted in the field. The systemic arterial pressure should be controlled at normal levels. Neither hypotension nor hypertension is acceptable, since the brain is adversely affected by either. Initial fluid infusion is usually with balanced salt solutions if blood loss is present. This may be changed to maintenance electrolyte solutions at three-fourths maintenance levels after blood losses have been replaced and the blood pressure and pulse have normalized.

The cerebral circulation is extremely sensitive to changes in the arterial carbon dioxide tension (PA_{CO_2}).[65] A significant amount of cerebral vasoconstriction can be produced by even mild hyperventilation, and this is a potent means of decreasing intracranial pressure. Children with severe head injuries (unconsciousness, deterioration in clinical signs, or GCS of 8 or less) should be intubated and hyperventilated (PA_{CO_2} = 25–28 torr).

When intubation is not possible, the arterial carbon dioxide tension can be temporarily controlled with bag and mask ventilation.

Because the use of steroids in patients with head injury has never been conclusively shown to be of benefit, we no longer recommend this therapy. Patients with open skull fractures or penetrating brain injuries should receive ampicillin (200 mg/kg) and methicillin (100 mg/kg). If a patient presents with a foreign body in the brain, the foreign body should not be removed. Instead the foreign body should be stabilized with dressings until it can be removed in the operating room.

Patients with scalp lacerations should have the wound probed carefully for bony defects or foreign bodies. Scalp lacerations should be closed only after they have been explored, debrided, and irrigated.

Persistent convulsions greatly increase brain oxygen requirements and should be treated with diphenylhydantoin in a dose of 10 mg/kg intravenously, which may be repeated in 30 minutes if the seizures continue (see Chapter 16).

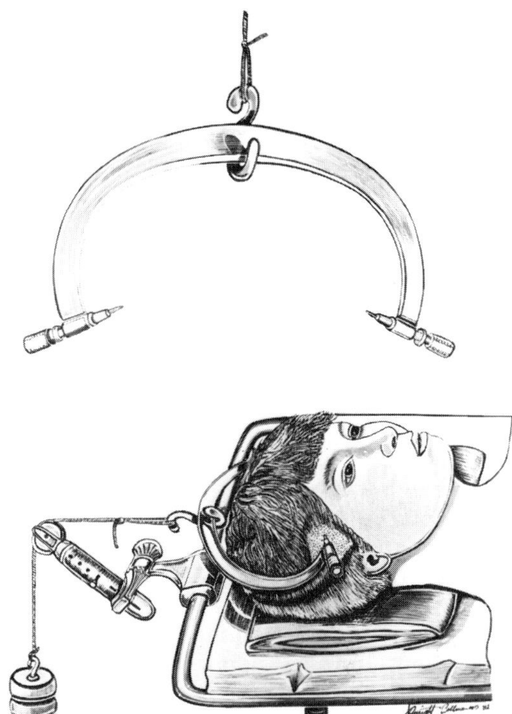

Figure 1–10. Patients with cervical spine fractures may need to be immobilized in Gardner-Wells tongs. The points of the tongs are inserted into the temporal ridge above the mastoid process. These tongs should not be used in neonates or infants or in patients with massive open or comminuted skull fractures, Paget's disease, or hangman's fracture when the mechanism of injury has been distraction.

Neck

Cervical spine injuries are rare in children under 12 years of age, but should be suspected in any child who has significant head or facial trauma, who is unconscious, who complains of neck pain, or who has injuries due to significant trauma of any type. The devastating consequences of neglecting such an injury and the subtle findings often associated with cervical spine fractures in children warrant this level of caution. In patients with unexplained, refractory shock, the possibility of spinal cord injury with spinal shock should be considered. Muscle flaccidity, deep tendon reflexes, and rectal sphincter tone should be assessed. Proper immobilization with sandbags, back boards, cervical collars, KED splints, or cervical tongs should be used to stabilize the cervical spine (Fig. 1–10). All spinal cord injuries in childhood should be considered reversible. They should be treated with immobilization, neurosurgical referral, and steroid therapy (dexamethasone 0.5 to 1.5 mg/kg). Of particular importance is the fact that up to 67 per cent of children with spinal cord injury have no radiographic abnormality demonstrated.[66] The majority of children with this syndrome of spinal cord injury without radiographic abnormality have symptoms of transient paresthesias, numbness, or subjective paralysis following the injury. Because of the devastating sequelae when such spinal cord injuries are neglected, any patient with such a history should remain in immobilization until evaluated by a neurosurgeon, even if the cervical spine radiographs are normal.

Penetrating injuries to the neck are uncommon in children but require careful evaluation for neurovascular and airway damage. Exploration of neck wounds should be carried out in the controlled conditions of the operating room. Neck wounds should *never* be probed in the emergency department.

Abdomen

The most important concern in patients with abdominal trauma is not to make a specific diagnosis of the exact type of injury, but to determine when acute abdominal injuries requiring surgery are present.[67] An orderly, efficient examination should be performed on all children, even those without abdominal trauma. This familiarizes the physician with the broad range of findings in children. Proficiency in examining the abdomen in children requires a thorough, systematic approach; experience; re-examination at frequent intervals; and reassurance to the child with each part of the examination. Serious abdominal injuries are often less obvious and are more difficult to diagnose than chest, head, or extremity injuries.

The dramatic findings of a tension pneumothorax require less diagnostic acumen than that required for accurate abdominal examination. In addition, the spectrum of findings in the abdominal examination is broad, from a child with hemoperitoneum, whose abdomen is rapidly filling with blood, to a child with more subtle, yet no less critical, injuries.

Hemorrhage is the most immediate threat to life in patients with abdominal trauma. Infection and intra-abdominal sepsis cause significant morbidity and mortality in patients who survive the initial injury, but hemorrhage constitutes the more immediate hazard.[68]

Examination of the abdomen should be approached thoroughly and carefully, since even minor changes may indicate crucial diagnostic information. The examination should be repeated at frequent intervals (at least every 15 minutes), since in many injuries, detectable signs evolve over the course of the initial examination and resuscitation.

In patients with shock and the possibility of abdominal injury, IV lines should be placed in the upper extremities, hematocrit and amylase levels should be obtained, and the child should immediately be typed and crossmatched for one fourth to one half the total blood volume.

The first step in examining the patient with abdominal trauma is to carefully note the vital signs, particularly the pulse and blood pressure; this should be repeated every 5 minutes during the initial phase of evaluation. A rising pulse and decreased pulse pressure may be the sole indicators of progressive intra-abdominal bleeding. In many cases, blood is not exquisitely irritating to the peritoneum, unless contaminated by bile, bowel contents, or pancreatic fluids. Therefore, the progressive development of shock may be the first indicator of significant abdominal organ injury.

Abdominal girth should be measured and recorded and the site of measurement marked with a pen (to insure that subsequent measurements are made at the same level). As noted previously, even small changes in abdominal girth may indicate major vascular depletion.

A double-lumen sump nasogastric or orogastric tube should be passed on all patients with abdominal trauma. This serves several functions, including (1) removing air from the stomach, which improves ventilation and lessens vagal stimulation; (2) emptying the stomach of liquid and particulate matter, thus decreasing the likelihood of aspiration and assisting preparation for anesthetic induction; and (3) providing diagnostic information concerning the presence of blood in the upper gastrointestinal tract.

All clothes should be removed before examination, with the important exception of MAST (see page 16). Rapid removal of MAST may result in profound and irreversible hypotension. Deflation of MAST should be delayed until a normal pulse and blood pressure have been attained, and then it should be accomplished gradually.

After checking the vital signs, placing a nasogastric tube, starting IV fluids, carrying out appropriate laboratory tests, and checking abdominal girth, the physician completes the examination by assessing the abdomen through (1) visual examination, (2) auscultation, (3) percussion, and (4) palpation. Visual examination identifies obvious injuries, whether in the form of bruises, hematomas, or penetrating injuries. With penetrating injury, it is particularly important to see if there are both entry and exit wounds. Auscultation reveals either presence or absence of bowel sounds. Rarely one may hear an abdominal bruit, with associated vascular injuries. On percussion, the abdomen may be normal, tympanitic, or dull. Tympany suggests gastric distention or free air from a perforated hollow viscus, whereas dullness is associated with hemoperitoneum or a full urinary bladder.

Palpation should be undertaken carefully and gently, starting at a location away from the site of injury. In conscious children, it is important to reassure them throughout the examination. It is often beneficial to have them place a hand on top of your examining hand to "help you," since this frequently reassures patients and allows a more thorough examination in frightened children. Point tenderness or generalized pain, with guarding, suggests peritoneal irritation, particularly when associated with rebound tenderness. Peritoneal irritation may be due to blood, bowel contents, or bile or pancreatic secretions. It is often difficult to distinguish abdominal wall pain from peritoneal irritation. In these cases, frequent examination, relaxation of the abdominal wall musculature, or peritoneal lavage (discussion follows) may be of assistance in making the diagnosis. Finally, the lower ribs and pelvis should be gently compressed to see if abdominal discomfort results, since this may reflect splenic, liver or pelvic injury.

Although many children with intra-abdominal organ injuries will have localizing signs of the injury, many other children have little in the way of physical findings other than unexplained shock. Conversely, in a frightened child, any manipulation may produce crying and mimic abdominal tenderness. The importance of frequent, gentle examinations and close monitoring of vital signs cannot be overemphasized.

Examination of other body areas may also give clues to abdominal injury. Shoulder pain in conjunction with left upper quadrant tenderness (Kehr's sign) indicates diaphragmatic irritation, frequently associated with splenic injury.[69] Rectal examination should be performed on all children with abdominal trauma. Presence of a cul-de-sac mass or pelvic rim tenderness may indicate peritoneal trauma. However, tenderness may be difficult to interpret owing to the anxiety created by the rectal examination.

Gentleness and reassurance greatly enhance the effectiveness of the examination. Pelvic examination may also be of value in detecting abdominal injury.

Peritoneal Lavage

When used appropriately, diagnostic peritoneal lavage may be of great benefit in detecting intra-abdominal injury. It is *never* a substitute for thorough physical examination of the abdomen. If physical examination reveals an acute surgical abdomen, peritoneal lavage is unnecessary and only delays definitive treatment.[70]

Specific indications for peritoneal lavage include altered level of consciousness due to alcohol intoxication or head injuries, spinal cord injury, lower rib or pelvic fractures, hematuria, and an abdominal examination that is not diagnostic but which leads to significant suspicion of abdominal injury remains.[30, 71, 72] Additionally, thoracic and other injuries that will require a long period of anesthesia necessitate peritoneal lavage.

This procedure is definitely contraindicated in patients with obvious indications for exploratory laparotomy and who have had multiple abdominal operations.[30] In the latter case, either four-quadrant paracentesis or laparoscopy may be diagnostic.

When peritoneal lavage is indicated, the surgeon who will be caring for the child should be consulted prior to the procedure. In some cases, the surgeon may request that the emergency physician or pediatrician proceed with lavage, but the surgeon should always be given an opportunity to examine the abdomen and perform the lavage. Details of the peritoneal lavage procedure are on pages 333–334.

Genitourinary Tract

Although genitourinary tract injuries occur frequently in children, the majority of these injuries are subtle in nature. Careful assessment is therefore necessary to make an accurate diagnosis. It is often easy to focus attention on a child with significant chest, head, or abdominal trauma and neglect consideration of the concomitant injuries to the genitourinary tract.

Any child with abdominal tenderness, pelvic fracture, perineal swelling, flank tenderness, or lower rib fractures should be considered to have some degree of genitourinary injury until proved otherwise. Inspection of the skin may be helpful in directing attention to injury. Abrasions, contusions, or ecchymosis over the flanks or lower abdomen should raise the suspicion of renal or bladder injury. Scrotal hematoma or perineal swelling raise the possibility of urethral injury. In patients who are conscious, inability to void despite the urge to do so indicates bladder or urethral injury. Palpation of the abdomen and flanks may cause pain at the site of injury or reveal the presence of a mass.

In all children in whom genitourinary injury is suspected, the bladder should be decompressed and urinalysis performed. Bladder decompression serves several purposes, including (1) providing a means of following urine output, (2) providing a sample for urinalysis, (3) decreasing risk of further complication in cases of urethral or bladder interruption by decreasing urinary extravasation, (4) preventing urinary obstruction that results from blood clots in the bladder, and (5) providing a route for contrast roentgenographic studies, when indicated. The most common means of bladder decompression is by urethral catheterization. An appropriate-sized, well-lubricated, soft

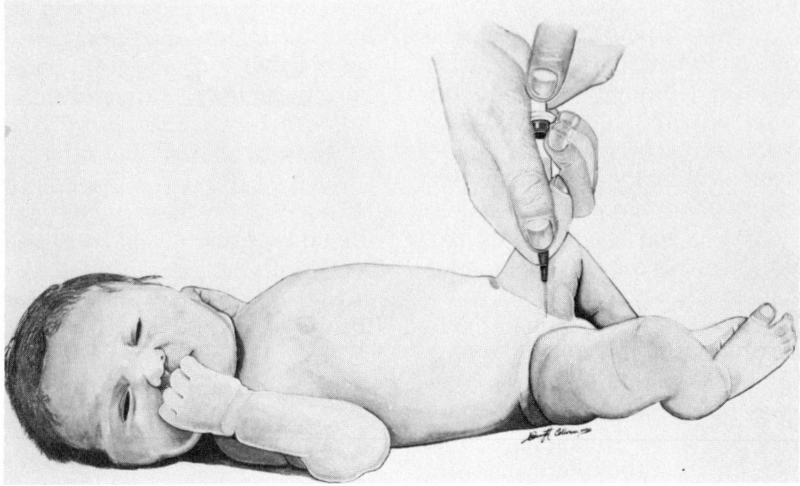

Figure 1–11. The bladder may be temporarily decompressed by percutaneous suprapubic catheterization. A plastic angiocatheter can be inserted just above the pubis in the midline at a 90-degree angle to the spinal axis. Aspiration of the syringe will produce urine when the bladder has been entered.

catheter should be placed under sterile conditions. Such a catheter should pass easily in children, and the procedure should be stopped if resistance is encountered. The contraindication to urethral catheterization is the possibility of urethral injury (scrotal hematoma, perineal swelling, blood at the urethral meatus, or inability to void). Forcing the catheter may convert a partial urethral tear into a complete one.[73]

An alternate method of temporarily decompressing the bladder is the use of percutaneous suprapubic decompression. Although suprapubic cystostomy may be indicated for more long-term care, a plastic angiocatheter can be temporarily inserted just above the pubis in the midline at a 90-degree angle to the spinal axis. Aspiration on a syringe will produce urine when the bladder has been entered (Fig. 1–11).

Gross or microscopic hematuria is present in most genitourinary tract injuries, but the degree of hematuria does not correlate with the severity of the injury.[74] Significant injuries may produce only microscopic hematuria, whereas minor injuries can result in gross hematuria.

The use of roentgenographic studies completes the examination and guides thorough evaluation of the genitourinary tract. However, these studies are seldom crucial in the initial, emergent phase of evaluation, except when renal artery injury is suspected. Detailed discussion of the uses and indications for these studies is in Chapters 8 and 21.

Renal Injuries. Most conscious children with renal injuries have some degree of localized tenderness. Flank pain, abdominal tenderness, and hematuria are classic signs of renal injuries, the majority of which are renal contusions.[75] A mass is less frequently encountered and is usually present only when perirenal hematoma or extrarenal extravasation occurs. Patients with lower rib fractures (particularly posterior rib fractures) should be suspected of having renal injury.

Nearly half of patients with renal injury have additional injuries.[76] Patients with abdominal, pelvic, or flank injuries may have additional genitourinary injury; conversely, patients with renal injury should be carefully evaluated for other injuries.

Bladder Injuries. Lower abdominal pain, inability to void, abdominal distention, and hematuria may be associated with bladder injuries. Additionally, nearly one fourth of patients with pelvic fractures have associated bladder trauma. Extraperitoneal bladder rupture may produce subtle physical findings but can be documented by cystogram. When bladder injuries are present, the urinary system should be decompressed until definitive repair can be provided.

Urethral Injuries. Urethral injury is seldom life-threatening but can produce significant morbidity if neglected and requires attention to the signs and symptoms it produces. Blood at the urethral meatus, scrotal hematoma, perineal swelling, history of perineal injury, high-riding prostate on rectal examination, and difficulty in urethral catheterization are all possible indicators of urethral injury.[77]

Urethral injuries are uncommon in females and are usually caused by direct trauma to the perineum.

Ureteral Injuries. Trauma to the ureter is uncommon, particularly in children, but should be suspected in patients with severe blunt trauma, penetrating trauma, or fracture of the lumbar spine transverse process. In patients with penetrating trauma, the disruption of the ureter may occur anywhere, but with blunt injury, the disruption is nearly always at the ureteropelvic junction.[78] An additional finding with ureteral injuries is the presence of an enlarging flank mass without signs of retroperitoneal bleeding, indicating extravasation of urine.

Skin and Extremities

Although only a limited number of skin and extremity injuries are life-threatening, the nature of these injuries, their diagnosis, and their sequelae are of a paradoxical nature, particularly in children. The most obvious injuries, which also frequently look quite painful, may have a relatively low potential for long-term morbidity. But many injuries with life-threatening potential are often much less obvious. For example, the physician's attention is easily drawn to a fully displaced fracture of the epiphysis at the wrist. A pelvic fracture, on the other hand, is often not readily apparent, yet carries a significantly greater threat to life. Thus, attention may be focused on some areas of gross deformity instead of on other musculoskeletal injuries that present in subtle ways. Therefore, all patients should be systematically evaluated for orthopedic injuries. Up to 25 per cent of patients admitted to major trauma centers have at least one missed diagnosis on their initial evaluation. Over 80 per cent of these missed diagnoses are orthopedic injuries.[44]

The two types of skeletal trauma that may be life-threatening are cervical spine injuries and bleeding produced by fractures. Evaluation of both requires a high degree of diagnostic acumen. (Since the threat to life in patients with cervical spine injuries results from the possibility of neurologic damage, this subject has been more fully addressed in that section, page 27). Even injuries that are not life-threatening in themselves may assume great importance in patients with multiple trauma, since the additional bleeding and stress of the orthopedic injury may compound other problems.

Two other factors necessitate that musculoskeletal injuries be carefully evaluated. First, although there are few life-threatening orthopedic injuries, there are a number of limb-threatening orthopedic problems. Major joint dislocations, amputations, development of compartmental syndromes, and open fractures may all result in the loss of a limb, a tragic outcome for a child. Second, significant sequelae may result from skeletal injuries, including deformity, infection, nerve damage, and limb inequality.[79]

All these facts underline the need for thorough evaluation for orthopedic injury at some point in the initial work-up of the injured patient. Skin and extremity trauma is usually assigned the lowest treatment priority, since stabilizing cardiorespiratory, neurologic, and abdominal injuries clearly takes precedence. However, even in the initial phase, when musculoskeletal injuries are not the top priority, a caveat is necessary. In simplest terms, the caveat is, "Primum non nocere," Hippocrates's warning to "First, do no harm." The importance of suspecting cervical spine injury in all injured patients deserves repetition. In all resuscitative measures, the spine *must* be protected, whether by traction, immobilization, or both. The warning also applies to all other areas of orthopedic injury. Any area of gross deformity should be splinted carefully so that alignment is maintained. Bleeding should be controlled by direct pressure, elevation and, when indicated, use of MAST trousers. Immobilization of injured areas and control of bleeding are the cardinal rules in preventing further damage to the patient with musculoskeletal trauma.

Evaluation of Injury

Evaluation of skeletal injuries should be thorough and systematic. The history may provide important information. Any injury involving high-energy trauma (motor-vehicle accidents, automobile-pedestrian collisions, falls from a significant height, etc.) carries a high risk of orthopedic injury. Certain types of trauma result in characteristic injury. Patients whose knees strike an automobile dashboard may suffer posterior dislocation of the hip, whereas those involved in falls may have both calcaneal fractures and lumbar spine injury. The history of tetanus immunization should be recorded in all patients.

General Principles

1
Active immunization against tetanus with tetanus toxoid plays a major role in markedly reducing the incidence of cases of this disease, and the resulting deaths.

2
Recommendations for tetanus prophylaxis are based on 1) the condition of the wound, especially as related to its susceptibility to tetanus, and 2) the patient's immunization history.

3
Regardless of the active immunization status of the patient, all wounds should receive immediate surgical treatment, using meticulous aseptic technique, to remove all devitalized tissue and foreign bodies. Such care is an essential part of prophylaxis against tetanus. (See *A Guide to Initial Therapy of Soft-Tissue Wounds*, American College of Surgeons.)

4 Warning:
The only contraindication to tetanus and diphtheria toxoids for the wounded patient is a history of neurologic or severe hypersensitivity reaction to a previous dose. Local side effects alone do not preclude continued use. If a systemic reaction is suspected to represent allergic hypersensitivity, postpone immunization until appropriate skin testing is performed later. If a contraindication to a tetanus toxoid-containing preparation exists, consider passive immunization against tetanus for a tetanus-prone wound.

Wound Classification

Clinical Features	Tetanus-Prone Wounds	Nontetanus-Prone Wounds
Age of wound	$>$ 6 hours	$\leq$ 6 hours
Configuration	Stellate wound, avulsion, abrasion	Linear wound
Depth	$>$ 1 cm	$\leq$ 1 cm
Mechanism of injury	Missile, crush, burn, frostbite	Sharp surface (eg, knife, glass)
Signs of infection	Present	Absent
Devitalized tissue	Present	Absent
Contaminants (dirt, feces, soil, saliva, etc.)	Present	Absent

Figure 1–12. Prophylaxis against tetanus. (From the Committee on Trauma, American College of Surgeons, April 1984. Reproduced with permission.)

Illustration continued on opposite page.

Evaluation of musculoskeletal injuries should be thorough and systematic. The patient should be fully undressed prior to evaluation, with the important exception of MAST trousers. The physician's major tool in evaluating orthopedic trauma is not the x-ray machine, but the hand. This is not to say that x-rays are unimportant, but only that their use should be guided by the history and physical examination. For example, any history of high-energy trauma to the upper body or to the lower extremities calls for radiographic evaluation of the cervical spine or pelvis, respectively. Other radiographs should be ordered on the basis of the physical findings.

Palpation of all bones and joints should be undertaken systematically. Progressing in a head-to-toe fashion and assessing each area is simple, requires little time, and assures that all areas are evaluated. Assessment of pulses, capillary filling, and neurologic status can be accomplished simultaneously with palpation. Motor and sensory functions of each major nerve can be quickly tested during this survey. If femoral fractures are suspected, the circumference of the thigh should be measured, since comparison with later measurements may indicate the amount of blood lost. The pelvis should be palpated over the wings of the ilium, over the pubis anteriorly, and posteriorly over the sacrum. Although pain is usually elicited in patients with pelvic fractures, any child with high-

Immunization Schedule

Verify a history of tetanus immunization from medical records so that appropriate tetanus prophylaxis can be accomplished.

Td: Tetanus and diphtheria toxoids adsorbed (for adult use)
TIG: Tetanus immune globulin (human)

History of Tetanus Immunization (Doses)	Tetanus-Prone Wounds		Nontetanus-Prone Wounds	
	Td[1]	TIG	Td[1]	TIG[2]
Uncertain	Yes	Yes	Yes	No
0 or 1	Yes	Yes	Yes	No
2	Yes	No[3]	Yes	No
3 or more	No[5]	No	No[4]	No

[1] For children less than seven years old, diphtheria and tetanus toxoids and pertussis vaccine adsorbed (or diphtheria and tetanus toxoids adsorbed, if pertussis vaccine is contraindicated) is preferable to tetanus toxoid alone. For persons seven years old and older, Td is preferable to tetanus toxoid alone.

[2] When administering TIG and Td concurrently, use separate syringes and separate sites.

[3] Yes, if wound is more than 24 hours old.

[4] Yes, if more than ten years since last dose.

[5] Yes, if more than five years since last dose. (More frequent boosters are not needed and can accentuate side effects.)

Disposition

Give each patient an appropriate written record describing treatment rendered and providing instructions for follow-up that outline wound care, drug therapy, immunization status, and potential complications. Arrange for completion of active immunization.

Give every wounded patient a wallet-sized card documenting immunization dosage and date received.

For further review of prophylaxis against tetanus, see *A Guide to Prophylaxis Against Tetanus in Wound Management,* available from the American College of Surgeons Trauma Department.

Figure 1–12 *Continued*

energy trauma to the torso or lower extremities should have a pelvic x-ray taken.

Pain on palpation or on movement of joints or extremities alerts the physician to the possibility of fractures. Sprains are relatively rare in young children, since the epiphyses are weaker than the surrounding ligaments at this age. Thus, pain, swelling, or gross deformity requires splinting until radiographs have been taken.

Treatment

During this initial phase, fractures are generally not reduced until radiographs have demonstrated the precise injury. The two exceptions to this rule are when distal neurovascular compromise is present or when impending skin necrosis is produced by bone fragments. When reduction is indicated, a single, gentle attempt is often successful. Repeated attempts are both traumatic and undesirable. Open fractures are generally not reduced until adequate debridement has been effected.[30, 80] Instead, careful splinting is the proper initial management.

Distal pulse and neurologic status should be assessed every 15 minutes with any fracture of the lower extremity. Although compartment syndromes are rare in children, they can result in amputation of the extremity. The classic signs of pain, paresis, paralysis, puffiness, pallor, and no pulse all herald increased pressure within the compartmental space. Loss of the pulse is a late finding; fasciotomy is usually required prior to its development. If a compartment syndrome is suspected, all constricting material should be loosened, the extremity should be elevated, and a surgeon should be consulted regarding fasciotomy.

Dislocations of the knee, hip, or elbow are emergent problems, since serious neurologic and vascular sequelae often follow these injuries.[81] The injured area should be immobilized and distal neurovascular status monitored, and an orthopedist must be consulted immediately.

Traumatic amputation may produce significant bleeding and can be a source of systemic infection. Bleeding should be controlled by direct pressure or elevation prior to debridement. Amputed parts should be cleaned, placed in sterile dressings moistened with normal saline, and then put in a plastic bag, which is then placed in ice. The patient should be transferred to the nearest replantation center when resuscitation is complete and if other major injuries do not preclude transport. Extremity replantation has provided remarkable results, and all children with amputation should be considered as possible candidates for this surgery.[82]

The care of soft-tissue injuries is outlined in Chapter 17. However, two facets of their care deserve emphasis here. First, any patient with a traumatic wound must have adequate tetanus immunization provided (Fig. 1–12). Adequate immunization is present if two injections of tetanus toxoid, at least 30 days apart, are followed by repeat injection every 5 years. Patients with adequate prior immunization who have a tetanus-prone wound should have adequate debridement of the wound. In addition, passive immunization with human immunoglobulin may be necessary if the wound is grossly contaminated or if extensive soft-tissue damage is present. Patients without adequate immunization should have debridement, tetanus toxoid, and passive immunization with human immunoglobulin. Regardless of immunization status, the cornerstone of tetanus prevention is careful irrigation and surgical debridement of the wound.

Second, *all* soft-tissue injuries should be irrigated and debrided, particularly when contamination is present. Bleeding should be controlled and clots removed from the wound prior to closure. Contamination should be treated with irrigation, debridement, and, in some cases, excision of the wound margins. All too often physicians rely on antibiotics to do what they could more effectively have done themselves—keep the wound clean.

PSYCHOLOGIC IMPACT OF PEDIATRIC TRAUMA

The final aspect of the initial evaluation and therapy of pediatric trauma victims is perhaps the least urgent, but it is as important as the life-saving measures listed earlier. Perhaps no other type of emergency creates more anxiety and emotional impact than does pediatric trauma. This impact affects not just the child suffering the injury but also the parents and companions, prehospital care personnel, nurses, ancillary health care assistants, and physicians involved in the care of the child. For this reason, all health care professionals should be aware of the psychologic factors present in pediatric trauma and be prepared to meet the challenge that these factors present.

Because of its sudden and unexpected nature, pediatric trauma is always both physical and psychologic in nature. Whether the injury is a simple laceration, a fall at home, or a major motor-vehicle accident, the child is immediately and precipitously placed in an environment that is often painful, unfamiliar, and anxiety-producing. Since injuries are always unexpected, the child is totally unprepared, for both the injury itself and the events following it. This is an extremely confusing time for a child for several reasons. Children's intellectual capacities and defense mechanisms are less well developed than are those of adults, and they tend to interpret the pain inflicted by the injury as punishment for wrongdoing. Particularly among school-age children, there is a tendency for the child to feel guilty for having been injured. This is further accentuated and complicated by the fact that the diagnostic and therapeutic processes of treating the child's injury often produce more pain and discomfort. Children often have difficulty in distinguishing the pain and discomfort of treatment from further punishment.

The child is immediately placed in an unfamiliar setting of the emergency department and is surrounded by strangers in white coats, bright lights, and strange machines. The result is an increasing amount of confusion and bewilderment about how to react to the situation. In this sense, the psychologic trauma involves not just the original pain and suffering inflicted by the injury but also a continuing cycle of distress for which few children are prepared.

To add to the confusion, the parents also undergo significant psychologic trauma. Immediately after a child has been injured, parents face a complex psychologic stress constituted by several emotions, including fear, anxiety, guilt, and anger. The predominating emotions early in the child's care are guilt and anger. Parents perceive the child's injury and their failure to prevent the injury as their fault. At the same time, the parents are angry at the child (although such anger is usually supressed) for having been injured. However, this anger produces even more guilt in the parents for having given in to this emotion. Parents are often edgy, unsure, and relatively unfamiliar with the surroundings of the emergency department. In many ways the parents are as confused by the experience as the child. It is extremely common for parents to displace their guilt and anger to the health professionals caring for their child. The depth of this anger can be striking. It is not uncommon for parents to express extreme hostility against nurses, laboratory and x-ray technicians, and physicians for perceived delays in treatment, pain caused by venipuncture or IV placement, injection of local anesthestics, and so on.

In addition, health professionals themselves also undergo a significant degree of psychologic trauma, particularly in cases of major injuries. Even for those who deal with pain, suffering, and death on a daily basis, very few professionals remain unaffected by the horror of a major injury to a child. Psychologically it is difficult to explain, rationalize, or distance oneself from such an injury. Simply stated, major pediatric trauma is perhaps the most graphic demonstration of one's own vulnerability and mortality. This invariably produces a certain degree of anxiety and tension among those caring for the child. The situation is further complicated by the fact that physicians and nurses often feel barely suppressed anger at the parents or guardians for failing to prevent the child's injury. Add to this situation a crying child, angry and anxious parents, and the relative rarity with which most emergency personnel care for major pediatric trauma, and it becomes apparent that psychologic trauma is a major factor for those caring for childhood injuries.

In view of the preceding, the following recommendations should be kept in mind when dealing with the psychologic and emotional factors involved in pediatric trauma.

1. The most important aspect for physicians, nurses, and other medical personnel is *preparation*. Familiarity with childhood injuries and the treatment of such injuries and an understanding of the psychologic factors involved for parents and children alike are invaluable.

2. Maintain a calm and organized approach to the care of the patient. This is best accomplished by familiarity with a protocol approach to the initial evaluation and therapy of injured children, as is outlined in this chapter. The use of such diagnostic and treatment protocols ensures that the child will be cared for in an organized fashion.

3. Always communicate clearly, simply, and frequently with the child. The best means of reassurance is a straightforward and simple approach. Always let the child know what you are doing and assure him that you are going to help. Explain each procedure to him carefully, so that he knows what's happening. Whenever possible, talk to the child while you are examining, treating, or suturing him. Asking the child about pets, friends, or favorite cartoon characters can all decrease the child's anxiety and help him remain calm and cooperative.

4. *Never* lie to a child or mislead him. If a procedure or manipulation is going to produce pain, tell the child this, even as you reassure him that it will not last long. Telling a child, "This won't hurt," when it will destroys all trust and ensures that all further treatment will be much more difficult. In addition, the child is likely to remember this breach of trust, and later encounters with physicians may be quite difficult as a result.

5. Be gentle in the approach to the child throughout the patient encounter. This gentleness includes the tone of voice used, palpation, use of surgical instruments, and application of dressings. Avoid sudden movements and loud tones of voice.

6. Decrease the waiting time between the explanation of a procedure and the procedure itself by careful preparation. This is particularly important when the procedure will be painful. Be sure all instruments, materials, and personnel needed for assistance are immediately available.

7. As soon as the procedure is completed, return the child to playful activity as soon as possible. This decreases the child's tendency to remember the pain and suffering of the procedure. Inflating surgical gloves into balloons, giving the child a piece of suture to play with, or making an empty syringe into a squirt gun may be of help.

8. Always adopt a nonjudgmental approach to parents, babysitters, or compan-

ions who may be at fault for the child's injury. Emergency physicians and pediatricians have a responsibility for legitimate counseling regarding child safety, but the appropriate time for such counseling is not during the initial diagnosis and treatment phase. A judgmental approach during this period complicates the child's treatment.

9. Provide emotional and psychologic support for the parents, family, and fellow health care personnel. Caring for an injured child may be emotionally difficult for all these people, and all require the physician's understanding and assistance.

10. Be careful of careless comments made during the care of injured children. Such comments are frequently misinterpreted by the child or parents and can interfere significantly with the communication necessary to provide optimal care.

11. Provide psychologic and emotional support early and often during the care of the child.

Attention to these psychologic and emotional factors can make the care of injured children much more satisfying and productive, as well as improve the experience for the child.

REFERENCES

1. Haller JA: An overview of pediatric trauma. *In* Touloukian RJ (ed.): Pediatric Trauma. St. Louis, J. Wiley and Sons, 1978.
2. Keddy JA: Accidents in childhood. Can Med Assoc J 91:675, 1964.
3. Baker SP, Dietz PE: The epidemiology and prevention of injuries. *In* Zuidema GD, Rutherford RB, Ballinger WF (eds.): The Management of Trauma. Philadelphia, W.B. Saunders Company, 1979.
4. Velcek FT, Weiss A, Di Maio DH, et al.: Traumatic deaths in urban children. J Pediatr Surg 12:375, 1977.
5. Heimlich HJ: First aid for choking children. Pediatrics 70:120, 1982.
6. Standards and guidelines for cardiopulmonary resuscitation (CPR) and emergency cardiac care (ECC). JAMA 244 (suppl):453, 1980.
7. Sodium bicarbonate in cardiac arrest (editorial). Lancet 1:946, 1976.
8. Roberts JR, Greenburg MI, Knowles MA, et al.: Blood levels from intravenous and endotracheal epinephrine administration. JACEP. 8:53, 1979.
9. McIntype KM, Lewis AJ (eds.): Textbook of Advanced Cardiac Life Support. Dallas, American Heart Association, 1981.
10. Gascho JA, Crampton RS, Cherwek M, et al.: Determinants of ventricular fibrillation. Circulation 60:231, 1979.
11. American Heart Association: Textbook of Advanced Cardiac Life Support, Dallas, 1983.

11a. Tocantins LM: Rapid absorption of substances injected into the bone marrow. Proc Soc Exp Biol Med 45:292, 1940.

11b. Arberiter HI, Greengard J: Tibial bone marrow infusion in infancy. J Pediatr 25:1, 1944.

11c. Quilligan JJ, Turkel H: Bone marrow infusion and its complications. Am J Dis Child 71:457, 1946.

11d. Heinild S, Sondergaard J, Tuvdad F: Bone marrow infusions in childhood: Experience from a thousand infusions. J Pediatr 30:400, 1947.

11e. Turkel H, Bethell FH: A new and simple instrument for administration of fluids through bone marrow. War Med 5:222, 1944.

11f. Tarrow AB, Turkel H, Thompson CS: Infusions via the bone marrow and biopsy of the bone and bone marrow. Anesthesiology 13:501, 1952.

11g. Meola F: Bone marrow infusions as a routine procedure in children. J Pediatr 25:13, 1944.

11h. Macht DI: Studies on intraosseous injection of epinephrine. Am J Physiol 138:269, 1943.

11i. Turkel H: Intraosseous infusion. JAMA 151:1108, 1953.

11j. Turkel H: Deaths following sternal puncture. JAMA 156:992, 1954.

11k. Hughes WT, Buescher ES: Pediatric Procedures. Philadelphia, W. B. Saunders Company, 1980, pp. 117–121.

11l. Berg RA: Emergency infusion of catecholamines into bone marrow. Am J Dis Child 138:810, 1984.

11m. Papper EM: The bone marrow route for injecting fluids and drugs into the general circulation. Anesthesiology 3:307, 1942.

12. Rutherford RB, Buerk CA: The pathophysiology of trauma and shock. *In* Zuidema GD, Rutherford RB, Ballinger WF (eds.): The Management of Trauma. Philadelphia, W.B. Saunders Company, 1979.
13. Blalock A: Experimental shock: The causes of the low blood pressure produced by muscle injury. Arch Surg 20:959, 1930.
14. Stede MW: Plasma volume changes in the neonate. Am J Dis Child 103:10, 1962.
15. Raffensberger JG: Pediatric surgical emergencies. *In* Beal JM (ed.): Critical Care for Surgical Patients. New York, Macmillan, 1982.
16. Sinclair JC, Driscoll JM, Heird WC, et al.: Supportive management of the sick neonate. Pediatr Clin North Am 17:163, 1970.
17. Moore FD: The effect of hemorrage on body composition. N Engl J Med 273:567, 1965.
18. Crenshal CA, Canuzaro PC, Shires GF, et al.: Changes in extracellular fluid during acute hemorrhagic shock in man. Surg Forum 13:6, 1962.
19. Lillehei RC, Longebeer JK, Block JA, et al.: The nature of irreversible shock: Experimental and clinical observations. Ann Surg 160:682, 1964.
20. Shires GT: Pathophysiology and fluid replacement in hypovolemic shock. Ann Clin Res 9:144, 1977.
21. Carey LC, Lowery ND, Cloutier CT: Hemorrhagic shock. Curr Prob Surg 3:48, 1971.
22. Poole GV: Comparison of colloids and crystalloids in resuscitation from hemorrhagic shock. Surg Gynecol Obstet 154:577, 1982.
23. Lucas CE, Ledgerwood AM, Higgins, RF: Impaired salt and water excretion after albumin resuscitation from hypovolemic shock. Surgery 86:544, 1979.
24. Weaver DW, Ledgerwood AM, Lucas CE, et al.: Pulmonary effects after albumin resuscitation for severe hypovolemic shock. Arch Surg 113:387, 1978.

25. Lucas CE: Hazards of colloid resuscitation in shock. *In* Najarian JS, Delaney JD (eds.): Emergency Surgery. Chicago, Year Book Medical Publishers, 1982.
26. Bowman DL, Weaver DW, Vega J, et al.: Effects of albumin on serum protein homeostasis after hypovolemic shock. J Surg Res 24:299, 1978.
27. Safar P: Resuscitation in hemorrhagic shock, coma, and cardiac arrest. *In* Cowley RA, Trump BF (eds.): Pathophysiology of Shock, Anoxia, and Ischemia. Baltimore, Williams and Wilkins, 1982.
28. Lewis HJ, Szeto HF, Bayer WL, et al.: Severe hemodilution with hydroxyethyl starch and dextran. Arch Surg 93:941, 1966.
29. Haupt MT: Colloid osmotic pressure and fluid resuscitation with hetastarch, albumin, and saline. Crit Care Med 10:159, 1982.
30. Committee on Trauma, American College of Surgeons: Advanced Trauma Life Support Course. Chicago, American College of Surgeons, 1984.
31. Committee on Trauma, American College of Surgeons: Early Care of the Injured Patient. Philadelphia, W.B. Saunders Company, 1982.
34. Shires GT: Crystalloid resuscitation in shock. *In* Najarian JS, Delaney JD (eds.): Emergency Surgery. Chicago, Year Book Medical Publishers, 1982.
33. Shires GT: Management of hypovolemic shock. Bull NY Acad Med 55:139, 1979.
34. Bivins MG: Blood volume displacement with inflation of anti-shock trousers. Ann Emerg Med 11:409, 1982.
35. Gaffney FA, Thal ER, Taylor WF, et al.: Hemodynamic effects of medical anti-shock trousers. J Trauma 21:931, 1981.
36. Hoffman JR: External counterpressure and the MAST suit: Current and future roles. Ann Emerg Med 9:419, 1980.
37. Abraham E: Pneumatic anti-shock trousers. West J Med 138:84, 1983.
38. Williams TM, Knopp R, Ellyson JH: Compartment syndrome after anti-shock trouser use without lower extremity trauma. J Trauma 22:595, 1982.
39. Brotman S, Brownor BD, Cox FP: MAS trousers improperly applied causing compartment syndrome in lower extremity trauma. J Trauma 22:598, 1982.
40. Cowley RA, Dunham CM (eds.): Shock Trauma/Critical Care Manual. Baltimore, University Park Press, 1982.
41. Freeland AE, Hughes JL Jr.: Early management of the severely injured extremity. *In* Hardy JD (ed.): Critical Surgical Illness. Philadelphia, W.B. Saunders Company, 1980.
42. Chan RN, Ainscow D, Sikorski JM: Diagnostic failures in the multiply injured. J Trauma 20:674, 1980.
43. Dove DB, Stahl WM, Del Guercio LRM: A 5 year review of deaths following urban trauma. J Trauma 20:760, 1980.
44. Johnson DG, Jones R: Surgical aspects of airway management in infants and children. Surg Clin North Am 56:263, 1976.
45. Mayer T, Matlak ME, Dixon J, et al.: Experimental subglottic stenosis: Histologic and bronchoscopic comparison of electrosurgical, cryosurgical, and laser resection. J Pediatr Surg 15:944, 1980.
46. Eichelberger MR, Randolph JG: Thoracic trauma in children. Surg Clin North Am 61:1181, 1981.
47. Richardson JD, Adams L, Flint LM: Selective management of flair chest and pulmonary contusion. Ann Surg 196:481, 1982.
48. Lindskog GE: Some historical aspects of thoracic trauma. J Thorac Cardiovasc Surg 42:1, 1961.
49. Jones KW: Thoracic trauma. Surg Clin North Am 60:957, 1980.
50. Mayer T, Matlak ME, Johnson DG, et al.: The modified injury severity scale in pediatric multiple trauma patients. J Pediatr Surg 15:719, 1980.
51. Mayer T, Walker ML, Johnson DG, et al.: Causes of morbidity and mortality in severe pediatric trauma. JAMA 245:719, 1981.
52. Bowers SA, Marshall LF: Outcome in 200 consecutive cases of severe head injury treated in San Diego County: A prospective analysis. Neurosurgery 6:237, 1980.
53. Becker DP, Miller JD, Ward JD, et al.: The outcome from severe head injury with early diagnosis and intensive management. J Neurosurg 47:291, 1977.
54. Bruce DA, Schut L, Bruno LA, et al.: Outcome following severe head injury in children. J Neurosurg 48:679, 1978.
55. Mayer T, Walker ML: Emergency intracranial pressure monitoring in pediatrics: Management of the acute coma of brain insult. Clin Pediatr 21:391, 1982.
56. Grossman RG: Treatment of patients with intracranial hematomas. N Engl J Med 304:1540, 1981.
57. Bruce DA, Raphaely RC, Goldberg AI, et al.: Pathophysiology, therapy, and outcome following severe head injury in children. Child's Brain 5:174, 1979.
58. Teasdale G, Jennett B: Assessment of coma and impaired consciousness: A practical scale. Lancet 2:178, 1974.
59. Jennett B, Bond MR: Assessment of outcome after severe brain damage. Lancet 1:480, 1975.
60. Jennett B, Teasdale G, Galbraith S, et al.: Severe head injury in three countries. J Neurol Neurosurg Psychiatry 40:291, 1977.
61. Gennarrelli T: Care of the head injured patient. Presented to the 67th Annual Clinical Congress of the American College of Surgeons, San Francisco, October 1981.
62. Bruce DA, Alavi A, Bilaniuk L, et al.: Diffuse cerebral swelling following head injury in children. The syndrome of "malignant brain edema." J Neurosurg 54:170, 1980.
63. Miller JD, Leech P: Effects of mannitol and steroid therapy on intracranial volume-pressure relationships in patients. J Neurosurg 42:4, 1975.
64. Wespic JG, Baker EP: Neurosurgical emergencies. *In* Wilkins EW (ed.): MGH Textbook of Emergency Medicine. Baltimore, Williams and Wilkins Company, 1978.
65. Enevoldzen EM, Jennsen FT: Autoregulation and CO_2 responsiveness of cerebral blood flow in patients with acute severe head injury. J Neurosurg 48:689, 1978.
66. Pang D, Wilberger JE: Spinal cord injuries without radiographic abnormalities in children. J Neurosurg 57:114, 1982.
67. Feins NR: Multiple trauma. Pediatr Clin North Am 26:759, 1979.
68. Anderson LB, Ballinger WF: Abdominal injuries. In Zuidema GD, Rutherford RB, Ballinger WF (eds.): The Management of Trauma. Philadelphia, W.B. Saunders Company, 1979.

69. Dunphy JE, Botsford TW: Physical Examination of the Surgical Patient. Philadelphia, W.B. Saunders Company, 1964.
70. Alyyono D, Perry JF: Value of quantitative cell count and amylase activity of peritoneal lavage fluid. J Trauma 21:345, 1981.
71. Goldberger JM: Selection of patients with abdominal stab wounds for laparotomy. J Trauma 22:476, 1982.
72. Moore JB, Moore EE, Markovchick VJ, et al.: Diagnostic peritoneal lavage for abdominal trauma: Superiority of the open technique at the infraumbilical ring. J Trauma 21:570, 1981.
73. Blandy J: Injuries of the urethra in the male. Injury 7:77, 1976.
74. Evins SC, Thomason WB, Rosenblum R: Non-operative management of severe renal lacerations. J Urol 123:247, 1980.
75. Morse TS, Smith JP, Howard WH, et al.: Kidney injury in children. J Urol 98:539, 1967.
76. Waterhouse K, Gross M: Trauma to the genitourinary tract: A 5 year experience with 251 cases. J Urol 101:241, 1969.
77. Waterhouse K: The surgical repair of membranous urethral strictures in children. J Urol 116:363, 1976.
78. Boston VE, Smyth BT: Bilateral pelvi-ureteric avulsion following closed trauma. Br J Urol 47;149, 1975.
79. Heppenstall RB (ed.): Fracture Treatment and Healing. Philadelphia, W.B. Saunders Company, 1980.
80. Gregory GF: Open fractures. *In* Rockwood CA, Green DP (eds.): Fractures. Philadelphia, J.B. Lippincott Company, 1975.
81. Chipman Clark (ed.): Emergency Department Orthopaedics. Rockville, Md., Aspen Publications, 1982.
82. Kleinert HE, Jablon M, Tsai T: An overview of replantation and results of 347 replants in 245 patients. J Trauma 20:390, 1980.

CHAPTER

2 Management of Hypovolemic Shock

THOM A. MAYER

This chapter has several purposes, the most important of which is to present a working definition of shock, as well as a general synopsis of the pathophysiology of shock in pediatric patients. However, this textbook focuses on pediatric *trauma* victims; therefore, the discussion will primarily address hypovolemic shock. More specifically, most of the discussion focuses on hemorrhagic shock, which is a specific subtype of hypovolemic shock. Interested readers are referred to other reviews of cardiogenic, obstructive, and distributive shock.[1–3] A second purpose of this chapter is to highlight the differences in shock in pediatric patients versus adult patients.

DEFINITION AND PATHOPHYSIOLOGY OF SHOCK

In many patients, the recognition and diagnosis of shock is straightforward. Few physicians would fail to diagnose shock in a patient with severe multiple injuries, a blood pressure of 80/40, a heart rate of 150 beats per minute, an altered mental status, gross external bleeding, and decreased urinary output. Similarly, a patient with a life-threatening cardiac arrythmia and grossly unstable cardiovascular parameters would also be recognized as suffering from shock (although the shock is of a different type). Some definitions of shock focus on the clinical signs and symptoms of the disease (cool, pale extremities; hypotension; tachycardia; altered mental status; diminished urine output, etc.). However, the blood pressure may be normal, the extremities warm and flushed, the pulse relatively normal, yet the patient may be in shock. As early as 1919, Archibald and McClean noted that, "While a low blood pressure is one of the most constant signs of shock, it is not the essential thing, let alone the cause of it. We have focused our attention far too much on blood pressure."[4]

The central factor in all patients with shock is a *generalized state of inadequate tissue perfusion, resulting in impaired cellular respiration.*[5–7] This working definition of shock encompasses the broadest possible range of the condition, as well as focuses on the essential defect that the patient experiences, since the clinical signs and pathophysiologic disturbances are summarized by generalized inadequate tissue perfusion.

Maintenance of adequate tissue perfusion requires a properly functioning pump (the heart) capable of delivering an adequate type and volume of fluid (blood) through appropriate vessels (arteries, veins, and capillaries) without obstruction to flow. Inadequate tissue perfusion may result from defects of the pump, fluid, or vessels or from obstruction to flow. Correspondingly, shock may be classified hemodynamically as resulting from *cardiogenic* (pump), *hypovolemic* (fluid), *distributive* (vessels), or *obstructive* (flow restriction) factors (Table 2–1).[8] Thus, an extremely wide array of pathologic states may result in the

Table 2–1. CLASSIFICATION AND CAUSES OF SHOCK

Class	Clinical Causes
Hypovolemic	Hemorrhage Burns Peritonitis Vomiting Heat loss
Cardiogenic	Myocardial infarction Cardiomyopathy Myocardial contusion Arrhythmias Valvular disease Heart failure
Obstructive	Tension pneumothorax Cardiac tamponade Flail chest Pulmonary embolus Hemo/pneumothorax Hypertension
Distributive	Spinal cord injury Anaphylaxis Septicemia Drugs Anesthesia

final disease process of shock, although the specific mechanism causing inadequate tissue perfusion differs. Whatever the cause of shock, the end result and common pathway are still the same—inadequate tissue perfusion.

However, during the intitial phase of care of the trauma patient, shock is nearly always hypovolemic in nature. Furthermore, the hypovolemia that the patient experiences is usually due to either external or internal hemorrhage. (However, patients suffering from major burns have hypovolemic shock in which plasma is the major volume constituent lost.) Therefore, hemorrhagic shock (as a subtype of hypovolemic shock) is given primary focus in the following discussion. In rare cases, shock that manifests during the initial phase of care of the pediatric trauma patient may be due to other factors. For example, occasional pediatric patients are seen with spinal cord injury resulting in distributive shock. In addition, some patients may present with pericardial tamponade or tension pneumothorax and thus have obstructive shock. However, in most cases, the initial cause of shock in the pediatric trauma victim is hypovolemia. In addition, many pediatric trauma victims have the complicating factor of *hypoxia*, which markedly worsens existing shock. In this sense, both hypovolemia and hypoxia are critical factors in the development of shock in pediatric patients.[9]

Hypovolemic Shock

The development of hypovolemic shock is an extremely dynamic process, with multiple homeostatic mechanisms responding to maintain adequate tissue perfusion. The mechanisms involved in maintenance of perfusion depend on the amount and rate of blood loss, which is dependent on the type and severity of the trauma but which is also modified by factors such as age, underlying diseases, medications, and cardiovascular reserve. The earliest, simplest response to blood loss involves local factors, including vasoconstriction and activation of the coagulation system. Vasospasm at the site of injury and release of tissue thromboplastins, serotonin, and other clotting factors are the body's initial responses to localized bleeding.

The body's first major homeostatic response to hemorrhage is a rapid increase in venous tone, partially intrinsic to the venous system and partially sympathetically mediated. This increase in tone diverts blood from the venous capacitance system to the effective circulation, where it is needed. In effect, this results in an autotransfusion of significant magnitude, since in the resting state up to 70 per cent of the total blood volume resides in the capacitance system (the veins and venules).[10] This is a very rapid response, and a vital one, but its ability to compensate for blood loss is understandably limited to the amount of blood that can be "transfused" from the capacitance system. When blood loss reaches approximately 15 per cent of total blood volume, the increase in venous vasomotor tone is maximal and the homeostatic value of increased venous tone is exceeded.[11] At the same time, extracellular fluid mobilization also begins, with movement of fluid from the interstitial to intravascular space (see below).[12, 13] This phenomenon is known as transcapillary refill and results both in an increase in the intravascular volume and a decrease in the interstitial fluid compartment.[14, 15] This process requires at least 6 to 12 hours to complete and therefore does not account for large volume changes in the earliest phases of the homeostatic process.

Although up to 15 per cent of the total blood volume has been lost, few physical signs or symptoms are present to indicate the development of shock. When the limits of venous autotransfusion are exceeded, the venous pressure falls slightly, and diastolic filling of the heart decreases, which may cause a slight fall in stroke volume. However, these effects are extremely short-lived and are usually undetectable by the clinician. This is because atrial, carotid, and aortic baroreceptors detect these abnormalities and relay the information to the afferent arm of the regulatory system, the hypothalamic regulatory centers in the vasomotor center in the medulla.[16] The efferent arm of the system is the sympathetic nervous system, including both alpha- and beta-adrenergic receptors. The former receptors are responsible for peripheral vasoconstriction, resulting in the shunting of blood from the skin and muscle to the viscera (with the heart and brain being the focus of maintenance of perfusion).[17] These responses, in conjunction with the increase in venous tone previously described, result in an increase in total peripheral resistance. *Thus, the earliest detectable sign of im-*

pending shock is an increase in diastolic pressure or a decrease in pulse pressure.[18, 19] Arterial blood pressure is maintained at a normal level, but it is critical to note that this results in depletion of residual compensatory mechanisms.

Beta-adrenergic stimulation results in inotropic and chronotropic effects on the heart and increased oxygen utilization. Additional clinical signs that quickly follow the increase in diastolic arterial pressure are a prolonged capillary refilling time (due to peripheral vasoconstriction) and a slight increase in the heart rate (secondary to beta-adrenergic stimulation).

At this stage of blood loss (15 to 25 per cent of total blood volume), the diastolic blood pressure is elevated, the pulse is slightly elevated, and a prolonged capillary refilling time may be present. The systolic arterial pressure is well maintained, further emphasizing the fact that blood pressure alone is an inadequate barometer of shock. However, at this point the patient's residual compensatory mechanisms are precariously low. Endocrine stimulation results in aldosterone and antidiuretic hormone release, with salt and water retention contributing to maintenance of adequate circulatory volume.[20] Additional signs of impending shock at this stage are restlessness or anxiety (secondary to adrenergic stimulation), thirst, and a mild increase in the respiratory rate, which may result in mild respiratory alkalosis.

At this point, up to 15 to 25 per cent of the total blood volume may have been lost, but blood pressure is maintained at a normal level. Increased total peripheral resistance, adrenergic stimulation, extracellular fluid mobilization, and endocrine responses have all been recruited and produce signs that the effective circulatory volume has been compromised. However, if the clinician is not attuned to these sometimes subtle signs and the pathophysiologic mechanisms that produce them, he cannot fully comprehend the patient's status, much less treat it effectively. Furthermore, the patient's homeostatic mechanisms are extremely labile at this point, and even small increases in blood loss or the continuation of blood loss may result in rapid and serious clinical deterioration.[21] At approximately 25 to 30 per cent blood loss, these mechanisms fail to more ostensible degrees, resulting in a fall in arterial blood pressure. At nearly the same level of blood loss, cellular respiration is compromised to the extent that anaerobic metabolism predominates and systemic acidosis results. This acidosis decreases myocardial contractility, decreases myocardial and vascular responses to catecholamines, and promotes intravascular clotting.[22] Thus, shortly after hypotension develops, the patient becomes acidotic and relatively more resistant to resuscitation because shock has been developing well before hypotension becomes apparent.

As tissue perfusion fails and anaerobic metabolism becomes the predominant source of energy production, several consequences result. Anaerobic metabolism is extremely inefficient, producing only 2 moles of adenosine triphosphate (ATP) per mole of glucose metabolized. Aerobic metabolism, on the other hand, produces 38 moles of ATP per mole of glucose metabolized through the tricarboxylic acid cycle. In addition to producing minimal amounts of ATP, excess lactate is produced and systemic acidosis may result.[23]

The most important result of anaerobic metabolism is the failure of the energy-dependent sodium-potassium pump. This pump is responsible for maintaining the normally low intracellular sodium by pumping it out against a gradient.[24, 25] In this sense, the sodium-potassium pump is responsible for maintaining the normal homeostatic environment in which the cell functions. Lysosomal and mitochondrial function, as well as membrane structure, are dependent upon the maintenance of this homeostasis. When the sodium pump fails, sodium and water move into the cell from the interstitial space and potassium moves out.[26, 27] This process results in marked depletion of interstitial fluid and increases in intracellular volume. Thus, the cell begins to swell as tissue perfusion fails.

Hemorrhagic shock therefore results in three major changes in the patient's total body water composition. First, there is a decrease in the effective circulatory volume or total blood volume. Second, as tissue perfusion falls there is an increase in the intracellular fluid volume as the sodium-potassium pump fails. Finally, as transcapillary refill occurs, fluid is drawn from the interstitial fluid compartment, resulting in a relative deficit in this space.

If inadequate tissue perfusion and oxygen deprivation persist for a long enough period of time, major cellular damage ensues.[28–30] As the cell swells and energy failure continues, mitochondria and lysosomes are injured, the cell membrane is disrupted, and the cell fails and dies. If enough cells are injured, tissue failure, organ failure, and/or death of the organism may result.

In addition to the cardiovascular, cellular, and subcellular changes present in shock, myriad other alterations have been noted, affecting virtually the entire organism, including the kidney,[31] liver,[32, 33] heart,[34] and central nervous, endocrine, immunologic, and hematologic systems.[35–37] Readers interested in exploring the multiple aspects of the pathophysiology of shock are directed to excellent, in-depth reviews of the subject.[38, 39]

In summary, the pediatric trauma victim in shock most often suffers from hypovolemic shock, usually secondary to hemorrhage, but which may be further complicated by the presence of hypoxia. In essence, shock is a generalized failure of adequate tissue perfusion, resulting in impaired cellular and subcellular respiration. However, the development of shock is a progressive and dynamic process, and one in which loss of up to 25 per cent of blood volume may be remarkably insidious. For this reason, clinicians must be aware of the pathophysiologic processes of shock, as well as the signs and symptoms that these processes produce. As hypovolemic shock progresses, three major alterations in body fluid composition are noted: a decrease in effective circulatory volume, an increase in intracellular fluid space as the sodium-potassium pump fails, and finally, a deficit in the interstitial fluid space as transcapillary refill occurs.

SHOCK IN THE PEDIATRIC PATIENT

Having established a working definition of shock and having defined the pathophysiology of the disease, a question still remains, "Is shock different in the pediatric patient?" The answer to this question is necessarily equivocal. To begin with, the types of shock are the same in adult and pediatric patients and may be classified as hypovolemic, cardiogenic, obstructive, or distributive. The pathophysiology of shock appears to be the same in the adult and pediatric patient, particularly at the cellular level.[40] Generalized inadequate tissue perfusion is the basis of shock regardless of the patient's age, and basic cellular responses appear to be identical. Although research models for pediatric shock have not been extensively developed or tested,[40, 41] it is nonetheless generally accepted that the general pathophysiology of the disease does not differ in adult and pediatric patients.

However, in several respects shock is quite different in pediatric patients. First, although pediatric patients may be subject to any one of the four types of shock, cardiogenic shock and, to a lesser extent, obstructive shock occur much less frequently in children. This is simply because children rarely suffer from diseases that predispose to the development of these types of shock. For example, myocardial ischemia or infarction, pulmonary embolism, systemic hypertension, and arrhythmias are rarely seen in children. Since trauma and infection are more common causes of morbidity and mortality in pediatric patients, it is not surprising that most cases of pediatric shock are hypovolemic or distributive in nature. Specifically, hemorrhagic shock and septic shock are the most common types of pediatric shock.

Second, there is a precariously thin margin for error in recognition and treatment of pediatric patients with serious injury. Because of their smaller total blood volume, children may lose the same amount of blood as an adult with a similar injury, but this amount represents a much larger percentage of total blood volume. For example, a scalp laceration may result in the rapid loss of large quantities of blood. In the adult patient, this blood loss would be well tolerated, whereas in the child it can represent a major hemorrhage.

Third, the types of injury differ in pediatric and adult patients. Data from several centers indicate that neurologic injury occurs more frequently in children, in part because the head accounts for a larger percentage of body surface area and weight.[42, 43] Furthermore, pediatric patients with head injury have anatomic and pathophysiologic differences in their response to head injury. Pediatric patients have a lower incidence of mass lesions and more often show diffuse cerebral swelling in response to severe head injury.[44] As an additional example, pediatric patients with abdominal trauma much more commonly experience paralytic ileus.[45] This fact is extremely important in the treatment of pediatric patients in shock because ileus may cause abdominal distention and subsequent diaphragmatic elevation, which may compromise pulmonary function.

Fourth, although adults have specific ranges for normal values for pulse, blood pressure, heart rate, and respiratory rate, these indices are developmental and age-related in pediatric patients. This fact requires the clinician to have a broader knowledge of the range of normal values in children (see Chapter 1). In addition, drugs and intravenous infusions are age and/or weight related in pediatric patients, as opposed to the relatively fixed dosages and volumes used in adult patients.

Fifth, patients below the age of 2 years, and even many older pediatric patients, are unable to verbalize adequately the severity and location of pain, rendering diagnosis much more difficult. This lack of verbal communication requires the physician to maximize use of his diagnostic skills.

Sixth, pediatric patients have a much more erratic homeostatic thermoregulatory response, particularly infants.[46] Adults tolerate being fully undressed for evaluation. However, exposure in a cold examination room or x-ray room and intravenous infusion of fluids below body temperature can often greatly compound shock in the pediatric patient, whose thermoregulatory mechanisms are much less effective.

Finally, infants classically present with signs and symptoms of shock that differ in important respects from those of either older pediatric patients or adults. Infants in shock may present with hyper- or hypoventilation, erratic cardiovascular parameters, skin mottling, glucose intolerance, metabolic instability, or progressive respiratory failure.[47] In many cases, the onset of shock in infants is insidious, requiring continual monitoring and frequent examination for timely recognition.

GOALS OF THERAPY FOR SHOCK

Chapter 1 presents a practical approach to the initial treatment of pediatric patients in shock, emphasizing the goals of restoring effective circulatory volume, maximizing oxygen delivery, and decreasing ongoing blood loss. The purposes of this section are to further delineate the rationale and conceptual basis for such therapy and to present data on the possibilities of future therapy for shock. In some cases, one form of therapy may assist in accomplishing more than one goal and is therefore listed under more than one heading.

Restoring Effective Circulatory Volume

Numerous clinical and laboratory studies verify that rapid expansion of the effective circulatory volume results in improved outcome for patients with hemorrhagic shock.[48–50] This is true regardless of whether the fluid infused is crystalloid, colloid, whole blood, blood components, or synthetic blood substitutes. A significant controversy continues concerning which of these solutions is *most* appropriate for the initial resuscitation of the shock patient (see later section), but all agree that restoration of volume is beneficial. Because the underlying defect in shock is failure of tissue perfusion, it is not surprising that restoration of perfusion per se is beneficial. The Fick equation, which quantitatively describes oxygen consumption, is readily used as a guide in understanding the priorities of therapy for shock.

$$V_{O_2} = Q \times 1.39\ Hb \times (Sa_{O_2} - Sv_{O_2})$$

There are three variables in this equation affecting oxygen consumption: blood flow, hemoglobin concentration, and fractional unloading of oxygen from the hemoglobin molecule. When conceptionalized in this manner, it is clear that even if hemoglobin and fractional unloading of oxygen remain constant, increasing blood flow independently increases oxygen transport. Thus, the first goal of therapy is to restore volume, either by *infusing* crystalloids or colloids or by *transfusing* blood or blood components.

Prior to experimental and clinical studies in the 1960s, most surgeons believed that the most important aspect of therapy in hemorrhagic shock was rapid transfusion of whole blood, since it was assumed that this was the central deficit. However, landmark studies by Moyer,[51] Shires,[52] and others[53] documented the phenomenon of transcapillary refill and the deficit in the interstitial fluid space. These studies and extensive clinical experience indicated that early use of colloids or crystalloids significantly benefited the trauma patient.[54–56] However, over the next 20 years an extensive debate developed between proponents of crystalloid infusion and those in favor of colloid infusion. The American College of Surgeons' Committee on Trauma recommends initial resuscitation with crystalloid solution (specifically, Ringer's lactate solution),[57, 58] but the controversy continues, and the reader can easily find conflicting recommendations in the literature regarding fluid resuscitation. The following is a brief summary of the laboratory and clinical studies used to justify both colloid and crystalloid infusion.

Colloids Versus Crystalloids

Proponents of colloid therapy for patients in hemorrhagic shock usually base their recommendation on two assumptions. First, as early as 1959, Guyton and Lindsey[59] demonstrated the role that plasma colloid osmotic pressure (PCOP) can play in the development of pulmonary edema, inasmuch as they showed that lowering PCOP in dogs resulted in lowering the threshold for development of pulmonary edema. Furthermore, a normal PCOP has been advocated to be a critical factor in both maintenance of an appropriate left ventricular filling pressure and an appropriate gradient between colloid osmotic pressure and hydrostatic pressure. In this sense, colloid therapy is said to be superior to crystalloid therapy because presumably it maintains a normal PCOP better (thereby improving optimal preload) and because a decrease in PCOP (supposedly occurring with the use of crystalloid solutions) would result in pulmonary edema.[60] The second assumption is that colloid resuscitation practically results in shorter resuscitation time, improved outcome, and less development of peripheral edema than crystalloid resuscitation.[61]

Although numerous laboratory and clinical studies[62–64] are cited to demonstrate the superiority of colloid over crystalloid resuscitation, most of these studies suffer from either a failure to assess resuscitation on the basis of cardiovascular parameters, such as left ventricular filling pressure or cardiac output (or both), or a failure to account for the larger volume of fluid required for crystalloid resuscitation (see later).

Supporters of crystalloid resuscitation base their arguments on several factors. First, left ventricular filling pressure and not PCOP is the most critical aspect of resuscitation in hemorrhagic shock. Although PCOP may be higher in patients who undergo colloid resuscitation, this has not been shown to affect response to resuscitation or outcome. Because of the effectiveness and extensiveness of pulmonary lymphatics, a decreased PCOP does not appear to play a significant role in the development of pulmonary edema or adult respiratory distress syndrome (ARDS) in the trauma patient.[65, 66] Esrig[67] and Kohler[68] have shown that sepsis and not decreased PCOP or crystalloid infusion is associated with the development of ARDS. In both multiple trauma patients[69] and patients undergoing major aortic reconstructions,[70] left ventricular filling pressure and cardiac output are the most accurate indicators of the adequacy of resuscitation and no difference in outcome was present in patients with colloid versus crystalloid resuscitation. Virgilio[70] noted both decreased PCOP and serum albumin in patients with crystalloid resuscitation, but there was no difference in intrapulmonary shunt, cardiac output, or pulmonary capillary wedge pressure. More importantly, he noted no difference in outcome in patients with crystalloid versus colloid resuscitation, despite the preceding changes.

Second, the interstitial fluid deficit described by Shires[52] and others[51, 53] requires resuscitation of the patient by infusion of a fluid that equilibrates with this space. The original studies showed that resuscitation with Hartmann's solution did equilibrate with this space and more effectively resuscitated laboratory animals.[51, 52] (Since that time, most clinicians have substituted lactated Ringer's solution for Hartmann's solution in treatment of the trauma patient.)

Third, because of equilibration and transcapillary refill, the volume of crystalloid solution infused is much greater than either the amount of blood lost or the amount of blood or colloid solution required for resuscitation. Moyer[51] estimated that three to four times as much balanced salt solution would be required for proper resuscitation in hemorrhagic shock, a figure remarkably close to the current recommendation of 3 ml of balanced salt solution infused for each milliliter of blood lost. Again, this recommendation is based on the fact that a significant degree of equilibration occurs, with the balanced salt solution replacing the interstitial fluid deficit described previously.

Fourth, detailed studies on trauma patients have demonstrated altered pulmonary[71] and renal function[72] in patients resuscitated with albumin solution as compared with those undergoing crystalloid resuscitation. In addition, changes in myocardial function and coagulation were implied by these data, although subsequent studies have been less clear concerning these effects. Weaver[73] and Moss[74] have noted prolonged ventilation time

(8 days in patients resuscitated with colloid solution versus 3 days in those resuscitated with crystalloid solution) and a higher $F_{I_{O_2}} - Pa_{O_2}$ ratio in patients treated with colloid solution. Lower glomerular filtration rates and lower sodium and osmolar clearance were also noted in patients resuscitated with colloid solutions.[72] Although these extensive studies indicate that there may be an increased incidence of complications in trauma patients resuscitated with colloid solutions, other clinical studies have failed to confirm these findings.[75]

Fifth, given the fact that resuscitation with albumin has not been shown to be superior to crystalloid resuscitation and may be associted with increased side effects, cost considerations assume significant importance. The average cost for patients resuscitated with albumin solutions is $1,040, compared with a resuscitation cost of $8.00 using crystalloid solutions.[76] For all the preceding reasons, most trauma surgeons recommend infusion of crystalloid solution for the initial resuscitation of the trauma patient.

Additional studies continue on alternate solutions for infusion therapy, including dextran,[77] hetastarch,[78] stroma-free hemoglobin,[79] and perfluorochemicals.[80] However, at present there is no justification for the use of these solutions in pediatric patients. Thus, the best means for initially restoring effective circulatory volume in the pediatric patient with hypovolemic shock is by initial infusion of crystalloid solution. The volume infused and strategy employed are detailed in Chapter 1.

Transfusion of Blood and Blood Components

Transfusion of blood or blood components also serves to restore effective circulatory volume but is reserved for the initial resuscitation of the trauma patient with exsanguinating hemorrhage. Patients in whom blood loss has been documented may require the immediate transfusion of type O negative or type-specific blood. Most pediatric trauma victims in hypovolemic shock can initially be resuscitated with crystalloid solution, with blood transfusion given after the blood has been typed and crossmatched. Details of transfusion therapy are listed later.

An additional means of increasing the effective circulatory volume is by autotransfusion from a hemothorax. Although this technique has been utilized widely on adult patients, there is very little experience with it in the pediatric age group. This is probably due to the fact that penetrating trauma and large hemothoraces are uncommon in children.

A final means by which effective circulatory volume may be increased is through the use of Military Anti-Shock Trousers (MAST). MAST do serve to increase the effective circulatory volume. However, it has been demonstrated that the major response to MAST use is from the nonpharmacologic increases in total peripheral resistance.[81, 82] The amount of autotransfusion resulting from MAST use is limited to 5 to 10 per cent of the total blood volume.[83] Thus, although MAST do result in minor increases in the effective circulatory volume, the major role that they play is in increasing the total peripheral resistance.

Maximizing Oxygen Delivery

Optimizing oxygen delivery is essential to the care of the patient in shock, since inadequate tissue perfusion affects both blood flow and oxygen delivery. Several specific aspects of therapy for shock assist the patient by maximizing oxygen delivery. Of prime importance is maintenance of an adequate airway with provision of humidified oxygen (see Chapters 1 and 3). Supplemental oxygen should be provided to *all* pediatric patients with signs or symptoms of shock, at least until arterial blood gases can be evaluated. Maintenance of a Pa_{O_2} of 90 to 100 is clearly beneficial, although there is no evidence that hyperoxemia is of benefit and it may even be harmful.[84]

In addition to providing an adequate airway and supplemental oxygen, transfusion may be required by many patients in hemorrhagic shock to increase the red blood cell mass, since this constitutes the major oxygen-carrying capacity. Transfusion with blood or blood components accomplishes all three goals of shock therapy, inasmuch as it increases the effective circulatory volume, increases oxygen delivery (assuming that red blood cells or whole blood is transfused), and may decrease further blood loss by replacing platelets and coagulation factors. For this reason, transfusion of blood or blood components constitutes the mainstay of major trauma resuscitation, and a clear understanding of transfusion therapy is essential.

In most patients with 25 per cent or more blood loss, or in patients with continuing signs of shock, blood replacement will usually be necessary.[85] The amount of red blood cells transfused depends upon the magnitude of blood loss present in any given patient. By observing the patient's signs and symptoms, a fairly accurate estimate of blood loss can be made (see Chapter 1, pages 13–15). Once the loss has been estimated, the red cell mass can then be restored via transfusion. Alternately, some clinicians prefer to empirically transfuse 10 to 15 ml/kg of packed red blood cells for patients with 25 per cent or less blood loss. Transfusion of this volume may be repeated if blood loss continues or if severe hemorrhage is present. Finally, some physicians transfuse trauma patients until a hematocrit of 35 is attained. However, because hemorrhage, transcapillary refill, and fluid equilibration are dynamic processes, this method may prove inaccurate.

Whole Blood Versus Component Therapy

As mentioned previously, for many years transfusion with whole blood was the "gold standard" for trauma patients, largely because it was assumed that whole blood infusion resulted in precise replacement of the fluid that had been lost. However, further experience and study showed that in addition to blood loss there was a deficit in the interstitial fluid compartment. With the advent in the 1950s of plastic blood bags that could be easily centrifuged, entered aseptically, and stored without altering the viability of the blood products, blood components became more widely utilized. This trend has continued, and over 40 per cent of all blood utilization today is by component therapy.[86, 87] One of the reasons for this has to do with the relative availability of fresh (less than 3 days old) donor blood and the "storage lesion," which occurs in all stored blood but is accentuated in blood stored for long periods (excellent reviews detail the components of the storage lesion).[88, 89]

Component therapy refers to the centrifugation and separation of blood into its component parts, with transfusion of relatively isolated components to match the individual patient's needs. Its specificity contrasts with the "shotgun" transfusion of whole blood, in which the patient often receives unnecessary components. The advantages of component therapy are better utilization of a scarce resource (one unit of blood may benefit several patients), less volume is transfused, component transfusions are generally more concentrated and have

Table 2–2. COMPONENT THERAPY

Component	Indications	Contents	Amount per Unit
Whole blood	Hemorrhage ≥100% TBV*	Red cells	230 ml
Type O negative	Exsanguinating hemorrhage	Plasma	220 ml
Type specific	Exsanguinating hemorrhage	Anticoagulants	63 ml
Typed and cross matched	Ongoing losses	Stable coagulation factors	
Packed red cells	Hemorrhage ≥25%	Red cells	230–250 ml
		Plasma	minimal
Platelets	Plt† count ≤20,000/mm³	Platelets	5.5×10^{10}
	Plt† count ≤30,000/mm³ + surgery	Stable coagulation factors	1–2%
	Plt† count ≤50,000/mm³ with bleeding		
Fresh frozen plasma	PT/PTT‡ >1.5 normal, or every 3–4 units PRBCs§	All coagulation factors	175–250 units
		Fibrinogen	500 mg
Cryoprecipitate	Hemophilia A	Fibrinogen	250 mg
	von Willebrand's disease	Factors V and VIII	80–100 units
	Hypofibrinogenemia		

*TBV = total blood volume.
†Plt = platelet.
‡PT/PTT = prothrombin time/partial thromboplastin time.
§PRBC = packed red blood cells.

greater biologic activity, and more specific therapy is provided (Table 2–2).

Whole Blood. Whole blood transfusion is now much less commonly used in trauma centers than previously. However, some surgeons argue that whole blood transfusion may be faster, more effective, and present less hepatitis risk in patients requiring massive transfusion (over ten units or one total blood volume transfusion). Nevertheless, most trauma surgeons argue that transfusion with components can more readily supply the specific elements of blood necessary, providing that appropriate laboratory testing is done (see later section).

A unit of whole blood consists of approximately 230 ml of red blood cells, 220 ml of plasma, and 63 ml of anticoagulant. Although fresh whole blood provides all stable coagulation factors, after 3 to 5 days of storage, it lacks the labile coagulation factors (factors V and VIII), platelets, and effective granulocytes.

Packed Red Blood Cells. Transfusion of red blood cells in a relatively isolated form has become the standard means by which red cell mass is increased in the trauma patient. Its advantages are that concentrated red blood cells are delivered, with fewer antibodies, electrolytes, anticoagulants and proteins and less volume than whole blood. The only significant disadvantage is slower infusion time, which can be easily corrected with the use of blood pumps and/or reconstitution with normal saline prior to transfusion. A unit of packed red blood cells consists of 230 to 250 ml of red blood cells, with minimal amounts of plasma. This is the same red blood cell mass in two thirds of the volume of whole blood. Although packed red blood cells have minimal amounts of platelets, fibrinogen, and other coagulation factors, this can easily be corrected with additional component therapy. In rare cases, the use of frozen, washed, irradiated, leukocyte-poor, or deglycerolized red blood cells may be preferable to the use of simple packed red blood cells.[90] The amount of packed red blood cells transfused depends upon the amount of previous blood loss, as well as anticipated blood loss. However, one of three approaches may be used to guide therapy: (1) the amount of blood loss should generally be replaced; (2) 10 to 15 ml/kg of packed red cells should be transfused; or (3) a hematocrit value of 35 should be attained (see pages 14–16).

Platelets. Platelet packs must contain at least 5×10^{10} platelets per pack, plus a small amount of plasma (totaling 50 to 70 ml), with an average pH of 6.0. Recent experience with platelet transfusion indicates that most patients requiring even major transfusions can be given platelets simply on the basis of their documented platelet count. Although leukemic patients are often able to tolerate platelet counts of 20,000/mm^3 without bleeding, many trauma patients have been noted to bleed with counts above 50,000/mm^3. We generally advocate the clinical strategy for platelet transfusion outlined by the Maryland Institute of Emergency Medical Services.[91] This protocol recommends transfusion for any patient with a platelet count of less than 20,000/mm^3, for patients with platelet counts of 30,000/mm^3 or less in whom there is no bleeding but surgery will be required, and for patients with platelet counts of less than 50,000/mm^3 in whom there is evidence of bleeding. Transfusing one platelet pack in a patient with a 5 L total blood volume usually gives a rise of 5,000 platelets/mm^3 and raises the level of stable clotting factors by 1 to 2 per cent. The amount of platelets transfused is generally based on this approximation. In a child with a total blood volume of 1 L, the use of one platelet pack would result in a rise in the platelet count of 25,000/mm^3.

Fresh Frozen Plasma. In whole blood, the stable coagulation factors are present at normal levels for up to 1 year of storage. However, labile coagulation factors (factors V and VIII) are not present in significant levels after 3 to 4 days of storage. A unit of fresh frozen plasma provides approximately 175 to 250 units of all stable and labile coagulation factors, as well as approximately 500 mg of fibrinogen and 250 ml of fluid. One disadvantage of the use of fresh frozen plasma is that it takes 30 to 45 minutes to thaw. Some surgeons have recommended the use of one unit of fresh frozen plasma for every 3 to 4 units of packed red blood cells transfused. However, this probably represents overtreatment of the trauma patient in hypovolemic shock. We recommend simply following the prothrombin and activated partial thromboplastin times, with transfusion of fresh frozen plasma when these values exceed 1.5 times the control value.

Cryoprecipitate. Ten to fifteen ml of cryoprecipitate delivers 250 mg of fibrinogen and 80 to 100 units of factors V and VIII. Cryoprecipitate is rarely needed in trauma patients but may be utilized in patients with hemophilia A or von Willebrand's disease or in patients with low fibrinogen.[92]

Additional Measures

Provision of airway, with supplemental oxygen, and transfusion represent the two most important means of maximizing oxygen delivery. However, other therapeutic efforts also serve to effect this goal. For example, some patients in hypovolemic shock require pharmacologic stimulation of myocardial contractility for treatment. The cardiac output is dependent upon both the heart rate and the stroke volume of the heart. Stroke volume of the heart depends on the preload of the heart (which is maximized by providing an adequate amount of fluid for the heart to pump), myocardial contractility, and afterload. Once an appropriate amount of fluid has been infused to provide an appropriate left ventricular filling pressure, some patients may require augmentation of contractility to treat shock.[93] The use of dopamine, isoproterenol, or dobutamine may be necessary in shock patients after provision of sufficient fluid to optimize the left ventricular filling pressure. However, it is critical to note that these inotropic agents should be used only after the adequate volume has been restored.

As indicated previously, MAST may also assist the trauma patient, probably by increasing total peripheral resistance. In this sense, this benefit is effected by enhancing the afterload against which the heart pumps.

Decreasing the patient's oxygen demands also serves to optimize therapy in shock. For example, temperature elevation of 1° C raises oxygen consumption by approximately 12 per cent. Similarly, hypothermia also places increased oxygen demands on the patient. Therefore, temperature control is important in the shock patient. Additional means of decreasing oxygen demands may include minimizing patient stimulation, controlling pain, and administering sedatives.

A number of elements of therapy for shock have been assessed in laboratory studies. All these methods serve to maximize oxygen and/or energy delivery. Several studies have attempted to assess the effect of providing adenosine triphosphate (ATP) to the patient in order to maximize energy utilization.[94–96] These studies have produced conflicting results; however, it appears that the use of ATP—magnesium[97] may result in decreased mortality in laboratory animals subjected to hypovolemic shock. Some researchers have proposed that provision of solutions containing glucose, potassium, and insulin (GKI) may also serve to maximize oxygen and energy utilization.[98, 99] However, GKI has not been widely used, and results of current studies do not generally support its use. Although steroids in pharmacologic doses have been proposed to be of benefit in hypovolemic shock, most data support their use only in specific patients with septic shock.[100]

Recent research broadens our understanding of the type and number of interactions present in shock, specifically with regard to the role played by beta-endorphins in hemorrhagic shock. Beta-endorphin is released from the anterior pituitary gland, along with adrenocorticotropic hormone (ACTH) under the stress of hemorrhagic shock. Endorphin receptors have been found in the central nervous system, heart, liver, kidney, and intestines. Although the specific role played by beta-endorphin in hemorrhagic shock is yet to be clarified, experimental evidence indicates that blockade of beta-endorphin with naloxone results in improved survival, at least in the laboratory animal.[101–102] In this sense, the use of naloxone also serves to maximize oxygen delivery. In addition to the possible beneficial effect of naloxone on patients in hemorrhagic shock, it may also benefit patients with head injury[103] and spinal cord injury.[104] However, further laboratory and clinical studies are necessary to determine whether naloxone will have any role in the treatment of humans with hemorrhagic shock.

Decreasing Ongoing Blood Loss

In addition to restoring effective circulatory volume and maximizing oxygen delivery, the final goal of therapy for shock is to decrease further blood loss. Stated simply, this goal of therapy is hemostasis. The specific elements of decreasing ongoing blood loss and attaining hemostasis are by general measures, MAST, surgical methods, or transfusion. General measures include placement of pressure dressings and elevation of bleeding sites, as well as cautious application of hemostats to spurting vessels. However, hemostats should be applied extremely cautiously, since major neurologic damage may result from their injudicious application. In general, we advise clamping blood vessels only under careful surgical control or on vessels on the scalp. Particular caution should be exercised in clamping vessels in the head and neck regions or in an extremity. The use of MAST may be indicated in lower extremity fractures, lower extremity bleeding, or pelvic fractures.

The mainstay of decreasing ongoing losses is through surgical hemostasis. Major bleeding may occur in the chest or abdomen or other sites. After restoration of effective circulatory volume and maximization of oxygen delivery, timely surgical therapy to treat bleeding should be carried out. For example, in the patient with a ruptured spleen, provision of lactated Ringer's solution, packed red blood cells, and oxygenation and ventilation is critical. However, it is also important to quickly determine that bleeding is present and that surgical therapy will be required.

Transfusion therapy may also serve to decrease ongoing blood losses by providing adequate levels of platelets and coagulation factors. As indicated previously, transfusion results in all three goals of therapy for shock, including hemostasis.

REFERENCES

1. Graber TW: Congestive heart failure and cardiogenic shock. *In* Rosen P, Baker FJ, Braen GR, et al. (eds.): Emergency Medicine: Concepts and Clinical Practice. St. Louis, CV Mosby Company, 1983.
2. Shoemaker WC: Pathophysiology, monitoring, and therapy of shock syndromes. *In* Shoemaker WC, Thompson WL (eds.): Critical Care: State of the Art. Fullerton, Ca., SCCM, 1980.
3. Hierro FR, Palomeque A, Calvo M, Torralba A: Septic shock in pediatrics. Paediatrician 8:93, 1979.
4. Cannon WB: Traumatic Shock. New York, D. Appleton and Co., 1923.
5. Rutherford RB, Buerk CA: The pathophysiology of trauma and shock. *In* Zuidema GD, Rutherford RB, Ballinger WF (eds.): The Management of Trauma. Philadelphia, W.B. Saunders Company, 1979.
6. Moore FD: Metabolic Care of the Surgical Patient. Philadelphia, W.B. Saunders Company, 1960.
7. Perkin RM, Levin DL: Shock in the pediatric patient. Part I. J Pediatr 101:163, 1982.
8. Houtchens BA, Wolcott MW, Clemmer T: Initial evaluation and treatment of major trauma. *In* Wolcott MW (ed.): Ambulatory Surgery and the Basics of Emergency Surgical Care. Philadelphia, J.B. Lippincott Company, 1981.
9. Mela L: Reversibility of mitochondrial metabolic response to circulatory shock and tissue ischemia. Circ Shock (Suppl) 1:61, 1979.
10. Alexander RS: Veno motor tone in hemorrhage and shock. Circ Res 3:181, 1955.
11. Moore FD: The effects of hemorrhage on body composition. N Engl J Med 273:567, 1965.
12. Shires T, Coln D, Carrico J, Lightfoot S: Fluid therapy in hemorrhagic shock. Arch Surg 88:688, 1964.
13. Campion DS, Lynch LJ, Rector FC, et al.: The effect of hemorrhagic shock on transmembrane potential. Surgery 56:1051, 1969.
14. Cunningham JN Jr, Shires FT, Wagner Y: Cellular transport defects in hemorrhagic shock. Surgery 60:215, 1971.
15. Hagberg S, Haljamas H, Rockert H: Shock reactions and skeletal muscle. III. The electrolyte content of tissue fluid and plasma during hemorrhagic shock. Ann Surg 168:283, 1961.
16. Hinshaw LB: Autoregulation in normal and pathological states, including shock and ischemia. Circ Res (Suppl 1) 28:46, 1971.
17. Alho A, Jaattela A, Lahdensuu M, et al.: Catecholamines in shock. Ann Clin Res 9:157, 1977.
18. Zeifach BW, Bronek A: The interplay of central and peripheral factors in irreversible hemorrhagic shock. Prog Cardiovasc Dis 18:147, 1975.
19. Trunkey DD, Sheldon GF: The treatment of shock. *In* Zuidema GD, et al. (eds.): The Management of Trauma. W.B. Saunders Company. Philadelphia, 1979.
20. Skillman JJ, Lawler DP, Hickler RB, et al.: Hemorrhage in normal man: Effect on renin, cortisol, aldosterone, and urine composition. Ann Surg 166:865, 1967.
21. Negovsky VA: Introduction reanimatology—the science of resuscitation. *In* Stephenson HE (ed.): Cardiac Arrest and Resuscitation. St. Louis, C.V. Mosby Company, 1974.
22. Hazard PB, Griffin JP: Sodium bicarbonate in the management of systemic acidosis. South Med J 73:1339, 1980.
23. Schumer W: Localization of the energy pathway block in shock. Surgery 64:55, 1978.
24. Illner H, Shires GT: The effect of hemorrhagic shock on potassium transport in skeletal muscles. Surg Gynecol Obstet 150:17, 1980.
25. Cunningham JN Jr, Shires GT, Wagner Y: Cellular transport defects in hemorrhagic shock. Surgery 60:215, 1971.
26. George BC, Ryan NT, Ullrick WC, Egdahl RH: Persisting structural abnormalities in liver, kidney, and muscle tissues in hemorrhagic shock. Arch Surg 113:239, 1978.
27. Holden WD, DePalma RG, Drucker WR, McKalan A: Ultrastructural changes in hemorrhagic shock. Ann Surg 162:517, 1965.
28. Trump BF, Berezesky IK, Cowley RA: The cellular and subcellular characteristics of acute and chronic injury with emphasis on the role of calcium. *In* Cowley RA, Trump BF (eds.): Pathophysiology of Shock, Anoxia, and Ischemia. Baltimore, Williams and Wilkins Company, 1982.
29. Janoff A, Weissman G, Zweifach BW, Thomas L: Pathogenesis of experimental shock. IV. Studies of lysosomes in normal and tolerant animals subjected to lethal trauma and endotoxemia. J Exp Med 116:451, 1962.
30. Trump BF: The role of cellular membrane systems in shock. *In* The Cell in Shock. Kalamazoo, Upjohn Company, 1974.
31. George BC, Ryan NT, Ullrick WC, Egdah RH: Persisting structural abnormalities in liver, kidney, and muscle tissues following hemorrhagic shock. Arch Surg 113:289, 1978.

32. Cowley RA, Hankins JR, Jones RT, Trump FB: Pathology and pathophysiology of the liver. *In* Cowley RA, Trump BF (eds.): Pathophysiology of Shock, Anoxia, and Ischemia, Baltimore, Williams and Wilkins Company, 1982.
33. Champion HR, Jones RT, Trump BF, et al.: A clinico-pathologic study of hepatic dysfunction following shock. Surg Gynecol Obstet 142:657, 1976.
34. Weidner MG, Albrecht M, Clowes GH: Relationship of myocardial function to survival after oligemic hypotension. Surgery 55:73, 1964.
35. Ryan N, George BC, Harlow CL, et al.: Endocrine activation and altered muscle metabolism after hemorrhagic shock. Am J Physiol 233:439, 1977.
36. Shoemaker WC: Pathobiology of death: Structural and functional interactions in shock syndromes. Pathobiol Annu 6:365, 1976.
37. Hardaway RM, Chun B, Rutherford RB: Histologic evidence of disseminated intravascular coagulation in clinical shock. Vasc Dis 2:254, 1965.
38. Chaudry IH, Baue AE: Overview of hemorrhagic shock. *In* Cowley RA, Trump BF (eds.): Pathophysiology of Shock, Anoxia, and Ischemia. Baltimore, Williams and Wilkins Company, 1982.
39. Shoemaker WC: Pathophysiology and therapy of hemorrhage and trauma states. *In* Cowley RA, Trump BF (eds.): Pathophysiology of Shock, Anoxia, and Ischemia. Baltimore, Williams and Wilkins Company, 1982.
40. Rowe MI, Arango A: Colloid versus crystalloid resuscitation in experimental bowel obstruction. J Pediatr Surg 11:635, 1976.
41. Rowe MI: Shock and resuscitation. *In* Welch KJ (ed.): Complications of Pediatric Surgery. Philadelphia, W.B. Saunders Company, 1982.
42. Mayer T, Walker ML, Johnson DG, Matlak ME: Causes of morbidity and mortality in severe pediatric trauma. JAMA 245:719, 1981.
43. Bruce DA, Ralphaely RC, Goldberg AI, et al.: Pathophysiology, treatment, and outcome following severe head injury in children. Child's Brain 5:174, 1979.
44. Bruce DA, Alavi A, Bilaniuk L, et al.: Diffuse cerebral swelling following head injuries in children: The syndrome of "malignant brain edema." J Neurosurg 54:170, 1981.
45. Rowe MI, Marchildon MB: Pediatric Trauma. *In* Shoemaker WC, Thompson WL (eds.): Critical Care: State of the Art. Fullerton, Ca., SCCM, 1981.
46. Oliver TK: Temperature regulation and heat production in the newborn. Pediatr Clin North Am 12:765, 1965.
47. Crone RC: Acute circulatory failure in children. Pediatr Clin North Am 27:525, 1980.
48. Lillehei RC, MacLean LC: Physiological approach to successful treatment of shock in experimental animals. Arch Surg 78:414, 1959.
49. Shires GT, Brown FT, Canisaro PC, Somerville N: Distributional changes in extracellular fluid during acute hemorrhagic shock. Surg Forum 11:115, 1960.
50. Shires GT, Coln D, Carrico CJ, Lightfoot S: Fluid therapy in hemorrhagic shock. Arch Surg 88:688, 1964.
51. Moyer CA: Fluid Balance. Chicago, Year Book Medical Publishers, 1954.
52. Shires GT: Pathophysiology and fluid replacement in hypovolemic shock. Ann Clin Res 9:144, 1977.
53. Carey JS, Scharschmidt BF, Culliford AT, et al.: Hemodynamic effectiveness of colloid and electrolyte solutions for replacement of simulated operative blood loss. Surg Gynecol Obstet 131:679, 1970.
54. Virgilio RN, Smith DE, Zurins CK: Balanced electrolyte solutions: Experimental and clinical studies. Crit Care Med 7:98, 1979.
55. Weil MH, Henning RJ: New concepts in the diagnosis and fluid treatment of circulatory shock. Anesth Analg 58:124, 1979.
56. Lucas CE: Resuscitation of the injured patient: The three phases of treatment. Surg Clin North Am 57:3, 1977.
57. Committee on Trauma, American College of Surgeons: Advanced Trauma Life-Support Manual, Chicago, 1980.
58. Walt AJ (ed.): Early Care of the Injured Patient. W.B. Saunders Company, Philadelphia, 1982.
59. Guyton AC, Lindsey AW: Effect of elevated left atrial pressure and decreased plasma protein concentration on the development of pulmonary edema. Circ Res 7:649, 1959.
60. Shoemaker WC, Schluchter M, Hopkins JA, et al.: Fluid therapy in emergency resuscitation: Clinical evaluation of colloid and crystalloid regimens. Crit Care Med 9:367, 1981.
61. Safar P: Resuscitation in hemorrhagic shock, coma, and cardiac arrest. *In* Cowley RA, Trump BF (eds.): Pathophysiology of Shock, Anoxia, and Ischemia. Baltimore, Williams and Wilkins Company, 1982.
62. Shoemaker WC: Effects of transfusion on surviving and nonsurviving postoperative patients. Surg Gynecol Obstet 142:33, 1976.
63. Brinkmeyer S, Safar P, Motoyama E, Stezoski W: Superiority of colloid over electrolyte solutions for fluid resuscitation. Crit Care Med 9:369, 1981.
64. Shoemaker WC, Hauser CJ: Critique of crystalloid versus colloid therapy in shock. Crit Care Med 7:117, 1979.
65. Demling RH, Manchar M, Will JA, Belzer FO: The effect of plasma oncotic pressure on the pulmonary microcirculation after hemorrhagic shock. Surgery 86:235, 1979.
66. Zarins CK, Rice CL, Smith DE, et al.: Role of lymphatics in preventing hypooncotic pulmonary edema. Surg Forum 25:267, 1976.
67. Esrig BC, Fulton RL: Sepsis, resuscitated hemorrhagic shock and "shock lung": An experimental correlation. Ann Surg 182:218, 1975.
68. Kohler JP, Rice CL, Zarins CK, et al.: Does reduced colloid oncotic pressure increase pulmonary dysfunction in sepsis? Crit Care Med 9:90, 1981.
69. Shah DM, Browner BD, Dutten RE, et al.: Cardiac output and pulmonary wedge pressure: Use for evaluation of fluid replacement in trauma patients. Arch Surg 112:1161, 1977.
70. Virgilio RW, Rice CL, Smith DE, et al.: Crystalloid versus colloid resuscitation. Is one better? Surgery 85:129, 1979.
71. Lucas CE, Ledgerwood AM, Higgins RF, Weaver DW: Impaired pulmonary function after albumin resuscitation from shock. J Trauma 20:446, 1980.
72. Lucas CE, Weaver D, Higgins RF, et al.: Effects of albumin versus non-albumin resuscitation on plasma volume and renal excretory function. J Trauma 18:564, 1978.
73. Weaver DW, Ledgerwood AM, Lucas CE, et al.: Pulmonary effects of albumin resuscitation for

severe hypovolemic shock. Arch Surg 113:387, 1978.

74. Lowe RJ, Moss GS, Jilek J, Levine HD: Crystalloid versus colloid in the etiology of pulmonary failure after trauma. Surgery 81:676, 1977.
75. Cogbill TH, Moore EE, Dunn EL, Cohen RG: Coagulation changes after albumin resuscitation. Crit Care Med 9:22, 1981.
76. Moss GS: Panel discussion on hypovolemic shock. Presented before the annual meeting of the American College of Surgeons, Chicago, 1982.
77. Gelin LE, Davidson I: Plasma expanders and hemodilution in the treatment of hypovolemic shock. *In* Cowley RA, Trump BF (eds.): Pathophysiology of Shock, Anoxia, and Ischemia. Baltimore, Williams and Wilkins Company, 1982.
78. Thompson WL: Hydroxyethyl starch. *In* Jamieson GA, Greenwalt TJ (eds.): Blood Substitutes and Plasma Expanders. New York, Alan R. Liss, 1978.
79. DeVenuto F, Friedman HI, Neville JR, et al.: Appraisal of hemoglobin solution as a blood substitute. Surg Gynecol Obstet 149:417, 1979.
80. Mitsuno T, Chyanagi H, Naito R: Clinical studies of a perfluorochemical blood substitute (Flusol—DA). Ann Surg 195:60, 1982.
81. Gaffney FA, Thal ER, Taylor WF, et al.: Hemodynamic effects of medical antishock trousers. J Trauma 21:931, 1981.
82. Goldsmith SR: Comparative hemodynamic effects of antishock suit and volume expansion in normal human beings. Ann Emerg Med 12:348, 1983.
83. Bivins HG, Knopp R, Tierran C, et al.: Blood volume displacement with inflation of antishock trousers. Ann Emerg Med 11:409, 1982.
84. Holbrook PR: Care of the Critically Ill Child. *In* Shoemaker WC, Thompson WL (eds.): Critical Care: State of the Art. Fullerton, Ca., SCCM, 1980.
85. Morse TS: Evaluation and initial management. *In* Touloukian RJ (ed.): Pediatric Trauma. New York, John Wiley and Sons, 1978.
86. Myhre BA, Harris GE: Blood components for hemotherapy. Clin Lab Med 2:3, 1982.
87. Hemphill BH: Blood collection and use by AABB institutional members (1976). Transfusion 19:365, 1979.
88. McCullough J, Yunis EJ, Benson SJ, et al.: Effect of blood bank storage on leucocyte function. Lancet 2:1333, 1969.
89. Collins JA: Problems associated with massive transfusion of stored blood. Surgery 75:274, 1974.
90. Myhre BA (ed.): A Seminar on Blood Components. Washington, D.C., American Association of Blood Banks, 1977.
91. Cowley RA, Dunham M: Shock Trauma—Critical Care Manual, Baltimore, University Park Press, 1982.
92. Borucki DT (ed.): Blood Component Therapy. 3rd ed. Washington, D.C., American Association of Blood Banks, 1981, pp. 55–57.
93. Driscoll DJ, Gillette PC, McNamara DG: The use of dopamine in children. J Pediatr 92:309, 1978.
94. Baue AE, Worth MA, Sayeed MM: Alterations in magnesium and sodium plus potassium-activated triphosphate in hemorrhagic shock. Surg Forum 21:8, 1970.
95. DiStazio J, Maley W, Thompson B, et al.: Effects of ATP-$MgC1_2$ administration during hemorrhagic shock. Adv Shock Res 3:153, 1980.
96. Chaudry IH, Sayeed MM, Baue AE: Evidence for advanced uptake of adenosine triphosphate by muscle of animals in shock. Surgery 77:833, 1975.
97. Chaudry IH, Sayeed MM, Baue AE: Effect of adenosine triphosphate—magnesium chloride administration in shock. Surgery 75:220, 1974.
98. Ryan NT, Clowes GHA: Metabolic effects of glucose-insulin-potassium infusion during experimental intraperitoneal sepsis. Circ Res 3:309, 1976.
99. Dennis RC, Harlow C, Egdahl RH, Hechtman H: Enhancement of myocardial function with glucose, insulin, and potassium. Surg Gynecol Obstet 151:185, 1980.
100. Schumer W: Steroids in the treatment of clinical septic shock. Ann Surg 183:345, 1976.
101. Faden AI, Holaday JW: Opiate antagonists: A role in the treatment of hypovolemic shock. Science 205:317, 1979.
102. Albert SA, Shires GT III, Illner H, Shires GT: Effects of naloxone in hemorrhagic shock. Surg Gynecol Obstet 155:326, 1982.
103. Hayes RL, Galinat BJ, Kulkasac P, Becker DP: Effects of naloxone on systemic and cerebral responses to experimental concussive brain injury in cats. J Neurosurg 58:720, 1983.
104. Faden AI, Jacobs TP, Holaday JW: Opiate antagonist improves neurologic recovery after spinal injury. Science 211:493, 1980.

CHAPTER

3 Ventilatory Therapy, Anesthesia, and Respiratory Support

ROBERT L. RAYBURN

If an injured child reaches a suitable emergency facility alive, his greatest risks of preventable death are from errors in managing ventilation and circulation or from failure to detect hidden injuries.[1] In this chapter, ventilatory therapy will be discussed in detail, and circulatory therapy will be mentioned as far as it pertains to resuscitation and preparation of traumatized pediatric patients for anesthesia.

INITIAL EVALUATION

The evaluation and treatment of multisystem trauma requires a team approach. The anesthesiologist has the responsibilities of providing life support, relief of pain, and satisfactory operating conditions for surgery.[2] Initial evaluation and management of most pediatric trauma begins at the site of the accident by emergency medical technicians or paramedics. This care is continued en route to the emergency room, where further evaluation and treatment are begun by a group of specialists, e.g., emergency physicians, anesthesiologists, surgeons, pediatricians, respiratory therapists, nurses, and laboratory personnel, and it is their combined expertise that hopefully will tip the scales in favor of survival for the injured. It is important for the anesthesiologist to be aware of all the findings and therapy connected with the patient, since it is his responsibility to further manage or correct these conditions when the patient undergoes surgical therapy.

It becomes necessary in a text to place events in a chronological order, even though in reality many aspects of the evaluation and therapy of the patient may occur simultaneously. However, looking at the patient from the standpoint of the anesthesiologist, certain aspects of care take priority, and others must understandably follow as rapidly as time and circumstance will allow.

Obviously of prime importance is the fact that there must be a viable patient. Therefore, the initial contact with the patient must involve a quick (seconds to minutes) overall evaluation of the patient, with priority placed on the airway (respiratory), cardiovascular, and neurologic status, essentially in that order. Quickly the question must be answered, "Is resuscitation necessary?" Resuscitation may require full cardiopulmonary resuscitation (CPR) or only simple airway management or fluid resuscitation.

If CPR is required, the steps recommended by the American Heart Association should be followed (see pages 2–9).[3] These initial activities may be carried out simultaneously with other resuscitative measures, such as providing relief of tension pneumothorax or control of active arterial bleeding.

In addition, a protocol approach to the trauma patient should always be followed.[4] The principles of both CPR and the initial evaluation and treatment of pediatric trauma victims are detailed in Chapter 1. The initial overall supportive phase may take place either prior to surgery or in the early stages of the delivery of anesthesia, depending upon the specifics of the individual case.

After the patient has been stabilized through resuscitation and has been assessed through a general physical examination and history, he must be reassessed. Decisions should now be made as to the urgency of further evaluation, diagnostic procedures, or definitive procedures such as surgery.

A complete present and past medical history should be obtained as soon as possible. If the anesthesiologist is involved in the initial resuscitation of a patient destined for surgery or in the intensive care unit (ICU), those not actively participating in the care of the patient should obtain information concerning the injury from observers, family members, or medical attendants at the scene.[5] Of pertinence to the anesthesiologist is a history of recent ingestions of food (although most patients are assumed to have a full stomach); trauma to the neck or airway; trauma to the thorax with the possibility of pneumothorax, hemothorax, or lung abnormality;[6, 7] and injuries to the cardiovascular system. It is also important to get a list of any therapy or drugs given at the scene that may influence further planned therapy for the patient. An estimation of blood loss, although many times inaccurate, may be helpful.

The past medical history is extremely important and should be obtained as completely as possible—certainly any history of allergies; medications taken within the past 6 months; previous surgical experience; other medical problems such as congestive heart disease, renal problems, or diabetes; and any family history of anesthetic complications must be obtained, unless the urgency of the operation mandates that the time spent obtaining the information would jeopardize the patient's well-being. Even in this instance ancillary personnel should seek information and pass it to the anesthesiologist while he continues the acute care of the patient.

In his haste to appropriately stabilize ventilation and circulation and to prepare the operating room (OR) for arrival of the traumatized patient, the anesthesiologist should not forget to perform a physical examination of the body areas that are pertinent to the delivery of life support and anesthesia and to the placement of monitoring devices. Under most circumstances, these areas of most importance are the respiratory, cardiovascular, central nervous, and genitourinary systems, as well as the extremities and ophthalmologic system. The importance of various abnormalities in these systems is discussed later.

PREANESTHETIC TREATMENT AND STABILIZATION

Preanesthetic treatment and stabilization of the child may take place in the emergency room or ICU or may occur in the OR either prior to or as part of the induction of anesthesia.

Respiratory System

The respiratory system is the first system to require attention in a trauma patient. The pediatric patient, and especially the neonate, is distinctly different from the adult anatomically, and many of the differences predispose these small patients to respiratory difficulties.[8–10] In the pediatric patient, the head is large and the neck short. The tongue is relatively large, and the nasal passages are narrow. The neonate is an obligate nasal breather. The glottis, trachea, and airways are of a small caliber, and there is abundant lymphoid tissue in the upper airways of many patients. The larynx is located more cephalad, usually between the C2 and C4 vertebral levels. The epiglottis is long and stiff and projects posteriorly at a 45 degree angle. The vocal cords have a lower attachment anteriorly, and the cricoid cartilage causes the narrowest constriction of the trachea. The ciliated columnar epithelium below the cords is loosely bound by areolar tissue, creating susceptibility to edema formation.

The ribs of the infant are horizontal, creating a cylindrical thorax, which causes the intercostal muscles to have little effect on respiration. For this reason, diaphragmatic breathing plays a greater role in pediatric patients, but this may be inhibited by abdominal distention, which may occur in traumatic injuries. Since the chest wall is more compliant and cartilaginous in the infant than in the adult, it is common to see inward or paradoxic motion of the rib cage during inspiration in neonates with stiff lungs or airway obstruction. Another factor that limits the neonate's ability to increase tidal volume is the almost horizontal insertion of the diaphragm, compared with the oblique insertion of the diaphragm in adults. This results in an inward pull on the lower rib cage compared with an upward pull in adults. For this reason, the neonate's diaphragm is less efficient in raising abdominal pressure, and so the small patient responds to respiratory distress with retractions and tachypnea, rather than hypernea.[11] It has also been shown that whenever significant distortion of the rib cage occurs in the newborn, the infant experiences respiratory muscle fatigue.[12] The oxidative capacity of human ventilatory muscles (hence resistance to fatigue) increases markedly from midgestation to early childhood.[13] Additionally, the oxygen utilization of a child on a per kilogram basis is twice that of an adult,[14] and therefore, in the face of respiratory obstruction, hypoxia will develop more rapidly in a child. These circumstances clearly demonstrate the urgency of paying particular attention to the respiratory system of the traumatized pediatric patient.

Initial Ventilation and Oxygenation

Initially, evaluate the patient to see if he is breathing. If he is, deliver a high concentration of oxygen by mask and proceed with further evaluation. If the patient is not breathing, he must be ventilated. The oropharynx should be quickly cleared and the airway opened by placing the patient in the head tilt–neck lift[3] or "sniffing" position (see Fig. 1–2, p. 3).[15] Prior to intubation, the patient must be ventilated so that oxygenation is improved, allowing time for intubation. This may be done by means of mouth-to-mouth ventilation (which delivers approximately 16 per cent oxygen) if no equipment is available[3] or by means of a bag and mask ventilation system.

If no oxygen source is available, it is necessary to use one of the various self-inflating bag-valve systems,[16–19] commonly referred to as "Ambu bags." These systems are extremely useful when no oxygen is available because they facilitate ventilation with 21 per cent oxygen in a patient who otherwise would have to receive mouth-to-mouth ventilation. These systems can be improved by means of supplemental oxygen and a reservoir, but they generally require at least 15 L/minute flow to approach 100 per cent oxygen delivery to the patient.[17–19] However, with some of the systems, if the patient breathes spontaneously, he may entrain air, or air and oxygen, instead of 100 per cent oxygen.[16] A number of systems with the oxygen reservoir are also very cumbersome, especially in the pediatric patient, and occasionally some are even prone to fall apart during use or cleaning.[18, 19] The peak inspiratory pressure is limited by the operator or by a valve that opens at various pressures with different models. Under certain conditions this may lead to either underventilation or overdistention of the lungs.[18, 19] Newer models* seem to have overcome some of these problems. Therefore, when an oxygen source is lacking, these self-inflating systems are extremely useful and are generally used in combination with an oral pharyngeal airway and a clear mask. The addition of an oxygen flow to these systems improves oxygen delivery. Once the patient is intubated with an endotracheal tube, these devices may continue to be used to provide ventilation.

The use of the bag and mask systems referred to as the "nonrebreathing systems" is probably preferable when an oxygen source is available. An advantage of these systems is that 100 per cent oxygen may be delivered at essentially any flow rate, and as opposed to the self-inflating bag-valve systems, the peak inspiratory pressure can be individually set for each patient by means of a relief or "pop off" valve. The physician may set the valve to deliver any desired positive end expiratory pressure (PEEP) by readjusting it after inspiration and keeping the reservoir bag distended. These systems are generally more convenient to use with a pediatric patient, and some are designed to decrease the dead space by bringing the oxygen delivery tube flush with the end that attaches to the endotracheal tube.† These systems require an operator with slightly more "educated hands," but because of their overall benefits, these systems are probably superior to the self-inflating bags, especially if reasonably long support of ventilation is required. With proper oxygen flow rates of at least 4000 ml/m^2/minute for the patient breathing spontaneously and 2500 ml/m^2/minute for the patient requiring controlled ventilation (Table 3–1), the arterial P_{CO_2} should remain normal and 100 per cent oxygen delivery can be assured.[20] (When used at these flow rates, these systems are more properly called partial rebreathing systems, since a controlled amount of rebreathing of expired carbon dioxide occurs.) In these systems, humidification is improved at these flow rates, as opposed to the self-inflating systems in which humidity is lost to the atmosphere. Likewise heat retention is improved,[21] which is frequently important in children. The addition of a heated humidifier to the inspiratory oxygen line is helpful in smaller patients. These partial rebreathing systems are also generally used with an oral pharyngeal airway and a clear mask, so that regurgitation and color of the lips can be seen. The partial rebreathing systems may also be used with the endotracheal tube once it is inserted or may be used with the newer esophageal obturator airways (EOAs) presently being developed (Fig. 3–1).

The recent development of oxygen-powered resuscitators provides another modality for supplying oxygen and ventilation to trauma patients. These resuscitators have a manually triggered valve, which is attached to a pressurized source of oxygen. The devices are portable and usually come in a kit containing a mask, oxygen source, and valve. They generally provide 100 per cent oxygen

---

*Puritan Bennett PMR-2 child self-inflating bag-valve-mask system (Puritan Bennett Corp., Kansas City, MO);

†CPRAM partial rebreathing system (KHI Associates, Frazer, PA).

Table 3–1. TABLE FOR APPROXIMATING FRESH GAS FLOW IN VARIOUS PATIENTS FOR A Pa_{CO_2} OF 40 TORR

Weight		Approximate	Surface Area	Spontaneous Respiration		Controlled Ventilation	
kg	*lb*	*Age*	*(m²)*	*Approx. Flow ml/kg/min*	*Patient Flow* ml/min*	*Approx. Flow† ml/kg/min*	*Patient Flow‡ ml/min*
3	6.6	Newborn	0.25	330	1000	180	625§
6	13	3 months	0.3	200	—‖	180	—‖
10	22	1 year	0.5	200	2000	180	1250
20	44	5.5 years	0.8	150	—‖	100	—‖
30	66	9 years	1.0	150	4000	100	2500
40	88	12 years	1.3	130	—‖	80	—‖
50	110	14 years	1.5	130	6000	80	3750
65	143	adult	1.7	100	—‖	60	—‖
70	159	adult	1.75	100	7000	60	4200
85	187	adult	1.9	100	—‖	60	—‖
100	220	adult	2.0	100	8000	60	5000

*Based on flow for spontaneous respiration of 4000 ml/m²/min.
†Greatest accuracy is achieved with a fresh gas flow of 2500 ml/m²/min.
‡Based on flow for controlled ventilation of 2500 ml/m²/min.
§Minimal flow is usually limited to 500 ml/min.
‖Flow should be individually calculated.

at flow rates of greater than 100 L/minute and have an inspiratory peak pressure safety relief valve set at 40 to 50 cm H_2O. They are also designed to operate at all temperature extremes in North America. They fit standard 15 mm/22 mm couplings for masks, endotracheal tubes, and EOAs, and most have a trigger positioned so that both hands of the rescuer can remain on the mask to hold it in place while supporting the head of the victim in the "sniffing" position (Fig. 3–2).[22–24] In addition, many oxygen-powered resuscitators allow the patient to receive 100 per cent oxygen while breathing spontaneously, and some have a separate oxygen port to attach a bag system should the resuscitator fail. A few also have a suctioning apparatus attached. The advantage of the resuscitators is that the rescuer can use both hands to support the airway while delivering oxygen. However, as with the self-inflating bags, exhaust gases are vented into the atmosphere, resulting in loss of heat and humidity; it is difficult to apply PEEP; and the preset inspiratory pressure relief setting may be exceeded in certain types of lung disease or CPR. It is probably wise to have a nonrebreathing (partial rebreathing) system as a back-up if any of these conditions should present problems.

Mechanical aids that are frequently useful in providing ventilation to comatose or apneic patients are oropharyngeal and nasopharyngeal airways. The oral pharyngeal airways come in various sizes, 000 to 5 for pediatric patients, and are inserted through the mouth to keep the tongue from falling back against the posterior pharynx. Naso-

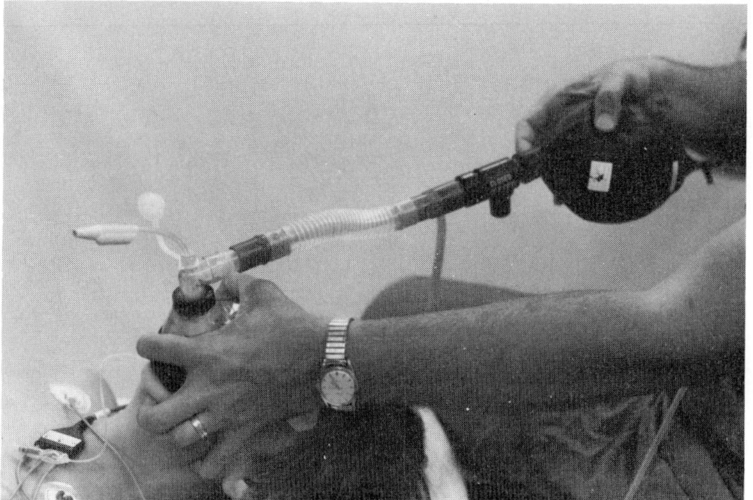

Figure 3–1. Partial rebreathing system attached to esophageal obturator airway.

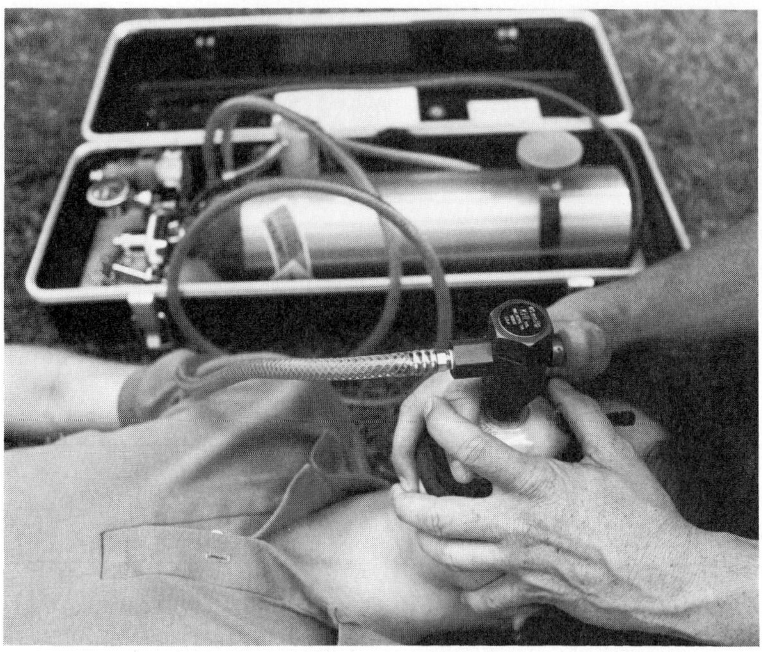

Figure 3–2. Proper use of an oxygen-powered resuscitator on older pediatric patient. (From KHI Association, Frazer, PA. Reproduced with permission.)

pharyngeal airways are used less commonly in children because bleeding may result from hypertrophied adenoid tissue. The nasopharyngeal airway is lubricated and inserted through the nose so that the tip lies behind the tongue in the posterior pharynx.

Maintenance of a Patent Airway

Once the patient has been initially oxygenated and ventilated by one of the preceding methods, it is appropriate to attempt to establish a more secure airway. If an experienced intubationist is available, it is best to secure the airway with an endotracheal tube. However, in adolescents and some pre-adolescents, the EOA may be an alternative if intubation is not successful or practical.

Esophageal Obturator Airway

The advantage of an EOA is that no visualization with a laryngoscope or other device is necessary in order to pass it into the esophagus. It does necessitate some prior training to do the insertion properly, but the skill required is less than that needed for intubation. The tube is only inserted into patients who are not breathing or who are deeply unconscious.[3] Present EOAs should not be inserted in small children, conscious or semiconscious patients, patients with

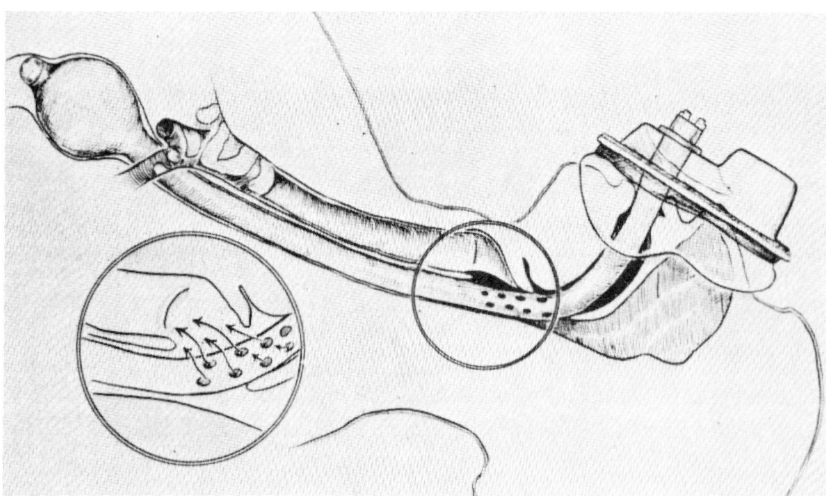

Figure 3–3. Proper placement of the esophageal obturator airway. (From Michael TA: The esophageal obturator airway. JAMA 246:1098, 1981. Copyright 1981, American Medical Association.)

known esophageal disease, or patients with known caustic poisoning.

The EOA consists of a cuffed tube mounted through a face mask. Several openings are present in the upper third of the tube, which allow air to pass into the upper esophagus, nasopharynx, and trachea. The distal tube and cuff lie in the distal esophagus when properly placed and, when the cuff is inflated, prevent ventilating gases from passing into the stomach (Fig. 3–3). The proximal portion of the tube fits through a face mask,

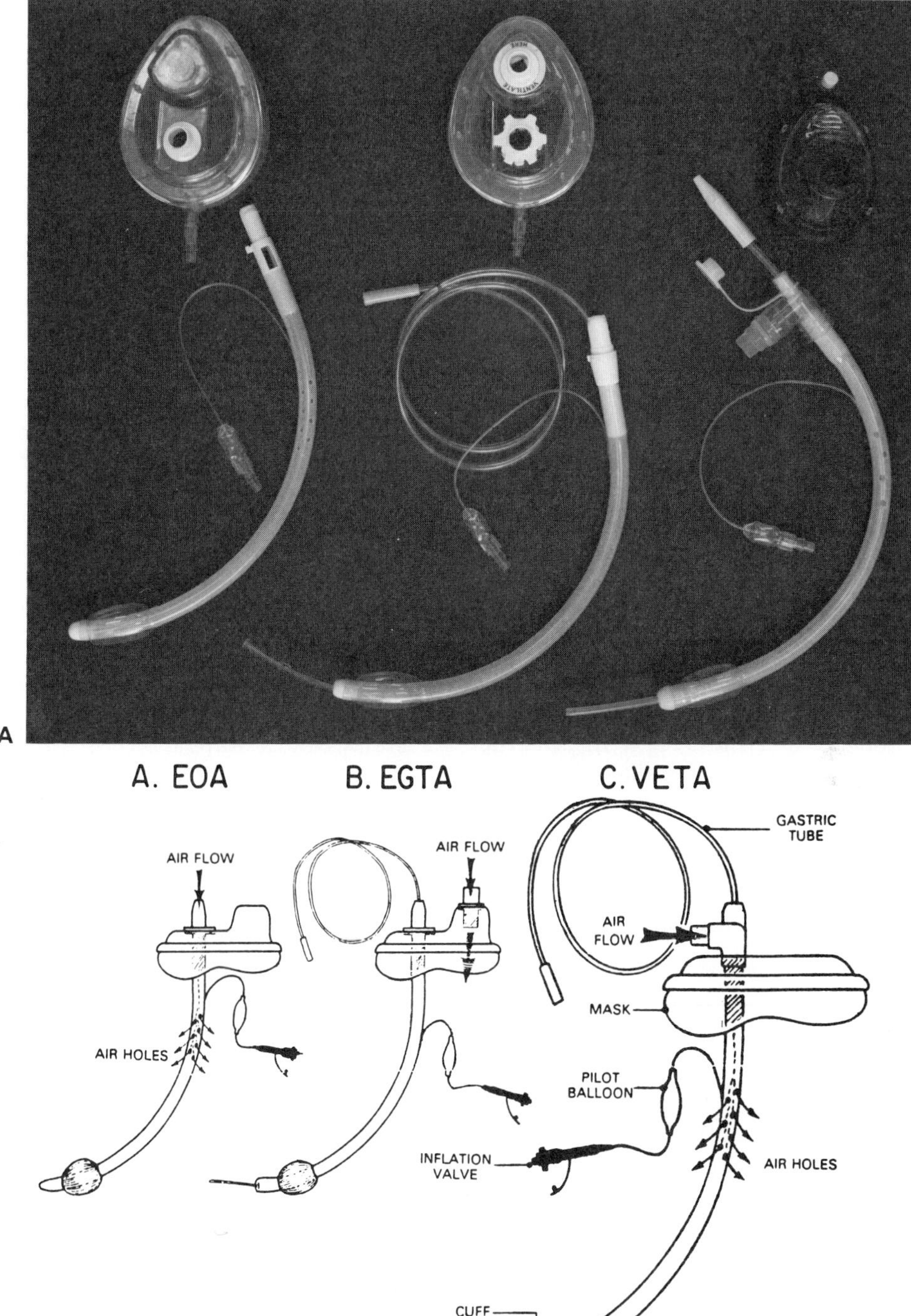

Figure 3–4. Photograph and schematic drawing of esophageal obturator airway (EOA), esophageal gastric tube airway (EGTA), and vented esophageal tube airway (VETA). (Adapted from Donegan JH: Cardiopulmonary resuscitation. *In* Miller RD (ed.): Anesthesia, New York, Churchill Livingstone, 1981, p. 1505.)

Table 3–2. MASKS

Age of Patient	Type
Premature and newborn	Rendell Baker 0
1 month to 1 year	Rendell Baker 1
1 year to 2 years	Rendell Baker 2
2 years to 10 years	Rendell Baker 3
Adolescent	2–4 adult masks

which is held sealed against the face to prevent gases from leaking out into the atmosphere.

The vented esophageal tube airway (VETA) has a central opening for passage of a gastric tube and an outer co-axial tube through which ventilation is provided into the upper airway from the openings in the upper third of the tube (Fig. 3–4). The VETA also has the advantage that it works with almost any size mask, thus allowing a better seal in pediatric patients.

The proper methods for insertion of the EOA are described in the literature.[3, 25] Complications do occur with the EOA. The most common situation is misplacement of the EOA, with the insertion into the trachea,[3, 25] which should be recognized promptly by the absence of breath sounds when ventilation is attempted. However, with the VETA, confirmation of tracheal insertion and adequate ventilation may be achieved by ventilating through the gastric tube port. Tracheal insertion is probably much less likely in pediatric patients owing to the smaller diameter of the trachea. The present EOAs are not indicated in patients less than 10 to 12 years of age.

Esophageal rupture has also infrequently been reported with EOAs, but the incidence seems to have decreased because the newer types have blunter ends and allow venting of the stomach.[25, 26] It is wise for the surgeon and anesthesiologist to be on the watch for signs of esophageal perforation in order to institute early diagnosis and treatment of this condition.[26] When receiving a patient with an EOA, the anesthesiologist must remember that if the patient remains unconscious, an endotracheal tube should be inserted before the EOA is removed. If the patient regains consciousness and is breathing spontaneously, the EOA may be removed. When it is to be removed, the patient should be turned on the side; the gastric tube, if present, should be suctioned; and the balloon should be deflated before attempting removal. Regurgitation may follow removal more commonly when EOAs without a gastric port are used.

Endotracheal Intubation

The most effective way of securing the airway and preventing aspiration of stomach contents is by endotracheal intubation. This is indicated in the trauma patient in the following circumstances: (1) if the rescuer is unable to provide adequate oxygenation with the previously mentioned methods; (2) if the patient is unable to protect his own airway owing to coma, areflexia, seizure activity, hypertonicity, or head, neck, or face injuries; (3) if there is a need for prolonged artificial ventilation or transport for any significant distance; or (4) if the patient requires immediate surgery in which general anesthesia must be delivered. It must be stressed that in a patient unable to protect his airway, it is mandatory that the trachea be protected with an endotracheal tube (or EOA) prior to venting the stomach with a gastric tube. Regurgitation is frequently associated with this procedure, and a patient without protective reflexes will likely aspirate.

Endotracheal intubation usually requires more time to effectively accomplish than the procedures mentioned thus far. For this reason, it is mandatory that oxygenation of the lungs by mouth-to-mouth ventilation or bag and mask ventilation precedes attempts at tracheal intubation. Because of the difficulties, delays, and complications in proper placement of an endotracheal tube,[27] it should be inserted only by medical personnel and professional allied health personnel who are highly trained and who either perform endotracheal intubation frequently or are retrained frequently in this technique.[3] In essence, placement of an endotracheal tube requires at least some experience and train-

Table 3–3. INTUBATION EQUIPMENT

Age of Patient	Laryngoscope Blades	Essential Extras
Premature and newborn	Miller 0	Stylets (wire or Teflon coated);
1 month to 1 year	Miller 1	lubricating ointment;
1 to 2 years	Wis Hipple 1½	Yankauer Tonsil Suction suction catheters;
2 years to small adult	Miller 2	Magill forceps, small and large;
Large adult	Miller 3	tongue blades; oral pharyngeal airways

Adapted from Johnson DG, Jones R: Surgical aspects of airway management in infants and children. Symposium on Pediatric Surgery. Surg Clin North Am 56:263, 1976.

Table 3–4. PEDIATRIC ENDOTRACHEAL TUBE DIMENSIONS*

Age of Patient	French Size	Internal Diameter† (mm)	Oral Length‡ (cm)	15 mm Male Connector Size mm ID	Suction Catheter (French)
Newborn (≤1.0 kg)	11–12	2.5–3.0	10	3	6
Newborn (≥1.0 kg)	13–14	3.0–3.5	11	3	6
1–4 months	15–16	3.0–3.5	11	4	6–8
4–8 months	17–18	3.5–4.0	12	4	8
8–12 months	19–20	4.0–4.5	12	5	8
12–36 months	21–22	4.5–5.0	13	5	8
3–4 years	23–24	5.0–5.5	14	6	10
5–6 years	25	5.5–6.0	16	6	10
6–7 years§	26	5.5–6.0	16–18	7	10
8–9 years§	26–28	6.5–7.0	18	7	12
10–11 years§	28–30	7.0–7.5	18–20	8	12
12–14 years§	30–32	7.0–7.5	20–22	8	14
≥ 16 years§	32–34	7.5–8.0	20–24	8	14

*Clear polyvinylchloride endotracheal tubes that satisfy the USP standard implant test and lightweight nylon connectors are recommended. One tube size smaller and larger should be available for individual variations.

†Formula([Age of patient (yr)]/4) + 4.0 = size of tube (inside diameter [ID]).

‡Add approximately 2 cm for nasotracheal tube length.

§Cuffed tubes should be used in children above 6 to 8 years of age.

ing. The rescuer should not interrupt ventilation for more than 30 seconds per attempt. If reasonable attempts at endotracheal intubation have been made without success, the rescuer should then perform one of the aforementioned methods of ventilation (i.e., use of EOAs; bag and mask ventilation, with various oral and nasal airways; or mouth-to-mouth ventilation) in order to ventilate the patient until personnel more experienced in airway management are available. Types of masks and the equipment necessary for intubation of the pediatric patient are listed in Tables 3–2 and 3–3, and proper size endotracheal tubes are shown in Table 3–4. Each trauma victim must be considered by the intubationist to have a full stomach. Therefore, it is imperative that if laryngeal reflexes are intact, they are not compromised lest aspiration occur. This will generally dictate that one of two techniques of endotracheal intubation will be necessary: awake intubation or a rapid-sequence intubation.

Both techniques require that the patient first be placed in the proper position for intubation. The sniffing position, used to align the oral, pharyngeal, and laryngeal axes (Fig. 3–5), is accomplished by elevating the back of the head and then extending the head at the atlanto-occipital joint. Occasionally in infants, the occipital region of the head will be prominent enough so that nothing will be needed to raise the head. However, placing a patient in the sniffing position is contraindicated if the patient has cervical spine injuries. It is wise to avoid extension or manipulation of the neck in this patient,

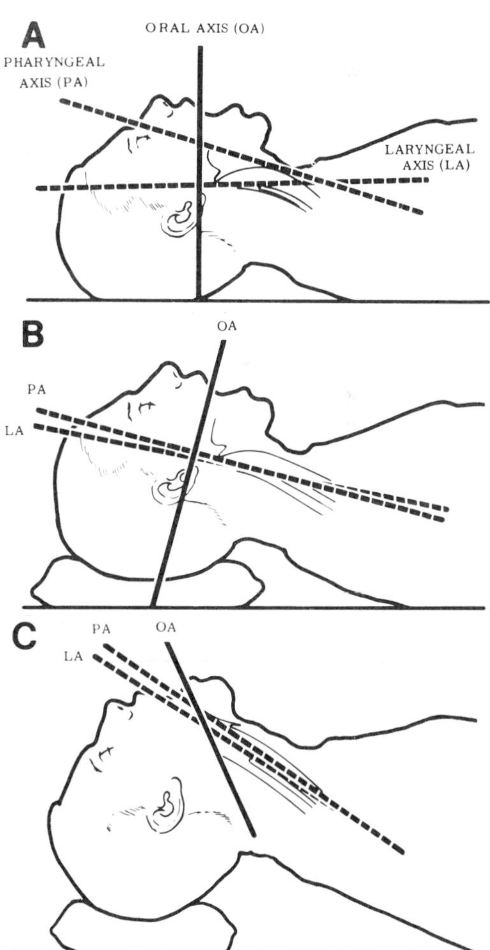

Figure 3–5. Schematic drawing showing oral, pharyngeal, and laryngeal axes in normal supine patient (*A*), with elevation of the head (*B*), and with extension at the atlanto-occipital joint (*C*). (From Stoelting RK: Endotracheal intubation. *In* Miller RD (ed.): Anesthesia. New York, Churchill Livingstone, 1981. Reproduced with permission.)

and management of the airway is best accomplished with an EOA; nasotracheal intubation; oral intubation, using muscle relaxants with an assistant holding the head to prevent extension; or, occasionally, tracheostomy.[28, 29]

Nasal and Oral Intubation

Intubation of the trauma patient may take place at the site of the accident, in the emergency department, or in the OR. Awake intubation should not be attempted in patients with increased intracranial pressure or penetrating wounds of the eye or the neck. Awake intubation may be performed using either the nasal or the oral route. However, in smaller children, the nasal route is usually much less effective. This is because uncuffed tubes are generally used in children less than 6 to 8 years of age, so the tube size relative to the trachea is much more closely approximated than in an adult, in whom a smaller tube with a cuff is used. Also the greater likelihood of the presence of hypertrophied lymphoid tissue (adenoids and tonsils) may preclude passage of the tube. Finally, the higher location of the larynx in the small pediatric patient causes a more acute angle from the nasopharynx, making successful intubation less likely.

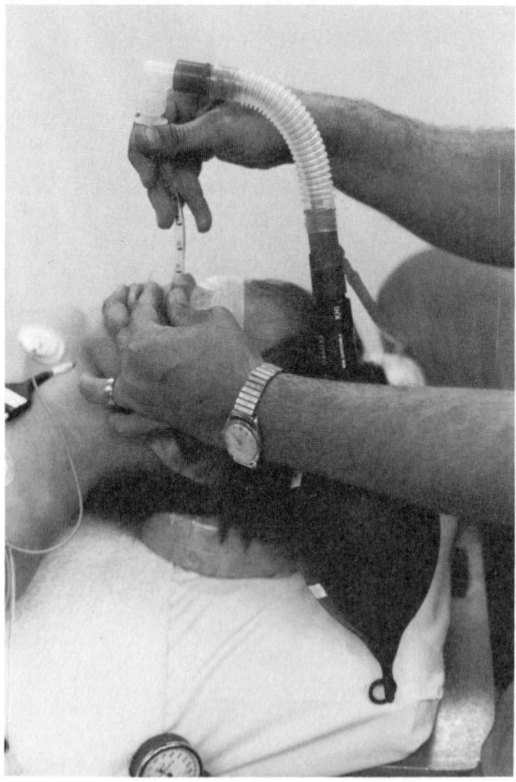

Figure 3–6. Nasal intubation with proper hand placement and supplemental oxygen by way of a partial rebreathing system.

However, in the adolescent or pre-adolescent patient, an awake nasal intubation may be a plausible choice. This technique is usually performed in a patient who still has spontaneous respiration. If time will allow, nasal intubation should be preceded with a topical vasoconstrictor to prevent bleeding from the nasal mucosa. Usually in children, phenylephrine 0.02 per cent (10 μg/kg) or xylometazoline 0.05 per cent nasal spray is effective, but in older or more alert children, cocaine 5 per cent (3 mg/kg) may be used. Passage first of a lubricated suction catheter or nasopharyngeal airway into the posterior nasopharynx may help to dilate the nasal passages.[16] Then, a small suction catheter passed through the nasal endotracheal tube and protruding about 3 cm beyond its tip will serve as a "leader" and prevent mucosal injury, submucosal tunneling, entry into a false passage, or entry of debris into the lumen of the tube.[30] Once the tube has passed into the oropharynx, the suction catheter can be removed.

It is usually helpful to attach a source of oxygen, for instance a nonrebreathing (partial rebreathing) bag system, to the tube once the suction catheter has been removed, since this will help prevent hypoxia and will also identify the inspiratory and expiratory cycles of respiration. The tube is advanced blindly, with the left hand used to hold the lips closed and also palpate the neck area for clues as to tube position (Fig. 3–6). It is believed by some that having the patient protrude his tongue or grasping the tongue and manually pulling it outward may facilitate nasotracheal intubation.[31] However, good control studies have not yet been carried out on this technique. The tube should be advanced into the trachea during inspiration. The respiratory motion of the reservoir bag will decrease or stop if the nasotracheal tube enters the esophagus or piriform sinus, but it is improved if successful intubation of the trachea occurs. Once the trachea is intubated, the cuff can be inflated and paralysis or induction of anesthesia may ensue if necessary.

In certain patients, in whom blind nasotracheal intubation is unsuccessful, direct vision through the mouth using a laryngoscope may be necessary. Usually a pair of Magill forceps are used to grasp the nasotracheal tube, which lies in the posterior oropharynx, and to place the tip into the trachea. The tube is then advanced into the trachea by pushing on the end of the tube that exits from the nose. A nasotracheal tube is generally more stable in the pediatric patient, but nasal intubation usually takes longer and should not be tried in patients who are not breathing or who have cranial, maxillary, or facial injuries. Nasal intubation is useful in seizure patients or patients who are too uncooperative to open their mouths and yet are breathing spontaneously. Prolonged nasotracheal intubation may be associated with sinusitis or deformity of the nose.[32]

"Awake" (i.e., not under anesthesia) oral tracheal intubation is most appropriate in the patient with respiratory arrest, simply because the patient is usually flaccid and oral intubation can be accomplished rapidly. Even though the procedure can usually be performed quickly by someone properly trained, adequate oxygenation of the patient should precede the attempt. The head is placed in the sniffing position, and a laryngoscope blade of proper size (see Table 3–3) is inserted into the right side of the mouth, sweeping the tongue to the left. The proper size endotracheal tube is placed through the cords a few centimeters, and bilateral breath sounds are auscultated. In order to more securely fix the tube, it is not uncommon to change the oral tube to a nasal tube as circumstances permit. This is usually done by deviating the oral tube to the left side of the mouth and having an assistant continue ventilation. A vasoconstrictor is applied to the nasal mucosa, and a well-lubricated straight tube is inserted through the nose as far as the posterior oropharynx. The nasal tube is then visualized by means of oral laryngoscopy and grasped 1 cm from the tip with Magill forceps. When the tube is positioned just to the right of the oral tube at the orifice of the larynx, the assistant removes the oral tube, and the nasal tube is inserted and advanced into the trachea. This process allows for quick resuscitation of a patient with an oral tube and transfer to a nasal tube with essentially no time for hypoxia or aspiration. In order to assure proper placement, the tube should be advanced until breath sounds are not heard on one side of the chest, indicating a mainstem bronchus intubation, and then the tube should be pulled back a centimeter or two. The head should be flexed because this will move the tube toward the carina, and breath sounds should be rechecked.[33] If ventilation is satisfactory, the tube should be taped securely and a chest x-ray should be taken as soon as possible.

It may become necessary to do an awake oral intubation in a trauma patient who is spontaneously breathing. This may be required for the induction of anesthesia in patients with impending respiratory failure or in smaller patients in whom nasal intubation was unsuccessful. In the pediatric population, it is unlikely that the intubationist can expect much cooperation from the patient. Such methods as application of lidocaine to the tongue and pharynx or intravenous sedation are usually of no distinct aid in performing the intubation. One should be exceptionally careful with sedation because, if overdone, reflexes may be obtunded and, upon regurgitation, the patient may aspirate. Therefore, in the smaller patient, usually less than 2 to 4 months of age, awake oral intubation usually is feasible, but for older patients, the rapid-sequence intubation (see Induction of Anesthesia) is generally the preferred method. The procedure for performing an awake oral intubation in the breathing patient should be the same as that described previously for carrying out oral intubation, but the addition of supplemental oxygen during laryngoscopy has been shown to be of benefit, since the patient is breathing spontaneously.[34] Laryngoscopes are available that have been modified for this purpose[35] (Fig. 3–7) and are especially beneficial in

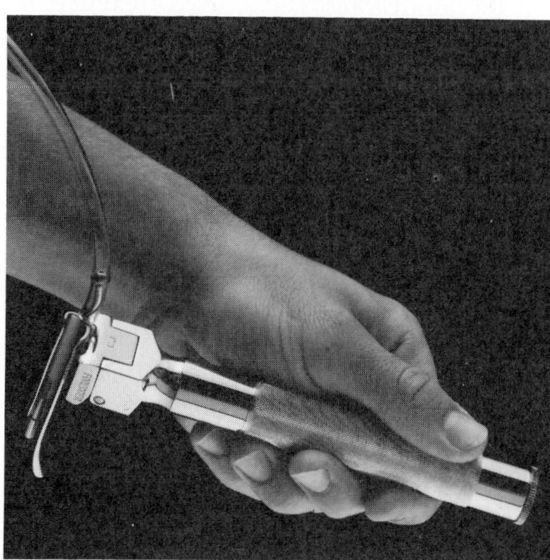

Figure 3–7. Oxyscope for delivering supplemental oxygen during intubation. (From Foregger Medical Division, Langhorne, PA. Reproduced with permission.)

preventing hypoxia in the more difficult intubation.

In certain cases of difficult intubation the pediatric flexible fiberoptic laryngoscope may be of help. Use of this instrument takes time, experience, and adequate equipment. For these reasons, the flexible fiberoptic laryngoscope should only be used after the patient has been initially stabilized by one of the more rapid methods described previously.

Obviously these procedures take time and are indicated only in special cases. They require experienced people and adequate equipment and, above all, should only be done after the patient has been initially stabilized by some of the more rapid methods described previously.

Surgical Opening of the Airway

Every effort should be made to improve or secure the airway with the preceding methods. However, if complete upper airway obstruction is present or if injuries to the larynx[36] prevent relief of obstruction by these methods, more heroic procedures are most certainly necessary. It will, however, be the extremely rare patient who will require one of the following procedures. Transtracheal catheter ventilation via cricothyrotomy may be successful in small children even with the small size of the trachea and small size of the catheter that must be inserted. In older children, pre-adolescent or adolescent, a large-bore intravenous (IV) catheter is placed through the cricothyroid membrane and directed caudally into the trachea. The plastic catheter is secured in place and connected to a system that permits ventilation of the lungs by means of intermittent jets of oxygen.[3, 37] In some institutions, high-frequency positive pressure ventilation (HFPPV) has been used successfully, but it is necessary that there be an exit route (e.g., through the upper airway) for venting of gases lest overpressurization of the lungs and barotrauma result.[38] In older patients, the cricothyroid membrane may be incised and a large-bore tube placed to secure the airway.

An emergency tracheostomy in children is rarely indicated.[15] Even acute mechanical obstruction secondary to a foreign body is more effectively managed by back blows, chest thrusts, abdominal thrusts (Heimlich maneuver), or bag and mask ventilation, followed by definitive management of the airway.[15, 39] Most tracheostomies will be required for head and neck or upper airway injuries and should be performed only after the airway has been secured with an endotracheal tube or bronchoscope. Tracheostomies are performed differently in children than in adults, and proper technique should be used to avoid long-term complications.[15]

Once ventilation has been assured by one of the preceding methods, the anesthesiologist will want to further assess the respiratory system. Evaluation of the upper airway should be completed, checking for foreign bodies, loose teeth, especially in the 6 to 12 age group, and sites of bleeding. The neck region should be examined for injuries to the larynx, trachea, and mainstem bronchi. Evidence of direct trauma or the presence of subcutaneous emphysema over the face, neck, and chest suggests injuries to these structures. Inspection of the chest may reveal paradoxic movements of the chest, indicating two or more rib fractures (a mainstem bronchus intubation should also be considered), and the possibility of lung contusion, which may require postoperative ventilatory support. Penetrating wounds may also be found, suggesting pneumothorax or hemothorax, which may require prompt tube thoracostomy.

Radiographic examination is mandatory in almost any trauma patient who requires respiratory support or who has evidence of facial or thoracic trauma. Confirming the presence or absence of foreign bodies, properly placed respiratory devices, aspiration, pulmonary contusion, hemothorax, pneumothorax, etc., will be important in the intra- and postoperative management of the patient.

Examination of arterial blood gases is also helpful in determining acid base status and oxygenation, both of which are important in the choice of the anesthesia technique for a patient destined for surgery.

Cardiovascular System

The cardiovascular system is the next system that requires stabilization in the trauma patient. Just as with the respiratory system, the anesthesiologist's skills may enhance the resuscitative efforts involving the cardiovascular system, especially in the areas of IV line placement and drug administration. Certainly if the anesthesiologist has not been available for the initial resuscitation and stabilization, he should be aware of what actions have been taken, since continuation of cardiovascular support will fall into his hands during surgery.

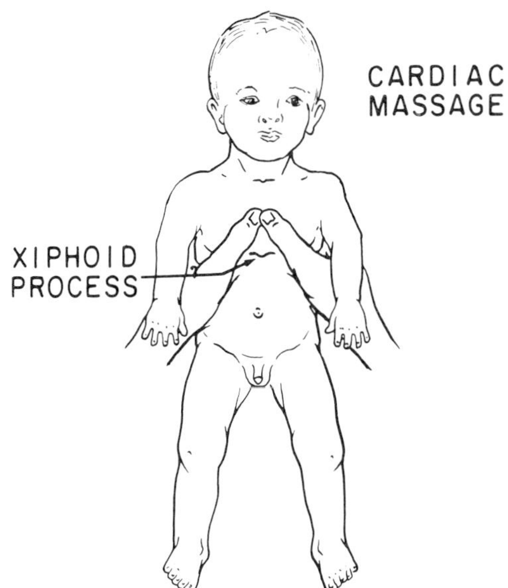

Figure 3–8. Proper placement of hands for infant cardiac compressions.

Cardiopulmonary Resuscitation

Initially, in the more severely traumatized patient, full cardiopulmonary resuscitation (CPR) may be necessary. While respiration is supported, external cardiac massage should be instituted. In the infant, the proper area for compressions is the midpoint between the nipples, and in the child, just above the xyphoid process. In infants and small children, the chest is quite pliable. Usually it is best to encircle the chest with the hands and use the thumbs to compress the sternum ½ to ¾ in. (1.3 to 2.5 cm) (Fig. 3–8).[5, 40] Compressions performed on the child will require more force. Therefore, the child should be placed on a hard surface. The heel of the hand should be used, and the sternum compression increased to 1 to 1½ in. (2.5 to 3.8 cm). Since the heart rate is inherently faster in infants and children, the rate of compressions should be 100 compressions per minute in infants and 60 to 80 compressions per minute in children. Whether one rescuer or two is providing CPR, the ratio of compressions to respirations is 5 to 1. There is some preliminary evidence that increasing abdominal pressure in the intubated patient by the use of military anti-shock trousers (MAST) or abdominal binders may be helpful in improving both systolic and diastolic pressures as well as blood flow to the brain during cardiac compression.[41–43] Owing to some reports of abdominal injury,[44] the technique cannot be recommended for routine use at this time, but it may have promise for the future. However, the anti-shock garment (MAST) is generally helpful in counteracting initial hypovolemia, provided it is not overinflated.[45]

Placement of Intravenous Lines

Once effective CPR has been instituted, the placement of adequate IV lines is mandatory. At the time IV therapy is being started, blood should be drawn and sent for type and crossmatch and for initial screening laboratory tests. In patients with abdominal trauma, it is wise to have the majority of the IV lines or, at the minimum, at least one IV line in the upper extremity. Inferior vena cava (IVC) compression from a distended abdomen may prevent adequate response from fluid or drug resuscitation through IV lines in the lower extremities. While detailed information on venous access is listed on pages 9–12, several points deserve emphasis. First, the IV line should be placed *rapidly*, whether by percutaneous peripheral cannulation, percutaneous central cannulation, or cutdown technique. Second, because underlying cardiovascular, pulmonary, or renal disease is more rare in children than in adults, rapid fluid administration is quite safe in the pediatric trauma victim. For this reason, in the initial phases of resuscitation, the ability to assess the central venous pressure (CVP) is less important in children. While CVP catheters may be of benefit in the ongoing resuscitation or intraoperative phases of care, it is not necessary to place a central venous line initially. Third, the IV line should be secured carefully to prevent dislodgment or infiltration. Chapter 34 details the appropriate means of taping and securing IV lines. Finally, if the child is not responding appropriately to adequate fluid or drug infusions, the IV line should be rechecked to assure that it is functioning properly.

Use of Drugs and Fluids

Once electrocardiogram (EKG) monitoring and a secure IV line are available, drugs may be given for resuscitation or support of the cardiovascular system. (Under certain circumstances in which an IV line cannot be promptly secured, epinephrine or lidocaine may be administered in the recommended IV dosage down the endotracheal tube. These drugs usually are well absorbed by this route, and this method should be tried before the

Table 3–5. DRUGS FOR PEDIATRIC RESUSCITATION AND CARDIOVASCULAR SUPPORT

Drug	Dose (intravenous)	How Supplied	Remarks
Atropine sulfate	0.01–0.02 mg/kg/dose	0.4 mg/ml, 0.4 mg/0.5 ml, 1 mg/ml	
Calcium chloride (10%)	20 mg/kg/dose	100 mg/ml	Give slowly
Calcium gluconate (10%)	60 mg/kg/dose	100 mg/mg	Give slowly
Dexamethasone sodium phosphate	1.5 mg/kg/dose initial for brain swelling, or 1.5 mg/kg/day	4 mg/ml	
Diazepam	0.1–0.3 mg/kg/dose	5 mg/ml	Give slowly (respiratory depression)
Phenytoin sodium	10–15 mg/kg/dose for seizure, then 5–10 mg/kg/day	50 mg/ml	
Dopamine HCl (infusion)	2–20 μg/kg/min	40 mg/ml	Alpha-receptor dominates at > 10 μg/kg/min
Epinephrine HCl (1:10,000)	0.1 ml/kg/dose (0.01 mg/kg/dose)	1:10,000 (0.1 mg/ml)	Should be given centrally
Epinephrine HCl (infusion)	0.05–1.0 μg/kg/min	1:1,000 (1 mg/ml)	Usual effect at 0.1 μg/kg/min
Fusosemide	1 mg/kg/dose	10 mg/ml	May repeat doubling dose
Isoproterenol HCl (infusion)	0.05–1.0 μg/kg/min	1 mg/5 ml	Usual effect 2–20 μg/kg/min
Lidocaine	1 mg/kg/dose	20 mg/ml	
Lidocaine (infusion)	30 μg/kg/min	20 mg/ml	
Mannitol	1 g/kg/dose	1 g/4 ml	
Naloxone	0.01 mg/kg/dose	0.4 mg/ml, 0.02 mg/ml	
Sodium bicarbonate	1–2 mg/kg/dose, or 0.3 × kg × base deficit	1 mEq/ml	Should be diluted in newborns
Sodium nitroprusside (infusion)	Start at 0.5 μg/kg/min	10 mg/ml	Usual effect at 1–10 μg/kg/min; keep dose as low as possible and watch for acidosis

intracardiac route is used.) Drugs and their dosages frequently used in pediatric resuscitation and cardiovascular support are shown in Table 3–5. These dosages are rough guidelines and should be individualized in each case. If defibrillation is required, usually a current at 2 to 5 watt/second (joules)/kg (beginning with the lower dose) is recommended, using well-lubricated, external paddles of the appropriate size.[47]

Since the weight of pediatric patients is so important in estimating the proper dosage of drugs and fluids to be given, we have found the Weech mnemonics to be of aid in the trauma situation in which a patient's age is known but the weight is usually not readily available (Table 3–6).

To avoid overloading the patient with fluid, infusions of epinephrine and isoproterenol are mixed using the following formula:

$$\text{Weight in kg} \times 60 = \mu\text{g of drug in 100 ml of fluid}$$

This is usually placed in a Metriset. Then an infusion of 1 drop/minute (pediatric dripper) or 1 ml/hour equals a dose of .01 μg/kg/minute.

For infusions of dopamine and nitroprusside, the following formula is used:

$$\text{Weight in kg} \times 6 = \text{mg of drug in 100 ml of fluid}$$

Table 3–6. WEECH MNEMONICS FOR APPROXIMATE HEIGHT AND WEIGHT OF INFANTS AND CHILDREN

At birth	Weight (W) in lb = 7 lb 6 oz (3.4 kg)
From 3 to 12 months	W (lb) = age (mo) + 11
From 1 to 6 years	W (lb) = (age [yr] × 5) + 17
From 6 to 12 years	W (lb) = (age [yr] × 7) + 5
At birth	Length = 20 in.
At 1 year	Length = 30 in.
From 2 to 14 years	Height (in.) = (age [yr] × 2½) + 30

From Vaughan VC III: Growth and development. *In* Vaughan VC III, McKay RJ (eds.): Nelson Textbook of Pediatrics. Philadelphia, WB Saunders Company, 1975, p. 25.

Then an infusion of 1 drop/minute (pediatric dripper) or 1 ml/hour equals a dose of 1 μg/kg/minute. Frequently, the nitroprusside is diluted to one-half strength. It should be remembered that the dosage of dopamine in small children may exceed the usual adult dosage before the characteristic increases in heart rate, blood pressure, and cardiac index are seen.[48, 49]

Examination and Monitoring

Once the initial resuscitation is completed, it is wise to perform a rapid examination of the cardiovascular system, which should include assessment of vital signs, examination of the heart and lungs, x-ray for heart size and pericardial fluid, and evaluation of peripheral pulses and perfusion. A history should also be taken concerning previous cardiac disease and drugs. With an eye toward further care in the ICU or intended surgical therapy, it may be appropriate to secure further monitoring at this time, or it may wait until transfer to the OR or ICU. A CVP line may be indicated in patients with large, sustained, or anticipated blood loss; patients who may require a prolonged convalescent course; and patients in whom fluid management will be critical. Although in our experience successful insertion of CVP catheters following trauma is more difficult in smaller patients, at least one study of relatively healthy patients shows no increase in failure rate for cannulation of the internal jugular vein in smaller patients.[50] It is generally believed that the incidence of complications from CVP catheter placement is higher in children than in adults, although most complications of CVP catheter placement are not life threatening if recognized.[50, 51] The CVP line may be placed more innocuously through an antecubital vein or from the femoral region. The external jugular route may be used with the aid of a J-wire.[52] The internal jugular route may also be used.[50, 51] The subclavian route is usually the last choice (see sections on intraoperative management and monitoring).

The pulmonary artery line is not used with great frequency in pediatric trauma, generally because the heart of the pediatric patient is usually "healthy," and once proper fluid status is achieved (monitored by CVP), the cardiac output is usually satisfactory. There are, however, specific patients in whom a Swan-Ganz catheter may be helpful, such as those who have undergone prolonged resuscitation, those who have had direct cardiac trauma, or those with pre-existing heart disease. Its insertion is generally by the same routes as the CVP line, with the femoral route being the more rarely used. Owing to the size of the Swan-Ganz catheter, a cutdown may be required.

In patients with unstable respiratory or cardiovascular status or with neurologic injury or patients destined for major surgery, the placement of an arterial line is recommended. This line gives the anesthesiologist continuous blood pressure monitoring, arterial blood gas monitoring, and ready access to blood for laboratory sampling. A more extensive discussion of CVP lines, pulmonary artery lines, and arterial lines follows in the section on intraoperative monitoring.

Central Nervous System

During the resuscitation and initial stabilization of the patient, the anesthesiologist and/or resuscitators should be ever mindful of the status of the central nervous system of the patient (Chapter 16). Certainly of primary importance is effective ventilation, with a high concentration of oxygen, and effective circulation. Following these initial steps, the rescuer's attention should turn to controlling intracranial pressure (ICP). Intracerebral hemorrhage and edema may increase ICP and potentiate life-threatening cerebral or cerebellar herniation. Steps should immediately be taken to decrease the ICP in head-injured or postanoxic patients. These steps should include hyperventilation with reduction of Pa_{CO_2} to approximately 25 torr. This can be accomplished by increasing the ventilation to approximately twice normal with the bag-valve or oxygen-powered resuscitation systems, or increasing the oxygen flow to approximately 5000 ml/m^2/minute, using a nonrebreathing (partial rebreathing) system. Ventilation with this flow rate should be rapid, i.e., at least twice the oxygen flow rate. Fluid is restricted to three-fourths maintenance (if appropriate in the context of the rest of the clinical situation), and steroids (dexamethasone 1.5 mg/kg/dose initially) may be given. Diuresis may be employed in certain cases but not routinely. Mannitol is potentially hazardous and should be administered as directed in Chapter 16. Elevation of the head is also helpful if the patient is not in shock.

Not uncommonly, it may be necessary to perform a diagnostic procedure, using, for example, CAT scans, x-rays, burr holes, or subarachnoid bolt placement in a semicomatose or agitated patient, prior to or in lieu of taking the patient to the operating room. Frequently, to lower ICP and to aid in the effective performance of the study, it may be necessary to anesthetize the patient. Usually a muscle relaxant such as pancuronium bromide (Pavulon) in a dose of 0.08 to 0.1 mg/kg, with or without a short-acting barbiturate, e.g., thiopental 2 to 4 mg/kg/dose, depending on consciousness of the patient, is sufficient to perform these procedures (see Intraoperative Management). Should the patient not require surgery, the muscle relaxant can usually be reversed within 45 minutes and the patient's neurologic status followed as necessary.

Extremities

The pre-anesthetic evaluation and stabilization of extremity injuries generally falls to the orthopedic surgeon. However, since the patient may ultimately require anesthesia for surgical therapy of the injured extremity, certain points need to be checked by the anesthesiologist. Fractures should be splinted, since the patient will need to be transported to the OR. Vascular injuries to extremities should be noted, since it is generally unwise to place monitoring devices in these extremities because further injury may occur or the anesthesiologist may not be able to obtain needed information on the patient's condition during surgery. Nerve injuries may present medical as well as legal problems. Most would believe it unwise to carry out regional anesthesia technique in an extremity that may have nerve injury. The performance of the block may be difficult (see section on regional anesthesia techniques) and the legal implications of nerve injury in a patient who has had a regional technique performed may be worrisome.[53]

Renal Function

The anesthesiologist taking the trauma patient to the OR will become responsible for the fluid maintenance and urine output of the patient. It is imperative that he is aware of the fluids the patient has received, finds out if any renal abnormalities or damage exists, and makes sure that a urinary catheter is in place in the comatose or complicated surgical patient.

Laboratory Values

In the preoperative period, the anesthesiologist needs to make sure that appropriate samples for laboratory tests have been sent, and he should be aware of any information received. Blood replacement in the OR will depend to some extent upon the hematocrit of the patient. Therefore, a complete blood count as well as a sample for type and crossmatch must be sent to the laboratory, and a check made with the blood bank to assure that blood is at least tentatively available. Arterial blood gases should be assessed in the more severely traumatized patient or in the patient whose respiratory function is compromised, and appropriate correction of values started prior to going to the OR. Laboratory values, such as ionized calcium levels in patients who have received large amounts of plasma, serum glucose in small patients, clotting studies in transfused patients, and baseline electrolyte and renal studies in severely traumatized patients, should be evaluated as soon as possible, since these will influence management and choice of anesthetic during surgery.

PREPARATION FOR SURGERY

Premedication

Once the patient has been resuscitated and stabilized, the anesthesiologist should determine the best ways to pharmacologically prepare the patient for the anesthetic that he plans to deliver. Under the category of premedication falls both medications designed to alleviate pain and anxiety as well as those designed to help prevent the serious effects of aspiration.

Certainly patients who are severely traumatized and have a precarious circulatory status or those who are already unconscious or disoriented do not need premedication with analgesic drugs. Premedication with sedatives is usually not beneficial and may be detrimental. Drugs such as scopolamine and barbiturates may cause excitement if analgesia is not adequate.[54] Other patients, such as those with head injuries and those with undetermined abdominal trauma, should most likely not be sedated until a definite plan for surgery is decided upon. On the other hand, it is inhumane to withhold analgesics from a patient in pain if the drugs can be administered safely and do not increase his risk from trauma or surgery. Usually the best policy is to administer small incremental doses of narcotics intravenously (Sublimaze 0.5 μg/kg/dose, morphine 0.05 mg/kg/dose) and titrate to effect, giving at least a few minutes after each dose to evaluate the patient's analgesia and cardiorespiratory status. Narcotics may cause hypotension resulting from a vasodilatory effect or a relief of pain-induced muscular rigidity,[29, 45] and naloxone should be available to reverse the narcotic should apparent overdose occur. The possibility of increasing ICP due to hypoventilation in patients with head injuries should be weighed against the possibility of worse damage from the patient's excitability or attempts used to control the patient.[55]

Anticholinergic drugs may frequently be given to small patients under 6 months of age prior to surgery to prevent vagal reflexes.[8] This can usually be done quite adequately by giving the anticholinergic intravenously just before the induction of anesthesia. Anticholinergics that are generally used are atropine 20 μg/kg/dose and glycopyrrolate 5 μg/kg/dose. Salem,[56] however, reported that glycopyrrolate 7.5 to 10.0 μg/kg/dose 1 hour before anesthesia reduced the gastric volume by one third in studied patients versus controls. Also a significantly greater number of patients in the glycopyrrolate-treated group had pH values above 2.5. (Both the pH values and the volume of gastric fluid are critical in aspiration. A pH of less than 2.5 or a volume of 0.4 ml/kg or greater is usually considered necessary to produce the aspiration syndrome.)[57] In adult patients, Stoelting found that glycopyrrolate 3 μg/kg/dose did not produce protective effects.[58] It appears then that a higher than usual dose is necessary and must be administered at least an hour before surgery. A possible argument against using anticholinergics are reports that show that all anticholinergic drugs cause a reduction of lower esophageal sphincter tone and therefore reduced protection against aspiration.[59, 60]

Cimetidine is a specific histamine (H_2 receptor) antagonist that inhibits the secretion and acidity of gastric fluids. It also appears to have little effect on the tone of the lower esophageal sphincter or rate of gastric emptying.[61] Goudsouzian showed that cimetidine in a dose of 7.5 mg/kg given between 1 and 4 hours prior to surgery reduced the volume of gastric contents to less than 0.4 ml/kg and increased the pH of these gastric contents to more than 2.5 in 95 per cent of the children studied.[62] Cimetidine is probably more effective if given parenterally, e.g., intramuscularly, and caution should be used in administering the drug to patients with renal or hepatic failure or a history of asthma.[61] Cimetidine also appears to decrease the clearance of diazepam and chlordiazepoxide* and should be used cautiously in the presence of these drugs. However, it should be remembered that in patients with a traumatic injury, gastric motility may cease at the time of injury, and the stomach may be filled with a large amount of food and gastric secretions, even though it may have been many hours since the patient last ate. Therefore, neither glycopyrrolate nor cimetidine will effectively prevent aspiration in these patients.

Two drugs that act by both having a central antiemetic effect and increasing emptying of the stomach and upper gastrointestinal tract are metoclopramide and domperidone. Reports on the effectiveness of these drugs are controversial,[63–65] and further studies are necessary. Metoclopramide appears more likely to cause toxic reactions in children than in adults[66, 67] and therefore should be used cautiously in children, especially in view of the controversy concerning its effectiveness.

Another approach to managing the full stomach is the use of pre-induction antacids. These are contraindicated in comatose patients with an unprotected airway or patients with injuries of the gastrointestinal tract. Stoelting found that antacids raised the pH above 2.5 in all his patients.[58] White studied the effects of Maalox® on adults requiring emergency surgery and found the pH to be greater than 2.5 in all patients.[68] The percentage of patients with gastric volumes greater than 25 ml was also less than that of controls. Wheatley showed that Milk of Magnesia 30 ml by mouth in adults raised the pH above 2.5 if given 10 to 80 minutes prior to induction of anesthesia.[69] Although antacids are effective, Gibbs showed in dogs that the induced aspiration of a mixture of particulate antacid and saline with a pH of 8.3 had similar effects on Pa_{O_2} and shunt fraction as did aspiration of hydrochloric acid at pH 1.8.[70] Also, the more prominent histologic findings were in the antacid group. However, sodium citrate, which is a nonparticulate antacid, appears to produce only transient hypoxia and minimal tissue changes when aspirated. It is more effective in neu-

*Physician's Drug Alert, July 1982.

tralizing an acid pH than particulate antacids and, in a dose of 30 ml by mouth in adult patients, provided a safe gastric pH in essentially all patients.[71] However, it does not reduce the volume of gastric contents.

In the face of the present evidence, it seems logical to use an anticholinergic (preferably glycopyrrolate), cimetidine (if an hour's delay prior to surgery is anticipated), and a nonparticulate antacid by mouth if not contraindicated in the premedication of a patient. Unfortunately, it is probable that when particles of food are aspirated, pulmonary problems may be prominent even in the face of a "safe" pH of the gastric contents. It therefore becomes evident that proper premedication of the patient may be helpful, but it does not eliminate the need for a careful and safe induction of anesthesia.

Transport to the Operating Room

Once the patient is stabilized and preoperative medications (if any) are given, it is time to plan for the transport of the patient to the OR. However, before the patient is transported, the anesthesiologist must insure that all facilities in the OR (including all surgical instruments and monitoring and anesthesia equipment) are ready for the arrival of the patient. There is rarely any justification for rushing to the OR before proper preparations have been made.

In the more critical cases (respiratory trauma, unstable cardiovascular system, or central nervous system trauma), the anesthesiologist should attend the transport. In the intubated patient, a device that will deliver 100 per cent oxygen during spontaneous or controlled ventilation should be used. My preference is a nonrebreathing (partial rebreathing) circuit (see section on preanesthetic respiratory treatment). Blood pressure monitoring should be available during transport, either by means of a portable blood pressure cuff with auscultation, portable oscillotonometer, automated oscillotonometer, blood pressure cuff and palpation of the artery, Doppler ultrasound, or transducer connected to a portable monitor if an arterial line is present. Also, a convenient device for portable monitoring mean blood pressure if an arterial line is in place is the Pressurveil connected to an aneroid manometer.[72] The EKG should also be monitored in transport. A precordial stethoscope is helpful to monitor respiration and also as a back-up for cardiovascular monitoring should there be interference with the EKG. In all patients, but especially in smaller patients, means should be provided to prevent heat loss while transporting the patient. This may be accomplished by humidifying inspired gases[21, 73]; covering the body with warm towels, blankets, or drapes[74]; or using portable warmers.

The patient should be transported as quickly and as carefully as possible. Emergency equipment for intubation or reintubation, as well as resuscitative drugs, should accompany the patient until he is safely within the confines of the OR.

INTRAOPERATIVE MANAGEMENT

The intraoperative management of the trauma patient includes adequate monitoring; safe induction and maintenance of anesthesia; support of respiration with adequate humidification, fluid maintenance, and blood replacement; and consideration of the patient's special anesthetic needs.

Monitoring

Monitoring of the pediatric trauma patient may range from routine to extensive, depending upon the severity of the case. Routine monitoring is monitoring that is applicable to all patients, regardless of their pathophysiologic status. Specialized monitoring is used for a particular pathologic problem (e.g., serum glucose in the diabetic patient), and extensive monitoring refers to the monitoring of all major systems in patients undergoing extensive surgery.[75]

Upon arrival in the OR, the patient should be placed on the operating table in such a fashion that further injury is not created and vulnerable portions of the body are protected. It is important for the anesthesiologist to make sure that eyes, ears, lips, teeth, tongue, and extremities are protected from burns, compression, or overextension.

Routine Monitoring

Routine monitoring, which is applied to any patient undergoing surgery, consists of the following elements. First, the most basic monitoring during anesthesia uses the so-called physical diagnosis aspects of monitoring (Table 3–7). This involves the inspection, palpation, and auscultation of various por-

Table 3–7. PHYSICAL DIAGNOSIS ASPECTS IN MONITORING OF ANESTHETIZED PATIENTS

Inspection
- Skin—color, capillary refill, rash, edema, hematoma
- Nail beds—color, capillary refill
- Mucous membrane—color, moisture, edema
- Surgical field—color of tissues and blood, rate of blood loss, muscular relaxation
- Position—potential for trauma (joints, nerves, circulation)
- Movement—purposeful or reflex (nonparalyzed patient), ventilation
- Eyes—conjunctiva (color, edema), pupils (size, direct and consensual reactivity, change with stimulation)

Palpation
- Skin—temperature, texture (e.g., papular rash), edema, hematoma, subcutaneous emphysema (crepitation)
- Pulses—fullness, rate and rhythm
- Muscle tone

Auscultation
- Ventilation—breath sounds (normal, pathologic, absent; distribution over lung fields)
- Heart sounds—rate, rhythm, extra sounds, murmurs
- Blood pressure—results of
- Location of nasogastric tube

Adapted from Hug CC: Monitoring in anesthesia. *In* Miller RD (ed.): Anesthesia. New York, Churchill Livingstone, 1981, p. 158.

tions of the body for clues to the patient's condition and anesthetic depth.

Other monitoring routinely done in the OR includes the use of the EKG and precordial or esophageal stethoscope[76] and the noninvasive measurement of blood pressure, using a cuff and one of the following methods: oscillation of the cuff pressure, auscultation of Korotkoff's sounds, ultrasonic detection of arterial wall motion under or distal to the cuff, or detection of pulse distal to the cuff by palpation.[75] It is important that the cuff be the proper size in order to get an accurate result. The present recommendation is that the width of the cuff be 40 per cent of the circumference of the arm or leg or 20 per cent wider than the diameter of the arm or leg. Preferably the bladder should encircle the arm or leg but not overlap, and under all circumstances, it should overlie the artery.[72, 77, 78] In children, ultrasonic detection is a very commonly used technique and has shown great accuracy.[79, 80] A number of automated devices are available for measurement of blood pressure in infants and children.* The relative merits and disadvantages of these devices are not among the topics of this chapter and are discussed elsewhere.[72, 76]

Since children have a very large surface area compared to mass,[76] temperature changes during anesthesia are quite common. The incidence of malignant hyperthermia is also much more common in children than in adults.[81] For these reasons, temperature should be monitored in every patient who receives an anesthetic. Where to measure temperature during surgery is a controversial issue. A measurement of core temperature using the rectal, esophageal, nasopharyngeal, tympanic, or axillary site appears to be satisfactory when the anesthesiologist understands the limitations of each location under certain surgical conditions.[76, 82] The tympanic temperature is thought by some to be the most accurate, but technical difficulties and complications have limited its use.[75, 76, 82] Since infants lose heat primarily by convection (if in a cold room), conduction (if in contact with a cold object), evaporation (of prep solutions), or radiation (if left uncovered), it is wise to prevent these conditions, since oxygen consumption is directly related to the gradient between skin temperature and environmental temperature.[83]

Monitoring of inspired oxygen concentration has now become routine in the OR, and alarms are usually set to warn the anesthesiologist if inspired oxygen concentration drops below a preset level (usually 30 to 35 per cent). Disconnect or low-pressure alarms as well as overpressurization or high-pressure alarms are frequently used in conjunction with ventilators in the OR to warn of any problems with ventilation of the patient when it is being done mechanically. Commonly, if muscle relaxants (to be discussed later) are used, a nerve stimulator monitors the degree of neuromuscular blockade. The percentage of neuromuscular receptors occupied by a muscle relaxant is monitored by single twitch stimuli, tetanic stimuli, or train of four stimuli. Proper use of these monitoring techniques is discussed in recent reviews.[84, 85]

Extensive Monitoring

Many trauma patients going to the OR will require more extensive monitoring because of the extent of their injuries and/or the probability of major changes occurring during the surgery. These conditions will require more sophisticated monitoring of the cardiorespiratory, central nervous, and urinary systems. Some of these monitors may have been

*Dinamap (Critikon, Tampa, FL); Arteriosonde (Hoffmann-LaRoche, Belleville, NJ); Doppler Ultrasound Flowmeter (Parks Electronics, Aloha, OR); Infrasonde sensor (Marion Scientific Corp., Kansas City, MO).

applied to the patient in the emergency room or ICU prior to transport to surgery and have already been mentioned.

Invasive Hemodynamic Monitoring

Probably one of the most useful invasive monitors in a critically ill infant or child is the arterial line. It has been repeatedly documented that arterial pressure is a good indicator of the volume status of a pediatric patient whose cardiopulmonary status is relatively normal.[86, 87] The arterial line consists of a catheter placed in an artery and connected by means of a fluid-filled line to a transducer for monitoring pressure. This line also provides quick access to blood for laboratory tests and blood gas measurements. The line is usually placed in an artery with good collateral flow, such as the radial, ulnar, dorsalis pedis, posterior tibial, or superficial temporal artery.[88] In patients in severe shock, these vessels may be extremely difficult to cannulate or may give inaccurate readings due to peripheral vasoconstriction. Therefore, initially a femoral or brachial line may be necessary, but we prefer to change to a more peripheral artery once resuscitation is completed. The more central catheter is removed, since complications from the central artery catheters are likely to be more devastating. Work done by Downs[89] would suggest that the catheter for arterial lines in children be nontapered, small relative to the size of the artery, and filled with heparinized saline. Automatic infusion devices such as the Intraflo* work well to maintain patency in larger patients.[72] In children who weigh less than 10 kg, we use microinfusion pumps such as the Razel† to maintain patency over long periods, thus avoiding fluid overload of the patient. Generally we use 22- or 24-gauge catheters in all our pediatric patients and have found patency to be good.

Complications are essentially nonexistent, provided catheters are not placed into arteries compromised by previous vascular injury or disease; pre-insertion tests for the presence of a complete palmar arch, with ulnar dominance and adequate collaterals, are performed; the catheter is promptly removed if transient ischemia is noted; and immediate embolectomy is performed when ischemic changes persist.[90] Flushing of arterial lines must be done carefully because retrograde flow and possible central embolization may occur.[89, 91] Guidelines for arterial cannulation in pediatric patients are presented in Table 3–8. Obviously these guidelines need to be individualized to each case.

Probably the next most useful invasive monitor in the pediatric trauma patient is the central venous pressure (CVP) catheter. A catheter inserted into the central venous circulation provides information concerning the right side filling pressure of the heart and reliable access to the venous system for administration of blood, fluids, or drugs. The CVP line is therefore both a monitor as well as a therapeutic modality. It should be placed as quickly as is feasible (see section on initial cardiovascular stabilization of the patient). Placement of this catheter prior to the onset of severe hypovolemia greatly enhances the success of its insertion. General indications for placement of the CVP line in the pediatric surgical patient are listed in Table 3–9. In most pediatric patients without cardiopulmonary disease, the CVP will provide an accurate reflection of the balances between blood volume, venous capacitance, and car-

Table 3–8. INDICATIONS FOR ARTERIAL CANNULATION IN PEDIATRIC SURGICAL PATIENTS

1. Requirement for extensive surgical procedures and/or supplemental oxygen in infants less than 45 weeks gestation (i.e., at risk for retrolental fibroplasia)
2. Most cardiac and major vessel surgery with the exception of uncomplicated patent ductus arteriosus ligation
3. Cardiopulmonary bypass surgery
4. Major anticipated blood loss (i.e., greater than 50 per cent of estimated blood volume)
5. Surgery with potential for rapid blood loss (i.e., greater than 10 to 15 per cent of estimated blood volume)
6. Significant cardiovascular disease, hemodynamic instability, or potential for sudden cardiovascular change
7. Deliberate hypotension, hypothermia, or hemodilution
8. Intracranial operations or the need for prolonged intraoperative hypocapnia
9. Severe respiratory disease or trauma, a Pa_{O_2} less than 300 torr on FI_{CO_2} 1.0, or requirement for postoperative ventilation
10. The need for repetitive arterial blood sampling
11. Inability to monitor blood pressure indirectly
12. Extensive trauma or surgery in which the duties of the anesthesiologist preclude continuous monitoring of blood pressure without an arterial cannula

Adapted from Hug CC: Monitoring in anesthesia. *In* Miller RD (ed.): Anesthesia. New York, Churchill Livingstone, 1981, p. 182, and personal communication from Eugene K. Betts, Children's Hospital of Philadelphia.

*Intraflo (Sorensen Research, Salt Lake City, Utah).
†Razel (Razel Scientific Instruments, Stanford, CT).

Table 3–9. INDICATIONS FOR CENTRAL VENOUS PRESSURE LINE IN PEDIATRIC SURGICAL PATIENTS

1. Lack of peripheral veins for cannulation
2. Pre-existing or anticipated intraoperative hypovolemia
3. Anticipated third space replacement to exceed 50 per cent of estimated blood volume
4. Site for rapid infusion of blood or fluids
5. Intravenous administration of drugs likely to injure peripheral vessels
6. Aspiration of air emboli (sitting craniotomies)
7. Removal or frequent sampling of venous blood
8. Cardiopulmonary bypass
9. Possible indications—congestive heart failure, deliberate hypotension, or hemodilution

Adapted from Hug CC: Monitoring in anesthesia. *In* Miller RD (ed.): Anesthesia. New York, Churchill Livingstone, 1981, p. 182, and personal communication from Eugene K. Betts, Children's Hospital of Philadelphia.

diac function. Placement of the central venous line in pediatric patients usually requires some skill. In order to achieve the highest rate of success, the line is placed percutaneously via the right internal jugular vein using the Seldinger technique[92] with one of the various approaches described in detail in the literature.[93–96] In patients to be heparinized in whom a carotid puncture would have dire consequences and in patients with abnormal necks due to trauma or surgery, another site must be chosen. Although it usually requires more time, external jugular vein cannulation has approximately a 60 per cent success rate in pediatric patients[52] and usually avoids the possibility of pneumothorax or carotid puncture. Other less successful sites may be used, such as the antecubital area of the arm, the left neck internal and external jugular veins, the femoral vein, and the subclavian vein. The subclavian vein is usually our last choice for a site for CVP line placement owing to the interference with care that may result from the positioning for insertion[97] and the possible complications resulting from unsuccessful puncture attempts.[98] It should probably be attempted only after other sites have been unsuccessful.[98] In pediatric trauma victims with head and neck trauma or those requiring immediate attendance to their airway, it is usually more efficacious to place a femoral CVP line initially. This line can be used for initial resuscitation, and if the tip is within the thorax, it can be used for CVP measurements during surgery. It also will allow resuscitation to proceed while other lines requiring more time are placed under less urgent circumstances. It is extremely unusual for the head-up position to be used during traumatic neurosurgery, so placement of the central line for extraction of air is usually not necessary. Proper techniques for placement of a CVP line for extraction of air can be found in the literature.[99–101]

In trauma patients who have pre-existing or have suffered from cardiopulmonary sequelae, the use of a pulmonary artery (Swan-Ganz) catheter may be of extreme value in measuring pulmonary artery and left heart filling pressures. In addition to providing a means for measuring central venous pressures, pulmonary artery pressures, and pulmonary capillary wedge pressures, the inclusion of a thermistor permits the measurement of cardiac output by thermodilution. Pulmonary artery catheters are indicated for patients with unstable circulation (e.g., those with massive trauma, burns, hypotensive shock, sepsis), certain types of heart disease (e.g., heart failure, pericardial disease, valvular disease), and severe respiratory problems. More extensive reviews on the subject of pulmonary artery catheters can be found in the literature.[72]

Measurement of Urine Output

Measurement of urine output is extremely important in any trauma victim. In all patients, except those who have minor trauma or probable urethral injuries (see Chapter 21) or who are to undergo exceptionally short procedures, a catheter should be inserted into the bladder for the evaluation of the urine and measurement of its volume. Infant renal function is somewhat decreased under a year of age, and particularly within the first month of life,[81] as a result of a reduced glomerular filtration rate, urea clearance, and concentrating ability. However, infants can concentrate urine if stressed, but this concentrating ability will not approach the adult level until between a month and 1 year of age. The capability of excreting a volume load also approaches adult levels between a month and 1 year of age.[81, 102] If proper fluid resuscitation and maintenance is given in the OR, pediatric patients should be expected to respond with a urine output of 0.5 to 2.0 ml/kg/hour. If this is not the case and appropriate fluid maintenance is thought to have been given, probably the first check should be to make sure the catheter and bag system are functioning properly. Air locks and kinks are common in the OR. If the catheter collection system is functioning properly, further evaluation should include assessment of the patient's vascular volume and possibly cardiac output by means of monitoring devices already mentioned. See Chapter 7 for further assessment of renal function. For patients with head injuries, monitoring of the intracerebral pressure (ICP) may be necessary. This may be accomplished by a ventriculostomy, subdural bolt, or epidural transducer. Generally only a small portion of patients will have ICP monitored in the OR. Whether ICP is monitored mechanically or visually (inspection of the brain at craniotomy), the influence of anesthetics, anesthetic techniques, position of patient, surgical manipulation, and dressings will be reflected (see Chapter 16).[103–106]

Monitoring of Intra-arterial Blood Gases

Continuous monitoring of intra-arterial blood gases during pediatric surgery is not commonplace, owing to mechanical and technical problems. However, continuous monitoring of arterial carbon dioxide may be approximated by monitoring either the end tidal carbon dioxide, using circle systems,[107, 108] or the mean expired carbon dioxide, using partial rebreathing anesthesia systems,[109] in patients without significant pulmonary disease. This monitoring may be accomplished by means of a mass spectrophotometer or an infrared carbon dioxide analyzer.* Some of these devices are small enough to be placed directly on anesthesia machines for convenient monitoring. In certain cases, such as in craniotomies or some pulmonary procedures, this continuous monitoring may be helpful in detecting problems should sudden changes occur.[110]

Measurement of Arterial Oxygen Tension

The arterial oxygen tension can be measured transcutaneously.† This may be accomplished by using a heated electrode on the skin, usually over the chest or abdomen. Correlation in children between the electrode and arterial Pa_{O_2} once the electrode has warmed (15 to 20 minutes) is good,[111] but unfortunately these devices are inaccurate when the arterial blood pressure falls two standard deviations below the mean, when the patient has persistent pulmonary hypertension, and in the face of certain anesthetics, such as halothane and nitrous oxide, but usually not enflurane or isoflurane.[112, 113] Membranes are now available that appear to decrease the effect of anesthetics. A new and extremely useful monitor for measuring arterial oxygen saturation is the pulse oximeter. This device will not create a burn, may be placed on any extremity, requires no warm up time, and can also monitor the heart rate.‡

Laboratory Monitoring

Laboratory monitoring of trauma patients during anesthesia is variable, being dictated by the case at hand. However, it is common to monitor arterial blood gases, acid base status, serum electrolytes, and hematocrit; in smaller patients, serum glucose and calcium are surveyed. It also may be necessary to evaluate blood clotting factors or platelets in patients needing large amounts of blood.

Induction of Anesthesia

Before the induction of anesthesia, the anesthesiologist should check all equipment (anesthesia machine, suction, monitors, airway equipment [Tables 3–2 to 3–4], IV fluids, and drugs). The induction of anesthesia in the pediatric trauma patient must take into consideration the special circumstances of each patient. In general, most patients will have full or potentially full stomachs, and many will have a potentially unstable cardiorespiratory status. The induction of anesthesia may be divided into two phases. The first phase is securing the airway, usually by means of an endotracheal tube, and the second phase is induction of anesthesia either by inhalation or intravenously. These two phases may occur simultaneously or one may precede the other. The first consists of safely securing the airway. In certain patients, the physician may elect to perform an awake intubation in order to maintain airway reflexes and avoid aspiration of gastric contents. Certain conditions such as open eye injuries, intracerebral hypertension, or some neck injuries are considered contraindications to this procedure. This technique is generally used only in unconscious, very small, or very unstable patients. The method for awake intubation has been discussed elsewhere.

A second approach to securing the airway for anesthesia is the rapid-sequence technique. This technique is used if the patient's status seems to justify it, i.e., the patient is awake and has reasonable cardiovascular stability. This is our most commonly used technique in trauma patients arriving in the OR

---

*Cavitron (Advanced Medical Systems, Anaheim, CA); Instrumentation Industries (Bethal Park, PA); Hewlett-Packard Co. (Waltham, MA).

†Radiometer American (Westlake, OH); Hewlett-Packard Co. (Waltham, MA); Novametrix Medical Systems (Wallingford, CT); Instrumentation Industries (Bethal Park, PA).

‡Nellcor (Hayward, CA); Marquest Medical Products (Englewood, CO).

unintubated. In this type of induction, the anesthesia and intubation occur almost simultaneously. There are essentially two forms of this technique. The first form is that described by Strept and Safar[114] and Levin.[8]

1. One hundred per cent oxygen is administered for 3 minutes by face mask. In uncooperative children who will not tolerate the mask, many times the mask can be held just above the face, and with oxygen being heavier than air, a higher percentage of oxygen may be inspired.

2. At the same time, administer a small dose of nondepolarizing muscle relaxant, e.g., pancuronium 0.01 to 0.02 mg/kg or *d*-tubocurarine 0.05 to 0.01 mg/kg intravenously (many report this is not necessary in children less than 3 to 5 years of age).[8]

3. Immediately following the use of the muscle relaxant, administer a small dose of an anticholinergic drug, e.g., atropine 0.02 mg/kg or glycopyrrolate 0.005 mg/kg intravenously.

4. After 3 minutes of preoxygenation or approximately 90 seconds after administration of the nondepolarizing muscle relaxant, thiopental 1 to 4 mg/kg or ketamine 1 to 2 mg/kg should be given intravenously. The smaller doses should be given in the hypovolemic or depressed patient. Many believe that the use of ketamine is preferable in the hypovolemic patient and that even smaller doses are indicated to prevent the cardiac depressant effects of the drug (0.35 to 0.7 mg/kg intravenously).[29] One or 2 ml of fluid (e.g., normal saline) should be given immediately afterward to flush the line, and then 1.5 to 2.0 mg/kg of succinylcholine should be given immediately. (The succinylcholine will cause a precipitate to form with the thiopental, and the flush helps to prevent this from occluding the small IV catheter. It is sometimes wise to flush the line after administering the succinylcholine as well.)

5. The Sellick maneuver[115] (cricoid pressure) is applied immediately upon cessation of spontaneous respiration. This is a firm antero-posterior pressure on the cricoid cartilage to occlude the esophagus. We prefer to put one finger on either side of the cricoid (being careful not to press on the carotids) and another finger directly on the cricoid in order to keep it pressed firmly against the anterior portion of the vertebral bodies of the neck.

6. The patient should not be ventilated by mask because this may inflate the stomach, causing regurgitation. When the patient relaxes, the trachea is quickly intubated orally.

7. The position of the tube should be confirmed by chest expansion and bilateral breath sounds before the cricoid pressure is released. Prior to performing the rapid-sequence procedure in a patient of questionable volume status, it may be wise to raise the head of the bed 30 to 40 degrees, wait a few minutes, and then take a blood pressure reading, comparing it with that of the patient in the supine position. A decrease in blood pressure may indicate hypovolemia. Usually we find it wise to infuse 5 to 10 per cent of the patient's estimated blood volume of crystalloid solution prior to induction with the rapid-sequence technique. A number of studies have also been done concerning whether the patient should be head up or head down for induction. The head up position does not prevent regurgitation and may cause hypotension during induction, and the head down position does not prevent aspiration. Therefore, most anesthesiologists prefer the level supine position.[76] However, in certain patients with bleeding from the oral cavity or nose, in whom mechanical difficulty with the intubation is not anticipated, a rapid-sequence procedure may be done with the patient on his side and a suction catheter in the down cheek so that blood does not pool at the airway. Caution should be used; this intubation is not for the inexperienced who have not previously done intubations with the patient in the lateral position.

An alternative to the previously described technique for rapid-sequence intubation is the technique reported by Bennett[116] and Brown.[117]

1. Preoxygenate as in step 1 of the first technique described.

2. After 3 minutes, administer pancuronium 0.15 mg/kg intravenously, followed immediately by either ketamine or thiopental in the doses mentioned previously.

3. Continue with cricoid pressure and intubation as mentioned earlier. This technique, in which thiopental is employed as the induction agent, is probably preferred over the previously mentioned rapid-sequence technique for patients with intracranial hypertension. This is because both ketamine and succinylcholine are avoided. Both these agents may increase intracerebral pressure.

It is debatable whether evacuation of the stomach preoperatively with a nasogastric (NG) tube is beneficial. Certainly evacuation of the stomach with a tube is no assurance that food and gastric contents will not be regurgitated and aspirated.[118] It is frequently quite difficult to pass an NG tube in frightened young patients, and unless there is another reason for doing so, I do not persist. If a hard-walled NG tube is down at the time of induction of anesthesia, it is left in place and cricoid pressure is applied. If it is a soft-walled tube (red rubber tube), it is removed. Certainly in any patient with a full stomach, after the induction of anesthesia and the securing of the airway with an endotracheal tube, an NG tube should be passed and the stomach suctioned.

In the rare event that an IV line cannot be secured in a patient, some would advocate an inhalation induction.[76, 118] It is true that in many cases this can be done without the patient regurgitating, but we prefer to use this technique only when all other possibilities have been exhausted. Anesthesia is usually induced with nitrous oxide and oxygen, to which halothane is added after 30 to 45 seconds in 0.5 per cent increments every 3 to 4 breaths. Once the patient is not moving, we prefer to have an assistant attempt to start an IV. Many times this will be successful, since the patient is not fighting and the veins may be more prominent from the effects of the halothane. If placement of an IV line is successful in patients over 3 years of age, we give pancuronium 0.01 mg/kg followed by atropine 0.02 mg/kg intravenously. The nitrous oxide is turned off, and the patient is maintained on halothane and oxygen. After 60 to 90 seconds, succinylcholine 1.5 to 2.0 mg/kg is given intravenously. When the patient ceases spontaneous respiration, cricoid pressure is applied and intubation is performed. This technique decreases the time between loss of reflexes and intubation and theoretically should decrease the chances for aspiration. It also avoids the cardiopulmonary depression that may be concomitant with a deep inhalation induction (since topical spray to the larynx and trachea is contraindicated in patients with full stomachs). An alternative would be to use pancuronium 0.15 mg/kg instead of succinylcholine.

If an IV line cannot be secured even after inhalation induction, this leaves no alternative but to carry the patient to a deep enough level of anesthesia with the halothane so that intubation can be performed. This means that the patient must be carried into the surgical stage of anesthesia in which laryngeal reflexes are diminished.[119, 120] This usually takes approximately 5 minutes if respirations are gently assisted. With experience this can be done without inflating the stomach or causing regurgitation. However, some anesthesiologists prefer to avoid assisting the respiration, allowing the patient to spontaneously breathe himself down to an adequate level of anesthesia, but this will take longer. Once the patient is determined to be at the proper plane of anesthesia (i.e., eyes centered, small pupils, relaxed abdomen, regular but shallow respiratory pattern, and decreased use of intercostal muscles for respiration), intubation can be performed. (Some children will not exhibit all these signs.) However, since the patient must be carried to a deep level of anesthesia and the airway is unprotected for a prolonged period, I am reticent to use this technique. I believe that it should only be used in certain selected patients, e.g., generally young patients with poor veins who have suffered trauma not associated with extensive blood loss.

Maintenance of Anesthesia

The maintenance of anesthesia in the trauma victim involves the continuation of all the procedures that have been mentioned thus far; factors of surgical and anesthetic insults must also be taken into consideration.

Drugs Used in Anesthesia

The choice of anesthetic agent is probably not as important as how it is given.[5] Anesthetic agents that may be used to treat the trauma victim may be classified into inhalation agents, IV agents, and local anesthetics. (The latter will be discussed in connection with local and regional anesthetic techniques.) In conjunction with the first two classes of agents, a muscle relaxant may be given either for surgical conditions or to facilitate the use of less anesthetic agent.

Inhalation Agents

There are essentially four inhalation anesthetics in current use, i.e., nitrous oxide, halothane, enflurane, and isoflurane. Each of these agents has special properties of its own. When used in combination with other agents, properties of these anesthetics may change. It is not the purpose of this chapter to give an exposé on the various attributes of these anesthetics, but it is pertinent to point out their major cardiorespiratory influences that may be crucial to the trauma victim. Much of the information involving anesthetic influences on the cardiovascular and respiratory systems is derived from animal models, and at present, it can only be assumed that the human, particularly the pediatric patient, responds in the same manner.

Nitrous oxide (N_2O) is probably the most frequently administered anesthetic, but since the MAC (minimal alveolar concentration necessary to produce anesthesia in 50 per cent of patients) is approximately 100 per cent,[121] it is commonly given in combination with another anesthetic. It produces a relatively mild direct myocardial depressant effect in the isolated heart.[122] In the intact healthy patient, the cardiac depressant effects of nitrous oxide are probably counteracted by sympathetic stimulation caused by the gas.[122] It might be surmised that in the severely traumatized patient who is "sympathetically depleted," the administration of nitrous oxide may allow the cardiac depressant effects to predominate. Luckily, nitrous oxide has a very short duration of action, owing to its low blood/gas solubility coefficient, and can quickly be discontinued if the patient does not seem to tolerate its administration. When nitrous oxide is administered to a patient who has already received 1 mg/kg of morphine, a marked decrease in cardiac output and blood pressure occurs.[123] When nitrous oxide is used in combination with potent inhalation anesthetics (halothane, enflurane, isoflurane) to produce the same MAC as those anesthetics alone, the result is less cardiac depression and improved blood pressure. (For this reason, the potent anesthetics are usually given in combination with nitrous oxide unless an unusually high inspired oxygen is necessary or there is fear of expanding trapped gas in a body cavity.) Nitrous oxide in combination with other anesthetics has been shown to decrease airway mucociliary flow, but almost all anesthetics,[124] many premedications, inhalation of dry gases,[125] high-inspired oxygen concentrations,[126] positive pressure ventilation,[127] and inflation of the endotracheal tube cuff[128] have this effect.

Owing to the very low blood/gas partition coefficients of nitrogen, hydrogen, and methane, nitrous oxide preferentially diffuses into bowel gas spaces, causing a 100 per cent increase in gastrointestinal volume in 2 hours. The magnitude of volume change is dependent upon the initial amount of bowel gas present, the concentration of nitrous oxide administered, and the duration of anesthetic exposure.[129] For these reasons, nitrous oxide is generally not administered in patients with intestinal obstruction or is used in low concentrations for short periods of time. In those conditions in which volume and/or pressure changes occur more rapidly, as with pneumothorax, intracerebral air, or venous air embolism, nitrous oxide inhalation is best avoided.[129]

Nitrous oxide probably has little effect on or may slightly increase pulmonary artery pressure in patients with pre-existing pulmonary hypertension.[130, 131] It has very little respiratory depressant effect either alone or in combination with low concentrations of more potent inhalation anesthetics.[132]

The other three inhalational anesthetics will be discussed together for reasons of comparison (Table 3–10). This discussion is necessarily brief, but more extensive reviews are available.[122, 133, 134] Halothane, enflurane, and isoflurane all decrease mean arterial blood pressure proportionate to their concentration.[135–138] With the first two agents, this is primarily due to a direct cardiac depressant effect, whereas with isoflurane this is due to vasodilation. This vasodilation may be ameliorated to some extent by surgical stimulation[122] and the use of low-dose isoflurane with nitrous oxide. Also the cardiac depressant effects of halothane and enflurane are less when used with nitrous oxide.[139] In patients who have suffered trauma and who may be marginally hypovolemic, isoflurane and, to a lesser extent, enflurane will cause severe hypotension due to a decrease in peripheral vascular resistance. In patients who have good fluid resuscitation and receive low-dose anesthesia, this effect should be minimal. Patients who have marginal cardiac output secondary to trauma or hypoxic injury are likely not to tolerate the more cardiac depressant anesthetics, i.e., enflurane and halothane, even though myocardial oxygen consumption is decreased. Patients with obstructive heart lesions, e.g., aortic stenosis, are probably less likely to tolerate the vasodilatory effects of isoflurane, whereas patients with congestive heart failure or mitral regurgitation might benefit from its use. Animal studies have indicated higher concentrations of halothane may not be as well tolerated during periods of decreased arterial oxygen content due to hypoxia but seem to be tolerated without untoward effects during periods of decreased arterial oxygen content due to anemia.[140, 141] One method of experimentally producing hepatotoxicity with halothane in animals is to

Table 3–10. COMPARISON OF POTENT INHALATION ANESTHETICS

	Halothane	Enflurane	Isoflurane
Direct cardiac depressant	Moderate	Severe	Mild to none
Effect on heart rate	None	Increase	Increase
Cardiac safety	Fair	Poor	Good
Decrease in cardiac output	Moderate	Severe	Mild
Decrease in arterial pressure	Mild*	Moderate*	Moderate†
Decrease in systemic vascular resistance	Mild	Moderate	Marked
Increase in blood flow to muscle	Little change	Little change	Marked increase
Stability of heart rhythm‡	Least	Good	Best
Dose of epinephrine for extrasystole§	2.1 μg/kg	> 10 μg/kg	6.7 μg/kg
Effect on pulmonary vascular resistance (PVR)‖	Mild decrease	Mild decrease	No change
Effect on hypoxic pulmonary vasoconstrictive response**	Probable inhibition	Probable inhibition	Probable inhibition
Left ventricle work and myocardial O_2 consumption	Decrease	Decrease	Decrease
Effect on ventilation	Mild decrease	Severe decrease	Moderate decrease
Ventilatory response to hypoxia	Decrease	Decrease	Decrease
Cerebral O_2 consumption	Decrease	Decrease	Decrease
Seizure activity	None	Present	None
Effect on cerebral blood flow (CBF)††	Marked increase	Mild increase	Little change
Enhancement of succinylcholine	Mild	Moderate	Moderate
Metabolized	Most	Intermediate	Least
Probable safety in face of enzyme induction or hypoxia	Least	Intermediate	Most
Effect on renal blood flow, glomerular filtration rate (GFR), urine flow	Decrease	Decrease	Decrease
Serum inorganic fluoride‡‡	Least	Most	Intermediate
Safety for kidney	Good	Probably good	Good
Mutagen, teratogen, carcinogen	No	No	No
May cause malignant hyperthermia	Yes	Yes	Yes
Effect on intraocular pressure	Decrease	Decrease	Decrease
Cost	Least	Intermediate	Most
Postoperative analgesia	Poor	Poor	Poor

*Decreases blood pressure by reducing cardiac output.
†Decreases blood pressure by decreasing total peripheral resistance.
‡With all anesthetics, stability of rhythm is more likely when lidocaine accompanies the injection of epinephrine.
§Dose to produce extrasystole in 50 per cent of patients at 1.25 MAC.
‖Clinically PVR may increase in response to a decrease in cardiac output produced by these agents.
**Some studies suggest that halothane and enflurane may not inhibit this response.
††At 1.0 MAC (at 0.5 MAC or less there is little increase in CBF with any of these agents).
‡‡None of the levels produced by these anesthetics appear to be detrimental.
Compiled from information contained in Eger EI II: Isoflurane: A review. Anesthesiology 55:559, 1981; and Hickey RF, Eger EI II: Circulatory pharmacology of inhaled anesthetics, and Pavlin EG: Respiratory pharmacology of inhaled anesthetic agents. Both in Miller RD (ed.): Anesthesia. New York, Churchill Livingstone, 1981, pp. 331–382.

pretreat with phenobarbital (enzyme inducer) and then cause the animal to become hypoxic.[142] Since these conditions may occur in trauma patients, if all other conditions are equal, it may be wise to choose an anesthetic with less metabolic breakdown (e.g., isoflurane). In patients with unstable heart rhythm due to cardiac drugs or due to injected epinephrine, isoflurane or enflurane would be better choices.

Controlled ventilation decreases cardiac output with all three anesthetics, but frequently it is necessary in trauma patients. However, if spontaneous ventilation is indicated, use of halothane seems preferable. All three anesthetics decrease the respiratory response to hypoxia, and all patients should be watched carefully after anesthesia until they awaken. Halothane seems to have the most pronounced bronchodilatory effect,[134] whereas isoflurane seems to be somewhat irritating to the airways and should probably not be used in asthmatics.[143] There is controversy concerning the pulmonary vascular response to these inhalational anesthetics. The direct effect of these anesthetics appears to be pulmonary vasodilation, but in a clinical setting, a decrease in cardiac output may produce a compensatory pulmonary vasoconstriction.[144, 145] In terms of the central nervous system, all three anesthetics decrease cerebral vascular resistance and autoregulator response. However, isoflurane stands out as a clearly superior anesthetic. It produces less increase in cerebral blood flow, decreases cerebral oxygen consumption, and does not cause seizures. One drawback is that isoflurane seems to be more irritating to the respiratory tract, causing an increased incidence of laryngospasm and coughing in the patient upon emergence from anesthesia, which could elevate intracerebral pressure.[143]

Decreasing arterial Pa_{CO_2} to approximately 25 torr will prevent the increase in cerebral blood flow with all agents, but it appears that better results are achieved if hyperventilation is instituted prior to the use of halothane.[146, 147] However, an impaired response to changes in carbon dioxide tension may be associated with extensive intracranial disease (anoxic injury, severe trauma, and widespread tumor).[148] Also, enflurane, halothane, and isoflurane do not prevent the cerebral edema or increase in intracranial pressure that follows a traumatic injury to the brain.[149]

All three anesthetics enhance the actions of muscle relaxants, but enflurane and isoflurane have more pronounced effects. The effects on the kidneys of each of these inhalation agents are similar. Each anesthetic (and this is generally true for IV anesthetics as well) causes depression of renal function, characterized by a redistribution of intrarenal blood flow. The glomerular filtration decreases less than the renal plasma flow so that the filtration fraction increases. The renal vascular resistance increases with or without a change in blood pressure. The total urine flow decreases and an antidiuretic state is created. Both solute and free water clearance decrease. These effects are transitory and are generally reversed by cessation of anesthesia. Although enflurane rarely results in peak free fluoride levels greater than 25 mm/L, it is potentially nephrotoxic and should be avoided in patients with renal dysfunction.[150]

In summary, the inhalation anesthetics have varied properties, and these properties appear to be more pronounced at the higher concentrations. It should be noted that the MAC of each of these agents is higher in children than in adults. When all is taken into consideration, there is very little to recommend enflurane in the pediatric population. The other inhalation anesthetics, when used to maximize their good properties and minimize their poor qualities, should be useful in the treatment of the pediatric trauma patient.

Intravenous Agents

The IV agents may be categorized as narcotic and non-narcotic drugs.

Narcotics

Narcotics may be classified into the naturally occurring (morphine, codeine, papaverine), semisynthetic (heroin, Dilaudid), and synthetic (levorphanol, methadone, pentazocine, meperidine, and fentanyl). Generally, only three of these narcotics play a major role in anesthesia. These are morphine, meperidine, and fetanyl. Two newer narcotics with mixed agonist-antagonist properties, i.e., butorphanol (Stadol) and nalbuphine (Nubain), have been available for only a short time, and few data are available on their use in pediatric patients.

Morphine is the drug by which most narcotics are measured. It has a rapid onset and a prolonged duration of action due to its retention in the central nervous system. Morphine is eliminated primarily by metabolism; it is converted to inactive or less active metabolites that are excreted by the kidney. Its elimination in patients with liver disease is prolonged, but it may or may not be prolonged in patients with decreased urine output.[151, 152]

Morphine is selective in its effects on the central nervous system, i.e., it causes intense analgesia but relatively poor amnesia. Morphine cannot achieve two of the primary objectives of anesthesia, that is, it does not produce muscular relaxation and does not reliably control autonomic responses.[151] For this reason, it is commonly used in combination with other anesthetics or muscle relaxants. Narcotics cause a marked reduction in responsiveness of the brain respiratory center to stimulation from carbon dioxide. Morphine, meperidine, and fentanyl in small doses decrease respiratory rate without changing tidal volume. Higher doses will decrease both. Morphine and meperidine can cause bronchoconstriction, and morphine (and probably other narcotics) decreases bronchial ciliary motion.[152] Patients who are sleeping (i.e., in the recovery room without a surgical stimulus) are most sensitive to the respiratory depressant effects of narcotics.

Morphine significantly increases pulmonary artery blood pressure and decreases pulmonary blood volume.[152] Morphine may also cause truncal rigidity, miosis, cough suppression, and nausea and vomiting. Truncal rigidity may dictate the need for muscle relaxants during surgery. The tendency for this narcotic to cause cough suppression as well as its propensity to promote nausea and vomiting may theoretically make aspiration more likely at the end of operation when the patient has a full stomach. It is wise to make sure that the patient is awake, with good airway reflexes, prior to extubation.

The hemodynamic effects of morphine are mainly venodilation, with a lesser and more transient arterial dilation. These stem from the histamine release associated with the administration of morphine and the respiratory depression, which causes hypercarbia and possibly hypoxia.[153] Hypotension can be minimized by (1) correcting hypovolemia, (2) maintaining the patient in the supine or Trendelenburg position, (3) limiting the IV dose rate of morphine (70 μg/kg/minute is probably satisfactory for children),[152] (4) limiting the total dose to less than 0.5 mg/kg,[152] (5) supporting ventilation to minimize hypercarbia and hypoxia, (6) treating bradycardia (vagal response to histamine), and (7) administering a vasopressor promptly if the preceding measures are not adequate.[151] Owing to the vasodilatory effects of morphine, there may be increased blood requirements during surgery,[154] but morphine may be beneficial in congestive heart failure patients. Morphine does not reliably block autonomic sympathetic responses to surgery even in high doses. The hypertension that may occur with these sympathetic responses is probably associated with incomplete amnesia.[155] Morphine causes a dose-dependent increase in the concentration of catecholamines in both blood and urine of humans. It is generally assumed that epinephrine is better tolerated during narcotic anesthesia, but recent studies in dogs showed the dose of epinephrine necessary to induce dysrhythmias to be no greater than that used during halothane, enflurane, or nitrous oxide anesthesia. However, the incidence of malignant dysrhythmias was less with narcotic–nitrous oxide anesthesia.[156]

There is controversy concerning the renal effects of morphine.[151, 152] It appears that although renal function may be decreased during narcotic anesthesia,[157] morphine and fentanyl probably do not stimulate antidiuretic hormone (ADH) release in man and in fact may depress the release of ADH in response to surgical stimulation.[158, 159] Morphine stimulates smooth muscle of the gastrointestinal and genitourinary tracts. Spasm of these tracts as well as the sphincter of Oddi may occur with use of morphine, fentanyl, or meperidine. Pain from spasm is effectively treated with these narcotics, and spasm may be relieved with nitroglycerin. Finally, all narcotics appear to decrease cerebral blood flow, intracranial pressure, and cerebral oxygen consumption.[152]

Frequently, as previously mentioned, morphine is used in combination with other agents. When nitrous oxide is combined with intravenously administered morphine, myocardial depression frequently occurs.[123, 160] One study showed nitrous oxide produced a concentration-dependent decrease in stroke volume, cardiac output, and arterial blood pressure, with an increase in systemic vascular resistance.[160] Heart rate is usually not affected by addition of nitrous oxide. Similar effects have been found with meperidine[161] and fentanyl.[162] Use of diazepam and barbiturates in combination with morphine has produced cardiac depression. However, scopolamine and droperidol do not appear to cause significant cardiovascular depression when combined with morphine.[163, 164] Potent inhalation agents have been combined with narcotics. Low to moderate concentrations of halothane given after large doses of morphine cause cardiac depression,[165] just as enflurane–nitrous oxide does when given with high-dose fentanyl.[166] However, lower doses of fentanyl produce few changes.[166]

Meperidine, because of its negative inotropic effects as well as its marked reduction of systemic vascular resistance, causes more profound hypotension than equal doses of morphine.[152] It is structurally similar to atropine, and therefore may cause tachycardia.[167] It is popular as a supplement in nitrous oxide–narcotic balanced anesthesia, but the cardiovascular depressant effects of nitrous oxide are present when used in combination with meperidine. It is our clinical impression that children have less respiratory depression after receiving meperidine, and it is commonly used in a balanced technique when patients are to be extubated at the end of the case. The tachycardia produced by this drug is usually well tolerated by children, or meperidine may be used in combination with low-dose fentanyl (to combine the bradycardia effects of fentanyl). Meperidine is generally not used in unstable or critically ill patients because of its negative inotropic effects.

Fentanyl, when administered in equipotent doses, is more potent and has a shorter time of onset and duration of activity than either morphine or meperidine. It is highly lipid soluble and is therefore rapidly redistributed from the central nervous system to other tissues, producing its short-lasting effect. With multiple doses, there is an accumulation of fentanyl in the storage tissues, less redistribution, and a more prolonged effect.[151] Fentanyl in anesthetic doses (50 to 100 μg/kg) as well as analgesic doses (5 to 10 μg/kg) produces moderate hypotension.[168, 169] This hypotension is thought to be primarily due to bradycardia. Like morphine, fentanyl in doses of 0.5 to 30 μg/kg causes a rise in blood catecholamines, but larger doses attenuate this response.[152] Fentanyl releases little or no histamine and appears not to increase fluid maintenance or blood replacement requirements. Except for possibly a smaller increase in pulmonary artery pressure,[152] the other effects of fentanyl are similar to those of morphine.

Non-Narcotics

Under this class of IV anesthetics, barbiturates, benzodiazepines, butyrophenones, and ketamine will be discussed.

The barbiturates have been classified for clinical purposes into four classes according to their duration of activity: long-acting, intermediate-acting, short-acting, and ultra short-acting, even though this classification does not correlate well with the elimination half-lives of the drugs.[170] Only the ultra short-acting barbiturates (e.g., thiopental, methohexital) are used for clinical anesthesia. These barbiturates depress the central nervous system, particularly the cerebral cortex and the reticular activating system.[152] In less than anesthetic doses, barbiturates seem to cause the patient to be more sensitive to somatic pain.[171] When given in anesthetic doses (thiopental sodium 2 to 6 mg/kg intravenously, or methohexital up to 2.0 mg/kg intravenously, in healthy children),[172, 173] the ultra short-acting barbiturates rapidly cross the blood-brain barrier and produce hypnosis in one circulation time. The barbiturates then rapidly redistribute into muscle, fat, and other body tissues so that within 5 minutes the brain levels are one half of the initial peak levels. It is because of this rapid removal from brain tissue that a single dose of thiopental is so short acting.[174] For this reason, barbiturates are generally used only for induction of anesthesia, for short procedures, or to supplement anesthesia in neurosurgical procedures.

In isolated mammalian hearts, barbiturates cause direct myocardial depression, which is dose related. Thiopental produces little change or a slight increase in total peripheral resistance but markedly increases venous vessel compliance with venous pooling. In unstimulated man, thiopental causes a dose-dependent decrease in arterial blood pressure, stroke volume, and cardiac output. Reductions in output vary from 10 to 50 per cent with a dose of 3 to 9 mg/kg.[152] Reflex tachycardia, compensatory increases in peripheral arterial resistance, and surgical stimulation may minimize the depressant effect of the barbiturates. Hypertensive and hypovolemic patients are more susceptible to marked decreases in cardiac output and blood pressure.[152] Also, the more rapid the injection, the more marked the cardiovascular derangements.[175] Thiopental increases coronary artery blood flow but also increases heart rate and myocardial oxygen consumption and may cause dysrhythmias during spontaneous ventilation.[152] Thiopental is a potent respiratory depressant and will produce apnea when the cerebral thiopental concentration is at its peak. Following apnea, shallow respirations resume, but in the absence of stimulation, severe respiratory depression may recur. Thiopental decreases the sensitivity of the medullary respiratory center to carbon dioxide.[176] The respiratory tract appears to be sensitive to stimuli during light thiopental anesthesia, causing a greater propensity for laryngospasm or bronchospasm.[177]

Thiopental decreases cerebral blood flow, but cerebral metabolism and oxygen utilization are decreased more.[152] For this reason, barbiturates have become desirable anesthetics for patients with marginally adequate cerebral perfusion or intracranial hypertension.[178, 179] Thiopental may cause some decrease in renal function in large doses, but these effects are readily reversible. Thiopental (pH 10.6 to 10.8) may cause tissue necrosis if injected intra-arterially or subcutaneously. The barbiturates should be avoided in any patient with a history of porphyria.

The benzodiazepines are classified as minor tranquilizers.[180] These compounds are administered by anesthesiologists for premedication, sedation, or induction of anesthesia. The benzodiazepines include diazepam, lorazepam, and recently midazolam. These agents produce sedation, amnesia, and mild muscle relaxation and have anticonvulsive effects. When these drugs are used alone the cardiovascular effects are mild, producing little change in ventricular contractility, heart rate, or systemic or pulmonary artery pressures.[181, 182] However, if given after large doses of narcotics, e.g., fentanyl or morphine, mild to moderate cardiovascular depression may occur.[163, 168] The benzodiazepines appear to produce moderate respiratory depression, although there is controversy in the literature.[183] This depression has been reversed with physostigmine[152] (with a reasonably high incidence of side effects) and with high-dose naloxone.[183] Midazolam is a newer benzodiazepine, which has promise. It is two to three times as potent as diazepam, has a shorter duration of action, and causes less thrombophlebitis but causes similar respiratory depression.[184] Diazepam is usually given in a dose of 0.1 to 0.3 mg/kg intravenously.

The butyrophenones are classified as major tranquilizers. The only one of clinical importance in anesthesia is droperidol, which owing to its long duration of action (8 to 12 hours) is usually used in combination with a narcotic (neuroleptanalgesia), nitrous oxide, or muscle relaxants as a form of balanced anesthesia. Droperidol causes the patient to be placid, sleepy, indifferent to the environment, and frequently amnesic.[152, 185] Droperidol does not produce analgesia alone but does seem to potentiate and prolong the effects of narcotics.[186] It also has significant postoperative antiemetic effects,[187] but in low doses, droperidol has little effect on the respiratory and circulatory systems. It may produce some degree of hypotension owing to its peripheral alpha-adrenergic blocking effects[188, 189] but also may cause hypertension in patients with pheochromocytoma.[189] Droperidol appears to protect against catecholamine-induced cardiac dysrhythmias and is a cerebral vasoconstrictor, but it does not affect cerebral metabolic rate.[152] The major concerns with droperidol in pediatric trauma patients are the possibility of hypotension in marginally hypovolemic patients and its prolonged postoperative sedative effects in patients with full stomachs.

Ketamine is an anesthetic that may be given intravenously or intramuscularly and produces a state of unconsciousness described as dissociative anesthesia. The onset of unconsciousness is rapid, usually taking place in 20 to 60 seconds when 1 to 2 mg/kg are given intravenously. The drug produces excellent amnesia and analgesia, which last 10 to 20 minutes with a single IV dose. The usual recommended dose of ketamine in children is 1 to 2 mg/kg intravenously and 5 to 10 mg/kg intramuscularly; however, neonates and small children may require a higher dose.

Ketamine has been considered the drug of choice for induction of anesthesia in patients with marginal cardiovascular status,[190, 191] but this view is being questioned.[191, 192] Certainly there is controversy concerning the effects of ketamine under various conditions.[152, 190–192] It is well documented that ketamine is a cardiovascular stimulant in the healthy or relatively healthy patient. Heart rate, arterial blood pressure, and cardiac output are usually increased, but these responses may be inhibited by other anesthetics. Use of ketamine during potent inhalation anesthesia renders the compound a severe cardiovascular depressant, probably owing to its direct negative effect on the myocardium.[152, 193] The cardiovascular stimulation of ketamine requires an intact peripheral sympathetic nervous system. Increases in plasma epinephrine and norepinephrine occur soon after IV ketamine. Whether ketamine causes release of catecholamines or prevents re-uptake is not conclusively known.[191] However, use of diazepam (0.1 to 0.2 mg/kg intravenously) in conjunction with ketamine (1 to 2 mg/kg intravenously) seems to ameliorate the cardiovascular stimulatory effects of ketamine, as well as prevent the ketamine-induced increases in intracranial pressure in some patients.[152, 194] Ketamine usually does not increase systemic vascular resistance but does increase pulmonary artery pressure, improve coronary blood flow, and increase myocardial oxygen consumption. However, some studies have shown that during severe preoperative stress or hemorrhage, cardiopulmonary parameters and oxygen transport may not be as well maintained with ketamine as with other anesthetics.[191, 192] However, this is controversial.[195] We generally avoid using ketamine in large doses in the severely traumatized patient and avoid it altogether in the patient with cyanotic or obstructive heart disease. In addition, ketamine is probably best avoided in patients who are severely hypertensive, patients with myocardial disease, or patients with increased intracranial pressure (owing to its effect of increasing cerebral blood flow and metabolic rate).

Ketamine produces mild respiratory depression,[193] but upper airway reflexes are usually maintained. However, aspiration can still occur, and patients with full stomachs should be intubated.[152] Ketamine may cause significant secretions, and use of an anticholinergic in conjunction with ketamine is usually indicated. Ketamine relaxes lower airway smooth muscle and antagonizes the effects of histamine.[152] Respiratory depression after succinylcholine is prolonged with ketamine. Postoperatively, ketamine may promote nausea and vomiting. It may also produce posthypnotic emergence phenomena, which are usually more common in the older patient but which may be decreased through the use of other drugs in conjunction with the ketamine.

Muscle Relaxants

The muscle relaxants may be divided into two groups, depolarizing and nondepolarizing. Muscle relaxants are used as adjuvants to either inhalation or IV anesthetics to allow a smaller dose to be used, to improve the surgical conditions, or to facilitate endotracheal intubation.

Depolarizing Muscle Relaxants

The only depolarizing muscle relaxant currently being used with any significant frequency is succinylcholine. The duration of action is short, owing to the fact that the compound is readily broken down by plasma pseudocholinesterase. Apnea produced by succinylcholine lasts approximately 3 minutes in the normal patient. The duration of action of the drug has been shown to be prolonged by certain factors, among which are liver disease, starvation, pregnancy, phenelzine (a monamine oxidase inhibitor), echothiophate (eye drops), organophosphorous insecticides, hexafluorenium (nondepolarizing muscle relaxant), cytotoxic drugs, acetylcholinesterase inhibitors, and low or atypical plasma cholinesterase.[85, 196] Succinylcholine may be administered to pediatric patients in a single dose of 1 to 2 mg/kg intravenously (the higher dose in the neonate or infant) and 2 to 4 mg/kg intramuscularly.[8, 197] If further doses should become necessary over a short time interval or if an IV infusion is required for an hour or more, it is wise to change to a nondepolarizing muscle relaxant to avoid a phase II block, which may be difficult to reverse.[85, 196, 198] Most pertinent to the discussion of depolarizing muscle relaxants in the trauma patient are the side effects and complications of these relaxants, which are, as a rule, more prominent in the pediatric patient.[85, 196] Succinylcholine stimulates the autonomic ganglia, which may cause cardiac dysrhythmias, bradycardia, or hypotension. This phenomenon is much more common when a second dose of succinylcholine is given approximately 5 minutes after the first. Many of these undesirable side effects are prevented by thiopental, anticholinergics (atropine, glycopyrrolate), ganglion blockers, and nondepolarizing muscle relaxants.[85, 196] A number of reports and studies have shown that succinylcholine produces an elevated serum potassium in patients with certain conditions or diseases. Burn patients have been reported to have had cardiac arrests secondary to a high serum potassium after receiving succinylcholine. The susceptibility appears to be from 10 to 60 days postburn and varies with the extent of the burn. Since pretreatment with a nondepolarizing muscle relaxant will not assure prevention of the response, administration of succinylcholine should be avoided in these patients.

Severely traumatized patients with massive tissue damage may also develop the hyperkalemic response to succinylcholine, which can occur between 1 week and 60 days postinjury or until adequate healing of muscle has taken place.[199, 200] In patients with neuromuscular disease (e.g., muscular dystrophy) and spinal cord injury (e.g., hemiplegia or paraplegia for the first 6 months following injury), the hyperkalemic response has been reported. The response has also been reported in patients with severe abdominal infections, renal failure, and certain cerebral diseases (e.g., cerebral vascular accidents, increased ICP, encephalitis, ruptured aneurysms, closed head injury).[85, 201] Succinylcholine causes an increase in intraocular pressure, which lasts approximately 6 minutes. There is controversy as to whether pretreatment with nondepolarizing muscle relaxants will prevent this response.

Succinylcholine inconsistently increases intragastric pressure (IGP) and therefore increases the risk of aspiration in patients with full stomachs. This IGP is probably due to fasciculations of the abdominal muscles and also possibly due to a direct vagal stimulation from the succinylcholine. For this reason, an anticholinergic and pretreatment with a nondepolarizing muscle relaxant (possibly pancuronium because of its vagolytic actions, but *d*-tubocurarine has proved effective) are recommended (see Induction of Anesthesia).[202] Postoperative myalgia may occur following administration of succinylcholine. It appears that prevention of fasciculation may attenuate, but not totally prevent, these muscle pains. However, when a nondepolarizing muscle relaxant is used prior to administration of succinylcholine, the dose of succinylcholine should be increased 30 to 50 per cent.[85] We do not pretreat children less than 3 to 4 years of age with nondepolarizing muscle relaxants because succinylcholine causes minimal fasciculations and little increase in IGP in children below this age.[203] Succinylcholine may produce contractures rather than relaxation in patients with myotonia congenita and myotonia dystrophica, malignant hyperthermia in susceptible patients, and myoglobinuria in patients with muscle dystrophy, crush injury, and glycogen storage disease.[196] The myoglobinuria seems to be exacerbated by halothane and attenuated by pretreatment with a nondepolarizing muscle relaxant.

Nondepolarizing Muscle Relaxants

The nondepolarizing muscle relaxants presently available in the United States are *d*-tubocurarine, pancuronium, metocurine, and gallamine. Newer drugs that have just been released are atracurium and vecuronium. They will be discussed at the end of this section. When injected intravenously into a patient, nondepolarizing relaxants are distributed in a volume not much larger than the blood volume; however, over time, some relaxants may diffuse into tissues.[204] Whether a large initial single dose should be administered or smaller doses should be given intermittently to produce the desired effect is controversial,[85, 205] but in either case, the muscle relaxants should be monitored using a nerve stimulator, with a 90 to 95 per cent reduction of switch height as the goal (see Monitoring). Renal failure will affect the relaxants. Gallamine is entirely dependent upon renal excretion for elimination. Metocurine depends heavily on renal excretion, and pancuronium is more dependent on renal excretion than *d*-tubocurarine, but probably less so than metocurine.[85, 204] Therefore, *d*-tubocurarine is probably the preferred nondepolarizing relaxant for patients without renal function.[85] Biliary or liver disease may decrease the rate of excretion of both *d*-tubocurarine and pancuronium, but patients with cirrhosis may require a larger initial dose for adequate relaxation. Subsequent doses should be smaller than normal. Pancuronium is metabolized and excreted by the liver, whereas *d*-tubocurarine is excreted unchanged. Hypothermia prolongs the neuromuscular block of pancuronium owing to decreased metabolism but does not significantly decrease or prolong the relaxation of *d*-tubocurarine in humans.[85, 206]

There is controversy as to the responses of infants and children to nondepolarizing muscle relaxants. Many investigators believe that the infant in the first 1 to 2 months of life may be more sensitive to these relaxants and suggest extreme vigilance when administering nondepolarizing relaxants to this age group.[81] However, if proper doses are given, the relaxants are easily and completely reversed (see Reversal Agents). In the older child, it appears that elimination of these relaxants may be faster than in the adult.[85] Although *d*-tubocurarine, pancuronium, and gallamine are bound to plasma proteins, this relationship does not seem to be markedly affected by disease states that alter plasma proteins. However, burn patients have recently been shown to require approximately twice the normal dose of *d*-tubocurarine. It has been postulated that spread of neuromuscular receptors in burned subjects may be the reason rather than alteration of plasma proteins.[207] Certain drugs, such as antibiotics, furosemide, and nitroglycerine, have been shown to potentiate nondepolarizing muscle relaxants.[85, 208]

Probably the most important effects of these muscle relaxants in the pediatric trauma victim are their interactions with the cardiovascular system. All four nondepolarizing muscle relaxants produce cardiovascular effects, but metocurine seems to produce the least. Hypotension is produced by *d*-tubocurarine from liberation of histamine, and in large doses, it can cause ganglionic blockade. Premedication with promethazine, an antihistamine drug, will attenuate *d*-tubocurarine-induced hypotension.[85] Use of light levels of anesthesia and low doses of *d*-tubocurarine will decrease the incidence of significant hypotension. Metocurine may cause hypotension, but the incidence and magnitude are less than that caused by *d*-tubocurarine. Pancuronium produces a moderate increase in heart rate and, to a lesser extent, cardiac output but no major change in systemic vascular resistance. This is probably due to a vagolytic effect, since the prior administration of atropine will attenuate the cardiovascular effects of pancuronium.[85] Gallamine increases heart rate by both vagolytic effects and sympathetic stimulation. Gallamine and *d*-tubocurarine reduce the incidence of epinephrine-induced dysrhythmias. In the presence of tricyclic antidepressants and halothane, pancuronium may increase the incidence of dysrhythmias.

For adequate surgical relaxation, pancuronium is usually given in a dose of 0.08 to

0.1 mg/kg, *d*-tubocurarine in a dose of 0.5 to 0.6 mg/kg, gallamine 1 to 2 mg/kg, and metocurine 0.3 to 0.4 mg/kg. When used in conjunction with potent anesthetics, these doses should usually be reduced.

Two newer drugs that have just become available are vecuronium and atracurium. Vecuronium has a duration of action of one third to one half that of pancuronium and minimal cardiovascular effects and appears ideal for patients with impaired renal function.[209, 210]

Reversal Agents

The nondepolarizing muscle relaxants require the use of anticholinesterases, usually neostigmine, pyridostigmine, or edrophonium, to reverse the neuromuscular blockade. These anticholinesterases antagonize a nondepolarizing neuromuscular blockade by increasing the availability of acetylcholine at the muscle endplate mainly by inhibition of acetylcholinesterase and, to a much lesser extent, by increased release of transmitter from the motor nerve terminals.[85] Because each of these reversal agents produces marked muscarinic effects, atropine 0.02 mg/kg or glycopyrrolate 0.015 mg/kg are injected either prior to or preferably in conjunction with the anticholinesterase. Glycopyrrolate has the advantage over atropine in that it protects against the muscarinic effects of the anticholinesterase for a longer time and, when used in combination with neostigmine, produces very little effect on heart rate. Glycopyrrolate essentially does not cause any central anticholinergic effects, since it is a quaternary ammonium compound and therefore minimally crosses the blood-brain barrier. However, the reversal agents occasionally can produce conduction disturbances, bradycardia, or cardiac arrest, but this is usually in geriatric or cardiac patients or patients on tricyclic antidepressants.[85] Certain situations, such as recent doses of muscle relaxant, respiratory acidosis, metabolic alkalosis, abnormalities in serum electrolytes, intake of certain antibiotics, increased serum magnesium, and possibly low serum calcuim levels may cause reversal to be prolonged or inadequate.[211] Generally in a trauma patient with a full stomach, if reversal is deemed to be inadequate at the end of the case, it is wise to place the patient on a ventilator and extubate only when good muscle function has returned. Deciding which of the anticholinesterases to use is largely a matter of preference and experience.

Pyridostigmine has the longest duration of action and longest onset of action and is intermediate in severity of muscarinic effects. Neostigmine is intermediate in onset and duration but has the most severe muscarinic effects (these appear to be adequately prevented by glycopyrrolate). Edrophonium has the shortest onset and duration and probably the least severe muscarinic side effects.[212, 213] All three agents adequately reverse all the nondepolarizing muscle relaxants and all seem equally effective in patients with renal disease.[195, 212, 213] Our preference is to use neostigmine and glycopyrrolate in children. Usual doses of the anticholinesterases are the following: neostigmine 0.07 mg/kg, pyridostigmine 0.2 to 0.3 mg/kg, edrophonium 0.5 to 1.0 mg/kg.

It is the responsibility of the anesthesiologist to select from the various anesthetic agents mentioned previously those agents and techniques that best suit the particular conditions required by each pediatric trauma victim. The anesthesiologist will be called upon to make decisions as to which of the following physiologic factors is more important (peripheral perfusion, pulse pressure, cardiac output, cardiac rhythm, kidney perfusion, cerebral perfusion, ICP, etc.) and then apply his agents appropriately. In some cases it may not be the drug but the method of administration that is most important. In marginally hypovolemic or inadequately resuscitated patients, it is wise to administer anesthetic agents slowly and in small amounts, allowing time for the full effects to become apparent before administering further drug. This, in many cases, will improve survival of these patients and also decrease the total drug dosage.[5] The anesthesiologist must be ever mindful of the effects, side effects, and drug interactions of administered anesthetic agents. This can only be done by having a thorough knowledge of the patients and the anesthetic agents.

Maintenance of Respiration

The maintenance of respiration during anesthesia for a pediatric trauma patient may become rather complex. As has already been pointed out, most anesthetics cause a depression of respiration, which is more pronounced at higher concentrations.[214] Likewise, the normal respiratory responses to hypercarbia or hypoxia are depressed by most anesthetics.[215] Position during surgery may also cause compromise of respiration.

Placing a patient in the supine position causes the abdominal contents to force the diaphragm cephalad and reduce lung volume. Placing a patient in the Trendelenburg position may increase the Zone 3 portion of the lung, elevating pulmonary artery pressures and increasing the chances of pulmonary edema. The prone position, lateral decubitus position, and lithotomy position may also decrease effective ventilation, especially in patients who may have abnormal lung compliance from trauma.[215] As a result, most patients with severe trauma will usually be mechanically ventilated during surgery and possibly afterward. However, mechanical ventilation should be instituted cautiously in the marginally hypovolemic patient, since marked decreases in blood pressure and cardiac output may result. This is usually correctable by proper fluid management and/or appropriate pharmacologic cardiac support. In addition, mechanical ventilation of the supine patient may also cause less effective ventilation to perfusion ratios in the lung when compared with spontaneous ventilation,[216] so an increased inspired oxygen concentration may be required. Mechanical ventilation helps to prevent atelectasis and decrease the work of breathing, which may be critical in a marginally hypoxic patient.

Under most circumstances, except when a patient has increased ICP, it is wise to make sure that the patient is well oxygenated and normocapnic. Pulmonary oxygen toxicity is essentially unheard of when the $F_{I_{O_2}}$ is less than 0.5, and its duration of administration is less than 12 hours.[215] Toxicity from high arterial P_{O_2} in the eyes, i.e., retrolental fibroplasia, is of concern in infants up to 44 weeks gestational age. Pa_{O_2} should not exceed 80 to 100 torr for more than a few hours.

Hyperventilation causes hypocapnia and respiratory alkalosis. This may decrease Pa_{O_2}, cardiac output, the hypoxic pulmonary vasoconstrictive response compliance (bronchoconstriction), serum ionized Ca^{++}, cerebral blood flow, and serum potassium, while increasing oxygen consumption and airway resistance, and produce postoperative apnea and a leftward shift of the oxyhemoglobin dissociation curve.[217, 218]

Hypoventilation with resultant hypercapnia causes a respiratory acidosis. This may increase serum catecholamines, dysrhythmias, blood pressure, pulmonary artery pressure, pulmonary vascular resistance, and serum potassium and produce a rightward shift of the oxyhemoglobin dissociation curve, vasodilation of skin vessels, and constriction of muscle vessels.[219]

Because of the preceding effects, which may be of considerable consequence during anesthesia (e.g., dysrhythmias during halothane anesthesia, difficulties with muscle relaxants due to electrolyte changes), it is the responsibility of the anesthesiologist to maintain normocapnia unless increased ICP should be a more urgent consideration. This may be accomplished by using a circle system and monitoring end tidal or arterial carbon dioxide[107, 108] or by using a coaxial system with the controlled partial rebreathing anesthesia method (CPRAM) and monitoring mean expired or arterial carbon dioxide.[109] The advantage of the latter method is that acceptable humidity is provided while the patient is maintained normocapnic.[21]

Humidification

Regulation of humidity during anesthesia also falls within the realm of responsibility of the anesthesiologist. When inspired humidity is less than 12 to 16 mg H_2O/L of inspired gases for longer than an hour, pulmonary damage may result.[220] Also, low-inspired humidity may decrease body temperatures in pediatric patients under anesthesia and decrease mucociliary flow in the trachea.[221] Acceptable humidity should probably be between 14 and 30 mg H_2O/L with the more optimum values in the upper portion of this range.[21] Many anesthesia systems and techniques do not provide humidity in this range without addition of heated humidifiers or auxiliary devices.[21] The devices generally do an acceptable job if used properly, maintained adequately, and cleaned frequently. Unfortunately, this is not always the case, and problems may result when they are used during a complicated case, such as may occur with trauma. For this reason, we have chosen CPRAM for its simplicity and adequate humidification.[21] Whatever system is chosen for the pediatric trauma patient, it should be safe and achieve results in the ranges mentioned previously.

Fluid and Blood Replacement

More than half the blood administered to patients is given in the surgical suite, mostly by anesthesiologists.[222] The trauma patient who is otherwise healthy will tolerate 10 to 15 per cent blood loss without major changes in perfusion. However, evidence of sympathetic influence will be noticeable. When approximately 15 to 25 per cent blood loss occurs, perfusion is decreased to nonvital areas, transcapillary refill begins, and hypotension is evident. With blood loss greater than 25 to 30 per cent, clinical "shock" occurs. This is manifest by a low cardiac output, hypotension, vasoconstriction, and anaerobic metabolism with acidosis. Dilation of precapillary sphincters but persistent constriction of postcapillary sphincters occurs with loss of intravascular fluid into the interstitial space. Decreased urine output, increased hematocrit, and ultimately death will result if these processes are not reversed.[5] The reversal process involves restoration of the intravascular volume as soon as possible before irreversible changes have taken place.

Initial resuscitation should probably consist of that fluid that is most appropriate and quickly available. This generally means a crystalloid (synthetic salt) solution because it can be administered without crossmatching, can be stored at room temperature, and rapidly increases intravascular volume. Since these solutions equilibrate quickly throughout the entire extravascular space, volumes infused will usually need to be approximately three times the volume of blood lost, but on occasion, more will be necessary. This may cause certain complications, such as anemia, hypoproteinemia, and pulmonary or peripheral edema,[30] but these sequelae subside in 48 to 72 hours when the fluid is mobilized and excreted.[5] Usually a balanced salt solution is chosen, either normal saline, lactated Ringer's, or Normosol R. Each of these solutions has minor imperfections but clinically produces no significant acid-base disturbances.[5]

At the time the first large-bore IV line is placed, a sample of blood should be drawn for type and crossmatch. However, in severe hemorrhage or anticipated severe hemorrhage, type-specific blood may be used. This is preferable to O negative (universal donor) blood, which may have high levels of anti-A or anti-B antibodies, which may cause hemolysis of the recipient cells if the patient is blood group A or B. Type O Rh-negative uncrossmatched packed erythrocytes may be used to avoid this problem, and reconstitution with 0.9 per cent saline or Normosol R pH 7.4 will facilitate faster transfusion. If time permits, a type and screen or partial crossmatch[222] may be done prior to infusion of the unit; a complete crossmatch is done later.

Fresh, crossmatched blood appears to be the ideal fluid for resuscitation in patients with large blood loss, but it is generally in short supply. Therefore, the second choice is banked blood because it contains colloid plus hemoglobin. Whole blood is usually stored in citrate phosphate dextrose (CPD) at 1 to 6° C. The useful life of a unit is 21 days, but with the addition of adenine (CPD with adenine), the storage life is increased to 35 days. Unfortunately, the older the unit of blood, the greater the complications, or at least theoretic complications, involved in its use. Studies with blood stored in acid citrate dextrose (ACD), which is no longer used, showed that infusion of blood 7 days old or older caused a leftward shift of the oxyhemoglobin dissociation curve. Low levels of 2,3-diphosphoglycerate (which aids in the release of oxygen to the tissues) have likewise been reported in blood after 7 days of storage. This also causes a shift in the oxyhemoglobin dissociation curve to the left. Alkalosis and hypothermia may also shift the curve in the same direction and add to the difficulty of delivering oxygen to the tissues.[5, 222]

Whole blood stored in CPD for more than 24 to 48 hours has only 5 to 10 per cent of the normal platelet activity. Thus, a dilutional thrombocytopenia may occur when blood greater than 24 hours old is transfused in cases of massive hemorrhage. When the platelet count decreases to less than 75,000 to 100,000 cells/mm^3, a patient with massive trauma is likely to have uncontrolled bleeding. It is therefore recommended that a platelet count be checked after infusion of blood equal to one third the patient's blood volume or that platelets be given empirically when one half to two thirds of the blood volume has been transfused.[30, 222] Platelets that are ABO compatible should be given through a large (170 μ) filter in a dose of 4 to 6 units/m^2 surface area, which will increase the platelet count by 50,000 to 100,000 cells mm^3.[222]

Whole blood that has been stored 21 days contains between 15 and 50 per cent of the normal amounts of clotting factors V and VIII. For this reason, it is common to give fresh frozen plasma to replace these factors. This practice is questionable, since only low levels (20 per cent of V and 30 per cent of VIII) are needed for hemostasis. However, if there is any possibility of low clotting factors, it probably does no harm to the patient to administer 10 ml/kg of fresh frozen plasma after one half to two thirds of the blood volume has been replaced. Another cause of diffuse oozing may be disseminated intravascular coagulation (DIC). DIC is recognized by a decrease in factors I, II, V, VIII, and platelets and an increase in fibrin split products.[222]

The citrate in banked blood binds calcium and theoretically can cause signs of hypocalcemia, i.e., hypotension, narrow pulse pressure, elevated intraventricular end-diastolic pressure, and elevated CVP. However, for this to occur, blood would need to be given at greater than 2 ml/kg/minute.[222] Most believe that hypocalcemia secondary to citrate is exceedingly rare, but when administering massive transfusions it is wise to monitor the serum ionized calcuim level. The serum potassium level of 21-day-old blood may be as high as 20 to 30 mEq/L; however, it is rare for hyperkalemia to occur in the transfused patient for this reason. Even so, it is wise to keep this possibility in mind and observe the EKG for signs of hyperkalemia.

Administration of unwarmed blood has been reported to produce cardiac arrest.[5] In shock states, the blood volume is predominately perfusing the heart and other central organs. Therefore, administration of cold blood may decrease the patient's temperature to approximately 30° C, which may result in ventricular irritability and arrest. In a patient who is unparalyzed, shivering may occur, which can increase oxygen consumption to four times more than normal. It is therefore wise to warm blood in approved warmers to approximately 37° C if any appreciable amount is to be given.

Although the addition of CPD to a unit of blood decreases the pH to 7.1 (after 21 days the pH of the unit may be 6.9), this is rarely a problem clinically. Many studies[5, 222] have shown that it is generally not necessary to routinely give bicarbonate to patients getting a blood transfusion, and in fact, this may be harmful owing to a leftward shift of the oxyhemoglobin dissociation curve. However, the pH of the patient's blood should be determined during transfusion and bicarbonate given for significant metabolic acidosis.

A debate still exists as to whether banked blood may be infused safely through a standard (170 μ) filter or whether a micropore (=40 μ) filter is necessary. It is thought that removal of microaggregates by the micropore filter decreases the incidence of lung disease post-transfusion. However, evidence supporting this theory is scanty. It also seems that the microaggregates of significance do not begin to appear in stored blood until day 10 of storage. In light of present data, it seems logical to apply the following plan:

1. Use either filter for administration of small amounts of blood.
2. Use a micropore filter in patients receiving blood equal to more than half their blood volume.
3. Use a micropore filter for blood older than 10 days.
4. Do not use a micropore filter if it will hinder adequate administration of blood to an exsanguinating patient.

Other possible complications of transfusions include transfusion reactions (usually manifest under anesthesia by hemoglobinuria, bleeding diathesis, and hypotension) and hepatitis (A, B, and "non A, non B"). The prevention and treatment of these conditions are discussed in recent texts.[222] The need to prevent complications associated with transfusion of whole blood and to develop a ready source of oxygen-carrying solution has led to studies in the area of acellular oxygen-delivering resuscitation fluids. These fluids consist of hemoglobin solutions, perfluorochemicals, and synthetic chelates.[223] Although these solutions are not yet available for clinical studies, their proposed advantages are that they have the ability to be stored for long periods of time, they require no crossmatching prior to infusion, and they can provide adequate oxygenation in the face of severe anemia.

In addition to crystalloids and blood, other solutions that may be used for fluid resuscitation are the colloids. Much debate exists concerning their indications for use. Single donor plasma is usually produced from stored, banked blood and, as compared with fresh frozen plasma (FFP), generally lacks the labile clotting factors. Both products carry a hepatitis risk and are generally not available for acute resuscitation because they require thawing. Both should be given through a 170-μ filter over a period of less than 6 hours. FFP may be indicated to replace coagulation factors. Plasma protein fraction (PPF) 5 per cent is heat-treated plasma that inactivates the hepatitis virus. Since it is shelf-stable for years and requires no crossmatching, it would appear ideal for rapid fluid resuscitation. However, it is expensive and may cause vasodilation and hypotension if infused rapidly. Human serum albumin (HSA) solutions come in either 5 or 25 per cent solutions. The incidence of hypotension with the use of these solutions is less, the cost is similar to PPF, and the 5 per cent solution may be infused rapidly for resuscitation. This is probably the solution to rival the crystalloids for use in initial resuscitation, although its advantages are minor. The more concentrated albumin solution is probably indicated only in cases of hypoproteinemia, such as in burn or peritonitis patients.[5, 222]

Special Considerations

An open wound of the eye in a patient with a full stomach presents a special dilemma for the anesthesiologist. On the one hand, the anesthesiologist wishes to carry out those procedures already discussed to prevent aspiration of gastric contents, while on the other hand trying to prevent increases in intraocular pressure (IOP) and extrusion of vitreous. The major conflict revolves around the use of succinylcholine, which has been shown to increase IOP. Likewise increases in blood pressure, hypoventilation, and intubation have been shown to increase IOP.[224] The increase in IOP due to intubation has been attenuated with topical laryngeal anesthesia, but this is generally contraindicated in a patient with a full stomach. It is usually agreed that one should do those things possible to decrease the acidity and volume of gastric contents (see Preparation for Surgery), after which one of the rapid-sequence techniques discussed earlier should be used, preferably using thiopental, although ketamine does not seem to appreciably increase IOP in children.[225] Since the use of small doses of nondepolarizing muscle relaxant as pretreatment will not reliably prevent the increase in IOP by succinylcholine, the use of only a nondepolarizing relaxant for intubation may be preferable. Most anesthetics cause either no change or a slight reduction in IOP, provided coughing or bucking is prevented,[224–226] and are generally safe for maintenance anesthesia. During anesthesia, vigilance should be maintained so that prompt treatment may be instituted should bradycardia develop from the oculocardiac reflex. Treatment consists of cessation of surgical manipulation and IV atropine.[227] At the end of surgery, the question facing the anesthesiologist is whether to avoid having the patient cough and buck by extubating while the patient is at a deep level of anesthesia or to awaken the patient with the endotracheal tube in place because of complications as a result of a "full stomach." With the eye now sutured and the risk of aspiration being more life threatening, I prefer to awaken the patient before extubation. However, I do try to use a technique that allows for rapid awakening.

As noted previously, the anesthesiologist must take special precautions when managing the burn patient. Burn patients present with a number of management problems, among which are difficult airway, scarce venous access, scarcity of places for monitoring, drug dependency, multiple anesthetics, hypothermia, blood loss, hyperkalemia with succinylcholine, and systemic effect of topical medications. The management of these problems is the topic of a recent review, and is discussed in Chapter 25.[228]

Patients with acute spinal cord lesions usually lose the autoregulatory mechanisms for the vascular system below the injury. The peripheral vascular bed is flaccid, and the patient cannot respond to blood loss with the typical increase in vascular resistance. These patients may require unusually aggressive fluid resuscitation. A week or so following injury, these patients may develop the syndrome of autonomic dysreflexia in response to a visceral stimulus, usually of the bladder or bowel. Vessels above the cord lesion will dilate in response to the hypertension produced, but the vessels below the lesion will not; therefore, hypertension persists with the possibility of cerebral complications. This syndrome is usually prevented by deep anesthesia, lower body region anesthesia (spinal, epidural), or treatment with drugs that reduce peripheral sympathetic tone.[5]

Anesthesia for Minor Trauma and Regional Anesthesia

Pediatric patients who suffer minor trauma may have little to distinguish them from the average surgical patient except in terms of the urgency of the procedure and consideration of the full stomach. In certain specific cases, regional anesthesia may be applicable. This suitability usually depends both upon the nature of the injury and the psychologic acceptance by the patient. It is also of extreme importance that all preparation for regional anesthesia be done prior to bringing the patient into the OR. Although the use of spinal and epidural anesthesia has been reported in children, they have not achieved great popularity and are rarely administered in children under the age of 10 years.[229] The only regional anesthetic techniques that are commonly employed at our hospital are brachial plexus block (usually the axillary approach, but also occasionally the interscalene technique), caudal block, and ankle block.

The axillary approach to the brachial plexus block is usually performed only in cooperative children above 6 to 7 years of age.[229] The patient is positioned with the affected arm abducted at a right angle, with the forearm and hand supinated. The elbow is flexed, with the hand under the head or in the salute position.[229, 230] The axilla is prepped and draped. A solution consisting of 50 ml of 1 per cent mepivacaine (or lidocaine) with 60 mg tetracaine and 0.20 ml epinephrine is prepared. The dose is 7 mg/kg of the mepivacaine (Carbocaine), i.e., 0.7 ml/kg of the solution.[229] The axillary artery is palpated at the level of the insertion of the pectoralis major muscle on the humerus. A 25-gauge needle attached to an IV extension set and syringe is used.[231] The physician makes a skin wheal over the artery and inserts the needle directly toward the artery while an assistant withdraws the plunger of the syringe. If a paresthesia that is transmitted to the hand is elicited, the appropriate dose may be injected. If, as is usually the case, paresthesias are not produced, the needle is advanced until the artery is encountered, as evidenced by a return of bright red blood into the IV extension tubing. The needle is further advanced carefully until the blood flow just ceases. Now the point of the needle should lie just beyond the artery but within the axillary sheath. Once this placement is clearly determined, one half the calculated dose is injected, while the fingers of the hand used to palpate the artery occlude the sheath distally. Then the needle is withdrawn with negative pressure on the plunger of the syringe until the point of the needle lies just proximal to the artery, as evidenced by a cessation of blood return as the needle is withdrawn through the artery.[230] At this point, the other half of the dose is injected. This method eliminates the subjectivity of paresthesias in the somewhat excitable pediatric patient. When done carefully, a good "sausage" develops and excellent anesthesia results, which sets up quickly (5 to 10 minutes) and lasts for 4 to 6 hours. When performing an interscalene block, the needle is inserted at the C6 vertebral level between the anterior and midline scalene muscles.[232] The needle is advanced until a paresthesia of the C5 to C6 dermatome is elicited, or a nerve stimulator may be attached to the needle to give objective evidence that the tip of the needle lies within the neurovascular sheath. Approximately two thirds of the dose recommended for axillary block is used in the interscalene technique.

The caudal anesthetic technique is usually performed for pain relief at the end of urologic, anal, or lower extremity surgery. The patient is placed on the left side, with the knees brought up to the chest, and the lower sacral region prepped. The sacral hiatus and the posterior iliac spine are located. The latter represents the level that is usually the lower extent of the arachnoid, but in children, the dural sac extends more caudally. Therefore, one does not want to advance the needle more than 1 cm into the sacral hiatus to avoid a subarachnoid injection. A 20-gauge needle is used to make a hole in the skin, and then a 22-gauge needle is passed through the skin hole at a 60 degree angle to the skin and advanced against the sacral bone. The angle is decreased until the needle is felt to pass through the sacrococcygeal ligament. Aspiration is carried out, and if no spinal fluid or blood is present, a dose of 0.5 ml/kg of 0.25 or 0.5 per cent marcaine gives good analgesia. The lesser concentration will produce a relatively low block without muscle paralysis, but 0.5 per cent may be used for a higher and more profound block. The patient is usually placed supine after the block to afford good spread of the anesthetic and to avoid a possible unilateral block. Other dosage regimens recommended are as follows:

(1) 0.1 ml per year of age per segment,[231]

(2) $$\text{Volume (ml)} = 4 + \frac{D - 15}{2}$$

where D = the distance in centimeters from the seventh cervical spinous process to the sacral hiatus.[229]

Ankle blocks are generally performed at the end of anesthesia for pain relief, and techniques for carrying out the procedures are described in standard texts.[231] The IV regional technique (Bier's block) is useful for hand and forearm injuries in older cooperative patients but generally has the potential for causing greater complications. For this reason, it is used infrequently at our institution. Proper performance of this block is discussed in the literature.[76, 230] A final block that may be used for certain patients is the femoral nerve, lateral femoral cutaneous nerve, and abductor nerve block (3 in 1 block).[233]

POSTOPERATIVE CONSIDERATIONS

Following anesthesia, the patient will either go to a recovery room or to the ICU. Wherever the patient is to go, it is important that the personnel there be notified in advance so that they can prepare for the patient's arrival. Prior to extubation, the stomach should be suctioned to remove as much of the gastric contents as possible. Although this cannot guarantee an empty stomach, it should decrease the volume of gastric contents regurgitated if the patient should vomit. It will also remove any gastric air, which may promote vomiting.

The patient with a potential full stomach should be placed on his side prior to extubation to prevent airway obstruction or massive aspiration of gastric contents in the event of vomiting. The patient should be alert and have airway reflexes intact before extubation is performed. The time for recovery of reflexes from inhaled anesthetics is a function of both the solubility coefficient of the agent and the level of alveolar ventilation of the patient.[234] Recovery from narcotics is frequently a function of the dose administered, time since last dose, and renal function.[234] It is important that one or two functioning large-bore suctions are available at extubation. Also, one must be absolutely certain that the patient is stable before transfer or extubation. Occasionally the change from mechanical to manual ventilation can cause a change in the patient's condition.[29] This should be checked prior to transport.

Extubation should be performed during inspiration and with positive pressure on the airway. This positive pressure causes a "gush" of air to vent around the tube as it is being removed, and blows debris, secretions, or blood away from the airway, which helps avoid obstruction. Vital signs are checked once again to make sure that the patient is stable. The patient is then transported to the recovery room on his side to prevent pooling of tracheal or gastric secretions at the airway.[234] The patient should maintain this position until awake.

Upon arrival in the recovery room, the anesthesiologist should give the nurse a full report on the patient. This should include the patient's name, medical problems, age, injuries, and allergies; surgical procedures performed; pre-operative medications given; anesthetic agents and methods used; and record of fluid and blood replacement, blood loss, urinary output, gastric output, and any complications.[234] It is usually wise to give oxygen by placing a loose-fitting face mask on most patients who have undergone fairly major surgery until they are fully alert. Vital signs should be monitored frequently, and a good stir-up regimen should be instituted.[235, 236] This generally includes deep breathing exercises, coughing, positioning, mobilization, and provision of analgesia.[236] Once the patient has been stable for a reasonable length of time, usually 40 to 60 minutes, he can usually be discharged from the recovery room by the anesthesiologist.

If the patient is to go directly to the ICU, extubation may or may not be performed. If it is, the precautions already mentioned should be observed. If the patient is to be ventilated postoperatively, transport by means of a system with an adequate supply of oxygen is necessary. A transport monitor should be used to monitor EKG, arterial pressure, CVP, and respiratory rate, as well as possibly pulmonary artery pressure during transport to the ICU. The monitoring necessary during transport should be individualized for each case. Monitoring systems should be available in advance in the ICU so that the patient is unmonitored for only a few seconds while converting to the ICU monitors.

Ventilation in the ICU should be provided by means of a ventilator,* which has the capability for intermittent mandatory ventilation (IMV).[237, 238] This method uses mechanical cycling at the lowest rate that, in combination with spontaneous breathing, maintains PA_{CO_2} and PH_a at normal levels. Positive end expiratory pressure (PEEP) or continuous positive airway pressure (CPAP) is employed as necessary to improve oxygenation. Undesirable cardiovascular depression is minimized both because of the lower rate of mechanical cycling and the maintenance of spontaneous respiration, which decreases mean intrapleural pressure.[239] When the pa-

*Bourns BP 100, Bear Medical Systems (Riverside, CA); Secrest (Anaheim, CA); Bennett 7200 (Overland Park, KS), Bourns Bear, Bear Medical Systems (Riverside, CA); Emerson IMV (Cambridge, MA).

tient is initially placed on the ventilator, the mechanical respiratory rate may need to be more rapid owing to residual paralysis from the muscle relaxants. As this wears off, the respirator rate may be decreased, and a smooth weaning process instituted.

The weaning procedure can begin when there is: (1) reversal of the muscle relaxation, (2) improvement in any pulmonary pathophysiological process, (3) cardiovascular stability, (4) adequate arterial blood gas values, and (5) a favorable clinical impression of the patient's status.[240] Weaning should progress slowly by first decreasing the inspired oxygen concentration to nontoxic levels ($F_{I_{O_2}} < 0.5$), then decreasing PEEP/CPAP and respiratory rate until the patient is breathing spontaneously on a CPAP of 3 to 4 m H_2O, and $F_{I_{O_2}}$ 0.3 to 0.4. If arterial blood gases remain acceptable, the patient may be extubated. It is important to make sure that the patient has not been fed recently and that the stomach is suctioned before extubation. In patients with neurologic trauma, it is important to make sure that the gag reflex is intact. Patients should not be fed for approximately 6 to 8 hours after extubation for two reasons. First, after prolonged intubation, airway reflexes may be abnormal,[241] and second, if the patient is going to require reintubation, this will usually occur within this time, and the need to contend with a full stomach will be avoided.

Following extubation, the patient will usually need supplemental oxygen. Usually adequate inspired oxygen can be provided by simple oxygen masks that deliver an $F_{I_{O_2}}$ of 0.35 to 0.60. However, if higher-inspired oxygen is necessary, a partial rebreathing or nonrebreathing mask may be used to deliver an $F_{I_{O_2}}$ of 0.8 to 1.0.[240] If further assistance is necessary after extubation, spontaneous PEEP or CPAP by mask has been shown to be effective in adults, but studies of these methods using pediatric patients are lacking.[240, 242] There are three major physiological differences between PEEP and CPAP: (1) work of breathing, (2) venous return and cardiac output, and (3) functional residual capacity (FRC). The PEEP system necessitates the generation of subambient pressure to inspire fresh gas. This maneuver increases the work of breathing but also may improve venous return to the right side of the heart and thus improve cardiac output.[240] CPAP, on the other hand, can usually be regulated so that the work of breathing is minimal, but CPAP creates a continuous positive intrapleural pressure, which may impede venous return and decrease cardiac output. Continuous flow CPAP systems generally have the advantage over demand CPAP systems in that they allow the capability of adjusting the necessary inspiratory effort.[240]

Other modalities that may be useful in postoperative respiratory care are intermittent positive pressure breathing (IPPB) and incentive breathing. The goals of postoperative respiratory therapy include inflation of collapsed alveoli, increased vital capacity, increased total lung capacity, increased functional residual capacity, and restoration of normal ventilation/perfusion relationships.[240] Significant postoperative atelectasis occurs in 20 to 40 per cent of patients undergoing abdominal or thoracic surgery.[240] This is usually due to "splinting" as a result of incisional pain. IPPB appears to have some efficacy in the treatment of atelectasis in postoperative patients,[240] but controversy surrounds this issue.[243] IPPB will usually need to be delivered by mask in patients less than 4 years of age, uncooperative patients, or weakened patients; patients over 5 years of age will frequently cooperate in using a mouthpiece. The Respiratory Care Committee of the American Thoracic Society has listed the indications and proper techniques for the administration of IPPB. IPPB should be used to improve delivery of aerosol medications in patients who are unable to coordinate the breathing pattern, to improve coughing and expectoration, to decrease rising $P_{A_{CO_2}}$, and to decrease pulmonary distress. The proper techniques require that (1) baseline measurements are taken of the patient's spontaneous tidal volume and maximum voluntary inspired volume, (2) the device is explained to the patient, (3) delivered volumes are measured to assure that IPPB tidal volume exceeds the patient's spontaneous tidal volume, (4) there is an inspiratory pause, (5) the therapeutic objectives are defined, documented, and periodically evaluated, and (6) a simpler and less costly treatment is used when feasible.[240] Incentive breathing is based on the observation that normal breathing patterns should facilitate a deep breath every 5 to 10 minutes to reverse or prevent alveolar collapse.[244] One of the most efficacious ways of doing this is by means of a sustained maximal inspiration. A number of devices are available that serve this purpose, but again most are useful in the patient 5 years or older. Studies have shown incentive breathing to be at least as effective as IPPB therapy in reversing or preventing postoperative pulmonary complications.[240]

Complications that may arise from postoperative mechanical ventilation and/or other postoperative respiratory modalities include pulmonary oxygen toxicity, pulmonary infections, decreased cardiac output, pulmonary barotrauma, increased extravascular lung water, and redistribution of pulmonary blood flow.[240] Pulmonary oxygen toxicity is related to the partial pressure of inspired oxygen and not the F_{IO_2}. However, at roughly one atmosphere (760 mm Hg) pressure, it appears unlikely that pulmonary oxygen toxicity develops in man at an F_{IO_2} of less than 0.5, even with prolonged exposure.[240] In infants, the combination of high-inspired oxygen delivered for prolonged periods by mechanical ventilation with high peak pressures may lead to a syndrome of pulmonary oxygen toxicity termed bronchopulmonary dysplasia.[240] Whether pulmonary infections result from respiratory equipment is a debatable issue in the literature, but it does seem wise to change the equipment every 12 to 24 hours, use sterile water for humidification, and possibly use filters at air intake ports and in the patient's breathing circuit. The decrease in cardiac output produced by decreases in airway pressure (specifically increased mean intrathoracic pressure) has already been mentioned. This decrease in cardiac output correlates with two factors. The first mentioned is the intrapleural pressure, which is determined by lung and chest wall compliance. Low compliance (stiff) lungs transmit less pressure and therefore allow less decrease in cardiac output. Cardiac depression is exacerbated by hypovolemia. Numerous studies have confirmed that most of the depressant hemodynamic effects of increased mean airway pressure can be minimized with adequate intravascular fluid support.[240] Pulmonary barotrauma (pulmonary interstitial emphysema, subcutaneous emphysema, pneumothorax, pneumomediastinum, and pneumoperitoneum), which is associated with positive pressure therapy, appears also to be lessened by proper intravascular volume expansion.[240] Available evidence seems to show that mechanical ventilation more than PEEP appears to be a contributing factor to the increase in extravascular lung water. In the case of overdistention of the alveoli with PEEP, increased pulmonary artery pressure may occur with shunting and increased ventilation/perfusion abnormalities.[240]

REFERENCES

1. Morse TS: Step by step with an injured child. Emerg Med 6:121, 1974.
2. Goldberg AI: Anesthesia and intensive care. *In* Toubukian RJ (ed.): Pediatric Trauma. New York, John Wiley and Sons, 1978, p. 105.
3. McIntyre KM, Parker MR: Standards and guidelines for cardiopulmonary resuscitation (CPR) and emergency cardiac care (ECC). JAMA 244:453, 1980.
4. Committee on Trauma, American College of Surgeons: Early Care of the Injured Patient. 2nd ed. Philadelphia, WB Saunders Company, 1976, p. 1.
5. Zimmerman BL: Uncommon problems in acute trauma. *In* Katz J, Benumof J, Kadis LB (eds.): Anesthesia and Uncommon Diseases: Pathophysiologic and Clinical Correlations. Philadelphia, WB Saunders Company, 1981.
6. Levison M, Trunkey PD: Initial assessment and resuscitation. Surg Clin North Am 62:11, 1982.
7. Lewis FR: Thoracic trauma. Surg Clin North Am 62:100, 1982.
8. Levin RM: Pediatric Anesthesia Handbook. Garden City, New York, Medical Examination Publishing Company, 1980.
9. Steward DJ: Manual of Pediatric Anesthesia. New York, Churchill Livingstone, 1979, p. 5.
10. Eckenhoff JE: Some anatomic considerations of the infant larynx influencing endotracheal anesthesia. Anesthesiology 12:401, 1951.
11. Muller NL, Bryan AC: Chest wall mechanics and respiratory muscles in infants. Pediatr Clin North Am 26:503, 1979.
12. Muller N, Gulston G, Cade D, et al.: Diaphragmatic muscle fatigue in the newborn. J Appl Physiol 46:688, 1979.
13. Keens TG, Bryan AC, Levison H, et al.: Development of fatigue-resistant muscle fibers in human ventilatory muscles. J Appl Physiol 44:909, 1978.
14. Lister G, Hoffman JIE, Rudolph AM: Oxygen uptake in infants and children: A simple method for measurement. Pediatrics 53:656, 1974.
15. Johnson DG, Jones R: Surgical aspects of airway management in infants and children. Surg Clin North Am 56:263, 1976.
16. Dorsch JA, Dorsch SE: Understanding Anesthesia Equipment: Construction, Care and Complications. Baltimore, Williams and Wilkins Company, 1975, pp. 174, 228.
17. White RD, Gilles BP, Polk BV: Oxygen delivery by hand-operated emergency ventilation devices. JACEP 2:105, 1973.
18. Carden E, Hughes T: An evaluation of manually operated self-inflating resuscitation bags. Anesth Analg 56:202, 1977.
19. Carden E, Friedman D: Further studies of manually operated self-inflating resuscitation bags. Anesth Analg 56:202, 1977.
20. Rayburn RL: Pediatric anesthesia circuits. American Society of Anesthesiologists Annual Refresher Course Lectures, 1981, p. 117.
21. Rayburn RL, Watson RL: Humidity in children and adults using the controlled partial rebreathing anesthesia method. Anesthesiology 52:291, 1980.
22. Mosenkis R (ed.): Health Devices 3:207, 1974.
23. Mosenkis R (ed.): Health Devices 8:24, 1978.
24. McPherson SP: Respiratory Therapy Equipment. New York, CV Mosby Company, 1981, p. 196.

25. Michael TA: The esophageal obturator airway. JAMA 246:1098, 1981.
26. Kassels SJ, Robinson WA, O'Bara K: Esophageal perforation associated with the esophageal obturator airway. Crit Care Med 8:386, 1980.
27. Stoelting RK: Endotracheal intubation. *In* Miller RD (ed.): Anesthesia. New York, Churchill Livingstone, 1981, p. 233.
28. Venes JL, Collins WF Jr: Spinal cord injury. *In* Touloukian RJ (ed.): Pediatric Trauma. New York, John Wiley and Sons, 1978, p. 262.
29. Weiskopf RB, Fairley HB: Anesthesia for major trauma. Surg Clin North Am 62:31, 1982.
30. Giesecke AH Jr: Anesthesia for trauma surgery. *In* Miller RD (ed.): Anesthesia. New York, Churchill Livingstone, 1981, p. 1250.
31. Adams AL, Cane RD, Shapiro BA: Tongue extrusion as an aid to blind nasal intubaton. Crit Care Med 10:335, 1982.
32. Knodel AR, Beekman JF: Unexplained fevers in patients with nasotracheal intubation. JAMA 248:868, 1982.
33. Todres ID, deBros F, Kramer SS, et al.: Endotracheal tube displacement in the newborn infant. J Pediatr 89:126, 1976.
34. Wung J, Stark RI, Indyk L, et al.: Oxygen supplement during endotracheal intubation of the infant. Pediatrics 59:1046, 1977.
35. Todres ID, Crone RK: Experience with a modified laryngoscope in sick infants. Crit Care Med 9:544, 1981.
36. Dalal FY, Schmidt GB, Bennett EJ, et al.: Fractures of the larynx in children. Can Anaesth Soc J 21:376, 1974.
37. Spoerel WE, Narayanan PS, Singh NP: Transtracheal ventilation. Br J Anaesth 43:932, 1971.
38. Klain M, Smith RB: High frequency percutaneous transtracheal jet ventilation. Crit Care Med 5:280, 1977.
39. Roberts LS, Rayburn RL, Matlak ME, et al.: A unique method for the anesthetic management of laryngeal foreign bodies. Anesthesiology 56:480, 1982.
40. Todres ID, Rogers MC: Methods of external cardiac massage in the newborn infant. J Pediatr 86:781, 1975.
41. Chandra N, Snyder LD, Weisfeldt ML: Abdominal binding during cardiopulmonary resuscitation in man. JAMA 246:351, 1981.
42. Redding JS: Abdominal compression in cardiopulmonary resuscitation. Anesth Analg 50:668, 1971.
43. Rudikoff MT, Maughan WL, Effron M, et al.: Mechanism of blood flow during cardiopulmonary resuscitation. Circulation 61:345, 1980.
44. Harris LC Jr, Kirimli B, Safar P: Augmentation of artificial circulation during cardiopulmonary resuscitation. Anesthesiology 28:730, 1967.
45. Holcroft JW: Impairment of venous return in hemorrhagic shock. Surg Clin North Am 62:25, 1982.
46. Talbert JL, Haller JA Jr: The optimal site for central venous measurement in newborn infants. J Surg Res 6:168, 1966.
47. Chameidis L, Brown GE, Raye JR, et al.: Guidelines for defibrillation in infants and children. Report of the American Heart Association Target Activity Group: Cardiopulmonary resuscitation in the young. Circulation 56 (suppl):502A, 1977.
48. Gregory GA: Newborn and neonatal emergency anesthetics. American Society of Anesthesiologists Annual Refresher Course Lectures, 1980, p 119.
49. Lang P, Williams RG, Norwood WI, et al.: The hemodynamic effects of dopamine in infants after corrective cardiac surgery. J Pediatr 96:630, 1980.
50. Coté CJ, Jobes DR, Schwartz AJ, et al.: Two approaches to cannulation of a child's internal jugular vein. Anesthesiology 50:371, 1979.
51. Prince SR, Sullivan RL, Hackel A: Percutaneous catheterization of the internal jugular vein in infants and children. Anesthesiology 44:170, 1976.
52. Humphrey MJ, Blitt CD: Central venous access in children via the external jugular vein. Anesthesiology 57:50, 1982.
53. Moore DC: Regional Block: A Handbook for Use in the Clinical Practice of Medicine and Surgery. Springfield, Illinois, Charles C Thomas, 1971, p 47.
54. Adams AK: Psychological preparation and premedication. *In* Gray TC, Nunn JF, Utting JE (eds.): General Anesthesia. Boston, Butterworths, 1980, p. 913.
55. Shapiro HM: Neurosurgical anesthesia and intracranial hypertension. *In* Miller RD (ed.): Anesthesia. New York, Churchill Livingstone, 1981, p 1089.
56. Salem MR, Wong AY, Mani M, et al.: Premedicant drugs and gastric juice pH and volume in pediatric patients. Anesthesiology 44:216, 1976.
57. Teabeault JR: Aspiration of gastric contents: Experimental study. Am J Pathol 28:51, 1952.
58. Stoelting RK: Responses to atropine, glycopyrrolate, and Riopan of gastric fluid pH and volume in adult patients. Anesthesiology 48:367, 1978.
59. Brock-Utne JG, Rubin J, Welman S, et al.: The effect of glycopyrrolate (Robinul) on the lower esophageal sphincter. Can Anaesth Soc J 25:144, 1978.
60. Lind JF, Crispin JS, McIver DH: The effects of atropine on the gastro-esophageal sphincter. Can J Physiol Pharmacol 46:233, 1968.
61. Manchikanti L, Kraus JW, Edds SP: Cimetidine and related drugs in anesthesia. Anesth Analg 61:595, 1982.
62. Goudsouzian N, Coté CJ, Liu LMP, et al.: Dose response effects of oral cimetidine on gastric pH and volume in children. Anesthesiology 55:533, 1981.
63. Korttila K, Kauste A, Auvinen J: Comparison of doperidone, droperidol, and metoclopramide in the prevention and treatment of nausea and vomiting after balanced general anesthesia. Anesth Analg 58:396, 1979.
64. Diamond MJ, Keeri-Szanto M: Reduction of postoperative vomiting by preoperative administration of oral metoclopramide. Can Anaesth Soc J 27:36, 1980.
65. Blumenthal I, Costalos C: The effect of metoclopramide on neonatal gastric emptying. Br J Clin Pharmacol 4:207, 1977.
66. Casteels-Van Daele M, Jaeken J, et al.: Dystonic reactions in children caused by metoclopramide. Arch Dis Child 45:130, 1970.
67. Low LCK, Goel KM: Metoclopramide poisoning in children. Arch Dis Child 55:310, 1980.
68. White FA, Clark RB, Thompson DS: Preoperative oral antacid therapy for patients requiring emergency surgery. South Med J 71:177, 1978.
69. Wheatley RG, Kallus FT, Reynolds RC, et al.: Milk of magnesia is an effective preinduction antacid in obstetric anesthesia. Anesthesiology 50:514, 1979.

70. Gibbs CP, Schwartz DJ, Wynne JW, et al.: Antacid pulmonary aspiration in the dog. Anesthesiology 51:380, 1979.
71. Gibbs CP, Spohr L, Schmidt D: The effectiveness of sodium citrate as an antacid. Anesthesiology 57:44, 1982.
72. Lindop MJ: Monitoring of the cardiovascular system during anesthesia. Int Anesthesiol Clin 19:1, 1981.
73. Graff TD, Benson DW: Systemic and pulmonary changes with inhaled humid atmosphere. Anesthesiology 30:199, 1969.
74. Besch NJ, Perlstein PH, Edwards NK, et al.: The transparent baby bag: A shield against heat loss. N Engl J Med 284:121, 1971.
75. Hug CC Jr: Monitoring. *In* Miller RD (ed.): Anesthesia. New York, Churchill Livingstone, 1981, p. 157.
76. Smith RM: Anesthesia for Infants and Children. St. Louis, CV Mosby Company, 1980, pp. 12, 192, 237.
77. Goldring D, Hernandez A: Hypertension in children. Pediatr Rev 3:235, 1982.
78. Blumenthal S: Report of the task force on blood pressure control in children. Prepared by the National Heart, Lung and Blood Institute's Task Force on blood pressure control in children. Pediatrics 59 (suppl):797, 1977.
79. Janis KM, Kemmerer WT, Kirby RR: Intraoperative Doppler blood pressure measurements in infants. Anesthesiology 33:361, 1970.
80. Hernandez A, Goldring D, Hartmann AF: Measurement of blood pressure in infants and children by the Doppler ultrasonic technique. Pediatrics 48:788, 1971.
81. Gregory GA: Pediatric anesthesia. *In* Miller RD (ed.): Anesthesia. New York, Churchill Livingstone, 1981.
82. Vale RJ: Monitoring of temperature during anesthesia. *In* Gerson GR (ed.): Monitoring During Anesthesia. Int Anesthesiol Clin, Vol. 19. Boston, Little Brown and Company, 1981, p. 61.
83. Adamsons K Jr, Gandy GM, James LS: The influence of thermal factors upon oxygen consumption of the newborn human infant. J Pediatr 66:495, 1965.
84. Lee APB: Monitoring the neuromuscular junction. *In* Gerson GR (ed.): Anesthesia. Int Anesthesiol Clin, Vol. 19. Boston, Little Brown and Company, 1981, p. 85.
85. Miller RD, Savarese JJ: Pharmacology of muscle relaxants, their antagonists, and monitoring of neuromuscular function. *In* Miller RD (ed.): Anesthesia. New York, Churchill Livingstone, 1981, p 487.
86. Wallgren G, Barr M, Rudhe U: Hemodynamic studies of induced acute hypo- and hypervolemia in the newborn infant. Acta Pediatr Scand 53:1, 1964.
87. Linderkamp O, Strohhacker I, Versmold HT, et al.: Peripheral circulation of the newborn: Interaction of peripheral blood flow, blood pressure, blood volue, and blood viscosity. Eur J Pediatr 129:73, 1978.
88. Amato JJ, Solod E, Cleveland RJ: A "second" radial artery for monitoring the perioperative pediatric cardiac patient. J Peditr Surg 12:715, 1977.
89. Downs JB, Rackstein AD, Klein EF Jr, et al.: Hazards of radial-artery catheterization. Anesthesiology 38:283, 1973.
90. Miyasaka K, Edmonds JF, Conn AW: Complications of radial artery lines in the pediatric patient. Can Anaesth Soc J 23:9, 1976.
91. Lowenstein E, Little JW III, Lo HH: Prevention of cerebral embolization from flushing radial artery cannulas. N Engl J Med 285:1414, 1971.
92. Seldinger SI: Catheter placement of the needle in percutaneous arteriography. Acta Radiologica 39:368, 1953.
93. English ICW, Frew RM, Pigott JF, et al.: Percutaneous catheterization of the internal jugular vein. Anaesthesia 24:521, 1969.
94. Daily PO, Griepp RB, Shumway NE: Percutaneous internal jugular vein cannulation. Arch Surg 101:534, 1970.
95. Hall DMB, Geefhuysen J: Percutaneous catheterization of the internal jugular vein in infants and children. J Pediatr Surg 12:719, 1977.
96. Rao TL, Wong AY, Salem MR: A new approach to percutaneous catheterization of the internal jugular vein. Anesthesiology 46:362, 1977.
97. Dudrick SJ, Wilmore DW, Vars HM, et al.: Can intravenous feeding as the sole means of nutrition support growth in the child and restore weight loss in an adult: An affirmative answer. Ann Surg 169:947, 1969.
98. Groff DB, Ahmed N: Subclavian vein catheterization in the infant. J Pediatr Surg 9:171, 1974.
99. Munson ES: Intracardiac catheters in neurosurgical anesthesia. Anesthesiology 50:67, 1979.
100. Sink JD, Comer PB, James PM, et al.: Evaluation of catheter placement in the treatment of venous air embolism. Ann Surg 183:58, 1976.
101. Martin JT: Neuroanesthetic adjuncts for surgery in the sitting position III. Intravascular electrocardiography. Anesth Analg 49:793, 1970.
102. Graves S: Fluid and electrolyte therapy in children. American Society of Anesthesiologists Annual Refresher Course Lectures, 1981, p 114.
103. Shapiro HM, Wyte SR, Harris AB, et al.: Acute intraoperative intracranial hypertension in neurosurgical patients: Mechanical and pharmacologic factors. Anesthesiology 37:399, 1972.
104. Magnaes B: Body position and cerebrospinal fluid pressure. J Neurosurg 44:687, 1976.
105. Jorgensen PB, Misfeldt BB: Intracranial pressure during recovery from nitrous oxide and halothane anesthesia in neurosurgical patients. Br J Anaesth 42:977, 1975.
106. Leech P, Barker J, Fitch W: Changes in intracranial pressure and systemic arterial pressure during termination of anesthesia. Br J Anaesth 46:315, 1974.
107. Whitesell R, Asiddao C, Gollman D, et al.: Relationship between arterial and peak expired carbon dioxide pressure during anesthesia and factors influencing the difference. Anesth Analg 60:508, 1981.
108. Nunn JF, Hill DW: Respiratory dead space and arterial to end-tidal CO_2 tension difference in anesthetized man. J Appl Physiol 15:383, 1960.
109. Rayburn RL, Graves SA: A new concept in controlled ventilation of children with the Bain anesthetic circuit. Anesthesiology 48:250, 1978.
110. Brechner VL, Bethune RWM: Recent advances in monitoring pulmonary air embolism. Anesth Analg 50:255, 1971.
111. Huch R, Huch A, Albani M, et al.: Transcutaneous PO_2 monitoring in routine management of infants and children with cardiorespiratory problems. Pediatrics 57:681, 1976.

112. Peabody JL, Gregory GA, Willis MM, et al.: Transcutaneous oxygen tension in sick infants. Am Rev Resp Dis 118:83, 1978.
113. McHugh RD, Epstein RM, Longnecker DE: Halothane mimics oxygen in oxygen microelectrodes. Anesthesiology 50:47, 1979.
114. Strept WJ, Safar P: Rapid induction/intubation for prevention of gastric-content aspiration. Anesth Analg 49:633, 1970.
115. Sellick BA: Cricoid pressure to control regurgitation of stomach contents during induction of anaesthesia. Lancet 2:404, 1961.
116. Bennett EJ, Bowyer DE, Giesecke AH Jr, et al.: Pancuronium bromide: A double blind study in children. Anesth Analg 52:17, 1973.
117. Brown EM, Krishnaprasad D, Smiler BG: Pancuronium for rapid induction technique for tracheal intubation. Can Anaesth Soc J 26:489, 1979.
118. Salem MR, Wong AY, Collins VJ: The pediatric patient with a full stomach. Anesthesiology 39:435, 1973.
119. Yakaitis RW, Blitt CD, Anguilo JP: End tidal halothane concentrations for endotracheal intubation. Anesthesiology 47:386, 1977.
120. Dripps RD, Echenhoff JE, Vandam LD: Introduction to Anesthesia: The Principles of Safe Practice. Philadelphia, WB Saunders Company, 1977, p. 234.
121. Hornbein TF, Eger EI II, Winter PM, et al.: The minimum alveolar concentration of nitrous oxide in man. Anesth Analg 61:553, 1982.
122. Hickley RF, Eger EI II: Circulatory pharmacology of inhaled anesthetics. *In* Miller RD (ed.): Anesthesia. New York, Churchill Livingstone, 1981.
123. Stoelting RK, Gibbs PS: Hemodynamic effects of morphine and morphine–nitrous oxide in valvular heart disease and coronary artery disease. Anesthesiolgy 38:45, 1973.
124. Forbes AR, Gamsu G: Mucociliary clearance in the canine lung during and after general anesthesia. Anesthesiology 50:26, 1979.
125. Hirsch JA, Tokayer Jl, Robinson MJ, et al.: Effects of dry air and subsequent humidification on tracheal mucous velocity in dogs. J Appl Physiol 39:242, 1975.
126. Wolfe WG, Ebert PA, Sabiston DC: Effect of high oxygen tension on mucociliary function. Surgery 72:246, 1972.
127. Forbes AR, Gamsu G: Lung mucociliary clearance after anesthesia with spontaneous and controlled ventilation. Am Rev Resp Dis 120:857, 1979.
128. Sackner MA, Hirsch J, Epstein S: Effect of cuffed endotracheal tubes on tracheal mucous velocity. Chest 68:774, 1975.
129. Munson ES: Transfer of nitrous oxide into body cavities. Br J Anaesth 46:202, 1974.
130. Hilgenberg JC, McCammon RL, Stoelting RK: Pulmonary and systemic vascular responses to nitrous oxide in patients with mitral stenosis and pulmonary hypertension. Anesth Analg 59:323, 1980.
131. Schulte-Sasse U, Hess W, Tarnow, J: Pulmonary vascular responses to nitrous oxide in patients with normal and high pulmonary vascular resistance. Anesthesiology 57:9, 1982.
132. Hornbein TF, Martin WE, Bonica JJ, et al.: Nitrous oxide effects on the circulatory and ventilatory responses to halothane. Anesthesiology 31:250, 1969.
133. Eger EI II: Isoflurane: A review. Anesthesiology 55: 559, 1981.
134. Pavlin EG: Respiratory pharmacology of inhaled anesthetic agents. *In* Miller RD (ed.): Anesthesia. New York, Churchill Livingstone, 1981, p. 349.
135. Deutsch S, Linde HW, Dripps RD, et al.: Circulatory and respiratory actions of halothane in normal man. Anesthesiology 23:631, 1962.
136. Eger EI II, Smith NT, Stoelting RK, et al.: Cardiovascular effect of halothane in man. Anesthesiology 32:396, 1970.
137. Calverley RK, Smith NT, Prys-Roberts C, et al.: Cardiovascular effects of enflurane anesthesia during controlled ventilation in man. Anesth Analg 57:619, 1978.
138. Stevens WC, Cromwell TH, Halsey MJ, et al.: The cardiovascular effects of a new inhalation anesthetic, Forane, in human volunteers at constant arterial carbon dioxide tension. Anesthesiology 35:8, 1971.
139. Smith NT, Calverley RK, Prys-Roberts C, et al.: Impact of nitrous oxide on the circulation during enflurane anesthesia in man. Anesthesiology 48:345, 1978.
140. Cullen DJ, Eger EI II: The effects of halothane on respiratory and cardiovascular responses to hypoxia in dogs: A dose-response study. Anesthesiology 33:487, 1970.
141. Loarie DJ, Wilkinson P, Tyberg J, et al.: The hemodynamic effects of halothane in anemic dogs. Anesth Analg 58:195, 1979.
142. Brown BR: Anesthetic hepatotoxicity. American Society of Anesthesiologists Annual Refresher Course Lectures, 1981, p. 138a.
143. Lewis GB: Clinical use of isoflurane in pediatric anesthesia, and Steward DJ: Isoflurane: Toronto Experiences. *In* Abstracts of 20th Annual Clinical Conference in Pediatric Anesthesiology. Los Angeles, Children's Hospital of Los Angeles.
144. Benumof J: Anesthesia and the pulmonary circulation. American Society of Anesthesiologists Annual Refresher Course Lectures, 1981, p. 211.
145. Marshall B: Anesthesia and the pulmonary circulation. American Society of Anesthesiologists Annual Refresher Course Lectures, 1980, p. 207.
146. Adams RW, Cucchiara RF, Gronert GA, et al.: Isoflurane and cerebrospinal fluid pressure in neurosurgical patients. Anesthesiology 54:97, 1981.
147. Adams RW, Gronert GA, Sundt TM Jr, et al.: Halothane, hypocapnia, and cerebrospinal fluid pressure in neurosurgery. Anesthesiology 37:510, 1972.
148. Newfield P: Anesthetic considerations in patients with increased intracranial pressure. American Society of Anesthesiologists Annual Refresher Course Lectures, 1981, p. 119.
149. Smith AL, Marque JJ: Anesthetics and cerebral edema. Anesthesiology 45:64, 1976.
150. Sladen R: Can we prevent post-operative renal failure intraoperatively? American Society of Anesthesiologists Annual Refresher Course Lectures, 1981, p. 129.
151. Hug CC Jr: What is the role of narcotic analgesics in anesthesia? American Society of Anesthesiologists Annual Refresher Course Lectures, 1980, p. 138.
152. Stanley, TH: Pharmacology of intravenous narcotic anesthetics. *In* Miller RD (ed.): Anesthesia. New York, Churchill Livingstone, 1981.
153. Hug CC Jr: Pharmacology—anesthetic drugs. *In* Kaplan JA (ed.): Cardiac Anesthesia. New York, Grune and Stratton, 1979, p. 19.
154. Stanley TH, Gray NH, Isern-Amaral JH, et al.:

Comparison of blood requirements during morphine and halothane anesthesia for open-heart surgery. Anesthesiology 41:34, 1974.

155. Lowenstein E: Morphine "anesthesia"—A perspective. Anesthesiology 35:563, 1971.
156. Puerto BA, Wong KC, Puerto AX, et al.: Epinephrine-induced dysrhythmias: Comparison during anesthesia with narcotics and with halogenated inhalation agent in dogs. Can Anesth Soc J 26:263, 1979.
157. Deutsch S, Bastron RD, Pierce EC Jr, et al.: The effects of anesthesia with thiopentone, nitrous oxide, narcotics and neuromuscular blocking drugs on renal function in normal man. Br J Anaesth 41:807, 1969.
158. Stanley TH, Philbin DM, Coggins CH: Fentanyl oxygen anesthesia for coronary artery surgery: Cardiovascular and antidiuretic hormone responses. Can Anaesth Soc J 26:168, 1979.
159. Philbin DM, Coggins CH: Plasma antidiuretic hormone levels in cardiac surgical patients during morphine and halothane anesthesia. Anesthesiology 49:95, 1978.
160. McDermontt R, Stanley TH: The cardiovascular effects of low concentrations of nitrous oxide during morphine anesthesia. Anesthesiology 41:89, 1974.
161. Stanley TH, Liu WS: Cardiovascular effects of meperidine-N_2O anesthesia before and after pancuronium. Anesth Analg 56:669, 1977.
162. Lunn JK, Stanley TH, Eisele J, et al.: High dose fentanyl anesthesia for coronary artery surgery: Plasma fentanyl concentrations and influence of N_2O on cardiovascular responses. Anesth Analg 58:390, 1979.
163. Stanley TH, Bennett GM, Loeser EA, et al.: Cardiovascular effects of diazepam and droperidol during morphine anesthesia. Anesthesiology 44:255, 1976.
164. Bennett GM, Loeser EA, Stanley TH: Cardiovascular effects of scopolamine during morphine-oxygen and morphine–nitrous oxide–oxygen anesthesia in man. Anesthesiology 46:225, 1977.
165. Stoelting RK, Creasser CW, Gibbs PS, et al.: Circulatory effects of halothane added to morphine anesthesia in patients with coronary artery disease. Anesth Anlag 53:449, 1974.
166. Bennett GM, Stanley TH: Cardiovascular effects of fentanyl during enflurane anesthesia in man. Anesth Analg 58:179, 1979.
167. King BD, Elder JD Jr, Dripps RD: The effects of intravenous administration of meperidine upon the circulation of man and upon the circulatory response to tilt. Surg Gynecol Obstet 94:591, 1952.
168. Stanley TH, Webster LR: Anesthetic requirements and cardiovascular effects of fentanyl-oxygen and fentanyl-diazepam-oxygen anesthesia in man. Anesth Analg 57:411, 1978.
169. Stoelting RK, Gibbs PS, Creasser CW, et al.: Hemodynamic and ventilatory responses to fentanyl, fentanyl-droperidol, and nitrous oxide in patients with acquired valvular heart disease. Anesthesiology 42:319, 1975.
170. Gilman AG, Goodman LS, Gilman A: Goodman and Gilman's The Pharmacological Basis of Therapeutics. New York, Macmillan Publishing Company, 1980, p. 357.
171. Robson JG, Davenport HT, Sugiyama R: Differentiation of two types of pain by anesthetics. Anesthesiology 26:31, 1965.
172. Steward DJ: A Manual of Pediatric Anesthesia. New York, Churchill Livingstone, 1979, p. 281.
173. Coté CJ, Goudsouzian NG, Lui LMP, et al.: The dose response of intravenous thiopental for the induction of general anesthesia in unpremedicated children. Anesthesiology 55:703, 1981.
174. Stanley TH: Pharmacology of intravenous non-narcotic anesthetics (excluding ketamine). American Society of Anesthesiologists Annual Refresher Course Lectures, 1980, p. 235.
175. Etsten B, Li TH: Hemodynamic changes during thiopental anesthesia in humans: Cardiac output, stroke volume, total peripheral resistance and intrathoracic blood volume. J Clin Invest 34:500, 1955.
176. Patrick RT, Faulconer A Jr: Respiratory studies during anesthesia with ether and pentothal sodium. Anesthesiology 13:252, 1952.
177. Harrison GA: The influence of different anesthetic agents on the response to respiratory tract irritation. Br J Anesth 34:804, 1962.
178. Marshall LF, Shapiro HM, Rauscher A, et al.: Pentobarbital therapy for intracranial hypertension in metabolic coma Reye's syndrome. Crit Care Med 6:1, 1978.
179. Marshall LF, Smith RW, Shapiro HM: The outcome with aggressive treatment in severe head injuries. J Neurosurg 50:26, 1979.
180. Greenblatt DJ, Shader RI: Benzodiazepines. N Engl J Med 291:1011, 1974.
181. Dalen JE, Evans GL, Banas JS Jr, et al.: The hemodynamic and respiratory effects of diazepam (Valium). Anesthesiology 30:259, 1969.
182. Soroker D, Barzilay E, Konichezhy S, et al.: Respiratory function following premedication with droperidol or diazepam. Anesth Analg 57:695, 1975.
183. Jordan C, Lehane JR, Jones JG: Respiratory depression following diazepam: Reversal with high-dose naloxone. Anesthesiology 53:293, 1980.
184. Forster A, Gardaz JP, Suter PM, et al.: Respiratory depression by midazolam and diazepam. Anesthesiology 53:494, 1980.
185. Morrison JD: Neurolept techniques. *In* Dundee JW, Wyant GM (ed.): Intravenous Anesthesia. New York, Churchill Livingstone, 1974, p. 207.
186. Morrison JD, Loan WB, Dundee JW: Controlled comparison of the efficacy of fourteen preparations in the relief of postoperative pain. Br Med J 3:287, 1971.
187. Loeser EA, Bennett G, Stanley TH, et al.: Comparison of droperidol, haloperidol, and prochlorperazine as postoperative anti-emetics. Can Anesth Soc J 26:125, 1979.
188. Whitwam JG, Russel WJ: The acute cardiovascular changes and adrenergic blockade by droperidol in man. Br J Anaesth 43:581, 1971.
189. Hyatt M, Muldoon SM, Rorie DK: Droperidol, a selective antagonist of postsynaptic α-adrenoceptor in the canine saphenous vein. Anesthesiology 53:281, 1980.
190. Chasapakis G, Kakis N, Sakkaklis C, et al.: Use of ketamine and pancuronium for anesthesia for patients in hemorrhagic shock. Anesth Analg 52:282, 1973.
191. Waxman K, Shoemaker WC, Lippman M: Cardiovascular effects of anesthetic induction with ketamine. Anesth Analg 58:355, 1980.
192. Weiskopf RB, Townsley MI, Riorden KK, et al.: Comparison of cardiopulmonary responses to graded hemorrhage during enflurane, halothane,

isoflurane, and ketamine anesthesia. Anesth Analg 60:481, 1981.

193. Way WL: Ketamine: What is fact or fantasy. American Society of Anesthesioloists Annual Refresher Course Lectures, 1980, p. 236.
194. Thorsen T, Gran L: Ketamine/diazepam infusion anesthesia with special attention to the effects on cerebrospinal fluid pressure and arterial blood pressure. Acta Anesth Scand 24:1, 1980.
195. Idvall J: Influence of ketamine anesthesia on cardiac output and tissue perfusion in rats subjected to hemorrhage. Anesthesiology 55:297, 1981.
196. Ali HH: Clinical pharmacology and monitoring of a succinylcholine neuromuscular blockade. American Society of Anesthesiology Annual Refresher Course Lectures, 1980, p. 134.
197. Liu LMP, DeCook TH, Goudsouzian NG, et al.: Dose response to intramuscular succinylcholine in children. Anesthesiology 55:599, 1981.
198. DeCook TH, Goudsouzian NG: Tachyphylaxis and phase II block development during infusion of succinylcholine in children. Anesth Analg 59:639, 1980.
199. Mazze RI, Escue HM, Houston JB: Hyperkalemia and cardiovascular collapse following administration of succinylcholine to the traumatized patient. Anesthesiology 31:540, 1969.
200. Birch AA, Mitchell GD, Playford GA, et al.: Changes in serum potassium response to succinylcholine following trauma. JAMA 210:490, 1969.
201. Iwatsuki N, Kuroda N, Amaha K, et al.: Succinylcholine-induced hyperkalemia in patients with ruptured cerebral aneurysms. Anesthesiology 53:64, 1980.
202. Muravchick S, Burkett L, Gold MI: Succinylcholine-induced fasciculations and intragastric pressure during induction of anesthesia. Anesthesiology 55:180, 1981.
203. Salem MR, Wong AY, Lin YH: The effect of suxamethonium on the intragastric pressure in infants and children. Br J Anaesth 44:166, 1972.
204. Brotherton WP, Matteo RS: Pharmacokinetics and pharmocodynamics of metocurine in humans with and without renal failure. Anesthesiology 55:273, 1981.
205. Donlon JD, Savarese JJ, Ali HH, et al.: Human dose-response curves for neuromuscular blocking drugs: A comparison of two methods of construction and analysis. Anesthesiology 53:161, 1980.
206. Ham J, Stanski DR, Newfield P, et al.: Pharmacokinetics and dynamics of *d*-tubocurarine during hypothermia in humans. Anesthesiology 55:631, 1981.
207. Savarese J: Update on muscle relaxants and their antagonists. American Society of Anesthesiologists Annual Refresher Course Lectures. 1980, p. 135c.
208. Sokoll MD, Gergis SD: Antibiotics and neuromuscular function. Anesthesiology 55:148, 1981.
209. Fahey, MR, Morris RB, Miller RD, et al.: Clinical pharmacology of ORG NC45 (Norcuron™): A new nondepolarizing muscle relaxant. Anesthesiology 55:6, 1981.
210. Son SL, Waud BE, Waud DR, et al.: A comparison of the neuromuscular blocking and vagolytic effects of ORG NC45 and pancuronium. Anesthesiology 55:12, 1981.
211. Cronnelly R: Update on muscle relaxants and their antagonists. American Society of Anesthesiologists Annual Refresher Course Lectures, 1980, p. 135a.
212. Morris RB, Cronnelly R, Miller RD, et al.: Pharmacokinetics of edrophonium and neostigime when antagonizing *d*-tubocurarine neuromuscular blockade in man. Anesthesiology 54:399, 1981.
213. Ferguson A, Egerszegi P, Bevan DR, et al.: Neostigmine, pyridostigmine, and edrophonium as antagonists of pancuronium. Anesthesiology 53:390, 1980.
214. Eger EI II: Anesthetic Uptake and Action. Baltimore, Williams and Wilkins Company, 1974, p. 126.
215. Benumof Jl: Respiratory physiology and respiratory function during anesthesia. *In* Miller RD (ed.): Anesthesia. New York, Churchill Livingstone, 1981, p. 681.
216. Froese AB, Bryan AC: Effects of anesthesia and paralysis on diaphragmatic mechanics in man. Anesthesiology 41:242, 1974.
217. Breivik H, Grenvik A, Millen E, et al.: Normalizing low arterial CO_2 tension during mechanical ventilation. Chest 63:525, 1973.
218. Utting JE: Hypocapnia. *In* Gray TC, Nunn JF, Utting JJE (eds.): General Anaesthesia. Boston, Butterworths, 1980, p. 461.
219. Prys-Roberts C: Hypercapnia. *In* Nunn JF, Utting JE (eds.): General Anaesthesia. Boston, Butterworths, 1980, p. 435.
220. Chalon J, Loew DA, Malebranche J: Effects of dry anaesthetic gases on tracheobronchial ciliated epithelium. Anesthesiology 37:338, 1972.
221. Chalon J, Ali M, Ramanathan S, et al.: The humidification of anesthetic gases: Its importance and control. Can Anaesth Soc J 26:361, 1979.
222. Miller RD, Brzica SM: Blood, blood component, colloid, and autotransfusion therapy. *In* Miller RD (ed.): Anesthesia. New York, Churchill Livingstone, 1981, p. 885.
223. DeVenuto F: Hemoglobin solutions as oxygen-delivering resuscitation fluids. Crit Care Med 10:238, 1982.
224. Donlon JV Jr: Anesthesia for eye, ear, nose and throat surgery. *In* Miller RD (ed.): Anesthesia. New York, Churchill Livingstone, 1981, p. 1265.
225. Ausinsch B, Rayburn RL, Munson ES, et al.: Ketamine and intraocular pressures in children. Anesth Analg 55:773, 1976.
226. Ausinsch B, Graves SA, Munson ES, et al.: Intraocular pressure in children duing isoflurane and halothane anesthesia. Anesthesiology 42:167, 1975.
227. Arthur DS, Dewar KMS: Anesthesia for eye surgery in children. Br J Anaesth 52:681, 1980.
228. De Campo T, Aldrete JA: The anesthetic management of the severely burned paient. Intensive Care Med 7:55, 1981.
229. Eather KF: Regional anesthesia for infants and children. Int Anesthesiol Clin 13:19, 1975.
230. Moore DC: Regional Block. Springfield, Illinois, CC Thomas, 1971, p. 243.
231. Murphy TM: Nerve blocks. *In* Miller RD (ed.): Anesthesia. New York, Churchill Livingstone, 1981, p. 605.
232. Winnie AP: Interscalene brachial plexus block. Anesth Analg 49:455, 1970.
233. Winnie AP, Ramamurthy S, Durrani Z: The inguinal perivascular technique of lumbar plexus anesthesia: The "3 in 1 block." Anesth Analg 52:989, 1973.
234. Feeley TW: The recovery room. *In* Miller RD (ed.):

Anesthesia. New York, Churchill Livingstone, 1981, p. 1335.

235. Bennett EJ, Bowyer DE: Principles of pediatric anesthesia. Springfield, Illinois, Charles C Thomas, 1982, p. 346.
236. Drain CB, Shipley SB: The Recovery Room. Philadelphia, WB Saunders Company, 1979, p. 228.
237. Kirby RR, Robinson E, Schulz J, et al.: Continuous-flow ventilation as an alternative to assisted or controlled ventilation in infants. Anesth Analg 51:871, 1972.
238. Downs JB, Klein, EF, Modell JH, et al.: Intermittent mandatory ventilation: A new approach to weaning patients from mechanical ventilators. Chest 64:331, 1975.
239. Kirby RR, Smith RA: The anesthesiologist and intensive care. *In* Miller RD (ed.): Anesthesia. New York, Churchill Livingstone, 1981, p. 1449.
240. Smith RA: Respiratory care. *In* Miller RD (ed.): Anesthesia. New York, Churchill Livingstone, 1981.
241. Hedley-Whyte J, Burgess GE III, Feeley RW, et al.: Applied Physiology of Respiratory Care. Boston, Little, Brown and Company, 1976, p. 5.
242. Hoff BH, Flemming DC, Sasse F: Use of positive airway pressure without endotracheal intubation. Crit Care Med 7:559, 1979.
243. Gold MI: Is intermittent positive pressure breathing therapy (IPPB RX) necessary in the surgical patient? Ann Surg 184:122, 1976.
244. Bartlett RH, Gazzaniga AB, Geraghty TR: Respiratory maneuvers to prevent postoperative pulmonary complications: A critical review. JAMA 224:1017, 1973.
245. Kirby RR, Smith RA: The anesthesiologist and intensive care. *In*: Miller RD (ed.): Anesthesia. New York, Churchill Livingstone, 1981, p. 1447.

Selected Readings

Dunbar BS, McGill WA, Epstein BS: Anesthesia for the injured child. *In* Randolph J, et al.: The Injured Child: Surgical Management. Chicago, Year Book Medical Publishers, 1979, p. 107. *This chapter is an overview of anesthesia for the injured child. Many of the differences in anesthetizing children who have suffered injuries versus adults are brought out well in this chapter.*

Furman EB (ed.): The anesthesiologist's role in pediatric acute care. Int Anesthesiol Clin 13:1, 1975. *This edition of the clinics covers almost all aspects of anesthesia for the pediatric patient requiring acute care. Chapters by recognized experts cover muscle relaxants, regional anesthesia, respiratory problems, fluid management, and anesthesia for the burned child.*

Giesecke AH Jr (ed.): Anesthesia for the surgery of trauma. Clin Anesthesia 11:3, 1976. *This book deals rather extensively with the subject of anesthesia for the surgery of trauma. Although written with the adult patient primarily in mind, it gives the reader a good understanding of preanesthetic, intraoperative, and postanesthetic care.*

Goldberg AI: Anesthesia and intensive care. *In* Touloukian J (ed.): Pediatric Trauma. New York, John Wiley and Sons, 1978, p. 105. *This chapter extensively covers most aspects of anesthesia and intensive care for the pediatric trauma victim. Included are initial resuscitation, preoperative considerations, induction procedures, intraoperative management, postoperative considerations, airway management, and anesthesia for minor trauma.*

Gregory GA: Pediatric anesthesia. *In* Miller RD (ed.): New York, Churchill Livingstone, 1981, p. 1197. *This chapter is included because it provides a recent comprehensive treatment of the subject of pediatric anesthesia by one of the recognized experts. It also presents a different viewpoint on several subjects, which is worthy of the reader's cognizance.*

McIntyre KM, Parker MR: Standards and guidelines for cardiopulmonary resuscitation (CPR) and emergency cardiac care (ECC). JAMA 244:453, 1980. *This article is must reading for anyone involved in cardiopulmonary resuscitation of children. It includes information on airway management, cardiac massage, and pharmacologic management of the arrested individual or patient in shock.*

Smith RM: Anesthesia for outpatient and emergency surgery. *In* Anesthesia for Infants and Children. 4th ed. St. Louis, CV Mosby Company, 1980, p. 513. *This is a good chapter to introduce the reader to various considerations of particular importance in the pediatric trauma patient. It is helpful largely from a practical and clinical standpoint.*

Steward DJ: Management of trauma, including acute burns and scalds. *In* Manual of Pediatric Anesthesia. New York, Churchill Livingstone, 1979, p. 207. *This chapter gives a short overall presentation of the most important concepts for the anesthetic management of the pediatric trauma patient.*

Tunell WP, Smith EI: Respiratory support in trauma. *In* Randolph J, et al.: The Injured Child: Surgical Management. Chicago, Year Book Medical Publishers, 1979, p. 59. *This short chapter describes the recognition, prevention, and treatment (including intubation and tracheostomy) of respiratory failure in pediatrics trauma victims.*

Weiskopf RB, Fairley HB: Anesthesia for major trauma. Surg Clin North Am 62:31, 1982. *This is a rather concise, but up-to-date overview of anesthesia for trauma patients, with the major emphasis placed on airway and fluid management.*

Zimmerman BL: Uncommon Problems in Acute Trauma. *In* Katz J, Benumof J, Kods LB (eds.): Uncommon Diseases: Pathophysiologic and Clinical Correlations, Philadelphia, WB Saunders Company, 1981, p. 635. *This is an excellent, up-to-date chapter on the complete subject of anesthesia for the trauma victim. The chapter is extensive, with over 200 references. Although written with the adult patient in mind, most of the basic principles apply to all trauma patients.*

CHAPTER

4 Fluid and Electrolyte Management

RICHARD L. SIEGLER

BODY VOLUME AND COMPOSITION

The objective of all fluid and electrolyte therapy is to establish and maintain the normal volume and composition of the body fluids. Approximately 60 per cent of the body weight of a child and adolescent is water; in infants, up to 75 per cent is water. Total body water (TBW) is composed of the intracellular fluid (ICF) and the extracellular fluid (ECF) (Fig. 4–1). The intracellular fluid compartment, which accounts for approximately 40 per cent of body weight and two thirds of TBW, is relatively free of sodium but very rich in potassium, phosphate, protein, and magnesium (Fig. 4–2). A sodium pump, located at the cell membrane, actively exchanges sodium for potassium.

The extracellular fluid (ECF), which accounts for approximately 20 per cent of body weight and one third of TBW, is in turn composed of the interstitial and intravascular compartments (Fig. 4–1). Sodium is the major cation in the extracellular compartment, and chloride and bicarbonate the major anions. Potassium is present in only modest quantities (Fig. 4–2). The electrolyte composition of the interstitial and intravascular fluids is almost identical, except for a lower concentration of Cl^- and HCO_3^- in the intravascular fluid to offset the negatively charged protein.

Because the concentration of intracellular electrolytes is relatively fixed, the distribution of total body water between the intracellular and extracellular compartments is largely determined by the osmolar concentration of sodium and its attendant anions. For this reason, a fall in the serum sodium concentration results in a shift of water from the extracellular to the intracellular compartment, and contraction of the extracellular compartment results in a contraction of its subcompartments, which include the intravascular space. Conversely, an increase in the extracellular sodium concentration effects a transfer of intracellular water to the extracellular compartment and results in an ex-

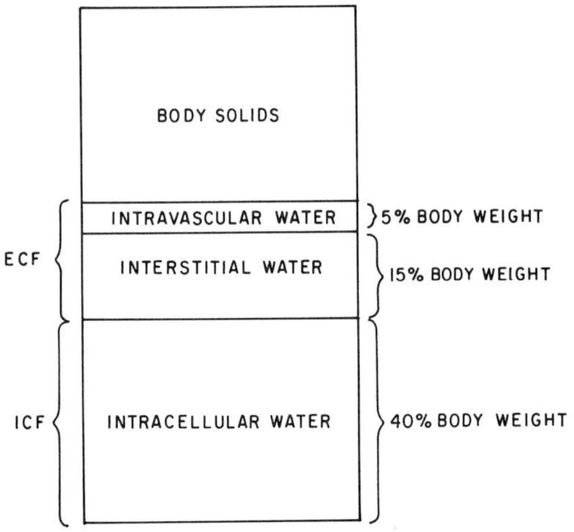

BODY SOLIDS
ECF: INTRAVASCULAR WATER — 5% BODY WEIGHT
ECF: INTERSTITIAL WATER — 15% BODY WEIGHT
ICF: INTRACELLULAR WATER — 40% BODY WEIGHT

Figure 4–1. Body fluid compartments.

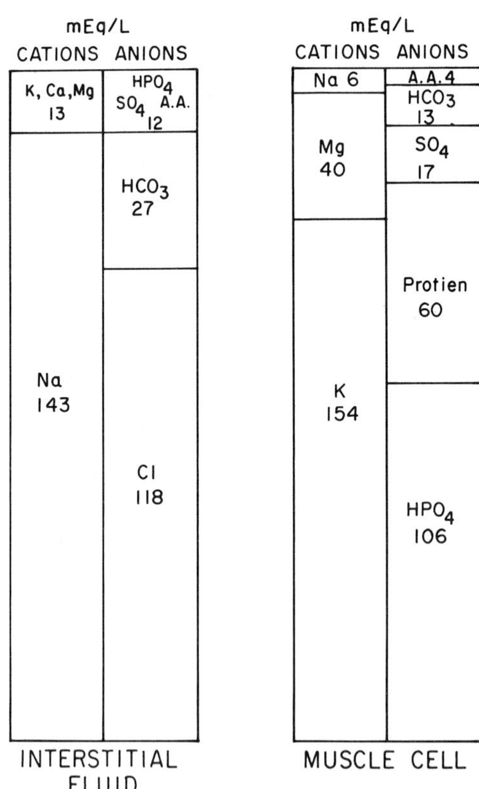

Figure 4–2. Body fluid electrolyte composition.

panded interstitial and intravascular volumes. Remember that body salt (sodium) is the major determinant of extracellular volume; therefore, if there is an abnormality in body volume (e.g., edema, dehydration), "think" salt, not water.

The distribution of extracellular water between the two subcompartments is largely determined by the differential concentration of the colloids, mainly albumin and the other proteins, between these two compartments. Gram for gram, albumin exerts four times more oncotic pressure than globulin. Even though there is more total albumin in the interstitial compartment because of its much larger volume, the concentration (g/dl) of albumin is higher in the intravascular compartment because it is retained within the capillaries. If the serum albumin concentration decreases, a greater percentage of the extracellular water will move to the interstitial compartment, and the intravascular (blood) volume will contract.

Although electrochemical principles dictate that the concentration of plasma anions equals that of the cations, the electrolytes customarily measured (Na^+, K^+, Cl^-, HO_3^-) reveal an anion gap (cations minus anions) of approximately 11 to 19 mEq/L. This "normal" gap is accounted for by unmeasured anions, largely by the negatively charged proteins, phosphates, and sulfates. Substantial increases in this gap, as will be discussed later, are seen in metabolic acidosis that is caused by the addition of acid.

With the exception of neonates, severely stressed individuals, and those with a renal or adrenal disorder, normal body volume and composition can be maintained despite wide variation in the intake or output of fluids and electrolytes (Fig. 4–3). This impressive water and electrolyte tolerance is due to the kidney's unique ability to modify the glomerular filtrate by selectively retaining (that is, reabsorbing) or rejecting (excreting) filtered water and electrolytes according to the needs of the body. This quantitative and qualitative filtrate modification occurs virtually throughout the length of the nephron.

In response to either an increase or decrease in the effective arterial blood volume (renal perfusion pressure), the proximal convoluted tubule either decreases or increases the isotonic reabsorption of filtered salt and water. The precise mechanisms responsible for this variable isotonic reabsorption of filtrate are uncertain but may be secondary to changes in the serum concentration of a "natriuretic factor" (a "third" factor) or to changes in the osmotic pressure of the colloids in the peritubular capillaries, or both. Under normal circumstances, about 65 per cent of the filtered salt and water are reabsorbed isotonically in the proximal tubule.

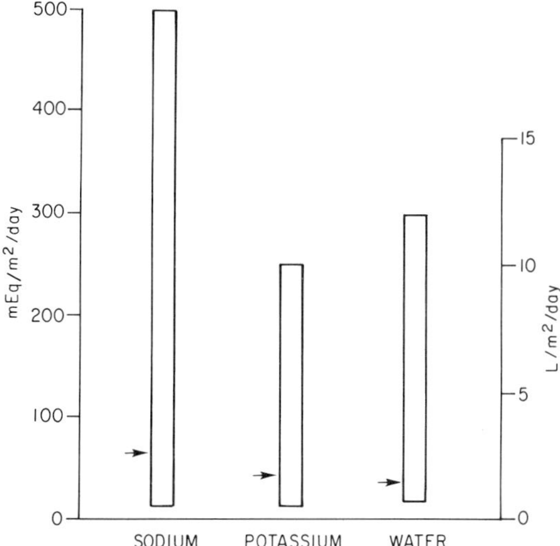

Figure 4–3. Limits of tolerance. Customary intake indicated by arrows. Under conditions of stress, minimum K^+ requirement may increase; maximum Na^+ and H_2O limits may decrease.

The ascending limb of Henle then modifies the filtrate by "actively" pumping an additional 25 per cent of chloride into the renal interstitium; this is followed by the passive transfer of sodium. This process contributes to the hyperosmolar composition of the renal medullary interstitium and makes free water (that is, water free of solute) available for excretion.

The distal nephron (i.e., the distal convoluted tubule and its collecting ducts) further modifies the filtrate by retaining or rejecting, by separate mechanisms, the remaining salt and water. Increases or decreases in the effective arterial blood volume either suppress or stimulate, respectively, aldosterone production, which modulates the reabsorption of the remaining 10 per cent of urinary sodium chloride. In addition, a fall in the effective arterial blood volume, as sensed by volume and pressure receptors in the left atrium and carotid sinus, or a rise in the serum osmolality (that is, in the serum sodium concentration), as detected by the osmoreceptors in the brain, stimulates the pituitary secretion of antidiuretic hormone (ADH, vasopressin). This hormone activates adenyl cyclase, which results in cyclic adenosine monophosphate (AMP) production and facilitates an increase in water permeability in the distal tubules and collecting ducts. The medullary interstitium is normally hyperosmotic (as high as 1400 [mOsm]/L) secondary to the active transport of salt in the ascending limb of Henle and to the passive diffusion of urea into the distal nephron. Therefore, in the presence of ADH, water passively diffuses down the concentration gradients, resulting in a urinary specific gravity as high as 1.036 (1400 [mOsm]/L).

Even though the kidney possesses an impressive ability to maintain homeostasis, that ability is limited. Imbalance will occur if the water or electrolyte intake or output is sufficient to exceed renal compensatory capabilities.

If 3 to 5 days are allowed for adaptive changes, an older infant or child can tolerate as little as 10 to as much as 500 mEq/m^2 of body surface area (BSA)* of sodium per day; however, under conditions of stress, a range of 50 to 250 mEq/m^2/day is a safer estimate. Amounts above or below these limits or tolerance result in edema or volume depletion, respectively.

Except when oliguria is present or changes in serum pH are occurring, potassium tolerance is approximately 10 to 250 mEq/m^2/day. Greater or lesser amounts cause hyper- or hypokalemia, respectively. Under conditions of stress, the excretion of potassium may increase and result in a higher than usual minimum requirement for normal maintenance.

The minimum requirements for water depends upon the insensible and sensible losses, upon the urinary solute load, and upon the ability to concentrate the urine. It is therefore not possible to give an absolute figure, but an estimate can be calculated. Assuming an average solute load and concentrating ability, the minimum figure is approximately 700 ml/m^2/day. With a limited urinary concentration ability, as seen in the very young infant, minimum water requirements are greater. Conversely, with a decreased solute load (i.e., an intake that is low in electrolytes and proteins), water requirements will be less. Insufficient water intake will cause hypernatremia (hyperosmolality), cell shrinkage, and dehydration.

*Values are expressed in terms of square meters (M^2) of body surface area. A 3-kg newborn is approximately 0.2 M^2, a 30-kg child, 1.0 m^2, and a 50-kg child, 1.5 M^2. Please refer to a normogram for more details.

Maximum water tolerance for a normal person is approximately 12 L/m^2 day. Values above this result in water retention, dilutional hyponatremia (hyposmolarity), and cellular swelling, a condition known as water intoxication. As will be discussed later, there are conditions that are characterized by an inability to form and/or excrete free water normally; these further decrease the affected individual's maximum water intolerance.

In summary, modification of the glomerular filtrate by the variable reabsorption of isotonic quantities of salt and water in the proximal tubule and by the independent retention or rejection of the remaining salt and water in the distal nephron maintains the body's salt and water balance unless intake or output exceeds limits of the body's tolerance.

FLUID THERAPY

Guidelines for resuscitation fluid therapy are covered in Chapter 1. The following discussion will assume that any depletion in volume will have been corrected during the resuscitation phase of therapy.

Maintenance Fluids

If a child already has normal body volume and composition, maintaining the balance requires that fluid and electrolyte intake (oral, enteral, intravenous [IV]) equals output (skin, lungs, gastrointestinal [GI], urinary). Although the kidney has an amazing ability to maintain the salt and water balance, the renal homeostasic mechanisms that regulate the limits of tolerance may be impaired in a stressed or traumatized child. Therefore, it is prudent that the fluids selected place little additional stress on the kidneys in making the compensatory adjustments. Table 4–1

Table 4–1. CUSTOMARY DAILY MAINTENANCE FLUID AND ELECTROLYTE REQUIREMENTS

	Per m^2 BSA	Per kg Body Weight	Per 100 kcal
Water (ml)	1200–1800	50†	100
Sodium (mEq)	30–60	1–2	3
Chloride (mEq)	30–60	1–2	3
Potassium (mEq)	20–40	0.75–1.5	2

*BSA-body surface area.
†Varies with size of child, 100 ml/kg for infants, 40 ml/kg for adolescents.

Table 4–2. REPRESENTATIVE WATER INTAKE AND OUTPUT IN A 30-kg CHILD

Intake	(ml/day)	Output	(ml/day)
Fluid	800	Urine	800
Water content of food	500	Skin	300
Water of oxidation	200	Lungs	250
		Stool	100
Total	1,500	*Total*	1,500

contains the customary fluid and electrolyte maintenance recommendations for well, nonstressed children. Even though one can usually deviate from these guidelines without upsetting the salt and water balance, deviation is imprudent given the difficulties in evaluating and quantifying renal compensatory capability in injured and stressed children.

Maintenance water requirements include replacement of insensible (skin and lung evaporation) as well as sensible (urine, GI, sweat) water losses. The actual volume requirements are less than the total losses because of the production of endogenous water (e.g., water of oxidation, preformed water). Table 4–2 illustrates customary intake and output in a 30-kg child. Maintenance water requirements can be related to body weight, body surface area, or caloric expenditure. Given even modest renal regulatory capability, any of these methods are sufficiently accurate for clinical purposes under normal conditions. All these methods provide sufficient free water (water free of electrolytes) to replace both the insensible water loss (which is electrolyte free) and water obligatorily excreted with the urinary solute. Failure to do so would result in hypernatremic dehydration.

It must be remembered that there are numerous conditions that either increase or decrease customary water maintenance requirements and require an adjustment in intake (Table 4–3).

Urinary electrolyte losses normally mirror

Table 4–3. WATER REQUIREMENT MODIFICATION

Factors That Increase Requirements	Factors That Decrease Requirements
Fever	Renal failure
Hyperventilation	Use of mist tent
Osmotic diuresis	Use of humidified oxygen
Sweating	Impaired renal free water excretion (e.g., SIADH*)

*SIADH = syndrome of inappropriate antidiuretic hormone.

intake. As with water balance, many factors influence electrolyte requirements. Abnormal GI losses (e.g., suction, vomiting) or "third spacing" of salt and water in instances of tissue trauma, burns, or ileus, temporarily increases electrolyte requirements.

Activation of the renin-angiotension-aldosterone system, which occurs in response to a decrease in effective arterial blood volume, an increase in circulating catecholamines, or elevations in the serum potassium concentration, stimulates sodium retention and potassium excretion.

Because approximately 98 per cent of total body potassium is located within the cell, its concentration within the cell is almost 40 times greater than in the extracellular compartment. Therefore, whenever there is any destruction of cells, including the red cells, a rapid and substantial rise in the serum potassium concentration should be anticipated. A very rapid transfer of intracellular potassium to the extracellular compartment also occurs as a response to acidosis. A 0.6 to 1.0 mEq rise in serum potassium for every 0.1 decrease in the serum pH should be expected. Conversely, with the correction of acidosis, a rapid cellular influx of potassium may result in severe hypokalemia.

Volume Monitoring

Invasive monitoring, using central venous or flotation catheters (Swan-Ganz catheters), provides an accurate assessment of intravascular (blood) volume. These techniques, coupled with cardiac output measurements (e.g., thermal dilution), permit manipulation pharmacologically of the preload (diastolic filling pressure) and afterload (systemic resistance) to maximize cardiac output and tissue perfusion while avoiding pulmonary edema.

In less critically ill children, who do not require invasive monitoring, accurate, daily weight measurements and periodic, careful physical examinations provide a reliable assessment of extracellular volume. Even though total body sodium is the major determinant of extracellular volume, the serum sodium concentration bears no predictable relationship to total body sodium and extracellular volume. For this reason, using the serum sodium concentration as an indicator of total body sodium is misleading. The serum sodium concentration merely reflects the relative concentrations of extracellular salt and water. An abnormality in the serum sodium concentration usually indicates an abnormality in total body water rather than in total body sodium.

Osmolar Monitoring

Measurements of the serum sodium concentration provide a practical estimate of osmolar balance. Unless severe azotemia or hyperglycemia is present, sodium and its attendant anions account for almost all extracellular osmolality. Serum osmolality can be estimated by multiplying the serum sodium concentration by two and adding 10 milliosmoles for the usual osmotic contributions of urea and glucose. Actual measurements of serum osmolality are rarely necessary.

A rising serum sodium concentration, that is, a rising osmolality, generally reflects a deficiency in total body water and, thus, the need for more water. Conversely, a falling serum sodium concentration in a nondehydrated patient indicates water retention and the need for fluid restriction.

In summary, although guidelines for fluid and electrolyte volume and composition are helpful in planning therapy, they do not replace the need for meticulous, periodic physical and laboratory assessments. Frequent examination of the child for signs of dehydration or edema, careful daily body weight determinations, serial measurements of the serum electrolytes, and, if appropriate, invasive monitoring will best serve to avoid major and potentially dangerous fluid and electrolyte problems.

Selecting the Proper Maintenance Solution and Route of Administration

A variety of commercially prepared oral and IV maintenance fluids are available. However, for short-term IV therapy, 0.2 per cent saline in 5 per cent dextrose with 20 to 30 mEq/L of potassium chloride suffices. The commercial maintenance solutions generally approximate this concentration of sodium chloride and potassium, but they also have the additional electrolytes necessary for longer periods of fluid support. Refer to Table 4–1 for maintenance fluid volume and composition guidelines. The use of these guidelines does not preclude the necessity of periodic physical and laboratory assessments. Recall that if a patient is not receiving sufficient calories, a daily weight loss approximating 1 to 1.5 per cent of the patient's weight should be expected. A weight loss of less than this amount generally indicates salt and water retention.

In a conscious stable patient with normal GI function, fluids may be given orally or, if the patient is anorectic but conscious, by nasogastric tube. Customarily, however, fluids are given intravenously. In stable, young infants, a small butterfly needle can usually be inserted into one of the scalp veins. In older infants and children, a small needle or IV catheter can be placed into a hand, arm, or foot vein. Occasionally, the external jugular vein will need to be catheterized or an IV cutdown procedure performed. Maintaining dependable IV access capable of accommodating a rapid volume infusion is imperative in unstable patients. Special care must be taken, particularly when utilizing the small vessels, that hyperosmotic or calcium-containing fluids do not extravasate into the subcutaneous tissue because this may result in severe tissue necrosis.

SPECIAL PROBLEMS

Hyponatremia

Hyponatremia, which is characterized by a low sodium concentration in the serum and interstitial fluid, causes a shift of water into the cells and results in cerebral edema. Although hyponatremia may be secondary to a decrease in total body sodium (owing to an inadequate replacement of GI sodium losses or to a shift of sodium into the cells), it is usually due to water retention (Table 4–4).

Many factors in addition to renal failure impair the kidney's ability to eliminate water. A decrease in the effective arterial blood volume (because of volume depletion, heart failure, hypoalbuminemia) causes increased isotonic reabsorption of filtrate in the proximal tubule. This increased reabsorption decreases the volume of the filtrate reaching the ascending limb of Henle, where free water is formed.

Even with the delivery of normal volumes of filtrate to Henle's loop, hypokalemia, hypercalcemia, and loop diuretics (e.g., furosemide) impair the loop's capacity to pump out salt and form free water.

And finally, even if normal amounts of free water are generated by the ascending limb of Henle, the inappropriate elaboration

Table 4–4. CAUSES OF HYPONATREMIA

Salt Depletion*
- GI losses (vomiting, diarrhea, suction, fistulas)
- Renal losses (diuretics, adrenal insufficiency)
- Skin losses (burns, sweating)

Sodium Shifts Into Cells (hypokalemia, "sick" sodium pump)

Dilutional Hyponatremia
- Shift of intracellular water to extracellular space (hyperglycemia)
- Excessive water administration
- Diminished free water generation
  - Renal failure
  - Decreased delivery of filtrate to loop of Henle secondary to increased proximal tubular reabsorption (hypovolemia, heart failure, shock, burns, sepsis, peritonitis)
  - Impaired loop function (loop diuretics, hypokalemia)
- Impaired free water excretion
  - ADH† secretion secondary to decreased effective arterial blood volume (shock, third spacing, volume depletion, heart failure)
  - Inappropriate secretion of ADH (SIADH‡)
  - Brain injury or infection
  - Lung disease (infection, atelectasis)
  - Drugs (opiates, barbiturates)

*Note that gastrointestinal (GI), renal, and skin fluid losses are almost always hyponatremic (i.e., contain more water than salt). Therefore, hyponatremia occurs only if these losses are replaced with fluids that contain even less salt.

†ADH = Antidiuretic hormone.

‡SIADH = Syndrome of inappropriate diuretic hormone.

of antidiuretic hormone (ADH) can cause a dilutional hyponatremia by facilitating an increase in the reabsorption of water in the distal convoluted tubules and collecting ducts. In traumatized patients, this occurs most often after a head injury or the administration of drugs (e.g., opiates and barbituates), which either potentiate or mimic the action of the ADH or cause its inappropriate release by the posterior pituitary gland. The diagnosis of the syndrome of inappropriate ADH (SIADH) secretion should not be entertained until (1) renal failure, (2) decreased effective arterial blood volume (EABV), (3) impaired loop function, and (4) hypoadrenalism have been excluded as explanations for the hyponatremia. ADH activity (as shown by urinary specific gravity > 1.004 to 1.006) in a volume-expanded hyponatremic patient is inappropriate and generally constitutes sufficient evidence for the diagnosis of SIADH. Supportive evidence includes a high (>40 mEq/L) urinary sodium concentration (which is evidence of volume expansion) and a low blood urea nitrogen (BUN), and a low serum uric acid concentration (which is secondary to volume expansion and hemodilution). Peripheral edema is usually minimal or absent. However, an elevated BUN and a low (< 10 mEq/L) urinary sodium concentration suggests impaired generation of free water caused by a decrease in the EABV.

Treatment depends on the cause and the magnitude of the hyponatremia. If the low serum sodium concentration is caused by a deficit in total body sodium, saline should be administered. Although hyponatremia because of salt depletion indicates the need for sodium in excess of water, administration of hypertonic saline is usually unnecessary, except in instances of severe water intoxication (as indicated by coma, seizures). Normal (0.9 per cent) saline generally suffices if it is also used for replacing insensible fluid loss. This procedure, in effect, provides salt in excess of water, promotes a positive sodium balance, and corrects the hyponatremia.

On the other hand, if the hyponatremia is dilutional, restricting fluids rather than administering sodium is the proper therapy. However, the fluid restriction must be sufficient to produce a negative water balance, which will be evident in weight loss. This necessitates fluid intake that is less than the ongoing losses. One convenient guide is to administer only enough water to replace the insensible water losses, thereby allowing urinary water excretion to produce a negative water balance and to correct the dilutional hyponatremia. It is actually necessary to cause a decrease in body weight to be assured that the patient is experiencing a negative water balance.

In addition, if the child is free of edema and if the urinary sodium loss is substantial (e.g., as in SIADH), the urinary sodium should be replaced in order to prevent eventual salt depletion. The administration of hypertonic (3 per cent) saline should be reserved for patients with severe hyponatremia (< 110 mEq/L) or for those with hyponatremic encephalopathy.

The development of encephalopathy is related both to the magnitude of the hyponatremia and to the rapidity of its development. Although an abrupt fall in the serum sodium concentration to 125 mEq/L may be sufficient to cause seizures, a slow decrease to 115 mEq/L may be well tolerated. However, serum levels below 110 mEq/L almost always cause central nervous system (CNS) signs and symptoms and should be considered life-threatening. Even under these circumstances, it is rarely necessary to raise the serum sodium concentration to more than 120 to

125 mEq/L. In calculating the sodium chloride dose, it is important to remember that its "effective" space of distribution is total body rather than extracellular water. Therefore, the appropriate quantity of sodium is calculated by multiplying the desired change in the serum sodium concentration by the space of distribution. For example, to increase the serum sodium concentration from 110 to 120 mEq/L in a 10-Kg child, the correct amount of sodium (mEq) would be as follows: 10 (the desired mEq/L change in sodium concentration) times 6 (the space of distribution in liters), or 60 mEq. The 3 per cent hypertonic saline solution contains approximately 0.5 mEq of sodium per milliliter. If the entire amount were infused rapidly, the serum concentration would rise transiently above 120 mEq/L because the immediate space of distribution is the extracellular compartment, which approximates 20 per cent of body weight and only one third of the eventual space of distribution. The distribution of the total body water from the intracellular to the extracellular compartment occurs fairly rapidly following an infusion of hypertonic saline, and the total amount can safely be infused over a 1-hour period.

Hypernatremia

Hypernatremia can result from an infusion of hypertonic sodium solutions e.g., sodium bicarbonate), but it more commonly occurs as a result of inadequate water replacement (Table 4–5). It is easy to fall behind with water replacement if a child has increased insensible losses because of fever or hyperventilation, GI losses from nasogastric suction, or urinary losses caused by posttraumatic diabetes insipidus or a mannitol-induced diuresis. Hypernatremia initially causes a transfer of intracellular water to the extracellular compartment and results in cell shrinkage. In the CNS, this can cause an initial contraction of the brain mass and produce CNS dysfunction or intracranial hemorrhage, or both. After a variable and uncertain period of time (from to 8 to 36 hours), compensatory mechanisms, which are poorly understood, such as the generation of idiogenic osmoles or the influx of additional potassium, or both, cause a re-expansion of the intracellular compartment to its previous volume. Because the osmolalities of the two compartments are now equal, the rapid infusion of hyponatremic fluids will decrease the extracellular osmolality and result in cerebral edema and seizures.

Table 4–5. CAUSES OF HYPERNATREMIA

Excessive Sodium Administration
Hypertonic sodium bicarbonate administration
Hypertonic saline infusion
Water Depletion (loss of water in excess of salt)
GI* tract (vomiting, diarrhea, suction)
Skin (sweating, fever, burns)
Lungs (hyperventilation)
Kidney (diabetes insipidus, osmotic diuresis, diuretics).

GI = gastrointestinal.

Assuming that large quantities of hypernatremic fluids (e.g., hypertonic sodium bicarbonate) have not been given and that there are no signs of an expanded extracellular compartment (as manifested by edema or an elevated central venous pressure), it can reasonably be assumed that the hypernatremia is caused by a deficiency in total body water. If the serum sodium concentrations are being carefully followed, early adjustments in the fluid regimen can correct the water deficit and avoid severe hypernatremia. However, if the hypernatremia is not discovered for 8 hours or more and if the serum sodium concentration is severely elevated (> 160 mEq/L), it is safer to decrease the serum sodium concentration slowly. A useful rule is to allow the sodium to fall no faster than 10 mEq/L/day). The amount of water needed to correct the hypernatremia can be estimated because the magnitude of the water deficit is proportional to the degree of hypernatremia, and the effective space of distribution for the sodium is the total body water. The following formula is useful in calculating the amount of free water required to lower the serum concentration to normal:

$$0.6 \times \text{body weight} \times \frac{(\text{plasma } [Na^+] - 1)}{140}$$

If, however, as is usually the cause, there is also a salt deficit (e.g., because of insufficient replacement of GI losses), some sodium chloride in the form of 0.2 to 0.45 per cent saline (plus potassium chloride) is required. Twice the volume of 0.45 per cent saline (one-half isotonic) is required to provide the same amount of free water. In order to avoid a precipitous drop in the serum sodium concentration, ongoing sodium losses must also be replaced. In some cases of hypernatremic dehydration, it has been noted that the urinary sodium concentration far exceeds that of the plasma once renal perfusion is improved. Therefore, because substantial amounts of sodium may be lost in the urine, the serum sodium concentration will fall much more rapidly than expected unless these losses are replaced. Although usually 0.2 per cent saline with 20 to 40 mEq Kc1/L is used as the repletion fluid, urinary sodium losses may require a net fluid sodium concentration approximating 0.45 to 0.9 per cent saline. The fluid should be given at a rate designed to lower the serum sodium concentration 10 mEq/L/day. That is, if the serum sodium concentration is 170 mEq/L, one third of the estimated free water deficit should be given on each of 3 consecutive days. To accomplish this, add the insensible loss replacement (350 [mL/M^2] per day) and the ongoing urinary and GI water and electrolyte losses.

In summary, although 0.2 per cent saline is generally satisfactory both for repletion and maintenance replacement, urinary and GI sodium losses need to be measured and replaced milliequivalent for milliequivalent if a rapid fall in the serum sodium concentration is to be avoided.

It is often especially difficult to maintain water balance in patients with head injuries. Although the inappropriate release of ADH (SIADH) and secondary dilutinal hyponatremia occur most often, central (pituitary) diabetes insipidus and hypernatremic dehydration occasionally develop. When using vasopressin (Pitressin) or desmopressin acetate (DDAVP), special care must be taken to decrease the infusion of water appropriately in order to prevent a precipitous fall in the serum sodium concentration.

Edema

Edema is defined as an increase in the volume of the interstitial compartment. The volume of this compartment is determined by the factors that affect the distribution of extracellular fluid between the intravascular and interstitial compartments and include capillary permeability, capillary hydrostatic and oncotic pressure, and interstitial hydrostatic and oncotic pressure. Under normal circumstances, there is a slight (0.5 mm Hg) filtration gradient favoring the passage of small amounts of intravascular fluid to the interstitial compartment. This fluid is normally returned to the vascular compartment via the lymphatic drainage.

Table 4–6. PATHOGENESIS OF EDEMA

Primary (Initiating) Factors
- Increased capillary permeability
  - Burns
  - Sepsis
  - Hypoxemia
  - Shock
- Decreased plasma colloid concentration
  - Transcutaneous protein loss (burns)
  - Catabolism
  - Malnutrition
- Increased capillary hydrostatic pressure
  - Expanded blood volume
  - Restricted venous return
  - Heart failure

Second (Amplifying) Factors
- Increased proximal renal tubular salt and water reabsorption
- Increased distal renal tubular salt reabsorption (aldosterone)
- Increased distal renal tubular water reabsorption (antidiuretic hormone [ADH])

Factors favoring increased transfer of intravascular fluid to the interstitial compartment include increased capillary permeability, elevated capillary hydrostatic pressure, and decreased plasma oncotic pressure. However, hypovolemic shock would preclude the development of clinically detectable edema if this transfer was not coupled with increased renal salt and water retention. Edema formation, therefore, requires both primary (initiating) and secondary (amplifying) factors (Table 4–6).

Primary (Initiating) Factors

Increased Capillary Permeability. Under normal circumstances, the capillary walls restrict the passage of colloids (albumin and the other proteins) while allowing the free passage of crystalloids (electrolytes). However, in response to burns, shock, hypoxia, or sepsis, the integrity of the capillary walls may be compromised. Under these circumstances, albumin and other proteins become more evenly distributed throughout the entire extracellular compartment. This results in decreased capillary oncotic pressure, increased interstitial oncotic pressure, and increased movement of plasma to the interstitial compartment.

Decreased Plasma Colloid Concentration. The capillary oncotic pressure falls in response to a decrease in the plasma concentration of protein. Although all plasma proteins contribute to the oncotic pressure of the plasma, albumin, because of its greater concentration and smaller molecular size, contributes more osmotically active particles than the other proteins.

In traumatized children, a fall in the concentration of plasma colloids occurs subsequent to burn-induced transcutaneous protein loss and after prolonged periods of catabolism or inadequate protein intake.

Increased Capillary Hydrostatic Pressure. Although there is an effective precapillary sphincter, which maintains a constant capillary hydrostatic pressure irrespective of changes in arteriolar pressure, there is no comparable autoregulatory mechanisms on the venous side of the capillary network. Therefore, any increase in venous pressure is transmitted to the capillary beds. Consequently, increased blood volume (because of excessive fluid administration), restricted venous return (e.g., hepatic vein thrombosis), or impaired cardiac accommodation of venous blood (e.g., heart failure) increases capillary hydrostatic pressure and initiates edema.

Secondary (Amplifying) Factors

The primary factors decrease the effective arterial blood volume and initiate a series of complex renal events that result in salt and water retention and a further increase in volume of the interstitial compartment. There is an increased fractional reabsorption of isotonic quantities of salt and water in the proximal convoluted tubule. The responsible mechanisms are only partially understood but include a decrease in the concentration of a circulating natriuretic factor (a "third" factor) and an increase in the peritubular capillary oncotic pressure. There is also increased reabsorption of salt and water in the distal convoluted tubules and in the collecting ducts subsequent to the increased secretion of aldosterone and ADH, respectively.

Treatment

Therapy should address both the primary and the secondary factors. If the edema is initiated by increased capillary permeability (e.g., hypoxia, shock, sepsis), treating the underlying condition obviously constitutes an important component of therapy.

If, on the other hand, the edema is initiated by a low plasma oncotic pressure caused by increased protein losses or decreased protein intake, the IV administration of albumin, amino acid, or protein hydrolysate may be necessary.

But, irrespective of the primary factors, the presence of edema indicates an excess in body salt and water. Because extracellular sodium (and its attendant anions) is the major determinant of extracellular volume, a negative sodium balance is the goal of therapy. This necessitates restricting sodium intake to less than output.

If renal homeostatic mechanisms are reasonably intact, a proportionate volume of water will usually be excreted. However, many conditions associated with edema formation are also characterized by an impaired ability to generate or excrete free water. This abnormality is expressed as a decrease in the serum sodium concentration (hyponatremia). An edematous child has a surfeit of body sodium, irrespective of the serum sodium concentration. If an edematous patient is also hyponatremic there is not only an excess of total body sodium, but also an even greater excess of total body water. In this circumstance, the child needs not only restriction of sodium but also restriction of water. This requires water restriction sufficient to produce a drop in body weight, necessitating the intake of less fluids than insensible and urinary losses.

A common error in the management of edematous hyponatremic patients is to increase the sodium intake. Although this may partially correct the hyponatremia, it does so at the expense of worsening the edema. *An edematous patient's sodium requirements are zero* irrespective of the serum sodium concentration, thus only sodium-free solutions should generally be given. Infusion of saline-containing solutions should be limited to the emergency treatment of hyponatremic encephalopathy (water intoxication) or hypovolemic shock.

Except for pulmonary edema, edema is rarely life-threatening. There may be times, however, when tense ascites or large pleural effusions impair ventilation. Under these circumstances, restriction of sodium may be insufficient and the use of diuretic agents may be necessary. Factors that initiate edema may also decrease effective arterial blood volume and the patient's responsiveness to diuretics. Effective diuresis may therefore require the use of potent loop diuretics (ethacrynic acid, furosemide). Because ototoxicity occurs less frequently with the use of furosemide (Lasix), this agent is preferred over ethacrynic acid. The customary starting dose is 1 mg/kg, given either orally or intravenously. Doses as high as 10 mg/kg can be given, although there is some risk of temporary and, occasionally, permanent hearing impairment. Ototoxicity appears to be less if the larger doses are given slowly over a period of 1 to 2 hours. Large doses given more than once a day must be administered cautiously in children with impaired renal function. If there is diminished plasma oncotic pressure, the diuretic response can be augmented by preceding the administration of furosemide with an infusion of albumin (1 g/kg of body weight) or by the use of metolazone (Zaroxolyn).

Acidosis

Acidosis, which is characterized by the retention of H^+ and a low serum pH, can be respiratory or metabolic in origin; the simultaneous occurrence of both respiratory and metabolic acidosis is particularly life-threatening.

Respiratory Acidosis

Acute respiratory acidosis, indicated by a low pH, an elevated P_{CO_2}, and compensatory renal HCO_1^- retention, occurs in traumatized patients who are retaining CO_2 because of injuries to the thoracic wall, airway obstruction, alveolar dysfunction, or CNS hypoventilation (Table 4–7).

The primary way to treat respiratory acidosis is to improve ventilation. If the acidosis is severe and cannot readily be controlled with ventilatory support, IV buffering agents may be necessary. However, if bicarbonate is administered, caution must be exercised because it results in the production of additional CO_2, which must also be removed by the lungs. If one is dealing with a "closed system" that provides no escape for the additional CO_2, the acidosis may worsen.

Table 4–7. CAUSES OF RESPIRATORY ACIDOSIS

Mechanical
Chest wall injuries
Airway obstruction
Central Depression
Drugs (e.g., opiates, barbiturates)
CNS* injury
Cardiac arrest
Pulmonary (Alveolar)
Respiratory distress syndrome (ARDS†, shock lung)
Pneumonia
Pulmonary edema

*CNS = central nervous system.
†ARDS = acute respiratory diseases.

Table 4–8. CAUSES OF METABOLIC ACIDOSIS

Addition of Acid
Lactic acidosis
Renal failure
Hyperalimentation
Loss of Bicarbonate
Diarrhea
Bowel fistulas

TRIS buffer (THAM) is an effective hydrogen ion acceptor that produces a fall in the P_{CO_2}. Otherwise, it offers no real advantage over sodium bicarbonate except in those instances in which sodium retention poses a problem. THAM can cause hypoglycemia, hyperkalemia, and respiratory depression; moreover, it is very irritating to tissues and requires good renal function for excretion. If THAM is used, it is customarily given according to the following formula over a period of at least one hour:

ml (0.3 M THAM = body wt in kg × base deficit (mEq/L).

Metabolic Acidosis

Metabolic acidosis, characterized by a low pH, a low HCO_3^-, and compensatory hyperventilation, can result from the addition of acid or from the loss of bicarbonate (Table 4–8). The loss of bicarbonate from the lower intestine (through diarrhea or a fistula) or kidney (because of renal tubular acidosis) is uncommon after trauma, but the acute addition of acid occurs frequently. The primary cause of the acid accumulation is a decrease in tissue perfusion and an inadequate delivery of oxygen to the tissues. The tissue hypoxia results in an increase in anaerobic metabolism and in lactic acid production. Contributing factors may include a decrease hepatic conversion of lactate, a decreased excretion of renal acid, and an increased production of inorganic acids from the catabolic breakdown of the sulphur-containing amino acids. If the metaboic acidosis is caused by the acute addition of acids (e.g., lactic acids), the concentration of unmeasured anions (e.g., lactate) will increase and result in an elevated (> 20 mEq/L) anion gap. On the other hand, if the acidosis is the result of bicarbonate loss, the kidney will retain chloride (hyperchloremia) and the gap will not change.

Although definitive therapy for metabolic acidosis requires treating the underlying cause (that is, the decrease in tissue perfusion, hypoxia), the cautious administration of an IV buffer (e.g., sodium bicarbonate, THAM) is generally necessary if the arterial pH is less than 7.2 to prevent: (1) arrhythmias, (2) a decrease in cardiac output, (3) pulmonary vasoconstriction, and (4) impaired cellular metabolism. Sodium bicarbonate is usually the buffer of choice. Although there is some uncertainty as to its actual space of distribution, all would agree that its "effective" space of distribution is greater than that of extracellular water but somewhat less than that of total body water. A convenient guide is to assume that its eventual space of distribution approximates 50 per cent of body weight. Because it takes up to 12 hours for it to equilibrate within this entire space, it is safer to assume its space of distribution to be 30 per cent of the body weight during the first hour of administration.

To calculate the dose of bicarbonate needed to raise the serum concentration from 5 to 10 mEq/L in a 40-kg child, recall that the eventual space of distribution will be 50 per cent of the body weight (20 L of body fluid). The appropriate dose (100 mEq) can be determined by multiplying the desired rise in serum bicarbonate (i.e., 5 mEq/L) times the space of distribution (i.e., 20 L). In an acid-base steady state, only about 50 per cent of the total HCO_3^- dose should be infused during the first hour. However, because of ongoing acid production, the actual rise in the serum HCO_3^- concentration will usually be less. Frequent reassessments of the HCO_3^- requirements are therefore necessary during treatment. Moreover, a rapid, complete correction of metabolic acidosis can be dangerous because it can decrease the respiratory drive and cause the P_{CO_2} to rise. And, because CO_2 diffuses into the cells and crosses the blood–brain barrier more rapidly than does HCO_3^-, this correction can result in a worsening of the intracellular and CNS acidosis.

Alkalosis

Alkalosis, which is characterized by a low H^+ concentration and an elevated pH, can, like acidosis, be either respiratory, metabolic, or both, in origin.

Respiratory Alkalosis

Respiratory alkalosis is characterized by an elevated pH, a low P_{CO_2}, and a fall in the serum HCO_3^-. The alkalosis is caused by hyperventilation resulting from hypoxemia, anxiety, hypermetabolism, or CNS diseae (Table 4–9). Initially, the fall in the HCO_3^- concentration follows the buffering of H^+ ions, which have moved from the cells to the extracellular fluid. Later, compensatory excretion of the HCO_3^- by the kidneys occurs.

Table 4–9. CAUSES OF RESPIRATORY ALKALOSIS

Central Nervous System
Anxiety
CNS* trauma or hemorrhage
Sepsis
Fever
Hypoxemia
Atelectasis
Pulmonary emboli
Interstitial pulmonary disease
Anemia

*CNS = central nervous system.

A moderate respiratory alkalosis, that is, a P_{CO_2} of about 25 mm Hg, may be beneficial to children with head trauma because it decreases cerebral blood flow and may lessen cerebral edema. However, severe hypocapnia, may cause excessive cerebral hypoperfusion that could possibly result in ischemic damage.

If children are on ventilators, respiratory alkalosis can easily be treated by decreasing the tidal volume or the ventilation frequency, or both. Treatment is otherwise rarely necessary. In very extraordinary instances, characterized by an extremely elevated serum pH and an inappropriately high serum HCO_3^- concentration, the cautious administration of acid may be necessary.

Metabolic Alkalosis

Metabolic alkalosis, characterized by an elevation in blood pH and bicarbonate concentrations and by a compensatory rise in the P_{CO_2} (caused by centrally mediated hypoventilation), may be generated by the addition of bicarbonate or by the loss of acid (Table 4–10). Although metabolism acidosis may occasionally result from the overzealous administration of buffering agents, it most frequently results from renal or GI loss of acid.

Even though both renal and upper GI acid secretion are coupled to HCO_3^- regeneration (that is, a rise in the serum HCO_3^- concentration), HCO_3^- should normally be excreted rapidly once the serum HCO_3^- concentration

Table 4–10. CAUSES OF METABOLIC ALKALOSIS

Generation of Alkalosis
Addition of buffer
Excessive HCO_3^- or THAM administration
Massive blood transfusion (citrate administration)
Loss of Acid (H^+)
Vomiting
GI* suction
Urinary loss (secondary aldosteronism, diuretics)
Intracellular transfer (LK^+ deficiency)
Maintenance of Alkalosis
Decreased effective arterial blood volume
Hypovolemia
Third spacing
Heart failure
Hypokalemia
Hypochloremia

exceeds the renal threshold of 22 to 24 mEq/L. Therefore, the perpetuation (i.e., the maintenance) of a metabolic alkalosis indicates an increased fractional reabsorption (i.e., reclamation) of filtered bicarbonate. Decreased effective arterial blood volume (that is, a decrease in renal perfusion), hypokalemia, and hypochloremia, all raise the threshold for bicarbonate reabsorption, which in turn results in an increase in bicarbonate reclamation and in the perpetuation of the metabolic alkalosis. For example, if metabolic alkalosis develops in a child on nasogastric suction, the loss of hydrochloric acid would be responsible for its generation, and volume depletion, hypochloremia, or hypokalemia, alone or in combination, would be responsible for its maintenance. Complete replacement of the GI water and electrolyte losses would facilitate continuous renal excretion of the accumulating serum HCO_3^- and would prevent or reverse the metabolic alkalosis.

Hyperkalemia

An elevated concentration of serum potassium can result from excessive administration of potassium, from decreased excretion of potassium (because of renal failure), or from a shift of cellular potassium as a result of acidosis or cellular damage (Table 4–11). Recall that 98 per cent of total body potassium is contained within the cells and that the concentration of potassium within the intracellular compartment is approximately 150 mEq/L, which is 40 times greater than that of the extracellular compartment. Therefore, even a modest transfer of potassium between these compartments can result in a substantial change in the serum potassium concentration. For every 0.1 fall in the serum pH, there will be a 0.6 to 1.0 rise in the serum potassium concentration. Moreover, cellular destruction from burns, crush injuries, hemolysis, or infection can result in the release of substantial amounts of intracellular potassium.

Table 4–11. CAUSES OF HYPERKALEMIA

Excessive Administration of K^+
Decreased Renal Excretion
Transfer of Intracellular K^+
Acidosis
Burns
Crush injury
Catabolism

The major danger from hyperkalemia is cardiotoxicity. The first electrocardiographic sign is usually a peaking of the T waves. This is followed by a widening of the QRS complex and a loss of the P waves. If corrective measures are not taken, a sine-wave configuration and cardiac arrest will follow. Hyponatremia, hypocalcemia, and acidosis may add to the cardiotoxic effects of hyperkalemia.

Although it is customary in young infants to measure the serum potassium concentrations by using the capillary (heel stick) method, this technique can yield unreliable and misleading results. The serum potassium concentration will be spuriously elevated if intracellular potassium is released from the cells because of any vigorous squeezing of the heel. Moreover, because the degree of trauma of the tissue is unpredictable, the measurement is not easily reproducible. For this reason, whenever an elevated capillary measurement is obtained, it is imperative that it be confirmed by a venipuncture sample as soon as possible. Moreover, it is imprudent to assume that the K^+ is elevated because of cellular damage or hemolysis. Indeed, if the capillary level is within the potentially lethal range ($>$ 7.0 mEq/L), it is best to obtain an immediate electrocardiogram (ECG) rhythm strip to insure that there are no electrocardiographic signs of genuine hyperkalemia.

Therapy for hyperkalemia depends upon its magnitude and the severity of the ECG changes (Table 4–12). If a value has been obtained from a nonhemolyzed venipuncture sample that is 6 mEq/L or greater, treatment is recommended. If the elevation is modest ($<$ 7 mEq/L), simply withholding potassium and giving a cation exchange resin (Kayexalate, 1 g/kg body weight) will usually lower

Table 4–12. TREATMENT OF HYPERKALEMIA

Membrane Anatagonism
- 10% Calcium gluconate (0.3 mL/kg)
- Calcium chloride (0.1 mL/kg)

Intracellular Transfer
- $NaHCO_3$ (1 mEq/kg)
- 10% Glucose (10 mL/kg) with insulin (1 unit/3 g glucose)

Removal from Body
- Cation (Kayexalate) exchange resin (1 g/kg plus 1 ml 70% sorbitol/g resin)
- Dialysis

the serum potassium concentration by approximately 1 mEq/L. If GI function is normal, it is preferable to give the resin orally or by nasogastric tube mixed with 70 per cent sorbitol (1 ml/g resin) to avoid constipation. If upper gastric administration is not advisable, the resin can also be given by retention enema; however, for it to be effective, the enema should be retained for 20 to 40 minutes. Irrespective of the presumed effectiveness of the cation exchange resin, it is important that a follow-up determination of the serum potassium measurement be obtained within a few hours. With patients who show more severe degrees of hyperkalemia (> 7 mEq/L), it is imperative that they be placed on a cardiac monitor. In patients with severe hyperkalemia or serious ECG changes, or both, more aggressive measures are necessary. The cardiotoxic effects of hyperkalemia may be immediately counteracted at the membrane level by cautiously giving IV calcium while carefully monitoring cardiac rhythm. This will cause a very rapid but transient improvement of cardiac conduction and may allow time to initiate additional emergency measures. Potassium can be "driven" into the cells by administering sodium bicarbonate intravenously or by infusing 10 per cent dextrose with or without insulin, or by giving both. The response to glucose and bicarbonate is not as rapid as that to calcium but it lasts longer. These measures may be sufficient if kidney function is reasonably normal. Frequently, however, life-threatening hyperkalemia occurs in the setting of acute renal failure (because of acute tubular necrosis), and the removal of sufficient amounts of potassium from the body requires dialysis. Please refer to Chapter 7 for further details.

Hypokalemia

In contrast to hyperkalemia, hypokalemia is rarely of sufficient magnitude to cause life-threatening cardiac arrhythmias. Even so, ileus, muscular weakness, paralysis, rhabdomyolysis, and fatal cardiac conduction abnormalities may occur. Hypokalemia may also occur because of inadequate potassium intake, enteric or urinary losses of potassium, or because of the movement of K^+ into the cells (Table 4–13). In conditions characterized by the transfer of intracellular potassium into the extracellular compartment (e.g., acidosis, thermal or crush injury, sepsis), the serum potassium concentration can be normal or elevated even though there may be a substantial total body deficit, which is the result of ongoing renal excretion. If generous amounts of potassium are not given once the serum potassium concentration returns to the upper range of normal, severe hypokalemia can occur as potassium moves into the cells in response to a rise in the serum pH or after its incorporation into new tissue.

Accurate estimates of total body K^+ deficits are not possible because the majority is in the cells and is not accessible for measurement. For this reason, only rough guidelines are possible. For mild hypokalemia (2.7 to 3.3 mEq/L), giving 3 to 4 mEq/kg of potassium per day by slow infusion is usually sufficient. For more severe hypokalemia, associated with muscle weakness, GI ileus, or cardiac abnormalities (a peaked P wave and a flat T wave and U wave), more aggressive therapy is necessary. Doses of 0.5 mEq/kg of body weight can be infused over a 1-to 2-hour period in conjunction with cardic monitoring. In the event of life-threatening cardiac arrhythmias (premature ventricular contractions [PVCs], ventricular tachycardia), as much as 1.0 mEq/kg body weight may need to be infused over a 1-hour period. The immediate increase in the serum potassium concentration after an infusion can be estimated by assuming the immediate space of distribution to be the extracellular water (20

Table 4–13. CAUSES OF HYPOKALEMIA

Inadequate Intake or Administration of K^+

Body Losses
- Vomiting
- Suction
- Fistulas

Renal Losses
- Diuretics
- Secondary aldosteronism (volume depletion, hypotension, heart failure)
- Antibiotics (carbenicillin, penicillin, cephalexin, gentamycin, amphotericin, polymyxin)

Intracellular Transfer
- Alkalosis
- Insulin administration

per cent of body weight). Therefore, in a 10-kg child, the infusion of 0.5 mEq/kg (5 mEq) could effect no more than a 2.5 mEq rise in the serum potassium level. However, in a potassium-depleted child, intracellular transfer would result in a much smaller increase. To avoid recurrent hypokalemia as the potassium continues to move into the cells, any rapid infusion (over a 1- to 2-hour period) should be followed by a constant modest rate of infusion (3 to 4 mEq/kg over 24 hours).

Acute Renal Failure

In the patient with acute renal failure and with the loss of renal homeostatic capability, the administration of fluids and electrolytes must be meticulous in order to prevent abnormalities in body volume and composition. Please refer to Chapter 7.

Burns

The fluid and electrolyte management of children suffering from severe and extensive burns presents a singular challenge. Thermal injury causes edema, and the subsequent loss of the skin integument permits massive transudation of water, electrolytes, and protein. Insensible water losses are also increased. Partially offsetting these losses is aldosterone- and antidiuretic hormone (ADH)–mediated renal salt and water retention. In addition, the thermal injury to the cells acutely raises the extracellular potassium concentration, but later, a total body potassium deficiency occurs, which is caused by the urinary excretion of potassium.

Moreover, given the kidney's temporary inability to excrete water normally and the tendency of sodium to move into the thermally injured cells, hyponatremia frequently occurs. If large volumes of hyponatremic fluids (e.g., 0.2 per cent saline) are administered, the likelihood of severe hyponatremia is increased. The intracellular transfer of sodium can be decreased by the administration of generous amount of potassium.

Although a precise determination of the fluid, electrolyte, and protein requirements for the burn patient is difficult, skin loss replacement requirements can be estimated by relating them to the burn area in terms of the percentage of damaged body surface.

Because of increased capillary permeability during the first 24 hours following a major burn, transfusion is limited to balanced salt solutions. During approximately the first 12 hours of the postburn period, there is a pronounced decrease in the amount of water and electrolytes excreted by the kidneys. During this oliguric phase, potassium should not be infused unless hypokalemia occurs. But after the oliguric period, generous amounts of potassium and insensible water replacement are usually required. A reasonable guideline is to infuse 3 ml/kg of lactated Ringer's solution per percentage of burn surface area during the first 24 hours. This regimen should be adjusted according to body weight determinations, urinary electrolyte and volume measurements, and serum electrolyte assessments. Monitoring the blood volume by means of a central venous catheter or a pulmonary flotation (Swan-Gantz) catheter can be invaluable in difficult cases. A low central venous pressure or low pulmonary capillary wedge pressure, or both, indicates the need for additional fluid, even if edema is present. If, on the other hand, the blood volume is normal, the administration of extra salt and water will only worsen the edema. Please see Chapter 25 for additional details.

SUMMARY

Approximately 60 per cent of the weight of the body is water. Two thirds of water is within the cells and the remainder is in the extracellular compartment. Three fourths of the extracellular fluid is in the interstitial space and the rest is in the intravascular compartment. Potassium and phosphate are the most abundant intracellular electrolytes, and sodium and chloride are the major electrolytes in the interstitial and vascular spaces.

The distribution of the extracellular water between the intravascular and interstitial compartments is largely determined by the plasma oncotic pressure. A fall in the serum albumin concentration, for example, favors the transfer of intravascular water to the interstitial compartment.

Children can normally maintain water and electrolyte balance in spite of wide variations in intake and output. This homeostatic capability is because of the kidney's unique ability to selectively retain or excrete filtered water and electrolytes, depending on the needs of the body. However, abnormalities in body volume and composition will occur if intake or output exceeds the limits of tolerance.

Although renal homeostatic mechanisms normally allow substantial latitude in prescribing maintenance fluids, renal homeostatic capability may be impaired in stressed or injured children. Therefore, it is prudent to approximate intake to match output.

Even though fluid administration guidelines are helpful, the effect of fluid therapy on body volume and composition must be assessed frequently. Because sodium chloride is the major determinant of extracellular volume, changes in body weight and evidence of edema or dehydration, or both, offer a practical and reliable way of monitoring sodium administration. Estimating the serum osmolality by measuring the serum sodium concentration provides a practical method of monitoring water administration.

Hyponatremia may be caused by sodium losses from the GI tract, kidney, or skin or by a shift of sodium into the cells as a result of hypokalemia or a "sick" sodium pump. In addition, hyponatremia may be dilutional following (1) a shift of intracellular water to the extracellular space, (2) excessive water administration, or (3) diminished renal free-water generation or excretion. Hyponatremia resulting from sodium deficiency should be treated with 0.9 per cent saline, whereas dilutional hyponatremia requires water restriction.

Hypernatremia can occur subsequent to excessive sodium administration or because of a loss of water in excess of salt loss from the gastrointestinal tract, skin, lungs, or kidney. It should be corrected slowly, using hyponatremic fluids.

Edema, that is, an increase in the volume of the interstitial compartment, can be initiated by increased capillary permeability, decreased plasma colloid concentration, or increased capillary hydrostatic pressure. Irrespective of the initiating factors, clinically detectable edema can only develop if coupled with increased retention of salt and water by the kidneys. Therapy should include treating the initiating factors, implementing sodium restriction, and using diuretics.

Respiratory acidosis, characterized by CO_2 retention, can be caused by mechanical factors that impede ventilation, by CNS depression of the respiratory center, or by alveolar dysfunction. Respiratory support is the mainstay of therapy.

Metabolic acidosis, characterized by a low serum HCO_3^- concentration, can be caused by the addition of acid (e.g., lactate) or by the loss of bicarbonate through the GI tract or kidneys. If severe, buffering agents should be given cautiously.

Respiratory alkalosis, characterized by a low P_{CO_2} level, results from hyperventilation that may be caused by anxiety, CNS trauma, sepsis, fever, hypoxemia, or anemia. Treatment is rarely necessary.

Metabolic alkalosis, characterized by an elevated serum bicarbonate concentration, can be initiated by the excessive administration of a buffer such as sodium bicarbonate or by the loss of acid from the upper GI tract or kidneys. However for metabolic acidosis to persist, there must be an increase in the renal tubular reabsorption of filtered bicarbonate. This occurs because of a decrease in the effective arterial blood volume or as a result of hypokalemia or hypochloremia. Treatment must address both the initiating and perpetuating factors.

Hyperkalemia can occur from excessive administration of potassium salts, from decreased renal excretion of potassium, or from a transfer of intracellular potassium to the extracellular compartment in response to acidosis, burns, crush injury, or catabolism. Therapy depends on the magnitude of the hyperkalemia and includes counteracting the potassium at the cell membrane, "driving" it into the cells, and removing it from the body.

Hypokalemia can result from inadequate intake of potassium, from excessive GI or renal losses of potassium, from an intracellular transfer of potassium as a result of alkalosis or insulin administration. Potassium replacement must be done slowly.

Special fluid management modifications are necessary in treating children with severe burns. The loss of the skin integument results in the massive transudation of water, electrolytes, and colloids. During the early postburn period, therapy is further complicated by the decreased renal excretion of salt and water.

Selected Readings

Bruck E: Fluid and electrolyte therapy. Pediatr Clin North Am 19:193, 1972.

Gruskin AB: Fluid therapy in children. Urol Clin North Am 3:277, 1976.

Immelman EJ: Routine, early postoperative fluid therapy. S Afr Med J 50:1663, 1976.

Shires GT: Postoperative, post-traumatic management of fluids. Bull NY Acad Med 55:248, 1979.

CHAPTER

5 Intensive Care Monitoring

THOM A. MAYER
ITZHAK I. SHASHA

The purpose of this chapter is to acquaint the physician with an overall approach to pediatric intensive care monitoring. The chapters on anesthesia and respiratory support, fluid and nutritional support, and posttraumatic renal failure address specific elements of caring for children as they relate to those topics. Further, each of the chapters on care of certain specific body areas also present additional details that relate to management of the patient in the intensive care unit (ICU).

CAVEATS

Any visitor to modern day ICUs can not help being impressed by the amount of monitoring equipment available. Using such equipment, the physician is able to generate sophisticated physiologic profiles on virtually any patient. However, the data generated must be integrated with the findings of a sound history and physical examination. The history and physical examination should be a daily part of the care of any hospitalized patient, including those in the ICU. Additional data generated by various methods of monitoring should be used to augment the care of the patient. In this sense, no monitor can *replace* the effectiveness of a nurse or physician who carefully follows the patient's course. However, monitoring can *enhance* the medical team's effort in many instances.

All aggressive monitoring of the patient should be tempered by experienced judgment and with the knowledge of the possible harmful effects of monitoring. Several questions should be raised each time invasive monitoring is ordered. First, what are the general indications for each form of monitoring and what information does this monitoring provide? Second, how will this information result in possible changes in the child's care? Third, what are the possible side effects or complications of monitoring and how should their possible development be followed?

Certain forms of therapy require invasive monitoring to adequately determine the effects of therapy. For example, when systemic arterial hypertension requires the use of a nitroprusside drip, the arterial blood pressure must be closely followed to ensure that these are not wide variations in mean arterial pressure.[1] Thus, the use of nitroprusside is a general indication for arterial pressure monitoring. The information on arterial pressure may result in changes in therapy for the child inasmuch as the rate of nitroprusside infusion varies directly with the response of arterial pressure. Use of indwelling arterial catheters may result in complications, including ischemia, embolic phenomena, and local bleeding (see later). Thus, measurement of pulse and neurovascular examination, and examination of the site of the arterial catheter should be part of the routine care.

"Monitoring the monitor" should be a part of any invasive monitoring procedure and includes three aspects. First, routine attention to the possible complications of monitoring should be a daily concern. Second, ICU personnel must be familiar with the use of each device, including normal tracings, as well as abnormal ones. Orientation of new personnel is critical in this regard. Third, ICU monitoring is almost always a serial process of monitoring, and isolated values must be viewed with caution. In any given circumstance, the *trend* of the value may be as important as any isolated measurement.

SYSTEMS APPROACH

Having noted the responsibility entailed in invasive monitoring of the patient, one further caveat is necessary. *ICU patients are multisystem disease patients.* A patient whose illness is of sufficient severity to warrant care in the ICU is likely to develop alterations in physiology of other body systems.[2-4] For example, a patient with a severe head injury may also develop alterations in cardiovascular respiratory, gastrointestinal (GI), or renal system, and these systems should be monitored. For this reason, intensive care management requires a *systems approach* to the daily care of the patient.

Each of the following systems should be assessed on a daily basis in every ICU patient: cardiovascular; respiratory; psychologic-neurologic; renal, including fluid intake and output and electrolyte balance; metabolic-nutritional; and gastrointestinal, including liver and pancreas. Sites of possible infection, coagulation, and skin and extremities

NAME ________ Age ____ Ht ____ Wght ____

CARDIOVASCULAR

Temp ____ CVP ____

Pulse ____ PCW ____

Bp ____ CO ____

EKG ____ CI ____

MAP ____ Lactate ____

Exam

RESPIRATORY

Res. Rate on ____ Qs/Qt ____

RR_{off} ____ Vt ____

FI_{O_2} ____ VC ____

pH ____ MIF ____

PO_2 ____ Compliance ____

PCO_2 ____ FEV_1 ____

T_cPO_2 ____ ECO_2 ____

PEEP ____

IMV ____

M_vPO_2 ____

Exam

CXR

NEUROLOGIC/PSYCHOLOGIC

Glasgow Coma Scale Eye ____ Motor ____ DTR ____

Verbal ____ Sensory ____ ICP ____

Motor ____ Cranial Nerves ____ EEG ____

Pupils R ____

L ____

COAGULATION

PT ____ FSP ____ Other ____

PTT ____ Fibrinogen ____

Plt ct ____

Exam

RENAL, FLUID, ELECTROLYTES

Fluid: IV ____

PO ____

NG ____

Other ____

Crystalloid ____

Colloid ____

Fluid Out: Urine ____

Insensible ____

GI ____

NG ____

Other ____

Na ____

Cl ____

HCO_3 ____

K ____

BUN ____

Urine ____

SG ____

U_{osm} ____

UUN ____

CrCl ____

Total In: ____ Total Out: ____

Wght ____

Figure 5–1. A useful form for recording the daily status of the intensive care unit (ICU) patient.

Illustration continued on opposite page

METABOLIC/NUTRITION			Exam
KCal IV ______	Glucose		
TPN ______	TIBC		
GI ______			
Albumin ______	Magnesium		
Po_4 ______			
Ca^{2+} ______			
GASTROINTESTINAL, LIVER, AND PANCREAS			Exam
Guiac ______	SGOT ______		
Hct/Hgb ______	Alk Po_4 ______		
Bilirubin ______	LDH ______		
	Amylase ______		
INFECTION	Cultures:		Exam
Temp ______	Blood ______		
WBC ______	Urine ______		
Diff ______	CSF ______		
Smear ______	Sputum ______		
	Drains ______		

SKIN EXTREMITIES ______

MEDICATIONS 1 ______ 3 ______ 5 ______ 7 ______
2 ______ 4 ______ 6 ______

TUBES
NG ______ CVP ______ Foley ______ Arterial ______ Drains ______
PCW ______ ET ______ Venous ______ Trach ______

Figure 5–1 *Continued*

should also be monitored. In addition, nurses and physicians should be aware of all the patient's medications and should make a daily list of the tubes, lines, and methods of invasive monitoring that are employed. Figure 5–1 is an example of a form that may be used in reviewing the daily status of ICU patients.

In some patients, each system is monitored, and a value is listed for each of the variables under that system; in other patients monitoring of only certain systems may be required. However, it is important to consider each system on a daily basis, even if some are not being monitored. Also, it is important for both the physician and the nurse to recognize why monitoring of a system is not required. Finally, the records in systems approach monitoring should include a listing not only of the values obtained by invasive monitoring but also the essential element central to patient care—the physical exam.

TEAM CONCEPT

ICU management is best delivered when all members of the team communicate frequently and clearly. Although in the past ICU directors were often anesthesiologists, today the chief physician in the ICU may be a surgeon, anesthesiologist, pediatrician, or internist with a particular interest in intensive care. Regardless of the subspecialty of the ICU director, there must be clear communication between the attending physician, ICU director, and any resident staff who may be called upon to care for the patient. All physicians responsible for the care of the ICU patient should meet at least daily to discuss the overall plan of care for the patient. It is absolutely critical to include ICU nurses in this discussion, both for the information they can impart on the patient's progress and so they can clearly understand the plan of therapy. Nurses spend more time with the patient than any physician possibly could, and their input on the patient's status should be actively sought. Further, they frequently communicate with the family to a much greater extent than the physician does, and for this reason should be included in any discussion of the patient's status or plan of therapy.

The patient's records should be readily available, whether in the form of a bedside chart or computer printout. Computerization of ICU records is becoming increasingly prevalent and is a welcome addition to patient care, so long as the information is readily retrievable. Members of the ICU team should make an effort to communicate clearly with their colleagues. Improved patient care is the result of this communication. An important byproduct of this increased communication among the ICU team members is the ability to speak in a clear, coherent manner to the patient's family. Often several different members in an ICU staff may communicate with family members on the patient's status and progress.

MONITORING SPECIFIC SYSTEMS AND PARAMETERS

Cardiovascular System

Vital Signs

All ICU patients should have frequent monitoring of the vital signs including temperature, pulse rate, blood pressure, and respiratory rate. This basic information can provide important data on critically ill patients. If subtle changes in the vital signs are noted and treated early, significant morbidity can be avoided. Changes in core body temperature can cause increased oxygen consumption. Raising the temperature 1° C for instance, causes a 12 per cent in overall oxygen consumption.[5] Similarly hypothermia can also cause increased oxygen consumption. Children are particularly sensitive to changes in body temperature owing to their small overall body weight and relatively increased body surface area.[6] All children in an ICU should be maintained in a neutral thermal environment. Most patients should have a rectal or esophageal probe placed to monitor core body temperature, and radiant heaters with thermocouplers are available for use for infants and small children. Every effort should be to made to decrease excessive air currents in the ICU in order to minimize heat loss. Large windows often need to be covered to decrease such air movement. Children with fever should usually be treated with antipyretics to decrease oxygen consumption and myocardial work.

Peripheral temperature should also be monitored as a general measure of peripheral perfusion. Thermocouplers attached to the extremities or temperature sensitive paper are available for this purpose, but examination by the nurse or physician is simpler and equally as accurate in assessing peripheral temperature.

Pulse, respiratory rate, and blood pressure should also be monitored, with the frequency of monitoring dependent upon the patient's illness. In patients who are unstable or who are in the immediate postoperative period, the vital signs may be monitored as often as every 15 minutes, but most ICU patients have vital signs recorded on an hourly basis.

Electrocardiogram

Literally every patient in the ICU and all seriously ill patients in the emergency department should have a 3-lead electrocardiographic monitor with oscilloscope display in place. This convenient, inexpensive monitor is essentially used to measure cardiac rate and rhythm. High- and low-rate alarms should be set at appropriate levels, depending upon the patient's age and diagnosis. The cardiac rhythm should also be monitored for abnormalities. Diagnoses that may manifest in the electrocardiogram (EKG) (hyperkalemia, hypocalcemia, bundle-branch-block) may be recognized on the oscilloscope display, but a 12-lead EKG tracing is usually advisable to confirm the diagnosis.

Arterial Blood Pressure

Arterial blood pressure should be followed at least hourly in all ICU patients. Patients with relatively normal pressure may be monitored by auscultation with the stethoscope and the use of an appropriate-sized blood pressure cuff. Cuff sizes appropriate at various ages are as follows: 12 cm for patients older than 14 years, 9.5 cm for patients 5 to 8 years, and 5 cm for patients less than 5 years. Infants, young children, and those with low blood pressures may require the use of Doppler ultrasound to determine blood pressure accurately.[7] Indwelling arterial catheters may also be used for continuous blood pressure monitoring.

The use of indwelling arterial catheters is indicated in (1) patients with labile blood pressure, in whom rapid drops in mean arterial pressure are possible; (2) patients in whom arterial pressure must be monitored to assess the effects of therapy; and (3) patients in whom multiple measurements of arterial blood gases are required. In adults, multiple percutaneous arterial samples may be drawn to accurately determine arterial blood gases. However, in children, the pain, crying, and hyperventilation that percutaneous arterial puncture produces may result in inaccurate blood gas determinations.

When an indwelling arterial catheter is indicated, several sites are available. In the newborn the most accessible site is the umbilical artery, which is a relatively safe site for monitoring.[8] Alternate sites include the superficial temporal,[9] femoral,[10] dorsalis pedis, and radial arteries. The first two of these sites have significant complications associated with them in children, and they should be used only as a last resort. The dorsalis pedis artery is a relatively small artery but is sometimes easily palpable in older children and can be cannulated percutaneously. The most common site for arterial catheterization is the radial artery. Complications of cannulation include distal ischemia,[11] proximal embolization,[12] and hemorrhage or infection at the catheter site.[13, 14] Whenever radial artery catheterization is necessary, it should be performed to insure sufficient ulnar artery flow to allow sufficient perfusion of the hand. The catheter may be placed percutaneously using the Seldinger technique (Fig. 5–2A) or under direct vision via cutdown (Fig. 5–2B). Indwelling arterial cannulation allows for constant blood pressure monitoring, provides accurate information on systolic and mean arterial blood pressures, and allows for frequent arterial blood gas monitoring. Extreme attention must be paid to monitoring the possible development of the complications mentioned earlier. If ischemia, embolization, or local complications develop, the catheter should be removed immediately.[11]

Central Venous Pressure

Central venous pressure (CVP) is commonly monitored in adult trauma patients as a means of assessing the adequacy of volume replacement in hemorrhagic shock. The tip of the CVP catheter lies at the level of the right atrium and reflects the right atrial pressure. The right atrial pressure is a measure of right ventricular preload and, as such, is a measure of the adequacy of volume replacement. A low CVP usually means that intravascular volume has not been maximally replaced. A high CVP, however, may indicate either maximal vascular volume or the inability of the right ventricle to pump the available preload. In adults, a high CVP may be an inaccurate measure of intravascular volume because many of these patients have coronary artery disease with isolated ventricular dysfunction, chronic obstructive pulmonary disease, or increased pulmonary vascular resistance, any of which may elevate the CVP.[15] In children these diagnoses are much less common, and the CVP is usually an adequate indicator of intravascular volume. However, children who have had right ventriculotomies (tetralogy of Fallot repair), those with congenital heart disease with right ventricular dysfunction (pulmonary stenosis, ventricular septal defect), and patients with increased pulmonary vascular resistance all may have sufficient right ventricular dysfunction to raise the CVP. In children with these specific diagnoses, an elevated CVP may be more indicative of right ventricular dysfunction than of the status of intravascular volume.

CVP monitoring is rarely necessary in children during the *initial* phase of trauma resuscitation.[16] Any child without underlying cardiac or renal disease has sufficient cardiac reserve to handle a large infusion of fluid during resuscitation of shock. However, CVP monitoring is indicated in the ongoing resuscitation of children in shock, particularly those with continued blood loss. In general, CVP monitoring is indicated in pediatric patients who have had greater than 50 per cent of their total blood volume transfused initially, those patients with major (greater than 50 per cent total body surface area) burns, and any pediatric patient who requires large volumes of fluid infusion to maintain cardiac output (Table 5–1). When CVP monitoring is indicated, the catheter is usually threaded through either the subclavian, internal jugular, external jugular, brachial, or common facial veins. Complications from CVP monitoring include those of percutaneous central venous catheterization (when that route is used for placement of the catheter), as well

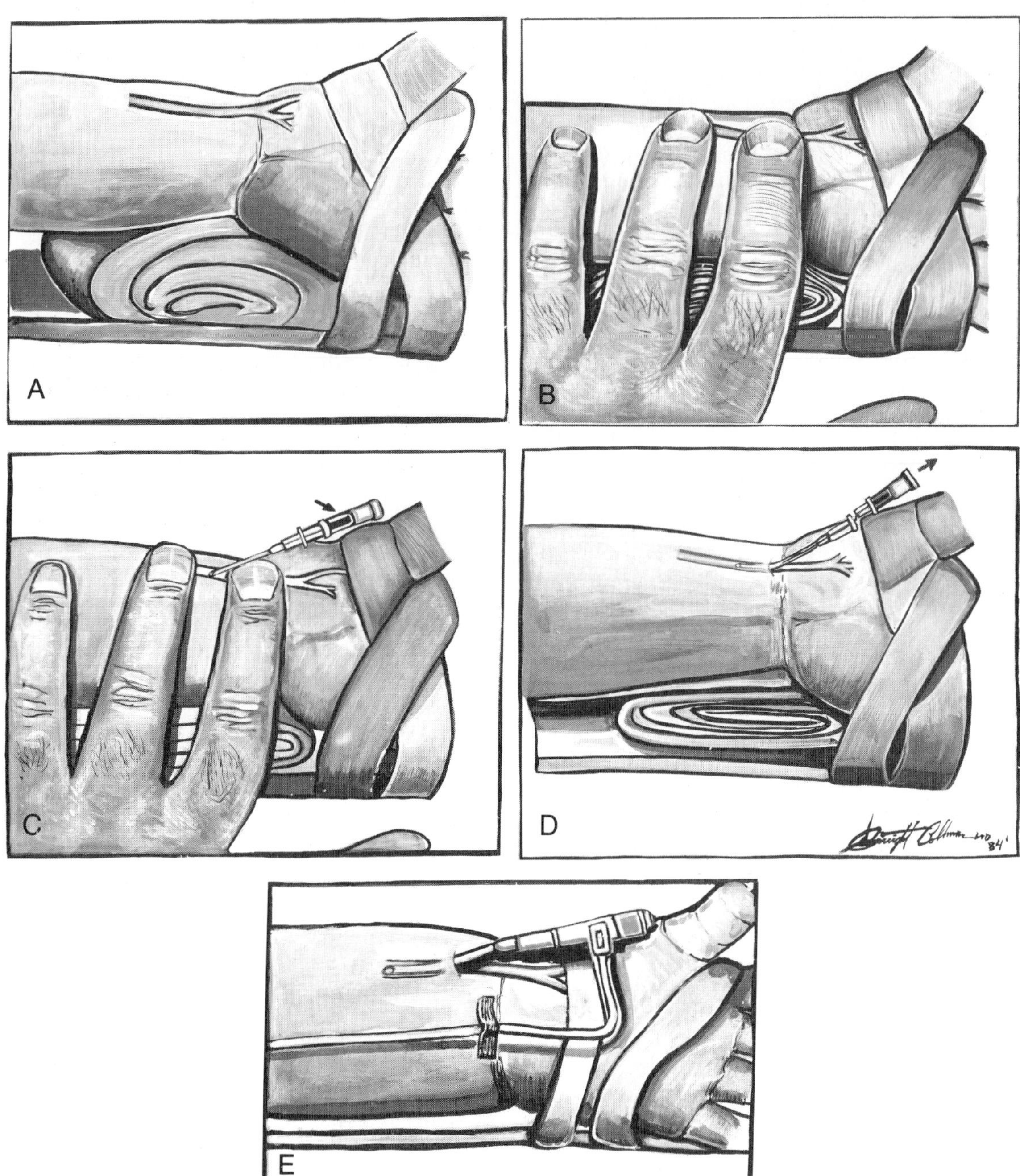

Figure 5–2. These drawings illustrate the technique for securing a radial artery catheter for arterial blood pressure monitoring. The technique illustrated is a modified Seldinger approach. The catheter can also be placed by direct vision by way of cutdown. *A,* The hand and arm should be firmly secured to an arm board, with a small roll of gauze placed underneath the wrist. *B,* The radial artery should be palpated carefully and an Allen test performed to confirm ulnar collateral flow. *C,* After flushing the catheter with heparinized saline, the artery is punctured. Confirmation of intra-arterial position is indicated by flow of arterial blood into the hub of the catheter (*arrow*). *D,* The catheter is advanced distally into the radial artery as the metal trocar is withdrawn (*arrow*). *E,* The indwelling arterial catheter is attached to a T-tube and monitoring system.

Table 5–1. INDICATIONS FOR CENTRAL VENOUS PRESSURE AND PULMONARY ARTERY MONITORING

Central Venous Pressure
Transfusion > 50% total blood volume
Burns > 50% body surface area
Ongoing monitoring of fluid therapy (surgery, ICU)
Pulmonary Artery Catheter
Poor peripheral perfusion despite maximal fluid therapy (high CVP*)
Pulmonary edema
Measurement of cardiac output or M_vPO_2† required
Acute renal failure

*CVP = central venous pressure.
†M_vPO_2 = mixed venous oxygen partial pressure.

as arrhythmias, incorrect pressure readings, and infection.[17] Patients who are receiving ventilatory assistance may have falsely elevated CVP readings if the ventilator is not disconnected during the recording of the CVP. In patients without right ventricular dysfunction, the CVP should be less than 12 cm of water. In patients with CVP readings below this level and in whom decreased cardiac output is suspected clinically, bolus infusion of fluid may be indicated empirically. Patients with CVP readings over 15 cm of water have either maximal fluid replacement, right ventricular dysfunction, or other obstruction to flow.

Pulmonary Artery Catheterization

In the early 1970s Swan and Ganz developed the balloon-tipped, flow-directed catheter for use in seriously ill patients.[18] The catheter is placed in an appropriate vein and advanced to the level of the right atrium. At this time, the balloon on the end of the catheter is inflated, allowing the flow of blood to direct the catheter through the circulatory system. By using this method, the catheter tip migrates through the right atrium into the right ventricle and out the pulmonary valve. Once the catheter has advanced through the pulmonary outflow tract, it is "wedged" into a small pulmonary artery. When pressure readings are taken at this position, they are indicative of the pressure in adjacent pulmonary veins. The pulmonary capillary wedge pressure is therefore an extremely accurate indicator of left atrial pressure. In patients with right ventricular dysfunction, the left atrial pressure is a more accurate indicator of left ventricular preload than is CVP. Another advantage of such catheters is their ability to measure cardiac output or mixed venous oxygen levels. In the vast majority of injured children, CVP monitoring is sufficient to allow accurate assessment of intravascular volume.[19]

However, in a limited number of patients in whom right ventricular dysfunction is present or in whom the monitoring of cardiac output or mixed venous oxygen levels are important, pulmonary artery catheterization may be indicated. This catheter is specifically indicated in (1) patients with inadequate peripheral perfusion in whom there is high CVP (*after* tension pneumothorax or cardiac tamponade have been excluded), (2) patients with pulmonary edema, (3) patients in whom cardiac output or other specific cardiovascular data must be monitored (e.g., with conditions such as septic shock, head injury requiring barbiturates, coma), or (4) patients with acute renal failure. When these indications are followed, the pulmonary artery catheter is seldom used in children because there is more commonly a relationship between the right and left atrial pressures in children, owing to the rarity of chronic lung disease and coronary artery disease in children.

Once a pulmonary artery catheter has been placed, additional cardiovascular data may be generated, including cardiac output, cardiac index, stroke-work index, systemic vascular resistance, and pulmonary vascular resistance, and so forth. In some centers, such data have been utilized to monitor children with severe trauma and may be utilized to predict outcome.[20] However, this level of sophistication in monitoring is not required by most pediatric ICU patients.

Respiratory System

In all ICU patients, careful monitoring of the respiratory status is necessary, beginning with a careful physical examination. This examination should include assessment of the patient's respiratory rate, ventilatory pattern, use of accessory muscles, and breath sounds, as well as comparison of the preceding parameters with previous examinations. A record should be kept on the chart of the last chest x-ray and its findings. In addition, physicians and nursing personnel should note the concentration of inspired oxygen (FI_{O_2}) and use of humidified oxygen.

The frequency of arterial blood gas determinations varies significantly according to the amount of inspired oxygen and the use of ventilatory assistance. In patients breathing room air, blood gases may be assessed once a day, or even less frequently. In patients receiving humidified oxygen ($FI_{O2} > 0.2$), but without ventilatory assistance, arterial blood gases may be assessed as often as every 4 to 8 hours (if the FI_{O2} is high or if the patient is being weaned from oxygen) or as infrequently as every 24 hours if low concentrations of oxygen are utilized. In patients who are intubated and receiving ventilatory assistance, blood gases are assessed more frequently (every 2 to 8 hours), again depending upon the severity of respiratory compromise and the need to assess continued therapeutic interventions.

Transcutaneous Oxygen Monitoring

The recent development of transcutaneous oxygen sensors has resulted in the ability to monitor oxygen tension at the skin surface in a continuous, noninvasive fashion.[21–23] The device consists of two basic parts—a heating coil to warm the skin to 45° C (thereby maximizing tissue capillary blood flow) and an oxygen sensor. It functions on the principle that oxygen diffuses readily from the dermal blood vessels to the skin surface when heat is applied. The transcutaneous oxygen sensor values correlate with oxygen delivery (defined as cardiac index times arterial oxygen content).

Under normal conditions, the arterial and transcutaneous oxygen concentration (T_cPO_2) are similar (correlation coefficient = 0.9).[24] However, in low flow states the T_cPO_2 falls more rapidly than does the arterial oxygen partial pressure (Pa_{O2}). Rowe and Weinberg[25] have shown that the T_cPO_2 can be an extremely sensitive indicator of low flow secondary to hemorrhage. Using a pig model, they found that the T_cPO_2 was a more sensitive indicator of hemorrhage than heart rate, blood pressure, cardiac output, or Pa_{O2}.

Simultaneous sampling of the T_cPO_2 and Pa_{O2} may assist the clinician. A low T_cPO_2 may be caused by low flow states or decreases in arterial oxygen concentration. A low T_cPO_2 and a normal Pa_{O2}strongly suggest that decreased flow or circulatory factors may be present as well.[26] Additional clinical studies are necessary to more sharply define the role of transcutaneous oxygen monitoring. However, preliminary evidence suggests that it may be beneficial when used in conjunction with arterial blood measurements.[27]

End-Expiratory Carbon Dioxide Partial Pressure (ECO_2)

The end-expiratory carbon dioxide partial pressure (ECO_2) is an approximation of the alveolar carbon dioxide partial pressure, assuming the anatomic deadspace has been flushed and gas distribution is uniform. When these two conditions are met, the ECO_2 is directly proportional to the arterial blood carbon dioxide partial pressure (PCO_2). The ECO_2 is measured by sampling expired gas by a pneumotachograph and is calculated as the average value of the maximum carbon dioxide partial pressure for each expiration over a 30-second period.

Although the ECO_2 is only an approximation of the PCP_2 it can provide a useful, accessible, noninvasive bedside means of estimation of ventilation. ECO_2 values greater than 45 mm Hg, for example, suggest carbon dioxide retention. This carbon dioxide retention may be the result of hypoventilation, reactive airway disease, collapsed alveoli, airway obstruction, etc.[28]

Ventilatory Assistance

When a patient has been intubated and is receiving ventilatory assistance, an increased level of monitoring is required. The amount of data generated and the variables assessed in the respiratory system vary, depending upon the type of ventilatory assistance, disease process, therapeutic interventions, etc. All patients should have the FI_{O2}, ventilatory rate (both on and off assistance), method of ventilation (spontaneous, intermittent mandatory ventilation, intermittent demand ventilation, etc.), and airway pressures and volumes recorded. In addition, minute ventilation, compliance, maximum inspiratory force, forced expiratory volume, and tidal volume are often assessed. Again, the therapeutic and prognostic significance of these values depends largely on the patient's condition and underlying pathologic problems.

Pulmonary Shunt

Under normal conditions, the majority of the blood pumped by the right ventricle to the lungs is oxygenated maximally and then pumped by the left ventricle to the systemic circulation. The extent to which the blood pumped by the right ventricle to the lungs is not oxygenated is expressed as the percentage of intrapulmonary shunt. Under normal circumstances, children oxygenate 95 per cent of the blood delivered to the lungs, resulting in a normal intrapulmonary shunt of 5 per cent or less. However, either anatomic or physiologic intrapulmonary shunting may develop during the course of a number of disease processes, including septic shock, pulmonary contusions, collapsed alveoli, or anatomic right to left shunts.

The percentage of intrapulmonary shunt (Q_s/Q_t) can only be accurately estimated when the mixed venous oxygen saturation is known, which requires the use of a pulmonary artery catheter. However, a reasonable approximation of the percentage of intrapulmonary shunt can be estimated by comparing the Pa_{O_2}/FI_{O_2} ratio. This ratio is normally 500, since the Pa_{O_2} is normally 100 and the FI_{O_2} on room air is 0.2. This corresponds to a normal intrapulmonary shunt of 5 to 6 per cent. A Pa_{O_2}/FI_{O_2} ratio of 300 represents approximately a 15 per cent pulmonary shunt, whereas a ratio of 200 represents a 25 to 30 per cent pulmonary shunt.[29]

Neurologic-Psychologic System

All ICU patients require assessment of the neurologic-psychologic system on a daily basis. Patients in ICUs are exposed to increased stress, abnormal hours of awake-sleep patterns, continual noise and lighting disturbances, and, in many cases, invasive monitoring. For this reason, even patients without any evidence of central nervous system disease should be assessed with regard to this system. In many cases, the patient's overall mental health is extremely important to recovery, even if there is no physiologic disturbance of consciousness.[30] Furthermore, alterations in other systems (metabolic, hemodynamic, etc.) may manifest themselves in the neuropsychologic examination.

The most important aspect of assessment of the patient's neuropsychologic status is the mental status examination. In children able to speak, the physician may be able to carry out a detailed mental status examination. However, a sensitive indicator of mental status in both verbal and nonverbal patients is the nurse's assessment of the patient's overall level of consciousness, alertness, and responsiveness. In small children in particular, nurses will usually be better able to assess these aspects because they spend significantly more time with the patient than do other hospital personnel.

In patients with an altered level of consciousness, an accurate, reproducible assessment of the level of consciousness is provided by the Glasgow Coma Scale (GCS) (see Chapter 1, Table 1–4).[31, 32] This scale measures the patient's response in eye opening, reaction to verbal commands, and motor response to pain.

Physician and nurse should frequently observe spontaneous movements, noting lateralized extremity weakness, hemiparesis, monoparesis, quadriplegia, etc. In patients with head injury, pupillary size and reactivity should be assessed regularly, with the frequency depending upon severity of injury. In patients with severe head injury (GCS $\leq$ 8), pupils should be assessed hourly, whereas in patients with more moderate injuries less frequent assessment is required. Assessment of deep tendon reflexes and cranial nerves and a complete neurologic examination may also be indicated in appropriate patients.

Intracranial pressure (ICP) monitoring is generally indicated in head-injured patients whose GCS is less than or equal to 8 or in those patients who are unable to follow commands or utter recognizable words following injury (see Chapter 16).[33–35] Once a neurologic insult has occurred, elevated ICP is clearly associated with outcome. Neither clinical examination nor alternative diagnostic means are able to give accurate information on ICP. When appropriate indications are present, ICP monitoring can greatly affect the patient's treatment and ultimate outcome.

Coagulation

Clinical examination is paramount in assessing defects of coagulation. The quantity, location, and quality of any blood loss should be noted. Blood loss may be indicative of an isolated injury (e.g., continuing hemothorax) or may be evidence of underlying defects of coagulation. The latter may be manifested as cutaneous petechiae or inordinate bleeding from wounds, vascular lines, GI tract, urinary catheters, etc. Any prolonged or abnormal bleeding should raise the suspicion of coagulation abnormalities.

Coagulation problems may arise from prior disease, such as hemophilia, thrombocytopenia, or von Willebrand's disease,[36] or may be due to the effects of trauma or sepsis, as occurs in disseminated intravascular coagulation.[37] Any patient who has generalized bleeding or in whom isolated bleeding persists despite adequate treatment for the specific injury should have coagulation parameters assessed. This should include the prothrombin time (PT), partial thromboplastin time (PTT), platelet count, and bleeding time. In patients with possible hereditary disorders or those in whom disseminated intravascular coagulation is suspected, other tests may be necessary, e.g., specific factors assays, fibrinogen, fibrin-split products (see Chapter 10).

Renal System Fluid Intake and Output and Electrolyte Balance

Assessment of renal status, fluid intake and output, and electrolyte balance is critical to effective care of ICU patients. In many respects, the maintenance of homeostasis depends on this area, since the composition of the body fluids constitutes the body's internal environment. The total amount of fluid given to a patient over a 24-hour period should be carefully recorded. This includes all fluids, whether infused by mouth, intravenous (IV) line, nasogastric tube, or feeding catheters, as well as all solutions used to flush lines, tubes, or catheters. Similarly, the type of fluid (crystalloid or colloid) should be noted. The patient's total fluid output also requires attention and should include urine output, insensible fluid losses, and losses from nasogastric tubes, fistulas, and the gastrointestinal tract. When severe electrolyte imbalances occur, fluid drained by urinary catheters, fistulas, or the GI tract may need to be analyzed for electrolyte content. Patients weight and net loss or gain of both weight and fluid should be recorded. Renal status is assessed by monitoring urine output, specific gravity, electrolytes, blood urea nitrogen, and creatinine. In some cases, it may be necessary to monitor urine osmolarity, urine sodium content, urine urea nitrogen, or creatinine clearance.

Metabolic-Nutritional System

The most important aspect of monitoring nutrition is an accurate account of the calories versus anticipated energy expenditures in the patient.[38] The calorie count must include all calorie resources, including IV fluid, parenteral hyperalimentation, and all calories supplied to the GI tract, whether by mouth, nasogastric tube, or feeding catheters.

The serum glucose should be closely monitored in ICU patients because glucose intolerance may develop during stress; this is extremely likely if the patient is septic, diabetic, or undernourished or is undergoing steroid therapy.[39] Both hypoglycemia and hyperglycemia should be controlled. Hyperglycemia may cause intracellular dehydration by osmotic diuresis. Although the serum transferrin level is perhaps the best indicator of the patient's overall nutritional status with regard to protein stores,[40] the test requires several days to process. The serum albumin is therefore more commonly used in the assessment of the patient's protein stores.[41] A low serum albumin implies inadequate nutritional support or liver dysfunction and samples should be obtained approximately once per week in the critically ill patient. In patients in whom nutrition is compromised, phosphate, calcium, magnesium, and additional elements may need to be evaluated.

Gastrointestinal System, Liver, and Pancreas

The physical examination provides a baseline assessment of the GI system. If a patient has a flat, soft abdomen with normal bowel sounds, this implies the presence of peristalsis; whereas passing flatus and/or stool implies that functional peristalsis is present. In patients with nasogastric tubes, the gastric pH should be assessed and controlled to prevent gastric and duodenal stress ulcerations. The presence of blood in the nasogastric aspirate or stool should be evaluated, and hematocrits should be followed in patients in whom GI bleeding is suspected.

Because shock and hypoxia may damage the liver, measurement of the serum bilirubin, alkaline phosphates, lactate dehydrogenase (LDH), and serum glutamic-oxaloacetic transaminase (SGOT) may be of value in assessing liver damage.[42] The serum amylase may also be of value in detecting pancreatic dysfunction.

Infection

Because sepsis is a constant threat to patients with multiple trauma, and particularly those who require invasive ICU monitoring, the possible development of infection should be carefully considered. The broadest, but least specific, manifestation of infection or sepsis is the development of physiologic instability.[43] This is often most notable in the cardiovascular system but applies to all body systems. Thus, physiologic instability in any body system suggests the possible development of sepsis or unrecognized infection. This is particularly noticeable in infants and neonates, in whom sepsis may be heralded by temperature instability, alteration in the white blood cell count, or unexplained cardiopulmonary variations.

Therefore, any patient who develops temperature instability, leukocytosis, leukopenia, or instability of other physiologic systems should be aggressively evaluated for the development of sepsis. As in other body systems, this evaluation should begin with a careful physical examination, which may localize the area of infection. Gram's stains of appropriate fluids or drainage sites, radiologic evaluation, or other diagnostic tests may also be indicated. Particular attention should be paid to any indwelling catheter or invasive means of monitoring as the possible source of infection. Sepsis may develop as a result from the use of urinary bladder catheters, IV or intra-arterial lines, chest tubes, or any other type of invasive monitoring equipment. The body temperature and white blood cell count should be frequently assessed in any seriously ill patient.

Because bacteremia and sepsis may stem from organisms that have colonized in the patient in the ICU, routine surveillance cultures may be useful. These cultures are usually taken from the urine, sputum, wounds, drains, and blood. Wounds and catheters sites should be inspected daily for any evidence of inflammation and specimens from drains or catheters that are removed from the patient should be cultured.

Skin and Extremities

The skin should be frequently examined to assess peripheral perfusion, which may be altered either as a result of the disease process (shock) or treatment (dopamine infusion). Capillary refill should be assessed at regular intervals in patients with any significant blood loss. Rashes should be noted and carefully described, since dermatologic abnormalities may be evidence of disease states, drug reactions, or nutritional deficiency. In patients who require more long-term care, the development of sores should be carefully noted.

The vast majority of undiagnosed injuries in multiple trauma patients are orthopedic in nature.[44] For this reason, the extremities should be carefully reassessed on a daily basis to assure that no orthopedic problems go undiagnosed.

MEDICATIONS

A complete list of the patient's medications and the dosages should be listed on a daily basis. In general, each medication should also be listed by the length of time the patient has been receiving this medicine. The physical examination and laboratory data should be correlated with the medication history.

INVASIVE MONITORING AND THERAPY

On a daily basis, both the medical and nursing staff must be aware of the degree of invasive monitoring that any patient is receiving. For this reason, these should be a complete list of tubes, lines, and drains being used. On some occasions, patients have had various forms of monitoring continued long past the necessary time period, simply because the staff has not been attuned to the length of time that this monitoring was utilized. As mentioned previously, whenever monitoring is utilized, it is imperative that the physician and nursing staff should assess for possible complications of such monitoring.

REFERENCES

1. Buchbinder N, Ganz W: Hemodynamic monitoring, invasive monitoring. Anaesthesiology 15:146, 1976.
2. Poticha SM: Management of patients with multiple injuries. *In* Beal JM (ed.): Critical Care for Surgical Patients. New York, MacMillan, 1982.
3. Houtchens BA, Wolcott MW, Clemmer T: Early management of major trauma. *In* Wolcott MW (ed.): Ambulatory Surgery. Philadelphia, JB Lippincott Company, 1980.
4. Hardy JD: Shock and cardiac arrest. *In* Hardy JD (ed.): Critical Surgical Illness. Philadelphia, WB Saunders Company, 1980.
5. Smith RM: Temperature monitoring and regulation. Pediatr Clin North Am 16:643, 1969.
6. Roe CF, Santulli TV, Blair CS: Heat loss in infants during general anesthesia. J Pediatr Surg 1:266, 1966.
7. Hill GE, Machin RH: Doppler determined blood

pressure recordings. Can Anaesth Soc J 23:323, 1976.
8. Kitterman JA, Tooley WH, Phibbs RH: Catheterization of the umbilical vessels in newborn infants. Pediatr Clin North Am 17:895, 1970.
9. Prian GW: Temporal artery catheterization for arterial access in the high-risk newborn. Surgery 82:734, 1977.
10. Johnson DG, Matlak ME: Ambulatory pediatric surgery. *In* Wolcott MW (ed.): Ambulatory Surgery. Philadelphia, JB Lippincott Company, 1980.
11. Mayer T, Matlak ME, Thompson JA: Necrosis of the forearm following radial artery catheterization in a patient with Reye's syndrome. Pediatrics 65:141, 1980.
12. Lowenstein E, Little JW III, Lo HH: Prevention of cerebral embolization from flushing radial artery cannulas. N Engl J Med 285:1414, 1971.
13. Bedford RF, Wollman H: Complications of percutaneous radial artery cannulation. Anesthesiology 38:228, 1973.
14. Mandel M, Dauchet PJ: Radial artery cannulation in 1,000 patients: Precautions and complications. J Hand Surg 2:482, 1977.
15. Swan HJC, Ganz W: The use of balloon flotation catheters in critically ill patients. Surg Clin North Am 55:501, 1975.
16. Harris BH, Eichelberger M, Haller JA, et al.: Symposium on trauma in children. Contemp Surg 22:123, 1983.
17. Herbst CA: Indications, management, and complications of percutaneous subclavian catheters. Arch Surg 113:1421, 1978.
18. Swan HJ, Ganz W, Forrester J, et al.: Catheterization of the heart in man with use of a flow-directed balloon-tipped catheter. N Engl J Med 283:447, 1970.
19. Rowe MI: Shock and resuscitation. *In* Welch KJ (ed.): Complications in Pediatric Surgery. Philadelphia, WB Saunders Company, 1982.
20. Pollick MM, Yeh TS, Ruttiman UE, et al.: Validation of the physiologic stability index (PSI) for critically ill infants and children. Crit Care Med 11:216, 1983.
21. Tremper KK, Shoemaker WC: Transcutaneous oxygen monitoring of critically ill adults with and without low flow shock. Crit Care Med 9:706, 1981.
22. Fenner A, Muller R, Busse HG, et al.: Transcutaneous determination of arterial oxygen tension. Pediatrics 55:224, 1975.
23. Harris TR, Nugent M: Continuous arterial oxygen tension monitoring in the newborn infant. J Pediatr 82:929, 1973.
24. Le Sonef PN, Morgan AK: Comparison of transcutaneous oxygen tension with arterial oxygen tension in newborn infants with severe respiratory distress. Pediatr 62:692, 1970.
25. Rowe MI, Weinberg G: Transcutaneous oxygen monitoring in shock and resuscitation. J Pediatr Surg 14:773, 1979.
26. Waxman K, Sadler R, Eisner ME, et al.: Transcutaneous oxygen monitoring of emergency department patients. Am J Surg 146:35, 1983.
27. Nolan LS, Shoemaker WC: Transcutaneous O_2 and CO_2 monitoring of high risk surgical patients during the perioperative period. Crit Care Med 10:762, 1982.
28. Powles ACP, Campbell EJ: An improved rebreathing method for measuring mixed venous carbon dioxide tension and its clinical application. Can Med Assoc J 118:504, 1978.
29. Cowley RA, Dunham CM (eds.): Shock Trauma/Critical Care Manual. Baltimore, University Park Press, 1982.
30. Mason EA: The hospitalized child: His emotional needs. N Engl J Med 272:406, 1965.
31. Jennett B, Teasdale G, Galbraith S, et al.: Severe head injury in three countries. J Neurol Neurosurg Psychiatry 40:291, 1977.
32. Langfitt T: Measuring the outcome from head injuries. J Neurosurg 48:673, 1978.
33. Mayer T, Walker ML: Emergency intracranial pressure monitoring in pediatrics: Management of the acute coma of brain insult. Clin Pediatr 21:391, 1982.
34. Marshall LF, Smith RW, Shapiro HM: The outcome with aggressive treatment. Part 1: The significance of intracranial pressure monitoring. J Neurosurg 50:20, 1979.
35. Venes J: Intracranial pressure monitoring in perspective. Child's Brain 7:236, 1981.
36. Myhre BA, Harris GE: Blood components for hemotherapy. Clin Lab Med 2:3, 1982.
37. Lanzkowsky P: Hematologic emergencies. Pediatr Clin North Am 26:909, 1979.
38. Michel L, Serrano A, Malt RA: Nutritional support of hospitalized patients. New Engl J Med 304:1147, 1981.
39. Levy JS, Winters RW, Heird WC: Total parenteral nutrition in pediatric patients. Pediatr Rev 2:99, 1980.
40. Kudsk KA, Stone J, Sheldon GF: Nutrition in trauma. Surg Clin North Am 61:671, 1981.
41. Wilmore DW, Kinney JM: Panel report on nutritional support of patients with trauma or infection. Am J Clin Nutr 34:1213, 1981.
42. Cowley RA, Hankins JR, Jones RT, Trump BF: Pathology and pathophysiology of the liver. *In* Cowley RA, Trump BF (eds.): Pathophysiology of Shock, Anoxia, and Ischemia. Baltimore, Williams and Wilkins, 1982.
43. Reimer SL, Michener WM, Steiger E: Nutritional support of the critically ill child. Pediatr Clin North Am 27:647, 1980.
44. Chan RNW, Ainscow D, Sikorski JM: Diagnostic failures in the multiply injured. J Trauma 20:684, 1980.

CHAPTER

6 Nutritional Support

RICHARD L. SIEGLER

NORMAL NUTRITIONAL REQUIREMENTS

Calories

Children require calories (i.e., energy) for growth, to support their activities, and to sustain their metabolic processes and body temperatures; the metabolism of food is the source of this energy. Normal energy requirements are equal to the sum of the kilocalories (kcal) needed to support the basal (resting) metabolic state, physical activity, and growth (Table 6–1). Basal resting requirements are approximately 0.6 kcal/m^2 body surface area/minute. The simple act of walking 1.5 miles/hour increases the body's caloric requirements to approximately 1.5 kcal/m^2 body surface area/minute, or 137 per cent above the basal rate.

If caloric intake exceeds expenditure, the excess calories are available for growth and for deposition as fat, glycogen, and protein. Conversely, if energy expenditures exceed intake, the body's stores of glycogen, fat, and protein are utilized to meet its energy requirements.

Carbohydrates customarily constitute the major source of energy; each gram supplies approximately 3.5 to 4.0 kcal. The most common carbohydrate energy source is glucose (dextrose); the other carbohydrates must first be metabolized by the body. Even though glucose can be manufactured from protein and the glycerol moiety of fat (i.e., gluconeogenesis), about 1.5 to 2.0 g/kg body weight/day are required to prevent ketosis.

In the average American diet, fats supply approximately 40 per cent of the calories.

Table 6–1. NUTRITIONAL REQUIREMENTS FOR NORMAL CHILDREN

Age (years)	Energy (kcal/kg/day)	Protein (g/kg/day)
3	100	2
4–10	80	1.5
11–18	50	1.0

However, only a few of the fatty acids cannot be synthesized by the body; they are therefore considered "essential" and must be supplied in the diet. For this reason the major advantage of dietary fat is its high caloric value. Fat, when metabolized, contributes approximately 9 kcal/g, whereas each gram of glucose and protein contributes less than 4 kcal. In addition, when fat is combined with carbohydrates as a source of energy, there may be better peripheral utilization of protein than when carbohydrates are used alone.

Protein

Protein, which forms skeletal muscle and visceral mass, is of vital nutritional importance. Even though protein is capable of supplying approximately 4 cal/g, for the most part, it is incorporated into lean body mass as long as sufficient nonprotein calories are provided. Although it is customary to think in terms of protein requirements (see Table 6–1), the actual requirement is based on the body's need for protein's substrate, the amino acids.

Amino acids are classified as either essential or nonessential. Essential amino acids are those that the body cannot produce and include leucine, isoleucine, valine, tryptophan, threonine, phenylalanine, methionine, and lysine. Histidine and arginine may also be essential during infancy and for patients in renal failure. We now know that even essential amino acid administration is unnecessary if the amino acid carbon skeleton is provided in the form of keto analogs. Nonessential amino acids can be synthesized by the body from nitrogen sources such as urea and ammonia. However, this synthesis does require an energy (caloric) source, and if sufficient calories are not provided, lean body mass (protein) will be sacrificed to support the body's metabolic needs. The amount of protein required depends on its essential amino acid content. Proteins that are high in

Table 6–2. DAILY VITAMIN REQUIREMENTS

	< 1 year	1–10 years	11–18 years
Water-Soluble Vitamins			
Ascorbic acid (mg)	35	45	50–60
Thiamine (mg)	0.3–0.5	0.7–1.2	1.1–1.4
Riboflavin (mg)	0.4–0.6	0.8–1.4	1.3–1.6
Niacin (mg)	6–8	9–16	14–18
Pyridoxine (mg)	0.3–0.6	0.9–1.6	1.8–2.2
Folic acid (mg)	30–45	100–300	400
Biotin (mcg)	35–50	65–120	150–300
Pantothenic acid (mg)	2–3	3–5	5–10
Cyanocobalamin (mcg)	0.5–1.5	2–3	3
Fat-Soluble Vitamins			
A (μg)	400–420	400–700	800–1000
D (μg)	10	10	10
E (mg)	3–4	5–7	8–10
K (μg)	12 20	15 60	71 140

Adapted from the recommendations of the Food and Nutrition Board, National Academy of Sciences-National Research Council.

essential amino acids are better able to maintain lean body mass (protein stores) than are proteins of low essential amino acid value.

Vitamins

Vitamins are a heterogeneous group of chemical substances that are necessary for health. They can be classified according to their solubility in fat and water. The four recognized, essential, fat-soluble vitamins are A (retinol), D (ergocalciferol, cholecalciferol), E (alpha tocopherol), and K. The recognized, essential, water-soluble vitamins include C (ascorbic acid), B_1 (thiamine), B_2 (riboflavin), niacin (nicotinic acid), B_6 (pyridoxine), folic acid (folacin), biotin, pantothenic acid, and B_{12} (cyanocobalamin).

Precise data regarding the minimum requirements, especially in infants and children, are lacking. The fat-soluble vitamins are stored in fat deposits and are, therefore, not rapidly depleted during periods of deprivation. In contrast, the water-soluble vitamins are lost rapidly from the body and need to be replaced on a daily basis. Reasonable daily allowances are listed in Table 6–2.

Minerals

Calcium and phosphorus are required for mineralization of the bone osteoid. Osteopenia will occur if the serum concentrations of calcium or phosphorus, or both, are below normal. Although it is common knowledge that tetany can result from hypocalcemia, it is not generally known that hypophosphatemia can cause blood cell (red blood cells [RBCs], white blood cells [WBCs], platelets) dysfunction, metabolic encephalopathy, and myopathy.

Hypermagnesemia causes depression of the central nervous system, and low levels of magnesium can cause nausea, anorexia, increased neuromuscular irritability, and encephalopathy.

The trace minerals (zinc, copper, manganese, chromium, cobalt, iodine, selenium, molybdenum) are also essential to health; however, precise, complete information about their importance has not yet been de-

Table 6–3. DAILY MINERAL REQUIREMENTS

	< 1 year	1–10 years	11–18 years
Calcium (mg)	360–540	800	1200
Phosphorus (mg)	240–360	800	1200
Magnesium (mg)	50–70	150–250	300–400
Iron (mg)	10–15	10–15	18
Iodine (μg)	40–50	70–120	150
Zinc (mg)	3–5	10	15

Adapted from the recommendations of the Food and Nutritional Board, National Academy of Sciences-National Research Council.

Table 6–4. EFFECT OF TRAUMA ON CALORIC AND NITROGEN BALANCE

Condition	Caloric Expenditure (increase above RME*)	Nitrogen/Protein Loss† (typical daily loss for 70-kg adolescent)
Multiple fractures	10%–25%	15 g/94 g
Infection	20%–50%	20 g/125 g
Extensive burns	100%–125%	40 g/250 g

*Resting metabolic expenditure (RME) = basal metabolic rate (BMR) + 10–15% for minimal physical activity.
†1 g of nitrogen = 6.25 g of protein.

termined. We do know zinc deficiency can lead to impaired wound healing and altered taste acuity. Copper deficiency causes anemia, and a deficiency in chromium can result in peripheral neuropathy, encephalopathy, and diabetes.

The normal nutritional requirements are summarized in Table 6–3.

NUTRITIONAL REQUIREMENTS OF INJURED CHILDREN

Trauma and infection affect the body's requirements for calories, protein, vitamins, and minerals; these effects are summarized in Table 6–4.

Calories

Trauma and its frequent companion, infection, both result in hypermetabolism. During the acute phase of trauma, oxygen and caloric consumption increases substantially. For example, a twofold or an even greater increase in energy expenditure may occur with severe burns. This hypermetabolic response is not confined to the injured organs but is a generalized phenomenon involving the entire body.

Protein

Trauma and infection also induce a state of negative nitrogen balance. The nitrogen loss is the result of a systemic response to stress and is characterized by the generalized release of amino acids from muscle tissue. After being transported to the liver, the amino acids are deaminated and converted to glucose (gluconeogenesis). The remaining nitrogen forms either nonessential amino acids or is converted to urea and excreted in the urine. This proteolysis and secondary gluconeogenesis probably result from autonomic nervous system and neuroendocrinologic signals that stimulate the secretion of glucocorticoids, glucagon, and catecholamines.

Vitamins and Minerals

It is not clear what effects stress, injury, and infection have on vitamin and mineral requirements. However, most accept the hypothesis that trauma and infection increase vitamin requirements. But with the probable exception of vitamin C, there are few data to support this contention.

NUTRITIONAL ASSESSMENT

The nutritional assessment provides the data base for deciding if and when nutritional support is needed. Moreover, once enteral or parenteral nutrition has been initiated, it provides the means for assessing the child's response to treatment.

The assessment should include anthropometric measurements (height, weight, relative body weight, triceps skinfolds, extrapolation of mid arm muscle circumference), a dietary history, calorie count, and simple tests of immunologic function. It is desirable that the dietary history, calorie count, and anthropometric measurements be performed by a trained nutritionist.

Dietary History and Calorie Count

The dietary history is particularly important if enteral nutritional support is planned. It should include a survey of any prior chronic problems, such as malabsorption, inflammatory bowel disease, or lactose intolerance, that might affect the child's ability to tolerate certain nutrients. Information from the child or the parent concerning certain dietary preferences or intolerances is also important in anticipation of a move from parenteral or enteral nutrition to a normal diet.

A baseline calorie count (of at least one and preferably three day's duration and including all sources of intravenous (IV) and oral nutrition) is needed to determine supplemental caloric and protein needs.

Fat Stores

Because approximately 50 per cent of body fat is situated in subcutaneous sites, an estimate of this compartment provides a reasonably reliable estimate of total body fat stores. Caliper measurements of the triceps or subscapular skinfold thickness are an easy and practical method for obtaining this information. Serial measurements should be performed by the same individual, as measurements made by different people have a large coefficient of variation. Reference values for normal skinfold thickness in children are available.

Protein Stores

Creatinine, the metabolic product of the muscle energy molecle creatine, is produced and excreted by the kidneys at a fairly predictable and constant rate and can, therefore, be used to estimate total body muscle mass. A guideline for estimating normal daily excretion of creatinine in children is as follows: excretion (mg/kg/body weight/day) = 15 + ½ age in years. An accurate assessment requires a carefully timed urine collection, which often necessitates the placement of a nonleaking bladder catheter. Because urinary catheters are often removed prior to considerations about total nutritional support, urinary creatinine measurements are, in actual practice, often impractical.

A more practical approach is to estimate the skeletal muscle mass by extrapolating the upper mid arm muscle circumference from measurements of the triceps skinfold and mid arm circumference. The measuement must be performed carefully and serial measurements should be conducted by the same individual. The upper arm muscle area may be a more accurate reflection of true skeletal muscle mass. This value can be derived from a nomogram.

There are no means of directly measuring the visceral protein mass in a living subject. But measurements of the serum concentrations of the hepatically synthesized, carrier proteins (albumin, transferrin, pre-albumin) can provide an indirect assessment. Serum albumin and transferrin measurements are easily made; however, determinations of pre-albumin are generally limited to research studies.

Even though serum albumin measurements are convenient, albumin's large body pool and 20-day serum half-life make this protein an insensitive indicator of recent changes in nutrition. Moreover, albumin levels can drop acutely and transiently in response to stress, and there is a delayed fall in the concentration of albumin following the onset of protein malnutrition. Conversely, as protein nutrition improves, the rise in the serum albumin concentration lags. Even so, albumin concentrations of less than 3g/L are evidence of protein malnutrition or liver dysfunction.

Transferrin, an iron-transporting globulin, has a shorter half-life (9 days) and a smaller body pool. Therefore, it more accurately reflects recent changes in protein nutrition. Values of less than 150 mg/dl generally indicate protein depletion.

Although not readily available in most clinical laboratories, pre-albumin, which is important in the transport of thyroxin, has a half-life of only 2 days and a small body pool. Therefore, its concentration reflects very recent changes in protein balance. Because it also changes very rapidly in response to infection or trauma, the interpretation of any change may be difficult. Levels below 15 mg/ml are generally considered to be below normal.

Measurements of transport protein concentrations are at best only indirect and imprecise indicators of total visceral protein stores. However, if they are used with circumspection, they can provide useful information.

Immune System

Severe protein malnutrition is associated with impaired immune responsiveness. Although many immunologic abnormalities have been described and many tests are available, the total lymphocyte count and simple tests of cell-mediated immunity are sufficient.

The total lymphocyte count is often depressed in children who have severe protein malnutrition. The count can be calculated by using the total and differential white blood cell counts: A total lymphocyte count of less than 2000 mm^3 is suggestive of malnutrition.

Assessment of delayed type hypersensitivity reactivity (DTHR), as determined by the body's responsiveness to common skin antigens (*Candida, Trichophyton,* mumps), is also useful. Anergy is commonly seen in malnutrition. A return of reactivity indicates improved nutrition.

DECIDING WHEN NUTRITIONAL SUPPORT IS NEEDED

During the first few days following trauma, the priorities are to stabilize the patient's cardiovascular and respiratory systems, to surgically attend to wounds and injuries, and to maintain normal body fluid volume and composition. However, the hypermetabolic response to trauma, coupled with the inability to provide sufficient calories, results in the depletion of glycogen stores and in the mobilization of fat and protein to provide the required fuel for the metabolic processes. Ideally, the child's total nutritional needs should be met from the first day of hospitalization; however, the morbidity and the time and expense commitments of total enteral or parenteral nutrition make this impractical.

We have little human data on the relationship of progressive malnutrition to morbidity and mortality. Losses of 40 per cent of body weight (one quarter of protein mass) are generally incompatible with life, and losses exceeding 20 per cent of body weight are associated with increased morbidity and mortality. Moreover, although specific trauma-related nutritional data in children are lacking, there is concern that nutritional deprivation during early childhood may have a permanent harmful effect on growth of organs, including the brain. For this reason, clinicians have taken an aggressive approach to nutrition.

Although nutritional assessment techniques (anthropometric measurements, serum protein determinations, immunologic assessments) are helpful, by themselves, they do not always provide a means for deciding when to begin full nutritional support. Most would agree that full nutritional support should be initiated when a previously well-nourished child has lost more than 10 per cent of his body weight, and sooner in a child who presents with poor nutrition. Although it may seem reasonable to attempt to provide full nutritional support prior to such a dramatic weight loss, there are no data to support this position. However, most clinicians begin consideration of nutritional support when a child has lost 5 to 10 per cent of body weight.

ENTERAL FEEDING

If a child is in need of nutritional support but is unable to ingest adequate quantities of food because of anorexia or an inability to swallow, the choice between enteral or IV feeding must be made.

If the gut is intact, enteral feedings are usually preferable because of their lower cost and greater safety. Moreover, the delivery of nutrients to the intestine may be necessary for maintaining its biochemical and histologic integrity. In addition, enteral feedings maintain the normal intestinal, hepatic, and metabolic sequence and, thus, deliver normally digested nutrients to the circulation. This latter advantage may be more theoretic than real, however.

Techniques

Traditionally, the nasogastric tube has been used for enteral feeding. The large-bore rubber or plastic tube has the disadvantage of being uncomfortable and of allowing gastroesophageal reflux and aspiration. More recently, small-bore catheters that have greater flexibility are being used. Nasogastric tubes are indicated for children who are alert and who have intact gag reflexes.

Delivering formula distal to the pylorus, using a duodenal tube or a jejunostomy, avoids the danger of gastroesophageal reflux and aspiration and is particularly advantageous in children who have poor gastric emptying. A Dobhoff tube (which is weighted with mercury) is designed to be passed through the pylorus. The tip of the tube should come to rest slightly past the ligament of Treitz. This can be facilitated by placing the patient on his right side so that peristalsis will propel the tube into the duodenum. If spontaneous placement does not occur within 24 hours, metoclopramide may be administered in an attempt to increase gastric peristalsis. Endoscopic and fluoroscopic guidance is also useful.

Irrespective of whether gastric or duodenal access is the choice, verification of the placement position is mandatory. If aspiration does not reveal gastrointestinal contents, radiologic verification should be obtained. Because these tubes are opaque, a plain film will usually suffice, but if there is any question regarding the tube position, small amounts of radiopaque dye (Gastrografin) can be injected.

Initiating Enteral Feedings

Formulas can be delivered into the stomach by either the intermittent bolus or continuous infusion method; intestinal feedings should be given by continuous infusion. Bolus feedings can be initiated by delivering 2 ml of formula/kg of body weight every 3 to 4 hours. If the gastric residual volume is less than 2 ml/kg at the time of the next feeding, the volume can be increased by 1 ml/kg per feeding until the desired volume has been achieved. Even though the stomach reservoir usually protects the child from intestinal distention and diarrhea, it is wise to use one-half strength formula on the first day of feeding. Continuous infusion feedings should begin with small volumes (1ml/kg/hour) of half-strength formula. If this is well tolerated during the first 24 hours, the volume can be increased by 0.5/ml/kg/hour until the desired volume is being delivered. Once the required volume has been achieved, the concentration can be increased gradually on a daily basis until full-strength formula is being delivered.

Choosing the Proper Formula

If the child has normal lipolytic and proteolytic intestinal activity, meal-replacement formulas can be used. Since these formulas contain intact starches, protein, and long-chain fatty acids (in the form of vegetable oil), they are relatively inexpensive and low in osmolality.

Diets are available that are composed of protein hydrolysates (casein, soybean, egg albumin), glucose polymers (oligosaccharides), and long-chain fatty acids. They too require intact lipolytic and proteolytic activity, provide 1 cal/ml, and are only slightly hyperosmolar. They can be delivered either into the stomach or the duodenum.

Elemental diets are useful for children who lack the ability to digest fats and proteins normally. These formulas utilize amino acids or peptides as the nitrogen source and glucose or oligosaccharides as the carbohydrate source and are usually very low in fat. Because of their low molecular weight, their osmolality is high.

Special formulas containing a single nutrient (e.g., fat, carbohydrate) can be added to provide the extra calories or a specific nutrient supplement. The fat additives are particularly helpful in providing additional calories to children who require water restriction. Table 6–5 summarizes the characteristics of some of the more popular enteral liquid formulas.

Complications

Whenever formula is introduced into the stomach, there is always the risk of regurgitation and aspiration. This risk can be lessened if obtunded, unconscious, or gag-reflex impaired children are excluded. The volume of the gastric residual should be always checked prior to the infusion of additional formula. A residual of greater than 2 ml/kg

Table 6–5. EXAMPLES OF ENTERAL HYPERALIMENTATION FORMULAS

	kcal/ml	Na/K (mEq/L)	mOSm/l	Carbohydrates (g/L)	Fat (g/L)	Protein (g/L)
Formulas Requiring Normal Digestion						
Isocal	1	23/34	300	132	44	34
Osmolite	1	24/26	300	145	39	37
Ensure	1	37/40	450	145	37	37
Sustacal	1	40/53	625	140	23	61
Elemental Diets						
Vivonex	1	20/30	550	231	1	22
Criticare HN	1	27/34	650	222	3	38
Caloric Additive Formulas						
Controlyte	2	0.8/0.4	598	286	96	Trace
Polycose	2	25/5	850	500	—	—
MCT Oil	7.7	—	Negligible	—	933	—

of body weight indicates the need to increase the time interval before feedings.

The use of formulas having an osmolality greater than plasma results in the transudation of plasma fluid into the intestinal lumen causing distention and diarrhea. Generally using small volumes of dilute formula in the beginning minimizes this problem.

TOTAL PARENTERAL NUTRITION

Indications for using total parenteral nutrition (TPN) rather than enteral nutrition include gut dysfunction or an unconscious or obtunded patient in whom duodenal tube (e.g., Dobhoff) placement is unsuccessful or aspiration is likely.

Intravenous Access

PERIPHERAL

Peripheral TPN offers the advantages of easier IV placement and a lower incidence of catheter-related complications. However, peripheral infusion of glucose in concentrations greater than 10 to 13 per cent produces hyperosmolar damage to the intima of veins and often results in phlebitis, sclerosis, and thrombosis. But if a fat emulsion is added, the caloric value of the IV fluid is markedly increased without substantially increasing the osmolality. Even so, the infusion of 10 to 13 per cent glucose, amino acids (2 to 4 g/kg/day), and lipids (3 to 4 g/kg/day) may not quite meet the nutritional needs of the younger catabolic patient. Moreover, when larger volumes of more dilute solutions are infused into sick children, their limits for water tolerance may be exceeded and hyponatremia may occur. If an infant is able to take some nutrition enterally or if an older child or adolescent has numerous peripheral veins in good condition and a normal ability to excrete free water, the peripheral venous route may be satisfactory.

CENTRAL

Because most severely injured infants and children require nutritional support for several weeks and because all their suitable peripheral veins may have been previously utilized, central TPN often becomes necessary. Moreover, if prolonged nutritional support is anticipated or if the initial number of usable peripheral veins is very limited, central placement of the catheter is generally indicated from the start. The standard percutaneous subclavian approach can generally be safely used (under controlled conditions) by experienced physicians in children who weigh more than 10 lb.

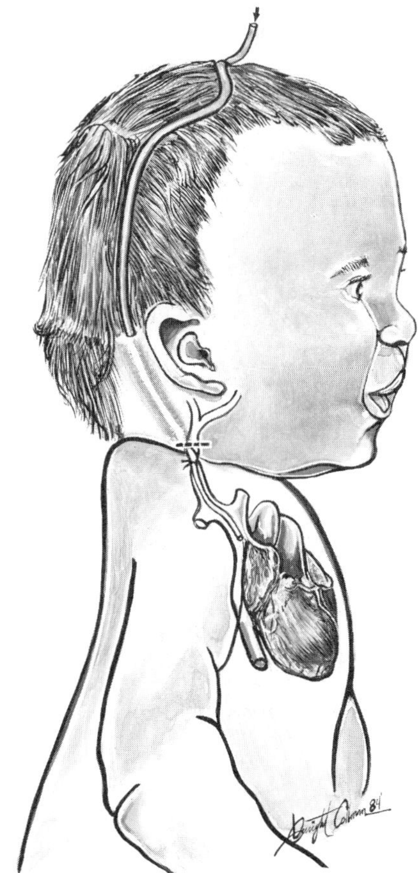

Figure 6–1. Customary position of central hyperalimentation catheter in young infant.

Experienced physicians may also percutaneously cannulate the internal or external jugular veins. Because of the small size of the subclavian and jugular veins and because of the relatively high position of the apex of the lung in very young children, central venous lines are usually inserted in the operating room by cutting down on the facial, external, or internal jugular vein. After the catheter is placed in the superior vena cava, the proximal end is often tunneled through the subcutaneous tissue and exited behind the ear (Fig. 6–1). This type of subcutaneous tunnel decreases the likelihood of infection and makes it more difficult for the infant to reach and dislodge the catheter.

Table 6–6. TOTAL PARENTERAL NUTRITION INFUSATE COMPOSITION

Calories*	< 10 kg: 120 kcal/kg/day 10–20 kg: 80 kcal/kg/day > 20 kg: 55 kcal/kg/day
Glucose	25–30 gm/kg day
Lipid†	1–4 g/kg/day
Protein‡	1.5–4 g/kg/day
Electrolytes and Minerals	
Sodium (as chloride)	2–4 mEq/kg/day
Potassium	2–4 mEq/kg/day
Calcium	1–3 mEq/kg/day
Phosphorus	1–2 mM/kg/day
Magnesium	0.2–0.3 mEq/kg/day
Iron (elemental)	1 mg/kg/day (max 15 mg/day)
Vitamins	
Multivitamin preparation (MVI_{12})	one ampule/day
Vitamin K	1 mg IM every 2 weeks
Trace Minerals	
(Zn, Ca, Mn, Cr)	one packet/day
Volume of Fluid	120–150 ml/kg/day
Heparin	0.5–1.0 u/ml infusate

*Caloric requirements may increase 50 to 100 per cent with severe stresses (e.g., trauma, infection).
†Only 0.5 g/kg twice/week will suffice to prevent fatty acid deficiency.
‡The higher amount is necessary with young infants and in patients with severe catabolism (e.g., sepsis, trauma).

Infusate Composition

Irrespective of the route (peripheral or central) of administration, the general goal of TPN is to provide enough calories (energy), protein, electrolytes, vitamins, and minerals to correct any existing nutritional deficiencies and to maintain a normal nutritional state (Table 6–6).

Glucose

The major source of calories in most parenteral solutions is carbohydrate, which supplies approximately 3.5 to 4 kcal/g. Although various carbohydrates, including fructose, have been used, most medical centers rely on glucose (dextrose). Even though concentrated glucose solutions are very hyperosmolar, they can be safely administered by central TPN because they are rapidly diluted if they are infused slowly into the superior vena cava. However, concentrations greater than 25 per cent are rarely necessary if an IV lipid is added to help meet the caloric requirements. With peripheral venous delivery, however, concentrations of 10 to 13 per cent are the maximum permissible because of the irritating nature of the more concentrated solutions.

Protein

Protein requirements range from between 1.5 to 4 g/kg/day. The protein can be either in the form of casein or fibrin hydrolysates or mixtures of crystalline amino acids. Only about 50 per cent of the nitrogen content of the hydrolysate mixtures is in the form of free amino acids; the remainder of the mixture is polypeptides. Moreover, the hydrolysates may contain ammonia, which can constitute a problem for very young infants or for children with impaired liver function. The extent to which the body can utilize these polypeptides to meet its nitrogen needs is uncertain. More protein hydrolysate than mixtures of amino acids is probably required to maintain nitrogen balance.

Sufficient calories (energy) must be available for nitrogen to be synthesized into body protein. Moreover, if sufficient calories are not provided, protein will be deaminated and metabolized for energy. The required calorie-nitrogen ratio is approximately 200:1; ratios as high as 400:1 may be necessary if catabolism is severe.

FAT

Essential fatty acid deficiency can occur in patients requiring parenteral nutrition for longer than 3 to 4 weeks if the diet is devoid of fat. Essential fatty acid deficiencies can be prevented by administering 0.5 g/kg/body weight of fat once or twice a week in the form of IV lipid emulsions, (e.g., 10 per cent Intralipid) or by the oral, rectal, or dermal application of modest quantities of vegetable oils.

Although greater amounts of lipid are unnecessary, their high caloric density (9 kcal/g) make them ideal for caloric supplementation. The ability of the body to metabolize fat emulsions depends upon the enzyme lipoprotein lipase. When the plasma triglyceride concentration exceeds 150 to 175 mg/dl, the enzyme system is customarily saturated and clearance of the emulsion is retarded. Administration of heparin results in an accelerated lipid clearance, suggesting that heparin increases lipoprotein lipase activity. The administration of as much as 4/kg/day of IV lipid is permissible as long as it does not provide more than 60 per cent of the total caloric intake and as long as hyperlipemia does not occur. The total daily amount should be delivered as slowly as possible, and bolus infusions should be avoided. Fat emulsions are unstable if mixed with hypertonic glucose, amino acid, or electrolyte mixtures. However, they can be administered through the same IV line, if they enter the system through a "Y" tube that is positioned immediately before the line enters the vein.

WATER, ELECTROLYTES, AND MINERALS

Water, electrolytes, and minerals should be provided in amounts sufficient to replace ongoing losses and to provide for repletion of body tissues.

Most of the sodium is provided in the form of sodium chloride. The body's chloride needs are therefore easily met. Potassium is customarily given in the form of potassium chloride. During periods of repletion, which are characterized by rapid new cell growth, substantial amounts of potassium will be incorporated into the new cells. This necessitates the provision of generous amounts of this electrolyte.

Calcium, in the form calcium gluconate or chloride, and phosphorus, in the form of sodium or potassium phosphate, should be provided in amounts sufficient to maintain a normal calcium-phosphorus product ($Ca \times PO_4$). A calcium-phosphorus product of 40 to 50 is ideal. Products of less than 30 are insufficient for normal bone mineralization; products greater than 65 or 70 result in metastatic calcification.

Magnesium should be provided in the form of magnesium sulphate.

If patients are on hyperalimentation for more than a few weeks, trace minerals should be given. Trace mineral packets, containing zinc, copper, manganese, and chromium, arc customarily added to the infusate.

Iron is not included in TPN solutions. If TPN continues for more than 2 weeks, oral, intramuscular, or IV administration will be required. Serum iron or ferritin measurements can be used to assess the need for supplementation.

VITAMINS

Since fat-soluble vitamins (A, D, E, K) are stored, they are not necessary for short-term parenteral nutrition. If therapy continues for more than 2 weeks, these vitamins should certainly be administered. On the other hand, the water-soluble vitamins (ascorbic acid, folic acid, pyridoxine, niacin, riboflavin, thiamine, pantothenic acid) are not stored in the body and should be given daily.

Initiation of TPN

The transition from routine IV fluid therapy to total parenteral nutrition should be done cautiously.

The dextrose concentration in the initial TPN fluid should be identical to the current IV fluid and electrolyte solution. The dextrose concentration can then be increased 3 per cent per day, until the caloric goal has been achieved. Small amounts of insulin can be also given if hyperglycemia and glycosuria occur.

Even though as much as 4 g/kg/day of protein may be required, it is prudent to start with only 1 or 2 g/kg/day. The concentration may be increased every few days as long as azotemia or hyperammonemia do not develop.

If fat emulsions are used as a calorie source, the customary daily starting dose of fat is one g/kg of body weight given as a continuous infusion. Remember that 100 ml of 10 per cent emulsion contains 10 g of fat!

Table 6–7. CATHETER-RELATED HAZARDS

Technical Problems
Pneumothorax
Hemothorax
Vascular laceration
Brachial plexus injury
Cardiac perforation and tamponade
Air embolism
Catheter malposition
Thoracic duct laceration
Thromboembolic Problems
Venous thrombosis
Atrial thrombosis
Pulmonary embolism
Septic emboli
Infection
Sepsis (bacterial, fungal)
Osteomyelitis
Septic arthritis
Endocarditis
Endophthalmitis
Miscellaneous
Hydrocephalus
Delayed perforation of heart or veins
Extravasation of fluid into thorax, mediastinum, pericardial or retroperitoneal space
Ascites
Fat embolism
Catheter fragment embolization
Skin slough

If hyperlipidemia (triglyceride level > 175 mg/dl) does not develop, the amount may be increased by a g fat/kg/day to a maximum dosage of 4 g/kg/day. If fat emulsions are given only to prevent essential fatty acid deficiencies, sufficient amounts (0.5 g fat/kg) can be administered over a 4-hour period once or twice a week. Emulsions should never be infused faster than 0.3 g fat/kg/hour.

Complications of TPN

CATHETER-RELATED HAZARDS

Complications related to the catheter include mechanical trauma resulting from technical problems, thromboembolism, and infection (Table 6–7).

Technical Problems. The technical complications related to the central insertion of a catheter can usually be prevented by reserving the percutaneous approach for infants weighing more than 10 lb. In smaller infants, the small size of the subclavian and internal jugular veins and the relatively high position of the lung apex increase the risk of pneumothorax, hemothorax, or injury to the subclavian artery, vein, and brachial plexus. If a catheter is to be inserted percutanously, it is mandatory that the physician have a thorough understanding of the anatomic relationships of the vessels and nerves. Moreover, if a guidewire is used, it is safer to keep the wire out of the heart.

Thromboembolic Problems. There is always a risk of thromboembolic complications. Catheter-related thromboembolic events may occur in as many as 20 per cent of patients, even if the catheter has been in place for only a few days. Even though thromboembolism, including pulmonary embolization, can occur, most thromboembolic events fortunately cause no detectable morbidity. Although it is usually impossible to ascertain the precise cause of the thrombi, they may result from intimal injury caused by the rotation of the catheter tip, from a reaction to the catheter materials, or from intimal injury that is subsequent to the hypertonicity of the infusate. Because of the possibility of atrial thrombi and perforation, it is best to keep the catheter tip out of the heart and within the superior vena cava.

Infection. The most common, serious, catheter-related complication is infection. Although organisms can be introduced during insertion, infections occur more frequently because of catheter violation (e.g., through the infusion of medications or blood by the extraction of blood samples). Even though it is theoretically possible to minimize this risk by maintaining meticulous technique when using the catheter for non-TPN purposes, it is prudent to limit the use of the catheter to TPN infusion. The migration of skin pathogens along the subcutaneous course of the catheter is another common cause of infection. Providing a subcutaneous catheter tunnel decreases this risk and meticulous care of the catheter exit site is also necessary. The catheter exit site should be cared for by a specially trained team of nurses: Several times a week the dressing should be changed, the exit site scrubbed, and iodinated antiseptic ointment applied.

The onset of catheter-related sepsis may be sudden or indolent. High-grade spiking or constant fevers may be preceded by several days of low-grade fever. A spiking fever probably indicates an intermittent release of organisms from the catheter tip, whereas a persistently elevated temperature probably indicates ongoing bacteremia. *Staphylococcus epidermidis* is the most frequent pathogen, but the common enteric organisms (*Escherichia coli, Pseudomonas,* enterococcus, and *Klebsiella*) can also infect. *Candida* infections continue to be a problem in the poorly nourished, immunosuppressed patient. It is often difficult to differentiate between *Candida* colonization and infection. *Candida* grown from a blood culture that is obtained distant to the catheter obviously implies fungemia, although not necessarily organ invasion. Testing for *C. precipitans* is helpful in making this distinction. If tests for *C. precipitans* are negative, deep-tissue invasion has not occurred. However, antibodies to the fungal protein indicate that tissue invasion has taken place.

If a child develops unexplained fever but does not otherwise look particularly ill, it is customary to change the nutrient solution and the tubing and filter and to obtain blood cultures. However, if the fever persists, the catheter should be removed and a specimen from the catheter tip cultured. Although the infection will usually resolve itself without the use of antibiotics once the catheter has been removed, most clinicians elect to begin broad-spectrum antibiotic coverage pending the results of the cultures. Amphotericin B is being replaced by the relatively nontoxic agent ketoconazole for treatment of invasive *Candida* infections.

Reinsertion of a new central catheter should be delayed temporarily because reseeding of the new catheter tip can occur if bacteremia is still present.

Because sepsis produces a catabolic state and increases the need for nutritional support, peripheral hyperalimentation should be started immediately. Post-infusion hypoglycemia can also occur if a dextrose infusion is abruptly discontinued. In 24 hours or so, after the fever and other signs of sepsis have subsided, a new central catheter can be inserted.

Metabolic Complications

Other TPN complications relate to the composition of the infusate or its rate of delivery (Table 6–8).

Table 6–8. METABOLIC COMPLICATIONS

Disorder	Clinical Manifestation
Electrolyte Imbalance	
Hypernatremia	CNS* dysfunction
Hyponatremia	CNS dysfunction
Hyperkalemia	Cardiotoxicity
Hypokalemia	Muscle weakness, ileus, cardiotoxicity
Metabolic acidosis	Kussmaul's respirations
Mineral Imbalance	
Hypercalcemia	Metastatic calcification, vomiting, diarrhea, hypertension, cardiotoxicity
Hypocalcemia	Tetany, rickets
Hyperphosphatemia	Metastatic calcification
Hypophosphatemia	Blood cell dysfunction, myopathies, rickets, CNS dysfunction
Hypomagnesemia	Muscle weakness, personality changes, tremors, tetany, seizures
Glucose Abnormalities	
Hyperglycemia	Polyuria, hypernatremia, dehydration, hyperosmolar coma
Hypoglycemia	Confusion, weakness, seizures
Protein-Related Problems	
Hyperammonemia	Encephalopathy (rare)
Azotemia	Uremia (rare)
Lipid Abnormalities	
Hypertriglyceridemia	Lipid vasculopathy, pulmonary, diffusion defect, reticuloendothelial cell defect, leading to infection, red cell and platelet clumping
Essential fatty-acid deficiency	Skin and hair abnormalities, intestinal and liver dysfunction
Liver Dysfunction	Cholestatic jaundice, hepatocellular injury, cirrhosis, liver failure
Miscellaneous	
Chromium deficiency	Encephalopathy, glucose intolerance, peripheral neuropathy
Zinc deficiency	Acrodermatitis
Vitamin K deficiency	Bleeding
Folic acid, vitamin B_{12}, copper deficiency	Anemia

*CNS = central nervous system.

Fluid, Electrolyte, and Mineral Imbalance. Hypernatremia and hyponatremia are common problems. Hypernatremia is usually the result of decreased total body water rather than increased total body sodium. This occurs when not enough free water is provided in the infusate. Young infants are particularly predisposed to develop hypernatremia and dehydration because they are less able to concentrate their urine and, therefore, have a greater obligatory urinary water loss. Hyponatremia usually occurs because of water retention (dilution) rather than salt depletion. Children with a decreased effective arterial blood volume (e.g., a low serum albumin concentration) have an impaired ability to excrete free water and are, therefore, prone to devleop hyponatremia. Most cases of hyper- and hyponatremia can be successfully treated by increasing or decreasing, respectively, the amount of free water in the infusate.

Abnormalities in the serum potassium concentration may also occur. Hyperkalemia may follow the release of large amounts of intracellular potassium in response to acidosis or catabolism (e.g., as in sepsis or fever). Hypokalemia may occur when replacement is insufficient to match the gastrointestinal or renal losses or when large amounts of potassium are being incorporated into new cells.

Care must be taken to maintain the calcium and phosphorus concentrations within normal limits. It should be remembered that substantial amounts of phosphorus are required during repletion therapy. In addition, in acidosis, glycosuria, and potassium depeltion, renal phosphate excretion is increased. Hypophosphatemia impairs blood cell (RBCs, WBCs, platelets) function, causes myopathies and central nervous system dysfunction, and eventually leads to rachitic bone disease.

Magnesium requirements increase during stress and during periods of new cell growth (repletion). If sufficient magnesium (0.2 to 0.3 mEq/kg/day) is not included in the TPN solution, personality changes, muscle weakness, tremors, tetany, and seizures may develop. Magnesium depletion also increases potassium and phosphate loss.

Glucose Abnormalities. Abnormalities in the serum glucose concentration occur frequently. Hyperglycemia occurs if the child cannot secrete endogenous insulin appropriately or if the rate of glucose administration is too rapid. Moreover, the onset of unexplained hyperglycemia in a previously normoglycemic child should be considered evidence of early sepsis. Although hyperosmotic nonketotic coma does not usually occur unless the serum glucose concentration exceeds 800 to 1000 mg/dl, lesser degrees of hyperglycemia can cause glycosuria and result in an osmotic diuresis, dehydration, and hypernatremia. Occasionally, in order to maintain caloric requirements, generous amounts of glucose must be continued in spite of hyperglycemia. In this situation, insulin should be given cautiously.

Hypoglycemia is a common problem if the infusion is abruptly discontinued. This occurs most often when a central venous catheter is removed and peripheral infusion of glucose is not started immediately.

Protein-Related Problems. Protein hydrolysates contain preformed ammonia and can cause hyperammonemia. Although crystalline amino acid solutions are ammonia-free, the earlier mixtures were deficient in arginine and thus tended to raise serum ammonia levels. Today's formulas contain more arginine, and hyperammonemia is rare.

Metabolic acidosis may occur when some of the crystalline amino acid mixtures are used, but it is rare unless more than 4 g/kg/day of protein equivalent is administered. It was a more common problem with the earlier amino acid solutions, and it probably cocurred because the amino acid hydrochloride salts were metabolized to hydrochloride acid. It now rarely occurs because acetate is used instead of chloride in the lysine salts.

Prerenal azotemia may occur if the urea production, resulting from the protein load, exceeds renal capability.

Abnormal plasma amino acid patterns are common and mirror the composition of the infusates. However, there have been no reports of ill effects as a result of these unusual amino acid profiles.

Lipid Abnormalities. The fat emulsions are customarily cleared by the enzyme lipoprotein lipase. However, when the serum triglyceride concentration exceeds 150 to 175 mg/dl, lipase enzyme activity is saturated, hyperlipemia occurs, and the reticuloendothelial (RE) system assumes a greater role in clearing the emulsion. This response may partially block the RE system and may predispose the child to infection.

Hypertriglyceridemia may also cause a vasculopathy, which is characterized by lipid droplets in the capillaries. This condition may produce a pulmonary diffusion defect.

Other side effects of hyperlipemia include erythrocyte membrane defects and increased red cell and platelet clumping.

Essential fatty-acid deficiency can occur during the long-term administration of fat-free solutions. Potential manifestations of essential fatty-acid deficiency include skin lesions, hair abnormalities, altered prostaglandin synthesis, and intestinal and liver dysfunction.

Liver Dysfunction. Hepatic dysfunction is a common complication of TPN. Cholestatic jaundice is the typical feature, but biochemical evidence of hepatocellular damage is also frequently seen. Cirrhosis or liver failure may occur occasionally. The pathogenesis is conjectural, and improvement may occur without discontinuation of the TPN. Because the putative causes include an excessive infusion of carbohydrate, fat and amino acid toxicity, and amino acid and essential fatty-acid deficiency, specific therapeutic recommendations are speculative.

Miscellaneous Complications. Other potential complications of TPN include encephalopathy and glucose intolerance resulting from chromium deficiency; acrodermatitis enteropathica, subsequent to zinc deficiency; bleeding because of vitamin K deficiency; anemia resulting from deficiencies of iron, folic acid, vitamin B_{12}, or copper; and a variety of other vitamin deficiency syndromes.

MONITORING THERAPY

Nutritional Assessment

Irrespective of whether or not caloric and protein administration goals have been achieved, the final determinant of successful enteral or parenteral therapy is documented evidence of improved nutrition. Therefore, anthropometric determinations (height, weight, fat stores, and somatic muscle mass measurements) and estimates of visceral protein stores (transferrin and albumin concentrations) should be performed weekly. Although changes in the child's weight should be a good nutritional parameter, the difficulty in obtaining valid (reproducible) weights in most hospitals makes this an unreliable indicator of nutritional status.

Biochemical Parameters

In addition to obtaining a baseline nutritional assessment, a baseline complete blood count and blood chemistry determinations (electrolytes, calcium, phosphorus, magnesium, ammonia, bilirubin, and liver enzymes) should be made. During the first week or two of therapy, serum electrolytes, blood urea nitrogen (BUN), and glucose concentrations sould be obtained daily; the other studies should be performed two or three times per week (Table 6–9). Thereafter, assuming there are no problems, electrolyte, glucose, and BUN concentrations can be measured three times weekly, and other studies can be performed once or twice a week. By periodically reviewing these data, the adequacy of the nutritional support can be assessed and many of the TPN complications avoided.

Table 6–9. BIOCHEMICAL MONITORING

Variable	Frequency	
	*Initially**	*Later*
Serum Electrolytes	daily	3 times/wk
Blood urea nitrogen (BUN)	daily	3 times/wk
Serum glucose	daily	3 times/wk
Serum ammonia	2 times/wk	weekly
Serum triglycerides†	2 times/wk	weekly
Serum calcium, phosphorus, magnesium	3 times/wk	2 times/wk
Hemoglobin	2 times/wk	2 times/wk
Liver function tests	weekly	weekly

*Until full strength formula is being infused and until the child is metabolically stable; usually requires one to two weeks.

†If using fat emulsion.

SUMMARY

The metabolism of food provides the energy (calories) to support work, body temperature, and metabolic processes. If the caloric intake exceeds these expenditures, the excess is available for growth and for deposition as fat, glycogen, or protein. If, on the other hand, caloric expenditures exceed intake, glycogen, fat, and protein will be utilized to satisfy caloric needs.

Carbohydrates and fat are the customary sources of energy. Fat, when metabolized, releases approximately 9 kcal/g, whereas carbohydrates contribute only 3.5 to 4.0 kcal/g. Although protein and carbohydrates are similar in their caloric value, protein is ordinarily utilized to form lean body mass as long as sufficient nonprotein calories are available.

Vitamins are a heterogeneous group of chemical substances that are vital to health. The water soluble vitamins are rapidly lost from the body and, therefore, should be provided frequently. The fat soluble vitamins are stored in fat depots and, therefore, do not need to be given frequently.

The body's minerals are involved in numerous physiologic processes. Normal calcium and phosphorus concentrations are required for mineralization of the bone osteoid, and magnesium concentrations influence central nervous system function. The trace metals (zinc, copper, manganese, chromium) also appear to be important to health, although not all of their roles are precisely known.

The hypermetabolic effect of trauma and infection increase caloric requirements and produce a state of negative nitrogen balance. A nutritional assessment is helpful in deciding if and when nutritional support is needed. The assessment should include anthropometric measurements (weight, fat, and protein stores), a dietary history and calorie count, an estimate of visceral protein stores (serum albumin and transferrin concentrations), and simple tests of immunologic function.

The indications for initiating full nutritional support are controversial. However, most would agree, that enteral or parenteral nutrition should be implemented if a child loses more than 10 per cent of his body weight. If intestinal function is normal, the enteral route is preferable because of greater safety and lower cost. If the child is obtunded or has an impaired gag reflex, the solution should be delivered directly into the intestine. Possible complications of using the enteral route include aspiration and hyperosmolar diarrhea.

If the child's gut is nonfunctional, IV therapy is necessary. Although peripheral veins can be used, it is difficult to provide sufficient carbohydrate calories without producing hyperosmolar damage to the veins. Therefore, the central IV route (i.e., the superior vena cava) is generally used for delivering total parenteral nutrition (TPN).

Irrespective of whether TPN is delivered peripherally or centrally, the goal is to provide sufficient calories, protein, electrolytes, vitamins, and minerals to correct any nutritional deficits and to meet the ongoing nutritional needs. Glucose is usually the major source of calories. Protein can be given in the form of protein hydrolysates or as mixtures of amino acids; sufficient amounts of nonprotein calories must also be provided. Although only small amounts of dietery fat are necessary to avoid essential fatty acid deficiencies, fat's high caloric density and low osmolality makes it an attractive source of calories. Water, electrolytes, minerals, and vitamins should be supplied in the customary amounts.

TPN should be initiated slowly, and the patient must be closely observed for complications. Catheter-related problems include pneumothorax, injuries to the subclavian artery, vein, or brachial plexus, thromboembolism, and infection. Metabolic complications include fluid and electrolyte imbalance, hyper- and hypoglycemia, azotemia, hyperammonemia, acidosis, hyperlipemia, and liver dysfunction.

In order to assess the results of nutritional therapy, anthropometric and blood chemistry measurements should be obtained on a frequent and regular basis.

Acknowledgment

I would like to thank Jan Pearson, R.D., M.S., for her help and assistance.

Selected Readings

American Academy of Pediatrics, Committee on Nutrition: Commentary on parenteral nutrition. Pediatrics 71:547, 1983.

Kudsk KA, Stone J, Sheldon GF: Nutrition in trauma. Surg Clin North Am 61:671, 1981.

Levy JS, Winters RW, Heird WC: Total parenteral nutrition in pediatric patients. Pediatr Rev 2:99, 1980.

Michel L, Serrano A, Malt RA: Nutritional support of hospitalized patients. N Engl J Med 304:1147, 1981.

Reimer SL, Michener WM, Steiger E: Nutritional support of the critically ill child. Pediatr Clin North Am 27:647, 1980.

Wilmore DW, Kinney JM: Panel report on nutritional support of patients with trauma or infection. Am J Clin Nutr 34:1213, 1981.

CHAPTER

7 Post-Traumatic Renal Failure

RICHARD L. SIEGLER

NORMAL RENAL FUNCTION

The kidneys normally receive 20 to 25 per cent of cardiac output, and almost all of this blood perfuses the renal cortex. Approximately 20 per cent of the blood plasma filters across the glomerular capillary walls and is collected in Bowman's space as ultrafiltrate. This process produces approximately 125 ml of ultrafiltrate for every 1.73 m^2 of body surface area/minute, or about 180 L/1.73 m^2/day.

Glomerular filtration is facilitated by the hydrostatic pressure within the glomerular capillaries and by the oncotic pressure within Bowman's space; it is inhibited by the hydrostatic pressure within Bowman's space and by the oncotic pressure within the glomerular capillaries.

The kidneys are able, by a process known as autoregulation, to maintain a normal glomerular filtration rate (GFR) over a wide range of renal perfusion pressures. A fall in the perfusion pressure causes dilatation of the preglomerular (afferent) arterioles and possibly some constriction of the postglomerular (efferent) arterioles, whereas a rise in the pressure produces preglomerular vasoconstriction and efferent arteriolar vasodilatation. This process maintains a normal glomerular intracapillary hydrostatic pressure in spite of changes in the renal artery pressure.

As the filtrate passes through the proximal convoluted tubule, through the loop of Henle, and through the distal convoluted tubule and collecting ducts, the water and electrolytes are selectively reabsorbed or rejected in accordance with the needs of the body. If a child is normovolemic and has an average intake and output of water and electrolytes, more than 99 per cent of the filtered salt and water will be reabsorbed and returned to the body. This will result in a urine volume of approximately 1 to 2 ml/kg of body weight/hour, with a sodium composition that approximates one-third to one-half normal saline (50 to 75 mEq/L).

However, renal tubular reabsorption of filtered salt and water does vary in response to the changes in the effective arterial blood volume (i.e., renal perfusion). Fractional reabsorption of the filtered sodium and water, that is, the percentage of filtered sodium and water that is reabsorbed by the proximal tubules, increases in response to renal hypoperfusion and decreases as a consequence of volume expansion. This variable reabsorption of salt and water may be related to changes in the blood concentration of a saluretic (a so-called "third") factor, or it may occur because of changes in the colloid pressure within the peritubular capillaries, or both. Salt and water reabsorption in the distal convoluted tubules and collecting ducts is also variable and is modulated by aldosterone and antidiuretic hormone (ADH, vasopressin) respectively. Renal hypoperfusion stimulates the renin-angiotensin-aldosterone system, which facilitates the reabsorption of sodium in the distal tubules; a decrease in the effective arterial blood volume provokes the release of ADH from the posterior pituitary gland and causes increased water reabsorption. Volume expansion, on the other hand, suppresses these hormones and results in a diuresis.

RENAL RESPONSE TO SHOCK

Autoregulation maintains a normal GFR in the adolescent until the mean renal perfusion pressure falls to less than 70 to 80 mm Hg. Below this pressure, efferent (arteriolar) vasodilatation is maximum, and the intracapillary hydrostatic pressure and GFR fall. In addition, blood is shunted from the outer cortex to the deep cortex and medulla. When the renal mean arterial pressure falls below 50 mm Hg in adolescents, glomerular intracapillary hydrostatic pressure becomes insufficient to overcome the oncotic pressure within the glomerular capillaries and the hydrostatic pressure within Bowman's space, and filtration ceases.

ACUTE RENAL FAILURE

Acute renal failure (ARF)—that is, an abrupt but reversible decline in the GRF—can be categorized as being prerenal, renal parenchymal, or postrenal in origin.

Pre-renal (Functional) Failure

If renal blood flow (renal perfusion pressure) is sufficiently depressed to overwhelm the renal autoregulatory mechanisms, GFR falls or ceases, and prerenal failure (azotemia) ensues. Prerenal azotemia results from inadequate renal perfusion rather than from renal parenchymal disease or dysfunction. In other words, the kidney responds appropriately to the signals it receives. The GFR is, therefore, depressed because of an inadequate intracapillary hydrostatic pressure, but the renal tubules continue to retain the filtered salt and water appropriately. If the renal hypoperfusion episode is short-lived, the pre- and postglomerular arterioles will relax as the renal perfusion pressure increases, and the GFR will return to normal.

There is no direct way to measure renal perfusion. Even a normal blood pressure, a normal central venous pressure (CVP), and a normal pulmonary wedge pressure do not absolutely assure normal renal perfusion. It is possible, therefore, that mild prerenal azotemia may occur even though the customary parameters of tissue perfusion are normal.

Acute Renal Parenchymal Failure

Severe or prolonged renal ischemic episodes usually cause acute renal parenchymal failure (ARPF). The pathogenesis of ARPF is incompletely understood. The term acute tubular necrosis (ATN), which has traditionally been used to describe this type of ARF, is not very useful because the histologic evidence of renal tubular cell necrosis can be found in only about 10 to 20 per cent of the cases. The newer term "vasomotor nephropathy" is also unsatisfactory, because although renal ischemia plays a role in the initiation of ARPF, its presence only partially explains the perpetuation of ARPF. For these reasons, the term ARPF will be used in this chapter.

The traditional hypotheses for the causes of ARPF have included (1) renal ischemia, characterized by a decrease in the total renal blood flow, by a shunting of blood from the cortex to the medulla, and by the prolonged intense vasoconstriction of the afferent arterioles; (2) mechanical blockage of the renal tubules by necrotic tubular debris; and (3) the blackflow of glomerular filtrate across the denuded tubular epithelium.

The bulk of the evidence suggests that prolonged and intense prerenal failure, characterized by afferent arteriolar vasoconstriction and by the shunting of blood away from the cortex, is the major factor responsible for the initiation of ARPF. There is some evidence that activation of the renin-angiotensin system plays a role in arteriolar vasoconstriction, but maneuvers designed to inhibit angiotensin II production do not protect experimental animals from developing ARPF. Moreover, plasma renin activity does not always remain elevated throughout the duration of the ARF. Although tubular obstruction does play a role in some experimental models of ARF, its role in man is uncertain. The importance of the back-flow of filtrate is even more conjectural and probably is not an important pathogenic factor, except perhaps in those patients who have true tubular cell necrosis.

The pigments hemoglobin and myoglobin do not appear to be sufficiently nephrotoxic to cause ARPF unless there are concurrent predisposing factors (e.g., volume depletion).

Prerenal azotemia and ARPF should be viewed as a continuum. Prerenal azotemia is the result of a decrease in renal perfusion of a sufficient magnitude to overwhelm the autoregulatory capabilities of the kidneys. But, if severe renal hypoperfusion persists for an hour or more or if less severe degrees of hypoperfusion are allowed to persist for hours to days, renal parenchymal damage will occur and ARPF will result. There is no precise instant that demarcates prerenal azotemia from ARPF. Instead, there appears to be a reversible transitional period between pure prerenal azotemia and ARPF. This period, which is characterized by evidence of renal parenchymal damage on urinalysis (hematuria, proteinuria, pyuria, renal tubular cells, granular casts) is generally reversible. However, if the causes of the early renal parenchymal damage are not identified and corrected, ARPF will generally occur.

Occasionally, direct renal trauma may be responsible for renal failure. Blunt trauma to the kidney can disrupt the intima of the renal artery and result in arterial thrombosis. Subsequently, prerenal azotemia, ARPF, or a complete renal infarction can occur, depending on the degree of arterial obstruction and on the extent of any collateral renal circulation from the superior mesenteric, spermatic, ovarian, or adrenal arteries.

Another uncommon cause of ARF resulting from trauma is disseminated intravascular coagulation (DIC). This can occur as a consequence of the trauma-induced release of thromboplastic factors. Gram-negative sepsis, a frequent complication of trauma, can also initiate DIC.

Postrenal Failure

ARF of the postrenal variety occurs not because of inadequate renal perfusion pressure or intrinsic renal damage but because of an obstruction to the outflow of urine. Postrenal failure should be suspected in a child who has sustained abdominal or pelvic trauma; this diagnostic possibility should receive special consideration in situations characterized by complete anuria. Glomerular filtration requires a positive transmembrane pressure differential between the glomerular capillaries and Bowman's space. With acute urinary tract obstruction, the increased hydrostatic pressure within the collecting system is transmitted in a retrograde fashion all the way to Bowman's space. When the hydrostatic pressure within Bowman's space equals that within the glomerular capillaries, glomerular filtration ceases.

Obstruction can also occur if there is bilateral occlusion of the renal pelvic outlet or the ureters or blockage of the bladder outlet or the urethra, by blood clots or edema. In a child with a solitary kidney, a unilateral, upper-tract obstructive process could obviously cause oliguric renal failure.

A ruptured bladder can also produce oliguria and azotemia because of the recycling of nitrogenous waste products back into the circulation after their reabsorption from the abdominal or pelvic space.

DIFFERENTIAL DIAGNOSIS OF ACUTE RENAL FAILURE

Distinguishing between post-traumatic prerenal, renal parenchymal, or postrenal failure is sometimes difficult. Most of the difficulty occurs in distinguishing between prerenal azotemia and ARPF. It goes without saying that in situations characterized by an obvious deficit in the effective arterial blood volume (e.g., hypotension, a low CVP, a low pulmonary wedge pressure), the restoration of tissue perfusion must be the first priority. If normalization of tissue perfusion does not result in a return of normal kidney function, renal diagnostic studies will be necessary.

Remember that in prerenal azotemia, the kidney is responding appropriately to the signals it is receiving. The normal renal response to decreased perfusion is to conserve sodium and water. Therefore, in prerenal azotemia, the urine is concentrated with the osmolality that is greater than 650 mOm/L (specific gravity >1.015) and a urinary sodium concentration that is low, usually less than 20 mEq/L. The calculation of the fractional sodium excretion,* that is, the percentage of filtered sodium that is excreted in the urine, offers even greater precision in estimating the degree of urinary sodium conservation and in distinguishing prerenal azotemia from ARPF. A fractional sodium excretion of less than 2 per cent in an infant or less than 1 per cent in an older child suggests prerenal failure. However, these guidelines are not reliable after a diuretic has been used (e.g., furosemide). These and the other features of prerenal azotemia are summarized in Table 7–1.

During the first 12 to 24 hours of emerging ARPF, the laboratory features that customarily distinguish prerenal azotemia from

*Fractional sodium (Na) excretion equals urine/plasma (U/P) Na concentration divided by U/P creat × 100.

Table 7–1. THE LABORATORY FEATURES OF ACUTE RENAL FAILURE

	Prerenal Azotemia	**Acute Renal Parenchymal Failure**
Urinary specific gravity	> 1.015	< 1.014
Urinary osmolality (mOm/L)	> 650	< 600
Serum BUN/ creatinine ratio	> 30:1	< 20:1
Urine-plasma urea ratio	> 20	< 10
Urine-plasma creatinine ratio	> 40	< 15
Urinary sodium concentration (mEq/L)	< 20	> 30
Urinary fractional sodium excretion	< 1%	> 2%
Urinalysis	Modest proteinuria, benign sediment	Hematuria, proteinuria, tubular epithelial cells and casts

ARPF may be equivocal. However, once ARPF is fully established, the damaged tubules will be unable to modify the glomerular filtrate substantially. Then, the osmolality of the urine will approach that of plasma (300 mOm/L), and the urinary sodium concentration will be greater than 30 mEq/L, and the fractional sodium excretion will be greater than 2 per cent. However, in cases of nonoliguric ARPF, the urinary sodium concentration and the fractional sodium excretion may be somewhat lower. In addition, the urinalysis should show evidence of parenchymal damage, as would be manifested by mild to moderate proteinuria, and by moderate to heavy hematuria; it should also show numerous renal tubular cells, white cells, and casts (tubular, white cells, granular). The other distinguishing features are summarized in Table 7–1.

Renal parenchymal failure caused by DIC is characterized by an elevated prothrombin time (PT) and partial thromboplastin time (PTT), a low fibrinogen concentration, positive fibrin split products, thrombocytopenia, and microangiopathic hemolytic anemia.

The presence of complete anuria suggests vascular injury. If renal pedicle trauma is suspected, isotope renography or renal arteriography, by either the conventional or digital subtraction technique should be performed. Renography is a reasonable screening procedure. It can be followed by arteriography, if necessary, to confirm the presence of a vascular injury.

An ultrasound examination will often be sufficient to exclude the signs of an obstruction, such as a dilated bladder, ureter, or renal pelvis. It is also adequate for visualizing pelvic collections of fluid, as can be seen with a ruptured urinary bladder. If one is in doubt about the presence of obstructive uropathy, cystocopy and retrograde pyelography must be performed. An isotope renogram cannot be depended upon to distinguish between ARPF and obstruction. Moreover, intravenous pyelograghy (IVP) should not be attempted under these circumstances because nonvisualization is to be expected and additional toxic damage to the kidney might occur.

GENERAL THERAPEUTIC CONSIDERATIONS

The treatment of ARF resulting from vascular injury, obstructive uropathy, or bladder rupture is usually fairly straightforward and is surgical in nature.

The therapeutic approach to DIC renal failure is more controversial, although all would agree that the initiating factors (e.g., sepsis) should certainly be addressed. The value of replenishing the consumed coagulation factors by administering fresh frozen plasma is less certain because it might even perpetuate the process. Although heparin therapy is often advocated for treating DIC, it is contraindicated in the early post-trauma period.

The therapy for "early" ARPF continues to be the subject of continuing discussion and debate. As discussed earlier, if the factors responsible for the prerenal azotemia (e.g., hypovolemia) are allowed to persist, ARPF can certainly evolve. It is during this transition period between prerenal azotemia and ARPF that therapeutic maneuvers may either abort the development of ARPF or at least convert oliguric ARPF to the nonoliguric variety. That is, the preglomerular vasoconstriction and intrarenal shunting of blood from the outer cortex to the deep cortex and the medulla can often be reversed before advanced renal parenchymal damage occurs. The first objective should obviously be to reestablish normal effective arterial blood volume (i.e., tissue perfusion). This can usually be accomplished by infusing fluid (e.g., blood, plasma, lactated Ringer's solution) or by administering adrenergic agents (e.g., dopamine) or vasodilators (e.g., sodium nitroprusside), or both, depending on the volume status, the cardiac output, and the systemic vascular resistance.

If oliguria persists in spite of conventional volume replacement, it may still respond to aggressive volume expansion (i.e., maximizing the preload). This technique requires the use of a pulmonary flotation catheter that is equipped to measure cardiac output. Colloid may be administered in spite of a normal or elevated CVP or pulmonary capillary wedge pressure (PCWP) as long as the volume expansion (preload) is increasing the cardiac output and not producing signs of early pulmonary edema (e.g., rales, radiographic signs, decreasing total lung-thorax compliance).

If normalization of the plasma volume does not result in the restoration of urinary output, IV mannitol (1 g/kg of body weight) or furosemide (up to 10 mg/kg given over 4 hours) may be tried. Both of these agents increase the renal blood flow and urinary solute excretion. Thus, they may be helpful in aborting incipient ARPF or in at least converting oliguric ARPF to the nonoliguric variety. However, there is no convincing evidence that these agents decrease the duration of established ARPF, the need for dialysis, or patient mortality. Furosemide may be preferable to mannitol because in the event of no diuretic response, it does not result in hyperosmolality. However, if used in high doses, furosemide may result in temporary and, at times, permanent hearing loss. Moreover, because a continuous infusion of furosemide (0.025 mg/kg/minute) is often required after the initial dose to maintain a diuresis, it is easy to achieve ototoxic serum levels, especially in the presence of renal failure. Again, it is important to replace any diuretic-induced urinary output with equal amounts of salt and water to avoid volume depletion. The risk-benefit ratio of using mannitol or furosemide therapy in treating incipient ARPF is at best marginal.

SPECIFIC MANAGEMENT PROBLEMS

Fluid and Electrolyte Principles

Children in acute renal failure (ARF) have lost their renal homeostatic regulatory capabilities and are, therefore, predisposed to water and electrolyte imbalance. However, the basic principles of fluid and electrolyte therapy still apply. Homeostasis demands that intake equal output. Moreover, if a deficiency in salt or water exists, appropriate repletion fluids must be administered in spite of renal failure. Conversely, if a child develops a surfeit of salt and water (edema), a negative balance must be achieved. It is clear, however, that with the loss of renal homeostatic capabilities, the management of fluids must be precise. Damaged kidneys may be unable to correct the therapeutic inaccuracies of the clinician.

The water requirements in renal failure obviously vary with the urinary output. The insensible water losses (water lost by skin and lung evaporation) and losses from the gastroinestinal tract (GI) or from perspiration must be added to the urinary volume. Because most children who develop post-traumatic ARF are hemodynamically unstable and thus are ill enough to justify the placement of an indwelling urinary catheter, the measurement of urinary output is easy. However, once the patient is out of shock and hemodynamically stable, the advantages of an indwelling catheter are outweighed by the risk of urinary tract infection and secondary sepsis. At this time, it is preferable to estimate urinary output in young children by using a urinary collection bag appliance or by weighing diapers. In the unconscious or obtunded older child or adolescent, a condom-type catheter can be used.

Net insensible water loss, that is, the true insensible loss minus the water of catabolism, approximates 350 ml/m^2 of body surface area per day. In a normovolemic child, that is, a child free of edema or volume depletion, the most convenient and precise method of determining free water requirements is to measure the serum sodium concentration. Irrespective of water guidelines (i.e., 350 ml/m^2/day), a rising serum sodium concentration indicates the need for more free water, whereas a falling serum sodium concentration in a nondehydrated patient indicates the need for water restriction. Moreover, unless the child is receiving adequate calories, a daily weight loss of less than 1 per cent indicates a positive fluid balance.

Likewise, electrolyte requirements parallel losses. Urinary electrolyte losses can be measured precisely by using timed urine collections. However, "spot" urinary electrolyte measurement is usually adequate. GI electrolyte losses can also be measured directly. Insensible loss, which by definition excludes perspiration, is electrolyte free. Because total body sodium chloride is the major determinant of extracellular volume, assessing body volume is a logical way of determining sodium chloride needs. If a child has a central venous or a pulmonary artery wedge catheter, measurements obtained from it can also be used to assess the child's need for salt. Although it might sound paradoxical, hyper- or hyponatremia most often reflects a deficit or an excess, respectively, in total body water rather than in total body salt (see page 146). If a child is not volume depleted but is anuric and has no GI fluid losses, electrolyte requirements are zero.

Although hyperkalemia is common in oliguric ARF, urinary postassium excretion can be substantial in the nonoliguric variety, and hypokalemia may even occur. Moreover, if there are substantial losses of electrolytes from the GI tract, as with nasogastric suction, a deficiency in total body postassium may occur even in the presence of oliguria. A hypokalemic child requires potassium repletion irrespective of renal function. However, repletion in this setting must be precise because life-threatening hyperkalemia can easily occur.

As the child begins to recover from ARF, the intake of water and electrolytes must mirror the increasing urinary losses. Accurate measurements of urinary water and electrolyte losses provide invaluable information. Urinary output usually increases in a fairly gradual fashion and is usually appropriate for the urinary solute (urea, electrolyte) load. However, glomerular filtration may sometimes improve faster than tubular function and result in a loss of salt and water that continues even after all excess water and solute have been excreted. A similar situation may occur following the resolution of a postrenal obstruction. In this situation, the obstructive uropathy leaves the kidneys with a temporary inability to conserve water and, in some instances, salt appropriately. In both of these polyuric situations, the continued replacement of ongoing losses is necessary in order to prevent salt and water depletion. Even though the tubular dysfunction and subsequent inappropriate polyuria and saluresis usually last for only a few days, they may occasionally persist for several weeks. With ongoing polyuria, the clinician is faced with the challenge of deciding whether or not the polyuria is being perpetuated by ongoing fluid administration or whether it is caused by persistent tubular damage. In these instances, it is appropriate to decrease fluid administration periodically to see whether the urinary output decreases proportionally. If it does not, any salt and water deficit must be replaced, and ongoing replacement of urinary water and electrolyte losses must be reinstituted. Every few days the kidneys can again be challenged by decreasing the administration of fluid.

Hyperkalemia

A potentially lethal but preventable complication of ARF is hyperkalemic cardiotoxicity. With oliguric ARF, the ability to excrete potassium is severely limited. Moreover, when ARF occurs as a consequence of trauma, massive quantities of intracellular potassium may be released from the cells as a consequence of a crush injury, catabolism, internal bleeding, and metabolic acidosis. The intracellular concentration of potassium is approximately 150 mEq/L, and the intracellular compartment accounts for approximately two thirds of total body water. Therefore, even a modest efflux of intracellular potassium to the extracellular compartment results in severe hyperkalemia. In addition, for every 0.1 fall in the serum pH, one can anticipate a 0.6 to 1.0 mEq rise in the serum potassium concentration. Hyperkalemia (Fig. 7–1) initially causes peaked T waves and a shortened Q-T interval. As the potassium concentration rises further, the QRS complex widens and the P wave disappears. Eventually, a sine wave and asystole occur. Although cardiac arrest usually occurs when the serum potassium concentration is greater than 8 or 9 mEq/L, death can occur with levels less than 7 mEq/L, especially if there is concurrent hyponatremia, hypocalcemia, or acidosis. Therefore, it is prudent to treat the patient when the serum potassium concentration is 6 mEq/L or greater. Earlier therapy is indicated if the potassium level is rising rapidly and approaching 6 mEq/L.

The approach to therapy (Table 7–2) depends on the magnitude of the hyperkalemia and the severity of the changes shown on the electrocardiogram (EKG). Mild to moderate hyperkalemia (i.e., a serum potassium concentration less than 7.0 mEq/L), with only a slight peaking of the T waves, can usually be treated by administering a cation exchange resin (e.g., Kayexalate). The customary Kayexalate dosage is 1 g/kg of body weight, given as often as every 4 to 6 hours. If the upper GI tract is intact and there is no ileus, it is best to give Kayexalate orally. To prevent severe constipation, it should be mixed with 70 per cent sorbitol (1 ml/g of resin). It can also be given rectally but must be retained

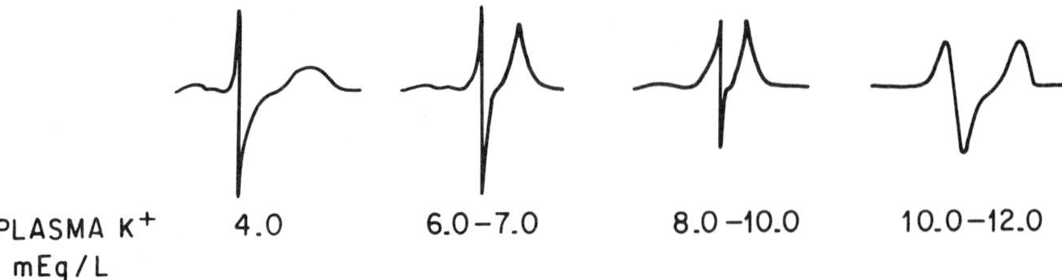

Figure 7–1. Depiction of the customary electrocardiographic changes seen with various degrees of hyperkalemia. However, hyponatremia, hypocalcemia, and acidosis may potentiate hyperkalemic cardiotoxicity and result in life-threatening arrhythmias in the presence of modest degrees of hyperkalemia.

Table 7–2. DRUG TREATMENT OF HYPERKALEMIA

Agent	Dose and Route of Administration	Action	Comments
Calcium gluconate (10%)	0.3 ml/kg body weight; slow IV push	Antagonizes the effect of hyperkalemia at the cell membrane	For life-threatening situations. Effect is rapid, but short-lived.
Sodium bicarbonate	1 mEq/kg body weight, IV	"Drives" K^+ into the cell	Can cause hypernatremia and hypervolemia
Glucose with insulin	1 gm/kg body weight with 1 unit insulin/3 g glucose; IV	"Drives" K^+ into the cell	Children in renal failure may be very sensitive to insulin
Cation exchange resin (e.g., Kayexalate)	1 gm/kg body weight mixed with 70% sorbitol (1 ml/g resin); po or retention enema.	Exchanges Na^+ for K^+, which is then excreted in the intestine	It will also bind with other cations and thus may cause hypocalcemia

for 20 to 40 minutes if an adequate potassium exchange is to occur. Even though Kayexalate primarily exchanges sodium for potassium, it also binds other cations (e.g., calcium).

Potassium can also be "driven" into the cell by the administration of sodium bicarbonate or glucose with insulin. If the child can tolerate the sodium load (i.e., is not in pulmonary edema) and is not hypernatremic, 1 mEq of sodium bicarbonate/kg of body weight can be given intravenously. In addition, glucose (1 g/kg of body weight) with insulin (1 unit/3 g glucose) can also be administered. These measures are usually adequate for the temporary management of moderate (i.e., K 6.5 to 7.0 mEq/L) hyperkalemia, as long as the ECG shows no more than peaked T waves. However, if the child is also in oliguric ARPF, treatment using dialysis is preferable.

Severe hyperkalemia, that is, a potassium concentration of 7 mEq or greater, or hyperkalemia associated with severe ECG abnormalities generally requires dialysis. While arranging for dialysis, it is often necessary to begin emergency measures. Because calcium can antagonize potassium at the cell membrane, administration of IV calcium usually results in a dramatic but short-lived improvement in the heart rhythm. This maneuver, coupled with the IV administration of sodium bicarbonate and glucose with insulin, can be repeated as necessary while arranging for dialysis. Either peritoneal dialysis or hemodialysis (HD) can be used; however, HD is much more efficient and may be required in highly metabolic or crush-injured patients.

Metabolic Acidosis

Normal kidneys participate in the regulation of acid-base balance by reabsorbing (i.e., reclaiming) filtered bicarbonate and by regenerating new bicarbonate (via titratable acid and ammonia formation). In ARPF, there is a quantitative defect in the ability to regenerate bicarbonate. Because of the ongoing production of acids from the metabolic breakdown of sulphur-containing amino acids and from the production of lactic acid (in instances of tissue hypoxia), metabolic acidosis should be anticipated. Children in shock who are producing large amounts of lactic acid and are in ARF are particularly at risk for developing life-threatening metabolic acidosis.

Most would agree that severe metabolic acidosis (pH < 7.1) should be treated with buffering agents. Tris buffer (THAM) is contraindicated because it requires renal excretion and the preparation contains some potassium. Sodium bicarbonate is, therefore, the usual mainstay of therapy. But it too should be administered cautiously to avoid a worsening of intracellular and central nervous system (CNS) acidosis and to avoid "overshoot" alkalosis. Overzealous administration can "turn off" the acidemia-induced hyperventilation and permit the P_{CO_2} level to rise. Because CO_2 is more diffusible than HCO_3, it enters the cells and the CNS more rapidly. Since CO_2 equilibrates with carbonic acid, it will lower the intracellular and CNS pH. Moreover, the lactic acid will eventually be metabolized to HCO_3 once the shock (tissue hypoxia) has been corrected. This phenomenon will add to the bicarbonate pool and can produce alkalosis. Therefore, it is prudent to administer only enough bicarbonate to keep the arterial pH > 7.2 and the serum HCO_3 above 10 mEq/L. Therapy with bicarbonate is often limited by a sodium-induced hypervolemia or hypernatremia, or both. Under these circumstances, dialysis will be required. Hour for hour, hemodialysis is much more efficient than peritoneal dialysis in correcting metabolic acidosis. If the child is on a ventilator, lowering the P_{CO_2} by increasing the respiratory rate is also helpful in minimizing the magnitude of the acidemia. Caution must always be exercised in the presence of a head injury and cerebral edema because hypocapnia decreases cerebral perfusion. Although modest hypocapnia (e.g., P_{CO_2} 25 mm Hg) is helpful in minimizing cerebral edema, severe degrees of hypocapnia may result in ischemic cerebral damage.

Volume Overload

In the presence of ARF of the renal parenchymal or postrenal variety, it is very easy to administer more salt and water than the kidney can excrete. Moreover, in burn patients, one can anticipate intravascular expansion when the excess extravascular (interstitial) fluids are mobilized. If ARF is present, this can result in severe intravascular expansion and pulmonary edema. With careful monitoring of body volume, it may be possible to decrease sodium and water administration before a severe fluid overload occurs. If a severe fluid overload occurs in the setting of ARF, dialysis is the only effective form of therapy. One should anticipate a 1 per cent loss of body weight per day unless the child is receiving full nutritional support. A weight loss of less than this generally indicates fluid retention.

Serum Sodium Concentration Abnormalities

Hyper- and hyponatremia generally indicate either a deficiency or an excess in total body water, respectively, rather than an abnormality in total body sodium. Therefore, if a child in renal failure develops hypernatremia, that is, an elevated serum sodium concentration, one can safely assume that the child is deficient in water. Conversely, if a nondehydrated patient develops hyponatremia—that is, a low serum sodium concentration—more stringent water restriction measures should be imposed.

A frequent error is to give increasing amounts of sodium chloride to a hyponatremic edematous child. One should equate edema with an increased total body sodium content, irrespective of the serum sodium concentration. An edematous hyponatremic patient has not only an excess in total body sodium but also an even greater excess in total body water. Salt should never be administered to an edematous child except in instances of hyponatremic encephalopathy or shock.

In summary, with rare exceptions, an abnormality in the serum sodium concentration indicates a need for readjusting the administration of water rather than sodium.

Phosphorus and Calcium Balance

One should anticipate hyperphosphatemia with ARF. Because the major route of phosphorus excretion is the kidney, a fall in the glomerular filtration rate (GFR) predictably causes a decreased clearance of phosphate. Moreover, because phosphorous is largely an intracellular ion, the extracellular phosphate pool will be increased in response to a crush injury and to catabolism. Hyperphosphatemia causes a reciprocal fall in the concentration of both total and ionized serum calcium.

In chronic renal failure, hypocalcemia also occurs because of the decreased gut absorption of calcium caused by the impaired hydroxylation of vitamin D. However, there is little information about the role of altered vitamin D metabolism in the hypocalcemia of ARF. Occasionally, the hypocalcemia may be severe enough to cause tetany or even seizures, and hypocalcemia tends to increase the cardiotoxicity of hyperkalemia.

The treatment of hyperphosphatemia in the setting of ARF differs from that in chronic renal failure. Customarily post-trauma patients ingest no phosphorus-containing foodstuffs; therefore, the use of phosphate binders (e.g., aluminum hydroxide gel) is of little value. Short-term hyperphosphatemia rarely requires specific therapy, and in and of itself, it is rarely an indication for dialysis.

The hypocalcemia should likewise be treated conservatively. Raising a child's serum calcium to normal in the setting of hyperphosphatemia may produce a calcium-phosphorus product in excess of 70 mg/dl. Although it is unlikely that detectable metastatic calcification will occur in the heart, nervous system, or skin during temporary renal failure, a high calcium-phosphorous product should be avoided. It is unnecessary to treat hypocalcemia unless it is causing signs or symptoms (e.g., tetany). If treatment is necessary, the serum calcium concentration should be raised only to levels sufficient to alleviate the hypocalcemic signs and symptoms while avoiding a calcium-phosphorus product in excess of 70 mg/dl.

Hyperuricemia

Uric acid excretion is always decreased as a consequence of impaired glomerular filtration. In addition, urate production is also increased whenever there is an increased destruction of nucleated cells. Short-term hyperuricemia rarely requires therapy. Even with levels in excess of 20 mg/dl, renal parenchymal damage or renal stones are virtually never seen. This renal-sparing effect is the result of the decreased delivery of urate to the renal parenchyma as a consequence of the low renal blood flow and GFR associated with ARF. In addition, clinical gout is exceedingly uncommon in children with renal failure–induced hyperuricemia. Uricosuric drugs, therefore, have no role in ARF, and xanthine oxidase inhibitors (e.g., allopurinol) are unnecessary.

Hypertension

Hypertension is rarely a problem in the early post-traumatic period, even in the setting of evolving ARPF. On the contrary, it is often a challenge to maintain a normal blood pressure. Later, once the shock or sepsis, or both, has been effectively treated, hypertension may occur.

In most cases, the hypertension results from an excess in total body volume (sodium). Even though expanding the extracellular compartment of a normal child produces little change in blood pressure, it can have a substantial effect on the blood pressure of a patient with severe renal parenchymal damage. This type of hypertension has been called renoprival hypertension, suggesting that the pathogenesis is linked to a deficiency in renal function. There is some evidence that the normal kidney responds to volume expansion by elaborating increased amounts of vasodilatory substances (e.g., prostaglandins, kinins). In the presence of renal damage, there may be an inability to elaborate these protective vasodilatory substances, and therefore even modest volume expansion may be sufficient to cause hypertension. Moreover, as the renin-angiotensin system is customarily very active, at least during the early stages of ARF, increased angiotensin II production may also contribute to the high blood pressure. Normalizing body volume, by restricting salt and water and by dialysis, customarily normalizes blood pressure. However, drug therapy may be necessary if the patient is not being dialyzed or if the blood pressure remains elevated in spite of salt and water restriction and dialysis. Systolic and/or diastolic readings above 130/80 in an infant, greater than 135/85 in a young child, above 150/95 in an older child, or more than 170/120 in an adolescent should probably be considered a hypertensive emergency and be treated with parenteral drugs. Lesser degrees of hypertension can be treated with oral medications as long as the patient is free of hypertensive signs or symptoms. Table 7–3 contains representative hypertensive medications.

Uremia

Uremia is the clinical expression of azotemia. That is, although azotemia is defined as the retention of nitrogenous waste products (e.g., urea, creatinine), the term uremia describes the signs and symptoms resulting from the accumulation of these toxic products. Even though uremia is undoubtedly largely caused by the retention of nitrogenous waste products, the identification and characterization of all the toxic products must await further investigation. Urea per se causes few if any symptoms unless the level is quite high (greater than 100 mg/dl), and even then the symptoms are usually quite mild. There are other substances, including methylguanidine and guanidinosuccinic acid and a host of so-called middle molecules, whose molecular weights range between 500 and 5000, which are probably also toxic. There is also some evidence that parathormone (PTH) is a uremic toxin. Although many of the classical signs and symptoms of uremia do not generally occur with short-term ARF, lethargy, somnolence, nausea and vomiting, and uremic encephalopathy, including seizures, are frequently seen.

Because it is uncertain which of the uremic toxins, alone or in combination, are responsible for these problems and because only urea and creatinine concentrations can be measured in the clinical laboratory, there is no precise way of predicting when uremia will occur. However, as a generalization, the

Table 7–3. TREATMENT OF HYPERTENSION

Hypertensive Emergencies

Drug	*Action*	*Dose and Route of Administration*	*Side Effects*
Hydralazine	Vasodilator	0.1–0.2 mg/kg body weight; IM or IV	Headache; tachycardia
Diazoxide	Vasodilator	5–10/kg body weight; rapid IV push	Hyperglycemia; fluid retention
Sodium nitroprusside	Vasodilator	0.5–8.0 μg/kg/min (1.0 μg/kg/min starting dose); IV drip; use infusion pump; monitor constantly	Cyanide poisoning

Nonemergency Therapy

Drug	*Action*	*Dose and Route of Administration*	*Side Effects*
Methyldopa	Central	10–40 mg/kg/day; IV or po, (2–4 divided doses)	Sedation; hemolytic anemia
Clonidine	Central	0.003–0.03 mg/kg/day; po (2 divided doses)	Sedation; rebound hypertension
Hydralazine	Vasodilator	1–3 mg/kg/day; po (2–4 divided doses)	Headache; palpitation
Prazosin	Vasodilator	0.01–0.3 mg/kg/day; po (2–3 divided doses)	Syncope; dizziness; headache
Minoxidil	Vasodilator	0.1–1.0 mg/kg/day; po (1–2 divided doses)	Hypertrichosis; tachycardia; fluid retention

blood urea nitrogen (BUN) level is more predictive of uremia than is the serum creatinine concentration. Uremic signs and symptoms are usually not seen with BUN levels of less than 100 mg/dl, but they can be anticipated if the BUN exceeds 150 to 200 mg/dl. Although the magnitude of the azotemia can be diminished and the uremia delayed with proper nutritional management (see next section), dialysis is the only definitive therapy.

NUTRITIONAL MANAGEMENT

There is general agreement that the provision of generous numbers of calories in the form of glucose has a protein-sparing effect, that is, the glucose decreases the breakdown of endogenous protein and consequently diminishes urea production. However, because renal failure causes peripheral insulin resistance, the administration of glucose is likely to cause hyperglycemia, and the cautious administration of insulin may also be necessary.

Moreover, the general consensus is that providing protein high in essential amino acid content will decrease the rate of urea synthesis. The traditional theory is that if essential amino acids and sufficient nonprotein calories are provided, the nonessential amino acids will synthesized. This is accomplished by using the urea nitrogen that is derived from the deamination of amino acids. Urea is first degraded in the intestine by the bacterial urease to carbon dioxide and ammonia; the ammonia is then reabsorbed into the portal system, where it is recycled into new amino acids. The importance of this phenomemon may have been somewhat overestimated, however. For although urea recycling is increased slightly in uremic patients, the nitrogen derived from this reaction contributes only a small, although nutritionally significant, additional amount of nitrogen to the protein pool.

Even though the customary minimum protein requirements for pediatric patients range from between 3 g/kg of body weight/day for infants to 1 g/kg of body weight/day for adolescents, one third of this amount may be sufficient (extrapolating from studies in adults) if the protein is composed almost entirely of the essential amino acids. There is some uncertainty as to what should constitute the full complement of essental amino acids in patients with renal failure. There is evidence that histidine is an essential amino acid in renal failure. Moreover, because the normal kidney synthesizes arginine, it should probably also be considered essential.

Keto amino acid analogs can be given in lieu of essential amino acids. Although they certainly improve the nitrogen balance and nutrition without adding to the nitrogen load, the keto analogs offer no clear-cut advantage over the free amino acids.

It is also uncertain whether providing some nonspecific (conventional) protein along with the essential amino acids is nutritionally advantageous over feeding the essential amino acids alone.

In patients with post-traumatic renal failure of the oliguric variety, it is usually impossible to give enough calories to meet even basal requirements, let alone the additional caloric requirements of a traumatized child, without exceeding the necessary fluid restrictions. In a larger child or an adolescent who is not particularly catabolic, one may come close to meeting the caloric requirements if one uses generous amounts of IV fat emulsion. However, because hyperlipidemia is frequently associated with ARF, it is difficult to give enough fat emulsion without causing the triglyceride level to rise above 175 mg/dl. At this serum concentration, the lipoprotein lipase activity is virtually saturated, and additional amounts of fat cannot be metabolized. And because of the need to restrict fluids, it is rarely possible to provide the oliguric, catabolic patient with full nutritional support without concurrent dialytic therapy. Once regular dialysis therapy has been initiated, it is possible to maintain the fluid balance by utilizing ultrafiltration or hemofiltration or by depending upon hypertonic (4.25% dextrose) peritoneal dialysis solutions to remove the excess fluid. The use of 4.25 per cent glucose in the peritoneal dialysate also adds additional calories. Moreover, essential amino acids can also be added to the peritoneal dialysate to promote a better nitrogen and caloric balance.

Therefore, once regular dialytic therapy has begun, either enteral or parenteral hyperalimentation can be started. If the gut is intact, enteral feeding should be used. Essential amino acid mixtures that also contain carbohydrates and vitamins are available. Carbohydrate, vegetable oil, or medium-chain triglyceride (MCT) oil can be added to increase the caloric density. Please refer to Table 7–4 for a summary of some representative enteral formulas.

However, if gut function is not normal, if the hyperosmolar nature of the formulas causes diarrhea or other unacceptable side effects, or if normovolemia cannot be maintained, central hyperalimentation must be used. Because of the ability to give fluids of a greater caloric density (e.g., 25 per cent glucose) through a central venous catheter, the child's caloric needs can be met with a smaller volume of infusate. Refer to Chapter 6 for details.

The safe use of either enteral or parenteral alimentation in the presence of ARPF requires an understanding of the impact of renal failure on the fluid and electrolyte balance. The volume must be limited to the amount of fluid that can safely be removed during dialysis. In many cases it may be necessary to dialyze daily to avoid peripheral and pulmonary edema. Although potassium and phosphate are required for new cell growth, it is best to leave these substances out of the hyperalimentation solution unless hypokalemia or hypophosphatemia develops. Because of the tendency to retain magnesium in renal failure, magnesium should

Table 7–4. ENTERAL ALIMENTATION IN ACUTE RENAL FAILURE

Formulas	**kcal/ml**	**Protein (g/L)**	**Carbohydrates (g/L)**	**Fat (g/L)**	**Na/K (mEq/L)**
Similac PM 60/40 (Ross)	0.67	15	69	37	7/14
SMA (Wyeth)	0.67	15	72	36	7/14
S-29 (Wyeth)*	0.67	17	101	23	0.4/8
Special Supplements Carbohydrate and Fat Preparations†					
Controlyte (Doyle)	2.0	Trace	286	96	0.8/0.4
Corn oil	8.4	—	—	933	—
MCT oil (Mead Johnson Nutritional)	7.7	—	—	933	—
Polycose liquid (Ross)	2.0	—	500	—	25/5
Sumacal (Organon)	2.0	—	500	—	7/6
Amino Acid Preparations	**kcal**	**Amino Acids**	**Carbohydrates**	**Fat (g/L)**	**Na/K (mEq/L)**
Amin-Aid (McGaw)	2.0/ml	19.4g/L	347g/L	64.7	6/6
Aminess tablets, (Cutter)	3.0/tab	0.69g/tab	0.05g/tab	0.02g/tab	Trace

*Since S-29 is low in sodium and calcium, these may need to be added.

†Because patients in renal failure often have hypertriglyceridemia, triglyceride levels must be monitored when using carbohydrate or fat preparations.

not be added unless hypomagnesemia occurs. Moreover, because the kidneys will be unable to excrete nitrogenous waste products and hydrogen ions normally, the use of protein is likely to result in a worsening of the azotemia and the metabolic acidosis. Giving the protein in the form of essential amino acids (Amin-Aid, Aminess, Nephramine, Aminosyn-RF) will lessen the azotemia. Finally, because of the tendency of patients with renal failure to develop hypertriglyceridemia, serum triglyceride levels must be checked frequently when using fats.

EFFECT OF ACUTE RENAL FAILURE ON DRUG USE

Because most traumatized patients in acute renal failure are given numerous pharmacologic agents, it is imperative that the clinician be aware of the major routes of drug excretion, the degree to which drug elimination is affected by renal failure, and the effect of azotemia on drug protein binding.

Drugs that are excreted by the kidneys have prolonged half-lives in the presence of ARF. One can modify drug dosing requirements by either decreasing the amount administered while maintaining the customary interval or by maintaining the customary dosage amount and increasing the drug dose interval. Although either method is usually satisfactory, it is well to remember that the dose interval modification method results in higher and longer peak serum concentrations as well as lower and longer drug trough level serum concentrations than does the dosage reduction method. A prolonged subtherapeutic trough concentration might be disadvantageous when dealing with rapidly multiplying organisms. A modification of this method is to give the customary dose and to follow it by the administration of half the normal dose every half-life. This avoids prolonged subtherapeutic blood levels. The decreased dosage method also avoids the problem of prolonged subtherapeutic blood concentrations and results in a more even (i.e., constant) serum concentration, with lower peak and higher trough serum drug concentrations. Some of the drugs used most commonly in injured children, the effect of ARF on the elimination of these drugs and dosage modification guidelines are detailed in Table 7–5. The dosing suggestions are only approximations; serum levels should be followed when possible.

Advanced azotemia also causes a decrease in the protein binding of many drugs. A greater percentage of these drugs are therefore present in their free (i.e., biologically active) form. This makes it difficult to interpret conventional serum levels, which measure only total (i.e., bound and unbound) concentrations. For example, what might ordinarily constitute a normal therapeutic serum level for total phenytoin (Dilantin) might, in fact, represent a toxic serum level because of increased concentrations of the free drug fraction. Therefore, free drug measurements may sometimes be necessary in the azotemic child.

DIALYSIS

Indications for Dialysis

Fluid overload and hyperkalemia are the most common reasons for beginning dialysis after trauma. Volume overload (edema) occurs frequently as a result of infusing large volumes of saline, or Ringer's, solutions. Crush injury, hypermetabolism, and acidosis all contribute to hyperkalemia. Severe metabolic acidosis, resulting from tissue hypoperfusion and impaired renal acid excretion, constitutes another common indication for dialysis. Moreover, severe or persistent posttraumatic metabolic acidosis may require the administration of massive quantities of sodium bicarbonate, which can result in a severe volume overload or in hypernatremia, or both. Hyperphosphatemia and secondary hypocalcemia can also contribute to the decision to begin dialysis.

Even if the child is fortunate enough to escape fluid and electrolyte problems, prophylactic dialysis should be begun before uremic symptoms (e.g., nausea, vomiting, encephalopathy) or life-threatening hemorrhage or infection occurs. Although (from a risk and cost/benefit perspective) there are no precise data indicating when to initiate dialysis, it is reasonable to take steps that will keep the BUN less than 100 mg/dl in all patients and the serum creatinine below 15 mg/dl in the adolescent, below 10 mg/dl in the child, and less than 5 mg/dl in the infant.

Selecting the Type of Dialysis

In past years, the use of hemodialysis was limited to larger children and adolescents.

Now, however, with the advent of pediatric blood lines and small volume, low-compliance dialyzers, infants can safely be hemodialyzed by experienced personnel.

Even so, peritoneal dialysis is usually preferred to hemodialysis in infants and small children for the following reasons. (1) The relatively larger peritoneal surface area of children increases the efficiency of peritoneal dialysis, and (2) peritoneal dialysis is easier to administer. In addition, in contrast to hemodialysis, heparinization is unnecessary and systemic bleeding is therefore not a problem.

Recent abdominal surgery is not an absolute contraindication to peritoneal dialysis. However, peritoneal dialysis should probably be avoided if there has been widespread bowel injury or if the nature of the abdominal injuries or surgery would cause severe leakage of dialysate. The presence of peritonitis is not a contraindication to peritoneal dialysis because antibiotics can be added to the dialysate, which may assist in treatment.

The efficiency of peritoneal dialysis is reduced in patients who are hypotensive because they experience a reduction in the splanchnic blood flow. However, these same patients are also at increased risk during hemodialysis because of their cardiovascular instability. Peritoneal dialysis may not be efficient enough for patients who are severely hypercatabolic and who are, therefore, experiencing rapidly rising urea, potassium, and acid levels.

In summary, the decision as to which dialysis modality to use depends largely on the availability of equipment, the interest and expertise of the dialysis personnel, and the clinical setting. Hemodialysis is more time-efficient and is preferable in instances of severe catabolism characterized by a rapid rise in the level of urea, potassium, and acid. Peritoneal dialysis, on the other hand, is safer in the hemodynamically unstable patient and offers the advantages of greater ease of administration in infants and small children and of continuous but gradual fluid and solute removal.

Peritoneal Dialysis

General Principles

Peritoneal dialysis utilizes the peritoneal surface as the dialyzing membrane. When the peritoneum is filled with dialysate (which approximates plasma, with the exception that it is free of protein and nitrogenous waste products), the nitrogenous waste products, phosphorous, and potassium move from the area of higher concentration (the plasma) to the area of lower concentration (the dialysate). Lactate, which is contained in the dialysate, buffers the inorganic acids. Dextrose (1.5 to 4.25 g/dl) increases the osmolality of the dialysate and facilitates the transfer of plasma and interstitial water to the dialysate. As a result, the nitrogeous waste products, as well as excess acid, potassium, phosphorus, and fluid, are removed from the patient.

Dialysis Procedure

Peritoneal dialysis requires the placement of a dialysis catheter, the selection of the appropriate dialysate mixture, and a calculation of the appropriate dialysate volume and dwell times.

Catheters are customarily inserted percutaneously at the bedside, although they can be placed in the operating room. Because they lack a subcutaneous tunnel, catheters inserted at the bedside are more likely to cause peritonitis if left in place for more than 72 hours. However, they have the advantage of being easily and quickly inserted and removed. The bedside placement of this type of temporary catheter (e.g., Trocath) is carried out as follows: the skin is appropriately cleaned, local anesthesia is provided, a cautious but generous stab wound through the skin and subcutaneous tissue is made with a number 11 Bard Parker blade, and then the catheter, with the trocar firmly positioned within the catheter, is pushed through the abdominal wall in the midline, a third of the distance down from the umbilicus to the pubic symphysis, with a pushing, twisting motion. A lateral approach can also be used if care is taken to avoid the inferior epigastric artery.

The possibility of penetrating a viscus is lessened if one third to one half of the calculated dialysate volume is infused through an 18-gauge needle or catheter before inserting the larger peritoneal trocar and catheter. This initial infusion of fluid causes the bowel to float and probably decreases the likelihood of perforating the bowel with the trocar. It also allows the operator to know when he has entered the peritoneal cavity because dialysate will flow up the catheter.

The possibility of penetrating a viscus is further lessened if the abdominal wall is lifted away from the bowel by an assistant. In addition, the operator should firmly fix one hand on the catheter close to the skin to prevent a sudden and deep penetration of the peritoneal cavity. The other hand must

Table 7–5. MEDICATION USE IN ADVANCED RENAL FAILURE*

Medication	Normal Half-life (hr)	Half-Life in Advanced† Renal Failure	Dosage Modification in Advanced Renal Failure	Removal with Hemodialysis (HD) and Peritoneal Dialysis (PD)	Comments
Narcotics					
Meperidine (Demerol)	3–7	(see comments)	None (see comments)	?	Patients in renal failure may be more "sensitive" to narcotics. The active metabolites of meperidine (Demerol) accumulate in renal failure and are toxic to the central nervous system.
Morphine	2–3	?	None (see comments)	HD, no; PD?	
Codeine	3	?	None (see comments)	?	
Sedatives and Anticonvulsants					
Chloral Hydrate	4–10	Same	None	HD, yes; PD?	May cause excessive sedation.
Paraldehyde	3.5–10	Same	None	?	
Phenobarbital	24–140	Same	None	HD, yes; PD?	
Phenytoin	24	Same	None	negligible	Because of decreased protein binding and increased free (biologically active) drug concentrations in uremia, therapeutic serum levels are achieved at a much lower total serum concentration. Measure free drug levels for precise information.
Antimicrobials					
Aminoglycosides 2–3 (gentamicin, tobramycin, amikacin, kanamycin)		30–48	Give one-half normal loading dose every 36–48 hr.	HD, yes: Give one-half normal loading dose after each 4-hour dialysis; PD, yes: Give one-half normal loading dose every 48 hr.	The initial (loading) dose is the same as with normal renal function. The concurrent use of penicillins, especially carbenicillin and ticarcillin, decreases the serum concentration of the aminoglycosides. This effect appears to be less with amikacin. The aminoglycosides are ototoxic and nephrotoxic; monitor serum concentrations (peaks and troughs).
Cephalosporins					
Cefamandole (Mandol)	1.0	8–12	Give one-half normal dose every 8–10 hr.	PD, ?; HD, yes; give one-half normal dose after each HD.	Because of the rapid proliferation of new cephalosporins, only selected cephalosporins have been included.
Cefoperazone (Cefobid)	1.5–2.5	Same	None	?	Dosage reduction necessary in the presence of combined renal and hepatic failure.
Cefotaxime (Claforan)	1.0–1.5	3–11	Give one-half normal dose every 12 hr.	PD, no; HD, yes: Give one-half normal dose after each HD.	
Cefazolin (Ancef, Kefzol)	1.5–2.0	18–48	Give one-half normal dose every 24–48 hr.	PD, no; HD, yes: Give one-half normal dose after each HD.	

Table 7–5. MEDICATION USE IN ADVANCED RENAL FAILURE* (*Continued*)

Medication	Normal Half-life (hr)	Half-Life in Advanced† Renal Failure	Dosage Modification in Advanced Renal Failure	Removal with Hemodialysis (HD) and Peritoneal Dialysis (PD)	Comments
Cephalosporins Continued					
Cephalothin (Keflin)	0.5–1.0	3–20	Give one-half normal dose every 8–12 hr.	PD ?; HD, yes: Give one-half normal dose after each HD.	
Moxalactam (Moxam)	2–4	20–40	Give one-half normal dose every 24–48 hr.	PD? HD, yes: Give one-half normal dose after each HD.	
Chloramphenicol	2–3	(see comments)	None	HD? PD, no.	Normal half-life for parent compound, but toxic metabolites may accumulate and cause central nervous system toxicity.
Penicillins					
Amoxicillin, ampicillin	1–2	5–20	Give one-half normal dose every 12 hr.	HD, yes: Give 0.5–1 normal dose after HD. PD, no.	Ampicillin contains 3 mEq sodium/g.
Carbenicillin	1–1.5	10–20	Give one-half normal dose every 12 hr.	HD yes, PD? Give one-half normal dose after each HD.	The concurrent use of carbenicillin with aminoglycosides will lower the serum concentration of the aminoglycoside.
Methicillin	0.5–1.0	4	Give one-half normal dose every 8–12 hr.	HD, no; PD, no.	
Nafcillin	0.5	1.0	None	HD, no; PD, no.	Dose must be reduced in combined hepatic and renal failure.
Oxacillin	0.5	.5–1	None	HD, no; PD, no.	
Penicillin	0.5	5–20	Give one-half normal dose every 12 hr.	HD, yes: Give normal dose after each HD; PD, no.	A maximum of 100,000 units/kg/day is recommended in order to avoid encephalopathy; 1.7 mEq of potassium and 2 mEq of sodium are contained in each gram of the respective penicillin salts.
Ticarcillin	1–1.5	10–15	Give one-half normal dose every 12 hr.	HD, yes: Give one-half normal dose after each HD; PD, no.	The concurrent use of ticarcillin with aminoglycosides will lower the serum concentration of the aminoglycosides; contains 5–6.5 mEq sodium/g.
Piperacillin	1–1.5	3–4	Give normal dose every 8–12 hr.	HD, yes: Give one-half normal dose after each HD; PD, no.	
Vancomycin	6–10	200–250	Give normal dose every 7–10 days or 2 mg/kg/day.	HD, no; PD, no.	Ototoxic; monitor serum concentration prior to each dose.

*Recommendations are presented only as rough guidelines.
†Glomerular filtration rate < 10 ml/min/1.73 m^2.

keep the trocar firmly engaged within the catheter or the cutting surface of the trocar will be lost. Once the peritoneum has been penetrated, the trocar should be retracted a centimeter or two, and the catheter gently advanced toward the peritoneal gutter or pelvis.

After adequate inflow and outflow have been documented, antimicrobial ointment and a dressing should be applied to the wound site and the catheter should be firmly taped in place.

The permanent-type catheter, on the other hand, is customarily inserted in the operating room and has the advantage of allowing repeated or continuous dialysis treatments through the same catheter. It is also associated with a lower incidence of infection. The Tenchkoff catheter, for example, has either one or two dacron cuffs. One is placed at the peritoneum, and the optional second cuff is placed subcutaneously close to where the catheter exists from the subcutaneous tunnel. This tunnel, containing one or two dacron cuffs, provides a fairly effective seal against the inward migration of skin pathogens.

The customary volume of dialysate ranges from between 25 to 50 ml/kg of body weight, and the customary dwell time (the time the dialysate is in contact with the dialyzing membrane) is usually 15 to 30 minutes. The dialysate must be warmed to body temperature, and because it contains no potassium, KCl (3.5 to 4.0 mEq/L) must be added. If the patient is hyperkalemic at the beginning of dialysis, no potassium needs to be added for the first three to six exchanges. It is customary to add 0.25 units of heparin/ml of dialysate to present occlusion of the catheter by fibrin. We customarily add a broad-spectrum antibiotic (e.g., Cefadyl) as prophylaxis against peritonitis. As an additional precaution, cell counts of the dialysate effluent should be performed every 12 to 24 hours. The presence of more than 100 cells/mm^3, with more than 50 per cent of them being polymorphonuclear cells, is presumptive evidence of peritonitis. One has the choice of using a dialysate containing 1.5, 2.5, or 4.25 per cent dextrose. Even though the 1.5 per cent dextrose mixture renders the dialysate slightly hyperosmotic relative to the plasma, the 2.5 or 4.25 per cent mixture must generally be used to cause appreciable fluid removal. However, caution must be exercised when using the more concentrated dextrose solutions because severe hypovolemia or hyperglycemia can occur. It is often appropriate to mix or alternate solutions to maintain the fluid balance.

Although there is rarely any difficulty in getting the dialysate to enter the peritoneal cavity, drainage problems are frequent. Poor drainage may occur because of problems related to the catheter's position, fibrin clots within the catheter, or obstruction of catheter drainage holes by omentum. If drainage problems occur, the patient's position can be changed, the catheter can be slightly rotated while taking care not to advance the contaminated external portion of the catheter into the peritoneal cavity, and heparinized saline can be vigorously injected into the catheter. The catheter should never be aspirated because omentum may be drawn into the catheter-drainage holes. If all these maneuvers fail to correct the drainage problems, the catheter must be removed and a new catheter must be inserted.

The dialysis treatment is usually continued until the fluid and electrolyte abnormalities have been corrected and the BUN approximates 50 mg/dl. If a temporary (acute) percutaneous catheter has been used, it should be removed within 72 hours of dialysis. The temporary-type catheters (e.g., Trocath) are customarily reinserted if and when a second dialysis is needed. The permanent-type catheter (e.g., Tenchkoff) is capped and reconnected to the dialysate tubing at the beginning of the next dialysis treatment. Meticulous sterile technique is mandatory.

Complications

Dialysis complications can be technical, metabolic, or infectious. The chance of perforating a hollow viscus when inserting a temporary-type catheter is remote if the technique described previously is used and if the child is free of abdominal adhesions. The risk of inducing serious bleeding is minimal if the temporary-type catheter is inserted midline along the linea alba because there are few blood vessels in this region. However, if a lateral approach is used, the risks are greater because the inferior epigastric artery parallels the lateral border of the rectus abdominis muscle. Slight intraperitoneal bleeding is common and is generally caused by the perforation of small capillaries. This bleeding customarily stops after a few dialysis exchanges.

The metabolic complications of peritoneal dialysis are related to the composition of the dialysate. Because all commercial dialysate solutions contain dextrose to make them hypertonic to plasma, they all have the potential of extracting water. Because the 4.25 per cent dextrose solution is very hyperosmotic, it can remove large quantities of fluid, which can thus result in volume depletion and hypernatremia. The dextrose also raises the patient's serum glucose concentration. The tendency toward hyperglycemia is accentuated by the peripheral insulin resistance characteristic of renal failure. Even so, severe hyperglycemia is unusual, and insulin administration is rarely necessary. Because the dialysate solution contains no potassium, severe hypokalemia can occur during prolonged dialysis treatments if potassium is not added to the dialysate.

The most frequent serious complication of peritoneal dialysis is peritonitis. If peritonitis is suspected or if a positive cell count is found (> 100 cells mm^3, with > 50 per cent polymorphonuclear cells), the dialysate should be gram-stained, culture and sensitivity studies should be obtained, and antibiotic therapy should be started. A positive cell count will usually precede the classical signs of peritonitis by many hours. Initial antibiotic selection should be based on an estimate of the most likely pathogens. Therapy should later be guided by the results of the culture and sensitivity studies. Most infections are caused by the *Staphylococcus,* usually *S. epidermidis* but often *S. aureus;* gram-negative organisms or the *Streptococcus* are less frequent pathogens. A cephalosporin antibiotic generally provides good broad-spectrum antibiotic coverage, pending the results of the culture and sensitivity studies. Negative cultures occur frequently, however. The antibiotic is customarily added to the dialysate, but a loading dose can also be given intravenously. If it is being added to the dialysate, adequate serum levels can be maintained, assuming that the dialysis is continuous and technically successful. Total duration of therapy is usually 7 to 10 days. It is also customary to double the dose of heparin in the dialysate to prevent occlusion of the catheter by fibrin.

HEMODIALYSIS

General Principles

Hemodialysis utilizes an artificial dialyzing membrane (e.g., Cuprophane) to separate the blood from the dialysate. Substances that are in higher concentration in the plasma, such as urea, creatinine, potassium, and phosphate, pass across the semipermeable dialyzing membrane to equilibrate with the dialysate. The dialysate is continually replaced, which maintains the high-concentration gradient between the plasma and the dialysate.

Excess body fluid is removed by ultrafiltration, which is accomplished by the creation of a positive transmembrane pressure gradient between the patient's plasma and the dialysate. This is generally accomplished by partially occluding the venous line that returns blood from the dialyzer or by applying negative pressure to the dialysate side of the system. Solitary ultrafiltration is an even more effective means of removing fluid. It is a dialysate-free system that provides very high transmembrane pressures by applying positive pressure on the blood side of the membrane and negative pressure on the other side.

Dialysis Procedure

Obtaining access to the circulation is obviously the first step, in the procedure. Although temporary access can be obtained by surgically placing percutaneous Scribner shunts, this has largely been superseded by the percutaneous placement of a femoral or subclavian catheter. A femoral or subclavian venous catheter can be inserted using the Seldinger technique, which utilizes a guidewire. The wire is threaded through a small needle that has been inserted into the vein percutaneously. Both femoral and superior vena cava catheters can be adapted to single-needle dialysis systems. Subclavian catheters especially designed for dialysis are available. When treating infants, it is safer to place the cathers in the operating room while using fluoroscopic control. In infants weighing less than 10 lb, subclavian catheters should be inserted through the internal or external jugular vein rather than through the subclavian vein. Even though percutaneous insertion into these vessels is possible, it is usually done by cutting down to the vessel. When using a guidewire, it is best to keep the wire out of the heart. It is safer to position the catheter so that the tip is in the superior vena cava rather than in the right atrium. Although femoral catheters are rarely left in place for more than a day or two, properly cared for superior vena cava catheters can be kept in place for several weeks.

The hemodialysis treatment must be planned in accordance with the size of the child. As a general rule, the volume of the dialyzer plus the dialysis blood lines should not exceed 10 per cent of the patient's blood volume (blood volume approximates 8 per cent of body weight), and the dialyzer surface area should approximate 75 per cent of the child's body surface area. Moreover, to decrease the likelihood of disequilibrium, which presumably results from the too rapid removal of osmotically active uremic toxins (e.g., urea), the urea should not be cleared any faster than 2 to 3 ml/kg of body weight/minute. By knowing the patient's weight and the clearance characteristics of the particular dialyzer (usually available in the package insert), one can calculate the blood flow (i.e., pump speed) necessary to accomplish the desired urea clearance. In addition, if the predialysis BUN is greater than 100 mg/dl, the dialyzed urea should be replaced with another osmotically active substance; mannitol, in a dose of 1 g/kg of body weight, should be infused during the course of dialysis. In the presence of renal failure, mannitol has a long serum half-life and is only very slowly metabolized by the liver. Care must, therefore, be taken to avoid causing hyperosmolality, which can occur if mannitol is given more than 2 days in a row. Some centers also add extra dextrose to the dialysate bath to cause a modest hyperglycemia (hyperosmolality) and thus further counteract the osmotic effect of removing the uremic toxins.

We customarily dialyze the patient for 3 hours on the first day, and 4 hours the following day. Thereafter, dialysis is usually performed every other day or three times per week. However, daily dialysis may be necessary to control the azotemia, hyperkalemia, hyperphosphatemia, and acidosis commonly seen in severely hypercatabolic patients.

Complications

Complications of hemodialysis can be either mechanical (technical), hemodynamic, or metabolic.

The insertion of femoral venous catheters can be complicated by hematoma, by thrombosis, by perforation of the femoral artery, or by damage to the femoral nerve. If a femoral catheter is left in place after completion of the dialysis, thrombophlebitis or thromboemboli can occur. Mechanical trauma to the vessels or to the heart, thromboembolism, and infection constitute the major potential complications of using the superior vena cava (SVC) for dialysis access. Even so, with proper care of the SVC catheter, it can be left in place and successfully used for 1 to 3 weeks. Moreover, a single catheter will generally suffice for the duration of the ARF.

Hemodialysis creates an arteriovenous (A-V) fistula and thus increases the demand on the heart. A young, healthy heart can increase its output appropriately and maintain normal blood pressure and tissue perfusion. However, an injured child suffering from severe lactic acidosis or sepsis may exhibit an impaired response to this form of cardiovascular stress. Moreover, hemodialysis increases the frequency of premature ventricular contractions, which may pose a particular risk to the severely injured patient. Aggressive fluid removal (ultrafiltration) is likely to cause hypotension, particularly if the cardiac output cannot increase in response to the hypovolemia. There is evidence that the traditional actetate dialysate mixture decreases cardiac output, at least in some patients. The use of a bicarbonate dialysis system, therefore, offers at least some theoretic advantages. Whenever dialyzing hemodynamically unstable children, it is also prudent to have IV lidocaine and other antiarrhythmic drugs at the bedside in the event of serious ventricular arrhythmias.

Encephalopathic complications (disequilibrium) include headache, nausea and vomiting, and occasionally, convulsions. Although the etiology is uncertain, they probably result from the rapid removal of urea and the other osmotically active particles from the extracellular compartment. This temporarily produces an osmotic concentration gradient between the intra- and extracellular compartments and causes water to move into the cells. The expansion of the cells in the central nervous system (CNS) causes cerebral edema and the disequilibrium syndrome. The likelihood of the disequilibrium syndrome can be decreased by taking the precaution to effect a gradual removal of urea by using a suitably sized dialyzer and appropriate blood pump speed and by infusing mannitol (1 g/kg/dialysis) intravenously to replace the osmotic particles being removed by dialysis. If mild disequilibrium symptoms occur (headache, nausea and vomiting), the pump speed (blood flow) can be slowed down. Serious disequilibrium (convulsions) generally responds to IV diazepam (0.1 mg/kg of body weight) when coupled with discontinuation of dialysis. IV mannitol may be helpful for reacalcitrant cases. Some patients experience less disequilibrium when switched from conventional acetate-containing dialysate to bicarbonate dialysis.

NATURAL HISTORY OF ACUTE RENAL FAILURE

In ARF, recovery of kidney function can be anticipated unless there is widespread cortical necrosis. Although the overall mortality of patients with trauma-related ARF is approximately 50 per cent, it is the extent of the trauma rather than the ARF that determines the outcome. With early prophylactic dialysis that keeps the BUN less than 100 mg/dl and with meticulous fluid and electrolyte management, few patients will succumb to the effects of the renal failure.

The duration of renal failure averages about 10 days, with a range of 3 to 30 days or more. Recovery is usually characterized by a gradual and progressive increase in the urinary volume and the GFR. The diuresis is usually appropriate for the prevailing solute and fluid load and usually terminates once the urea level has returned to normal and the excess salt and water have been excreted. Occasionally, however, an inappropriate polyuria may persist for days to weeks because recovery of tubular function lags behind recovery of glomerular filtration.

Once recovery begins, renal function sufficient to avoid the need for dialysis usually occurs within a week. Slow continued improvement may take place for up to 6 months. In approximately one third of adults, renal function never returns to normal, although virtually all regain enough function to be free of uremic signs or symptoms. The outcome in children appears to be even better, with virtually all children regaining normal or near-normal glomerular and tubular function.

SUMMARY

The kidneys normally receive 20 to 25 per cent of cardiac output, and 20 per cent of the blood plasma filters across the glomerular capillaries. A major factor responsible for glomerular filtration is the hydrostatic pressure within the glomerular capillaries. By a process known as autoregulation, normal kidneys are able to maintain a normal and constant GFR is spite of changes in kidney perfusion pressure. The glomerular filtrate is modified as it traverses through the tubular system by the selective reabsorption or rejection of water and electrolytes.

If, as a result of shock, the renal perfusion pressure drops to less than 70 to 80 mm Hg, the autoregulatory renal mechanisms are overwhelmed and glomerular filtration begins to drop. When this occurs, the patient experiences prerenal failure (azotemia). If the factors causing the prerenal failure (e.g., hypovolemia, sepsis) are corrected early, renal perfusion returns to normal and the azotemia is resolved.

However, if these factors are allowed to persist, acute renal parenchymal failure (ARPF), i.e., acute tubular necrosis (ATN), occurs. Although the pathogenesis of ARPF is only partially understood, there is general agreement that prolonged and intense renal hypoperfusion is responsible for its initiation. Persistent renal ischemia, perhaps complicated by mechanical blockage of the renal tubules by necrotic tubular debris and the backflow of filtrate across the denuded tubular epithelium, may also be a contributing factor.

Postrenal failure, that is, azotemia resulting from an obstruction to the outflow of urine, may occur as a result of occlusion of the renal pelvic outlet or the ureters, blockage of the bladder outlet, or bladder rupture.

Distinguishing between prerenal failure and renal parenchymal failure is sometimes difficult. In prerenal failure, kidney function is impaired not because of intrinsic renal parenchymal disease or damage but because of inadequate renal perfusion. Therefore, in prerenal azotemia, the kidney responds normally to decreased perfusion and avidly retains sodium and water. In this case, the urine is concentrated and the urinary sodium concentration is low. This can most accurately be determined by calculating the fractional sodium excretion. On the other hand, in ARPF (ATN), the tubules have been damaged, and they inappropriately reject filtered sodium and water. The urine is therefore isosthenuric, with a specific gravity of approximately 1.010. Because the tubules cannot retain sodium, the urinary sodium concentration is elevated, and the fractional sodium excretion is usually greater than 2 per cent.

Therapy for early or evolving ARPF should always include an attempt to normalize the effective arterial blood volume (renal perfusion). The use of mannitol or furosemide intravenously may also be beneficial.

However, once ARPF is firmly established, the management of fluids and electrolytes.

becomes paramount. Even though the basic principles of fluid and electrolyte management still apply, the loss of renal homeostatic ability demands precision. Maintaining normal body salt and water composition requires that intake be linked to output (urinary volume, insensible losses, GI losses). Hyperkalemia is a potentially lethal, but preventable, complication of ARF. Life-threatening hyperkalemia can be temporarily counteracted by infusing calcium. Maneuvers designed to drive the potassium into the cell include the administration of sodium bicarbonate and IV glucose with insulin. Potassium can be removed from the body by the oral or rectal administration of exchange resins (Kayexalate). The definitive therapy for severe hyperkalemia is dialysis.

Because normal kidneys participate in acid-based balance by reclaiming (reabsorbing) filtered bicarbonate and regenerating new bicarbonate, one should anticipate metabolic acidosis in all patients with ARF. In the setting of trauma, with its associated hypercatabolism and tissue hypoxia, the acidosis may be life-threatening. Sodium bicarbonate, administered in doses sufficient to keep the arterial pH above 7.2, and dialysis are the mainstays of therapy.

Volume overload (edema) commonly develops in traumatized children who have required generous volumes of salt-containing resuscitation fluids. In the presence of renal failure, dialysis offers the only means of normalizing body volume.

Abnormalities in the serum concentration of sodium also occur frequently in the traumatized child. As a general rule, hypernatremia indicates a need for more free water. On the other hand, hyponatremia in a nondehydrated patient indicates an excess of water and the need to impose water restriction.

Phosphate retention (hyperphosphatemia) and secondary hypocalcemia are anticipated complications of renal failure. Hyperphosphatemia causes a reciprocal fall in the serum calcium concentration, and the cautious administration of IV calcium may be necessary.

Hyperuricemia is also to be anticipated in children with ARF. It requires no specific therapy.

Hypertension may occur during the course of ARF. It usually responds to the dialytic removal of excess fluid. The administration of a vasodilator or a centrally acting antihypertensive agent may also be necessary.

Uremia, the clinical expression of azotemia, can produce nausea and vomiting, somnolence, lethargy, and seizures. These signs and symptoms may occasionally occur before the BUN reaches 100 mg/dl and should be anticipated when the BUN exceeds 150 to 200 mg/dl.

Nutritional support, in the form of generous amounts of carbohydrate calories, has a protein-sparing effect and diminishes the production of uremic toxins. Although fats are calorically dense, the hyperlipidemia of ARF usually prevents their utilization. Moreover, unless nutritional support is coupled with dialysis, it is not usually possible to give enough nutritionally rich fluids without exceeding the required fluid restrictions.

Renal failure frequently affects medication dosages. For agents customarily eliminated by the kidneys, either the dose must be decreased or the dose interval increased. Moreover, since azotemia decreases the protein binding of some drugs and therefore increases the biologically active or free component of the drug, the interpretation of total serum drug levels may be difficult.

Dialysis may be required because of fluid overload, hyperkalemia, metabolic acidosis, or uremia (e.g., nausea, vomiting, encephalopathy). Although hemodialysis can now be performed even on infants, the difficulty of acquiring vascular access in young infants makes peritoneal dialysis more attractive for this age group. Peritoneal dialysis, which utilizes the peritoneal surface as the dialyzing membrane, requires the cautious placement of the dialysis catheter, the selection of the proper dialysate fluid, and the determination of the appropriate dialysate volume and dwell time. The major complication of peritoneal dialysis is peritonitis. It can be detected early by the periodic examination of the dialysate effluent for the presence of white blood cells. Peritonitis, most often caused by the staphylococcus organism, does not require the discontinuation of dialysis and can be treated by adding antibiotics to the dialysate fluid. Hemodialysis has the advantage of being much more time-efficient in removing toxic waste products and excess electrolytes. Temporary circulatory access can be obtained by inserting catheters in the femoral or subclavian vein. The major complications of hemodialysis include mechanical trauma to the veins as a consequence of catheter insertion, hypotension from the rapid removal of intravascular fluid, and disequilibrium resulting from the rapid removal of osmotically active nitrogenous waste products.

Although the usual mortality of patients with trauma-related ARF is approximately 50 per cent, the seriousness of the trauma, which is responsible for the renal failure, actually determines the outcome. With early dialysis and meticulous fluid and electrolyte management, death from renal failure should be uncommon. Unless there is widespread cortical necrosis, kidney function should begin to improve within 3 to 30 (average 10) days, and complete or nearly complete recovery of kidney function can be anticipated.

Acknowledgements

I gratefully acknowledge the assistance of Sue Holmes, R. D., and Robert Reilly, Pharm. D., for their help with the nutrition and drug sections, respectively.

Selected Readings

Danielson R: Differential diagnosis and treatment of oliguria in post-traumatic and postoperative patients. Surg Clin North Am 55:697, 1975.

Ellis E, Gartner JC, Galvis AG: Acute renal failure in infants and children: Diagnosis, complications, and treatment. Crit Care Med 9:607, 1981.

Gonick HC, Barker WF: Maintenance of renal function following major trauma. Symposium on nonpenetrating thoracoabdominal injuries. Surg Clin North Am 52:783, 1972.

Hodson EM, Kjellstrand CM, Mauer SM: Acute renal failure in infants and children: Outcome of 53 patients requiring hemodialysis treatment. Pediatr 93:756, 1978.

Schrier RW (principal discussant): Acute renal failure. Kidney Int 15:205, 1979.

Shin B, Mackenzie CF, McAslan C, et al.: Postoperative renal failure in trauma patients. Anesthesiology 51:218, 1979.

CHAPTER

8 Radiographic Evaluation of the Injured Child

GEORGE W. NIXON
RICHARD B. JAFFE

Proper management of the injured child presents an unsurpassed challenge. Although the radiographic evaluation is only one aspect in the overall evaluation of such a patient, it is important to be skillful in ordering and evaluating these studies, as they may offer invaluable information concerning diagnosis and assist in planning therapy. Improperly ordered examinations, unnecessary studies, and technically poor studies may result in unnecessary delay in diagnosis, erroneous diagnosis, unnecessary movement of the patient, unjustified radiation exposure, and exorbitant costs. This chapter presents a basic working approach concerning the utilization of radiographic studies.

Common injuries of infants and children will be stressed in this chapter. Radiologic evaluation of trauma in older patients and of conditions not unique to the pediatric age group is well discussed elsewhere.[1] The major emphasis will be on utilization of conventional radiographs in the initial evaluation of the traumatized child. Computerized tomography (CT) is a well-established procedure for the initial evaluation of head trauma and has been reported to be useful in the evaluation of vertebral fractures,[2] acetabular fractures,[3] and abdominal injuries.[4] Other special diagnostic methods (ultrasonography, radionuclide scans, and angiography) are occasionally useful, and their use will be discussed when appropriate.

The initial priority in the diagnosis of the injured child is the history and physical examination. Radiographic studies of the severely injured child should not be done prior to thorough examination and institution of initial treatment to stabilize the patient's condition. Careful physical examination is the most important aspect of the evaluation of musculoskeletal trauma. It enables the primary care physician to determine if radiographic examination is necessary and, if so, which particular examination or examinations are indicated. When radiographic studies are ordered without the patient being examined initially, unnecessary or inappropriate studies may result. For example, a child or parent may state that the foot hurts when the site of injury is actually the lower leg (Fig. 8–1).

Although physical examination should be the initial method of localizing the site of

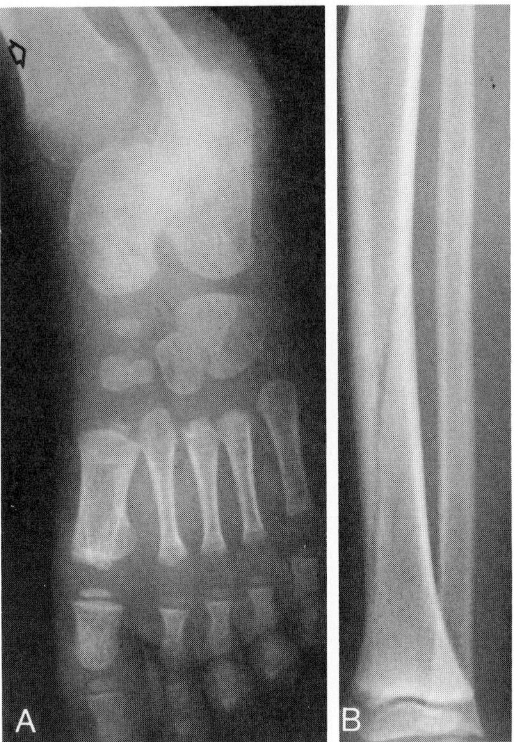

Figure 8–1. This 3-year-old child complained of pain in his foot following a fall from a tricycle. Foot films were ordered without examining the child. *A,* At the periphery of this oblique foot film there is a suggestion of a fracture in the distal tibial metaphysis *(arrow).* The patient was then clinically examined and noted to have localized physical findings in the midportion of the lower leg. *B,* Appropriate filming of the tibia and fibula shows a long oblique fracture involving the tibial diaphysis and extending into the distal metaphysis. This case illustrates the principle that physical examination should always precede radiographic evaluation.

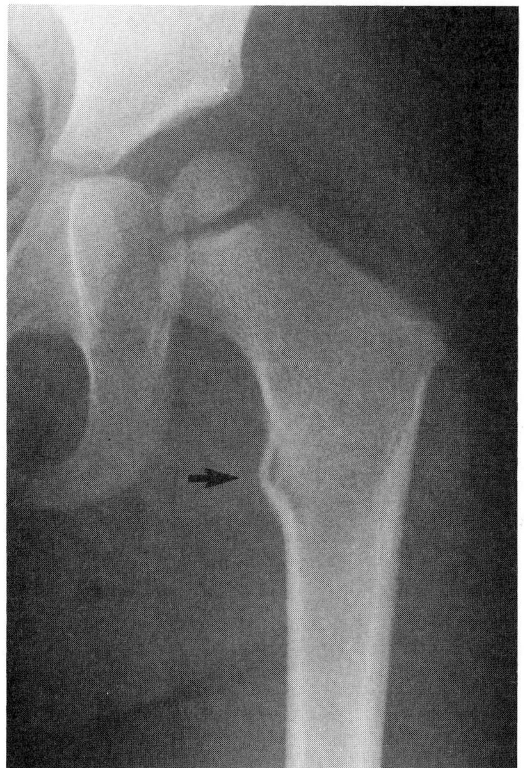

Figure 8–2. The site of injury may be difficult to localize in the young child. This 2-year-old boy refused to bear weight after a fall. He was very uncooperative and difficult to examine, and after initial physical examination, it was believed that the site of injury was below the knee. After the film findings of the tibia proved negative, additional films were done because of the persistent symptoms. An incomplete, cortical buckle fracture *(arrow)* involving the medial aspect of the proximal femur was demonstrated.

trauma, there are exceptions to this statement in the pediatric age group. In the comatose, delirious, or mentally retarded patient, it may be difficult to specifically identify the site of trauma and screening films may be justified. Also, it is notoriously difficult to examine a toddler and accurately determine the specific site of injury (Fig. 8–2). Infrequently, one must revert to a "shotgun" approach and obtain radiographs of an entire extemity. Careful, time-consuming examination often results in patient rapport and enables one to localize the problem. Reassessment during subsequent hours and days, especially in the severely injured patient, is crucial. Injuries not detected during initial evaluation may become apparent later. A hurried "get the kid to x-ray" approach is inappropriate.

Proper positioning, immobilization, and exposure factors are required to obtain films of good technical quality, and this is often a major challenge when dealing with a traumatized child. Detailed texts devoted to these aspects of pediatric radiologic care are recommended.[5, 6] If films are of poor quality, whenever possible, new studies should be done. A false sense of security results from overlooking abnormalities that may not be apparent on technically poor radiographs.

The radiology department should be alerted about their possible involvement in the evaluation of critically injured patients. This enables the radiology staff to prepare a room and material for the necessary examinations and, thus, decrease the total time necessary to perform these studies. Radiologists should be utilized as consultants during initial evalution and management, providing input concerning the type of examinations and techniques that would be of greatest value and least risk. If the volume of patients with severe trauma warrants, conventional radiographic equipment can be installed in the emergency department. Otherwise, radiographic evaluation should be performed in the x-ray department whenever possible because more sophisticated equipment will be available, enabling higher quality studies. Transfer from the emergency department is often impossible in the critically injured child, and in such cases portable examinations are acceptable. Whenever a critically injured patient is transferred to the radiology department, a physician or nurse should attend to monitor and care for the patient; this should not be the radiology technologist's responsibility. The role of the radiologic team is to peform roentgenographic studies; monitoring and caring for the critically injured patient is the job of the attending physician and nursing personnel.

All radiographic studies essential to the initial evaluation of the critically injured patient should be ordered at one time. This minimizes the number of times a patient is moved and decreases the total time spent in performing these studies. Studies should be prioritized so that the films of the most vital areas and those that are most important to patient management are done initially. If the patient's status deteriorates and radiographic evaluation must be discontinued, the more important examinations will have been performed. Lateral cervical spine and frontal chest films are usually the most urgent radiographic studies in the initial evaluation of the critically injured child, but depending on the type and location of the trauma, other studies may be more important. In caring for the severely injured patient, it is often good practice to defer certain radiologic studies (facial bone and extremity films) that will not alter immediate management. Also, certain examinations (mandible, facial, and orbital studies) are time-consuming and may require positioning that is not desirable during this period of initial treatment and evaluation.

The x-ray requisition form should be viewed as a request for radiologic consultation[7] rather than merely an order to do a certain procedure. Appropriate information should be supplied on this form to aid the radiologist in helping determine if the appropriate examination is requested and if additional studies or specific views might be helpful and in reaching proper radiographic interpretation. Whenever possible, films from the emergency room should be immediately reviewed by the radiologist, preferably in consultation with the emergency physician. This facilitates discussion to correlate history and physical findings with radiographic changes and enables proper decisions concerning diagnosis and the possible need for additional films.

Clinicians, in general, should not be concerned with ordering specific views but rather should merely request radiographs of the areas of concern (right wrist, left femur, chest, etc.). The radiology department should have routine views for each area that are appropriate in most situations. Occasionally supplemental views may be necessary after the initial routine films are reviewed.

A basic principle in obtaining radiographic studies is that only those films that will modify patient care should be done. For example, since the radiographic demonstration of a fracture in the lower sacrum or coccyx does not specifically modify treatment, films of this area are unnecessary. Also many clinicians manage nasal trauma entirely on physical findings rather than on whether a fracture of the nasal bones is demonstrated on radiographs; therefore, nasal bone films should not be done routinely. Since rib fractures are usually treated symptomatically, chest films rather than rib films should be obtained, since pneumothorax, hemothorax, and other changes that may require therapy are more readily identified on chest films. Radiographic studies should be done only for medical indications. If such studies would not modify the patient's medical care, there should be no medicolegal justification for them.

Every emergency and radiology department should have a system that enables the radiologist to compare his film interpretation with the findings of the primary care physician in those cases that are not discussed initially. If a discrepancy occurs, the clinician should be immediately notified so that patient care can be appropriately modified.

RADIOGRAPHIC EVALUATION OF MUSCULOSKELETAL TRAUMA

When radiographs of the injured area are obtained, it is generally recommended that the joint area proximal and distal to the site of trauma be x-rayed. When a fracture of the diaphyseal portion of a long bone is suspected, it is crucial that the proximal and distal joint areas are visualized, since an associated dislocation or fracture at the end of the bone occasionally occurs in association with a diaphyseal fracture (Fig. 8–3). Furthermore, the proximal and distal joint areas

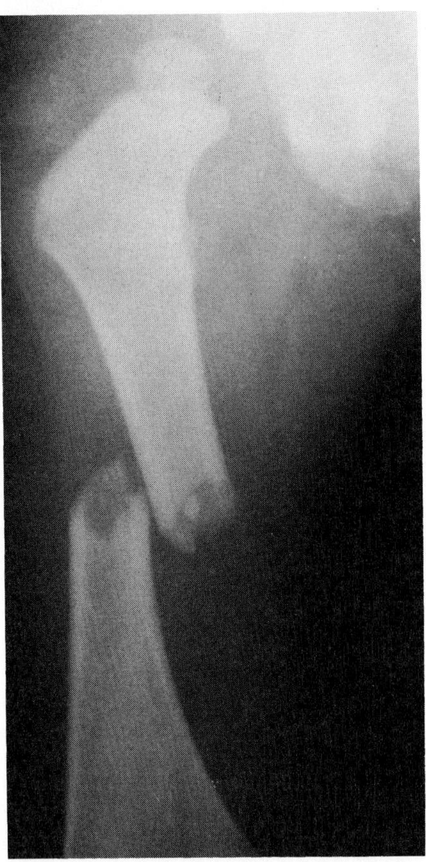

Figure 8–3. It is mandatory that the joint areas proximal and distal to a diaphyseal fracture be visualized radiographically. In addition to the mid femoral diaphyseal fracture, the femoral head is dislocated from the acetabulum.

are more difficult to evaluate on physical examination in the presence of a diaphyseal fracture. However, it is proposed that in certain cases, this approach of always filming the proximal and distal joint areas can be modified. When the patient is alert, signs and symptoms are confined to the metaphyseal, metaphyseal-diaphyseal, or epiphyseal area; and on physical examination there are no abnormal findings in the region of the opposite end of the bone; it is proposed that localized films (wrist or elbow rather than forearm) of the area of involvement be obtained. For example, if a child complains of pain in the region of the distal radius, has localized physical findings in this area, and is alert and cooperative and there are no abnormal findings in the region of the elbow, then the appropriate study would be a wrist rather than a forearm examination. Occasionally, there are symptoms and physical findings at both ends of a long bone (especially the wrist and elbow areas), and it is tempting to order forearm films to evaluate the wrist and elbow areas in a single examination. Usually on careful physical examination, one area can be excluded, but if not, separate examinations of both the wrist and the elbow areas rather than the forearm films should be ordered, as this enables optimal examination of the areas of major interest. This approach is recommended because of the radiologic principle that there is less detail, greatest distortion, and greatest magnification at the periphery of a film. Thus, wrist and elbow films in the preceding example enable optimal examination of the areas of major interest, whereas a forearm study would best delineate the diaphyseal area.

In general, diaphyseal fractures result in more impressive physical findings compared with those involving the ends of long bones. Careful examination for local tenderness, swelling, deformity, and pain with motion will usually result in accurate predictions of fractures in diaphyseal areas, and these are readily confirmed radiographically. Conversely, the presence of fractures in the metaphyseal, metaphyseal-diaphyseal, epiphyseal growth plate, and epiphyseal site is much more difficult to predict because these fractures often result in minor physical findings. Optimal films localized to the area of interest are often necessary to demonstrate fractures in these areas.

Severely injured extremities should be immobilized with a nonmetallic splint prior to radiographic study. The injured limb should be moved as little as possible to prevent additional pain and further injury. Radiologic technologists should move the radiographic equipment rather than the child's limb.

Radiographs of the injured area should routinely be obtained in two projections perpendicular to one another. It is not unusual for a fracture to be visualized on a single projection. If films show motion, improper technique, or poor positioning, new studies should be done, since errors are frequently made in interpreting poor studies.

Conventional views should be done whenever possible, but occasionally deformity or the presence of an immobilization device precludes this. In this situation, oblique views at right angles to each other should be sufficient. However, interpretation of nonstandard projections may be more difficult, particularly in the regions of the joints and ends of the long bones.

The clinical impression should always be correlated with any questionable radiographic change. If there are no physical findings in the region of possible radiographic abnormality, a fracture is very unlikely. Normal features and variants of the growing skeleton can be misinterpreted as traumatic change. Growth plates, irregular ossification of epiphyses, sesamoid and accessory bones, and pseudoepiphyses in short tubular bones may all be misinterpreted as fractures. Illustrations of the more frequently encountered normal variants are available in other textbooks,[8, 9] and should be available for reference.

Comparison films of the opposite extremity should not be routinely done, since this results in unnecessary radiation exposure and expense. Comparison films should be limited to those cases in which the diagnosis is questionable on the films of the injured side. It has been reported that the comparison views are seldom necessary.[10] One can often use adjacent bones on the injured side for comparison rather than resorting to comparison views. For example, it is as useful to compare the appearance of adjacent phalanges, metacarpals, or metatarsals as to compare those of the opposite hand or foot (Fig. 8–4). Also, one must realize that mimimal deformity in the cortex is often the only radiographic abnormality noted in incomplete fractures in children (Fig. 8–5). This type of fracture often involves the metaphyseal, metaphyseal-diaphyseal junction area. The normal metaphysis has a smooth and gradual flaring configuration, and any alter-

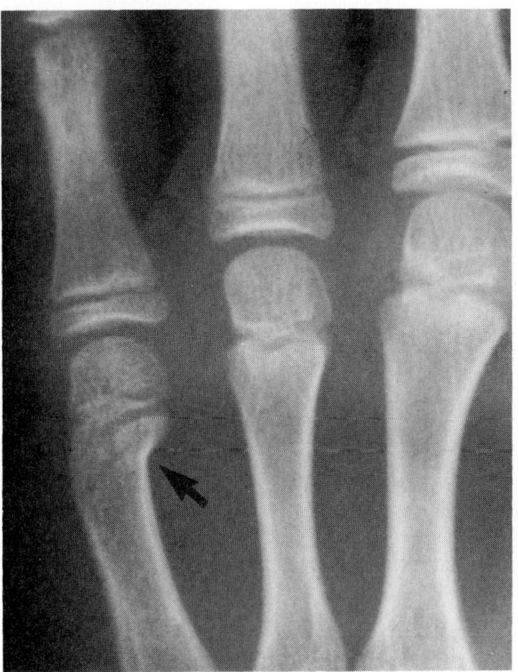

Figure 8–4. An incomplete cortical buckle fracture *(arrow)* involving the lateral aspect of the metaphysis of the fifth metacarpal (boxer's fracture). Comparison filming of the opposite hand is unnecessary because one can use the adjacent metacarpals of the injured side for comparison.

ation in this contour indicates the presence of an incomplete fracture. The metaphyseal areas should be closely scrutinized on all views for any disruption of this normal pattern.

An important management decision arises in cases in which physical findings are impressive but a fracture is not demonstrated radiographically. Radiologists often recommend follow-up films in 2 to 3 weeks to evaluate for evidence of a healing fracture. However, this is often of little practical help to the clinician, since it is necessary to reach a decision earlier concerning patient care. A more efficient approach is to initially immobilize the injured part and clinically re-examine it in 3 to 5 days. If there are no complaints or findings, treatment can be terminated. Persistent signs and symptoms justify further treatment. Follow-up films should only be carried out when they will specifically alter management.

Injuries in infants and children are considerably different from those in adults owing to special features of the immature skeleton. Several anatomic differences form the basis for these differences. It is obvious that fractures involving the epiphyseal growth plate are unique to the pediatric age group, but other factors are also important. Ligaments and other periarticular soft tissues are stronger than the neighboring epiphyseal growth plate, and therefore, serious ligamentous injury and dislocations are uncommon in children as compared with adults. Bone tissue is less brittle in children than in adults, and as a result, fractures are usually incomplete and infrequently comminuted. Children's bones are much more flexible than those of adults, and acute plastic bowing deformity occasionally occurs. In infants, the periosteum is firmly attached at the metaphyseal-epiphyseal growth plate junction and loosely attached along the diaphysis. This predisposes to metaphyseal corner fractures in the battered child syndrome. Fractures of the femoral neck, ribs, vertebral bodies, and carponavicular are much more common in adults than in children. Conversely, fractures of the clavicle, femoral diaphysis, and supracondylar portion of the humerus are much more frequent in the pediatric age group. Fractures may differ in the two age groups even when similar trauma is inflicted. For example, with similar trauma to the elbow, an adult commonly suffers a radial head fracture, whereas a supracondylar fracture of the distal humerus is the most frequent type of fracture in a child. Also, a radiographic sign may have a different implication in the two age groups. The presence of a positive fat pad sign in the elbow is strongly suggestive of an occult fracture of the radial head in an adult, but in a child, the incidence of any occult fracture in this setting is much lower.[11]

When an emergency room physician discusses the radiographic appearance of a fracture with an orthopedic surgeon via the telephone, certain aspects should specifically be described. These items are as follows:

- I. Type of fracture
  - A. Complete
    - 1. Transverse
    - 2. Oblique
    - 3. Spiral
  - B. Incomplete
  - C. Avulsion
- II. Which bone
- III. Which part (diaphysis [shaft], metaphysis, growth plate, or epiphysis)
- IV. Specify if growth plate is involved
  - A. If growth plate is involved, use Salter-Harris classification
- V. Comminution (no, yes)

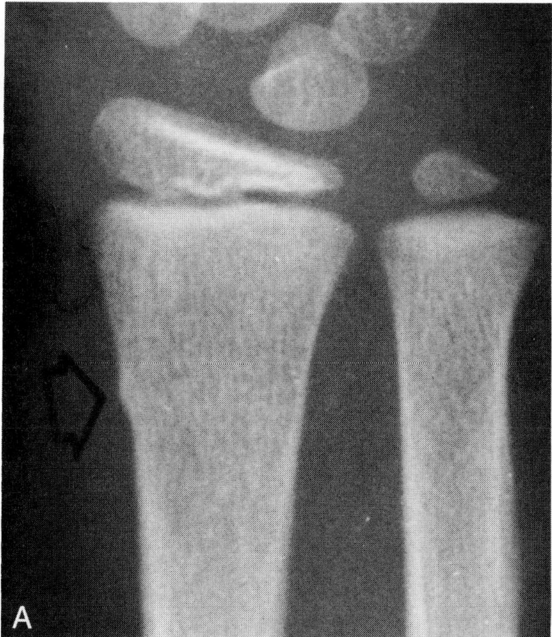

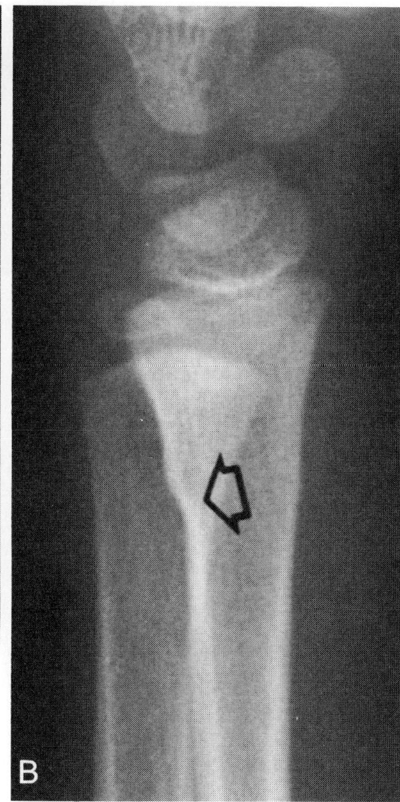

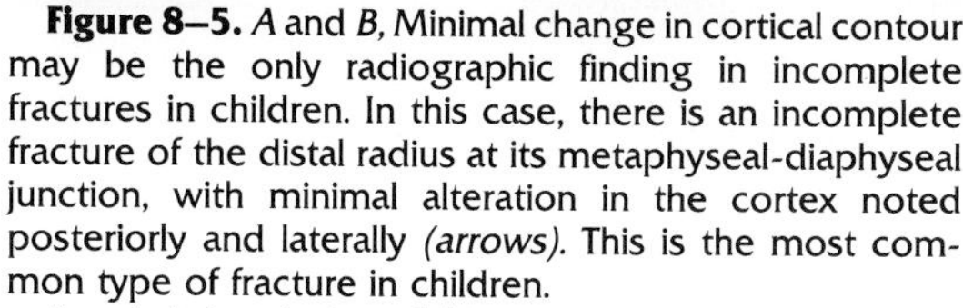

Figure 8–5. *A* and *B*, Minimal change in cortical contour may be the only radiographic finding in incomplete fractures in children. In this case, there is an incomplete fracture of the distal radius at its metaphyseal-diaphyseal junction, with minimal alteration in the cortex noted posteriorly and laterally *(arrows)*. This is the most common type of fracture in children.

A verbal description of this injury would be as follows: There is an incomplete cortical buckle fracture involving the distal radius at its metaphyseal-diaphyseal junction. There is mild cortical buckling posteriorly, but no significant angulation is noted. The growth plate is spared. The ulna appears intact. There are no findings to suggest that this is a pathologic fracture.

VI. Displacement (no, yes)
   A. Direction
   B. Degree
   C. Overriding

VII. Angulation (no, yes [which direction is apex of fragments directed])

VIII. Is there evidence of a predisposing bone abnormality (pathologic fracture)

Examples of verbal descriptions are included in Figures 8–5 and 8–8.

TYPES OF FRACTURES

Complete Fracture

Complete fractures may be transverse, oblique, or spiral in configuration. They usually involve the diaphyseal portion of a bone (see Fig. 8–3), although the metaphyseal region may also be involved. These fractures are usually suspected clinically and are seldom difficult to diagnose radiographically and therefore will not be described in detail. Complete fractures are less common than incomplete types, with the clavicle, femur, radius, and ulna being the most frequent sites of involvement.

Incomplete Fracture

Incomplete fractures (Figs. 8–2, 8–4, 8–5, 8–15) are the most common variety of fracture occurring in children. This type of fracture occurs when bone is subjected to a force and buckles or breaks at one cortical margin and bends at the other, without complete loss of bone continuity. This condition is variously described as a greenstick, torus, buckle, cortical buckle, or cortical impaction fracture. These fractures are most commonly seen in the medium-sized long bones (distal radius and ulna, distal humerus, clavicle, and the metacarpals and metatarsals) and almost always involve the metaphyseal or metaphyseal-diaphyseal areas. These fractures may re-

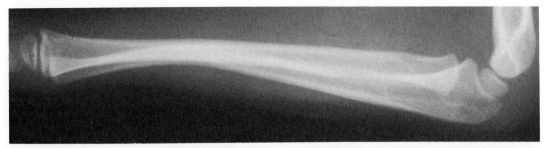

Figure 8–6. Defotmity of the forearm was noted in this 8-year-old boy after a fall. Mild acute plastic bowing of the radial and ulnar diaphyses is present, with the apices of the bowing directed anteriorly.

sult in limited clinical findings and minimal radiographic change. Each cortical margin on every view should be carefully inspected, and any abrupt change in the smooth gradual flaring configuration of the metaphysis implies that an incomplete fracture is present. Correlation with clinical findings is extremely useful in diagnosing this type of fracture.

Plastic bowing is essentially unique to long bones in children (Fig. 8–6).[12] This is an infrequent type of incomplete fracture that usually involves the radius and ulna, although involvement of the femur and fibula has also been reported. A longitudinal compressive force may result in bending of a long bone, and if this force exceeds the elasticity of the bone and is released before a fracture occurs, a bowing deformity of the shaft results. Multiple microfractures on the concave side of the bowed bone may result in the bowed deformity. The minor forms of this type of fracture may be difficult to diagnose, and comparison films of the opposite extremity in precisely the same position may be necessary for diagnosis. Isotope bone scanning has been reported to be useful in differentiating acute from chronic deformity.[13]

Epiphyseal Plate Fractures

Approximately 15 per cent of fractures in children involve the epiphyseal growth plate. The weakest portion of the bone in this area is at the junction of the metaphysis and epiphyseal plate (in the zone of hypertrophic cartilage adjacent to the provisional zone of calcification). Thus, when a fracture extends parallel along the epiphyseal plate, the growth plate cartilage remains attached to the epiphyseal rather than the metaphyseal fragment. The classification of Salter and Harris[14, 15] regarding epiphyseal growth plate fractures is widely used and has implications with respect to prognosis and required treatment as well as the mechanism of injury. These fractures are diagramatically illustrated in Figure 8–7.

A Type I fracture extends transversely along the entire epiphyseal plate, without extending into the metaphysis or epiphysis (Fig. 8–8). This fracture usually affects infants and younger children and is recognized by displacement of the epiphysis relative to the metaphysis. Comparison views are occasionally useful when there is little displacement. Diagnosis of a nondisplaced Type 1 fracture is very difficult. One should look for adjacent

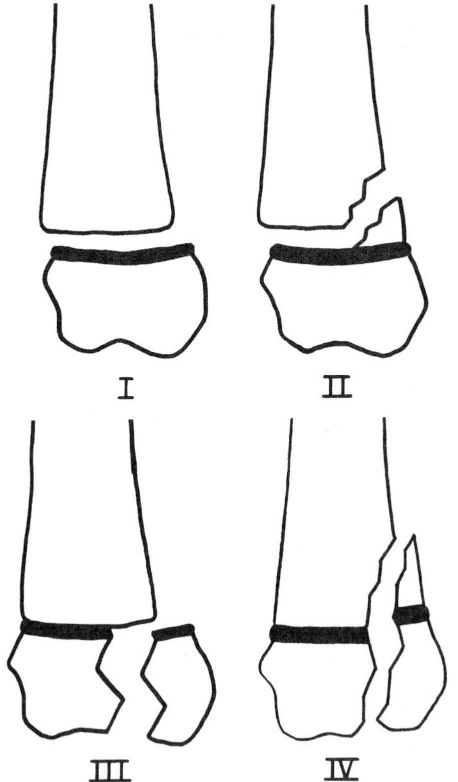

Figure 8–7. Diagram of the Salter-Harris classification of epiphyseal growth plate injuries.

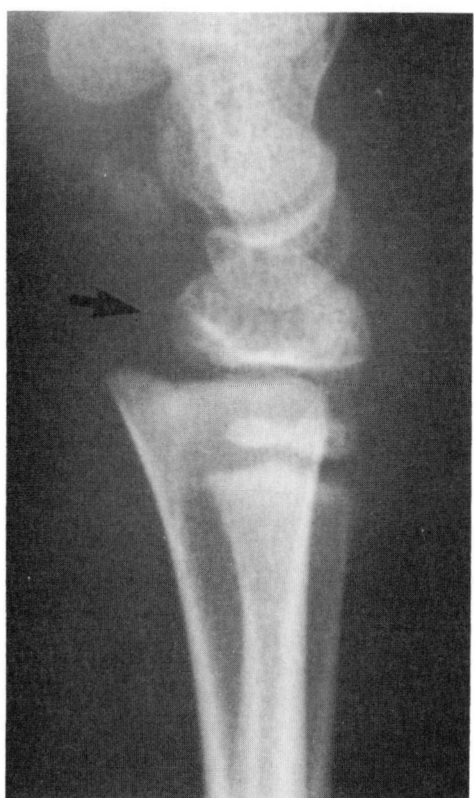

Figure 8–8. A Salter Type I fracture of the distal radius is present in this film of a 12-year-old boy. The epiphysis *(arrow)* is mildly displaced posteriorly.

An adequate verbal description of this fracture would be as follows: There is a Salter Type I fracture involving the distal radius, with mild posterior displacement of the distal fragment. There is no angulation. No predisposing bone abnormality is noted.

soft tissue swelling and correlate with clinical findings. Stress views in such a case may result in displacement or widening of the growth plate and confirm the diagnosis.

The Type II epiphyseal plate fracture is by far the most frequent variety of fracture that involves the epiphyseal plate and usually occurs in the older child. Anatomically, the fracture extends transversely through the growth plate and then extends obliquely through the metaphysis (Fig. 8–9). The size and configuration of the triangular metaphyseal fragment varies. This type of fracture is closely related to the Type I variety, and fractures that have been diagnosed as Type I fractures may actually have a tiny metaphyseal fragment.

The Type III epiphyseal growth plate fracture extends horizontally through a portion of the growth plate and then extends vertically through the epiphysis into the joint surface (Fig. 8–10). This fracture is uncommon and usually involves the distal tibia.

The Type IV epiphyseal plate fracture extends from the joint surface through the epiphysis, growth plate, and metaphysis (Fig. 8–11). The distal tibia, distal humerus, and phalanges of the hand are the most frequent sites involved. If the fracture line extends in continuous obliquity, this is an unstable situation, and there is often lack of continuity of the fragments of the growth plate and offset at the joint surface. Lack of continuity of the growth plate fragments results in healing across a portion of the growth plate. Thus, partial closure of the growth plate and subsequent angular deformity develop. Occasionally, the fracture line extends obliquely through the metaphysis, horizontally through a portion of the growth plate, and then vertically through the epiphysis.

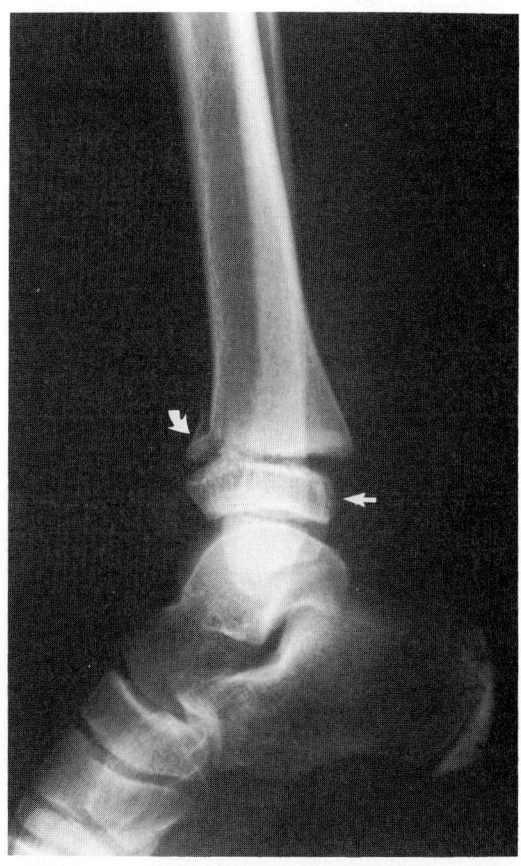

Figure 8–9. Salter Type II fracture of the distal tibia. Note the triangular metaphyseal fragment anteriorly *(curved arrow)*, which remains attached to the epiphysis *(arrow)*. The Type II fracture is the most common variety that involves the epiphyseal growth plate.

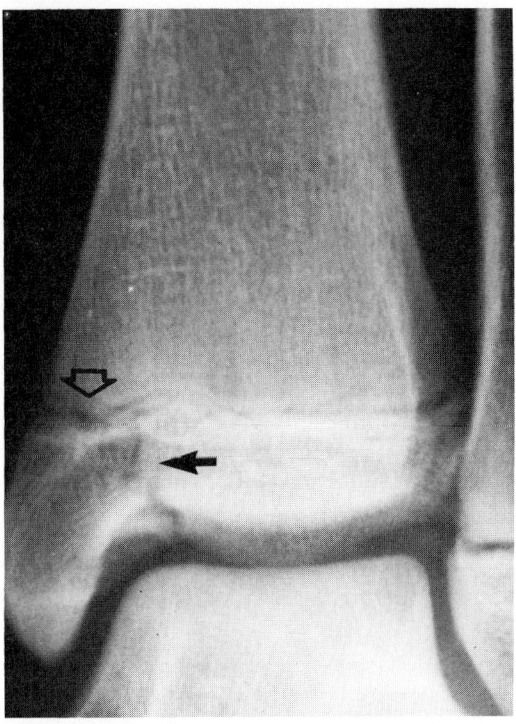

Figure 8–10. Salter Type III fracture involving the medial malleolar portion of the distal tibia. The fracture line extends through the epiphysis *(closed arrow)* to the growth plate and then extends medially along the growth plate *(open arrow).*

The prognosis in this unusual Type IV fracture is good, since the fragments are in a stable relationship and therefore the growth plate fragments are maintained at the same level.

A bone fragment bridging a portion of the growth plate may result in bony union of a portion of the growth plate. This and not merely the fact that the fracture is of a Salter Type IV variety, signals the potential for a growth distubance problem. This principle is illustrated in Figure 8–12, in which a small fracture fragment is located adjacent to the growth plate. This could represent a Type III or IV fracture, or this segment could represent a fragment fom the epiphysis and may not involve the growth plate. Regardless of its classification, this configuration should be recognized as a potential problem.

The Type V epiphyseal plate fracture is caused by a compression force resulting in damage to the cartilage of the epiphyseal plate. Radiographically, no bone abnormality is noted. There may be soft tissue swelling adjacent to the growth plate. This type of injury is seldom diagnosed acutely and becomes apparent with subsequent growth disturbance. The growth disturbance may be either an angular deformity if only a portion of the growth plate was damaged or generalized shortening if the entire growth plate was damaged.

Pathologic Fracture

Pathologic fractures are infrequent in pediatric patients. Meningomyelocele or other neurologic disorders with secondary undermineralization are the most common predisposing abnormalities. Other conditions causing pathologic fractures include simple bone cyst, fibrous dysplasia, histiocytosis X, metastatic disease, and osteogenesis imperfecta.

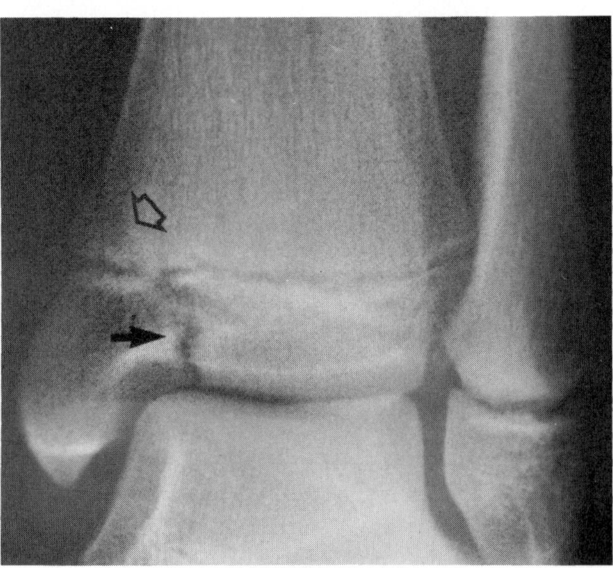

Figure 8–11. Salter Type IV fracture of the distal tibia. The fracture line extends through the metaphysis *(open arrow)*, growth plate, and epiphysis *(closed arrow).*

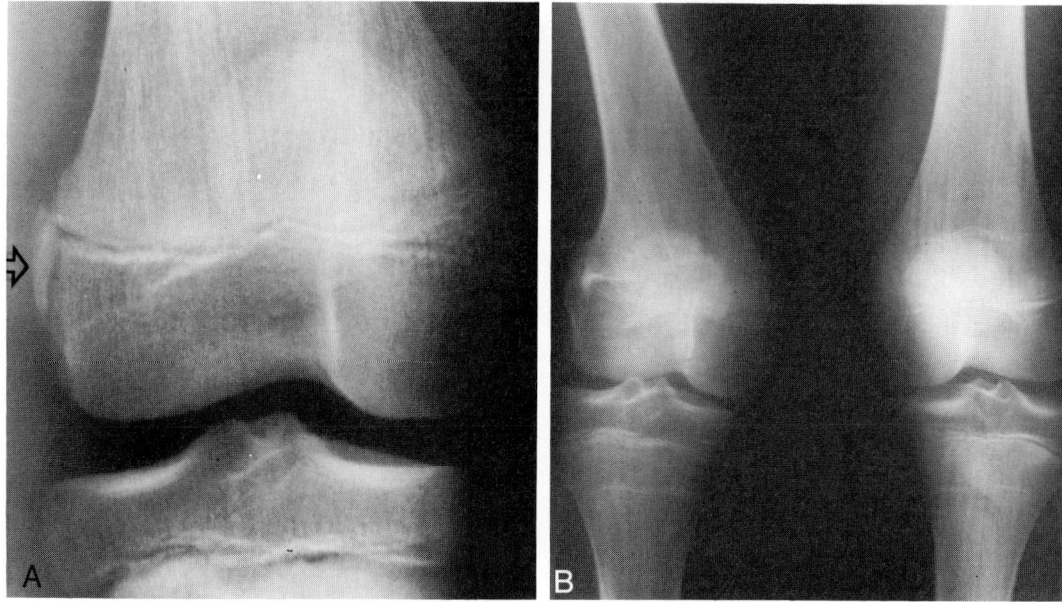

Figure 8–12. This 12-year-old boy was injured playing football. *A*, The radiograph shows a small fracture fragment along the lateral aspect of the distal tibia *(arrow)*. It cannot be definitely determined whether this represents a Salter Type III or IV fracture or a displaced fragment of the epiphysis in which the fracture does not involve the growth plate. There is a potential for growth disturbance with angular deformity because the bony fragment is located adjacent to the growth plate. *B*, Eighteen months later there is considerable valgus deformity at the knee because of growth retardation laterally. The fracture fragment healed, bridging the metaphysis and epiphysis. Operative management should have been done with internal fixation or removal of the fracture fragment.

RADIOGRAPHIC EVALUATION OF SPECIFIC AREAS

In this section the various anatomic areas will be very briefly discussed. There will be no attempt to cover all fractures; those that are easily detected radiographically will not be discussed. Rather, there is emphasis on injuries that may be difficult to detect or in which radiographic changes have specific management implications. Methods of examination, specific normal variants that are most commonly confused with fractures, and situations in which injuries or radiographic findings in children are different or have different implications than in adults will also be noted. Injuries of the immature (prior to epiphyseal growth plate closure) skeleton will be emphasized.

Hand

Routine radiographic examination of the hand consists of frontal and oblique views. The oblique projection is with the forearm in pronation, and it is necessary to separate the digits so that they are not superimposed upon each other. If the trauma involves an individual digit, an additional lateral view of this area is valuable and is readily obtained by flexing the uninvolved digits.

Cortical irregularity and incomplete cartilage clefts in the proximal portions of the second through fifth metacarpals are the most frequent normal variants confused with a fracture in this portion of the skeleton. Also, incomplete cartilage clefts in the distal aspects of the first metacarpal may occasionally mimic a fracture.

Except for crush injuries of the distal phalanges, fractures and dislocations of the hand are less common in children than in adults. The most frequent site of fracture in the hand is the phalanges. Fractures of the tips of the distal phalanges, incomplete fractures in the metaphyseal areas, and the various types of growth plate fractures are relatively common in the phalanges. Phalangeal and metacarpophalangeal dislocations are very uncommon. An incomplete fracture of the metaphysis of the fifth metacarpal is a relatively frequent fracture in older boys and has been termed a "boxer's fracture" because of the usual mechanism of injury (see Fig. 8–4).

Wrist and Distal Forearm

The routine radiographic examination of the wrist and distal forearm areas consists of frontal and lateral projections. In children, oblique views are seldom of value. The distal radius is the most frequent site of incomplete metaphyseal fracture, and the distal radial growth plate is the most frequent location for Type II epiphyseal growth plate injury. The incomplete fractures usually result in cortical buckling posteriorly, with angulation with the apex directed anteriorly. Occasionally, the cortical buckling involves the anterior surface of the radius, and it is of interest that this pattern is almost always seen in girls. With either an incomplete or an epiphyseal plate fracture involving the distal radius, there is often an associated fracture of the ulna at its metaphyseal region or avulsion of the ulnar styloid portion of the distal ulnar epiphysis. The incidence of carpal fractures and dislocations and dislocation of the distal radioulnar joint is extremely rare in children. However, fractures of the navicular occasionally do occur in teenagers. When clinically suspected, a navicular view (frontal projection with the hand in maximum ulnar deviation) should be obtained.

Mid Forearm

Routine radiographic examination of the forearm consists of frontal and lateral projections. Additional views are seldom necessary. The proximal and distal ends of the radius and ulna are better visualized with views centered over the wrist or elbow.

When there is an angulated fracture of either the radius or the ulna in its diaphyseal portion, the other bone must be affected. This can be either as a fracture, dislocation, or plastic bowing. A fracture of the ulnar diaphysis combined with dislocation of the proximal radius (Monteggia's fracture-dislocation) is an important injury (Fig. 8–13).[16] Unfortunately, the dislocation component of the injury is often unrecognized, and this results in permanent disability.

Elbow

The elbow is adequately examined with anteroposterior (AP) and lateral views. It is crucial that the films are done with the elbow in true frontal and lateral positions. Oblique views are rarely useful. Because of the multiple epiphyseal growth plates and traction epiphyses in the elbow region, comparison views are more useful in this area than in any other body region. Although some radiologists stress the importance of the times of ossification of the various ossification centers in the elbow region, this is of little practical value. However, it is crucial to remember that the medial epicondyle always ossifies before the trochlea (medial condyle). This is important because if there is calcific density visualized in the region of the trochlea and the medial epicondyle is not visualized, one must suspect that there has been avulsion of the medial epicondyle, with subsequent distraction into the joint.

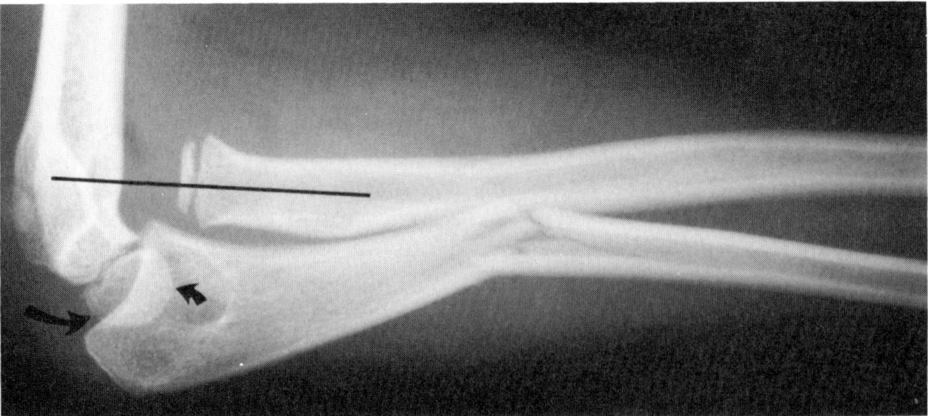

Figure 8–13. Monteggia's fracture-dislocation. There is an angulated fracture of the ulnar diaphysis. The proximal radius is dislocated anteriorly. Normally, a line extending through the axis of the radius should extend through the central portion of the capitellum *(arrows)*.

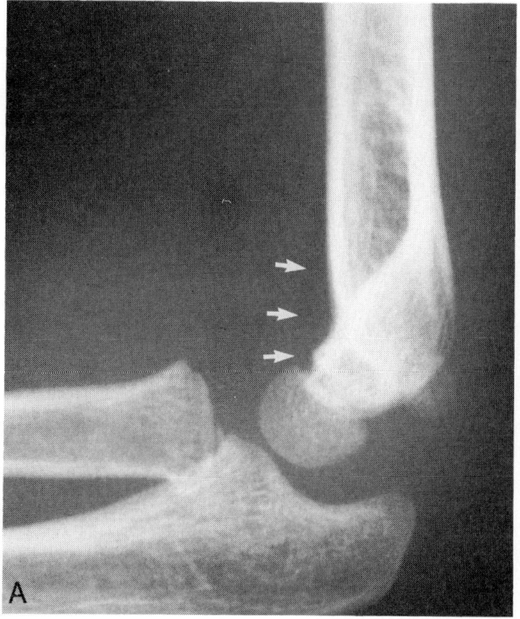

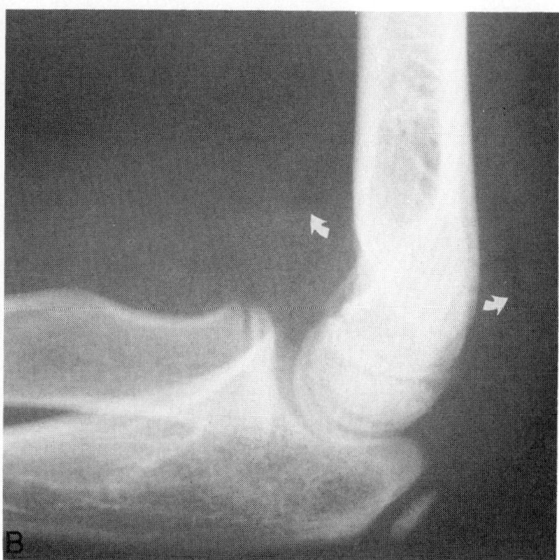

Figure 8–14. *A*, Radiograph shows the normal appearance of the anterior elbow fat pad in a 3-year-old child. The fat pad *(arrows)* parallels the anterior margin of the distal humerus. There is no fat density visualized posteriorly. *B*, Fluid in the elbow joint results in anterior and superior elevation and displacement of the anterior fat pad so that its lower margin is perpendicular to the long axis of the humerus *(anterior arrow)*. The posterior fat pad is displaced posteriorly *(posterior arrow)*.

Elbow trauma differs considerably in children as compared with adults. With the same mechanism of trauma, the radial head is frequently fractured in adults. In contrast, an incomplete supracondylar fracture is infinitely more common than a radial head fracture in young children. Fluid identified in the elbow joint by elevation of the anterior and/or posterior fat pad (Fig. 8–14) is presumptive evidence of a fracture in an adult. An occult radial head fracture is the most likely abnormality when a fracture is not visualized on conventional films. In contrast, when a fracture is not identified on conventional AP and lateral views in a child in whom there is radiographic evidence of fluid in the elbow joint, an occult fracture is usually not present, and additional oblique views in this setting are not justified.[11] Appropriate management is best determined by clinical evaluation. In this setting, the patient should be immobilized for approximately 5 days and then re-evaluated. If the patient is asymptomatic at this time, it can be assumed that a fracture is not present. If localized symptoms persist, appropriate immobilization therapy is recommended. Additional follow-up films are of limited value in management decisions.

The "jerked" or pulled elbow is a frequent injury in young children. In this condition, there is no abnormal alignment of the bony structures. The terms dislocated or subluxed radial head sometimes used to describe this lesion are misleading. Occasionally there is elevation of the elbow fat pads, indicating fluid in the elbow joint.

A fracture involving the distal metaphyseal portion of the humerus is commonly described as a supracondylar fracture. This is the most frequent fracture in the elbow region in children and almost always occurs between the ages of 3 and 9 years. The fracture may be complete or incomplete. With a complete fracture, the distal fragment is displaced posteriorly, and with an incomplete fracture, the apex of the fragments is directed anteriorly. The subtle forms of this injury may be difficult to detect radiographically (Fig. 8–15). The use of the anterior humeral line may be assistance in detecting this fracture.[17] In children over 2.5 years of age, this line should pass through the middle third of the capitellum. If this line extends through the anterior third or anterior to the capitellum, an incomplete supracondylar fracture is suggested. Proper positioning with a true lateral film is mandatory.

Fractures of the proximal radius are infrequent in children. They are usually of the

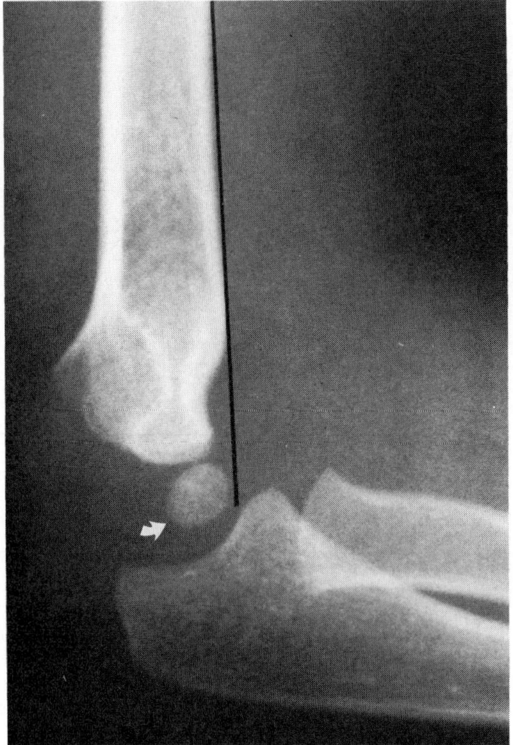

Figure 8–15. Minimal incomplete supracondylar fracture in a 4-year-old girl. A line extending along the anterior surface of the distal humeral diaphysis should normally extend through the middle third of the capitellum *(arrow).* In this instance, the anterior humeral line extends anterior to the capitellum, indicating the presence of a supracondylar fracture with mild angulation and the apex directed anteriorly.

Type II epiphyseal plate variety, although incomplete metaphyseal cortical buckle fractures occasionally occur.

Avulsion of the medial epicondyle is an important, but infrequent, childhood injury (Fig. 8–16).[18] This often occurs in association with posterior dislocation of the elbow. As noted earlier, the medial epicondyle ossifies prior to the trochlea, and intra-articular distraction of an avulsed medial epicondyle should be considered when there is ossification in the region of the trochlea and failure to visualize ossification in the medial epicondylar area. Since the medial epicondyle is located slightly posteriorly, minimal oblique views may show the medial epicondyle to be of normal appearance when it is not visualized on a true frontal projection.

Fracture of the lateral condylar area (capitellum) of the distal humerus is relatively common in children. This usually represents a Type IV epiphyseal plate fracture, with the fracture line extending through the epiphyses medial to the capitellum and across the epiphyseal plate and exiting through the metaphysis.

The elbow is the most frequent site of dislocation in children. There may be complete dislocation of the elbow, with the radius and humerus dislocated posteriorly. This type of dislocation is readily diagnosed radiographically. However, it should be remembered that there is often associated avulsion of the medial epicondyle, and following reduction of the elbow dislocation, radiographic evaluation must be done to determine if there has been avulsion of the medial epicondyle (see Fig. 8–16). Dislocation of the radial head also occurs and is usually in association with an angulated fracture of the ulnar diaphysis (Monteggia's fracture-dislocation) (see Fig. 8–13).[16] This is often missed because of the failure to note the normal anatomic relationship between the radial

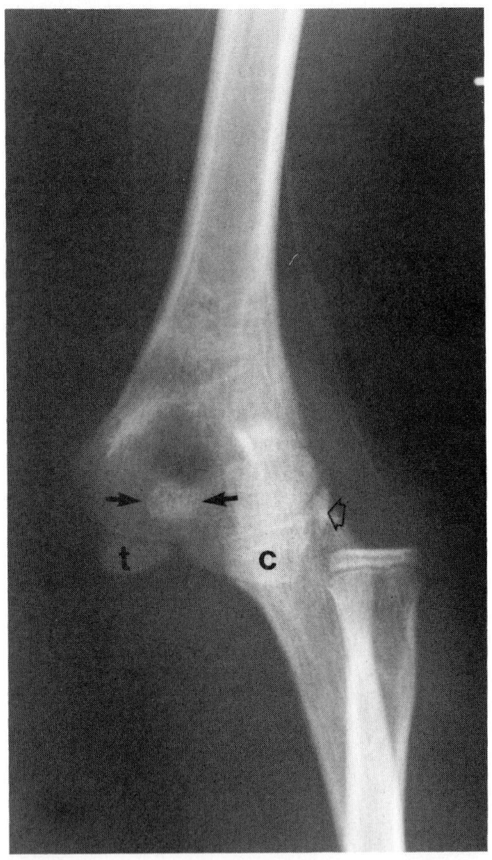

Figure 8–16. Fracture dislocation of the elbow. The radius and ulna are displaced laterally from the capitellum (c) and trochlea (t). The medial epicondyle *(closed arrows)* has been avulsed and displaced laterally. The lateral epicondyle *(open arrow)* is positioned normally.

head and capitellum (lateral condyle). The radial head should always be opposite the capitellum, and a line extending through the long axis of the proximal radius should always project through the capitellum. Acute dislocation of the proximal radius results in the radial head being displaced anterior to the capitellum in contrast to congenital dislocation in which the radius is usually posteriorly dislocated.

Humeral Diaphysis

The humeral shaft occasionally fractures in children. Its midportion is usually involved, and the fracture can be either of a transverse, spiral, or oblique variety. The radiographic detection of this type of fracture is seldom a problem when frontal and lateral radiographs are obtained.

Shoulder

Frontal radiographs with the humerus in internal and external rotation are routinely made for studying the shoulder. The rotation of the upper extremity results in visualization of the proximal humerus in two views approximately 90 degrees from one another. Since the soft tissues (ligaments, capsules, etc.) are stronger than the osseous structures at the end of the bone, dislocation of the shoulder essentially does not occur prior to closure of the growth plate of the proximal humerus. Therefore, axillary views to evaluate for dislocation are seldom necessary in young children. If a scapular fracture is suspected, a frontal view as well as a tangential view of the scapular area should be done.

A common error in the radiographic evaluation of the proximal humerus is to misinterpret a portion of the growth plate as a transverse fracture. The posterolateral portion of the proximal humeral epiphyseal plate extends distally beyond the rest of the growth plate, and on the external rotation view, this projects as a horizontal lucency in the metaphyseal area. In early childhood, ossification of the proximal humeral epiphysis begins in two separate areas, and this should not be misinterpreted as a fracture through the epiphysis.

Epiphyseal plate fractures are relatively common in the proximal humerus and are usually a Salter Type II variety, although Type I fractures occasionally occur. Although these fractures are usually readily evident, occasionally there may be only subtle widening of the epiphyseal line and the metaphyseal corner fragment may be small or difficult to recognize. Incomplete fractures also affect the area and are usually located in the proximal humeral metaphyseal area.

Clavicle

Radiographic evaluation of the clavicle consists of two frontal views, one straight AP and the other, angulated 15 degrees cephalically. If one is specifically concerned about a sternoclavicular dislocation, a special projection (Heinig view) or CT examination is necessary.[19]

The clavicle is the most commonly fractured bone in young children. The fracture is usually in the midportion of the clavicle and may be either complete or incomplete. With rotation, the normal curvature of the clavicle may be exaggerated and mimic a fracture. Occasionally, no radiographic abnormality is demonstrated, but if there are localized clinical findings indicating a clavicular fracture, it should be assumed that a minimal incomplete fracture is present and appropriate immobilization should be instituted. Follow-up films are probably not indicated, since they would not alter management, although they often demonstrate callus formation, confirming that an incomplete fracture was initially present.

Acromioclavicular separations are very uncommon in children although an equivalent injury occurs.[20] Because of the strong ligaments at the acromioclavicular joint, a fracture occurs through the distal clavicle, and the clavicular periosteum at the attachment site of the coracoclavicular ligament is detached from the bone (Fig. 8–17).

Foot

Conventional radiographic evaluation requires AP, lateral, and oblique views. If the calcaneus is the major site of trauma, a tangential view of this structure is necessary for definitive evaluation.

Several normal variants are often confused with fractures in the foot. The most frequent variants occur at the base of the fifth metatarsal. The normal apophysis (traction epiphysis) lies parallel to the lateral aspect of the proximal portion of the fifth metatarsal,

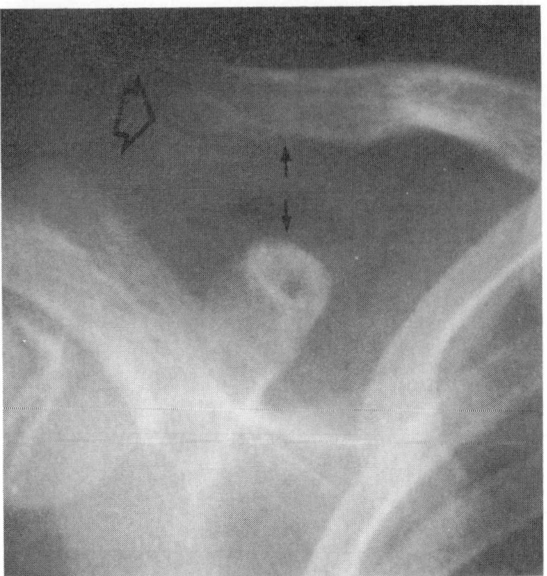

Figure 8–17. Radiograph shows a fracture *(open arrow)* through the distal clavicle and increased separation between the coracoid process of the scapula and the clavicle *(arrows)*. In children, this injury rather than acromioclavicular separation occurs.

and in contrast, nearly all fractures in this region extend transversely across the bone (Fig. 8–18). The normal apophysis may appear a surprising distance lateral to the remainder of the metatarsal, but comparison views usually show a similar pattern on the companion side. As in the equivalent structures in the hand, there is routinely considerable irregularity of the cortical margins in the bases of the second throgh fifth metatarsals. Correlation with clinical findings is urged before diagnosing a fracture in these areas. The calcaneal apophysis is often sclerotic and irregularly ossified, and this normal pattern should not be confused with a fracture or effects of avascular necrosis. Considerable variation exists in the appearance of the distal phalanges, and clinical correlation is often useful in determining the significance of such a finding.

A variety of fractures can affect the metatarsals and phalanges of the foot. Involvement of the epiphyseal plate is less frequent in the foot than in the hand. Except for the calcaneus, the tarsals are rarely fractured.

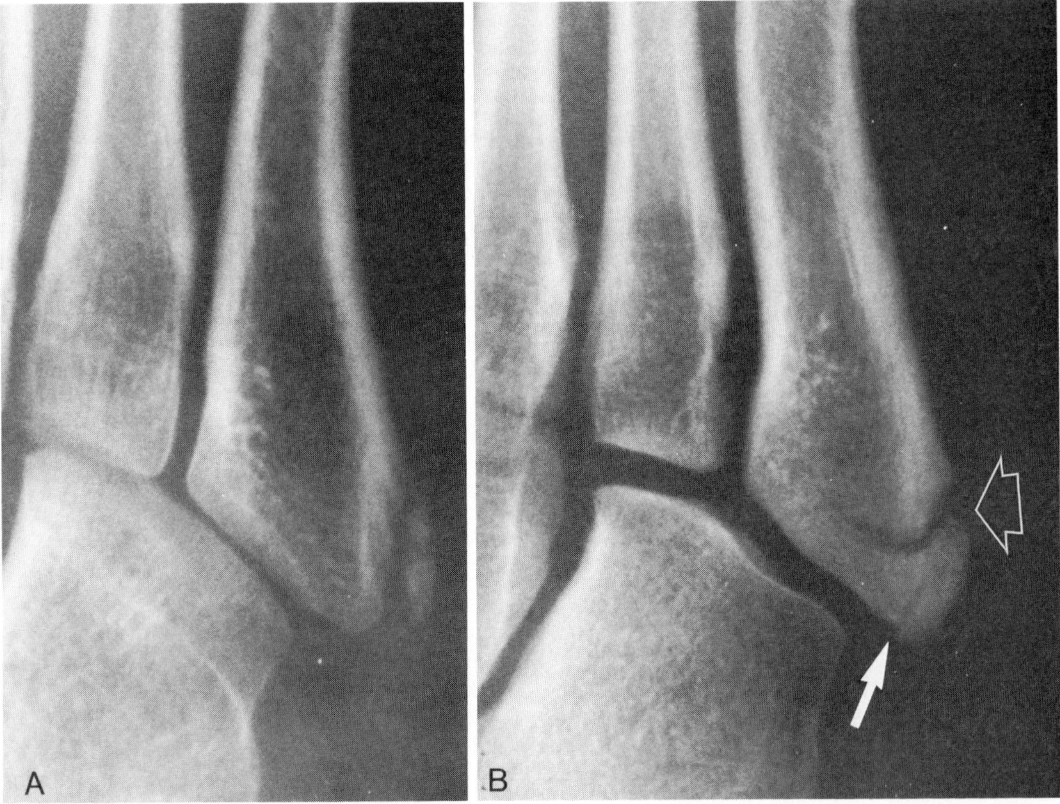

Figure 8–18. *A*, Normal appearance of the proximal portion of the fifth metatarsal. The growth plate for the ossification center parallels the long axis of the bone. *B*, In contrast, a fracture *(open arrow)* extends transversely through this portion of the metatarsal. A remnant of the growth plate is noted *(arrow)*.

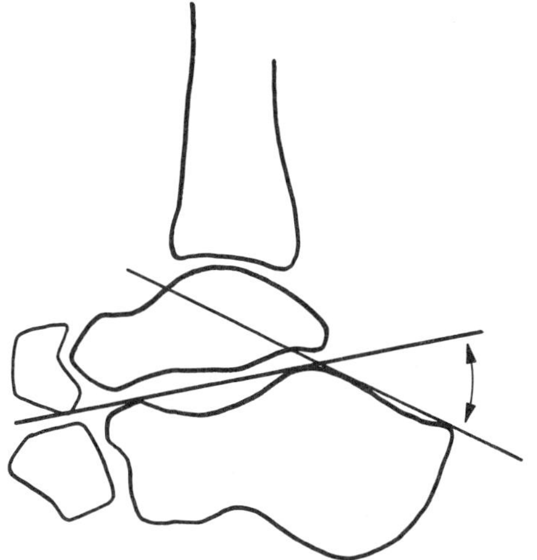

Figure 8–19. Diagram depicting Boehler's angle for evaluation of a calcaneal fracture. This angle normally measures 30 degrees to 35 degrees. An angle of less than 28 degrees indicates a calcaneal fracture.

Calcaneal fractures are often difficult to recognize. A tangential view often demonstrates the fracture best. An indirect method of confirming a calcaneal fracture is to determine Böehler's angle (Fig. 8–19).[21] If this measures less than 28 degrees, a calcaneal fracture is strongly suggested.

Opaque foreign bodies (usually needle fragments) are relatively common in the soft tissues of the feet in children. Removal under fluoroscopic control is encouraged because otherwise removal can be very difficult (Fig. 8–20). After the areas has been cleaned and draped, a small incision is made and blunt dissection done. Then, under fluoroscopic control, the object is grasped and removed. Careful attention to coning and exposure will result in minimal radiation to the patient and physician.

Ankle

The ankle is routinely filmed in AP, lateral, and internal oblique projections. If conventional films show no abnormality and physical findings are impressive, stress views in inversion and/or eversion can be obtained to demonstrate widening of the epiphyseal plate, which indicates a Salter Type I injury; in older children after closure of the epiphyseal plate, widening of the joint space implies ligamentous disruption.

Accessory ossicles are very common at the distal ends of the medial and lateral malleoli and are often misinterpreted as avulsion fractures. Another normal finding (which is occasionally misinterpreted as a Salter Type I fracture) is the apparent lateral offset of the distal fibular epiphysis, which is most confusing on the oblique view. Normal irregularity of the medial surface of the distal fibular metaphysis may mimic an incomplete fracture.

Occasionally incomplete fractures involve the distal tibial or fibular metaphyseal area,

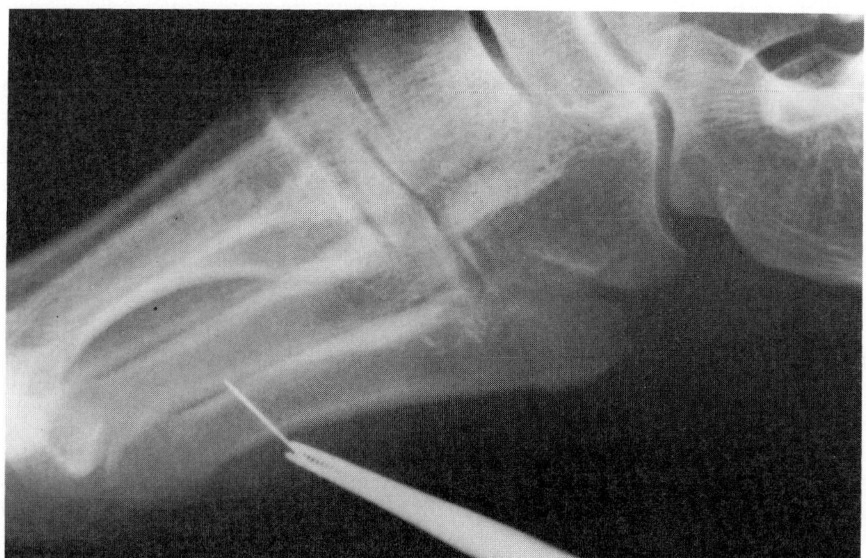

Figure 8–20. Opaque soft tissue foreign bodies are most easily removed under fluoroscopic control.

but most fractures in this region involve the epiphyseal plates of the distal tibia and fibula. Salter Type I fractures usually involve the distal fibular region, and the Type II usually affect the distal tibia. Type III fractures are relatively frequent in the distal tibia and can involve either the medial malleolar or anterolateral portion of the epiphysis.[22] The latter location is only affected in older children when the growth plate is partially closed. Type IV injuries also involve the distal tibia.

Fluid in the ankle joint can be detected radiographically.[23] This finding along with a history of trauma indicates an intra-articular injury. This is demonstrated on the lateral view, in which the margin of the capsule is normally identified anteriorly and has a concave configuration. With fluid distention, this capsule has a convex configuration. Normally, there is soft-tissue prominence posteriorly, and this should not be viewed as evidence of fluid in the joint.

Mid Tibia and Fibula

Certain fractures in this region are readily identified. A common fracture is the so-called toddler's fracture,[24] which characteristically is spiral, involves the mid and lower tibial diaphysis, and is often difficult to demonstrate (Fig. 8–21). If conventional films fail to show this fracture, high detail films and oblique views will often be useful in demonstrating this abnormality. Radionuclide scanning may occasionally be necessary to confirm or exclude this fracture.

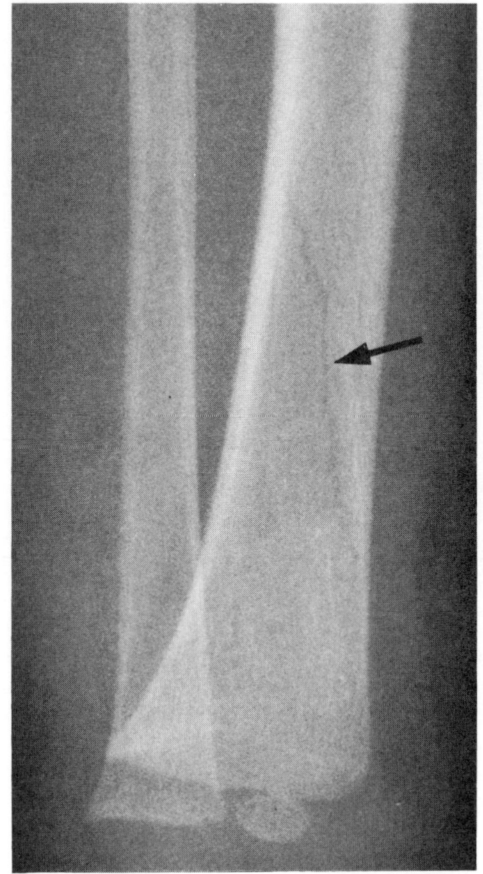

Figure 8–21. This 9-month-old child would not bear weight and there was localized tenderness elicited over the distal tibial diaphysis. A faint nondisplaced nonangulated oblique fracture line *(arrow)* is demonstrated in the distal tibial diaphysis.

Knee

AP and lateral views of the knee are usually sufficient to demonstrate any significant bone abnormality in this region. Oblique and tunnel views are seldom useful in evaluating the knee in children. In fact, the tunnel view is often confusing because it displays normal irregular ossification of the distal femoral epiphysis. This normal variant can be very prominent posteriorly in the non–weight-bearing areas, which is shown ideally on the tunnel view. Another normal variant that may mimic a fracture in this region is the lower margin of the tibial tubercle, which projects as a transverse lucency on the frontal view below the major portion of the proximal tibial epiphyseal plate. Benign fibrous cortical defects are commonly seen in the distal femoral and proximal tibial metaphyseal areas and are of no clinical significance. Cortical irregularity, which also represents a normal variant, is seen in older children along the posterior aspect of the distal femoral metaphysis, and on the frontal view, this may project as an area of relative lucency.

Fluid in the knee joint is radiographically detectable, as the suprapatellar bursa becomes distended.[25] This is seen on the lateral film as a widening of the soft tissue density posterior to the quadriceps tendon, or with greater fluid accumulation, the superior margin of the suprapatellar bursa is seen as an area of soft tissue density with a convex upper margin. Most fractures about the knee involve the epiphyseal growth plates. These are usually of the Type I and II varieties. Incomplete fractures and transverse fractures occasionally involve the metaphyseal and metaphyseal-diaphyseal areas of the distal femur and proximal tibia. A part of the tibial spine portion of the proximal tibial epiphysis can be avulsed at the cruciate ligament attachment site. The anterior cruciate ligament is usually involved. Patellar fractures are rare in the pediatric age group. Lateral patellar dislocation occasionally occurs in the adolescent age group; this is best demonstrated on a tangential (sunrise) view.

Femoral Diaphysis

Oblique, spiral, or transverse fractures may involve the mid femoral diaphysis. Mild comminution in this area is not unusual. These fractures are almost always readily demonstrated on routine radiographic evaluation, which consists of frontal and lateral views.

Pelvis and Hips

Routine radiographic evaluation consists of frontal films obtained in neutral and frog leg postions. The frog leg position is merely an AP view of the pelvis and a lateral view of the proximal femurs. There are multiple apophyses (traction epiphyses) about the pelvis (ischial, iliac spine, and crest apophyses) and proximal femurs (lesser and greater trochanters), which are often irregularly ossified and may be misinterpreted as fractures. The ischiopubic synchondroses may appear asymmetric.

Femoral neck fractures are rare in children and are usually readily detectable. Traumatic dislocation of the hip is also infrequent, but posterior dislocation occasionally occurs. The pelvis is also fractured much less often in children than in adults. Although major fractures of the pelvis are readily detectable, minimal incomplete cortical buckle fractures are relatively common and often missed. Careful comparison between the two sides of the pelvis is useful in avoiding this. Fractures into the acetabulum are often difficult to completely delineate on conventional radiographic evaluation. CT examination has been reported to be much more accurate in completely delineating such a fracture and in evaluating for fragments in the joint space.[3] The various apophyses about the hip may be traumatically avulsed (Fig. 8–22).[26] This usually occurs in adolescents engaging in athletic activities. The anterosuperior iliac spine, anteroinferior iliac spine, and ischial apophysis are the most common sites of apophyseal traumatic avulsion, although any of the apophyses of the pelvis or proximal femur may be involved.

Fluid in the hip joint can be detected radio-

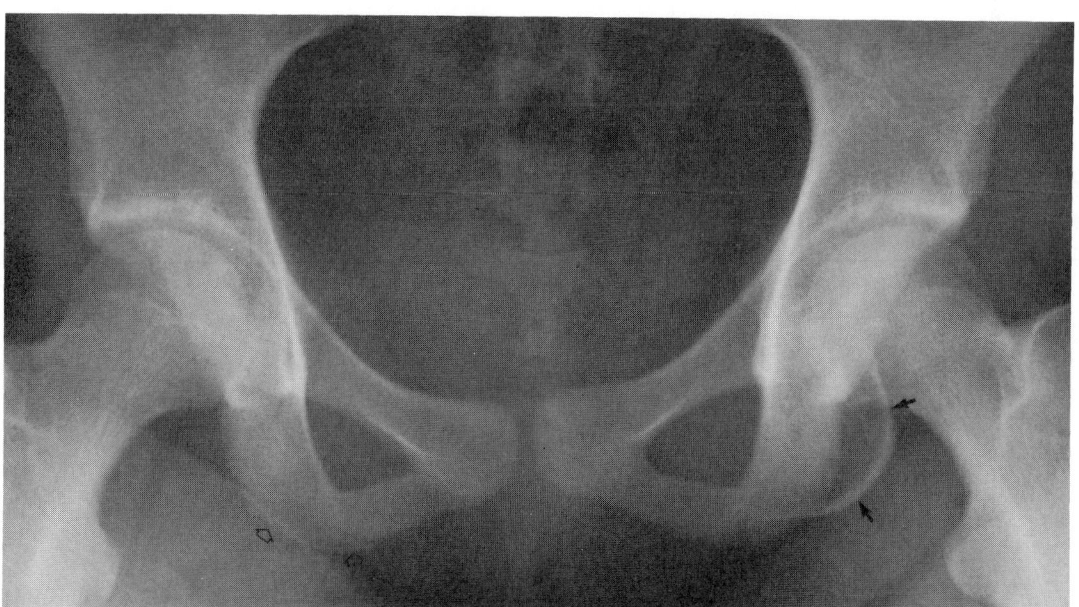

Figure 8–22. Severe left groin pain acutely developed in this 13-year-old boy while he was running. The left ischial apophysis has been avulsed and is displaced laterally and superiorly *(closed arrows)*. The right ischial apophysis *(open arrows)* is normal in appearance.

graphically, and this implies the presence of a hemarthrosis when there is a history of trauma. The diagnosis of fluid in the hip joint is made when the medial joint space is widened as compared with its companion side. Asymmetry of 2 mm or more indicates abnormal joint space widening. Correct positioning is crucial for this determination. The pelvis cannot be rotated, and the lower extremities must be positioned identically. Fat planes about the hip joint have been used to evaluate for joint fluid but are of limited value because they are remote from the hip joint capsule.[27]

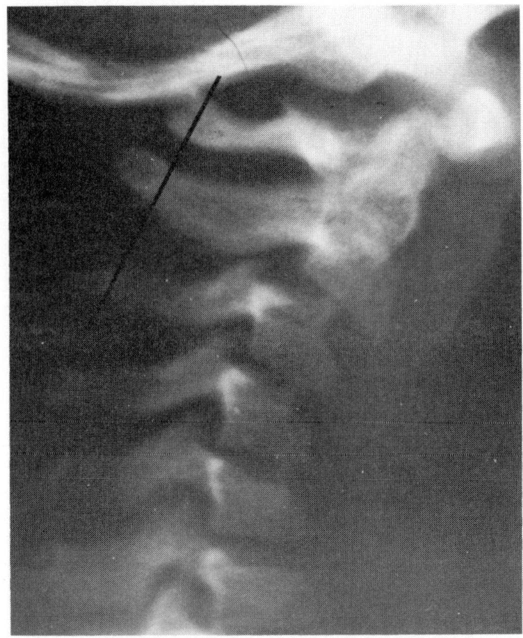

Figure 8–23. A common normal variant (physiologic pseudosubluxation of C2 on C3) is often misinterpreted as a C2–C3 dislocation. This is normally the area of maximum movement in the cervical spine in young children, and considerable mobility at this level is a normal variant and is seen when the head is flexed. The posterior spinal line is demonstrated. This line extends between the posterior margins of the neural canal of C1 and C3. The posterior margin of the neural canal of C2 should not be displaced more than 2 mm from this line.

Spine

Fractures and dislocations involving the vertebral column are very uncommon in young children. This is presumably related to the increased mobility and elasticity of the child's cervical spine as compared with that of the adult. Conventional radiographic studies are utilized in the initial evaluation of these injuries. CT is useful for more detailed evaluation concerning (1) the extent of complex fractures, (2) posterior element involvement, or (3) the presence of fragments within the spinal canal.[2] This method will not be described in greater detail because it is seldom used in the initial work-up and should be interpreted by specialists experienced in these studies. Also, conventional tomography or myelography will occasionally be useful in evaluating spinal injuries.

Cervical Spine

Reported indications for filming the cervical spine of trauma patients are predominantly derived from experience with adults. These film studies are indicated in patients who have suspected cervical spine injury, who are unconscious, and who have suffered head trauma. Because of the major implications of cervical spine injuries, this approach cannot be criticized, but those caring for the acutely injured child should realize that the incidence of fractures and dislocations in the cervical spine is extremely infrequent prior to adolescence unless there are focal signs or symptoms. The incidence and types of fractures in teenagers are probably similar to those in adults.

The method of radiographic evaluation is dictated by the patient's condition. In the unconscious patient or the child with clinical evidence of cervical spine injury, the head and neck should be immobilized and a horizontal beam lateral radiograph obtained without moving the patient. The entire cervical spine downward through C7 must be well visualized. This lateral film should be reviewed before further studies are done. If no abnormality is demonstrated, the patient can be transferred to a conventional x-ray table for additional studies unless contraindicated by other injuries. The patient is often transported with a cervical collar in place, which remains for the initial screening lateral view. After this film is evaluated and no abnormality is demonstrated, the collar can be removed and the lateral film repeated if the collar is opaque enough to preclude definitive evaluation. If the patient's condition warrants, AP and open mouth views should also be obtained. In the ambulatory or less severely injured child, oblique or AP pillar views can be obtained to evaluate the lateral articular masses.[28]

A systematic approach is recommended when evaluating spine films. Vertebral alignment, the relationship of adjacent vertebrae, the configuration of the vertebrae, and the appearance of the adjacent soft tissue structures must be analyzed. It is useful to compare the appearance of structures at adjacent levels. Alignment evaluation requires assessment of the anterior and posterior margins of the spinal canal as well as examination of the anterior vertebral body margins.

There are many normal variants encountered in the radiographic evaluation of the pediatric cervical spine that are commonly confused with the effects of trauma. Misinterpretation of normal variants is more common than actual cervical spine injuries in young children.

The most frequent normal variant that is confused with a serious cervical spine injury is normal mobility at the C2–3 level (Fig. 8–23). This common variant occurs in children up to approximately 10 years of age and is most often seen when the head is flexed or when the patient is lying supine and horizontal beam lateral filming is done. This normal variant is commonly called physiologic pseudosubluxation of C2. This anterior position of C2 relative to C3 is physiologic and attributed to normal laxity of the ligaments in this age group. It has been proposed that this normal variant can be evaluated by a line (Fig. 8–23) connecting the posterior cortical margin of the neural canal of C1 and C3 (the posterior spinal line).[30] If the posterior cortex of C2 is not displaced more than 2 mm posterior to this line, the relationship is normal. If the body of C2 is anteriorly positioned and the posterior cortex of its neural canal is more posterior to the spinal line, a bilateral pedicle fracture of C2 is inferred.

The thickness of the soft tissues in the prevertebral region should be evaluated with caution in infants and young children.[29] These tissues are redundant and mobile and, with flexion of the head, flexion of the spine, or expiration, normally appear very prominent (Fig. 8–24). Fluoroscopy can be done to determine if the posterior margin of the airway approximates the spine during inspiration.

Radiographically, the odontoid appears separated from the body of C2 by a cartilaginous line, which closes by about age 6. This should not be misinterpreted as a fracture at the base of the odontoid. A portion of the synchondrosis may remain unfused anteriorly and mimic a fracture in older children.

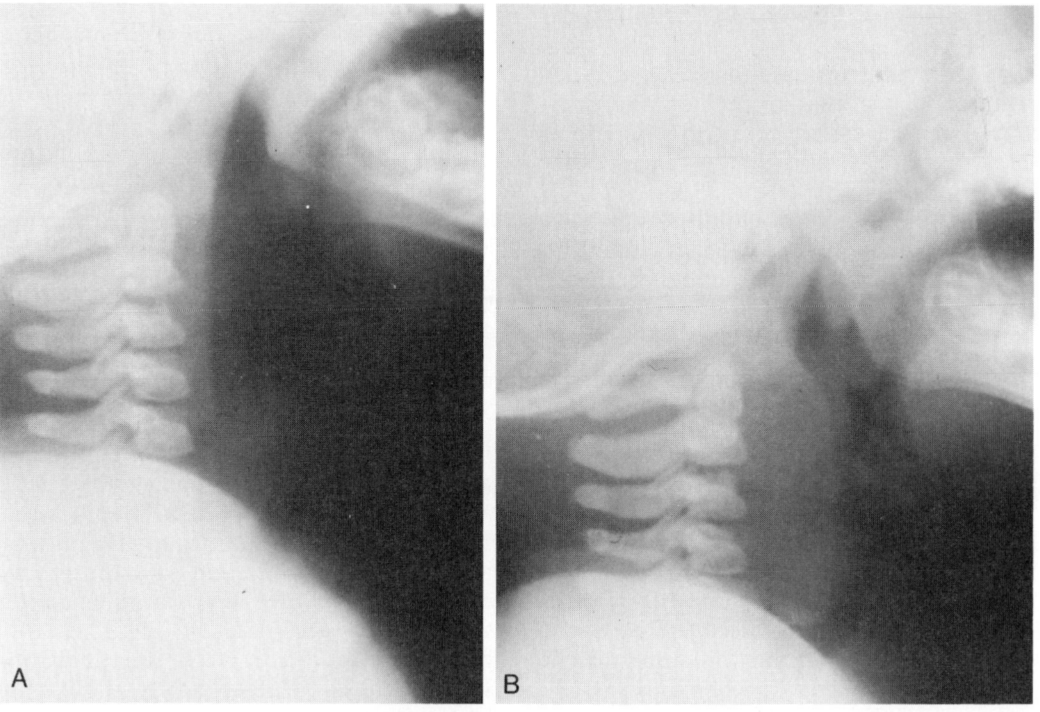

Figure 8–24. During respiration, considerable fluctuation in the thickness of the prevertebral soft tissues normally occurs in the infant and young child. *A*, During inspiration, the anterior margin of the soft tissues is in close approximation to the bony structures. *B*, During expiration, the soft tissues normally bulge forward. This pattern is also exaggerated by flexion of the head and neck.

Odontoid fractures usually occur at the odontoid base. The odontoid is usually displaced posteriorly, and there is angulation with the apex of the odontoid and C2 body directed anteriorly. A tilted odontoid implies a fracture.

Other normal variants in the cervical spine can also be confused with effects of trauma.[29] The vertebral bodies are wedge shaped in childhood, and this finding should not be misinterpreted as a fracture. If all the cervical vertebral bodies have the same configuration, this implies normal variation. Loss of the normal lordotic curvature of the cervical spine occurs as a normal variant and does not specifically imply effects of muscle spasm. With extension, the anterior arch of C1 normally becomes positioned superior to the odontoid. The distance between the odontoid and anterior arch of C1 may appear prominent on flexion views and, in the child, can normally measure up to 4 mm. Partial ossification in the end-plate apophyses that occurs in teenagers at the anteroinferior margin of the vertebral bodies should not be misinterpreted as an avulsion fracture.

Fractures of the C1 ring result from vertical compression forces. This is called a Jefferson fracture. The major radiographic finding described in this condition is lateral displacement of the lateral masses of C1 with respect to the lateral masses of C2. However, this finding is of limited value in children under 7 years of age because of incomplete ossification of the lateral aspect of the C2 lateral masses.[31] Using a ratio of the distance between the medial and lateral edges of C1 (less than 0.55 in normal children) has been suggested as a method of distinguishing the normal C1 ring from the Jefferson fracture.[31]

Bilateral pedicle fracture of C2 is commonly referred to as the hangman's fracture, but in children, the etiology is usually related to an automobile accident resulting in a hyperextension injury. Forward dislocation of C2 on C3 nearly always results in an abnormal posterior spinal line.

Fractures of the cervical spine below the C2 level are infrequent prior to adolescence. Compression fractures of vertebral bodies, fractures of the neural arch, dislocation, unilateral and bilateral interfacetal dislocation, and pillar compression fractures rarely occur in childhood.

Rotary subluxation at the C1–2 level is a controversial subject. This condition should be suspected when there is a persistent asymmetric relationship of the lateral masses of C1 to the odontoid process on open mouth views with rotation of the head in both directions. The spinous process of C2 is on the same side of midline as the mandible points. Some authors state that the odontoid-C1 distance must be widened[32] to make this diagnosis; others disagree.[33]

THORACOLUMBAR SPINE

Fractures involving vertebrae in the thoracolumbar region are much less frequent in children than in adults. Radiographic evaluation consists of AP and lateral views, although oblique views are occasionally helpful.

Normal variants are occasionally confused with fractures in the thoracolumbar spine. In infants and young children, there are normally central notches in the anterior margin of the vertebral bodies. In older children, there is irregularity in the anterior margin of the vertebral bodies superiorly and inferiorly, and as these end-plate areas ossify, this can be misinterpreted as small fracture fragments. There is normally minimal anterior wedging of the thoracic vertebrae, but each vertebral body appears the same as those adjacent to it.

Compression fractures of the vertebral bodies are the most frequent form of trauma involving the thoracolumbar spine. Radiographic signs include the wedge-shaped deformity noted on the lateral film with reduced height anteriorly. Involvement of multiple vertebral bodies may occur. Fractures and dislocations occasionally occur in the lumbar area. Other forms of fractures (transverse process and seat belt fractures) rarely occur in childhood.

Skull

The radiographic evaluation of skull trauma in children remains a controversial area.[34] Debate continues concerning indications for skull radiographs, significance of the presence of a fracture, management implications by the location of skull fractures, and indications for CT scanning. Efficacy studies have resulted in identification of high-yield criteria for the identification of skull fractures.[35] Utilization of these criteria to select patients needing skull radiographic examination has resulted in reduction in the number of studies performed and significant improvement in the yield of positive findings. However, the validity of these criteria in children has been questioned.[36] Rather than discussing these areas of controversy in further detail, a general philosphic approach utilized at our institution will be presented in this section.

There is limited correlation between the status of intracranial contents and plain skull film findings.[37] Absence of a skull fracture certainly does not imply that there has not been significant injury to the brain or adjacent meninges and vascular structures. Skull films merely evaluate damage to the calvarium, and although certain implications exist with specific fractures, the value of this method in evaluating patients with head trauma is limited. CT scanning has become extremely important in the evaluation of head trauma because it demonstrates the status of the intracranial structures. Epidural hematoma, subdural hematoma, intracerebral hemorrhage, intraventricular hemorrhage, subarachnoid hemorrhage, and cerebral edema can be demonstrated with CT scanning. Indications for this procedure are discussed in Chapter 16. Interpretation should be done by those with expertise in this area rather than by the emergency physician and, therefore, will not be discussed further.

The site and type of fracture, rather than merely the presence of a fracture, are what determine the seriousness of an injury. The major contribution of conventional skull films is to exclude or confirm certain types and locations of fractures that require specific therapy or are associated with an increased incidence of intracranial complications. Depressed fractures are of specific significance, since surgical correction is indicated unless displacement is minimal. Compound fractures (those communicating with paranasal sinuses or mastoid areas or those with an associated scalp laceration) have an increased likelihood of developing intracranial infection. Fractures that cross the middle meningeal artery or one of the venous sinuses are associated with an increased incidence of intracranial bleeding. Fractures of the posterior fossa need close clinical observation, since intracranial complications in this area can result in rapid deterioration. In addition to demonstrating and localizing a fracture, skull films can also show pneumocephalus or a foreign body in the calvarium or overlying soft tissues.

Although detailed listings of criteria for obtaining skull x-rays in trauma patients have been published, a more simplified list of criteria is adequate. These indications include (1) documented loss of consciousness, (2) neurologic findings, (3) penetrating or open wounds, and (4) focal injury. Additionally, all infants are evaluated radiographically because of the probable increased incidence of complications in skull fractures in this younger age group.[38]

The basic radiographic evaluation of the skull should include anteroposterior and Towne's (occipital) projections and each lateral projection. It is crucial that the films be done without rotation, since sutures, which are midline or symmetrically paired structures, are much more likely to be misinterpreted as fractures on improperly positioned studies. A horizontal beam lateral projection is useful in older children to evaluate for air-fluid levels in the paranasal sinuses, which would suggest communication between the sinus and the meninges. If a depressed skull fracture is suspected by history or physical findings or suggested on initial conventional films, localized tangential films of this area can be done to confirm the presence of depression and to determine the degree of depression. Occasionally, fluoroscopy is most helpful in evaluating for the presence and degree of depression.

Care must be taken not to misinterpret normal structures as fractures. Primary care physicians should become more familiar with the normal vascular grooves and sutures that are most often confused with fractures in childhood.[39] Correlation with physical findings is useful because fractures occur at the site of trauma; the contrecoup phenomenon that occurs with brain injury does not occur in the skull. Linear fractures appear as a discrete lucent line, which is usually quite straight. Except in the stellate-type fracture, there is seldom branching. In contrast, suture lines generally have serrated edges, are in specific locations, and, except for the midline sutures (sagittal and metopic), are symmetrically paired. Vascular grooves in the frontal region are often quite conspicuous on lateral views and are often more prominent in children than in adults. An unfused metopic suture is often confused with a midline fracture. This is most easily differentiated on the Towne's view, in which the metopic suture line will project over the foramen magnum (Fig. 8–25). A midline occipital fracture, in

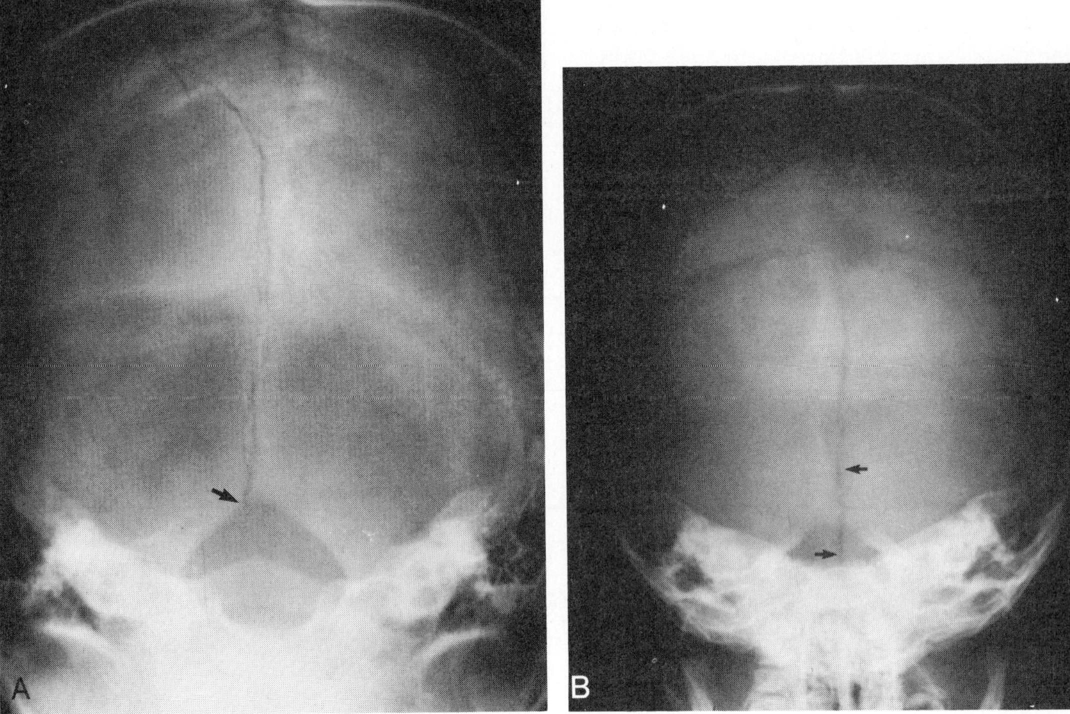

Figure 8–25. *A,* Towne's (occipital) view showing an occipital fracture that extends to the foramen magnum *(arrow). B,* This fracture is mimicked by an unfused metopic suture *(arrows).* This line projects beyond the margin of the foramen magnum.

contrast, will terminate at the margin of the foramen magnum (see Fig. 8–25).

TYPES OF SKULL FRACTURES

Linear Skull Fracture

Linear skull fractures are most frequent and most often involve the parietal or occipital bone. These fractures occasionally extend across a suture line. Also, the fracture may extend along the suture line, resulting in acute spreading of the suture (Fig. 8–26). This is called a diastatic suture fracture and is much more frequent in children than in adults. This diagnosis should be considered when a suture that is in continuity with a fracture is separated when compared with its companion suture. Unusually wide separation of fracture fragments should be noted because these cases are more likely to have subsequent development of a leptomeningeal cyst.

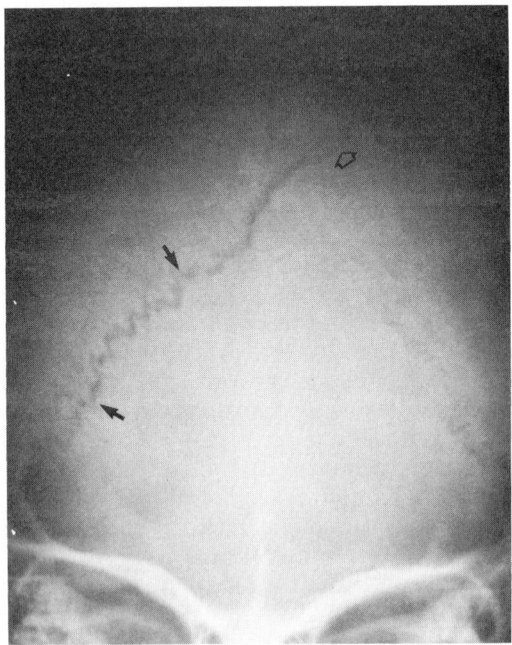

Figure 8–26. Diastatic suture fracture. The right lambdoid suture *(closed arrows)* is widened as compared with the normal left lambdoid suture. It extends into the left parietal bone as a linear fracture *(open arrow).*

Basilar skull fractures are usually not demonstrated on plain films of the skull. Unilat-

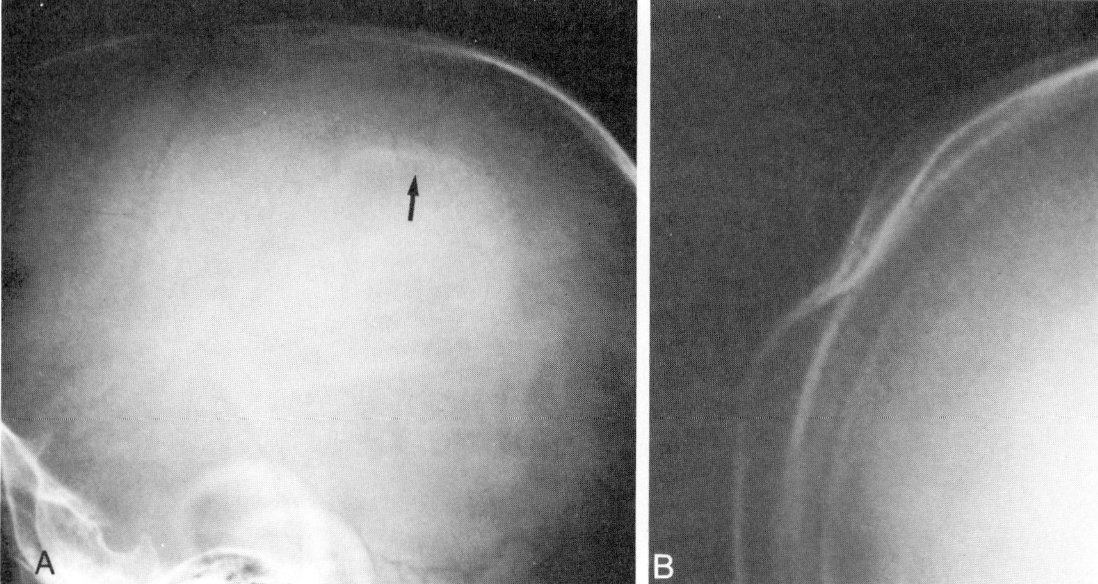

Figure 8–27. Depressed right parietal fracture. *A*, There is minimal change noted on the lateral film. A faint, linear area of increased density *(arrow)* is present. The possibility of a depressed fracture should be considered whenever a localized area of increased density is visualized. *B*, This frontal view readily demonstrates the localized area of depression.

eral opacification of a mastoid area is suggestive of a basilar fracture in a patient that has had trauma.

Depressed Skull Fracture

A depressed fracture is present when one or more fragments of bone are displaced into the cranial cavity (Fig. 8–27). These fractures are often the result of localized trauma causing a stellate fracture, with multiple fractures radiating outward from a central point. Depressed fractures result in overlapping of fragments, and the radiographic pattern is that of areas of increased density. Any opaque line in an area of trauma should be suspected of being a depressed fracture, and additional radiographic examination is justified for more definitive evaluation. Views tangential to the site of trauma usually will confirm the presence of depression and demonstrate the degree of displacement. Occasionally, fluoroscopy with spot films will be necessary for more definitive evaluation. The so-called "ping-pong" fracture is a form of a depressed skull fracture that is unique to the neonate and young infant. In this condition, there is localized depression without actual break in the continuity of the bone. Also, in infants in whom there is considerable mobility of sutures, a fragment may be elevated rather than depressed. There is a high incidence of underlying dural and cerebral injury in this situation.

FACIAL TRAUMA

Prior to adolescence, fractures in the mid facial area are extremely unsual.[40] The incidence and types of fractures occurring in adolescents are similar to those occurring in adults. Mandibular fractures occur more commonly although still considerably less frequently in children than in adults. Although all forms of mandibular fractures can occur, the most frequent type of fracture in the young child is an incomplete fracture of the mandibular neck (Fig. 8–28). The fracture fragments remain in apposition, with the apex of the fracture fragments usually directed posterolaterally. This is usually an isolated fracture, with the mandible being intact elsewhere. This is best demonstrated on a Towne's projection, in which the lateral angulation is apparent when compared with the companion side. Oblique views will also demonstrate the fracture but are often more difficult to interpret. Panorex views are ex-

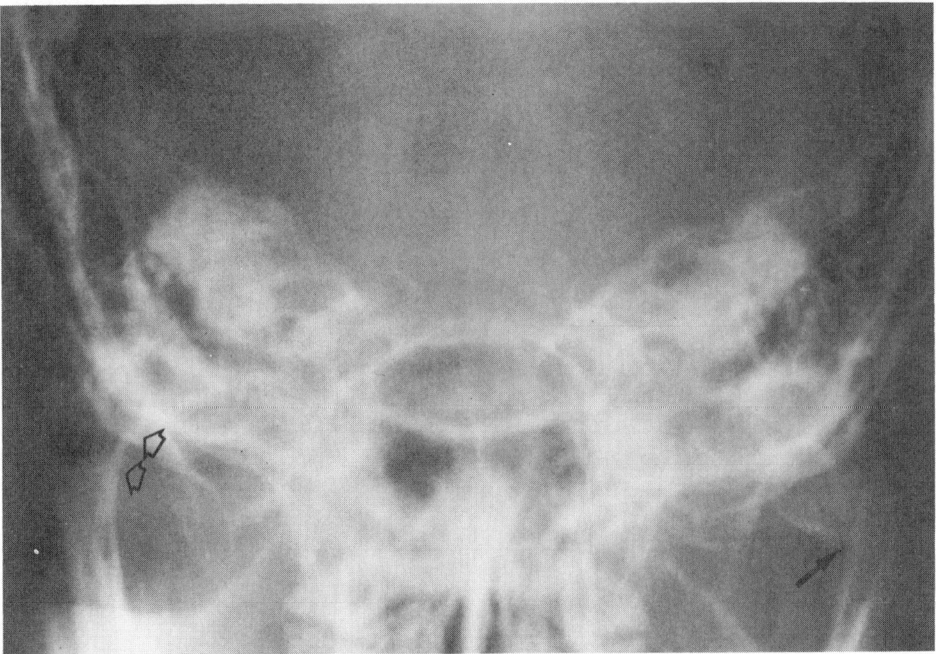

Figure 8–28. Incomplete fracture of the left mandibular neck *(closed arrow)*, demonstrated on a Towne's projection. Localized angulation at the fracture site is apparent when compared with the smooth curvature of the companion side *(open arrows)*.

tremely useful in evaluating mandibular and facial trauma if this modality is available.

THORACIC TRAUMA

Chest trauma in children occurs from blunt or penetrating injury and varies in severity from minor, inconsequential injuries to life-threatening emergent problems. Chest injuries are most frequently due to vehicular and auto-pedestrian accidents and are often a major contributing factor in fatal accidents.

A child who is ambulatory after trauma should have upright frontal and lateral chest radiographs taken. A patient with more severe injury can adequately be evaluated with an AP supine radiograph after initial stabilization. If the patient's condition permits, an upright chest radiograph should be obtained. In this position, pleural fluid is more easily recognized, air-fluid levels are more readily detected, free intraperitoneal air is easily seen beneath the diaphragm, and the mediastinum is more easily evaluated. If an upright view is not possible, decubitus films or a cross-table lateral film may be helpful to better delineate these abnormalities. Since each decubitus film gives different information, both right and left decubitus films are sometimes justified. The degree of pleural fluid is best demonstrated when the ipsilateral side is in a dependent position, whereas pneumothorax is best demonstrated when the side of concern is superiorly positioned. Additional chest views are rarely critical to the management of the patient, and if obtained, significant time should not be expended so that the patient's clinical condition is compromised.

Differentiation of extraventilatory air (pneumothorax, pneumomediastinum) from pleural fluid, atelectasis, or pulmonary contusion is not difficult. The lung with extraventilatory air will always appear more radiolucent than the adjacent normal lung. In contrast, the lung with pleural fluid, atelectasis, or pulmonary contusion has increased density as compared with the adjacent normal lung.

Chest structures in children may appear different or respond differently to trauma as compared with those of adults. The thymus is normally prominent in infants and young children and is accentuated on an AP supine view, and this normal variant must be considered in the evaluation of the mediastinum. Rib fractures are infrequent because of the resiliency of young bone but may be associated with additional injury. Injury to the thoracic vasculature, particularly the aorta, is extremely rare in children as compared with adults.

Soft Tissue and Skeletal Injuries

Soft Tissues

Superficial contusions with edema of the chest wall may disrupt the normal appearance of the soft tissue planes. Larger hematomas may project over the lung, and the increased density may simulate pulmonary injury.

Penetrating injuries may result in interstitial emphysema and even air-fluid levels in the soft tissues, and this too can be confused with pulmonary injury on a single view. Interstitial emphysema in the soft tissues of the chest wall, neck, and supraclavicular region usually occurs in association with pneumothorax and/or pneumomediastinum.

Rib Fractures

As mentioned earlier, rib fractures are infrequent in children but may signal underlying injuries. The initial chest radiograph is usually sufficient for the evaluation of rib injury, and additional rib views are not indicated.

Fractures of the first and second ribs are usually indicative of severe trauma. Earlier reports[41, 42] emphasized that these fractures may be a clue to underlying tracheobronchial injury or damage to the thoracic vasculature. However, more recent studies emphasize that fractures of these ribs by themselves are not an indication for arteriography.[43] Arteriography should be considered if the chest radiograph demonstrates widening of the superior mediastinum or right paratracheal stripe, displacement of the trachea or nasogastric tube to the right, widening of the right or left paraspinous line, or an enlarged or indistinct aortic knob.[41, 43] Fractures of the lower rib cage may provide a clue that the injury has been of sufficient force to lacerate the underlying liver, spleen, or kidney.[44]

Sternal Fractures

Fractures of the sternum are rare, usually involve the body, and result from a crush injury, such as hitting the dashboard during a vehicular collision. This fracture should serve to alert the clinician to the possibility of associated serious intrathoracic injury.[1] A lateral view of the sternum is usually sufficient to diagnose this injury.

Retrosternal Dislocation of the Clavicle

Traumatic retrosternal dislocation of the clavicle at the sternoclavicular joint and a Salter I fracture of the medial clavicle are rare problems but may be life threatening because the displaced clavicle can impinge upon the trachea and vascular structures. It is frequently difficult to diagnose on conventional radiographs, and special views (Heinig projection) may be required.[19] This lesion may be easily demonstrated by CT (Fig. 8–29).

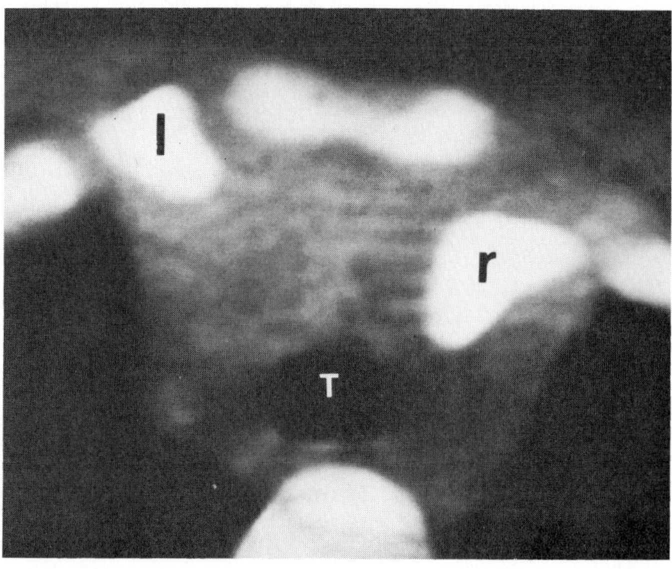

Figure 8–29. Right sternoclavicular dislocation in an 8-year-old boy involved in a motor vehicle accident. A computerized tomogram demonstrates the relationship of the proximal left clavicle (l) to the manubrium and of the posteriorly displaced right clavicle (r) to the trachea (T).

PULMONARY INJURIES

Pneumothorax and Pneumomediastinum

A traumatic pneumothorax is often caused by a fractured rib puncturing the pleural space and lung or by direct penetrating injury. However, these forms of extraventilatory air are not infrequent in children in whom rib fractures are not identified. Significant pneumothorax is usually recognized on an erect chest radiograph as an area of radiolucency adjacent to the collapsed pleural margin of the lung. In films taken with the patient in the supine position, a pneumothorax is more easily overlooked because the free pleural fluid air in children tends to collect anterior and medial to the lung.[45] A medial pneumothorax may cause superolateral displacement and compression of the lingular portion of the left lung and may produce a confusing localized density adjacent to the lateral aspect of the hemithorax.[46] A pneumothorax may also localize between the lung and hemidiaphragm, and this is termed a basilar pneumothorax (Fig. 8–30).[47] Other radiographic findings suggesting a basilar pneumothorax include a "double" appearance of the hemidiaphragm as air outlines the anterior costophrenic sulcus and unusually distinct visualization of the cardiac apex and pericardial fat tags.[47] A decubitus film, with the side of concern positioned superiorly, or a cross-table lateral view is suggested if an anterior, medial, or basilar pneumothorax is not easily recognized on a supine view. The presence of skinfolds, bandages, and clothing may simulate a pleural margin of the lung and suggest a pneumothorax, but close attention will usually indicate that these densities extend beyond the margin of the thoracic cage.

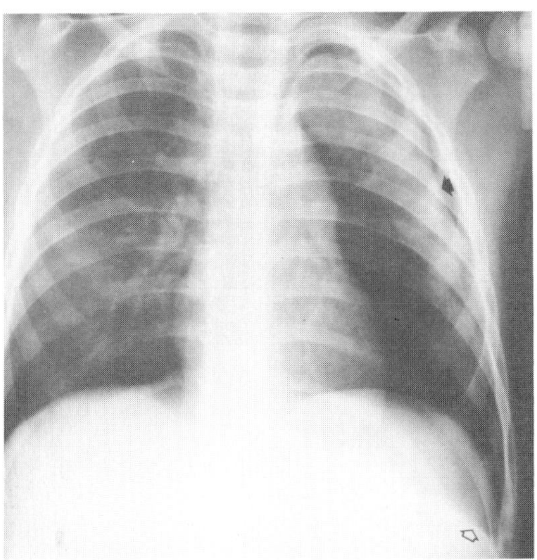

Figure 8–30. Pulmonary contusion and pneumothorax in a 3-year-old boy following auto-pedestrian trauma. Fractures of the left second, third, and fourth ribs laterally are not well visualized on this film. Increased density in the left upper lung is secondary to pulmonary contusion. A moderate left pneumothorax is present with air in the lateral pleural space outlining the margin of the visceral pleura of the lung *(closed arrow)*, in the basilar region outlining the anterior costophrenic sulcus *(open arrow)*, and medially, with hyperlucency adjacent to the left heart margin.

A tension pneumothorax may develop when the pleural defect permits air to enter the pleural space during inspiration but not escape during expiration. With time, the underlying lung becomes compressed and the cardiovascular and mediastinal structures shift to the opposite side. If not treated, ventilatory and circulatory compromise may ensue.

Serial chest radiographs in patients with severe chest trauma may be helpful if the patient's condition is unstable or if signs and symptoms are changing. A small pneumothorax may be missed on an initial supine radiograph and may subsequently develop into a tension pneumothorax and/or pneumomediastinum, especially when the patient is treated with positive pressure ventilation. It is also important to recognize that penetrating wounds in the neck and upper abdomen may penetrate the pleural space and produce a pneumothorax.

Pneumomediastinum is common in children following chest injury and frequently accompanies a pneumothorax. Gas from ruptured alveoli may dissect along peribronchial planes to the hilum and enter the mediastinum. As the air dissects into the mediastinum, it displaces the medial pleural margin laterally and often outlines the thymus (Fig. 8–31). In the lateral projection, an extrapulmonary collection of gas outlining the thymus is characteristic of a pneumomediastinum (Fig. 8–32*A*). Air may also dissect into the posterior mediastinum, outlining the descending aorta (Fig. 8–32*B*), or extend into the neck and soft tissues of the chest wall. It is important to recognize that a pneumomediastinum in children may extend into the abdomen and produce a pneumoperitoneum. If the extraventilatory air is not recognized within the chest, a serious intra-abdominal injury may be erroneously suspected.

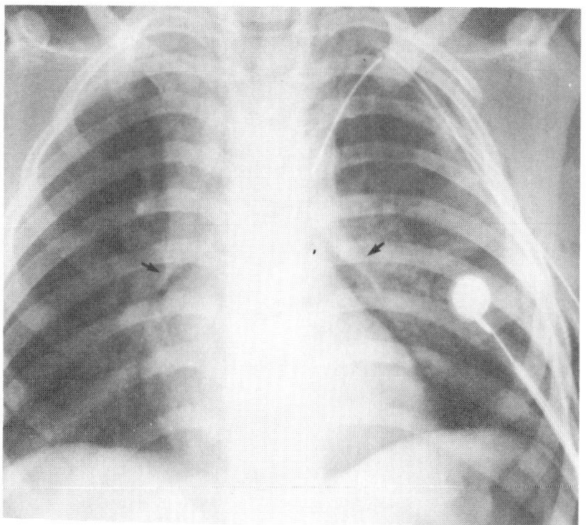

Figure 8–31. Hemopneumothorax and pneumomediastinum in a 5-year-old boy following a motor vehicle accident. Fractures of the left second to sixth ribs are present laterally and posteriorly. The hemopneumothorax has been treated with a left chest tube; subcutaneous emphysema is seen in the lateral soft tissues. A pneumomediastinum outlines the right and left lobes of the thymus *(arrows)*.

Differentiation of an anteromedial pneumothorax from a pneumomediastinum may be difficult on the supine radiograph. A decubitus view, with the ipsilateral side superiorly positioned, will differentiate the two by demonstrating the mobility of the free pleural air from the fixed position of mediastinal air.

Hemothorax

Blood may enter the chest cavity following disruption of vessels in the chest wall, pleura, lung, diaphragm, or mediastinum.[44] The exact site of bleeding cannot be readily determined from radiographic examination. As a general rule, hemothorax that is increasing on serial chest radiographs indicates bleeding from sites other than the lung.[44] If bleeding into the pleural space is from pulmonary or bronchial vessels, the expanding hemothorax tends to compress the soft tissues of the lung, producing hemostasis.[48]

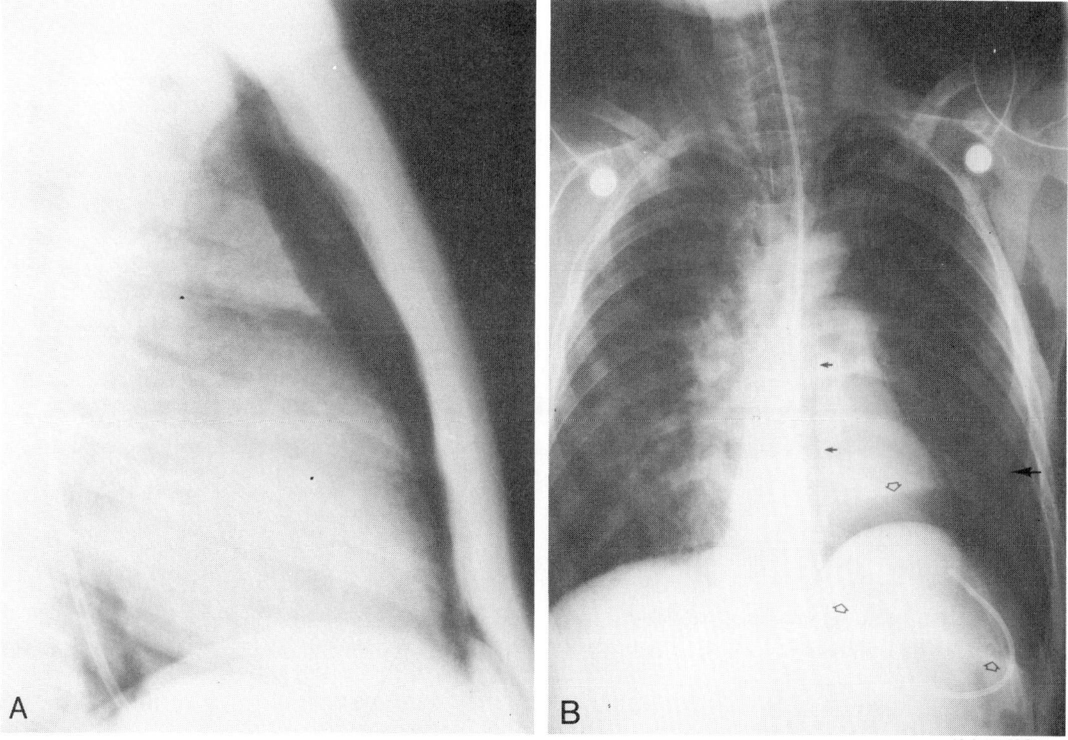

Figure 8–32. Subcutaneous emphysema, pneumothorax, and pneumomediastinum in an 8-year-old boy following motor vehicle accident. *A,* A lateral chest film demonstrates a pneumomediastinum, with air in the anterior mediastinal space outlining the thymus. *B,* An anteroposterior (AP) supine chest film demonstrates a moderate basilar pneumothorax *(open arrows)*, a lateral pneumothorax *(single closed arrow)*, and a pneumomediastinum, with air outlining the descending aorta *(two small closed arrows)*. Air has also dissected into the neck and left axillary region, producing extensive subcutaneous emphysema. Pulmonary density predominantly in the right lower lung is probably secondary to aspiration. A mid diaphyseal right clavicular fracture is also present.

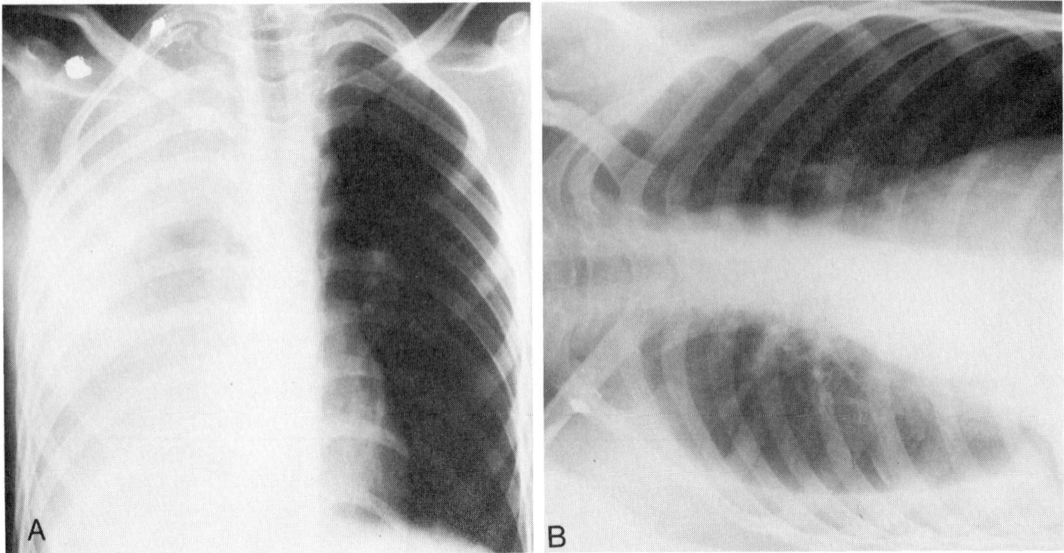

Figure 8–33. Hemothorax following a gunshot wound in a 9-year-old boy. *A*, Initial AP supine film demonstrates a large right hemothorax enveloping the lung, with the increased density noted laterally in particular. Posterior right rib fractures of the second and third ribs and retained metallic fragments are also seen. *B*, Three days later a decubitus film with the right side dependent demonstrates a moderate residual, mobile hemothorax. On the upright chest film, the fluid was predominantly localized in the subpulmonic pleural space.

Blood in the pleural space is usually freely movable. In the upright position, a small to moderate hemothorax initially produces blunting of the costophrenic angle and then widening of the paravertebral line. Significant amounts of blood may be present in the subpulmonic pleural space and may only be recognized if either an apparent elevation of the hemidiaphragm or an altered contour to the hemidiaphragm with a more lateral position of the diaphragmatic apex or "hump" is produced. If the subpulmonic effusion is on the left, the distance between the air-filled gastric fundus and base of the lung may be increased. Small amounts of fluid may also be present in the pleural fissures. An air-fluid level on the upright films indicates a hemopneumothorax.

With the patient in the supine position, blood tends to collect in the most dependent portion of the thorax. With a supine film, a small hemothorax is easily overlooked. As the hemothorax increases, one gradually is able to recognize an increase in density of the involved hemothorax. Larger effusions widen the paravertebral stripe in a supine position and gradually envelop the lung, producing increased density around the lung, particularly laterally (Fig. 8–33). A decubitus film, with the side of concern dependent, is helpful to better evaluate the amount of free pleural fluid (Fig. 8–33) and can better demonstrate pleural fluid when it is predominantly in the subpulmonic pleural space.

Chylothorax

A chylous pleural effusion may occur following an injury to the thoracic duct from either penetrating or nonpenetrating injury of the chest or upper abdomen. Crush injuries to the upper abdomen and lower thorax tend to cause disruption of the thoracic duct just above the diaphragm, and a lesion at this level typically produces a right chylothorax. Injuries to the upper part of the thoracic duct or neck may result in a left-sided chylous effusion.[49] Initially the extravasated chyle is confined to the posterior mediastinum (Fig. 8–34), but as the collection increases, it usually ruptures into the pleural space. The volume of fluid may be large but cannot be differentiated with radiographs from other causes of pleural effusion. CT may demonstrate high fat content, indicating chylothorax (Fig. 8–34).

Tracheobronchial Injury

Fracture of the bronchus or the intrathoracic portion of the trachea is usually caused

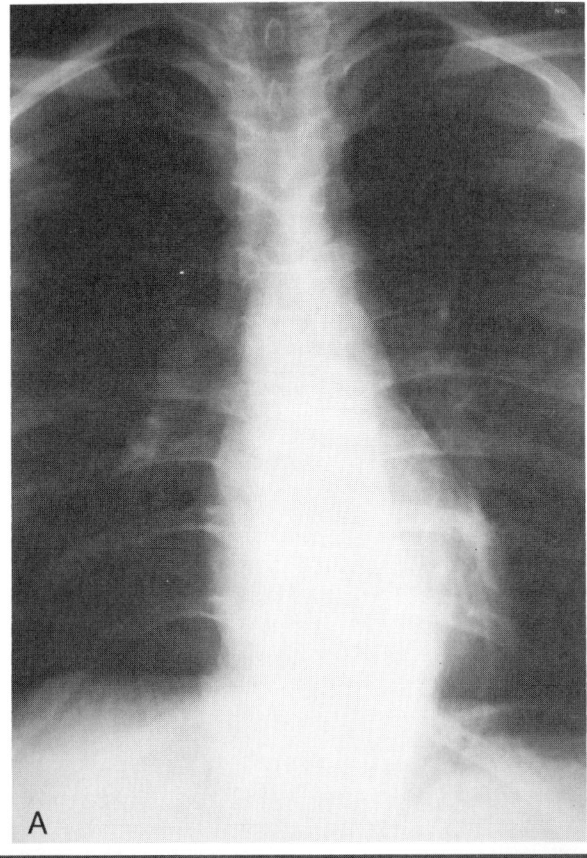

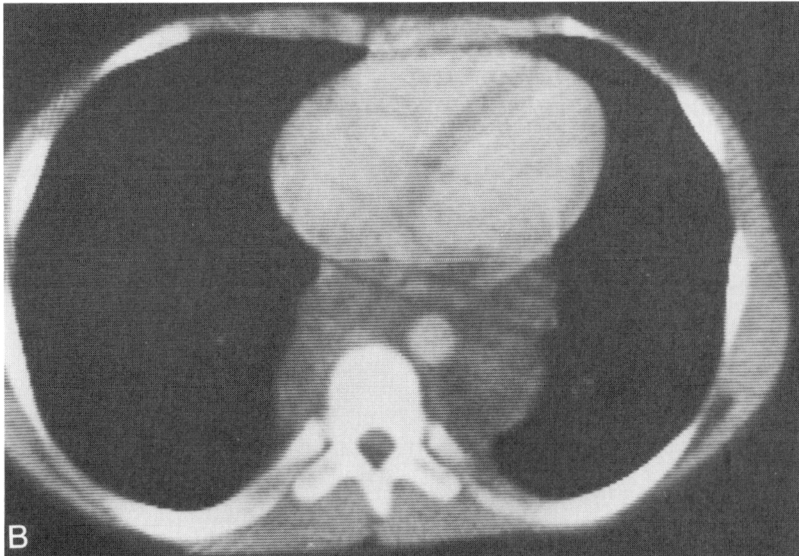

Figure 8–34. Traumatic thoracic duct laceration in a 14-year-old boy injured while playing football. Upright chest film *(A)* and computerized tomogram *(B)* demonstrate a loculated chylous effusion confined to the posterior mediastinum. *B,* The contrast-enhanced aorta is seen anterolateral to the vertebral body on the left. Density measurements of the chylous effusion indicated high fat content.

by blunt trauma to the anterior chest during vehicular accident and is a rare problem in children. Most injuries are located in the mainstem bronchi near the carina.[50] This injury is difficult to recognize radiographically, but the diagnosis should be considered with fractures of the upper three ribs, pneumomediastinum and pneumothorax that do not respond to aspiration or catheter drainage, and persistent subcutaneous emphysema.[44, 51] Later, atelectasis of the lung distal to the bronchial injury usually develops. On an upright view, the unsupported lung is demonstrated in the dependent inferomedial portion of the hemithorax rather than collapsing towards the hilum.[50]

Pulmonary Contusion

Pulmonary contusion or bruise of the lung is the most common radiographic finding in blunt chest trauma.[52] It usually presents as a nonsegmental patchy or homogeneous area of consolidation and is often located in the periphery of the lung (Fig. 8–35). This problem develops within 6 hours of injury. Differentiation from aspiration is not always possible. Resolution of pulmonary contusion is usually rapid and begins within 72 hours after injury, with complete clearing in 3 to 10 days.[44] Failure to show some resolution within 72 hours implies continued parenchymal bleeding or the development of associated pneumonia or atelectasis.[50]

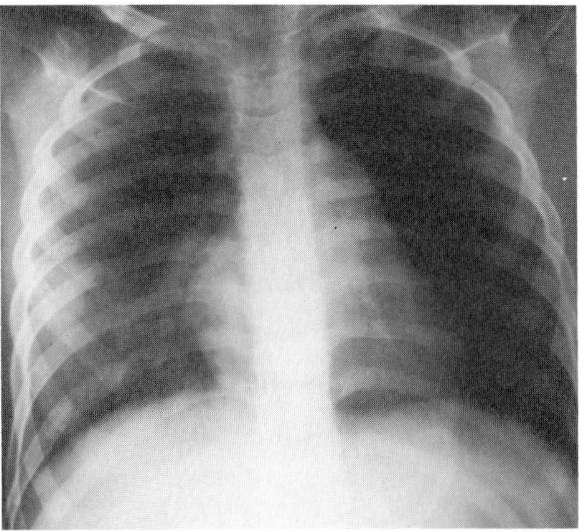

Figure 8–35. Pulmonary contusion in a 6-year-old boy following auto-pedestrian trauma. Mild to moderate parenchymal density is seen in the periphery of the right lung, typical of pulmonary contusion. Nondisplaced fractures of the right seventh and ninth ribs are also seen.

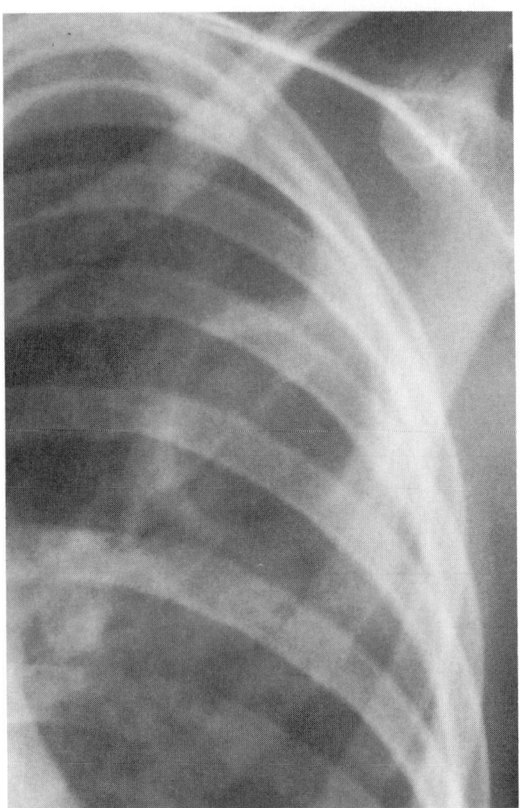

Figure 8–36. Pulmonary contusion and pulmonary laceration in the left upper lobe in a 5-year-old boy hit by a tractor. A close-up of the left upper lobe 3 days after injury demonstrates the pulmonary laceration as an area of radiolucency within the lung parenchyma (traumatic pneumatocele), surrounded by the changes of pulmonary contusion. No rib fractures are seen.

Pulmonary Laceration

Blunt or penetrating trauma to the chest may result in pulmonary laceration. Initially, only radiographic findings of lung contusion may be evident. With the clearing of the changes related to lung contusion, the laceration becomes visible as an area of radiolucency within the lung parenchyma, and this has been termed traumatic pneumatocele (Fig. 8–36). An air-fluid (blood) level may be present (Fig. 8–37). The traumatic pneumatocele may be single, multiple, unilocular, or multilocular and of variable size (Fig. 8–38). Typically they assume an elliptic, spheric, or lobular shape within the surrounding area of pulmonary contusion.[50, 53] The lesions usually decrease in size and completely resolve within several weeks.

Occasionally, the parenchymal defect from the pulmonary laceration fills with blood, resulting in a pulmonary hematoma. Hema-

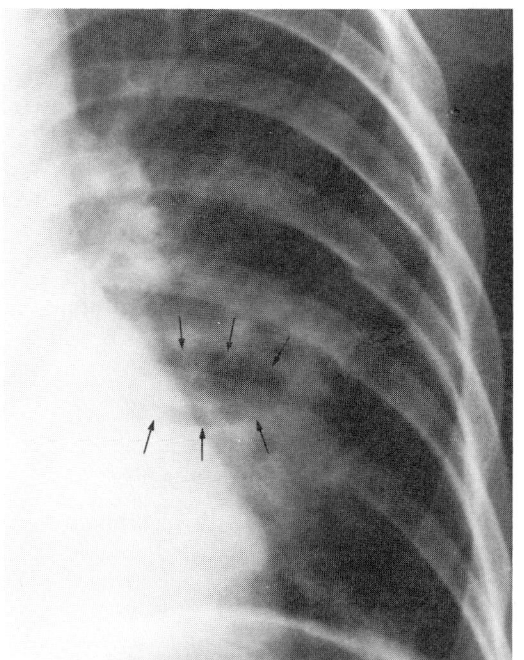

Figure 8–37. Pulmonary laceration in a 1½-year-old boy involved in an auto accident. A close-up of the left lung reveals fractures of the sixth to eighth ribs, with pulmonary laceration and contusion in the left lower lobe. Air-blood level is seen on this upright film.

tomas are generally well-defined, spindle-shaped, or spherical densities with sharp marginations. If blood is coughed up, the cystic nature of the pulmonary laceration becomes evident. The pulmonary hematoma

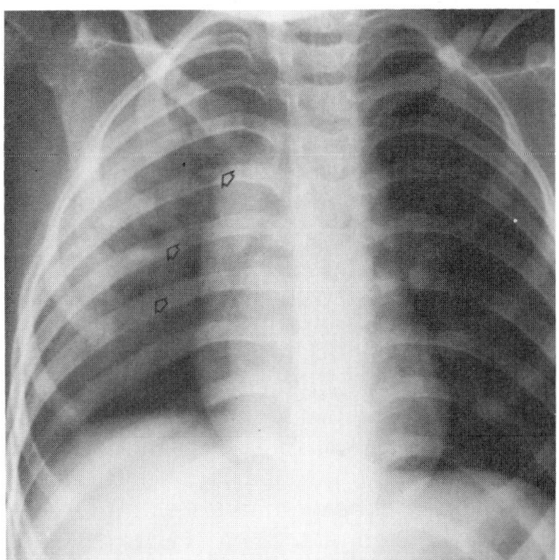

Figure 8–38. Pulmonary contusion with multiple pulmonary lacerations of the right lung in a 3-year-old boy thrown from a horse. Fractures of the right sixth to ninth ribs are present, with associated pulmonary contusion laterally and three areas of pulmonary laceration in the midportion of the lung *(arrows)*.

usually resolves in 5 weeks but may clear in as little as 3 weeks or as long as 1 year.[50]

Atelectasis

Post-traumatic atelectasis of a subsegment, segment, lobe, or entire lung may result from bleeding within pulmonary tissue; bronchial compression from peribronchial hemorrhage; and bronchial obstruction from blood clots, mucous plugs, or aspirated material.[50] These areas of atelectasis typically present as areas of increased density and may show displacement of a fissure and an air bronchogram. With major collapse, there may be a shift of the cardiovascular and mediastinal structures to the involved side and hyperinflation of the contralateral lung. When significant atelectasis persists, bronchoscopy may be necessary to evaluate the cause and exclude bronchial fracture.

MISCELLANEOUS

Esophageal Injury

Disruption of the intrathoracic esophagus may be produced by penetrating wounds or blunt trauma to the chest or abdomen. When the esophagus is damaged by blunt trauma, the location of the injury is largely determined by the site of impact. Trauma to the lower chest or upper abdomen may cause traumatic rupture of the distal esophagus. A crushing force to the upper thorax may lacerate the esophagus at this level. Radiographic findings of esophageal rupture include pneumomediastinum, interstitial emphysema in the neck, widened mediastinum, left lower lobe atelectasis, and left-sided pleural fluid. An esophagram with water soluble contrast material is necessary to show extravasation into the mediastinum and/or pleural space.[54]

Aortic Laceration and Rupture

Injury to the aorta and brachiocephalic vessels by blunt trauma is extremely rare in infants and young children but may be more common in teenagers. Arteriography should only be considered in the presence of widening of the superior mediastinum or right paratracheal stripe, displacement of the trachea or nasogastric tube to the right, apical pleural fluid, or an enlarged indistinct aortic knob.[41, 43, 55] Differentiation of the normally prominent thymus from widening of the upper mediastinum from hemorrhage is often impossible in infants and young children. As in adults, the most likely site of injury is at the junction of the mobile and fixed portions of the thoracic aorta near the ligamentum arteriosum, but injury to the proximal ascending aorta may also occur.

Diaphragmatic Injury

Diaphragmatic injuries may develop from penetrating wounds or blunt trauma to the lower thoracic and upper abdomen. In blunt trauma, it is most often the dome of the left hemidiaphragm that is injured.[56] The right diaphragm tends to be protected by the liver. The chest radiograph may show hemothorax; elevation of the hemidiaphragm; contralateral mediastinal shift; or herniation of the stomach, bowel, or mesentery into the chest.[57] Instillation of air into the stomach through a nasogastric tube will demonstrate if the stomach is herniated into the chest. A barium examination may be necessary to confirm herniated bowel into the chest, whereas a radionuclide examination can confirm herniated liver or spleen through a tear in the diaphragm.

ABDOMINAL AND GENITOURINARY TRAUMA

Abdominal and genitourinary trauma is common in children and is often present with multisystem injury. Although clinical evaluation is most important, radiographic investigation may be beneficial.

Plain film evaluation is a simple procedure but seldom provides definitive information. A supine film can demonstrate moderate intraperitoneal hemorrhage. Peritoneal fluid initially collects in the pelvis and paracolic gutters, and this may be apparent radiographically as increased density projecting over the pelvis or separating the ascending or descending colon from the properitoneal fat stripe. If perforation of the gastrointestinal (GI) tract is suspected, an upright film, which must include the hemidiaphragms; a cross-table lateral view,[58] or a left lateral (left side down) decubitus film is necessary to evaluate for pneumoperitoneum. Failure to visualize the psoas margins is of limited significance in young children. There is little retroperitoneal fat to demarcate these structures and overlying bowel gas further precludes visualization.

In recent years, intravenous (IV) urography, radionuclide scanning, ultrasonography, and angiography have been utilized to evaluate for suspected injury to specific organs. Often, however, clinical evaluation is nonspecific, and also multiple organs may be damaged. Computerized tomography (CT), therefore, is rapidly becoming more popular in the work-up of abdominal and genitourinary trauma.[4] This modality can comprehensively evaluate intra- and retroperitoneal structures.

Liver

Trauma to the liver from blunt or penetrating injury is associated with a high morbidity and mortality rate.[59] There is a broad spectrum of hepatic injuries, which includes subcapsular hematoma; parenchymal contusions; parenchymal and capsular lacerations; parenchymal rupture with hematoma formation; and vascular injuries that may result in laceration of vessels, arteriovenous fistulas or pseudoaneurysms.[60]

Plain film evaluation of liver injury is not reliable. Signs of bleeding into the peritoneal cavity may be present, with blood in the lateral flank separating the colon from the properitoneal fat line. Blood in the pelvis may be present as symmetric densities on either side of the bladder. Indirect signs suggesting the possibility of hepatic injury include fractures of the right lower ribs, elevation of the right hemidiaphragm, right pleural effusion, loss of the psoas and/or hepatic margin, and hepatic enlargement.[56, 59] Adynamic ileus may also be present. If the patient's condition is stable or can be stabilized, correct diagnosis of hepatic injury is dependent upon special radiographic investigation. The modality employed depends upon the expertise of the radiologist and equipment available and may include arteriography, radionuclide scan, or CT (Fig. 8–39). The last two modalities have the advantage of being noninvasive and usually can be performed in a short period of time. Angiography is more time-consuming, but can provide better delineation of vascular injury and aid the surgeon in segmental anatomy.

Spleen

The spleen is the most frequently injured organ in blunt abdominal trauma.[61] Conser-

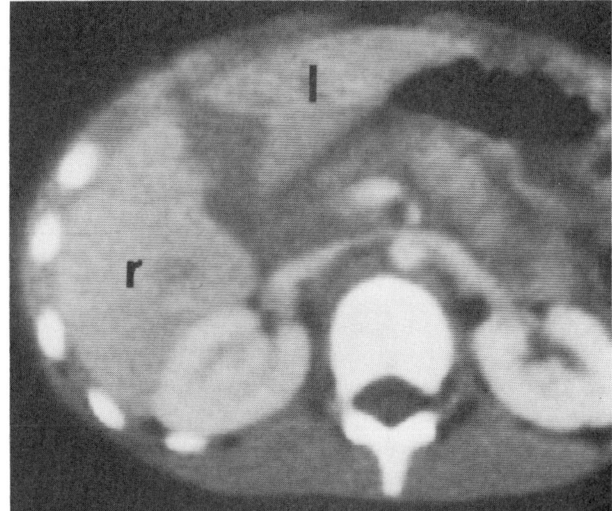

Figure 8–39. Laceration of the liver in a 9-year-old girl following auto-pedestrian trauma. Plain film of the abdomen was normal. Emergency computerized tomography demonstrates a laceration of the liver, with low density hematoma between the right (r) and left (l) lobes of the liver. The kidneys and retroperitoneum are normal. Additional scans demonstrated hematoma and edema adjacent to the head of the pancreas and mesentery. The spleen was normal. The lacerated liver was repaired and the hematoma was drained at operation.

vative management of splenic trauma, with total or partial preservation of the spleen, is now practiced in many institutions. Therefore, prompt and accurate evaluation of the degree of splenic injury is imperative. As with liver injury, plain film findings of splenic trauma are insensitive and inaccurate. Fractures of the left lower ribs, left pleural effusion, medial displacement of the stomach and/or left colon, obliterated psoas and peritoneal fat lines, and signs of peritoneal bleeding are occasionally present. The modality employed to recognize splenic injury is dependent upon available equipment and the expertise of the examining radiologist. Arteriography in the diagnosis of splenic injury has largely been replaced by radionuclide scanning which is both sensitive and accurate in the detection of significant splenic trauma.[62, 63]

The diagnosis of splenic laceration is based on the demonstration of a linear or wedge-shaped defect in splenic contour, whereas a subcapsular hematoma may be identified by a flattening of the normal splenic contour. Undoubtedly, CT will be employed more in the future to diagnose splenic injury because of its noninvasive nature, high degree of accuracy,[4, 64] and capability of simultaneously evaluating the other abdominal and retroperitoneal structures (Fig. 8–40).

Gastrointestinal Tract

The GI tract may be affected by blunt or penetrating trauma. The colon and stomach are much less frequently involved than the small bowel.

Trauma to the duodenum may result in perforation or intramural hematoma. The

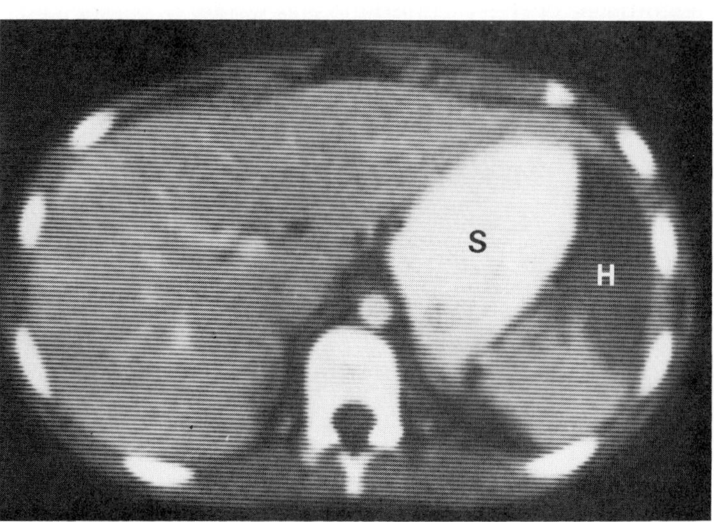

Figure 8–40. Splenic hematoma in a 12-year-old boy following abdominal trauma. Computerized tomography following intravenous injection of contrast medium clearly demonstrates the low-density hematoma (H) adjacent to the contrast-enhanced splenic parenchyma. The stomach (S) has been filled with contrast material by nasogastric tube. This scan also demonstrates normal appearance of the liver. The patient was managed conservatively and discharged 1 week after injury.

duodenal injury is seldom diagnosed during the initial evaluation of the traumatized child. Plain films are seldom diagnostic. Perforation is usually posteriorly directed into the retroperitoneum, and therefore, free intraperitoneal air is seldom seen. Retroperitoneal air around the right kidney and psoas muscle is infrequently demonstrated. A water-soluble contrast upper GI study will easily demonstrate the site of perforation.

Intramural duodenal hematoma is more common than duodenal perforation in children that have had blunt abdominal trauma. In this condition, plain films are of limited value but occasionally show gastric and proximal duodenal distention. Upper GI examination using a barium mixture will show an intramural mass, with thickened and distorted mucosal folds, and varying degrees of obstruction.

The jejunum and ileum may also be affected by trauma, with resultant perforation or intramural hematoma. The proximal jejunum is the most common site of perforation in children who have had blunt abdominal trauma. Pneumoperitoneum may be present, but small bowel perforation is certainly not excluded when free intraperitoneal air is not demonstrated.

Pancreas

Pancreatic injury is relatively common in children having abdominal trauma. This important injury is seldom diagnosed early. Plain film radiographic evaluation is seldom useful in the initial stages of assessment. Plain film changes are nonspecific although adjacent loops of bowel may be mildly dilated (localized ileus). CT may show edematous or hemorrhagic change. Ultrasound and CT are useful modalities in evaluating for the development of a post-traumatic pancreatic pseudocyst.

Kidney

Renal injury is rather common following blunt abdominal trauma. Varying degrees of renal contusion, renal laceration, and renal pedicle injury can occur. Renal injuries are more common in children with a previously unrecognized abnormality. Hydronephrosis is the most common predisposing problem.

Flank pain and hematuria clinically suggest renal injury; however, clinical examination, urinalysis, and findings on a plain abdominal radiograph do not allow one to reliably predict which patients will show urographic abnormalities. The degree of hematuria does not correlate well with the severity of renal injury, and major damage, especially that involving the renal pedicle, may be present in the absence of hematuria. It has been the traditional approach to investigate all patients with any signs and symptoms suggesting renal trauma with excretory urography. However, it has been our policy not to perform this procedure in clinically stable, asymptomatic patients with only minor hematuria. We have found, as have others,[65] that the findings on excretory urography rarely alter the clinical management of these patients. Excretory urography is best reserved for those children with persistent abdominal and/or flank pain or moderate to marked hematuria. IV urography is also recommended in patients undergoing exploratory laparotomy following trauma to exclude retroperitoneal injury and evaluate for possible pre-existing urinary tract abnormality, such as unilateral renal atresia.

IV urography has been the traditional radiographic method of investigating patients with suspected renal trauma. A satisfactory study in children consists of a scout film of the abdomen, and after a bolus injection of urographic contrast medium at a dose of 1 ml/lb, AP films are obtained at approximately 1 and 5 minutes after completion of the injection. Additional delayed or oblique views are occasionally useful. Infusion urography has received much publicity, but the slower injection is unnecessary and only results in needless prolongation of the procedure.

The radiographic findings are variable in renal contusion. The study is often normal in mild degrees of renal contusion. Diminished excretion of contrast medium with incomplete visualization of the collecting system often indicates more serious contusion (Fig. 8–41). Enlargement of the kidney is frequently demonstrated. Blood clots may be recognized as radiolucent filling defects within the renal collecting system and may cause ureteropelvic or ureterovesical obstruction with resultant proximal dilatation (Fig. 8–42).

Renal laceration may result in disruption of the pyelocalyceal system and cause extravasation of contrast material into the renal parenchyma and surrounding perirenal tissues (Fig. 8–43). Severe renal lacerations may be demonstrated as radiolucent fissures or separation of segments of functioning renal tissue (Fig. 8–44).

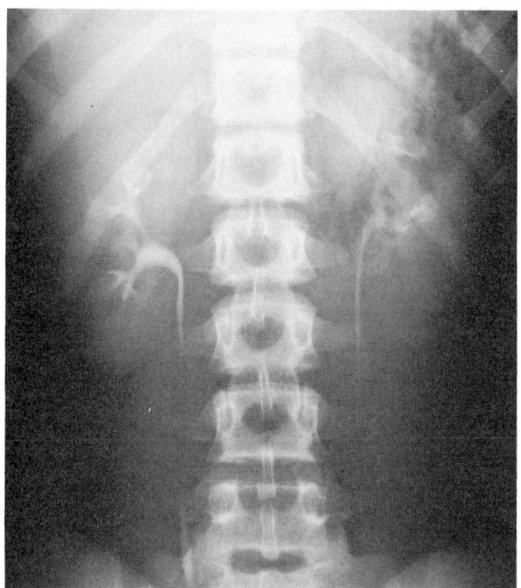

Figure 8–41. Renal contusion in a 12-year-old girl following abdominal trauma. An intravenous pyelogram (IVP) demonstrates mild enlargement of the left kidney, with diminished excretion in the lower pole region and distortion of the collecting system. The right kidney was normal. The patient was managed conservatively, and the follow-up IVP 3½ months later was normal.

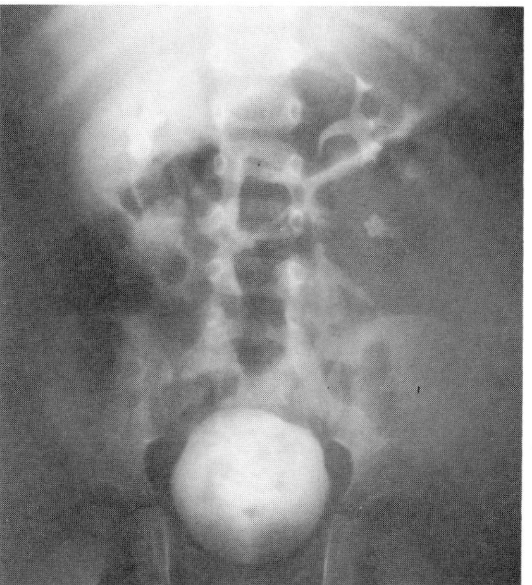

Figure 8–42. Renal contusion with transient ureteral obstruction from blood clots in a 2½-year-old boy who fell onto his right flank while playing. A short time later, his mother noted the passage of bright red blood and "clots" from his urethra. This IVP film at 30 minutes following injection of contrast medium demonstrates a prolonged nephrogram with mild caliectasis on the right. The left kidney is normal. The patient continued to pass clots per the urethra, and the 1-hour film was normal. The findings are believed to represent transient obstruction from the blood clots, which were dislodged by the hyperosmotic load of the contrast medium.

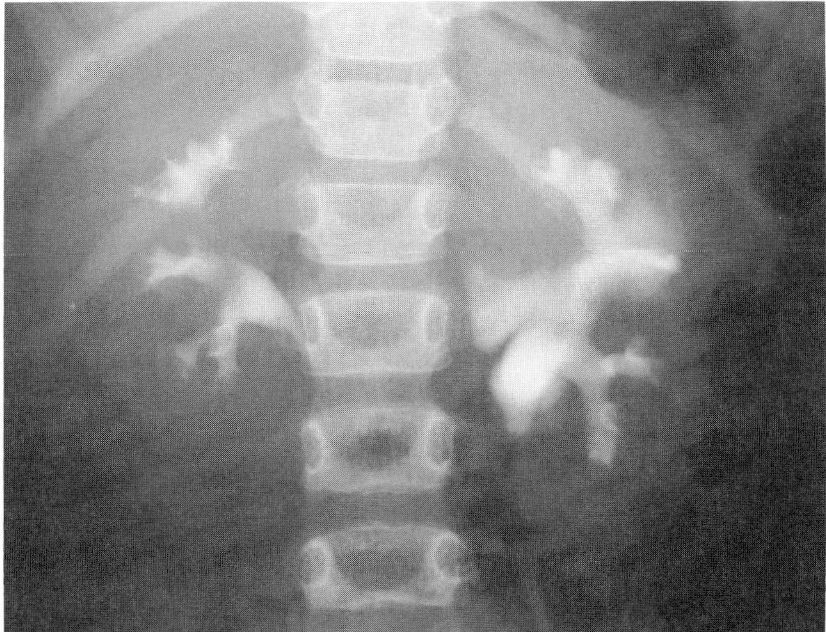

Figure 8–43. Renal laceration with disruption of the left pyelocalyceal system in a 5-year-old boy hit by an automobile. Urinalysis demonstrated moderate hematuria, and a plain film of the abdomen demonstrated fractures of the left tenth and eleventh ribs posteriorly. An IVP film 40 minutes after injection of contrast medium demonstrates mild enlargement of the left kidney, with extravasation of contrast medium around the renal pelvis, extending into the upper pole. The right kidney is normal.

The patient was managed conservatively. A follow-up IVP 3 months after injury demonstrated excellent renal function, with mild narrowing at the left ureteropelvic junction.

The major justification for IV urographic evaluation in trauma is to attempt to identify patients who have had injury to the renal artery. This injury is very uncommon in children. It is stressed that if the kidney is to be preserved, diagnosis of arterial occlusion must be made within a few hours of injury.[66] Unilateral nonvisualization on excretory urography suggests renal artery occlusion or disruption and is an indication for immediate arteriography (Fig. 8–45).[67] Before arteriography is performed, ultrasonography is suggested to exclude those rare patients with congenital absence of one kidney.

Occasionally following trauma, an excretory urogram will demonstrate a dense persistent bilateral nephrogram with incomplete visualization of the collecting systems. This

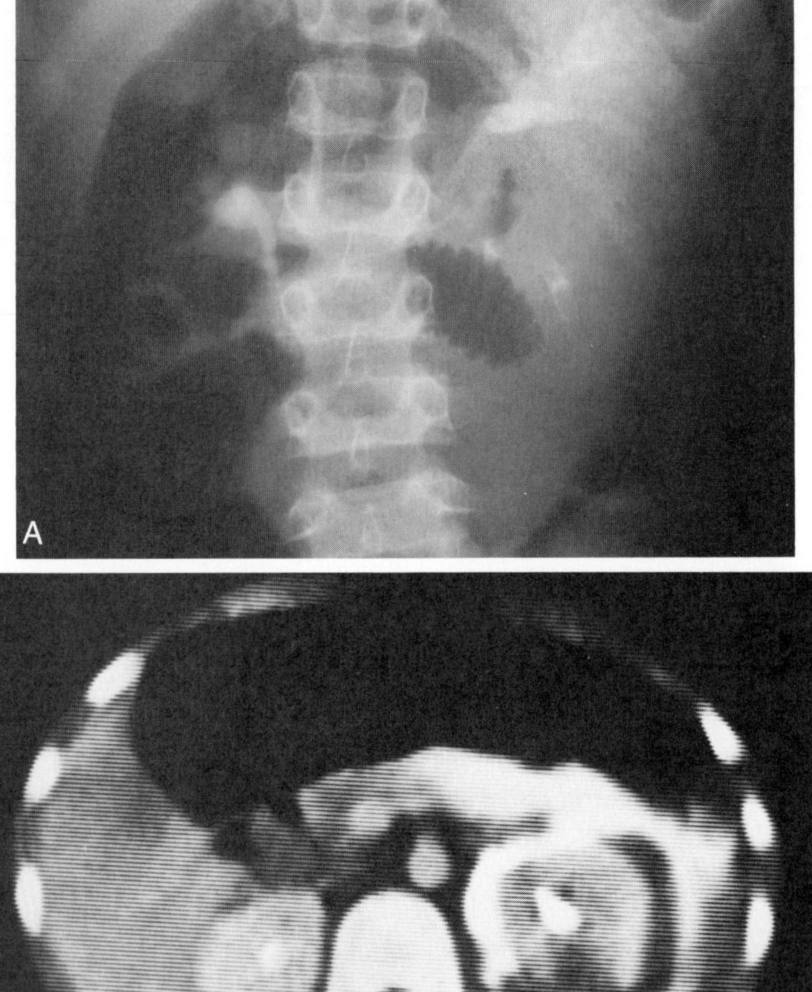

Figure 8–44. Severe renal laceration in a 9½-year-old boy who fell onto his left side while playing on the "monkey bars." *A*, IVP demonstrates on the 5-minute film bilateral excretion of contrast medium, with normal appearance of the right kidney and separation of the left kidney into functioning upper and lower pole segments. *B*, Computerized tomogram at the approximate level of L1 demonstrates extravasation of contrast medium into the anterior pararenal space and medially. Function of the upper pole fragment is seen with hematoma posteriorly. The upper pole of the right kidney is normal.

Illustration continued on opposite page

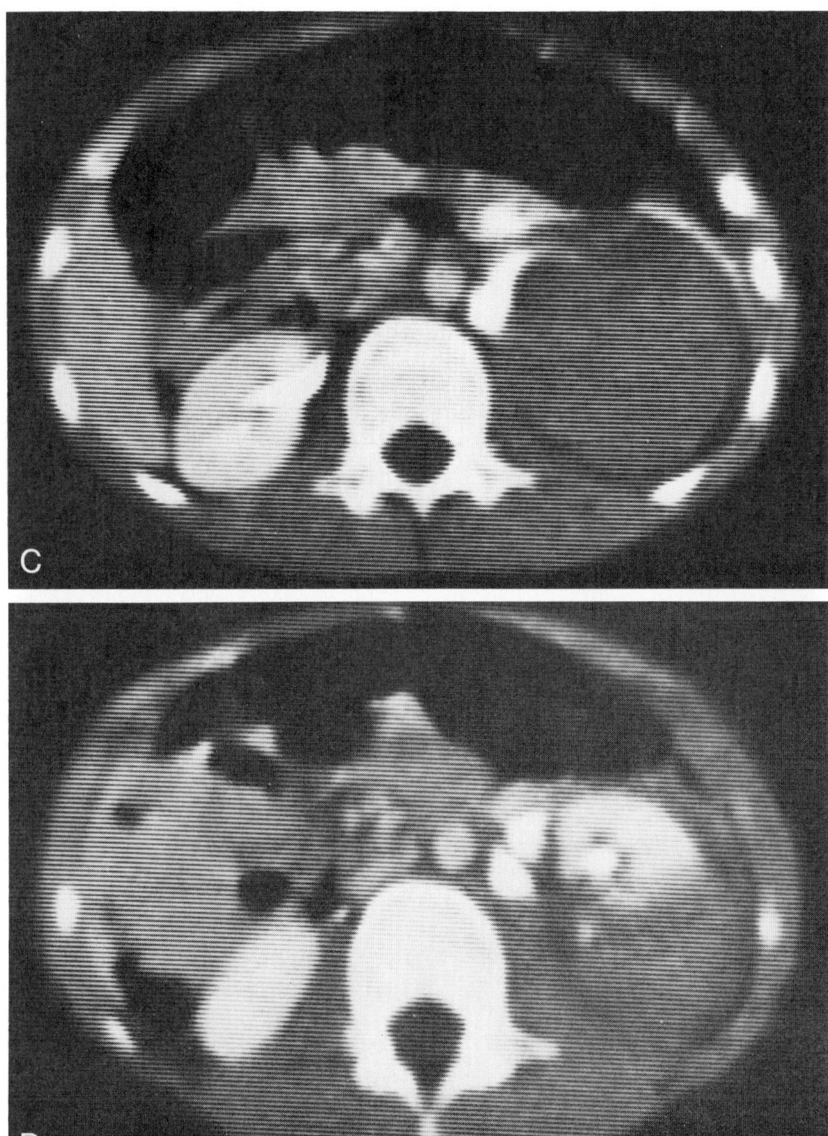

Figure 8–44 *Continued. C,* Computerized tomogram at the approximate level of L2 demonstrates that the large hematoma between the functioning upper and lower poles is confined to Gerota's fascia. Extravasated contrast medium is seen medial to the hematoma and lateral to the aorta. The mid portion of the right kidney is normal. *D,* Computerized tomogram at the approximate level of L3 demonstrates the functioning lower pole fragment and hematoma posteriorly and extravasated contrast medium medially. The lower pole of the right kidney is normal.

The patient remained stable, was managed conservatively, and was discharged 12 days after injury.

pattern suggests decreased renal perfusion secondary to hypotension, and following stabilization and correction of the pressures, the nephrogram clears and repeat studies, if performed, are usually normal.[68]

In the future, CT will be employed more for the evaluation of renal and abdominal trauma. Compared with excretory urography, CT not only provides better delineation of extensive renal damage (see Fig. 8–44) but also provides information concerning other abdominal organs and the retroperitoneum.[4]

Ureter

Ureteral injury in children secondary to blunt trauma is rare. Sudden hyperextension

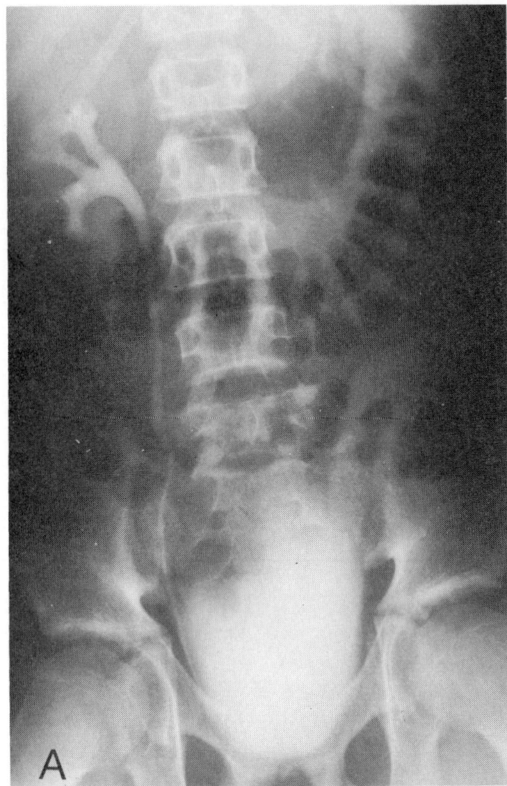

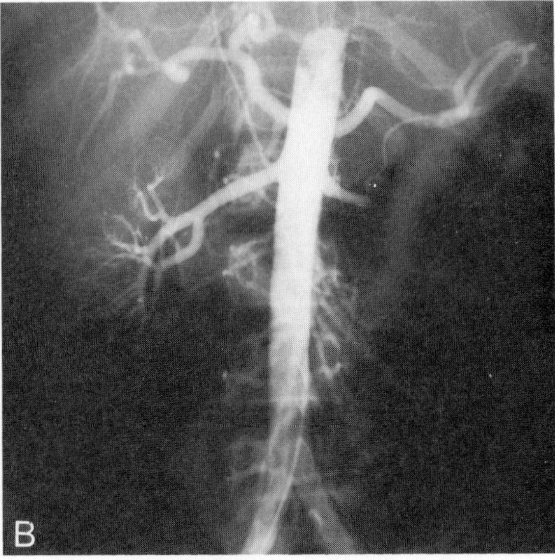

Figure 8–45. Traumatic left renal artery occlusion in a 13½-year-old boy involved in a motorcycle accident. *A,* After he developed left flank pain, an IVP performed in an outlying hospital demonstrates nonvisualization of the left kidney, an indication for an immediate arteriography. *B,* Following transfer, an emergency aortogram demonstrates occlusion of the mid left renal artery 2 cm distal to its origin. At operation, the kidney was infarcted and could not be salvaged.

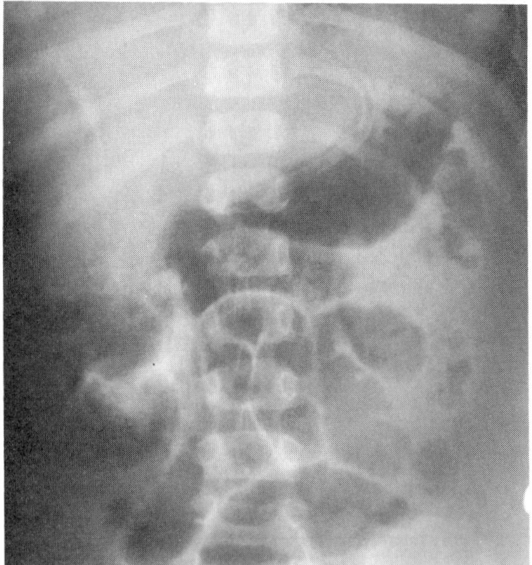

Figure 8–46. A 3½-year-old girl with laceration of the liver and avulsion of the right ureter at the ureteropelvic junction following trauma from an automobile accident. An IVP film 20 minutes after injection of contrast medium demonstrates extravasation around the lower pole of the right kidney. A linear collection of contrast medium in the right lobe of the liver indicates a parenchymal laceration. The patient was studied prior to the advent of computerized tomography, and arteriography was performed. This confirmed the laceration in the right lobe of the liver and normal appearance of the right kidney. At operation, a laceration of the right lobe of the liver was repaired. The ureter was found to be avulsed at the ureteropelvic junction and was repaired.

of the thoracolumbar spine associated with abrupt deceleration may cause disruption of the ureter at or near the ureteropelvic junction.[69] Extravasation of contrast material from the ureter may be seen on IV urography (Fig. 8–46). Other patients may show varying degrees of obstruction. Retrograde pyelography may be necessary for definitive study of ureteral injury.[70]

Bladder

Bladder injuries may result from blunt or penetrating trauma and are commonly associated with pelvic fractures.[71] The child with bladder trauma usually complains of lower abdominal pain and dysuria, may be unable to void, and may have hematuria of varying degree.[56] Plain abdominal radiographs typically show pelvic fractures and may demonstrate fluid in the peritoneal cavity. Excretory urography should be performed to evaluate renal function and cystography to evaluate the degree of bladder injury. Differentiation of intraperitoneal and extraperitoneal rupture can usually be made by cystography. Patients with bladder contusion and perivesical hematoma typically show elevation and deviation of the bladder out of the pelvis, with a

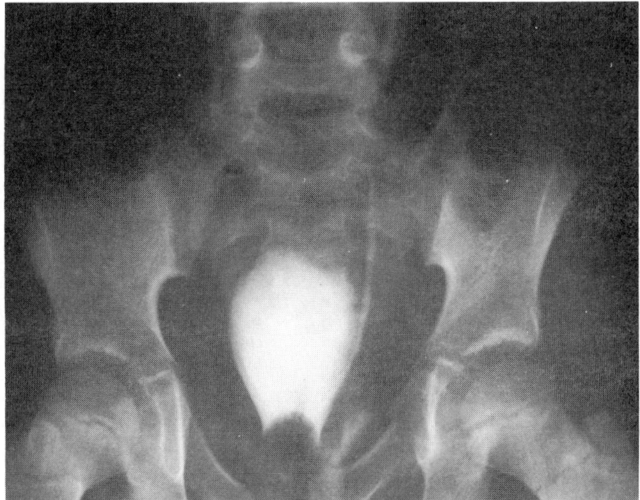

Figure 8–47. Perivesical hematoma in an 8½-year-old boy following auto-pedestrian trauma. This close-up film of the pelvic region on the 5-minute IVP film demonstrates fractures of the left inferior pubic ramus, left ischium, and left femoral neck. A perivesical hematoma is present, with the typical "teardrop" configuration to the bladder. Extravasation of contrast medium into the extraperitoneal tissues is seen also at the left base of the bladder.

"tear drop" configuration to the bladder (Fig. 8–47). Those with extraperitoneal and intraperitoneal rupture will show extravasation of contrast material outside the bladder, which may be confined to the pelvis or extend into the peritoneal cavity with intraperitoneal rupture (Fig. 8–48).[72]

Urethra

Urethral trauma, seen nearly exclusively in males, may occur secondary to a blow to the perineum or, more commonly, to a "straddle injury," such as falling astride the top of a fence. Incomplete tears are more common than total severance of the urethra.[73] The most common injury is disruption of the posterior urethra at the prostatomembranous junction.

Urethral injuries should be suspected in any child with pelvic fracture and inability to void. A drop of blood may be seen at the urethral meatus. It is critical that a retrograde urethrogram be performed before catheterization of the bladder is attempted (Fig. 8–49). This is best done with fluoroscopy. In this way, it is possible to recognize an incomplete tear with extravasation of contrast material, thus avoiding conversion to complete disruption during catheterization.[72] Evaluation of the bladder can then be carried out

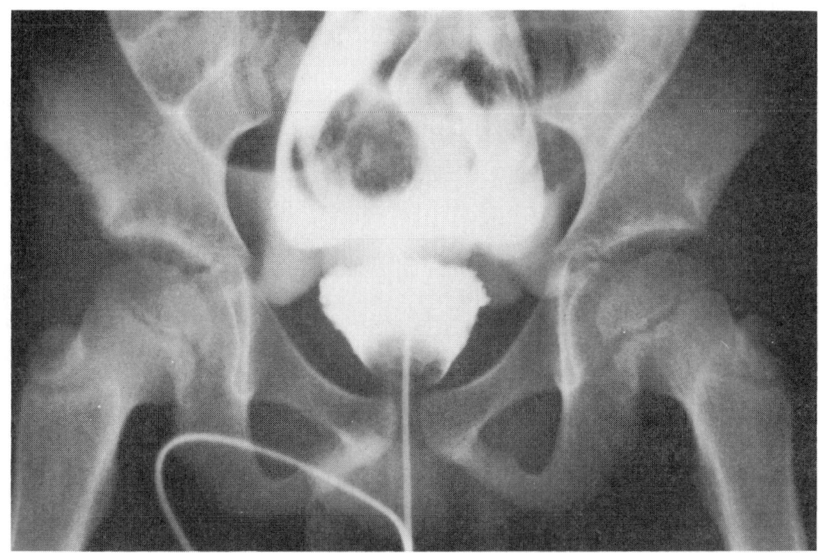

Figure 8–48. Intraperitoneal rupture of the bladder in a 7½-year-old boy who fell on a large rock. Computerized tomography of the abdomen revealed large amounts of intra-abdominal fluid. A cystogram demonstrates a small bladder, with extravasation of contrast medium into the peritoneal cavity filling the cul-de-sac and outlining loops of bowel.

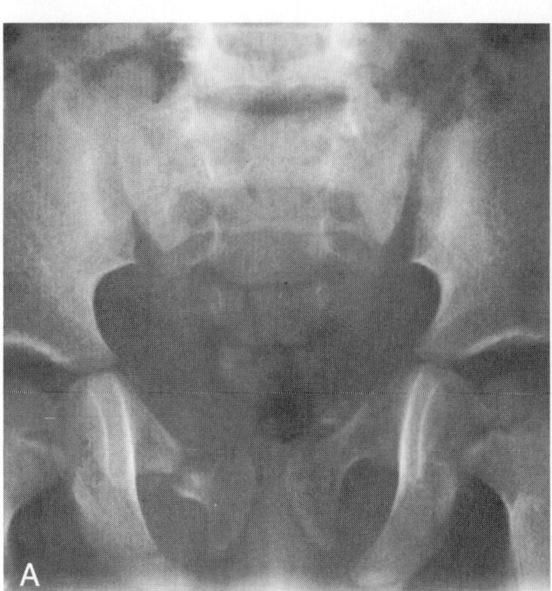

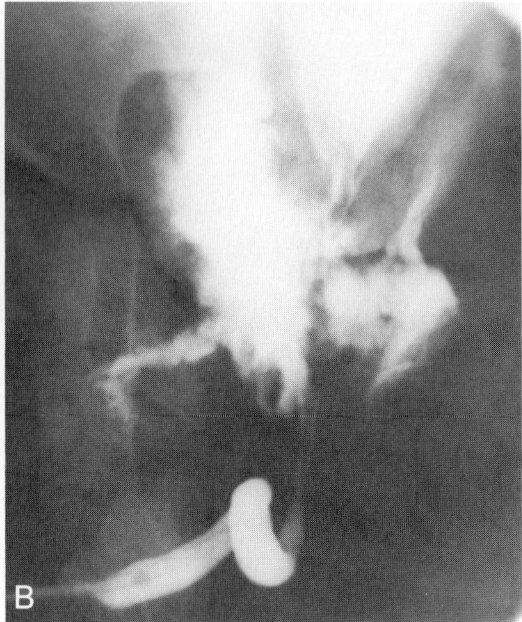

Figure 8–49. Partial disruption of the posterior urethra at the prostatomembranous junction in a 3-year-old boy run over by a slow-moving vehicle. *A*, Preliminary film of the pelvis demonstrates fractures of the right and left superior pubic rami. *B*, Retrograde urethrogram demonstrates an incomplete urethral tear, with extravasation of contrast medium at the prostatomembranous junction.

by excretory urography or cystography performed by suprapubic catheterization.[74]

BATTERED CHILD SYNDROME

Radiographic changes may confirm the diagnosis of the battered child syndrome in certain patients in whom this diagnosis is suspected or may lead to the diagnosis when an infant is being examined for a totally unrelated condition. Radiographic findings that reflect multiple episodes of trauma or specific types of trauma suggest that a child has been battered.

When the battered child syndrome is suspected, a skeletal survey examination is indicated. This consists of AP views of all of the long bones, hands and feet, pelvis, and ribs and lateral views of the spine and skull. A single total body film is not sufficient in this situation because the skeletal changes may be very minor and missed on a total body single film study, which would result in unnecessary magnification, distortion, and lack of detail. Also, films confined to areas in which there is physical evidence of trauma are unacceptable, since radiographic changes are commonly identified in areas in which there are no physical findings. Radionuclide bone scanning may be useful in the evaluation of this condition. CT scanning of the head is indicated if intracranial injury is suspected.[75]

Skeletal injuries are the most common radiographic abnormality in the battered child syndrome. Shaking or twisting type of trauma may result in unique radiographic findings.[9] The periosteum in infants is loosely attached along the diaphysis but firmly attached at the metaphyseal-growth plate junction area. Torsional forces cause avulsion of small metaphyseal fragments (Figs. 8–50 and 8–51). Metaphyseal corner fractures are virtually diagnostic of the battered child syndrome. This results in immediate radiographic evidence of trauma. In the ensuing days, subperiosteal new bone formation will develop along the metaphyseal and adjacent diaphyseal areas. The periosteal reaction may be very prominent. Its appearance may differ in various sites, which would suggest multiple episodes of trauma. Periosteal reaction may be seen as a single finding or in combination with metaphyseal avulsion fractures (Figs. 8–50 and 8–51). The metaphyseal fractures are most characteristic of the battered child syndrome, but all types of fractures can occur. Oblique, transverse, and Salter Type I and II fractures are not infrequent and occur when blunt or twisting trauma is inflicted. Multiple fractures in varying states of healing, a combination of subdural hematoma and a long bone fracture, or fractures of the posterior ribs in infancy are other radiographic findings that strongly suggest this diagnosis.

Other conditions are occasionally confused with the skeletal changes of the battered child syndrome. These include physiologic subperiosteal calcification, Menke's (kinky hair) syndrome, syphilis, birth trauma, and accidental trauma. Physiologic periosteal reaction is easily differentiated by its appearance. This is seen as a normal variant in infants, usually under 6 months of age, and is confined to the diaphyseal portions of the larger long bones,[76] whereas the periosteal reaction in the battered child is predominantly metaphyseal. Menkes' syndrome and syphilis should be excluded with careful physical examination and appropriate laboratory studies. Other forms of trauma can be excluded by history.

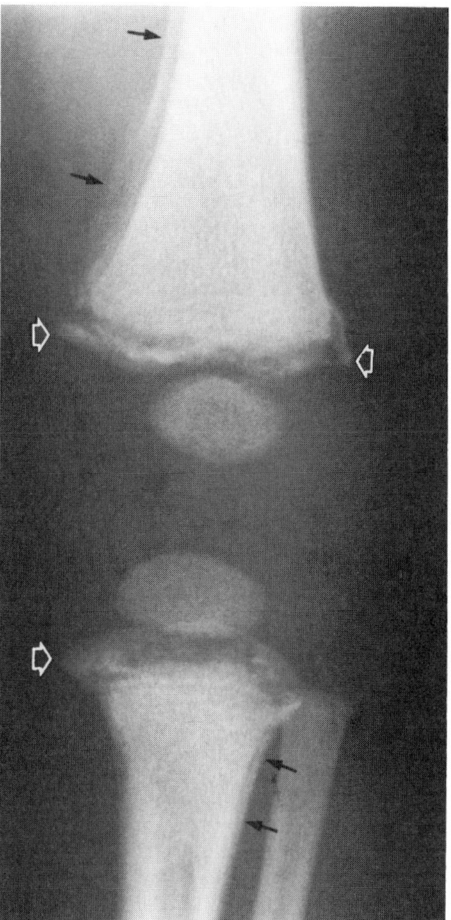

Figure 8–51. Multiple metaphyseal avulsion fractures are noted in the distal femur and proximal tibia. Periosteal reaction *(arrows)* is present in the metaphyseal portions of the distal femur and proximal tibia. This combination of findings is characteristic of the battered child syndrome.

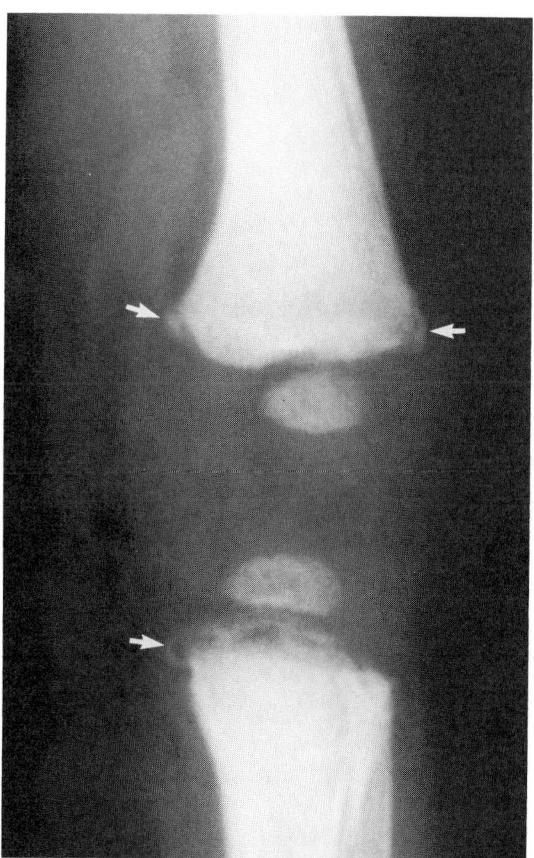

Figure 8–50. Typical bony changes of the battered child syndrome are demonstrated in this 2-month-old infant. Multiple metaphyseal corner fractures *(arrows)* are demonstrated in the distal femur and proximal tibia.

Absence of radiographic bone changes does not exclude child abuse. In fact, skeletal survey examinations are seldom abnormal in this condition in patients who are over 2 years of age. This is probably related to a combination of factors, which includes the fact that as the bony structures become larger and stronger, the periosteum becomes more firmly attached throughout the length of the bone, and also as the child grows, it becomes physically more difficult to inflict these same types of trauma.

Although long bone and craniocerebral trauma results in the majority of the radiographic changes in this condition, it should be noted that virtually all conceivable types of injury to the spine, chest, and abdomen have also been reported.

REFERENCES

1. Harris JH, Harris WH: The Radiology of Emergency Medicine. 2nd ed. Baltimore, Williams and Wilkins, 1976.
2. Handel SF, Lee Y: Computed tomography of spinal fractures. Radiol Clin North Am 19:69, 1981.
3. Mack LA, Harley JD, Winquist RA: CT of acetabular fractures; analysis of fracture patterns. AJR 138:407, 1982.
4. Kuhn JP, Berger PE: Computed tomography in the evaluation of blunt abdominal trauma in children. Radiol Clin North Am 19:503, 1981.
5. Darling DB: Radiography of Infants and Children. 3rd ed. Springfield, Charles C Thomas, 1979.
6. Poznanski AK: Practical Approaches to Pediatric Radiology. Chicago, Year Book Medical Publishers, 1976.
7. Homer, MJ: A radiologist's point of view. JAMA 246:2581, 1981.
8. Keats TE: An Atlas of Normal Roentgen Variants that May Simulate Disease. 2nd ed. Chicago, Year Book Medical Publishers, 1979.
9. Caffey J: Pediatric X-ray Diagnosis. 7 ed. Chicago, Year Book Medical Publishers, 1978, pp. 1335–1351.
10. McCauley RGK, Schwartz AM, Leonidas JC, et al.: Comparison views in extremity injury in children: An efficacy study. Radiology 131:95, 1979.
11. Nixon GW: The significance of joint fluid in children with elbow trauma. Presented at the American Roentgen Ray Society Meeting, San Francisco, 1981.
12. Borden S IV: Roentgen recognition of acute plastic bowing of the forearm in children. AJR 125:524, 1975.
13. Miller JH, Osterkamp JA: Scintigraphy in acute plastic bowing of the forearm. Radiology 142:742, 1982.
14. Rogers LF: The radiography of epiphyseal injuries. Radiology 96:289, 1970.
15. Salter RB, Harris WR: Injuries involving the epiphyseal plate. J Bone Joint Surg 45A:587, 1963.
16. Peiro A, Andres F, Fernandez-Esteve F: Acute Monteggia lesions in children. J Bone Joint Surg 59A:93, 1977.
17. Rogers LF, Malave S Jr, White H, et al.: Plastic bowing of torus and greenstick supracondylar fracture of the humerus: Radiographic clues to obscure fractures of the elbow in children. Radiology 128:145, 1978.
18. Chessare JW, Rogers LF, White H, et al.: Injuries of the medial epicondylar ossification center of the humerus. AJR 129:49, 1977.
19. Lee FA, Gwinn JL: Retrosternal dislocation of the clavicle. Radiology 110:631, 1974.
20. Reed MH: Coracoclavicular fracture separation—the pediatric equivalent of acromioclavicular separation. AJR 132:307, 1979.
21. Lusted LB, Keats TE: Atlas of Roentgenographic Measurement. 4th ed. Chicago, Year Book Medical Publishers, 1978, p. 193.
22. MacNealy GA, Rogers LF, Hernandez R, et al.: Injuries of the distal tibia epiphysis: Systemic radiographic evaluation. AJR 138:683, 1982.
23. Towbin R, Dunbar JS, Towlin J, et al.: Teardrop sign: Plain film recognition on ankle effusions. AJR 134:985, 1980.
24. Dunbar JS, Owen HF, Nogrady MB, et al.: Obscure tibial fracture of infants. The toddler's fracture. J Can Assoc Radiol 15:136, 1964.
25. Hall FM: Radiographic diagnosis and accuracy in knee joint effusions. Radiology 115:49, 1975.
26. Fernbach SK, Wilkinson RH: Avulsion injuries of the pelvis and proximal femur. AJR 137:581, 1981.
27. Brown I: A study of the "capsular" shadow in disorders of the hip in children. J Bone Joint Surg 57B:175, 1975.
28. Vines FS: The significance of "occult" fractures of the cervical spine. AJR 107:493, 1969.
29. Cattell HS, Filtzer DL: Pseudosubluxation and other normal variations in the cervical spine in children. J Bone Joint Surg. 47A:1295, 1965.
30. Swischuk LE: Anterior displacement of C2 in children: Physiologic or pathologic? Radiology 122:759, 1977.
31. Suss R, Adler D, Leeds NF, et al.: Pseudo-spread of the lateral masses of C1: A false sign of burst (Jefferson) fracture of C1 young children. Presented at the American Roentgen Ray Society Meeting, San Francisco, 1981.
32. Shapiro R, Youngberg AS, Rothman SLG: The differential diagnosis of traumatic lesions of the occipito-atlanto-axial segment. Radiol Clin North Am 11:505, 1973.
33. Fielding JW, Hawkins RJ: Atlanto-axial rotatory fixation (fixed rotatory subluxation of the atlanto-axial joint). J Bone Joint Surg 59A:37, 1977.
34. Leonidas JC, Ting W, Binkiewicz A, et al.: Mild head trauma in children: When is a roentgenogram necessary. Pediatrics 69:139, 1982.
35. Bell RS, Loop JW: The utility and futility of skull examination for trauma. N Engl J Med 284:236, 1971.
36. DeSmet AA, Fryback DG, Thornbury JR: A second look at the utility of radiography skull examination for trauma. AJR 132:95, 1979.
37. Harwood-Nash DC, Hendrick EB, Hudson AR: The significance of skull fractures in children; a study of 1,187 patients. Radiology 101:151, 1971.
38. Walker ML, Storrs BB: Personal communication, 1982.
39. Swischuk LE: The growing skull. Sem Roentgenol 9:115, 1974.
40. Waite DE: Pediatric fractures of jaw and facial bones. Pediatrics 51:551, 1973.
41. Fisher RG, Ward RE, Ben-Menachem Y: Arteriography and the fractured first rib: Too much for too little? AJR 138:1059, 1982.
42. Wilson JM, Thomas AN, Goodman PC, Lewis FR: Severe chest trauma: Morbidity implication. Arch Surg 113:846, 1978.
43. Woodring JH, Fried AM, Hatfield DR, et al.: Fractures of first and second ribs: Predictive value for arterial and bronchial injury. AJR 138:211, 1982.
44. Reynolds J, Davis JT: Injuries of the chest wall, pleura, pericardium, lungs, bronchi and esophagus. Radiol Clin North Am 4:383, 1966.
45. Moskowitz TS, Griscom NT: The medial pneumothorax. Radiology 120:143, 1976.
46. Riggs W, Tonkin ILD: Lingular collapse with medial pneumothorax: Puzzling image in children. AJR 137:919, 1981.
47. Ziter FMH Jr, Westcott JL: Supine subpulmonary pneumothorax. AJR 137:699, 1981.
48. Doubleday LC: Radiologic aspects of stab wounds of the heart. Radiology 74:26, 1960.

49. Ross JK: Review of surgery of the thoracic duct. Thorax 16:12, 1961.
50. Crawford WO Jr: Pulmonary injury in thoracic and non-thoracic trauma. Radiol Clin North Am 11:527, 1973.
51. Burke JF: Early diagnosis of traumatic rupture of the bronchus. JAMA 181:682, 1962.
52. Williams JR, Stembridge VA: Pulmonary contusions secondary to nonpenetrating chest trauma. AJR 91:284, 1964.
53. Fagan CJ, Swischuk LE: Traumatic lung and paramediastinal pneumatoceles. Radiology 120:11, 1976.
54. Goodman LR, Putman CE: The S.I.C.U. chest radiograph after massive blunt trauma. Radiol Clin North Am 19:111, 1981.
55. Woodring JH, Pulmano CM, Stevens RK: The right paratracheal stripe in blunt chest trauma. Radiology 143:605, 1982.
56. Stanley P, Gwinn JL: Urinary tract trauma: Diagnostic Imaging in Pediatric Trauma. New York, Springer-Verlag, 1980.
57. Hill LD: Injuries of the diaphragm following blunt trauma. Surg Clin North Am 52:611, 1972.
58. Seibert JJ, Parvey LS: The telltale triage: Use of the supine cross table lateral radiograph of the abdomen in early detection of pneumoperitoneum. Pediatr Radiol 5:209, 1977.
59. Franken EA, Jr, Smith JA: Roentgenographic evaluation of infant and childhood trauma. Pediatr Clin North Am 22:301, 1975.
60. DeFore WW, Mattox KL, Jordan GL, et al: Management of 1590 consecutive cases of liver trauma. Arch Surg 11:493, 1976.
61. Fitzgerald JB, Crawford ES, DeBakey ME: Surgical considerations of nonpenetrating abdominal injuries: An analysis of 200 cases. Am J Surg 100:22, 1960.
62. Gilday DL, Anderson PO: Scintigraphic evaluation of liver and spleen injury. Semin Nuclear Med 4:357, 1974.
63. Lutzkor L, Koenigsberg M, Meng CH, et al.: The role of radionuclide imaging in spleen trauma. Radiology 110:419, 1974.
64. Mall JC, Kaiser JA: CT diagnosis of splenic laceration. AJR 134:265, 1980.
65. McDonald EJ, Korobkin M, Jacobs RP, et al.: The role of emergency excretory urography in evaluation of blunt abdominal trauma. AJR 126:739, 1976.
66. Clarke DE, Georgitis JW, Ray FS: Renal arterial injuries caused by blunt trauma. Surgery 90:87, 1981.
67. Stables DP: Unilateral absence of excretion at urography after abdominal trauma. Radiology 121:609, 1976.
68. Korobkin MT, Kirkwood R, Minagi M: Nephrogram of hypotension. Radioilogy 98:129, 1971.
69. Richter MW, Lytton B, Myerson D, et al.: Radiology of genitourinary trauma. Radiol Clin North Am 11:593, 1973.
70. Carlton CE: Injuries to the ureter. Urol Clin North Am 4:33, 1977.
71. Montie J: Bladder injuries. Urol Clin North Am 4:59, 1977.
72. Sandler CM, Phillips JM, Harris JD, et al.: Radiology of the bladder and urethra in blunt pelvic trauma. Radiol Clin North Am. 19:195, 1981.
73. Garrett RA: Pediatric urethral and perineal injuries. Pediatr Clin North Am 22:401, 1975.
74. Corriere JN, Harris JD: The management of urologic injuries in blunt pelvic trauma. Radiol Clin North Am 19:187, 1981.
75. Zimmerman RA, Bilaniuk LT, Bruce D, et al.: Computed tomography of craniocerebral injury in the abused child. Radiology 130:687, 1979.
76. Shopfner CE: Periosteal bone growth in normal infants—a preliminary report. AJR 97:154, 1966.

SECTION

II Trauma to Children with Chronic Disease

CHAPTER

9 Injuries to Children with Chronic Cardiac Disease

GARTH ORSMOND

Congenital heart disease occurs in approximately 0.8 per cent of live births in the United States. About 40 to 50 per cent of children with congenital heart disease have severe enough problems to require cardiac surgery. There has been an increasing tendency to perform corrective surgery on children when they are very young. As a result many children will have already had their cardiac defect corrected by the end of the first year of life. Residual anatomic abnormalities and postsurgical myocardial dysfunction or arrhythmias may remain as long-term problems in some of these children. With other congenital lesions, early corrective surgery is not advisable or not necessary. In a few children only palliative surgery is possible. There are, therefore, a significant number of children with congenital heart disease who have chronic underlying cardiac problems that may require special management when the child is injured.

Acquired heart disease in children is less frequent than the congenital form. In many parts of the United States chronic rheumatic heart disease is becoming uncommon, but it remains a significant problem in underdeveloped countries and in certain population groups. Cardiac rhythm disturbances, cardiomyopathies, myocarditis, and hypertensive heart disease make up the remainder of the common acquired lesions seen in children.

A general understanding of the pathophysiologic abnormalities in children with chronic cardiac disease is necessary because these children may pose special management problems after major injuries. In addition, the trauma itself may adversely affect the cardiovascular system and add to the pre-existing abnormal circulatory function.

EFFECTS OF TRAUMA ON THE CARDIOVASCULAR SYSTEM

This section addresses only some of the important effects of local chest, central nervous system (CNS), and multiple organ system trauma on the cardiovascular system. These effects are particularly important in the child with an already compromised cardiovascular system. Furthermore, it may be difficult to separate the effects of the trauma on the cardiovascular system from the underlying cardiac problem itself.

Effects of Local Chest Trauma

Chest trauma can result in direct injury to the heart and great vessels.[1] When there is sharp tissue injury or laceration in the region of the heart, the possibility of cardiac or great vessel injury is readily apparent. With blunt, nonpenetrating, or crush injuries to the chest, the possibility of myocardial injury is often not considered and needs re-emphasis.

Major myocardial contusion, with consequent myocardial dysfunction, is probably more common with major blunt chest injuries than is generally realized. It has received little attention in the pediatric literature, probably because there is usually sufficient cardiac reserve to make up for any deficit caused by the injury. When there is chronic cardiac disease, this may not be the case, and the additional burden of myocardial contusion may be life-threatening unless it is recognized and its effects considered in overall patient management. Other important cardiac effects from closed trauma include hemopericardium and, in the recovery phases after chest trauma, post-traumatic pericarditis syndrome.

After sustaining a major chest injury, the patient should have a careful cardiac examination, chest x-ray, electrocardiogram (EKG), and myocardial enzyme determination. Specifically, the MB fraction of creatinine phosphokinase, or CPK, should be measured, since this is a good indicator of major myocardial damage.[2] In addition, two-dimensional echocardiography is very valuable in the diagnosis of pericardial fluid and may also allow for recognition of ventricular wall motion abnormalities or assessment of overall myocardial function. Clinical evidence of cardiac failure; electrocardiographic evidence of myocardial ischemia, such as S-T segment depression and T-wave changes; elevation of the MB fraction of CPK or abnormal radionuclide scanning suggest major myocardial contusion.[1]

In the management of patients with such disorders, a central venous or pulmonary artery wedge pressure line should be inserted early because it is helpful in determining the safe amount and rate of volume replacement that can be tolerated. In addition, inotropic drugs, such as digoxin and sympathomimetics (e.g., dopamine), may be necessary if there is significantly decreased myocardial function and hypotension, particularly after adequate fluid replacement. If the myocardial contusion is extensive, as judged by clinical, electrocardiographic, serum enzyme, and echocardiographic changes, then prolonged bed rest to decrease cardiac work is advisable, and the patient may need to be treated like an adult with a myocardial infarction. Careful ECG monitoring and treatment of arrhythmias may be necessary in the occasional patient.

Hemopericardium with tamponade is an obvious consequence of puncture wounds of the heart, but it may also occur after blunt chest trauma and in such circumstances, may not be easily recognized. When there is preexisting myocardial dysfunction or when there is a decrease in circulating blood volume, a moderate-sized effusion can have major effects, producing hypotension and decreased cardiac output. In patients with chest injuries in whom unexplained cardiomegaly or hypotension persists after local injuries and blood loss have been attended to, the possibility of a pericardial effusion should be considered. Echocardiography is diagnostic. The usual signs of cardiac tamponade—hypotension, elevated jugular venous pressure, hepatomegaly, muffled heart sounds, and pulsus paradoxus—can be masked by other underlying injuries. Persistent hypotension and shock may be the only findings. Early pericardiocentesis may be necessary if the relative effects of a moderate-sized effusion are uncertain. When there is a large effusion, urgent pericardiocentesis and thoracic surgery consultation is necessary.

In the recovery phase, often several weeks after chest trauma, post-traumatic pericarditis may occur.[3] It is characterized by fever, pericardial type chest pain, a pericardial rub, cardiomegaly, and, rarely, tamponade. Usually the disease is self-limited, but it may require treatment with anti-inflammatory drugs, such as aspirin, indomethacin, or steroids.

Effects of Central Nervous System Trauma

Head injuries, with their consequent cerebral contusion or intracranial hemorrhage, can have major effects on the cardiovascular system. These effects include (1) sinus bradycardia and hypertension secondary to raised intracranial pressure, (2) marked sinus tachycardia, (3) atrial or ventricular arrhythmias,[4] (4) electrocardiographic abnormalities,[5] (5) peripheral vasoconstriction, and (6) neurogenic pulmonary edema. The secondary cardiovascular effects can be very confusing, since they are often attributed to primary cardiac problems, particularly in the child with chronic cardiac disease. They are one of the more frequent reasons that a cardiologist is consulted in cases of major trauma.

Sinus bradycardia and hypertension are well-known effects suggesting increased intracranial pressure. Their significance is addressed elsewhere. Sinus bradycardia may sometimes be secondary to disturbed parasympathetic control of the heart secondary to head injury without there being raised intracranial pressure. On the other hand, if the child has had previous atrial surgery, e.g., the intra-atrial baffle operation for transposition, sinus node dysfunction may already exist and previous EKGs may be useful in detecting this. The presence of previous hypertension secondary to renal disease or coarctation should be easy to exclude by reviewing the patient's history or clinical notes.

Other arrhythmias may occur after head injury, and they are not infrequent.[4] Sinus tachycardia, with rates as high as 180 to 220 beats per minute, may persist even after volume replacement and control of pain and temperature. The mechanism is presumably excessive sympathetic nerve stimulation. Occasionally, digoxin is needed to slow the heart rate, but usually no treatment is necessary. Atrial arrhythmias (ectopic beats, fibrillation, flutter, or supraventricular tachycardia), ventricular arrhythmias (ectopic beats, ventricular tachycardia, or fibrillation), and abnormalities in atrioventricular conduction may all occur after major head trauma, particularly if there is subdural or epidural hemorrhage. These arrhythmias may require cardioversion or drug treatment.

Electrocardiographic changes seen with head injuries include S-T segment displacement, T-wave flattening and inversion, and other abnormalities that may mimic myocardial contusion or infarction. The mechanism of production is not understood, but the ECG changes are not secondary to raised intracranial pressure.

A less common but very important problem seen after head injury is the development of neurogenic pulmonary edema. The onset of pulmonary edema, particularly when there has not been excessive fluid administration, can be particularly confusing in the patient who already has underlying heart disease. In patients with major head injury, the possibility that the pulmonary edema may be neurogenic in origin must always be considered. It is thought that major shifts in peripheral blood result from abrupt increases in sympathetic activity, with fluid overload of the heart and the development of pulmonary edema.[6] Usually this is self-limiting, but it may add to the underlying respiratory distress and oxygenation problems and may require intermittent positive pressure ventilation with positive end-expiratory pressure and, occasionally, diuretic administration.

Effects of Hemorrhage and Hemorrhagic Shock

The management of hemorrhage and hemorrhagic shock is dealt with in detail in Chapter 1. Only the facets of the problem that pertain to the cardiovascular system are outlined here.

Major blood loss or volume depletion has significant effects on myocardial function as a result of the following mechanisms:

Decreased Preload. Inadequate circulating blood volume with inadequate filling pressure results in a decrease in preload, with a decrease in ventricular end-diastolic volume. Stroke volume decreases (Starling's law of the heart). Tachycardia may compensate for the decreased stroke volume and preserve normal cardiac output. When the patient has underlying cardiac disease, the adverse effects of reduced preload may be much greater than in a normal patient.

Peripheral Vasoconstriction or Increased Afterload. Peripheral vasoconstriction or increased afterload occurs in an attempt to reduce the total vascular bed in order to maintain adequate filling pressure or preload. Vasoconstriction is often selective—involving skin, muscle, and splanchnic bed—with cerebral and coronary blood flow being preserved. Although the increased peripheral resistance is an important compensatory mechanism in maintaining adequate venous return in the face of hypovolemia, the increased peripheral resistance or afterload can be deleterious if there is already decreased myocardial function or major left-sided valvular disease, such as aortic or mitral insufficiency. Adequate restoration of blood volume is necessary in these patients, and some of them may require administration of inotropic drugs to maintain adequate cardiac output. In a few selected patients, the peripheral resistance may need to be decreased by vasodilator drugs such as nitroprusside.

Decreased Contractility. Many factors serve to decrease cardiac function in hemorrhagic shock. The decreased preload and increased afterload have been mentioned previously. In addition, there may be a decrease in contractility or heart muscle function secondary to acidosis, electrolyte imbalance, and hypocalcemia (which may occur especially after massive blood replacement). More controversial, but generally accepted, is the experimental evidence that decreased splanchnic blood flow secondary to selective vasoconstriction and hypovolemia can result in cellular damage with release of lysosome hydrolase and other substances. Lysosome hydrolase may act on endogenous protein fragments, producing small protein fractions that depress myocardial function (myocardial depressant factor).[7] In septic and hemorrhagic shock, particularly when the latter does not respond rapidly to control of hemorrhage and volume replacement, it may be advisable to administer high-dose steroids (20 to 30 mg/kg of methylprednisolone) early in the disease because steroids can act as a cell membrane stabilizer, decreasing cell breakdown and production of lysosome hydrolase and myocardial depressant factor.[8] Digoxin and other inotropic drugs may be needed in patients with hemorrhagic shock who show clinical or echocardiographic evidence of myocardial dysfunction, with persistent hypotension and low cardiac output.

In addition, it is important to realize that hemorrhage results in loss of hemoglobin and, therefore, oxygen-carrying capacity. This is of particular importance in the child with cyanotic congenital heart disease and is discussed in the following section.

CARDIAC PATHOPHYSIOLOGIC ABNORMALITIES AFFECTING MAJOR TRAUMA

Children with congenital or acquired heart disease can have many different anatomic or functional abnormalities. A detailed description of each lesion is not possible or necessary in this book, but it is advisable for anyone managing such a child to consider the basic functional problems associated with any particular lesion and review them if necessary in a standard pediatric cardiology text or discuss them with a cardiologist. This section emphasizes the general pathophysiologic problems that need to be considered in a child with cardiac disease who has suffered major trauma. A brief overview of cellular oxygen supply and demand is provided, followed by discussion of the various pathophysiologic problems seen in patients.

Tissue Oxygen Supply and Demand

Individual cell survival, in the absence of direct cell injury, is dependent on cellular oxygen demands being met. Certain cell areas, e.g., the splanchnic bed, skin, and muscle, are less crucial for immediate survival, but they nevertheless must have adequate oxygen to meet their needs or they will be irreversibly damaged. Irreversible shock is the state in which cell death has occurred. In the management of any patient in shock, it is essential to try to increase tissue oxygen supply while reducing oxygen demands.

For the body as a whole, *tissue oxygen supply* is determined by (1) cardiac output, which is dependent on heart rate and stroke volume; (2) arterial oxygen content and the oxygen-hemoglobin dissociation curve; and (3) distribution of blood flow. *Oxygen demand or oxygen consumption* is determined by (1) temperature; (2) physical activity; (3) needs of individual organs to maintain vital functions; and (4) stress caused by sepsis, trauma, or healing.

It is important in any form of shock to consider the balance between oxygen supply and demand. In many patients, replacing blood volume or making minor adjustments in oxygenation or pressor medication may supply adequate oxygen to the tissues. In other patients, even on maximum therapy, adequate oxygen cannot be supplied. However, the patients can be kept alive until their overall state improves through reduction of total oxygen demands by controlling temperature, decreasing physical activity, taking over ventilation with artificial ventilation, and treating sepsis.

Altered Oxygen-Carrying Capacity and Oxygen Content in Cyanotic Congenital Heart Disease

Arterial oxygen content is a function of (1) hemoglobin (Hb) (2) oxygen-hemoglobin dissociation curve, and (3) arterial Po_2 and consequent oxygen saturation. Our general concept of thinking of oxygenation in terms of arterial Po_2 needs to be replaced by the concept that oxygenation depends upon arterial oxygen content and blood flow. Arterial oxygen content (ml of O_2/dl of blood) = Hb g/dl $\times$ 1.36 (each g Hb can hold 1.36 cc O_2) $\times$ O_2 saturation + 0.003 $\times$ Po_2 mm HG (dissolved O_2). Dissolved oxygen can be ignored at normal arterial Po_2 (70 to 100 mm Hg), but its contribution increases as the arterial Po_2 becomes higher.

The normal arterial oxygen content is approximately 15 to 20 ml of oxygen/dl blood. For example, at a hemoglobin concentration of 12 to 15 g/dl (which would be usual in children), an arterial Po_2 of 75 mm Hg, and an arterial oxygen saturation, with a normal oxygen-hemoglobin dissociation curve of about 95 per cent, the arterial oxygen content is equal to hemoglobin concentrations or: (12 to 15.5 mg/dl) × 1.36 × 0.95 (arterial O_2 saturation) = 15.5 to 19.4 ml O_2/dl blood. In infants, the arterial oxygen content may be lower because of the physiologic anemia that occurs during the 3- to 9-month stage.

In uncorrected cyanotic congenital heart disease, there is an intracardiac right-to-left shunt. Even after palliative surgery, such as a systemic-pulmonary shunt (e.g., Blalock-Taussig shunt for tetralogy of Fallot), there is still a large intracardiac right-to-left shunt. The arterial Po_2 in children with cyanotic congenital heart disease generally ranges from 35 mm Hg to 50 mm Hg. At a Po_2 of 35 mm Hg, only about 65 to 70 per cent of hemoglobin is saturated. At a Po_2 of 50 mm Hg, nearly 80 to 85 per cent of hemoglobin is saturated with oxygen. For the child to maintain an adequate arterial oxygen content, there has to be an increase in either the oxygen-carrying capacity, i.e., hemoglobin concentration, or a major increase in the cardiac output. It is almost always the hemoglobin concentration that increases. For example, if the arterial Po_2 is 40 mm Hg and the oxygen saturation is approximately 75 per cent, a hemoglobin concentration of 17.6 g/dl is required to achieve an arterial oxygen content of 18 ml of O_2/dl blood. In a child with cyanotic congenital heart disease, providing that there is no iron deficiency, the hemoglobin concentration increases to the level necessary to satisfy the general oxygen requirements of the body without a major increase in the cardiac index. The best way to determine the hemoglobin concentration that needs to be achieved in a child who has suffered major blood loss is to review his pre-existing hemoglobin level (provided that there has not been prior iron deficiency). It is essential that blood (often packed cells) replacement is continued until an adequate hemoglobin concentration is achieved. Once the hemoglobin reaches levels of 19 to 20 g/dl, tissue oxygen delivery may start to decrease because of increasing viscosity.

In patients with cyanotic congenital heart disease, it is usually the rule that an increase in inspired oxygen concentration does little to increase the arterial Po_2, arterial oxygen saturation, and oxygen content because there is an obligatory intracardiac right-to-left shunt.[9] However, this is not always true. Especially when there is co-existing lung disease produced either by lung trauma, ventilatory problems, pneumonia, or lung diffusion defects as seen with a shock lung, there may be an additional intrapulmonary right-to-left shunt with a further reduction in arterial oxygen saturation and content. Increasing the inspired oxygen concentration or improving ventilation with intermittent positive pressure ventilation, often with the addition of positive end-expiratory pressure, may improve ventilation and oxygen diffusion and increase the arterial Po_2. Even minor increases in the arterial Po_2 can be critical when a child has cyanotic congenital heart disease. For instance, an increase in the arterial Po_2 from 30 to 40 mm Hg generally results in an increase of oxygen saturation from about 55 to 75 per cent, and at a hemoglobin concentration of 17 g/dl (which would be common in cyanotic congenital heart disease), the increase in oxygen content would be 4.6 ml of oxygen/dl blood or 36 per cent. Thus, in any patient with critical oxygenation, even if it is thought unlikely that the Po_2 would change with increasing Fi_{O_2}, high Fi_{O_2} and possibly ventilator assistance should always be tried because there may be unexpected increases in arterial Po_2 and saturation.

Cardiac Lesions Requiring Increased Preload or Increased Atrial Filling Pressure

In terms of basic muscle physiology, preload is the degree of stretch or tension induced by a load on an individual muscle fiber, which results in a particular degree of contraction of that fiber. In terms of the whole ventricle, preload is generally thought of as being the ventricular end-diastolic volume, which is related to ventricular end-diastolic pressure. For practical purposes, ventricular end-diastolic pressure is usually measured in terms of right atrial pressure for the right ventricle and left atrial or pulmonary wedge pressure for the left ventricle. With certain cardiac lesions, increased filling pressure or preload may be required to achieve adequate cardiac output. Even the normal heart responds to increased preload by increasing contractility and ejection fraction and, therefore, stroke volume and cardiac output. In the abnormal heart, increased preload may be necessary to provide even normal cardiac output. Hypovolemia from blood or fluid loss results in decreased venous return and decreased preload. Peripheral vasoconstriction may compensate for the hypovolemia and maintain adequate filling pressure, or the body may be unable to compensate and stroke volume may be reduced and the only mechanism of maintaining or increasing cardiac output may be an increase in heart rate.

Left and right ventricular filling pressures, or preload, need to be considered independently even though in some conditions similar problems may affect both ventricles. In addition to ventricular muscle problems requiring increasing preload for effective function, atrioventricular valve stenosis may require an increased atrial pressure in order to develop sufficient ventricular end-diastolic pressure to maintain normal cardiac output.

Right ventricular preload is best assessed by central venous or right atrial pressure. Increased right ventricular wall thickness (hypertrophy) results in a decrease of right ventricular compliance so that increased preload is required to achieve normal cardiac contraction and stroke volume.[10] Examples of lesions with marked right ventricular hypertrophy include moderately severe or severe pulmonary stenosis and pulmonary hypertension. In these lesions, ventricular contractility is well preserved, and, provided adequate preload is present, ejection fraction and stroke volume will be normal.

Tricuspid stenosis presents a more complicated problem. Isolated tricuspid stenosis is rare in children and usually occurs as part of the hypoplastic right heart syndrome, consisting of pulmonary valve atresia and a small but thick-walled right ventricle. Currently, patients with this condition are treated in the immediate neonatal period by a pulmonary valvotomy, often with associated systemic-pulmonary shunt. Ventricular size may grow with time, but these patients usually have a markedly thickened noncompliant ventricle and associated tricuspid valve stenosis or hypoplasia. They may require both an increased atrial pressure to provide a pressure head to get blood across the stenotic tricuspid valve as well as an increase in the right ventricular end-diastolic pressure or preload in order to achieve any reasonable right ventricular stroke volume. It is important in any right-sided obstructive lesion, with either right ventricular hypertrophy or tricuspid valve stenosis, to realize that right atrial or central venous pressure may need to be maintained well above the normal range of 0 to 5 mm Hg. In fact, it may need to be as high as 15 to 20 mm Hg to maintain a normal cardiac index.

Another example of tricuspid obstruction is tricuspid atresia. Here there is no forward flow across the tricuspid valve, and in the uncorrected state, an atrial septal defect is necessary for survival. If the atrial septal defect is in any way restricted, high right atrial pressures will be necessary to get systemic venous return into the left heart. A systemic pulmonary shunt will usually have been performed in early infancy to provide pulmonary blood flow. At present, the mode of treatment of patients in middle childhood with this condition is to join the right atrium, either directly or by means of a valved conduit, onto the pulmonary artery (Fontan operation). The right atrium functions as the chamber, providing pulmonary blood flow, and very high right atrial or central venous pressure is necessary to generate adequate pulmonary blood flow, i.e., a right atrial pressure being in the region of 15 to 20 mm Hg. Even then, resting cardiac index is below normal in these patients, and adequate filling pressure is essential to their survival.[11]

Left ventricular preload is usually assessed by pulmonary artery wedge pressure, since direct measurement of left atrial or left ventricular end-diastolic pressure is usually not possible. When there is left ventricular hypertrophy secondary to either left-sided obstructive lesions, such as aortic stenosis or coarctation, or occasionally secondary to long-standing hypertension, then the hypertrophied left ventricle is less compliant than normal and requires greater than normal preload or atrial pressure to achieve a normal stroke volume.[10] Systolic contraction is usually normal, and the ejection fraction may even be increased. Patients with marked left ventricular hypertrophy often require a higher than normal left atrial or pulmonary wedge pressure to maintain adequate cardiac output.

When there is major myocardial dysfunction, such as occurs with cardiomyopathy, previous myocarditis, or sometimes after cardiac surgery, the end-diastolic volume in the left ventricle may be significantly increased and the ejection fraction low. A high left ventricular end-diastolic volume is necessary to maintain normal stroke volume (the stroke volume increases with increasing preload or end-diastolic pressure even in the abnormal heart). In patients with this condition, excess fluid administration may not be as well tolerated as it is in patients with ventricular hypertrophy and no systolic ventricular dysfunction. Pulmonary edema may ensue if excessive volume is administered too rapidly. The measurement of pulmonary wedge pressure may be important in the management of these patients.[12]

Mitral stenosis is an uncommon lesion in children. It too requires high atrial pressures, not because there are problems with ventricular compliance but because there is a need for a pressure gradient across the mitral valve to maintain adequate ventricular filling pressure or preload. Volume replacement in these patients has to be carried out very cautiously, and measurement of pulmonary wedge pressure is again helpful in the safer management of these patients in order to prevent pulmonary edema.

It is often difficult to achieve a balance between the preload necessary to achieve adequate cardiac output and excessive preload, which can exceed colloid osmotic pressure and result in right-sided or left-sided congestion. Right-sided congestion is less of a problem, since the hepatic congestion and peripheral edema do not have major deleterious effects in the immediate resuscitation period. Left-sided, or pulmonary, congestion results in pulmonary edema, with increasing respiratory distress and hypoxia. In any patient with left-sided disease requiring increased preload for effective myocardial function, caution must be used in volume administration. However, this does not mean that an adequate circulating volume is not necessary. Insertion of a Swan-Ganz catheter and measurement of pulmonary wedge pressure and occasionally the use of a thermodilution catheter, which allows measurement of cardiac output as well as pulmonary artery pressure and wedge pressure, should be considered in these patients. In addition, drugs that increase contractility may be necessary to temporarily improve cardiac function until a more stable state is reached.

Cardiac Lesions Sensitive to Increased Afterload

Peripheral and splanchnic vasoconstriction, with an increase in the total peripheral resistance, is a natural compensatory mechanism that attempts to maintain adequate venous return in hypovolemia. Most patients with cardiac disease will tolerate significant increases in peripheral resistance without deleterious effects. Certain patients will be adversely affected. For example, if there is severe mitral or aortic regurgitation, the regurgitation will increase with increased afterload. Of lesser importance, if there is a left-to-right shunt, it will also increase if systemic resistance increases without a corresponding increase in pulmonary resistance. In the occasional patient with markedly decreased myocardial function, increased afterload or systemic resistance is not tolerated, and there is a drop in cardiac index.

In general, it is unnecessary to do something about the peripheral vasoconstriction that occurs in the injured patient with hypovolemia. Once adequate circulating blood volume is restored and the cardiac output consequently increases, the peripheral resistance will fall. Rarely, a vicious cycle is set up because the elevated peripheral resistance decreases cardiac output, which results in the continuation of the peripheral vasoconstriction. Blood pressure in some patients with this condition may be normal or above normal, and once adequate preload is established, there will be a few patients in whom peripheral resistance requires reduction. Ideally, thermodilution measurement of cardiac output and measurement of blood pressure should be done to allow calculation of total peripheral resistance. If it is markedly elevated and if adequate preload has been assured, then cautious vasodilation with drugs like nitroprusside may actually improve cardiac output with improved stroke volume in the face of decreasing afterload.[13] There are also occasional patients with CNS disease who have markedly elevated peripheral resistance related to altered sympathetic activity. It is rarely necessary to treat these patients with vasodilators, but again the occasional need for it may occur, and it is always important to consider the role afterload is playing in the patient's problems.

Lesions Associated With Markedly Decreased Contractility

Cardiac lesions associated with markedly decreased myocardial function or contractility are uncommon in children. Examples of such lesions include cardiomyopathies and postmyocarditis myocardial dysfunction. Patients with such lesions may have a dilated heart and are functioning with a high end-diastolic volume and high end diastolic pressure as a means of maintaining adequate stroke volume. Their ejection fraction may be low and their ability to compensate for blood loss by increasing stroke volume may be minimal. The heart usually responds to stress by tachycardia, which on its own may not be sufficient to supply adequate cardiac output.

Most of these patients require higher than normal filling pressures to generate better myocardial contraction and maintain a normal stroke volume. Therefore, adequate preload should be supplied, and it is usually necessary to think of this in terms of the left ventricle, which is the dominant functioning ventricle, since isolated right ventricular myocardial dysfunction secondary to myocardial damage is unusual. The measurement of pulmonary wedge pressure is useful in deciding the amount of fluid that can be given without the patient developing pulmonary edema.

The early administration of inotropic agents such as digoxin, which unfortunately takes many hours to have maximal effect, and sympathomimetics, such as dopamine or dobutamine, is necessary in these children when they are critically injured and require an increase in myocardial function.[14, 15] In the occasional patient, the increase in afterload imposed by peripheral vasoconstriction may be counterproductive to overall blood supply, and the use of peripheral vasodilators such as nitroprusside may be necessary once the filling pressure or preload of the ventricle is adequate and when methods of increasing myocardial function with inotropic agents have not been sufficient.[13] Once peripheral vasodilators have been used, there is usually an additional need for volume replacement because of the expanded total vascular bed. Careful regulation of the peripheral vasodilator, circulating blood volume, and contractility is necessary in some of these patients to insure survival.

Lesions Associated With Altered Blood Flow Distribution—The Problem of Coarctation of the Aorta

Coarctation of the aorta is a frequent lesion in children. Although it has usually been corrected by the time the child is 4- to 5-years old, there may be residual coarctation after surgery or, in younger children, the coarctation may not yet have been repaired. In such patients, the pathophysiology is such that there is an increase in blood pressure in the upper extremities, which maintains adequate perfusion pressure particularly to the kidneys and to the lower extremities. Careful attention may need to be paid to maintaining a higher blood pressure in the upper extremities in order to maintain adequate renal perfusion. A systolic blood pressure of 130 to 150 mm Hg in the upper extremities in a patient with coarctation is not unusual. It is important to follow lower limb blood pressures and urine output and to try to maintain systolic blood pressures of 70 to 100 mm Hg in the lower extremities together with adequate urine output and renal function before considering the patient out of shock.

Disturbances of Cardiac Rate and Rhythm

Tachyarrhythmias and bradyarrhythmias may occur in the patient who has had trauma to the CNS. They may also occur when there has been direct myocardial injury. Furthermore, tachycardia occurs as a compensatory mechanism in an attempt to maintain adequate cardiac output when stroke volume is reduced because of inadequate preload secondary to hypovolemia. In certain lesions, the rapid heart rate may not allow time for ventricular filling and may, in fact, be counterproductive, e.g., mitral stenosis. In some patients, previous rhythm abnormalities may be aggravated by the trauma, and they present as an arrhythmia during resuscitation.

Supraventricular tachycardias may require electrical cardioversion followed by administration of either digoxin (Lanoxin) or propranolol. Intravenous (IV) verapamil is also effective in breaking a supraventricular tachycardia. Digoxin would be a preferred long-term medication, since it increases myocardial function, in contrast to propranolol, which may decrease myocardial function and, in addition, interferes with sympathetic reflexes that are protective in hypovolemic shock.

Ventricular arrhythmias are uncommon in children, but they may occur in the postoperative child with tetralogy of Fallot and may also be seen in patients with other postsurgical lesions. They may occasionally occur after localized chest or CNS trauma or even in the presence of an otherwise normal heart. Although occasional ventricular ectopic beats can be tolerated if they do not interfere with myocardial function or cardiac output, the presence of ventricular tachycardia is an emergency and should be treated by electrical cardioversion or IV lidocaine in doses of 1 mg/kg given slowly over 2 to 3 minutes.

Bradyarrhythmias may be very important in the presence of major blood loss, since they interfere with the compensatory sinus tachycardia necessary to maintain adequate cardiac output when decreased circulating blood volume decreases stroke volume. Most patients in shock should have a sinus tachycardia. The presence of bradycardia should be a clue of either major CNS problems such as raised intracranial pressure or problems of sinus node function or atrioventricular conduction. Atrioventricular block can easily be distinguished from sinus bradycardia by the EKG. If there is sinus bradycardia present, then the underlying cause, such as increased intracranial pressure, should be treated. If this is not possible, then certain drugs such as atropine or isoproterenol may be useful in the emergency situation. If atrioventricular block is present, then it is uncommon for atropine to significantly increase the heart rate. Isoproterenol may be more effective but may not make a dramatic difference when there is already maximum sympathetic stimulation secondary to trauma. In patients with complete atrioventricular block or even second-degree block with significant bradycardia, it may be necessary to insert a temporary pacemaker in order to establish more rapid ventricular pacing and maintain higher cardiac output when there is decreased stroke volume. Such circumstances may arise in patients with congenital or acquired post-surgical heart block who suffer major trauma and blood loss.

Pathophysiologic Changes Induced by Cardiac Drugs

The common drugs used in children with chronic cardiac disease include digoxin; diuretics, such as furosemide; antiarrhythmic agents, such as propranolol, quinidine and procainamide; and antihypertensive drugs, such as hydralazine, alpha-methyldopa, and minoxidil. If a patient is on these drugs, then their effects should be considered when the child is injured.

In the case of digoxin, continued administration of the drug is probably advantageous unless there is a major decrease in renal function or hypokalemia, which would result in digoxin toxicity. The effects of long-term propranolol administration may be more important, since it is a beta-blocker and may significantly interfere with the normal sympathetic response to major trauma or blood loss. The effects of propranolol can be overcome with a beta-receptor stimulator, such as isoproterenol. Other antiarrhythmic drugs, such as quinidine and procainamide, may result in significant myocardial depression, and unless the child has been suffering from a major life-threatening arrhythmia, their use should be stopped until cardiovascular homeostasis is established. Similarly the antihypertensive drugs may result in a block of the normal reflex response to hypovolemia, and they should be discontinued until adequate blood pressure is obtained with adequate cardiac output and renal perfusion. Occasionally, it may be necessary to overcome the peripheral vasodilator effects of some antihypertensive drugs by administering epinephrine or other peripheral vasoconstrictors until adequate blood pressure and circulating blood volume have been established. The long-term use of diuretics is not that frequent in children, but they may be administered in those with chronic congestive heart failure. Those diuretics that produce potassium loss of a major degree, such as furosemide, should always be administered with simultaneous daily potassium supplementation. However, it is possible that marked hypokalemia may occur with chronic administration, and careful attention should be given to electrolyte balance, particularly serum potassium levels.

APPROACH TO THE INJURED CHILD WITH UNEXPLAINED HEART MURMUR

Heart murmurs are frequent in childhood, being present in as many as 50 to 60 per cent of healthy children. The majority of these are innocent murmurs, being either an innocent systolic murmur of childhood ("vibratory" systolic murmur or Still's murmur), a pulmonic flow murmur, a venous hum, or a carotid bruit. Combinations of these may occur in some children. In the case of the venous hum, a characteristic continuous murmur is heard in the upper right sternal border, and it should disappear with compression of the right side of the neck or with turning the neck to the left side. The murmur should also decrease significantly when the child lies down. It should not be confused with the murmur of a patent ductus arteriosus because it has a different location and because of the various changes that result from the maneuvers outlined previously.

The other three common murmurs in children are all systolic ejection murmurs and are usually less than Grade 3 intensity. These murmurs may be accentuated by tachycardia, fever, or increased cardiac output. However, they can generally be distinguished from murmurs of aortic or pulmonary stenosis by their lack of an ejection click, the presence of a normal second heart sound, and the intensity, radiation, length and character of the murmur. If there is any doubt, then a cardiologist should be consulted to determine if this is an innocent or pathologic murmur. When the murmurs have any of the following characteristics, they are clearly pathologic and early consultation is advised: a holosystolic murmur, which indicates regurgitation through an atrioventricular valve or ventricular septal defect; an ejection murmur greater than Grade 3, i.e., associated with a thrill, which usually indicates significant aortic or pulmonic stenosis; a murmur associated with an ejection click or abnormality of the second heart sound; a late systolic murmur, which indicates mitral valve prolapse; any diastolic murmur; continuous murmur other than the venous hum. In addition, it is obvious that any patient who has major cardiomegaly, diminished heart sounds, or evidence of right- or left-sided heart failure should be regarded as having major cardiac problems regardless of the type of murmur.

PREVENTION OF BACTERIAL ENDOCARDITIS

Bacterial endocarditis is rare in children, but it may occur with acquired valvular or congenital heart defects. However, when there is uncontrolled septicemia, endocarditis may occur with a normal heart. The result can be major residual sequelae, with increased valvular dysfunction or death.

No controlled trial exists that shows that antibacterial prophylaxis prevents bacterial endocarditis. However, bacteremia occurs frequently after dental work, oropharyngeal surgery, urinary tract instrumentation, and gastrointestinal surgery. Bacterial endocarditis is more frequent after these procedures, and the organisms involved in the endocarditis correspond to those expected in the particular area. Antibiotic prophylaxis against bacterial endocarditis is, therefore, advised in patients with acquired valvular or congenital heart defects who are undergoing elective surgery, and the therapeutic regimens are outlined in a report by the American Heart Association.[16]

The use of prophylactic antibiotics after trauma is questionable unless the trauma involves extensive injuries with contamination or there is major abdominal, genitourinary, or gastrointestinal trauma.[17] With major open head injuries, antibiotics are also often advised. In each of these, the antibiotic is given more because of the underlying contamination, with expectation that actual infection has or will occur. The indication for the antibiotic and the length of administration is determined by the extent and the site of the trauma.[17] Thus, with major contaminated wounds, the common organisms involved are *Staphylococcus aureus,* Group A *Streptococcus,* and *Clostridium.* Antibiotic coverage usually includes a penicillinase-resistant penicillin and penicillin G, the latter being used because it is more effective against *Clostridium.* With abdominal, intestinal, and genitourinary trauma, the major organisms involved are enteric gram-negative bacilli, anaerobic bacteria, and Group D streptococci. Most frequently, parenteral antibiotics will be used in these patients, and either a cephalosporin or ampicillin with gentamycin is advised. The length of administration again depends upon the degree of organ damage or contamination. If major viscus rupture occurs, then occasionally clindamycin is added to the therapy. In the case of contaminated open wounds of the CNS, the combination of a penicillinase-resistant penicillin such as nafcillin and aqueous penicillin G or ampicillin is also advisable because the common organisms are *S. aureus,* Group A streptococci, and *Clostridium.*

With all injuries, careful cleaning of the wound is essential as is follow-up examination to exclude secondary infection. The role of antibiotic prophylaxis in many situations is controversial, and at present, it is advisable to follow the commonly accepted indications for the use of antibiotics when there is major contaminated trauma, instrumentation of the genitourinary system, or surgery on the oropharyngeal area.[16, 17] It seems unlikely that controlled trials will ever clarify this issue because of ethical and practical problems concerned in the patient who has underlying acquired valvular or congenital heart disease. Although the risks of endocarditis with bacteremia in these situations is probably low, it is generally agreed that antibiotic administration is advisable.

SUMMARY

Trauma may pose additional hazards to the child with chronic cardiac disease. There may be local or general effects on the cardiovascular system from the trauma itself, or the underlying cardiovascular abnormalities may require special attention during management of major or minor trauma. In the case of minor trauma, the main decision that needs to be made is whether antibiotic administration is necessary to prevent bacterial endocarditis. The choice of antibiotic is generally dictated by the local risks for infection and the risks of bacteremia, which depend upon the type of trauma and the site of infection. In some cases, additional instrumentation, like urinary catheters, may be needed during the management of the child, and this needs to be considered in antibiotic prophylaxis.

When there is major trauma, it is important to consider the effect of the underlying anatomic and pathophysiologic cardiac abnormality in the child. Control of bleeding and blood volume replacement is necessary in all children if they have suffered major blood loss. In the case of children with cyanotic congenital heart disease, it is important to replace adequate hemoglobin to compensate for the lowered oxygen content secondary to the intracardiac right-to-left shunt. In other cardiac patients, attention needs to be paid both to supply of oxygen to the tissues as well as to oxygen demands. A physiologic approach involving consideration of heart rate and control of arrhythmias; attention to the factors affecting stroke volume such as preload, afterload, and contractility; and consideration of the distribution of blood flow is essential. In addition to increasing the supply of oxygen and blood to the tissues, attempts should be made to reduce the overall oxygen consumption or oxygen demand by controlling temperature, unnecessary physical activity, respiration, and infection.

Chronic cardiac drug therapy may prove disadvantageous during major trauma. This is particularly the case with beta-blocking agents or peripheral vasodilators, but generally the effects of these can be overcome with other drugs.

Injuries pose a major threat to any child, but because of the underlying cardiovascular problems inherent in complex or major congenital or acquired heart disease, children with cardiac problems may require more extensive monitoring and consultation than other children suffering trauma.

REFERENCES

1. Symbas PN: Traumatic heart disease. Curr Probl Cardiol 7:1, 1982.
2. Roberts R, Sobel BE: Creatine kinase isoenzymes in the assessment of heart disease. Am Heart J 95:521, 1978.
3. Tibatznik B, Isaacs JP: Postpericardiotomy syndrome following traumatic hemopericardium. Am J Cardiol 7:83, 1961.
4. Vander Ark GD: Cardiovascular changes with acute subdural hematoma. Surg Neurol 3:305, 1975.
5. Abildskov JA, Millar K, Burgess MO, Vincent W: The electrocardiogram and the central nervous system. Prog Cardiovasc Dis 13:210, 1970.
6. Theodore J, Robin ED: Speculations on neurogenic pulmonary edema (NPE). Am Rev Resp Dis 113:405, 1976.
7. Lefer AM, Martin J: Origin of myocardial depressant factor in shock. Am J Physiol 218:1423, 1970.
8. Sheagren JN: Septic shock and corticosteroids. N Engl J Med 305:456, 1981.
9. Shannon DC, Lusser M, Golbla HA, Bunnel JB: The cyanotic infant—heart disease or lung disease. N Engl J Med 287:951, 1972.
10. Covell JW, Ross J Jr: Nature and significance of alterations in myocardial compliance. Am J Cardiol 32:449, 1973.
11. Shachar GB, Fuhrman BP, Wang Y, et al.: Rest and exercise hemodynamics after the Fontan procedure. Circulation 65:1043, 1982.
12. Swan SJC: The role of hemodynamic monitoring in the management of the critically ill. Crit Care Med 3:83, 1975.
13. Guiha NH, Cohn J, Mikulic E, et al.: Treatment of refractory heart failure with infusion of nitroprusside. N Engl J Med 291:587, 1974.
14. Driscoll DJ, Gillette MD, MacNamara DG: The use of dopamine in children. J Pediatr 92:309, 1978.
15. Perkin RM, Levin DL, Webb R, et al.: Dobutamine: A hemodynamic evaluation in children with shock. J Pediatr 100:977, 1982.
16. Kaplan EL, Anthony BF, Bisno A, et al.: Prevention of bacterial endocarditis. Circulation 56:139A, 1977.
17. Antimicrobial prophylaxis for surgery. The Medical Letter 21:73, 1979.

Selected Readings

Hurst JW (ed.). The Heart. 5th ed. New York, McGraw-Hill, 1982. *An excellent general text on all aspects of cardiology, including pediatric heart disease.*

Keith JD, Rowe R, Vlad P (eds.): Heart Disease in Infancy and Childhood: 3rd ed. New York, Macmillan, 1978. *Detailed pediatric cardiology text, expecially good for anatomy and physiology in relation to congenital heart disease.*

CHAPTER

10 Injuries to Children with Hematologic Disorders

RICHARD T. O'BRIEN
JOANN L. ATER

Hemostatic mechanisms play a critical role in our response to injury. They represent a complex surveillance system that responds with remarkable speed and precision to preserve vascular integrity and to limit the immediate effects of local injury. This system is carefully regulated, allowing for repair of bleeding sites even while uninterrupted blood flow is maintained. Patients with disorders of hemostasis have an important handicap when faced with trauma, and special knowledge and skill are required for their optimal management. There is probably no other chronic disorder in which trauma poses such a serious threat to patients.

NORMAL HEMOSTATIC MECHANISMS

Normal hemostasis is the product of a complex interaction of blood vessels, platelets, and plasma coagulation factors. We generally consider blood vessels, platelets, and plasma clotting factors separately, but it is important to understand their interrelation (Fig. 10–1). Because of their critical role in both the initiation and localization of hemostasis, the contribution of blood vessels deserves emphasis. The vascular response includes vasoconstriction, collagen exposure, and thromboplastin release (see later). Following local injury, normal hemostasis is initiated by the exposure of collagen from the blood vessel to circulating platelets. Platelets have the capacity to adhere to collagen and in doing so release adenosine diphosphate (ADP), which induces platelets to aggregate into a primary platelet plug. It is this sequence of events that we assess functionally with measurement of bleeding time. Both quantitative and qualitative disorders of platelets result in a prolongation of the bleed-

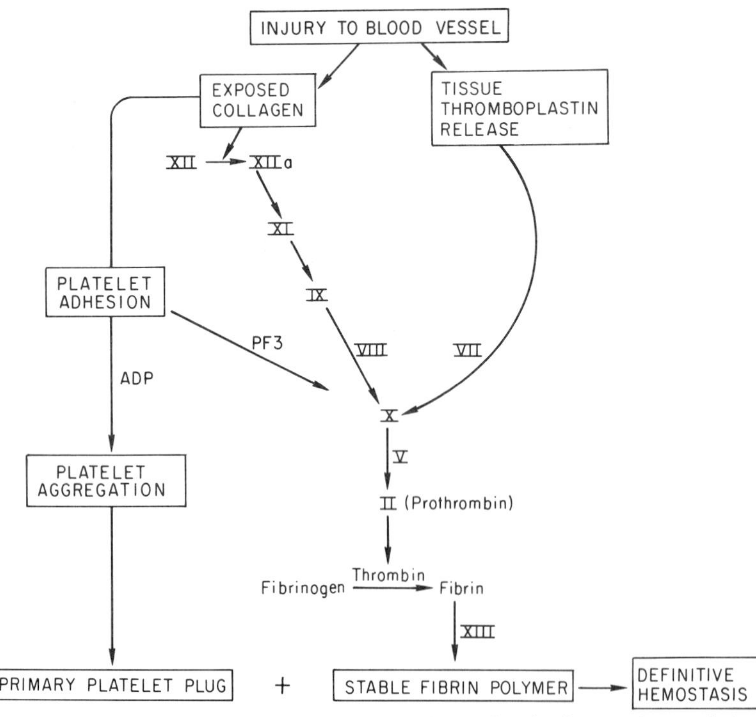

Figure 10–1. A representation of the interaction among blood vessels, platelets, and coagulation factors in normal hemostasis.

ing time. When platelets adhere to collagen, they also release a phospholipid, which plays a role as a cofactor in the cascade of coagulation factors.

Exposure of collagen from vessel walls provides yet another triggering mechanism, which localizes hemostasis to the site of injury in that it activates Factor XII, thereby initiating the cascade of clotting factors to fibrinogen and a fibrin clot. A final mechanism that contributes to normal hemostasis results from the local release at the site of an injury of a substance called tissue thromboplastin, which, in the presence of Factor VII and calcium, bypasses a number of coagulation factors and results in a fibrin clot.

Hemostasis is often a confusing and intimidating subject for the clinician, particularly when the complexities of the reactions among coagulation factors are presented in great detail. Fortunately, many of the details can be deleted without significantly jeopardizing an understanding of hemostasis sufficient for everyday clinical evaluation and management. Figure 10–2 represents a practical schema of the coagulation factor cascade and its evaluation. Basically, we assess the functional adequacy of clotting factors with two common screening tests—the activated partial thromboplastin time (PTT) and the prothrombin time (PT), the specific factors involved in each are noted in Figure 10–2. Each of the coagulation factors can be quantified individually when it is necessary to document specific factor deficiencies. Minor deficiencies of specific factors may not be detected by the screening tests, but minor deficiencies are generally not associated with significant bleeding problems. Therefore, normal values for PT and PTT usually indicate that the patient has adequate functional activity of all plasma coagulation factors necessary for normal hemostasis. All the coagulation factors, except for Factor VIII, are made in the liver, and vitamin K is necessary for the synthesis of Factors II, VII, IX, and X. These general remarks should provide a framework for a rational and practical method of evaluation and management of trauma in patients with disorders of hemostasis.

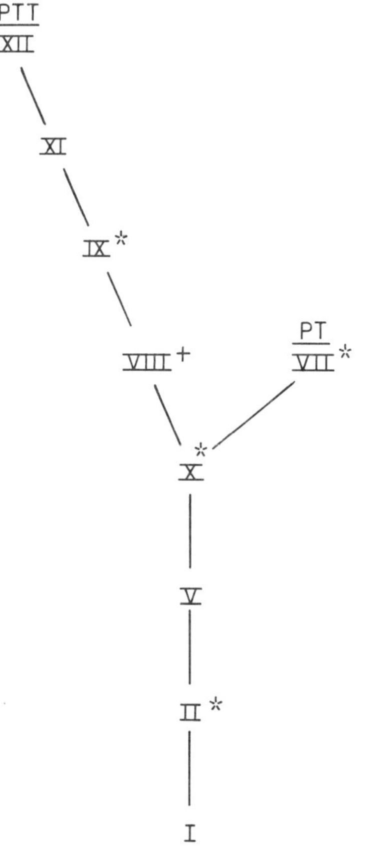

Figure 10–2. A simplified schema of the coagulation factor cascade and its evaluation. * indicates factors requiring vitamin K for their synthesis. + indicates the only factor not made by the liver, Factor VIII.

EVALUATION OF ABNORMAL BLEEDING

The extent of the evaluation necessary in any given patient depends on the physician's previous medical knowledge of the patient. Patients with well-documented hemostatic disorders (such as hemophilia) require little or no diagnostic evaluation, so one can proceed promptly to management decisions, which are discussed later. The traumatized patient with abnormal bleeding and no previous diagnosis requires prompt diagnostic evaluation. The clinical tools of history and physical examination, supplemented by *selected* laboratory studies, provide the basis for accurate diagnosis and direct appropriate management.

The history provides some of the most useful clues to the diagnosis of abnormal bleeding, but it must be elicited with specific questions. What is the personal history for bleeding with circumcision, intramuscular injections, dental work, lacerations, surgery, and so on? Have there been any problems with easy bruising, epistaxis, or menstrual bleeding? Petechiae, bruising, and mucous membrane bleeding suggest platelet disorders, whereas hemarthroses are characteristic of hemophilia. The family history should be taken with awareness of the sex-linked recessive pattern of classic hemophilia and Christmas disease and the autosomal dominant pattern of von Willebrand's disease, since these three diseases constitute the vast majority of congenital deficiencies of coagulation factors. A medication history should be assessed, since numerous drugs can cause abnormal bleeding. Aspirin, dipyramidole, sulfinpyrazone, and phenylbutazone are examples.

All patients should receive a full physical examination, with particular attention paid to the skin and mucous membranes, since these areas are frequently the first in which bleeding problems become evident. Deep bruises or hemarthroses are characteristic of hemophilia, whereas superficial bruises and petechiae suggest platelet dysfunction or deficiency. Equally important is whether abnormal bleeding occurs from a single site or multiple sites. *The most common cause of abnormal bleeding is a vascular defect that is too large for normal hemostatic mechanisms to control.* An isolated bleeding site suggests that cause. Although laboratory studies ultimately provide a specific diagnosis of hemostatic disorders, the intelligent and expedient use of the laboratory frequently derives from the clues provided by the history and physical examination.

The laboratory evaluation can be conveniently divided into two stages—screening and definitive studies (Table 10–1). A negative screening evaluation is strong presumptive evidence against a hemostatic disorder but does not exclude it. Screening studies should include a PT, PTT, and platelet count, at a minimum, and measurement of bleeding time, if practical. Fresh citrated plasma may be frozen and reserved for possible further studies as necessary. Although most of these tests are relatively simple laboratory procedures, the collection of the blood specimen can pose several difficulties. Falsely prolonged values may result from traumatic venipunctures, obtaining blood from lines containing heparin, or inadequate filling of tubes that contain a fixed volume of anticoagulant.

Under the circumstances of acute hemorrhage, practical management often limits the extent of the diagnostic evaluation to screening procedures plus a limited number of diagnostic studies. In practice, this approach is generally adequate. *When faced with serious bleeding, expectant therapy should never be withheld to await the results of diagnostic studies.*

Table 10–1. LABORATORY EVALUATION OF DISORDERS OF HEMOSTASIS

Screening Studies
Prothrombin time (PT)
Partial thromboplastin time (PTT)
Platelet count
Bleeding time
Definitive Studies
Specific factor procoagulant assays
Specific factor antigen assays
Clot solubility in 5 M Urea
Inhibitor assays
Platelet adhesiveness
Platelet aggregation studies
Ristocetin cofactor assays
Fibrinogen degradation products

MANAGEMENT OF PLATELET AND VASCULAR DISORDERS

Table 10–2 outlines the details of treatment for thrombocytopenia, platelet function abnormalities, and inherited and acquired defects of coagulation. This table should be referred to throughout the following discussion.

Thrombocytopenia

Petechiae, ecchymoses, and mucous membrane bleeding, such as epistaxis are clinical hallmarks of thrombocytopenia. Gastrointestinal (GI) bleeding may occur, but central nervous hemorrhage poses the greatest threat to life, particularly with trauma. Menorrhagia is common in postpubertal females with thrombocytopenia.

The risks of bleeding are directly related to the severity of the thrombocytopenia. Platelet counts above 70,000/mm^3 are generally not associated with an increased risk of bleeding, provided that the platelets function normally, whereas platelet counts under 20,000/mm^3 may be associated with spontaneous bleeding. Children typically tolerate thrombocytopenia much better than adults, and serious bleeding in the absence of trauma is very uncommon even when the thrombocytopenia is severe.

The management of thrombocytopenic hemorrhage depends on the mechanism for the thrombocytopenia as well as the location and severity of the bleeding. Minor bleeding

Table 10–2. EMERGENCY TREATMENT TO THE INJURED CHILD WITH A HEMOSTASIS DISORDER

Category	Type of Injury and/or Evidence of Bleeding	Initial Therapy
Thrombocytopenia		
Impaired production (e.g., leukemia, aplastic anemia, etc.)	Minor (epistaxis, lacerations, soft tissue trauma)	Local measures, such as compression for 15–20 minutes, are generally sufficient
	Major*	Platelet transfusions 1 unit/6 kg body weight (1 unit for infant to 10 units for adult)
Autoimmune (e.g., ITP† or SLE‡	Minor (petechiae, bruises, mucous membrane bleeding)	Prednisone 2 mg/kg/day or equivalent for maximum of 3 weeks
	Major (CNS,§ GI,‖ or other life-threatening bleeding)	Prednisone 2 mg/kg/day, exchange transfusion with fresh whole blood and emergency splenectomy
Platelet Function Abnormality		
Von Willebrand's disease	Hemarthrosis, soft tissue injury, hematuria, mucous membrane bleeding*	Fresh frozen plasma, 10–15 ml/kg IV or cryoprecipitate 2 bags/10 kg IV
	Life-threatening (CNS, retropharyngeal, retroperitoneal, GI) bleeding*	Fresh frozen plasma, 10–15 ml/kg IV or cryoprecipitate 3 bags/10 kg IV
Chronic disorders (e.g., uremia, diabetes, etc.)	Any	Correction of underlying disorder, e.g., dialysis
Inherited Deficiencies		
Factor VIII deficiency (classical hemophilia)	Hemarthrosis, soft tissue injury, hematuria, mucous membrane bleeding*	Factor VIII concentrate 20–25 units/kg IV
	Life-threatening (CNS, retropharyngeal, retroperitoneal, GI) bleeding*	Factor VIII concentrate 40–50 units/kg IV
Factor VIII deficiency with known inhibitor	Hemarthrosis, soft tissue injury, mucous membrane	Factor IX concentrate 75 units/kg IV
	Life-threatening (CNS, retropharyngeal, retroperitoneal, GI) bleeding*	Factor VIII concentrate 100 units/kg IV or greater, Factor IX concentrate 75 units/kg IV, or Autoplex 50–100 units/kg IV (product of choice for high titer inhibitor)
Factor IX deficiency (Christmas disease)	Hemarthrosis, soft tissue injury, mucous membrane bleeding,* or hematuria	Factor IX concentrate 20–25 units/kg IV
	Life-threatening (CNS, retropharyngeal, retroperitoneal GI) bleeding*	Factor IX concentrate 40–50 units/kg IV
Other congenital factor	Any	Fresh frozen plasma 15 ml/kg IV; concentrates of Factors I, II, VII, and X are also available, if needed.
Acquired Coagulopathies		
Vitamin K deficiency	Any	Vitamin K_1 1 mg/IV (may give more if liver disease)
Liver disease	Any	Fresh frozen plasma 10–15 ml/kg IV
DIC**	Mild (epistaxis, lacerations, soft tissue and mucous membrane bleeding)	Treat underlying causes
	Life threatening bleeding*	Treat underlying cause and transfuse fresh frozen plasma 10–15 ml/kg IV and platelets 1 unit/6 kg IV

*More than one dose of therapy may be needed.
†ITP = idiopathic thrombocytopenic purpura.
‡SLE = systemic lupus erythematosus.
§CNS = central nervous system.
‖GI = gastrointestinal.
**DIC = disseminated intravascular coagulation.

such as ecchymoses or epistaxis generally responds to simple local measures. Compression of the involved area is usually sufficient to stop bleeding. In disorders in which the thrombocytopenia is due to impaired platelet production, such as leukemia, aplastic anemia, or drug-induced thrombocytopenias, platelet transfusion provides the best management. The appropriate dose is 1 unit/6 kg body weight (providing from 1 unit of platelets for a neonate to 10 units of platelets for an adolescent). In order to obtain maximum therapeutic affect, platelets must be freshly acquired and carefully handled, under which circumstances they generally survive for a number of days. With repeated transfusion of random donor platelets, sensitization to platelet antigens occurs, resulting in antibodies that ultimately limit the usefulness of subsequent platelet transfusions.[1]

Management is often difficult in cases in which thrombocytopenic bleeding is due to increased platelet destruction. Examples of this include autoimmune conditions (such as idiopathic thrombocytopenic purpura[2] and systemic lupus erythematosus[3]), hypersplenism, hemolytic-uremic syndrome, and disseminated intravascular coagulation. Transfused platelets generally have markedly shortened survival in these disorders. In fact, their survival may be so short that one cannot achieve any significant rise in platelet count.

Idiopathic thrombocytopenic purpura is one of the most common causes for severe thrombocytopenia in children.[4] The antibody in that disease is a pan-platelet agglutinin directed against some ubiquitous platelet antigen, rendering platelet transfusion of little value. Serious bleeding, particularly central nervous system (CNS) bleeding, requires aggressive management. An exchange transfusion with fresh whole blood may yield a transient improvement in the platelet count. Corticosteroids (equivalent to 2 mg/kg/day of prednisone) may also be of benefit because of their vascular effects and because they may improve platelet survival by inhibiting the phagocytosis of antibody-coated platelets.[5] Under life-threatening circumstances, such as CNS bleeding, an emergency splenectomy may result in sufficient improvement in the platelet count and hemostasis to permit a life-saving neurosurgical procedure to be safely performed.[6] The management of serious thrombocytopenic hemorrhage generally requires consultation with a hematologist.

Platelet Functional Abnormalities and Vascular Abnormalities

Abnormalities in platelet function are associated with the same types of bleeding noted in thrombocytopenic individuals.[7] Defects in platelet function may be due to either intrinsic or extrinsic factors. Intrinsic disorders of platelet function, such as Glanzmann's disease or storage pool disease, are very uncommon and usually can be managed quite effectively with platelet transfusions.[8]

Platelet function abnormalities are more commonly due to extrinsic causes, a classical example of which is the impairment in platelet function induced by aspirin or other medications.[9] Aspirin affects platelet function by inhibiting the secondary phase of platelet aggregation, which results in a prolongation of the bleeding time.[10] The ingestion of a single dose of aspirin affects the function for the life span of the exposed platelets (about 10 days) and does not seem to be a dose-related phenomenon. This functional defect in hemostasis generally does not cause clinical bleeding problems, which is fortunate because no specific therapy is available.

Another relatively common extrinsic platelet functional defect is that of von Willebrand's disease, an autosomal dominant inherited condition characterized by both a deficiency of Factor VIII and platelet dysfunction.[11] There are a number of variants of von Willebrand's disease, but the classical and most common variant is characterized by a prolonged bleeding time, abnormal platelet adhesiveness, abnormal platelet aggregation induced by ristocetin, and a variable but generally mild deficiency of both Factor VIII procoagulant and antigenic activity. Infusion of either fresh frozen plasma (10 to 15 ml/kg) or cryoprecipitate (2 to 3 bags/10 kg) will correct this extrinsic defect. However, the correction of the defect in platelet function lasts only a few hours, which limits the effectiveness of replacement therapy in this condition. Fortunately, life-threatening bleeding is uncommon in von Willebrand's disease.

There are a variety of vascular disorders that may be associated with bleeding, particularly purpura.[12] Henoch-Schönlein purpura is an excellent example of an acquired non-thrombocytopenic purpura due to vascular disease. There are also a number of uncommon inherited disorders, such as Ehlers-Danlos syndrome and osteogenesis imperfecta, which also may be associated with purpura. There is no known specific therapy for these conditions, but bleeding is generally mild. In addition, a large number of chronic disorders, such as uremia, diabetes, and a host of other systemic conditions are associated with platelet dysfunction.[13] Correction of the underlying disorder results in an improvement in platelet function.

MANAGEMENT OF COAGULATION FACTOR DISORDERS

Inherited Deficiencies—The Hemophilias

At least 95 per cent of all inherited deficiencies of coagulation factors are accounted for by deficiencies of Factor VIII (hemophilia A) or Factor IX (hemophilia B or Christmas disease).[14] Both of these are inherited as sex-linked traits. A large majority of patients with deficiencies in Factor VIII and Factor IX are classified as having clinically severe diseases and have less than one per cent procoagulant activity. For those patients, the diagnosis of hemophilia is almost invariably made during the first year of life. Hemarthroses are the clinical hallmark of the disease, but hemorrhage may occur at any site, particularly in association with trauma. CNS bleeding is a major threat, as are GI and retroperitoneal hemorrhage. The latter site of bleeding may present diagnostic problems, since it is not uncommon for patients with retroperitoneal bleeding to complain initially of pain referred to a distal site, such as the hip or knee. A high index of suspicion and a careful physical examination are needed to make the diagnosis, which can be confirmed with an intravenous pyelogram or abdominal computerized tomography (CT) scan.

The key to the successful management of bleeding in hemophilia is the prompt and adequate use of factor replacement therapy.[15–16] Fresh frozen plasma is useful, but volume considerations limit the amount of specific factor that can be administered by this route. As a result, various concentrates of Factor VIII or Factor IX are routinely used, which permit the administration of very large doses of specific coagulation factors. These concentrates are derived from pooled plasma, so they carry a significant risk for hepatitis.[17] Nonetheless, the risk/benefit ratio, particularly when significant trauma has occurred, greatly favors their use. In fact, *the patient with hemophilia who has sustained a significant injury should receive specific factor replacement therapy immediately, even before a complete evaluation of the injury has been carried out.* Any delay in the correction of the hemostatic defect in the injured patient with hemophilia is hazardous.

The dose and frequency of factor replacement therapy in the hemophilia patient depends on the site and extent of the bleeding. The more common bleeding episodes, such as hemarthroses or soft tissue hemorrhage, respond quite predictably to a single dose of specific factor replacement. A dose of 20 to 25 units/kg of Factor VIII raises the level of that procoagulant to 40 to 50 per cent activity. The same dose of Factor IX yields 30 to 35 per cent activity. Such doses also provide for adequate hemostasis needed for minor surgery, such as suturing lacerations or a cut-down procedure.

Epistaxis or oral bleeding also responds quite predictably to the same dose of Factor VIII or Factor IX replacement. However, a single dose is often inadequate in these circumstances. Bleeding may reoccur a few days later when the blood clot in the nose or mouth can be dislodged after the plasma coagulant activity has returned to baseline low values. Consequently, a series of three doses of factor replacement given 36 to 48 hours apart is often needed for mucous membrane bleeding in hemophilia. An effective alternative is a single dose of specific factor replacement along with the oral administration of the antifibrinolytic agent ϵ-aminocaproic acid (Amicar) 100 mg/kg/dose qid for 7 days.

Life-threatening hemorrhage in a patient with hemophilia requires more intensive replacement therapy.[18] The patient should promptly receive 40 to 50 units/kg of Factor VIII or Factor IX and should be monitored closely, making certain that the PTT remains normal. Laboratory analysis to quantify factor levels may also be very helpful in the management of severe bleeding. The frequency of doses of replacement therapy depends on the half-life of the infused factor. *The risk of undertreatment far outweighs any small theoretic risk from overtreatment.* A 12-hour dosage schedule has proved practical for us, at least during the first few days in the management of life-threatening bleeding. Alternately, a continuous infusion of Factor VIII may be used.[19] A similar dosage schedule is recommended for elective surgery. Normal hemostasis should be maintained by a regular schedule of replacement therapy for at least 7 days and often longer. A hematologist should participate in the daily management of serious bleeding in a patient with hemophilia.

Approximately 15 per cent of patients with Factor VIII deficiency develop an inhibitor or an immunoglobulin that inactivates infused Factor VIII,[20] rendering management extremely difficult, particularly when serious bleeding occurs. The level of an inhibitor generally diminishes with time provided that there is no further antigenic stimulus. Low titer inhibitors can usually be overcome by large doses of Factor VIII, the specific dose depending on the titer of the inhibitor. This is a clear instance in which the support of a sophisticated coagulation laboratory is necessary for optimal management. A few days of relatively normal hemostasis may be lifesaving and can usually be achieved. However, a secondary antibody response may occur, and the titer of inhibitor often rises to levels that cannot be overcome even with massive doses of Factor VIII. Inhibitors of high titer porcine Factor VIII, an extremely potent allergen, have been used, as well as so-called "activated" coagulation products. Concentrates of the vitamin K–dependent clotting factors, which are used in the treatment of hemophilia B, have been found useful in the treatment of patients with Factor VIII deficiency who have developed an inhibitor.[21] Autoplex has been developed specifically for such circumstances and is the drug of choice for life-threatening hemorrhage in patients with Factor VIII deficiency and an inhibitor of high titer.[22, 23]

All other congenital factor deficiencies are inherited as autosomal recessive traits. Fresh frozen plasma contains all clotting factors and, in a dose of 15 ml/kg, provides adequate hemostasis under most circumstances of bleeding in these less common coagulopathies. In addition, there are concentrated products available for the treatment of deficiencies in Factors I, II, VII, and X if needed. The recommended frequency of replacement therapy should depend on the severity of the bleeding episode and also on the half-life of the deficient factor that is being infused (Table 10–3).

Table 10–3. BIOLOGIC HALF-LIVES OF THE PLASMA COAGULATION FACTORS

Factor VII	1.5 to 5 hours
Factor VIII	9 to 18 hours
Factor V	15 to 20 hours
Factor IX	20 to 24 hours
Factor X	1 to 2 days
Factor XI	1.5 to 3.5 days
Factor XII	2 days
Factor II	2.8 to 4.4 days
Factor I	3.2 to 4.5 days
Factor XIII	4.5 to 7 days

Acquired Coagulopathies

Acquired coagulopathies may be broadly divided into two groups, depending on whether the deficiency is due to impaired production or increased destruction or utilization of the clotting factors. All the coagulation factors, except for Factor VIII, are synthesized by the liver and many (Factors II, VII, IX, and X) require vitamin K for synthesis. Liver disease and vitamin K deficiency, therefore, are obvious causes for decreased production of coagulation factors.

Vitamin K is a fat-soluble vitamin, deficiency of which may result from any condition that interferes with fat absorption, such as liver, gallbladder, small intestine, or pancreatic disease. Coagulopathies due to vitamin K deficiency respond rapidly to an injection of vitamin K_1. Although a dose of 1 mg is generally adequate, many recommend higher doses when faced with coexistent liver disease. The IV administration of a single dose of vitamin K_1 to a deficient patient typically results in cessation of bleeding within a few hours, followed by improvement in the activities of the vitamin K–dependent factors within 24 hours.

Adequate liver function is critical for normal hemostasis, since the liver is the site of synthesis of plasma coagulation factors and inhibitors of coagulation. The liver is also responsible for the clearance of activated coagulation factors. Liver disease, therefore, may be associated with a variety of defects in hemostasis and at times more than one mechanism may be operative concurrently. Treatment of clinical bleeding in patients with liver disease should include the parenteral administration of vitamin K and replacement therapy with fresh frozen plasma in a dose of 10 to 15 ml/kg. Platelet transfusions may also be indicated if severe thrombocytopenia occurs.

The management of coagulopathies in which the mechanism is increased destruction or utilization of clotting factors may be more difficult. Disseminated intravascular coagulation (DIC) is the most common example of this type of coagulopathy. It is important to remember that DIC is not a disease but rather a relatively common pathophysiologic mechanism associated with many disorders. Conditions in which DIC may occur include Rocky Mountain Spotted Fever, meningococcemia, trauma, sepsis, snakebite, and neoplasms. Although heparinization can reliably interrupt the consumption of platelets and coagulation factors characteristic of DIC, it is rarely necessary. The optimal management of DIC depends on the successful treatment of the underlying disease.[24, 25]

RED BLOOD CELL DISORDERS

Anemia may result from either decreased production or increased destruction (hemolysis or hemorrhage) of red blood cells. Regardless of the cause, the body compensates in a rather uniform way for the effects of anemia through both intraerythrocytic and cardiovascular changes. Virtually all causes of anemia are associated with a shift in the oxygen dissociation curve to the right due to increases in the concentration of 2,3-diphosphoglycerate (2,3 DPG) within the red cell.[26] Functionally, this results in a decrease in hemoglobin-oxygen affinity, thereby enhancing oxygen delivery to the tissues. In many chronic anemias this mechanism alone may be sufficient to provide full compensation for even moderate degrees of anemia. When this mechanism is insufficient, cardiovascular compensatory changes occur. They include an initial increase in cardiac output and, when necessary, a redistribution of blood flow to vital organs. This compensatory effect is remarkably efficient. For example, patients with severe but chronic anemia (hemoglobin concentration = 3 to 5 g/dl) are usually completely asymptomatic when at rest.

Management of the traumatized patient with acute anemia is straightforward, assuming that the clinician is reasonably certain that the acute blood loss is the cause of the anemia. In these circumstances, provision of adequate circulatory volume is paramount (see Chapter 1, pages 14–16). Vascular volume may be replaced with packed red blood cells, whole blood, colloid, crystalloid, or other plasma expanders, depending upon clinical circumstances. The management of the individual with chronic anemia who experiences trauma should be influenced by the severity of the anemia, the injury itself, and the planned management of the patient. Most patients with chronic anemia are well compensated, and transfusion for the anemia per se is generally not indicated. However, if either the injury or its management (such as surgery) might exacerbate the anemia, then blood replacement may be necessary. Successful surgical management of trauma in children with chronic anemia often requires red blood cell transfusion, even in cases in which it might not otherwise be necessary. In chronic anemias, packed red blood cells should be given. A rule of thumb practical for estimating the amount of blood needed is that the number of milliliters per kilogram of packed red blood cells administered will raise a patient's hematocrit by approximately the same number. For example, 10 ml/kg of packed red blood cells will raise the hematocrit by 10 percentage points; 15 ml/kg will raise it by 15.

A patient's chronic compensatory response to anemia may also contribute to the risks associated with trauma. Hemolytic anemias are typically characterized by both medullary and extramedullary erythroid compensation. Medullary compensation consists of expansion of the red marrow, which in severe hemolytic processes may be associated with overt radiographic bone changes. Such bone changes may be sufficient to produce an increased risk of fractures, even with relatively minor trauma and at times may be extreme, such as in patients with thalassemia major (Fig. 10–3).[27] The extramedullary compensation is characterized by hepatosplenomegaly, and an enlarged spleen may be associated with an increased risk of rupture when there is trauma.

Finally, there are a number of causes for anemia that potentially can be aggravated by trauma or its management. Inadequate fluid management in sickle cell disease may contribute to a painful or vaso-occlusive crisis.[28] Oxidant drugs may induce an acute hemolytic episode in an individual with glucose-6-phosphate dehydrogenase deficiency. Consultation with a hematologist may be helpful in the management of a patient with chronic anemia who has a serious injury.

NEOPLASTIC DISORDERS

The prognosis for children with cancer has improved dramatically over the past two decades so that today cure is a realistic goal for the vast majority of patients.[29] The course of the disease has been transformed from an

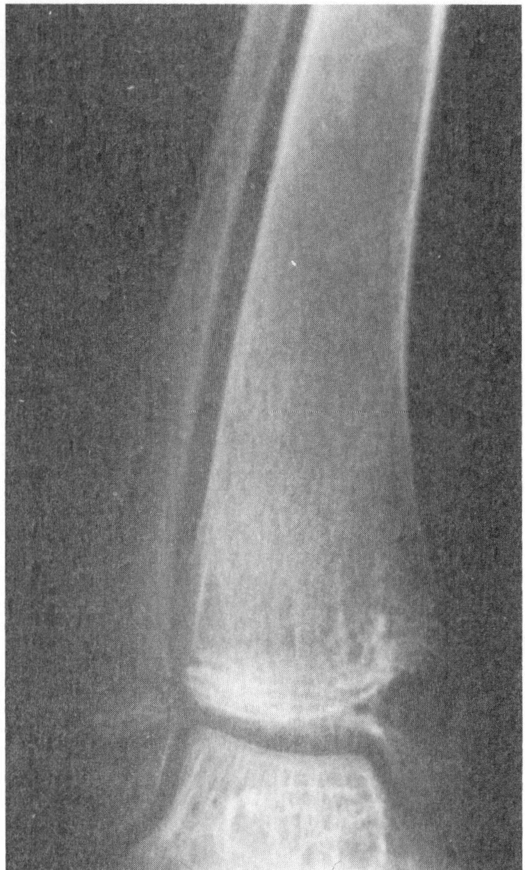

Figure 10–3. Marked thinning of the bone cortex secondary to medullary expansion in a patient with thalassemia major.

acute to a chronic process. This improved prognosis has been largely the result of an aggressive, multi-disciplinary approach to both the evaluation and management of the child with cancer. This intensive therapy, although effective for a majority of patients, has a relatively narrow therapeutic index. Consequently, the potential risks of the therapy are considerable. Injury to a child with neoplastic disease, therefore, may be associated with an increased risk of complications either because of the clinical manifestations of the underlying disease or its therapy.

The patient with cancer may have an increased chance of experiencing an injury or of developing significant complications once the injury occurs. The child with a tumor of the CNS, for instance, may have weakness or cerebellar dysfunction, which might predispose to injury because of the neurologic deficit. Trauma to a child with neoplastic disease who has proptosis, hepatosplenomegaly, or airway compression may place him at an increased risk for developing complications. Perhaps the best example is the child with bone metastases, in whom the risk of a fracture is considerably enhanced (Fig. 10–4).

Rather than the disease itself, it is more likely that the treatment of the child with cancer would affect the risks associated with trauma. Typically the management of cancer involves a combined approach utilizing surgery, radiation therapy, and chemotherapy. Each of those therapeutic modalities may influence the potential effects of an injury. It is important that the details of the patient's cancer treatment is known to the physicians caring for his injury. The child with one kidney because of nephrectomy in the management of Wilms' tumor may require special

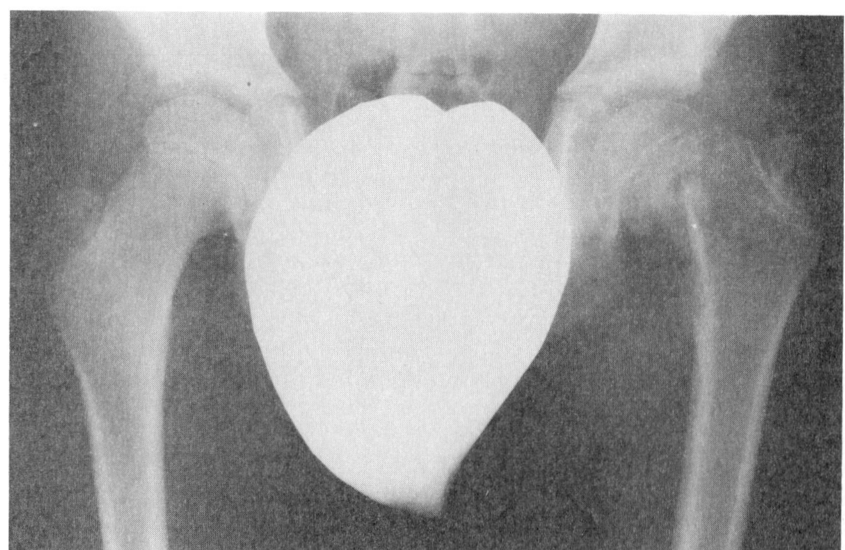

Figure 10–4. Pathologic fracture through the neck of the femur in a patient with metastatic neuroblastoma.

consideration in the evaluation and management of trauma to the abdomen. Likewise, radiation therapy may have long-lasting effects on the tissues within the radiation field. Thus the risk of fracture may be greatly increased in bone that has been subjected to such therapy.

Chemotherapy imposes perhaps the greatest risks to a child with cancer who sustains an injury because chemotherapy usually is administered for a protracted period of time and is associated with a large number of potential acute toxicities, which might be of significance in face of trauma. The greatest risk of chemotherapy is associated with bone marrow suppression. Although neutropenia is the most common myelosuppressive effect of chemotherapy, thrombocytopenia is not uncommon and is of critical importance to the management of such a patient. Management of injury to a child with neoplastic disease may be facilitated by consultation with a pediatric oncologist. Any patient with malignant neoplastic disease who experiences significant trauma should have a complete blood count and platelet count obtained promptly. If the risk of the injury is significant, such as a head injury, and the platelet count is less than 70,000/mm^3, the patient should promptly receive a transfusion of platelets. (In addition, chemotherapeutic agents such as 1-asparaginase may induce a coagulopathy by interference with the synthesis of clotting factors in the liver.)[30]

REFERENCES

1. Dutcher JP, Schiffer CA, Aisner J, et al.: Alloimmunization following platelet transfusion: The absence of a dose response relationship. Blood 57:395, 1981.
2. Karpatkin S: Autoimmune thrombocytopenic purpura. Blood 56:329, 1980.
3. Karpatkin S, Strick N, Karpatkin MB, et al.: Cumulative experience in the detection of antiplatelet antibody in 234 patients with idiopathic thrombopurpura, systemic lupus erythematosus and other clinical disorders. Am J Med 52:776, 1972.
4. McWilliams NB, Maurer HM: Acute idiopathic thrombocytopenic purpura in children. Am J Hematol 7:87, 1979.
5. Handlin RI, and Stossel TP: Effect of corticosteroids on the phagocytosis of antibody coated platelets by human leukocytes. Blood 51:771, 1978.
6. Woerner SJ, Abildgaard CR, French BN: Intracranial hemorrhage in children with idiopathic thrombocytopenic purpura. Pediatrics 67:453, 1981.
7. Huebsch LB, Harker LA: Disorders of platelet function. West J Med 134:109, 1981.
8. Weiss HJ: Congenital disorders of platelet function. Semin Hematol 17:228, 1980.
9. DeGaetano G, Donati MB, Garattini S: Drugs affecting platelet function tests. Thromb Diath Haemorrh 34:285, 1975.
10. Schwartz AD, Pearson HA: Aspirin, platelets and bleeding. J Pediatr 78:558, 1971.
11. Bloom AL: The von Willebrand's syndrome. Semin Hematol 17:215, 1980.
12. Nydegger WE, Miescher PA: Bleeding due to vascular disorders. Semin Hematol 17:178, 1980.
13. O'Brien RT: Hematologic manifestations of chronic systemic disease. *In* Miller DR, Pearson Howard: (eds.): Blood Disease of Infancy and Childhood. St. Louis, CV Mosby Company, 1978, pp. 451–462.
14. Buchanan GR: Hemophilia. Pediatr Clin North Am 27:309, 1980.
15. Jones P: Developments and problems in the management of hemophilia. Semin Hematol 14:375, 1977.
16. Biggs R: Recent advances in the management of haemophilia and Christmas disese. Clin Haematol 8:95, 1979.
17. Spero JA, Lewis JH, Fisher SE, et al.: The high risk of chronic liver disease in multitransfused juvenile hemophiliac patients. J Pediatr 94:875, 1979.
18. Eyster ME, Gill FM, Blatt PM, et al.: Central nervous system bleeding in hemophiliacs. Blood 51:1179, 1978.
19. McMillan CW, Webster WP, Roberts HR, et al.: Continuous intravenous infusion of Factor VIII in classic haemophilia. Br J Haematol 18:659, 1970.
20. Shapiro SS: Antibodies to blood coagulation factors. Clin Haematol 8:207, 1979.
21. Lusher JM, Shapiro SS, Palascak JE, et al.: Efficacy of prothrombin-complex concentrates in hemophiliacs with antibodies to Factor VIII. N Engl J Med 303:421, 1980.
22. Abildgaard CF, Penner JA, Watson-Williams EJ: Anti-inhibitor coagulant complex (Autoplex) for treatment of Factor VIII inhibitors in hemophilia. Blood 56:978, 1980.
23. Sjamsoedin LJ, Heijnen L, Mauser-Bunschoten EP, et al.: The effects of activated prothrombin compplex concentrate (FEIBA) on joint and muscle bleeding in patients with hemophilia A and antibodies to Factor VIII. N Engl J Med 305:717, 1981.
24. Corrigan JJ: Heparin therapy in bacterial septicemia. J Pediatr 91:695, 1977.
25. Gross SJ, Filston HC, Anderson JC: Controlled study of treatment for disseminated intramuscular coagulation in the neonate. J Pediatr 100:445, 1982.
26. Oski FA, Delivoria-Papadopoulos M: The red cell 2,3-diphosphoglycerate and tissue oxygen release. J Pediatr 77:941, 1970.
27. Pearson HA, O'Brien RT: The management of thalassemia major. Semin Hematol 12:255, 1975.
28. Pearson HA, Diamond LK: The critically ill child: sickle cell disease crises and their management. Pediatrics 48:629, 1971.
29. Mauer AM, Simone JV, Pratt CB: Current progress in the treatment of the child with cancer. J Pediatr 91:523, 1977.
30. Land VJ, Sutow WW, Fernbach DJ, et al.: Toxicity of 1-asparaginase in children with advanced leukemia. Cancer 30:339, 1972.

CHAPTER

11 Injuries to Children with Endocrine and Metabolic Disease

BRUCE A. BUEHLER

The treatment of chronic endocrine and metabolic diseases has advanced rapidly, and with the advent of improved therapy, many pediatric patients now lead very active lives. Unfortunately, this increased activity has led to the potential for traumatic injury. The purpose of this chapter is to briefly review the more common chronic endocrine and metabolic disorders that may require acute management after trauma.

DIABETES MELLITUS

Diabetes can be thought of as three different disease states: (1) juvenile diabetes, which requires daily insulin therapy; (2) chemical diabetes, in which the hyperglycemia occurs only during pregnancy; and (3) adult-onset diabetes, which can be partially controlled by dietary management. In the pediatric age group, the majority of diabetic patients have insulin-dependent or juvenile diabetes. They may present major therapeutic dilemmas for the physician dealing with multiple trauma.

Long-term care for most insulin-dependent diabetics is provided at home, and it is very seldom that insulin-dependent diabetics require hospitalization, unless an acute event precipitates diabetic ketoacidosis. Unfortunately, trauma is one of those events that can initiate a major episode of ketoacidosis.

At initial examination, the insulin-dependent diabetic with traumatic injury may appear to be in good "control," with no signs of hyperglycemia or ketosis. It is in the first 24 hours after injury that the potential for severe hyperglycemia and ketoacidosis can occur. Therefore, when examining the diabetic child in the emergency room, it is important to obtain a history of the exact insulin schedule used daily and determine baseline serum glucose and serum and urine ketones.

Most insulin-dependent diabetics utilize a combination of neutral protamine Hagedorn (NPH) insulin and regular insulin on a single or twice daily dosage regimen. NPH insulin is a long-acting insulin, with expected peak action at 6 to 8 hours postinjection and continued insulin activity for approximately 12 hours. (Note: The exact peak time and half-life of a dose of insulin are greatly variable among individuals, and therefore, these times are only guidelines.) The effect of regular insulin is more rapid in onset than NPH, with a 1 to 2 hour peak time and 4 to 6 hours of total insulin activity. Most insulin schedules are established to create a smooth curve of insulin dosage over an 8 to 12 hour period after each injection, but acute trauma may drastically change the response to previously adequate maintenance of glucose homeostasis. Because of this potential, the clinician must closely monitor the diabetic patient for the first 24 hours after trauma.

If the patient has received his daily insulin dose prior to injury, he may initially have excess exogenous insulin with inadequate calories, since he may be unable to eat for several hours. In this situation, it is necessary to provide adequate calories in order to utilize the insulin already administered to the patient. Routine utilization of intravenous (IV) fluids containing 5 per cent glucose provides only minimal calories and may be inadequate. This will depend on the proximity of food intake prior to trauma and the specific point in time after insulin dosage that the patient is injured. In most instances, hypoglycemia will be the major early event in the traumatized insulin-dependent diabetic. Hourly monitoring of glucose will indicate whether adequate calories are being provided. If there is a trend toward hypoglycemia, 10 per cent glucose with electrolytes can be utilized. It is also important to remember that insulin drives potassium intracellularly, and therefore, the administration of potassium may be necessary if the patient has adequate urinary output (Table 11–1).

If hypoglycemia and hypokalemia are not encountered in the first few hours following trauma, the next critical point is when the pre-existing dose of insulin has been metabolized. The clinician must be aware of when to add insulin to the therapeutic regimen after trauma. For example, if the patient arrives at the emergency room with multiple fractures and had received his routine maintenance dose of NPH insulin 6 hours prior to trauma, the patient has approximately 4 to 6 hours before becoming insulin deficient. During the first 4 to 6 hours, hypoglycemia can occur, but after this time the likelihood of hyperglycemia, increased urinary glucose output, and then ketoacidosis increases rapidly. In order to prevent this cycle, insulin must be introduced, and a good indicator of insulin need is a blood glucose of 250 mg/dl or more in the presence of maintenance glucose. It must be remembered at all times that withholding insulin for extended periods will lead to hyperglycemia and possible acidosis.

Table 11–1. MANAGEMENT OF DIABETICS WITH TRAUMA

Criteria for Initiation of Insulin Therapy
- BS* > 300 mg/ml
- BS < 300 mg/ml with ketosis
- Serum osmolality > 290 mOsm/L

Intravenous Fluids
- Initially NS† or LR‡ at 20 ml/kg or greater§ for 1 hour
- Follow by D_5½NS if BS < 300 mg/dl

Potassium
- If urinary output normal (1–2 ml/kg/hr) → 3–4 mEq/kg/24 hr
- Monitor potassium and glucose every 4 hr
- If potassium increases or BS < 300 mg/ml, reduce to 2–3 mEq/kg/24 hr

Bicarbonate
- Use only if pH ≤ 7.10 or serum bicarbonate ≤ 10 mEq/L
- Dose = serum bicarbonate × body wt (kg) × 0.3 × ½ OR raise pH to 7.15
- Avoid overdosage (paradoxical acidosis)

Insulin
- Begin therapy when BS > 300 mg/dl
- BS > 300 mg/dl, but < 500 mg/dl, give 0.25 units regular insulin every 2–4 hr
- BS > 500 mg/dl, but < 750 mg/dl, give 0.5 units regular insulin every 2–4 hr
- BS > 750 mg/dl, give 1–2 units regular insulin every 2–4 hr

*BS = blood sugar.
†NS = normal saline.
‡LR = lactated Ringer's.
§If shock is present.

The patient *must* receive insulin while hospitalized in order to prevent these conditions.

When the patient is treated with subcutaneous regular insulin, IV therapy is imperative until the patient can take a regular diet. The IV fluid should contain glucose if the initial blood glucose is less than 300 mg/dl. Maintenance therapy of D_5 ½ normal saline or D_5 Ringer's lactate is an excellent initial therapy. Potassium requirements on a daily basis are 2 to 3 mEq/kg/day, which should be added to the fluid if the patient has adequate urinary output. Potassium should be withheld or lowered in amount if the patient is anuric or oliguric. Initial therapy should maintain the blood sugar level at greater than 100 but less than 300 mg/dl. Bicarbonate therapy is not necessary unless the pH is less than 7.10, and then only small doses should be administered until pH is greater than 7.15. Excess bicarbonate may cause a paradoxical intracellular or cerebrospinal fluid acidosis if used to completely return pH to 7.40; therefore use it very cautiously! If blood glucose begins to increase (greater than 250 mg/dl) or ketosis increases, the clinician should consider giving 0.25 to 0.5 units regular insulin/kg, subcutaneously. Unless ketones are 3 to 4 plus in urine or serum, or glucose is greater than 500 mEq/dl, the 0.25 unit dose should be adequate. This dose should be given every 4 to 6 hours, depending upon the exact level of glucose in the serum (see Table 11–1).

Therefore, determination of serum glucose, sodium, potassium, ketones and pH every 1 to 2 hours is mandatory during the initial phase of therapy. It is also useful to test all urine output for ketones and glucose. The most sensitive urinary test is the Clinitest tablet test, as opposed to the standard urine dipstick method. A marked increase of urinary glucose output should warn the physician of impending hyperglycemia and lack of adequate insulin. The development of ketosis without hyperglycemia is an indication that inadequate calories are being given to the patient, whereas the development of hyperglycemia and ketosis is associated with inadequate insulin. If serum glucose is less than 300 mg/100dl, there are negative or trace serum ketones, and normal serum electrolytes have been maintained, then 4 to 6 hour subcutaneous doses of regular insulin at 0.25/units/kg should maintain the patient in good control. It is not imperative in the post-traumatic patient that the blood sugar be as tightly controlled as recommended for chronic care; therefore, there is no need to give excessive amounts of insulin to maintain the sugar at 100 mEq/dl, but there must be adequate insulin to maintain the sugar below 300 mEq/dl.

When the patient is stable and is eating and the blood sugar level has stayed below 300 mg/ml without ketosis, it is best to return the patient to his previous daily schedule of insulin. The blood sugar of hospitalized diabetics may not appear to be as tightly controlled as that of the patient who is active; but in most instances, adequate calories with the previous insulin dosage will maintain the patient in a clinically stable condition. Continue to monitor urine glucose and ketones as well as A.M. and P.M. blood glucose. If there has been severe trauma to the kidney or if the patient is unable to take oral fluids, then the clinician may be forced to stay with the IV therapy and regular insulin therapy until the patient is more stable. It is always wise to consult with the patient's primary physician in order to arrive at an individualized maintenance schedule for the patient until normal function returns, especially if it appears that the patient cannot be stabilized within the first 24 hours. Each diabetic is unique in his response to therapy, and the physician who has been dealing with the patient's diabetes is probably best suited to address the special needs of his patient.

Subcutaneous insulin is probably the safest method of insulin dosage, but a recently developed low-dose IV insulin protocol can be utilized. The utilization of low-dose continuous IV insulin has been suggested as a more physiologic method in treatment of ketoacidosis, but it requires very close monitoring. Many recent review articles detail this method.[1-3] Basically this procedure consists of constant infusion of low-dose regular insulin in saline IV fluid. The dosage and method are summarized in Table 11–2. Utilization of this method requires continual monitoring of glucose, serum pH, and serum ketones. One advantage of this method is that bicarbonate therapy is rarely required in spite of initial low pH or low serum bicarbonate level. Once initiated, this therapy requires at least hourly monitoring of serum glucose and acetone, and in the initial phases, monitoring every half hour is recommended. The critical points in therapy are when the blood glucose begins to fall rapidly and approaches the 300 mg/dl value. At that point, glucose must be added to the IV infusion fluid and IV insulin therapy should be discontinued if the blood glucose falls below 200 mg/dl. Also, if the pH corrects itself to 7.35 or better without the use of bicarbonate, the IV infusion of insulin should be discontinued and subcutaneous injection of regular insulin should be instituted on the dosage schedule suggested in Table 11–1. The great value of this therapy appears to be the maintenance of constant insulin levels as opposed to the erratic absorption of subcutaneous insulin under conditions of shock or hypoperfusion. The disadvantage of IV insulin therapy is the rapidity of falling glucose with resultant hypoglycemia if the patient is not closely monitored.

In recent studies, it appears that the use of human albumin in the constant infusion pump is not necessary to prevent insulin from adhering to the syringe or tubing, but it is recommended that a plastic syringe be utilized instead of glass.[1, 2] It is also imperative that the physician is available throughout therapy and that the staff is closely briefed on the critical points in therapy. In a university hospital we have found this therapy invaluable and very acceptable, but we have the advantage of continual house staff coverage throughout therapy. When constant physician monitoring is unavailable, it is probably wisest to employ the slower but more predictable method of using subcutaneous insulin as opposed to constant infusion owing to the large time commitment required in the initial phases of the latter therapy.

Table 11–2. PROTOCOL FOR CONSTANT IV INSULIN THERAPY

Indications
- BS* ≥ 500 mg/dl
- BS < 500 mg/dl, but ketosis present

Requirements
- Physician supervision
- Initial monitoring of BS, ketones, pH
- Infusion pump system

Initial Preparation
- Regular insulin 0.25 units/kg in 50 cc plastic syringe plus 0.45% NS†
- Begin infusion at 0.06 units regular insulin/kg/hr

Ongoing Therapy
- BS = 300 mg/dl → add glucose to IV‡ fluids
- Serum pH = 7.35 → discontinue IV insulin, begin SQ§ insulin every 2–4 hr
- Continue IV fluids + SQ insulin until oral feeding normal

*BS = blood sugar.
†NS = normal saline.
‡IV = intravenous.
§SQ = subcutaneous.

In summary, treatment of diabetics after major trauma is based on close monitoring of serum glucose, pH, and ketones. If the clinician is acutely aware that the diabetic can become hyperglycemic rapidly after trauma and that therapy must be initiated in the early phases of treatment for trauma, the management of diabetes is quite successful. Unfortunately, the clinician often becomes so involved in the treatment of the trauma that by the time monitoring of diabetes has begun, the patient is already in mild to moderate ketoacidosis. Once the patient is stable and has resumed oral intake along with his routine daily dosage of insulin, he should no longer be considered at high risk for other problems. The well managed diabetic patient in good condition is not more susceptible to infection or poor healing than other individuals. Infection and healing are usually a consequence of poor diabetic control and long-standing hyperglycemia with microvascular disease. In general, most juvenile diabetics receiving adequate medical attention are quite able to handle the stress of trauma and to repair injuries at a normal rate. If there is concern about previous diabetic control, the utilization of a hemoglobin (Hb)-A_{1c} determination may alert the physician to a potentially compromised patient. Hb-A_{1c} is a good marker of sustained hyperglycemia and suggests poor control prior to trauma, which may make the patient a poorer surgical risk. If there is marked elevation of Hb-A_{1c}, the chronic control of the diabetes should be attended to as soon as the patient is stable, and an attempt to achieve "tight" diabetic control is necessary to aid in the healing process. It is rare in the pediatric age range to see severe diabetic renal disease, but in the patient with poor control of blood sugar or inadequate medical care, kidney status should be evaluated. Finally, the best therapy for diabetes is for the patient to return as quickly as possible to a routine activity level, with normal food intake, and previously prescribed insulin dosage.

HYPOGLYCEMIA

The two broad categories of hypoglycemia in children are ketotic and nonketotic hypoglycemia. Nonketotic hypoglycemia is indicated by increased insulin levels or abnormal pituitary function, whereas it is postulated that ketotic hypoglycemia is a defect in peripheral release of amino acids and decreased gluconeogenesis.[4] In general, children with nonketotic hypoglycemia are treated with oral diazoxide, a drug that appears to counteract the peripheral effects of insulin. This drug is very effective in its oral form in treating hypoglycemia, but when given intravenously it can cause severe hypotension and has a very poor effect on glucose maintenance. Therefore, in the rare case in which a child is being treated for trauma and requires diazoxide therapy, the drug should be given only in its enteral form and not intravenously. Many children with nonketotic hypoglycemia require partial or total pancreatectomy early in life.[5] These children are at increased risk for developing diabetes. In dealing with any patient who has had a pancreatectomy, the physician should be alert to changes in blood glucose, which may precipitate a diabetic ketoacidosis.

The major form of therapy for ketotic hypoglycemia is provision of multiple high calorie meals throughout the day. On rare occasions, children with this condition require steroid therapy in order to mobilize peripheral amino acids for gluconeogenesis. If the physician encounters a child with ketotic hypoglycemia who has significant trauma, he should probably utilize IV therapy with glucose and monitor blood glucose closely. Because of the side effects of steroid therapy in acute trauma, it is probably best not to use IV or oral steroids during the immediate post-traumatic period. If the child has been on long-term steroid therapy that may have suppressed adrenal function, then the physician must continue administration of steroids either intravenously or orally. If a continual infusion of IV glucose is established and routine blood glucose measurements obtained, it should be easy to maintain a blood glucose level between 80 and 100 mg/dl. Ketosis is not a metabolic blockade but a result of chronic hypoglycemia, and if blood sugar is maintained in the normal range, there should be no evidence of ketosis. If the child is mildly ketotic, no therapy is required as long as blood glucose is maintained in the normal range. As soon as oral intake is established, most children with ketotic hypoglycemia will do quite well on approximately a six meal per day diet schedule, and the family will in most cases have a specific dietary plan that has been worked out with their physician.

In both ketotic and nonketotic hypoglycemia, if blood glucose is maintained in the normal range, healing and resistance to infection should be normal. Recently there has been an increased tendency for physicians to diagnose hypoglycemia based on an abnormal Glucose Tolerance Test (GTT) when, in fact, the patient has never been clinically hypoglycemic and by history has not been ketotic. In this instance, it is always difficult to decide whether or not therapy is required, but it would be prudent to follow blood sugars and to maintain IV therapy for the first 24 hours. The immediate post-traumatic period is when a child with hypoglycemia is most likely to show severe symptoms. In general it is not necessary to provide a protein source or other calorie source for the patient other than IV glucose.

GALACTOSEMIA AND FRUCTOSEMIA

Galactosemia and fructosemia are hereditary deficiencies of the enzymes required to utilize galactose and fructose, respectively. Galactose is the reducing sugar that is normally associated with glucose as the complex sugar lactose. Fructose and glucose are normally associated as the complex sugar sucrose. If the diagnosis of galactosemia has been made, then the child will be on a lactose- and galactose-free diet, whereas in fructosemia, the child will be on a sucrose- and fructose-free diet. In both instances, the presence of the specific sugar causes severe hypoglycemia and ketosis. The treatment of choice is to remove the offending sugar and utilize IV glucose therapy. If the child has no intake of galactose in galactosemia or fructose in fructosemia, there will be no symptoms. On glucose therapy, the patient should maintain normal blood glucose levels and will do quite well without oral intake. When the patient starts intake, then the offending sugar should be removed from his diet; the parents in most cases are very aware of specific foods that the child can have. During the immediate post-traumatic period, unless exposed to the offending sugar, the child should not have an increased incidence of hypoglycemia or ketosis, and the only necessity is a calorie source to maintain normal blood sugar.

In both galactosemia and fructosemia, it is important for the clinician to remember that children with these disorders, during exposure to the offending sugar, will show a positive Clinitest reaction, in the urine, which can be misinterpreted as spilling glucose. Therefore, any child who presents with a positive Clinitest reaction in the urine for whom a history is not available should be tested with a urine dipstick utilizing glucose oxidase prior to any therapy. Clinitest tablets will detect the presence of all reducing sugars, including galactose and fructose, but the urine dipstick will only react with pure glucose. Therefore, if the Clinitest reaction is positive and the urine dipstick test results are negative, it is possible that the child has galactosemia or fructosemia. It is especially important that this is determined so that the clinician does not attempt to treat a positive urine sugar with insulin in the case of galactosemia or fructosemia. In most instances, when children are spilling these abnormal sugars, their blood glucose may already be quite low and the use of insulin will create a state of severe hypoglycemia. When an injured child is brought into an emergency room and there is no medical history available, it is routine procedure to carry out urine tests using a Clinitest tablet and a urine dipstick on the first voiding to ascertain if any reducing sugars are being spilled in the urine. It is also important to obtain a blood glucose on a child brought in who is unable to give a history.

THYROID DISEASE

Most children with thyroid problems have hypothyroidism, and it is very rare to see hyperthyroidism in the young child. Hyperthyroidism is more associated with the post-pubertal individual. Clinically, children with hypothyroidism or hyperthyroidism can have palpable goiters, and therefore, physical examination alone cannot document which disease state is present.

In general, hypothyroid children are on synthetic thyroid or desiccated thyroid. This oral medication can be missed for 1 to 2 days, but it is advisable to treat within 48 hours of last dosage. The physicians of patients on replacement thyroid therapy should measure serum thyroxine (T_4) concentration at initial examination to verify adequate prior therapy, even if they plan to maintain present dosage. Measurement of thyroid stimulating hormone (TSH) is probably not necessary unless the physician plans to adjust dosage. Children with adequate thyroid hormone replacement should have low TSH levels owing to suppression of the pituitary by normal serum thyroid levels. On adequate thyroid medication, the child will do well in spite of trauma and needs no further therapeutic modality in order to enhance healing.

Hyperthyroidism can be treated surgically or by utilizing thyroid suppressant medicine, such as propylthiouracil. This medication works by binding iodide and preventing excess production of free thyroid. In the case of surgical intervention, most patients remain euthyroid after surgery, but occasionally they become hypothyroid and require medication as noted earlier. There is a possibility that patients under medical therapy with suppressant medication may develop thyroid storm. This can be a true medical emergency and can lead to cardiac arrhythmias and death. In general, impending thyroid storm is heralded by severe tachycardia with or without hyperthermia. This tachycardia can become quite severe and cause a decreased cardiac output with secondary manifestations of poor peripheral perfusion. If the physician suspects impending thyroid storm, a thyroid level can be obtained but usually is not available rapidly enough to be utilized as a diagnostic criterion in the early phase. In most instances the physician will be forced to make the diagnosis on clinical grounds.

The drug of choice for thyroid storm is oral or IV propranolol. The peak effect after oral administration occurs within 1 to 2 hours and the half-life is approximately 3 hours, whereas the peak effect of IV propranolol occurs in a few minutes and the half-life is only 10 minutes. With the use of IV propranolol, there will be rapid control of the tachycardia, but usually heart rate does not return to normal, remaining slightly elevated even after adequate therapy. Propranolol is a beta-adrenergic blocker and therefore should not be used in any patients who have congestive heart failure, severe reactive airway disease, or heart block (second degree or greater) or who are pregnant. It should also not be given in conjunction with other myocardial depressant medications, such as procainamide or quinidine. The dosage used for IV or oral administration should be calculated using body weight with the aid of a pharmacist or pharmacy handbook. Adult dosages should not be given to children owing to the profound side effects of overdosage.When giving propranolol, the physician should be aware that a major complication of its beta-adrenergic blockage is severe hypoglycemia. Therefore, during and after therapy, blood glucose should be monitored closely. Throughout the time that oral propranolol is being utilized, routine blood glucose measurement should be obtained. The severity of hypoglycemia can be quite marked, and it is advisable to be providing IV glucose during therapy.[5] In any patient who is hyperthyroid, cardiac monitoring should be maintained and tachycardia should be followed closely. Partially treated hyperthyroidism can be a major emergency, and the physician should be continually aware of impending thyroid storm throughout the initial phases of therapy for trauma. It is advisable to keep patients with this condition in an intensive care unit until they are stable and there is no evidence of tachycardia or excessive serum thyroid levels, as measured quantitatively. Once the patients are able to take oral medications, they should be placed back on their thyroid suppressant medication.

ADRENAL DISEASE

Chronic diseases of the adrenal glands including congenital adrenal hypoplasia and Addison's disease, require the chronic administration of steroids for maintenance of normal homeostasis. In the case of severe trauma, all patients with chronic adrenal disease, require the addition of excess steroids in order to get through the critical post-traumatic period. In general, the clinician can administer large quantities of steroids for short periods of time without the patient developing serious side effects. Therefore, when a patient comes in for trauma and is on chronic steroid therapy, it is advisable to use a large dose of steroids for up to 3 days and then discontinue the dose. It has been shown that a short-term 3-day dose of steroids does not suppress the adrenal glands adequately to cause major problems, and the dose can be returned to the previous level or discontinued. If the patient is on chronic steroid therapy, it is wise to return to the chronic level and then reduce it if necessary or maintain previous therapeutic regimens. In general, in our emergency room we utilize a dose of 100 mg of hydrocortisone sodium succinate (Solu-Cortef) intravenously immediately and a dose of 100 mg of Solu-Cortef intravenously twice daily for 2 days. Following this dosage, we return to the previous dose employed prior to trauma and do not utilize a schedule of tapering steroids. Serum sodium and potassium should be closely monitored. Sodium replacement by the IV route and steroid replacement should prevent hyponatremia and hyperkalemia. Following initial IV therapy, the patient should be returned to any mineralocorticoid therapy previously used.

AMINOACIDOPATHIES

The aminoacidopathies most commonly seen in children include phenylketonuria, homocystinuria, tyrosinemia, and other disorders of single amino acids. In all instances of aminoacidopathies, the acute treatment of choice is to remove proteins containing the offending amino acids and to maintain adequate calorie balance. Therefore it is recommended that patients be started immediately on IV glucose in order to maintain adequate blood sugar level without added proteins. If patients are maintained on adequate calories, they will not go into negative nitrogen balance and will be well controlled by glucose alone. If patients are given *inadequate* calories, they will go into negative nitrogen balance and break down their own amino acids, causing a secondary problem with the enzyme blockade. When patients are alert and awake and able to take oral fluids, they should resume their previous diet as described by the parents. In general, these patients do very well if given IV fluids but do poorly if they are not allowed to have adequate calories.

ORGANIC ACIDEMIAS

The more common organic acidemias include maple syrup urine disease, methylmalonic acidemia, nonketonic hyperglycinemia, and isovaleric acidemia. All these diseases are hallmarked by acidosis and elevated organic acids in the urine when patients are not on adequate dietary therapy. If these patients suffer acute trauma, the major danger is acidosis. In order to prevent the onset of acidosis, the clinician should remove all protein intake and begin IV therapy with adequate maintenance calories. In general, if adequate sugar is given intravenously, the patient will remain nonacidotic and will not go into negative nitrogen balance, utilizing stored peripheral amino acids. The best laboratory values to follow are the pH, bicarbonate and base deficit, and blood urea nitrogen, looking for negative nitrogen balance. If these are maintained in the normal range with adequate calories and no protein source, the patient can go several days with just IV therapy. The addition of hyperalimentation or an oral protein source can precipitate an acute attack in these patients, and therefore it should be avoided until they are stable. As soon as the patients are stable and can resume oral intake, they should be returned to previous diet as prescribed. In most instances, the family will have specific dietary requirements, or the hospital nutritionist or dietician can supply the diet specific for the disease being treated. Under even the most severe conditions, the removal of protein source and the supplementation with adequate glucose calories will prevent the side-effects of organic acidemias on an acute basis.

REFERENCES

1. Perkin R, Marks J: Low-dose continuous insulin infusion in childhood diabetic ketoacidosis. Clin Pediatr 18:540, 1979.
2. Veeser T, Glines M, Niederman L, Monteleone J: Low-dose intravenous insulin therapy for diabetic ketoacidosis in children. 131:308, 1977.
3. Mauseth R: Treatment of diabetic ketoacidosis. J Clin Endocrinol Metab 21:33, 1979.
4. Gardner L: Is propranolol alone really beneficial in neonatal thyrotoxicosis? Am J Dis Children 134:819, 1980.
5. Mayer T, Matlak ME, Lowry SL, et al.: Protean manifestations of neonatal hyperinsulinism. Ann Surg 194:140, 1981.

CHAPTER

12 Injuries to Children with Chronic Renal Disease

RICHARD L. SIEGLER

NORMAL WATER AND ELECTROLYTE TOLERANCE LIMITS

Individuals with normal kidney function can maintain water and electrolyte balance in spite of wide variations in their intake and output (see Fig. 4–3). Sodium balance can be maintained with intakes as low as 10 mEq/m^2/body surface area/day or as high as 500 mEq/m^2/day. Tolerance limits for potassium are customarily 10 to 250 mEq/m^2/day, and water tolerance limits range from 0.7 to 12 L/m^2/day. Salt (that is, volume) depletion occurs only if salt intake falls below the lower limits of tolerance, and salt excess (edema) develops only if the upper limits of tolerance are exceeded. Similarly, hyperkalemia and hypokalemia do not occur unless the body's upper and lower tolerance limits of potassium are exceeded, respectively. Moreover, water depletion (hypernatremia) only occurs if the intake is less than the lower limits of tolerance; water intoxication (hyponatremia) is seen only if the upper limits of tolerance are exceeded.

THE EFFECT OF KIDNEY DISEASE ON TOLERANCE LIMITS

However, children with chronic renal disease have much narrower limits of tolerance. They are predisposed to abnormalities in body volume and composition, especially during episodes of trauma or illness. Chronic renal disease can be divided into two major categories (Table 12–1). Glomerular disease is characterized by abnormalities that predominantly affect the glomeruli. Tubulointerstitial disease, on the other hand, is distinguished by the abnormal structure and function of the tubules and the connective tissue (interstitium) that occupies the spaces between the nephron units. Patients with glomerular diseases have different limits of tolerance than those with tubulointerstitial diseases (Fig. 12–1).

Children with glomerular disease (e.g., glomerulonephritis, membranous glomerulopathy, focal segmental sclerosis, minimal change disease) tend to have lower maximum limits of sodium tolerance and therefore are predisposed to develop an excess of salt, which results in edema unless salt intake is restricted. Moreover, these patients often develop hypoalbuminemia, which in turn results in a contracted effective arterial blood volume and an inability to generate and excrete free water normally. Since water intake normally exceeds that of sodium (i.e., the sodium concentration of the diet is less than 140 mEq/L), these children tend to retain water in excess of their salt intake and develop hyponatremia, or water intoxication.

On the other hand, patients with tubulointerstitial disease (e.g., obstructive uropathy, reflux nephropathy, interstitial nephritis) but not in renal failure, tend to have higher than normal minimum limits of sodium and water tolerance. That is, because of their tubulointerstitial disease, they have an impaired ability to conserve salt and water appropriately. This predisposes them to salt and water depletion, especially during periods of decreased salt and water intake or during episodes of increased loss (e.g., gastroenteritis, nasogastric suction). On occasion, an inability to respond to aldosterone appropriately causes an impaired distal tubular sodium-potassium and sodium-hydrogen exchange and results in hyperkalemia and renal tubular acidosis (Type IV RTA).

Moreover, although patients with glomerular disease tend to be sodium retainers and those with tubulointerstitial disease tend to be salt and water losers, advanced renal failure usually converts both groups into fluid and electrolyte retainers; that is, once the glomerular filtration rate (GFR) drops much below 5 per cent of normal, any tendency of the tubules to reject salt and water inappropriately is offset by the very limited filtration of water and electrolytes. At this point, retention of water, salt, potassium, magnesium, and phosphate can be antici-

Table 12–1. CLINICAL CHARACTERISTICS OF CHRONIC RENAL DISEASE

	Glomerular Disease	Interstitial Disease
Pathophysiology	Low sodium tolerance Albumin loss Sodium retention	Failure to conserve sodium Normal albumin Free water deficit
Clinical Findings	Edema Hypoalbuminemia Short stature Anemia	Decreased total body water Short stature Anemia
Urinalysis	Proteinuria Red blood cells Casts	No proteinuria Normal sediment Dilute urine (sp gr* < 1.010)
Fluid Therapy	Fluid overload common	Fluid requirements increased
Implications	Monitor fluid therapy closely Monitor sodium closely Early monitoring of PCWP†	Large volumes may be necessary Inappropriate polyuria Early monitoring of PCWP

*Sp gr = urine specific gravity.
†PCWP = pulmonary capillary wedge pressure.

pated unless the intake of these substances is appropriately restricted.

IDENTIFYING AND ASSESSING CHILDREN WITH CHRONIC RENAL DISEASE

If the abnormalities in fluid and electrolyte balance described previously are to be avoided, it is important that the traumatized child who also happens to suffer from chronic renal disease be identified promptly.

Physical Characteristics

Children with long-standing severe renal disease tend to be short and thin; those with glomerular disease, especially those with heavy proteinuria (nephrotic syndrome) may present with edema. The edema is usually most prominent in the periorbital areas, the pretibial region, and the ankles. Occasionally there may be total body edema (anasarca). The child may be cushingoid as a consequence of the use of glucocorticoids. If the child has renal insufficiency (azotemia), a (normochromic, normocytic) anemia will usually be present, but the chronic anemia may be difficult to detect in a traumatized child who has been bleeding. If the child has been on hemodialysis, scars and needle tracks resulting from fistula construction and use should be obvious on either the arms or the legs. Blunt trauma or hypovolemia often causes such fistulas to clot and results in a loss of the characteristic bruit. If the child is currently being treated with chronic peritoneal dialysis there will be a peritoneal cath-

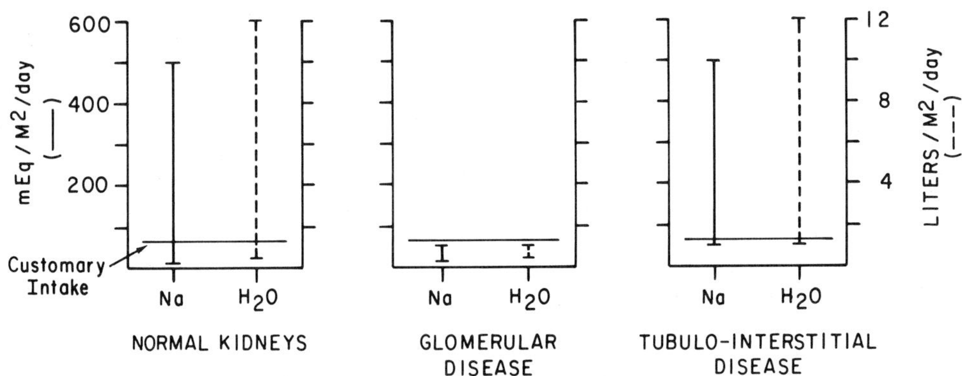

Figure 12–1. Depiction of the customary intake of sodium and water, as well as the upper and lower limits of tolerance for normal children and for those with glomerular and tubulointerstitial disease. Salt and water retention occurs if intake exceeds maximum (upper) tolerance limits; salt and water depletion occurs if intake is less than the minimum limits of tolerance.

eter (e.g., Tenckhoff) exiting from the abdominal wall. A post-renal transplant patient will have a generous scar on the lower abdomen. Scars in the region of the bladder or the flank should alert the physician to the likelihood of reflux nephropathy or hydronephrosis, respectively. Children, especially young children, with long-standing renal insufficiency may have obvious osteodystrophy, manifested by distal flaring of the long bones, bowed legs, valgus deformities of the knees, or osteotomy scars.

Laboratory Features

The urine of children with glomerular disease usually contains substantial amounts of protein (3 to 4 plus); red and white cells and casts are customarily present with glomerulonephritis. Red cell casts may also be seen.

However, children with tubulointerstitial disease may have little or no proteinuria and an unremarkable urinary sediment, in spite of advanced renal parenchymal damage. A dilute urine (specific gravity [sp gr] < 1.010) may be the only clue of an underlying renal problem for these children.

A serum creatinine concentration greater than 1.0 mg/dl is usually abnormal in a girl or a preadolescent boy and indicates an impaired GFR (i.e., renal insufficiency). This value may be difficult to interpret in a traumatized child who may also be experiencing prerenal azotemia or early acute renal parenchymal failure (ARPF), i.e., acute tubular necrosis. If the injury precedes the serum creatinine determination by only a few hours or so, the serum creatinine concentration should still be nearly normal in spite of the more recent renal hemodynamic changes. In these circumstances, serum creatinine values greater than 1.5 to 2.0 mg/dl should constitute presumptive evidence of pre-existing renal disease. Moreover, even though isosthenuria (sp gr 1.010 to 1.012) is characteristic of fully established ARPF, one would not expect isosthenuria to be present during the first few hours of an evolving ARPF, and it should suggest pre-existing renal damage. The presence of a hyperchloremic metabolic acidosis should lead one to suspect chronic renal failure or renal tubular acidosis. The acidosis seen with trauma and tissue hypoperfusion (lactic acidosis) is associated with a normal, rather than an elevated, serum chloride concentration.

Estimating the Magnitude of Chronic Renal Failure

Reviewing any recent pre-trauma laboratory medical records is the most accurate way of assessing the magnitude of any pre-existing chronic renal damage. Recall that a normal serum creatinine concentration is 0.5 to 0.7 mg/dl in a young child. A serum creatinine concentration of 1 to 1.4 mg/dl, therefore, translates into a corrected GFR of only 50 per cent of normal. Moreover, a serum creatinine value of 2.0 mg/dl in a young child translates into a GFR of approximately 25 per cent of normal. However, this relationship between the serum creatinine concentration and the GFR only holds true if the child is in a steady state at the time of the measurement, i.e., the rate of creatinine excretion is equal to the rate of production. A traumatized child is obviously in a very dynamic non–steady state. Therefore, it is impossible to use a single post-traumatic serum creatinine measurement to accurately assess the magnitude of renal insufficiency.

FURTHER DETERIORATION OF RENAL FUNCTION FOLLOWING TRAUMA

A chronically diseased kidney may be less able to autoregulate in response to variations in the renal perfusion pressure; that is, although a normal kidney is able to maintain a constant GFR over a wide range of perfusion pressures, the GFR in a diseased kidney is likely to fall with even modest decreases in renal perfusion pressure. Therefore, after trauma, one should anticipate a much greater rise in the blood urea nitrogen (BUN) level and serum creatinine concentration in a child with chronic renal disease than in a child with normal kidneys.

Individuals with chronic renal insufficiency are also predisposed to develop superimposed acute renal failure (ARF) when given iodine-containing radiographic contrast materials. Although there are times when intravenous pyelography (IVP) or angiography is clearly needed, ultrasound or computerized tomography (CT) scanning should be used instead whenever possible.

EFFECT OF TRAUMA ON HOMEOSTASIS

Even if the trauma does not result in a further deterioration in kidney function, the effect of trauma, secondary infection, and hypercatabolism can cause profound changes in the body's urea pool, in the acid-base balance, and in the serum electrolyte and mineral concentration (Table 12–2).

The hypercatabolism subsequent to trauma and infection can substantially add to the urea nitrogen pool. Therefore, one should anticipate additional prerenal azotemia in children with chronic renal insufficiency because of their limited ability to filter the increased nitrogen load. This prerenal azotemia is most pronounced in children with extensive burns and in those whose course is complicated by sepsis.

Because of the high intracellular concentration of potassium (150 mEq/L), crush injuries, burns, acidosis, and sepsis cause the release of massive amounts of potassium into the extracellular compartment. In addition, the reabsorption of red blood cell potassium, resulting from hematomas or GI bleeding, will cause a similar rise in the serum potassium concentration. Therefore, one should be on the alert for life-threatening hyperkalemia in children with chronic renal insufficiency who also have sustained trauma.

The intracellular compartment also contains generous quantities of phosphate (40 mEq/L), which is released into the extracellular compartment after cellular damage. In the presence of renal insufficiency, this results in hyperphosphatemia and secondary hypocalcemia. For this reason, the serum calcium and phosphorus concentrations should be carefully monitored in children sustaining severe tissue damage (e.g., crush injuries, burns).

Whereas the normal kidney responds to metabolic acidosis by increasing the secretion of hydrogen ions, the diseased kidney has an impaired ability to respond to this challenge. One should then anticipate a more severe and prolonged metabolic acidosis subsequent to the decreased tissue perfusion that usually follows trauma.

Table 12–2. EFFECTS OF TRAUMA ON RENAL FUNCTION

Hypercatabolism (trauma, burns, sepsis)
Increased nitrogen load (prerenal azotemia)
Increased potassiumn load (acidosis, burns, crush injuries, sepsis)
Increased phosphate load with secondary hypocalcemia
Prolonged acidosis (impaired hydrogen ion secretion)

RESUSCITATION FLUID THERAPY IN CHILDREN WITH CHRONIC RENAL DISEASE

The general principles of resuscitation fluid therapy are identical for all patients irrespective of renal function. However, in the presence of renal disease, one has to be precise when administering water and electrolytes because of the kidney's limited ability to make appropriate compensatory adjustments. Thus, it is necessary to monitor both body volume and composition closely during resuscitation (see Table 12–1).

Children with chronic tubulointerstitial disease (e.g, hydronephrosis, reflux nephropathy) who have not yet progressed into advanced renal failure have an impaired ability to conserve salt and water in spite of volume depletion. These children may therefore continue to have an inappropriate polyuria and saluresis that can worsen the hypovolemia.

Children with glomerular disease and children with advanced renal failure have an impaired ability to excrete any excess salt or water that might be administered during resuscitation. As a result, these children are predisposed to hypervolemia. It is therefore advisable to insert central venous pressure lines or pulmonary artery flotation (Swan-Ganz) catheters in these children to monitor preload accurately.

Renal disease also predisposes children to abnormalities in the serum sodium concentration (i.e., hyper- or hyponatremia). Children with tubulointerstitial disease fail to conserve water, and children with glomerular disease and those in advanced renal failure have an impaired ability to excrete a water load. Therefore, children who have sustained trauma may present with either hyper- or hyponatremia. However, serum sodium concentration abnormalities will be minimized if appropriate resuscitation fluids (e.g., 0.9 per cent saline, lactated Ringer's solution, blood components) are used.

The serum potassium concentration must also be monitored closely. Although the amount of potassium contained in Ringer's lactate solution, blood, and plasma should not elevate the serum potassium concentration appreciably, resuscitation fluids containing unphysiologic concentrations of potassium (i.e., > 4.0 mEq/L) should certainly be avoided. If a child presents with hyperkalemia, which can be anticipated following the type of severe cellular damage seen with crush injuries and burns, it is preferable to give potassium-free solutions. This should result in a modest decrease in the serum potassium concentration as a result of expanding (that is, diluting) the extracellular compartment.

Hyponatremia (serum sodium < 130 mEq/L) in a hypovolemic patient indicates a need to give salt in excess of water. As traumatized children generally already have a metabolic acidosis, this can be accomplished by infusing hypertonic sodium bicarbonate solutions or by adding sodium bicarbonate to saline solutions. However, one must be cautious in administering hypertonic sodium chloride or sodium bicarbonate to children with renal insufficiency because they excrete excess sodium or bicarbonate very slowly. The risks of producing metabolic alkalosis, hypervolemia, or hypernatremia are substantial.

MAINTENANCE FLUID AND ELECTROLYTE THERAPY

One's latitude in prescribing maintenance fluids following resuscitation depends on the type and magnitude of the chronic renal disease. As indicated in Figure 12–1, until advanced renal failure occurs, patients with tubulointerstitial disorders tend to lose salt and water inappropriately. Conversely, children with glomerular diseases tend to retain salt and water. Therefore, patients with tubulointerstitial disease may require more than the usual amount of salt and water to maintain homeostasis, whereas those with glomerular diseases may require salt and water restriction (see Table 12–1).

Total body sodium is the major determinant of extracellular volume. Therefore, performing periodic assessments of the extracellular volume by measuring the body weight, by examining the child for the presence or absence of dehydration or edema, and, in some cases, by monitoring the central venous or pulmonary artery wedge pressure offers means for determining the need for sodium chloride. A contracted extracellular volume indicates the need for additional sodium chloride, whereas an expanded extracellular compartment (e.g., edema) indicates the need for salt restriction.

Measuring the serum sodium concentration offers a reliable means for determining the need for water. A serum sodium concentration that is falling below normal in a nondehydrated patient indicates a need for water restriction, whereas a serum sodium concentration that is rising above normal indicates a need for increasing the administration of free water.

If a child develops hypokalemia, potassium needs to be given, irrespective of the degree of renal insufficiency. Although mild to moderate hypokalemia should be treated cautiously (0.05 to 0.1 mEq/kg/hour), potassium doses as high as 0.5 to 1.0 mEq/kg/hour can be administered in instances of life-threatening hypokalemia. These large doses should only be given if the patient is under constant cardiac monitoring and is having the serum potassium concentration checked frequently. The margin of safety is obviously much less in children with advanced renal insufficiency, since the kidney will be unable to excrete any excess potassium appropriately.

Calcium, phosphorous, magnesium, and bicarbonate needs should be determined by monitoring the serum concentrations.

If one is uncertain as to the degree of renal insufficiency, if the patient remains oliguric following fluid resuscitation, or if the patient is known to have advanced renal disease, it is safest to match the volume and composition of the infusate to the child's water and electrolyte output. Net insensible free water loss, that is, evaporative loss from the lung and skin, minus the water of oxidation, equals approximately 350 ml/m^2/day. To this, one must add any urinary and intestinal losses. The volume and composition of urinary and intestinal losses should be measured to permit accurate replacement. Even when following these guidelines, periodic assessments of the extracellular volume and the serum electrolyte concentrations are necessary to avoid upsetting the fluid and electrolyte balance.

THE CHILD ON MEDICATIONS

Children with kidney disease may be on a variety of medications, including diuretics, antihypertensives, glucocorticoids, and immunosuppressives. Although children on high-dose steroids will have an obvious cushingoid appearance, there is no reliable way of identifying children on diuretic, antihypertensive, and immunosuppressive agents unless one has access to the child's medical records or has an accurate drug history. If there are physical signs of dialysis treatments or transplantation, one should assume multiple medication use.

The ingestion of a diuretic agent immediately prior to trauma will temporarily impair the kidney's ability to conserve salt and water and, as a consequence, to respond to hemorrhage. Antihypertensive agents, particularly the longer-acting central agents (e.g., methyldopa, clonidine) and the beta-adrenergic blocking agents (e.g., propranolol) may inhibit the normal cardiovascular response to hypovolemia by causing vasodilatation, a decreased sympathetic outflow from the brain, or a reduced cardiac output. Although the renin-angiotensin system normally plays little or no role in blood pressure control, it appears to be important in maintaining the blood pressure in the hypovolemic individual. Therefore, children on drugs that inhibit the release of renin, which include the beta-adrenergic blocking agents and the central-acting antihypertensives, may experience exaggerated hypotension following blood loss. Patients taking the angiotensin-converting enzyme inhibitor captopril may be particularly predisposed to hypotension following blood loss because of an impaired ability to convert angiotensin I to the powerful vasoconstrictor angiotensin II.

Children who have the nephrotic syndrome or glomerulonephritis or who have received a kidney transplant may be receiving immunosuppressive agents (e.g., cyclosporin, azathioprine, chlorambucil, cyclophosphamide). These agents will predispose the child to post-traumatic infection because of their inhibition of cellular or humoral immunity.

Children on therapeutic doses of glucocorticoids will begin to experience adrenal suppression within the first week of therapy. And the hypoadrenalism may persist for as long as 6 to 12 months after discontinuation of therapy. Therefore, if a child has been on glucocorticoids during the past year, it is prudent to administer physiologic stress doses of the glucocorticoid during the immediate post-traumatic period (e.g., hydrocortisone 1 to 1.5 mg/kg of body weight every 6 hours). Note that the physiologic stress doses are much lower than those recommended for the treatment of shock. The dosage should be tapered to a maintenance schedule (e.g., hydrocortisone, 0.3 mg/kg/day) as soon as possible because high doses impair wound healing and predispose patients to infection.

MEDICATIONS AND RENAL FAILURE

Chronic renal failure can affect the serum half-life of those medications excreted by the kidneys and can increase the serum concentration of the free (biologically active) fraction of protein-bound drugs. Therefore, in cases of renal failure, drug dosage modification is often necessary. Therapeutic guidelines for dosage modification are summarized in Table 7–5. The table is not intended to be extensive, and only approximate serum half-life and dosage modification guidelines are given.

THE CHILD ON HEMODIALYSIS

Although the incidence of end-stage renal disease (ESRD) is low in the pediatric population (1 to 3 cases/million population/year), it is important that dialysis patients be identified as soon as possible after their injury.

In addition to the previously discussed problems that should be anticipated in any child with advanced renal disease, children on hemodialysis are likely to experience special problems. Access to hemodialysis is almost always via a subcutaneous fistula. These fistulas are customarily constructed in the left upper or lower arm, although occasionally they may be in the dominant (right) arm or in the inner surface of the upper thigh. Although native arteries are customarily anastomosed to adjacent veins, synthetic materials (e.g., Gortex) or bovine grafts are sometimes used. The patency of a fistula is threatened if it has sustained trauma or if the patient develops shock. The absence of a bruit, best noted by auscultation over the fistula, indicates a loss of patency. Patency sometimes can be re-established by direct infusion of low doses of streptokinase (2500 to 5000 units/hour) into the downstream edge of the thrombus or by removal of the clot with a Fogarty catheter. If the fistula remains nonfunctional, a femoral or a subclavian catheter can be inserted to obtain temporary vascular access.

The traumatized child generally requires more frequent dialysis and is more likely to experience dialysis-related complications. Initiating a dialysis treatment opens a large arterial-venous shunt, which customarily requires an increase in cardiac output. If the patient is already hypovolemic from blood loss and is already experiencing a compensatory increase in cardiac rate and stroke volume, the additional strain of hemodialysis can cause circulatory collapse. Moreover, because of the intrinsic resistance in the venous side of the fistula, which produces a transmembrane pressure differential, a certain amount of ultrafiltration (fluid removal) is usually inevitable. This, too, may intensify hypovolemia and can cause hypovolemic shock. In the severely injured child, it is imperative that ongoing cardiovascular monitoring, preferably with a pulmonary artery flotation catheter, be performed during hemodialysis. Dialysis should be started cautiously. The volume of the system (dialyzer plus blood lines) should not exceed 10 per cent of the child's blood volume, the pump speed should be slow, and a modest-sized dialyzer (dialysis surface area $<$ 75 per cent of the patient's body surface area) should be used. The dialysis team must be supplied with generous amounts of both crystalloid (normal saline) and colloid (plasma, albumin) to treat any changes in blood pressure or circulatory volume.

The composition of the dialysate may need to be tailored to the individual. If hyperkalemia is present, the potassium concentration in the dialysate should be decreased (e.g., 1 mEq/l) and sometimes eliminated. Although discussion continues regarding the advantages of using bicarbonate in place of acetate as the dialysate buffer, acetate may impair cardiac performance and cause vasodilatation. For this reason, it is prudent to use bicarbonate dialysis in severely injured children.

Total body heparinization is customarily used during dialysis to prevent occlusion of the dialyzer by fibrin. Obviously, it is dangerous to give heparin to a bleeding patient. Moreover, azotemic patients already have a qualitative platelet defect characterized by impaired platelet adhesiveness. Therefore, every effort should be made to avoid systemic anticoagulation in a child who has experienced bleeding within the past 24 hours; dialysis can be conducted using regional heparinization. This requires the infusion of heparin into the arterial (inflow) arm and protamine sulfate into the venous outflow side. This limits heparin's action to the extracorporeal system and prevents it from entering the patient's circulation. However, the process is technically difficult, and the administration of excess protamine can also have anticoagulant effects. Regional citrate anticoagulation, and the infusion of prostacyclin have also been used successfully in lieu of heparin. An additional, and simpler, method to maintain dialyzer patency without heparin is simply to flush a hollow-fiber dialyzer every 15 minutes with normal saline. Although this adds to the patient's extracellular volume, the excess volume can be removed by ultrafiltration.

Because of the injured child's hypercatabolic state and the resulting accentuated azotemia, acidosis, hyperkalemia, and hyperphosphatemia, daily dialysis is generally necessary. The duration of the individual dialysis sessions ranges from between 3 and 5 hours. The frequency and length of the dialysis therapy should be designed to keep the predialysis blood urea nitrogen (BUN) levels less than 100 mg/dl, and the predialysis potassium concentrations less than 6 mg/dl. Please refer to Chapter 7 for additional suggestions.

THE CHILD ON PERITONEAL DIALYSIS

Peritoneal dialysis (PD), performed either as chronic ambulatory peritoneal dialysis (CAPD) or nightly, as continuous cyclic peritoneal dialysis CCPD), is becoming increasingly popular. Peritoneal access is obtained through the use of a permanently placed catheter. Catheter insertion through the anterior abdominal wall incorporates a subcutaneous tunnel, which is designed to inhibit the inward migration of bacteria and thus prevent peritonitis. If a child on PD sustains abdominal trauma, the catheter can be used to assess internal bleeding. Moreover, dialysis can be performed in spite of abdominal injuries, although the presence of intra-abdominal hemorrhage is likely to occlude the catheter. Although heparin is customarily added to the dialysate, its addition to the dialysate of a child suffering from severe abdominal trauma and hemorrhage is unwise. For these reasons, serious internal bleeding should be controlled before PD therapy is started.

PD is never as efficient as hemodialysis in removing potassium and nitrogenous waste products. Its efficiency will be further compromised in the presence of hypovolemia or septic shock. These conditions often impair splanchnic blood flow and, thereby, impair the clearance of nitrogenous waste products and electrolytes from the patient's circulation. In addition, severe tissue injury (e.g., crush injury, burns) and the hypercatabolism resulting from trauma or sepsis may add urea, potassium, phosphate, and acid to the extracellular pool faster than they can be removed with PD. Under these circumstances, hemodialysis will be necessary.

THE POSTRENAL TRANSPLANT PATIENT

Kidney transplants (allografts) are now being performed in children weighing as little as 15 to 20 lb. In the very small child, the donor kidney is placed in the right retrocolic position and attached to the aorta and inferior vena cava. In the larger child and adolescent, the kidney is placed in the pelvis and anastamosed to the inferior epigastric artery and vein. The donor ureter is customarily reimplanted into the native bladder, although occasionally it may be inserted into an ileal conduit. In either position, the kidney is sufficiently anterior and exposed to sustain damage in instances of abdominal trauma. Blunt trauma to the graft can result in a ruptured vascular pedicle with rapid exsanguination. Trauma can also cause renal laceration. Diagnostic studies such as renal ultrasound, IVP, angiography, and retrograde pyelography should be performed whenever allograft trauma is suspected. Rapid intervention may allow salvage of the graft as well as the patient.

Another important consideration to remember is that all post-transplant patients receive immunosuppressives (e.g., azathioprine, cyclosporin A) and steroids (e.g. prednisone). Azathioprine or cyclosporin A may need to be withheld after trauma when complicated by infection, but stress doses of steroids must be administered to avoid hypoadrenal shock.

CHAPTER

13 Injuries to Children with Chronic Lung Diseases

JOHN L. COLOMBO

It is estimated that there are over 10 million children in the United States with chronic respiratory illness. This represents approximately two thirds of all children under 17 years of age with any type of chronic illness. Many of these children have relatively minor illness, such as chronic sinusitis or hay fever. However, approximately 20 per cent, or 2 million of these children have asthma. Because children with cystic fibrosis (CF) now live longer than previously, there are a larger number of children with this disease. Bronchopulmonary dysplasia is more common today than in the past because of the improved survival of extremely premature babies with hyaline membrane disease.

Although these disorders are quite diverse as to etiology, prognosis, and treatment, they share one important feature: Children with chronic respiratory disease have less pulmonary reserve and are therefore at risk for development of acute respiratory failure when there is relatively minor insult to the lung. Some general factors of pediatric lung pathophysiology will be discussed in this first section. Problems pertaining to the most common specific disease processes will then be considered.

PATHOPHYSIOLOGY

Respiratory pathophysiology involves disorders of four major areas: (1) ventilation, (2) perfusion, (3) diffusion, and (4) control of ventilation. Frequently more than one of these is disturbed in a child with chronic lung disease.

Ventilation disorder is probably the most common abnormality seen, particularly in the pediatric age group. This relates partly to airway size, which, in turn, correlates with airway resistance.

Airway resistance is inversely proportional to airway radius to the 4th power. A 1 mm reduction in diameter in the adult trachea produces approximately a 25 per cent decrease in cross-sectional area. However, the same amount of narrowing in the infant trachea produces a 75 per cent reduction in cross-sectional area. Although not as dramatic, the narrower airway diameter extends throughout the bronchi, bronchioles, and alveoli. This inherent smallness is most likely the primary explanation for why the acute syndromes of croup and bronchiolitis are largely found in young children. The child who has the additional burden of chronic lung disease is at extremely high risk for acute ventilatory failure. The chronically ill child with respiratory disease may be unable to compensate with increased ventilation if his metabolic needs are increased, regardless of direct acute lung insult.

Abnormalities in the ventilation-perfusion relationship account for most of the hypoxemia seen with lung disease. Although hypercapnia is not uncommon in the child with chronic lung disease, hypoxemia is far more frequently seen. The carbon dioxide content of the blood varies linearly with Pa_{CO_2}, reflecting the fact that well-ventilated groups of alveoli hyperventilate and compensate for poorly ventilated groups of alveoli, thus producing a normal arterial carbon dioxide tension. However, the oxygen content of the blood increases proportionately with Pa_{O_2} only up to approximately 60 mm Hg; thereafter there is very little increase in oxygen content in spite of increasing partial pressure. Thus arterial oxygen cannot be significantly increased by compensation from hyperventilation of alveoli when there are large numbers of poorly ventilated alveoli.

The amount of oxygen necessary to prevent tissue hypoxia is determined by the oxygen-hemoglobin dissociation curve, hemoglobin concentration, and cardiac output. Because of the steep portion of the oxygen dissociation curve below Pa_{O_2} of 60 mm Hg, it is desirable to maintain the Pa_{O_2} in the range of 60 to 100 mm Hg. Because 99.98 per cent of the oxygen content is hemoglobin-bound oxygen, it is important to consider the hemoglobin concentration when dealing with a child with chronic or acute respiratory disease. The child with chronic lung disease may not have developed a compensatory polycythemia because of the short duration of his illness or nutritional factors.

Also, the child with cystic fibrosis rarely becomes polycythemic. Although the child may have adapted by other mechanisms to the chronic nature of his hypoxemia, a small amount of acute blood loss may cause critical decompensation in the tissue oxygen delivery.

Brief mention of the lack of utility of cyanosis as a physical sign should be made. The normally lower hemoglobin concentration of the young child, as well as the lack of polycythemia, make cyanosis a very late sign in the hypoxemic patient. Most observers do not perceive cyanosis, even in the normal adult, until arterial oxygen saturation is 80 per cent or lower. Therefore, measurement of arterial blood gases is probably more often indicated in the child with respiratory disease than in the adult. The choice of site for arterial puncture is similar to that in the adult, with the radial and then brachial arteries as first and second choices. Physicians should not let the small size of an artery disuade them from obtaining arterial blood gases whenever there is suspicion of abnormal gas exchange. When evaluating the child with underlying respiratory disease, measurement of arterial blood gases is the single most informative study to determine present status.

BRONCHOPULMONARY DYSPLASIA

Bronchopulmonary dysplasia is a syndrome of chronic lung disease that develops in infants with hyaline membrane disease. Various etiologic factors have been proposed, including positive pressure ventilation, high inspired oxygen tensions, endotracheal intubation, patent ductus arteriosus, and excess fluid administration. Probably the most important factors relate to the use of high positive pressures and high oxygen concentrations. Estimates of incidence of bronchopulmonary dysplasia range from 11 to 21 per cent in infants with severe hyaline membrane disease treated with positive pressure ventilation and supplemental oxygen for greater than 24 hours.[1] The overall incidence in infants with hyaline membrane disease ranges from 1 to 8 per cent.[2]

The degree of disability in children with bronchopulmonary dysplasia is quite variable. Some children have normal chest x-ray films and no clinical problems other than mild lower respiratory tract symptoms when they develop a viral upper respiratory infection (URI). At the other end of the spectrum are children with marked pulmonary disability. Chest radiographs show varying degrees of atelectasis (usually subsegmental) and areas of hyperinflation. Pulmonary function studies of surviving children with bronchopulmonary dysplasia show obstructive disease, which is often partially reversible with bronchodilator therapy. They also show bronchial hyperreactivity to methacholine challenge.[3] It has been reported that 37 per cent of infants surviving with severe bronchopulmonary dysplasia become clinically normal by 3 years of age.[4] It is not likely that this group of children will present with any major respiratory problems related to or associated with trauma. However, even children in this group may behave much like those with asthma, and this should be appreciated.

Other children with bronchopulmonary dysplasia are not so fortunate to have only mild or occasional respiratory dysfunction. Many have very borderline adequate pulmonary function. Respiratory rates of 60 to 80 breaths/minute in the quiet child are common. These children are chronically hypoxemic and sometimes hypercarbic. There is frequently significant cor pulmonale, and many of these children are on chronic supplemental oxygen therapy at home. Most of these children are on chronic diuretic therapy, and resultant electrolyte imbalance should be considered in any such child presenting to the emergency room. Chronic bronchodilator therapy is also used in most patients with significant bronchopulmonary dysplasia. Because of the borderline respiratory status of some patients, it is very important to obtain a history of such therapy and to continue it while managing the child's other acute problems. Steroid therapy is occasionally used for such patients and this should be ascertained for any such child presenting with acute trauma. If no history is available, it is probably best to administer steroids in a pharmacologic dose. Appropriate dosage is hydrocortisone 6 to 7 mg/kg initially, followed by 2 to 3 mg/kg every 4 to 6 hours.

The degree of chest abnormality shown radiographically frequently does not correlate well with the current clinical condition of the patient. It is not uncommon for the chest film to continue to show significant abnormality, with generalized hyperinflation and areas of infiltrates (atelectasis), cysts, and localized emphysema, when the clinical status of the child is actually mild or even normal. These chest film changes can be mistaken for congenital lobar emphysema, pneumonia, contusion, and even pneumothorax. The opposite end of this clinical spectrum is less common, but patients with relatively mild changes on chest film may have very significant ventilation-perfusion mismatching and/or reactive airway disease causing significant hypoxemia. It is important to assess the child clinically with a good physical examination and measurement of blood gases, paying particular attention to the serum pH. Old chest films for comparison can be very useful.

ASTHMA

Asthma is generally less serious and certainly less productive of multi-organ involvement than cystic fibrosis. However, it is nevertheless very important to be familiar with this disorder because of its extremely high incidence and potential seriousness in children. Estimates of the incidence of asthma in childhood range from 3 to 5 per cent or greater.[5, 6] Mortality of children with asthma is low (estimated 1 in 20,000 asthmatic children/year).[7] However, the risk of death in the severely asthmatic child is real, particularly if the degree of severity of the asthma is not recognized.

The purpose of this section is not to discuss in detail the diagnosis and treatment of asthma. However, since trauma or stress may precipitate an asthma attack, a brief discussion of physical signs and their relationship to the degree of airway obstruction is warranted. Recognition of these signs should serve as a warning signal that the patient's asthma, in addition to coexisting problems, warrants prompt attention. Commey and Levinson[8] studied 62 asthmatic children and showed only two physical findings that clearly correlated with severity of airway obstruction. These were sternocleidomastoid contraction and supraclavicular indrawing. These two findings were invariably associated with pulmonary function values indicative of moderately severe or greater airway obstruction. Sternocleidomastoid contractions correlated with the greatest degree of impairment. Pulsus paradoxus has also been shown to be an extremely valuable physical sign, correlating with the degree of airway obstruction and blood gas alteration. A pulsus paradoxus measurement of 10 mm Hg or greater has been found to be correlated with moderate to severe asthma. A pulsus paradoxus of 20 mm Hg or greater is highly suggestive of carbon dioxide retention and ventilatory failure.[9] The value of pulsus paradoxus in assessing the child with status asthmaticus is difficult to overstate. A brief mention of methodology for obtaining pulsus paradoxus in the rapidly breathing child is probably necessary. The blood pressure is taken in the usual manner, but since it is usually not possible to accurately correlate a particular pressure with a phase of the respiratory cycle, the following modification is useful. The systolic pressure reading of first sounds heard when irregular fading pulse begins is noted. Then the cuff is deflated very slowly until the sounds become uniform in intensity. The difference between these two systolic pressure readings gives the value of pulsus paradoxus.

The preceding physical findings are highly suggestive of moderately severe or greater airway obstruction from asthma. Finding them in the patient with asthma who has suffered trauma would suggest the need for further evaluation and treatment, including measurement of arterial blood gases.

For initial treatment of severe asthma in the child, there are two generally accepted modes of initial therapy. Drugs and dosages are listed in Table 13–1. The initial treatment of choice in some institutions is the use of an aerosolized bronchodilator such as isoetharine (Bronkosol) or metaproterenol. Isoproterenol is sometimes preferred in severe cases; fortunately the beta 1 cardiac side effects are much less likely to be harmful in the child who normally has good coronary artery supply.

The mainstay of therapy at many institutions remains epinephrine 1:1000, 0.01 ml/kg, up to a maximum of 0.5 ml. This can be given subcutaneously and, if some response is noted, can be repeated two times at 20-minute intervals. Depending on the type of trauma and the condition of the patient, there obviously may not be optimal time for aerosol treatments and this would make the use of epinephrine advantageous. At the same time IV aminophylline should be started. It is best to obtain a stat theophylline level and base initial therapy on this level. Usual desired therapeutic level is in the range of 10 to 20 μg/ml. A fairly accurate rule of thumb for estimating the loading dose of aminophylline based on serum levels is as follows: A dose of 1 mg/kg raises the blood level approxi-

Table 13–1. DRUG THERAPY OF ACUTE ASTHMA IN CHILDREN

Drug	Dosage
Epinephrine 1:1000	0.01 ml/kg/dose (max. 0.5 ml) subcutaneous may repeat × 2 in 20 minute intervals
Epinephrine suspension 1:200 (Susphrine)	0.005 ml/kg/dose (max. 0.2 ml), subcutaneous
Aminophylline	Loading dose: 7 mg/kg IV over 20 minutes, with initial maintenance dose based on age as follows: 2–6 months, 0.5 mg/kg/h; 6–12 months, 0.9 mg/kg/h; 1–9 years, 1.1 mg/kg/h; 9–16 years, 0.9 mg/kg/h; greater than 16 years, 0.7 mg/kg/h
Isoetharine 1%	0.25–0.5 ml in 3 ml saline by aerosol q 1–6 h
Isoproterenol 0.5%	0.25–0.5 ml in 3 ml saline q 1–6 h
Metaproterenol 5%*	0.1–0.25 ml in 3 ml saline q 2–6 h
Albuterol 0.5%*	0.2–1 ml in 3 ml saline q 2–6 h
Atropine 1 mg/ml†	0.1 mg/kg, max 1 mg, in 3 ml saline (by aerosol)
Hydrocortisone	Loading dose: 7 mg/kg IV, maintenance dose 2–3 mg/kg q 4–6 h IV
Prednisone	2 mg/kg/day

*Not approved by United States Food and Drug Administration (USFDA) for use in children under 12 years of age.

†Not approved by USFDA for aerosol use.

mately 2 μg/ml. If the patient shows no signs of toxicity and it is uncertain as to whether he has been receiving a theophylline preparation, it is reasonable to give a partial loading dose of 3 mg/kg if his condition warrants. A full loading dose otherwise should be given of 7 mg/kg, over a 20- to 30-minute period. In the asthmatic with major trauma, unless a certain history of no prior steroid use can be obtained, corticosteroid coverage should be given.[10] Even with minor trauma such as a laceration, if there is a history of steroid use for 2 weeks or longer in the past 6 months, steroid coverage should be given. Steroid use in these cases should be given regardless of whether the patient is having active asthma at the time seen in the emergency room. Steroid dose necessary to prevent adrenal insufficiency is lower than that necessary for treatment of acute asthma. The latter dose is 6 to 7 mg/kg of hydrocortisone for a loading dose and 2 to 3 mg/kg every 4 to 6 hours for maintenance. To prevent adrenal insufficiency, 3 mg/kg as a total daily dose of hydrocortisone is adequate. If the patient is able to take oral therapy, a comparable dose of prednisone is 1 mg/kg daily.

Any patient presenting with more than mild asthma (with or without trauma) deserves oxygen therapy after measurement of initial arterial blood gases is obtained. There is no reason to remove oxygen from the patient with significant distress to obtain gases "on room air." You can conclude that this patient will be hypoxemic without supplemental oxygen and it is not advisable to leave him without the oxygen so unnecessarily. Oxygen may be delivered by nasal cannula, starting at 3 to 4 L/minute. However, most younger children do not tolerate this as well as a mask. It is preferable to give oxygen by Venturi mask if there is significant distress because more reliable oxygen concentration can be delivered. Frequently it is necessary to use a croup tent or oxygen hood for the infant. The important point is to give supplemental oxygen to the acutely hypoxemic patient to prevent metabolic acidosis and relieve distress and anxiety, which may further aggravate the asthma.

CYSTIC FIBROSIS

When first recognized as a clinical entity in the late 1930s, cystic fibrosis (CF) was believed to be a rare disease uniformly fatal in infancy. A combination of significantly improved treatment and diagnosis of milder cases now allows us to see otherwise healthy-appearing children and adults who nevertheless have significant pulmonary and other organ-system involvement. The median life expectancy is now approximately 20 years of age. The major cause of morbidity and approximately 95 per cent of the mortality is the pulmonary disease. However, CF is a multi-system syndrome, which is characterized by generalized dysfunction of the exocrine glands.

CF appears to be transmitted as an autosomal recessive trait. This can only be assumed at this time, since there is no accurate means of detection of the carrier state. It is estimated that 1 in 20 Americans carry the gene for CF. The disease, most common in whites, does occur in all races. Estimates are that there are well over 20 thousand patients affected with CF in the United States.[1] An additional 800 to 1000 new cases are diagnosed annually. Because of the significant numbers of patients with this disease and the potential for multi-organ involvement and clinical manifestations, it is imperative that the physician concerned with emergency care is familiar with these abnormalities and potential complications.

One extremely important point to remember is that the disease is highly variable in regard to severity of different organ involvement. For instance, although the severity of pulmonary disease usually significantly affects the overall well-being of patients there are frequent cases of patients with very significant pulmonary disease who still have the appearance of relatively good health. Ten to fifteen per cent of patients with CF have adequate pancreatic function to maintain normal body weight and, in fact, sometimes may even be significantly overweight. These patients tend to have the mildest pulmonary disease but have complications such as pancreatitis. Other patients may have their major manifestation and potential problems resulting from biliary cirrhosis and portal hypertension, with resultant hypersplenism and esophageal varices. Therefore this discussion will describe the aspects of CF believed to be most important in emergency care in a systematic approach. These aspects are outlined in Table 13–2.

Table 13–2. SPECIAL PROBLEMS AND CONSIDERATIONS OF TRAUMA IN CYSTIC FIBROSIS PATIENTS

Pulmonary	Hemoptysis common in older age group
	Chronic CO_2 retention (caution with uncontrolled high inspired oxygen concentation in advanced disease)
	Pneumothorax, spontaneous bleb rupture not uncommon in moderate to advanced disease
	Reactive airway disease in many patients
	Sputum, frequently copious, can resemble bile or pulmonary edema
	Lungs colonized with *Staphylococcus aureus* and *Pseudomonas aeruginosa* as well as other *pseudomonas* species and occasionally other gram-negative rods
Gastrointestinal	Fatty liver changes, focal fibrosis
	Biliary cirrhosis, severe enough to cause cirrhosis and esophageal varices in 3% of patients
	Exocrine pancreatic insufficiency requiring enzyme replacement therapy with food in 90% of patients
	Diabetes mellitus in 8–15% of patients (ketoacidosis unusual)
	Meconium ileus equivalent with increased incidence of intussusception
	Pancreatitis
Infections	Higher doses of antibiotics necessary
	Not more susceptible to nonpulmonary infection
Fluid and Electrolytes	Increased sodium, chloride needs especially in infant, hot weather (acute salt loss)
	Hyponatremia, hypochloremia, hypokalemia secondary to SIADH,* cor pulmonale, CO_2 retention
Miscellaneous	Prolonged prothrombin time
	Cor pulmonale in advanced disease

*SIADH = syndrome of inappropriate antidiuretic hormone.

Pulmonary Disease

The pulmonary involvement of patients with CF is highly variable. Various pulmonary lesions include dilatation and hypertrophy of the bronchial glands, followed by mucous plugging of the small airways. This produces obstructive pulmonary disease and eventually infection and bronchiectasis. No matter what degree of trauma has been suffered, the increased metabolic needs may precipitate aggravation of already existing hypoxemia or hypercarbia. Measurement of arterial blood gases is indicated in any patient manifesting chest retractions or an altered state of consciousness. A significant number of patients with advanced disease will have chronic carbon dioxide retention. Oxygen must be administered to these patients with some degree of caution, as in the adult with chronic obstructive pulmonary disease. However, one is more likely to run into problems by withholding oxygen than by administering oxygen in low concentrations. The occurrence of increased carbon dioxide retention is readily reversible, whereas the damage done by hypoxia may be permanent.

The most rapidly potentially fatal complication of cystic fibrosis is pneumothorax. This occurs spontaneously in nearly 20 per cent of cystic fibrosis patients.[12] It is most common in the teenage or adult patient. If the patient with cystic fibrosis suffers even minor trauma, particularly of the type that would produce internal organ jarring, it is logical to assume that he has an even higher risk for spontaneous pneumothorax. A small to moderate-sized pneumothorax, even without tension, can produce severe symptoms in the patient with diffuse pulmonary disease. It is almost always necessary to treat any but the smallest pneumothoraces with chest tube drainage. Later in the course, pleural sclerosis should be considered because this treatment has been shown to reduce the recurrence rate from 63 to 12.5 per cent.[13]

In contrast to pneumothorax, hemoptysis can usually be treated with conservative therapy.[14] The incidence of hemoptysis in older patients with CF is as high as 76 per cent.[15] It is quite likely that with increased coughing, stress, and hypertension induced by trauma, hemoptysis may be induced or aggravated. However, unless there is strong suspicion or evidence to suggest major thoracic injury, overly invasive diagnostic or therapeutic procedures should be avoided. It is also advisable to avoid excessively rapid fluid replacement because this can prolong or even aggravate pulmonary bleeding in the CF patient.

Should pulmonary hemorrhage be massive and the patient appear to be in danger of asphyxiation, definitive treatment has been successful with several approaches. If the patient needs to undergo thoracotomy for other reasons, lobectomy or bronchial artery ligation may be indicated.[16] A major problem is localization of the site of bleeding. Occasionally the patient can describe a sensation of tingling or warmness from the area of bleeding. Bronchoscopy can be successful in localizing bleeding although this can be difficult to carry out during rapid, massive bleeding. Another option is arteriography of the bronchial arteries, which occasionally can show the extravasation of contrast material and certainly will show the location of the most tortuous bronchial artery collaterals. This can also be a definitive method of treatment when combined with embolization of the bronchial artery.[17] Special caution must be taken by the angiographer to observe closely for any spinal artery that might originate from the bronchial artery. However, again, it should be emphasized that conservative therapy is successful in the vast majority of cases even with massive (greater than 250 ml) hemoptysis. The reader is referred to the excellent review by Stern and associates.[14] It is also important to remember that a few CF patients are at high risk of hematemesis because of esophageal varices. This disorder must be differentiated from hemoptysis and is discussed in the next section.

The sputum from patients with CF is frequently copious, green, and sometimes frothy. This author has seen physicians, inexperienced with CF patients, mistake the sputum for either biliary secretions or pulmonary edema. Needless to say, it is important to find the true origin of such secretions.

Gastrointestinal Disease

Gastrointestinal (GI) disorders are the second most common manifestation of CF. Pancreatic insufficiency occurs in 85 to 90% of patients and is the most common GI problem. However, there are a variety of other GI problems, varying from mild to severe, which are important to consider in the patient with acute trauma. Fatty infiltration of the liver and focal biliary fibrosis occur in the majority of patients. These do not usually present clinical problems; however, it is worth noting that many patients with these disorders will have elevation of liver enzymes. A small proportion of these patients (approximately 3 per cent of all CF patients) will have severe complications of their liver disease, including hepatic failure, portal hypertension, bleeding esophageal varices, and hypersplenism.[11] These patients may be found to have thrombocytopenia and hematemesis.

Another complication of potential significance for hemostasis is prolonged prothrombin time. This can be secondary to vitamin K deficiency because of fat malabsorption as well as chronic antibiotic therapy. Chronic liver disease can further aggravate this problem. Therefore, in the patient with CF presenting with active bleeding, it is advisable to administer parenteral vitamin K.

Other GI complications that are probably of less potential significance in the situation of acute trauma include occasional acute pancreatitis, which mainly occurs in adolescents and young adults who have some exocrine pancreatic function. This rarely has serious clinical significance but must be remembered in the differential diagnosis of unexplained abdominal pain. Another condition causing abdominal pain and intestinal obstruction is referred to as meconium ileus equivalent. This occurs secondary to obstruction from the combination of malabsorption and abnormal bowel mucus. It is important to differentiate this from intussusception, which also has an increased frequency in patients with CF.[18]

Diabetes mellitus, usually in a mild form, occurs in up to 15 per cent of patients with CF. (Approximately half of these patients have glycosuria requiring insulin treatment.) Like most complications, this is more common in the older patient. However, ketoacidosis is an unusual occurrence in this group of patients.

Infections

The abnormally thick, viscous mucus produced in the respiratory tract of CF patients results in decreased mucociliary clearance and secondary bronchitis and bronchiectasis, with chronic colonization by bacteria. The most common organisms involved include *Staphylococcus aureus* and *Pseudomonas aeruginosa*. There is ample evidence in the literature supporting the effectiveness of antimicrobial therapy in improving lung function in CF.[19, 20] Fortunately, patients with CF appear to be no more susceptible than others to infections outside the respiratory tract. However, the CF patient suffering acute trauma who would otherwise require antibiotic therapy or who is likely to require prolonged bed rest or major surgery or appears to have borderline pulmonary function would usually benefit from the institution of antibiotic therapy against the organisms isolated in their sputum.

It is important to know that studies in CF patients have shown that for most antibiotics studied, larger than usual doses are necessary. The most commonly used antibiotics and doses recommended are listed in Table 13–3. Chest physiotherapy is generally believed to be very useful in reducing airway obstruction. Therefore, if possible, depending on type of trauma, it is recommended that this therapy be utilized, particularly if the patient will have decreased activity.

Table 13–3. MOST COMMONLY USED ANTIBIOTICS AND SUGGESTED STARTING DOSES IN CYSTIC FIBROSIS[21–23]

Antibiotics	Dosage
Gentamicin or tobramycin	10 mg/kg/day IV divided q 6 h
Carbenicillin	600 mg/kg/day divided q 4–6 h
Ticarcillin	400 mg/kg/day divided q 4–6 h
Nafcillin	200 mg/kg/day divided q 6 h
Ampicillin	200 mg/kg/day divided q 6 h
Clindamycin	40 mg/kg/day divided q 6 h

Fluid and Electrolytes

It was the knowledge that patients with CF had difficulty dealing with heat that led to the recognition of abnormal sweat electrolytes and ultimately their measurement as the major diagnostic test for the disease. Now there are several mechanisms recognized as contributing to fluid and electrolyte disturbance in CF patients. These are well outlined in a paper by di Sant' Agnese.[24]

The most urgent condition likely to be of consequence to the trauma patient involves acute salt loss. This can occur over a very short period because of massive salt loss through sweating. Severe circulatory changes can be seen, including vascular collapse and death. The serum sodium with such condition is rarely below 126 mEq/L because of the large amount of fluid lost. Rapid replacement with volume expanders (normal saline is ideal) is urgently needed in this condition. Subacute or chronic salt loss is also observed, particularly in infants. These patients frequently will present with hypochloremia, hypokalemia, and metabolic alkalosis unassociated with significant dehydration or other symptoms.[25] Hyponatremia is less serious than those complications mentioned previously. However, it is important to recognize that it is not an uncommon finding in an infant with CF, particularly in hot weather. Other causes of hyponatremia and hypoelectrolytemia include the syndrome of inappropriate antidiuretic hormone (SIADH), which is found in patients with severe pulmonary involvement. These patients may develop low serum sodium chronically, which may worsen acutely (less than 115 mEq/L, not uncommon). Usually the pH is normal and the blood urea nitrogen (BUN) is low. The extracellular fluid volume is significantly expanded, and fluid restriction is necessary. In addition, the administration of diuretics and saline infusion may be required. Chronic carbon dioxide retention with resultant hypochloremia and hyponatremia may be found and may be further complicated by hemodilution secondary to cor pulmonale. It is not unusual to have a combination of two or more of these pathologic mechanisms contributing to abnormal fluid balance.

In summary, when seeing a patient with CF, the necessity of being cognizant of the multiple-organ involvement and the implications for management cannot be overemphasized. The challenge is obvious, and the physician forewarned is forearmed to meet this challenge.

REFERENCES

1. Edwards DK, Dyer WM, Northway WH Jr: Twelve years experience with bronchopulmonary dysplasia. Pediatrics 59:839, 1977.
2. Truog WE, Prueitt JL, Woodrum DE: Unchanged incidence of bronchopulmonary dysplasia in survivors of hyaline membrane disease. J Pediatr 92:261, 1978.
3. Smyth JA, Tabachnik E, Duncan WJ, et al.: Pulmonary function and bronchial hyperreactivity in long-term survivors of bronchopulmonary dysplasia. Pediatrics 68:336, 1981.
4. Northway WH: Observations on bronchopulmonary dysplasia. J Pediatr 95:815, 1979.
5. Holsclaw DS: Pediatric pulmonary disease: An overview. Pediatr Ann 6:7, 1977.
6. Smith JM: Incidence of atopic disease. Med Clin North Am 68:3, 1974.
7. Bierman CW, Pearlman DS: Asthma. *In* Kendig EL, Chernick V (eds.): Disorders of the Respiratory Tract in Children. WB Saunders Company, 1983, p. 498.
8. Commey JO, Levison H: Physical signs in childhood asthma. Pediatrics 58:537, 1976.
9. Galant SP, Groncy CE, Shaw RC: The value of pulsus paradoxus in assessing the child with status asthmaticus. Pediatrics 61:46, 1978.
10. Melby JC; Pituitary-adrenal function consideration in asthma. *In* Weiss EB, Segal MS (eds.): Bronchial Asthma Mechanisms and Therapeutics. Boston, Little, Brown and Company, 1976, pp. 759–771.
11. Wood RE, Boat TF, Doershuk CF: Cystic Fibrosis: State of the art. Am Rev Respir Dis 113:833, 1976.
12. Holsclaw DS: Directions in pediatric respiratory disease. Clin Chest Med 1:407, 1980.
13. McLaughlin JF, Matthews WJ, Strieder DJ, et al: Pneumothorax in cystic fibrosis: Management and outcome. J Pediatr 100:863, 1982.
14. Stern RC, Wood RE, Boat TF, et al.: Treatment and prognosis of massive hemoptysis in cystic fibrosis. Am Rev Respir Dis 117:825, 1978.
15. Shwachman H, Kowalski M, Khaw KT: Cystic fibrosis: A new outlook. Medicine 56:129, 1977.
16. Levitsky S, Lapey A, Di Sant-Agnese PA: Pulmonary resection for life-threatening hemoptysis in cystic fibrosis. JAMA 213:125, 1970.
17. Schuster SR, Fellows KE: Management of major hemoptysis in patients with cystic fibrosis. J Pediatr Surg 12:889, 1977.
18. Holsclaw DS: Intussusception in patients with cystic fibrosis. Pediatrics 48:51, 1971.
19. Parry MF, and Neu HC: A comparative study of ticarcillin plus tobramycin vs. carbenicillin plus gentamicin for the treatment of serious infections due to gram-negative bacilli. Am J Med 64:961, 1978.
20. Wientzen R, Prestidge CB, Kramer RI, et al: Acute pulmonary exacerbations in cystic fibrosis: A double-blind trial of tobramycin and placebo therapy. Am J Dis Child 134:1134, 1980.
21. Kearns GL, Hilman BC, Wilson JT: Dosing implications of altered gentamicin disposition in patients with cystic fibrosis. J. Pediatr 100:312, 1982.
22. Kelly HB; Pharmacokinetics of tobramycin in cystic fibrosis. J Pediatr 100:318, 1982.
23. Huang NN, Schidlow DV, Palmer JJ: Antibiotics in pediatric respiratory diseases. Clin Chest Med 1:385, 1980.
24. di Sant' Agnese PA: The sweat defect in CF. *In* Warwick WJ (ed.) 1000 Years of Cystic Fibrosis Collected Papers. 1981.
25. Beckerman RC, Taussig LM: Hypoelectrolytemia and metabolic alkalosis in infants with cystic fibrosis. Pediatrics 63:580, 1979.

SECTION

III Specific Types of Trauma

CHAPTER

14 Spinal Cord Injury

BRUCE B. STORRS
MARION L. WALKER

Spinal cord injuries are fortunately an infrequent occurrence in pediatrics.* The outcome of these injuries often depends on a high index of suspicion and prompt recognition of neurologic problems.

Emergency management of the suspected spinal cord injury should follow the same guidelines as that for adults.

1. Assume any unconscious patient has a spinal cord injury until proved otherwise.
2. All multiply injured patients should be transported as if they had a spinal cord injury.
3. The cervical spine must be protected during airway management.
4. The neurologic examination is an important part of the complete trauma assessment.
5. Cervical spine radiographs must be taken in all unconscious and multiply injured patients.

The evaluation and resuscitation of the patient with spinal cord injury are identical to those of the trauma patient in general with the following notable exceptions:

1. Respiratory function may progressively deteriorate in the patient with cervical spinal cord injury.[2] Adequate ventilation on arrival does not guarantee continuation of adequate function.
2. Patients with upper thoracic and cervical injuries may behave physiologically as if they were sympathectomized, e.g., bradycardia with severe hypotension, warm dry skin with hypotension, and capacitance vessel pooling of blood.[3] Resuscitation in these situations may require pharmacologic manipulation as well as fluid and blood administration.
3. Hypothermia is common in severely injured children and is compounded in spinal cord injury secondary to the loss of vascular tone and pooling.[4]
4. Disturbance of motor and sensory levels may lead to misinterpretation of the physical examination, e.g., extremity fractures may cause no pain, intra-abdominal trauma may be severe without guarding or rebound tenderness, and severe chest injuries may elicit no direct complaint from the patient.
5. Acute urinary retention is very common in spinal cord injury. It may cause respiratory distress in the patient whose entire respiratory effort is from the diaphragm and may cause hypotension secondary to compression of the vena cava.[5]

DIAGNOSIS

A careful neurologic examination will disclose evidence of spinal cord dysfunction in the majority of patients with spinal cord injury.[6] Observation is an important tool and can be used while the immediate resuscitative efforts are being carried out. Visual inspection may demonstrate the typical "see-saw" respirations of the patient with paralyzed intercostal muscles secondary to cervical or upper thoracic spinal cord injury. Spontaneous movement of the patient may

*Spinal cord injuries occur with a frequency of 1/100,000 in children under age 14 and 3/100,000 in patients 14 to 16 years. By contrast, head injury occurs in 250/100,000 pediatric patients.[1]

give clues to the level of involvement; the paraplegic patient will only move his arms, will offer no resistance to bladder catheter placement or femoral puncture, and may not respond to manipulation of obvious fractures. The patient with cervical spinal cord injury may demonstrate movement of some arm muscles and paralysis of others. These are segmental and present in recognizable patterns.

C4 level. No arm movement, diaphragmatic paralysis.
C5 level. Deltoid and weak biceps function.
C6 level. Strong biceps, hands across chest.
C7 level. Triceps function, hand extension, weak hand flexion.
C8 level. Intrinsic hand function.

After the initial resuscitation has been completed, a mini-neurologic examination must be performed. This includes assessment of the level of consciousness, verbal and motor responses; ocular examination; limited cranial nerve examination; and motor, sensory, and reflex testing.

RADIOLOGIC EXAMINATION

The initial radiologic study should be a cross-table lateral of the cervical spine.[7] This is usually performed in the emergency department and should be supervised by the physician in charge. All extraneous material that may obscure the film should be removed. This does not include the immobilization device. Gentle axial traction exerted on the arms may help in visualizing the lower cervical or upper thoracic vertebrae. Acceptable radiographs should include all the cervical vertebrae and preferably the cervicothoracic junction. If no fracture or dislocation is present and if the patient is stable enough,

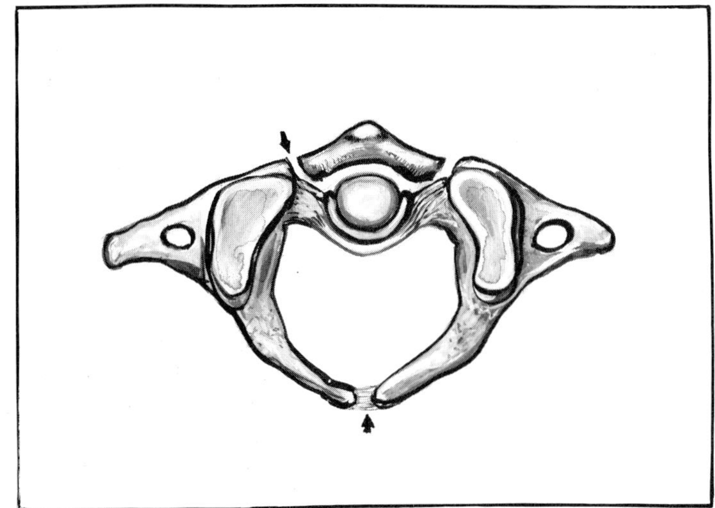

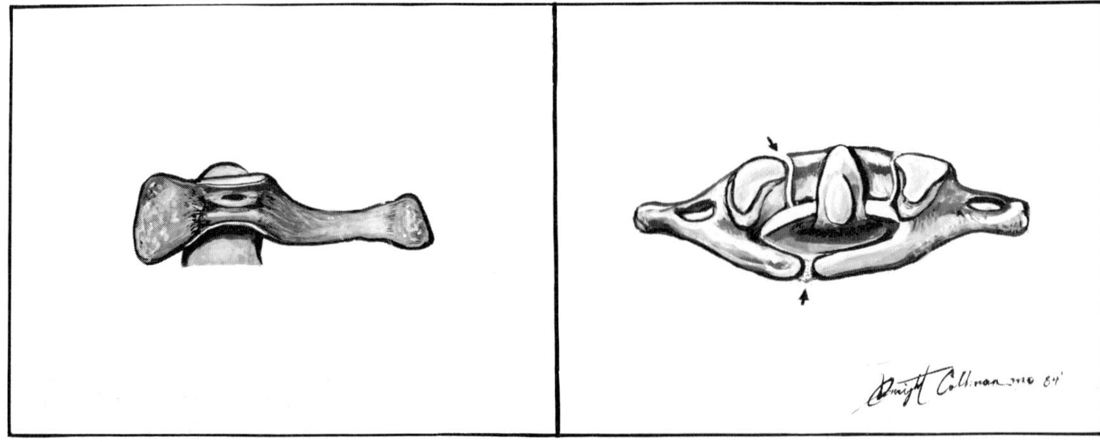

Figure 14–1. C1 anatomy. The figures demonstrate the relationship of the body to the neural arch of the first cervical vertebra. The arrows indicate the location of synchondroses in this vertebra.

a complete cervical spine series should be carried out in the x-ray department. If fracture or dislocation is diagnosed on the lateral film, additional therapy may be required prior to completion of the radiographic examination.

Proper interpretation of spine radiographs in children requires an understanding of the basic embryologic components of the spine as well as normal variations and peculiarities of the pediatric spine i.e., hypermobility, incomplete ossification, and variable soft tissue thicknesses. Nowhere are these factors more complex and difficult to interpret than in the region of C1 and C2. Figures 14–1 and 14–2 are schematic representations of the normal vertebral anatomy of C1 and C2, and the approximate dates of fusion of the synchondroses are shown on the diagrams. It is apparent from these diagrams that significant clefts are present in the C1-2 anatomy up to the age of 6 years, and these sites of bony apposition are points of weakness for fractures to occur into adult life.[8, 9] Distinguishing a fracture from normal variation at these epiphyseal lines may be quite difficult and can require a fair amount of experience in interpreting radiographs of the cervical spine. However, in cases in which fracture or dislocation of the C1-2 complex is suspected, it is safer to immobilize the patient first and obtain help in interpreting the radiographs later.[10]

Pitfalls in interpreting the cervical spine radiographs of children are as follows:

1. The vertebral bodies of the infant and child are not rectangular as in the adult. They have a normal biconcave appearance, which may be confused with compression fracture. However, comparison with the neighboring vertebrae often alleviates this suspicion because all the vertebral bodies appear the same.

2. Angulation in the infant spine is much more extreme than that in adults and owing to the laxity and high cartilage content of the cervical spine, offsets of vertebral bodies are normal rather than abnormal. These are particularly obvious at the C2-C3 level and are often misinterpreted as subluxations.[11] Using the width of the prevertebral soft tissues as an indication of cervical spine trauma may provide false-positive information. The retropharyngeal soft tissues of the child may change dramatically with inspiration and expiration as well as with crying and are affected by flexion and extension as well. So, although the appearance of the soft tissues may be quite useful in interpreting adult x-rays, the condition of the patient must be considered when trying to interpret them in the pediatric patient.

3. Because of the laxity of the ligamentous structures and the high cartilage content of the cervical spine in the infant and child, severe angulation may occur with no apparent bony or ligamentous disruption. The syndrome of spinal cord injury without radiographic abnormality as reported by Pang and Wilberger[12] is a frequent occurrence in pediatric practice. Infants and children may sustain very severe spinal cord injuries without any evidence of radiographic abnormality.[13, 14] These lesions may be progressive and generally carry a poor prognosis for functional recovery.[12] Hence, *spinal cord injury cannot be excluded on the basis of normal appearing plain radiographs of the spine.*

Further, a significant number of patients with spinal cord injury without radiographic abnormalities have delayed onset of neurologic manifestations. Since the majority of

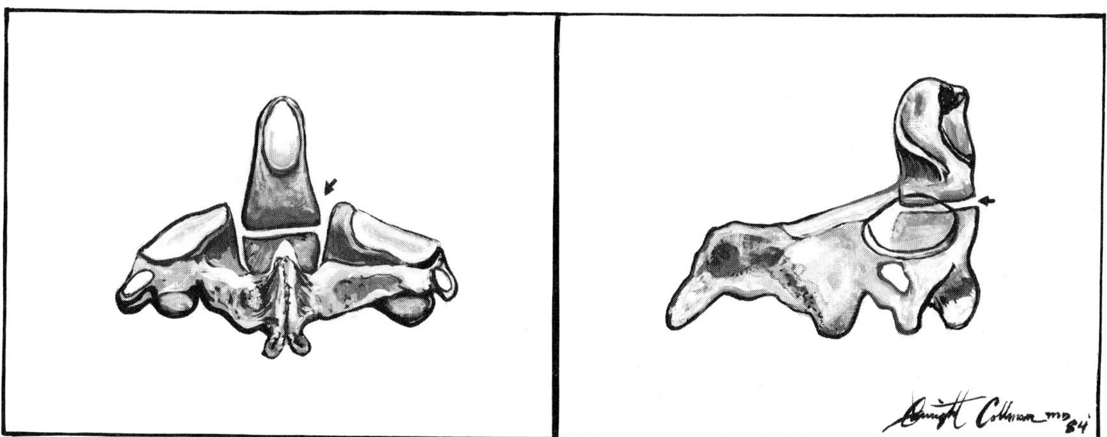

Figure 14–2. C2 anatomy. The arrows indicate the dates of fusion of the synchondroses, which occur at 3 to 6 years of age. Clefts in the C1–C2 anatomy may be present up to 6 years of age. Further, these are common sites for fractures, even into adult life.

these patients have transient symptoms initially, all such children should be evaluated very carefully.

The most important tools for the physician evaluating spinal injuries in children are an understanding of the normal embryologic and developmental peculiarities of the cervical spine and experience in viewing normal cervical spine films in children of various ages. Please refer to Chapter 8 for examples of pediatric spine radiographs.

THERAPY

The basic tenets of therapy of spinal cord injury are to prevent further injury, maximize the recovery potential of the neural tissue, and, in the case of persistent deficit, provide for early rehabilitation.

The spinal cord, like other neural tissue, has a high dependence on oxygen tension. Serum glucose concentration and arterial P_{CO_2} are critical determinants of metabolism and blood flow, respectively. With this in mind, the same precautions that exist in the head-injured patient apply to those with spinal cord injuries. Hypoxia, hypercarbia, anemia, and hypotension all adversely affect the function of the injured spinal cord.[15] Initial resuscitation is then the first step in treating the spinal cord injury. The maintenance of normal blood pressure, $P_{A_{O_2}}$, $P_{A_{CO_2}}$, and hemoglobin concentration will insure that no further injury will occur as a result of aberrations in these values.

Experimental and clinical studies suggest that steroids may be of benefit in spinal cord injury by preserving blood flow.[16] Some recommend dexamethasone (0.5–1.5 mg/kg) as an initial bolus. Recent laboratory data suggest that naloxone may also prove beneficial in augmenting spinal blood flow.[17]

Reduction of bony malalignment permits the spinal canal to assume a more normal shape if there are no intervening masses, e.g. bone, disc material, or hematoma. This is best accomplished with axial skeletal traction. Cervical dislocations and fracture-dislocations should be immobilized in traction if available.[18] There are numerous designs of skull tongs that may be utilized. In our experience, the Gardner-Wells variety has served well. They may be applied in the emergency department with local anesthesia, do not require any additional equipment (e.g., drills or wrenches), and good axial traction may be established in minutes.

The patient with a partial injury or the patient who has a progressive deficit presents special problems. These patients should be studied to evaluate the possibility that some potentially correctable factors may be at play. Myelography, with or without computerized tomography (CT) scanning, is difficult to carry out in injured patients but if the indications are present, it should be performed.[19] It is our practice to perform metrizamide myelography either from the lumbar or lateral cervical (C1-2) approach and to supplement it with CT scanning if we believe it would be useful. In this group of patients, the discovery of a surgically correctable lesion usually leads to operative intervention.[20]

The patient with an immediate and complete lesion is not subjected to myelography or CT scanning but is initially managed through appropriate cervical immobilization.

REHABILITATION

Of all the aspects of care of the patient with spinal cord injury, none has more far-reaching implications than that of rehabilitation. Unfortunately, the other aspects of spinal cord injury care receive much more attention than rehabilitation does. Pediatric rehabilitation has some very special requirements, necessitating an experienced, multidisciplinary team consisting of physical medicine and rehabilitation specialists as well as physical and occupational therapists, psychotherapists, and the educational specialists.

In addition to rehabilitation planning by the preceding specialists, it is also necessary for careful longitudinal follow-up of the pediatric patient with spinal cord injury to be undertaken by both neurosurgical and orthopedic specialists. They may be able to alleviate long-term progressive deformity or progressive spinal cord compression with worsening of the neurologic deficit. This follow-up must be carried out for many years.

SUMMARY

Pediatric spinal cord injury is fortunately an infrequent occurrence. There are some specific considerations in the management of the pediatric patient relative to size, embryologic and developmental vagaries, and long life expectancy following spinal cord injury. Recuperative and restorative powers of the infant and child are legendary and provide hope in situations that may otherwise be quite grim.

REFERENCES

1. Bruce DA: Neurologic injuries in pediatric patients. Symposium on Pediatric Trauma. Presented to the 68th Clinical Congress of the American College of Surgeons, Chicago, 1982.
2. Campbell J, Bonnett C: Spinal cord injury in children. Clin Orthop 112:114, 1975.
3. Hachen HJ: Spinal cord injury in children and adolescents: Diagnostic pitfalls and therapeutic considerations in the acute stage. Paraplegia 15:55, 1977.
4. Hubbard DD: Injuries of the spine in children and adolescents. Clin Orthop 100:56, 1974.
5. Kewalramani LS, Kraus JF, Sterling HM: Acute spinal cord lesions in a pediatric population: Epidemiological and clinical features. Paraplegia 18:206, 1980.
6. Sherk HH, Schut L, Lane JM: Fractures and dislocations of the cervical spine in children. Orthop Clin North Am 7:593, 1976.
7. Committee on Trauma, American College of Surgeons: Advanced Trauma Life Support Manual. Chicago, 1980.
8. Von Torklus D, Gehle W: The Upper Cervical Spine. New York, Grune and Stratton, 1972.
9. Dailey DK: The normal cervical spine in infants and children. Radiology 59:712, 1952.
10. Baker DH, Berdon WE: Special trauma problems in children. Radiol Clin North Am 4:289, 1966.
11. Burke DC: Spinal cord trauma in children. Paraplegia, 9:1, 1971.
12. Pang D, Wilberger JE: Spinal cord injury without radiographic abnormalities in children. J Neurosurg 57:114, 1982.
13. Melzak J: Paraplegia among children. Lancet 2:45, 1969.
14. Audic B, Maury M: Secondary vertebral deformities in childhood and adolescence. Paraplegia 7:11, 1969.
15. De la Torre JC, Johnson CM, Goode DJ, et al.: Pharmacologic treatment and evaluation of permanent experimental spinal cord trauma. Neurology 25:508, 1975.
16. Young W, Flamm ES: Effect on high-dose corticosteroid therapy on blood flow, evoked potentials, and extracellular calcium in experimental spinal injury. J Neurosurg 57:667, 1982.
17. Faden AI, Jacobs TP, Holaday JW: Opiate antagonist improves neurologic recovery after spinal injury. Science 211:493, 1980.
18. Anderson MJ, Schutt AH: Spinal injury in children. A review of 156 cases seen from 1950 through 1978. Mayo Clin Proc 55:499, 1980.
19. Burke DC, Murray DD: The management of thoracic and thoracolumbar injuries of the spine with neurological involvement. J Bone Joint Surg 58:72, 1976.
20. Andrews LG, Jung SK: Spinal cord injuries in children in British Columbia. Paraplegia 17:442, 1979.

CHAPTER

15 Thoracic Trauma

KENT W. JONES

Approximately 25 per cent of the 100,000 annual civilian traumatic deaths in this country result directly from chest injuries, and in another 25 to 50 per cent, chest injuries contribute significantly to the lethal outcome. Although chest trauma in children is not as common as it is in adults in most series, it poses a number of specific problems in diagnosis and management. Boys are twice[1] to three[2] times more susceptible to chest injury. Most chest injuries in children occur concomitantly with abdominal or head trauma.

Major advances in the rapid transportation of the injured, including helicopter retrieval,[3, 4] and the training and use of skilled paramedical personnel have resulted in the survival of many seriously injured children who previously would have died. This, in turn, has placed increased responsibility on the emergency room staff to act quickly and correctly in the management of patients with these serious injuries, since their delayed or incorrect diagnosis or treatment may contribute significantly to the morbidity and mortality of these children. It has been estimated, from an analysis of over 600 traumatic deaths occurring *after* the patients' arrival at the hospital, that one sixth of the deaths could have been prevented by prompt diagnosis and an additional one sixth could have been salvaged by institution of correct treatment.[5]

Since only 15 per cent of thoracic injuries require thoracotomy, every physician, specialist, and generalist should be prepared to diagnose and treat such injuries because they often occur in a location remote from a medical center, and without immediate availability of a thoracic surgeon. The fate of many of these children is determined by the response of the physician first attending them.

PATHOPHYSIOLOGY

Chest injuries are classically divided into two major categories—penetrating and non-penetrating (blunt) injuries. This basic separation has major clinical importance, since specific injuries fall almost entirely into one or the other group.

In non-penetrating injury, there is no communication between the organs of the chest and the outside as a result of the primary impact. It represents the commonest type of chest injury in children, most occurring from automobile or auto-pedestrian accidents. Smyth[1] found that 86 of 94 children sustaining chest trauma had received a non-penetrating type of injury. The majority of these injuries are associated with trauma to other organ systems outside the chest.

Penetrating injuries occur less commonly in children than in adults. They result from rib or clavicular fractures rather than from weapons or missiles. Some mechanisms of iatrogenic injury are unique to children, most being inflicted by the mechanical apparatus of patient care: (1) ventilators, (2) nasogastric tubes, (3) thoracostomy tubes, and (4) suction catheters.[6]

PATIENT EVALUATION AND TREATMENT

Many injuries to the thorax are capable of causing *severe* cardiorespiratory embarrassment *soon* after injury, the result being fatal if prompt and accurate evaluation and treatment are not undertaken. This requires a rapid, thorough patient assessment, followed by institution of appropriate therapy, based on the initial evaluation. Periodic reassessment of the patient's condition, and adjustment of therapy, when indicated, is also mandatory.

Diagnosis

Initial patient evaluation during the primary survey (see Chapter 1) consists of assessing the adequacy of *ventilation* and *circulation*. Assurance of a patent and adequate airway is paramount. The examiner can easily determine the condition of the airway by placing his ear close to the child's mouth and nose and listening to the exchange of air. Chest wall stability and prominence, the relationship of the trachea to the midline, the presence of subcutaneous emphysema, and the evaluation of the breath sounds bilaterally can all provide rapid, helpful information.

Simultaneously, a gross assessment of the circulation can be attained. Both the frequency and intensity of the extremity pulse are helpful guides to the evaluation of cardiac output, the presence of shock, and great vessel injury. The fullness of the neck veins, the blood pressure, and the quality of the heart sounds can all be readily assessed, and the presence of external hemorrhage should be investigated.

This approach is designed to detect only lesions of sufficient magnitude to result in early respiratory or cardiac decompensation. Mild cardiorespiratory disorders and other conditions having less acute impact may be missed while a search is made for major threats to a child's life. Lesser injuries can be detected during the secondary survey when time allows a more extensive and thorough examination.

Initial Resuscitation

The institution of initial resuscitative measures is dictated by the injuries uncovered during the evaluation. Its purpose is to provide adequate ventilation and restore circulation. As mentioned earlier, assurance of a patent and adequate airway is paramount. Its restoration depends upon the etiology of the obstruction. Foreign bodies require evacuation, whereas endotracheal intubation may be required in unconscious patients, those sustaining facial injuries, or those with laryngeal spasm. Emergency cricothyroidotomy should be reserved for specific conditions of mechanical obstruction, such as severe facial or laryngeal trauma, in which endotracheal intubation is not possible. Emergency tracheostomy can be a dangerous and time-consuming procedure when carried out under suboptimal conditions. Stabilizing a flail segment of chest wall or covering an open, sucking chest wound will improve ventilation significantly. The rapid insertion of an intravenous (IV) needle into the involved pleural space will quickly eliminate the lethal potential of a tension pneumothorax, allowing equilibration of the entrapped air with that of atmospheric pressure.

Children with extensive blood loss into the pleural space require immediate restoration of blood volume. Only then can the blood lost be safely evacuated with a chest tube. External blood loss should be replaced appropriately. Cardiac tamponade may require pericardiocentesis (see Fig. 1–9) or thoracotomy to restore appropriate hemodynamic parameters. Parenteral use of inotropic and vasopressor agents may also be required to provide adequate cardiovascular support, especially in those with direct myocardial injury. Such drugs should only be used when adequate volume replacement has been provided, as assessed by central venous or pulmonary artery pressure monitoring.

Whenever possible, children sustaining significant chest trauma should be admitted to a facility where skilled personnel and adequate monitoring equipment are available. Appropriate monitoring devices should provide a continuous display of the electrocardiogram (EKG) and blood pressure. Equipment for measuring pulmonary arterial (and wedge) pressure and cardiac output should be provided. Urine output and arterial blood gases should be closely monitored, and facilities for obtaining, developing, and viewing portable x-rays should be readily available. Specific diagnostic studies will be discussed with specific organ trauma.

Reassessment

Following initial evaluation and resuscitation, the injured patient's cardiorespiratory status should be continually reassessed to determine whether the condition has responded satisfactorily to the treatment instituted or has deteriorated. Continuous monitoring with the most sophisticated equipment and personnel available is mandatory in detection of early trends that indicate either an improvement or a worsening of the patient's condition. Repeated physical examination and roentgenographic evaluation are essential in this assessment. If response to treatment is only temporary, or deterioration continues in spite of resuscitation, exploratory thoracotomy may be necessary.

Indications for Early Thoracotomy in Infants and Children

The majority of thoracic injuries in children require prompt and accurate diagnosis and institution of appropriate resuscitative therapy. However, most (85 per cent or more) can be managed without thoracotomy. Reul and associates[7] performed emergency thoracotomy in only 91 of more than 900 patients, 27 being done in the emergency room because of refractory shock or cardiac arrest.

The following are relative indications for early thoracotomy in infants and children:[6,8]

1. No pulse with closed chest massage.
2. Heart fails to show response after 5 minutes.
3. Penetrating wound of the heart.
4. Cervical spine injury in which cardiac massage is necessary.
5. Massive or continuous intrapleural hemorrhage.
6. Cardiac tamponade following pericardiocentesis.
7. Widened mediastinum with left hemothorax or aortogram confirming aortic transection.
8. Ruptured esophagus.
9. Open pneumothorax with major defect in chest wall.
10. Massive pleural air leak suggestive of ruptured bronchus.
11. Traumatic diaphragmatic hernia.
12. Valvar or septal cardiac injury with resultant heart failure.

Unique Features of Children in Relationship to Chest Trauma

The compliance of the thorax in children is a result of the extremely flexible, elastic ribs and sternum. This elasticity makes fracture of these supportive structures less common in children than in adults, but allows internal injury to the thoracic organs to occur without external manifestations. The mediastinum is freely mobile and capable of wide anatomic shifts, causing the potential life-threatening situations of dislocation of the heart, angulation of the great vessels, pulmonary compression, and angulation of the trachea and major bronchi. Children sustaining any type of major trauma experience aerophagia. This, in turn, results in gastric dilatation, which limits diaphragmatic excursion, results in reflex ileus, and can lead to perforation of the upper gastrointestinal (GI) tract, leading to massive pneumoperitoneum.

Children's high metabolic needs allow the physician little time for deliberation and consultation when there is hypoxemia or hypotension. Their blood volume represents approximately 8 per cent of the total body weight, and a relatively small volume loss may result in hypovolemia and shock. Difficult venous access may restrict volume resuscitative efforts (see Chapter 1).

SPECIFIC INJURIES

Thoracic Cage

Soft Tissue

Although in and of themselves soft tissue injuries of the chest wall are not a usual cause of major morbidity or mortality, they frequently provide a clue to underlying, life-threatening thoracic trauma. General management of injuries to the soft tissues of the chest wall is similar to that of injuries of musculocutaneous tissues elsewhere in the body.

Subcutaneous Emphysema

Although subcutaneous emphysema is an important sign following chest trauma, the condition itself may be of little significance. It occurs when air is forced into the subcutaneous tissues and dissects along musculocutaneous planes, which provide little resistance. Air is capable of reaching these planes by one of three routes: (1) by major disruption of the pleura and intercostal muscles; (2) as an extension of mediastinal emphysema, or (3) by direct communication with an external wound (Fig. 15–1).

Treatment of subcutaneous emphysema should be directed toward its underlying cause, since the condition will reverse gradually once its source is controlled. Inhalation of high concentrations of oxygen will enhance the reabsorption of subcutaneous air by washing nitrogen from the blood and improving its diffusion from the subcutaneous tissues back into the circulation.

Clavicular Fractures

Isolated clavicular fractures from blunt thoracic trauma are unusual in children because of their compliant, elastic bony skeleton (their treatment is discussed in Chapter 22). If they do occur, sharp fragments from these

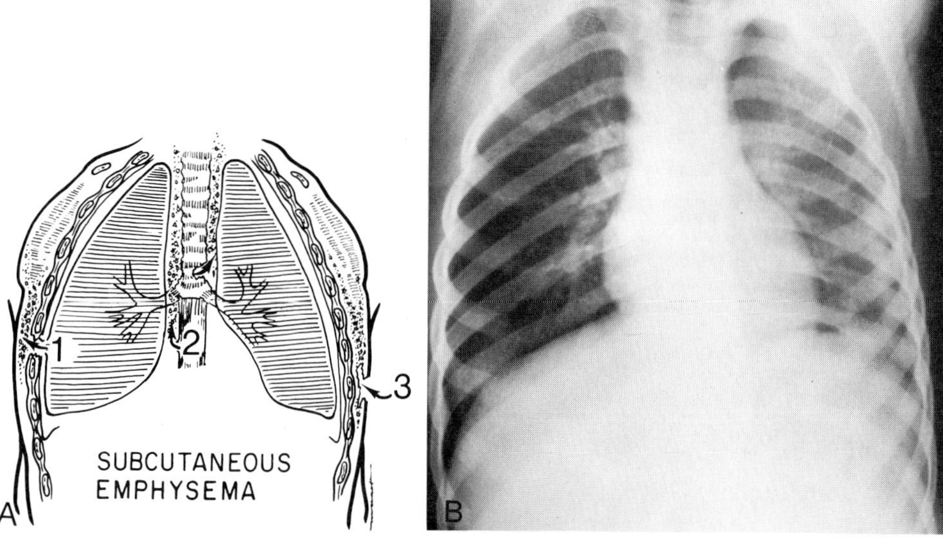

Figure 15–1. *A*, Subcutaneous emphysema results from one of the following mechanisms: (1) major disruption of the pleura and intercostal muscles, (2) extension of mediastinal emphysema, or (3) direct communication with an external wound. *B*, Chest roentgenogram demonstrating post-traumatic pneumomediastinum and chest wall subcutaneous emphysema.

fractures may cause injury to the subclavian vessels, brachial plexus, or apex of the lung.

Rib Fractures

Although most accounts of pediatric chest trauma show a low incidence of rib fracture, Smyth[1] cited an incidence of 47.8 per cent in 94 children and Levy[9] described fractures in 44 of 51 children (86 per cent) following crushing chest injuries. Thomas notes that "in infants, undisplaced fresh rib fractures may be difficult or impossible to see" (Fig. 15–2).[10]

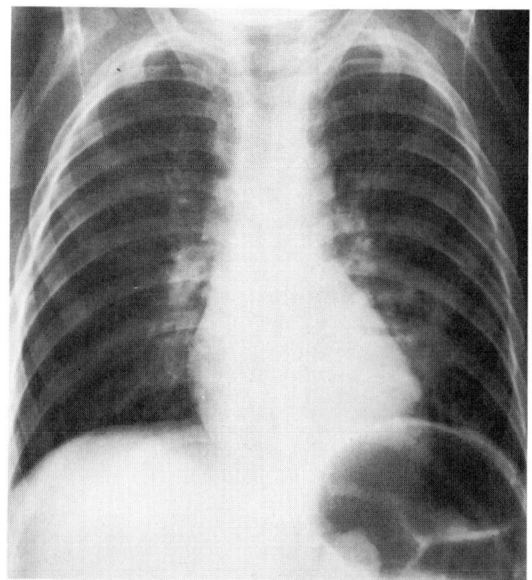

Figure 15–2. Chest roentgenogram demonstrating multiple rib fractures, pulmonary contusion, and left lower lobe pulmonary laceration with air/blood level.

First rib fractures from severe trauma should alert the clinician to possible significant injury within the chest or abdomen and dictate thorough evaluation of the thoracic aorta, tracheobronchial tree, and neurovascular structures of the upper extremities.[11, 12]

Treatment of rib fractures consists of rest and adequate pain relief to allow frequent cough and deep breathing. Intercostal nerve block may assist in providing this necessary analgesic.

Flail Chest

The fracture of several ribs on both sides of the point of impact often results in the intervening rib segments losing their continuity with the remainder of the rigid thorax. This unstable area responds to intrapleural pressure changes, resulting in paradoxical movement of the chest wall during respiration. The reduced ventilatory efficiency, leading to increased ventilatory work, and the underlying pulmonary contusion often lead to progressive respiratory insufficiency. Segmental fractures of three or more ribs located anteriorly and laterally are most apt to result in "flail" segments, the posterior ribs being protected and stabilized by the paraspinous muscles and the scapula. The paradoxical chest wall motion may be especially severe if there is an associated transverse fracture of the sternum.

In the past, *pendelluft*, a ventilatory phenomenon referring to "pendulum-like" movement of a portion of the lung's tidal volume back and forth between the lung on the injured side and the lung on the uninjured side, was thought to be the cause of the physiologic derangement in flail chest. It is now believed that the paradoxical movement of the segment of involved chest wall and crippling of its normal bellows function, underlying lung damage, and hypoventilation from chest pain are much more important factors in the development of respiratory insufficiency (Fig. 15–3).

Any child sustaining severe blunt thoracic trauma should be evaluated for an unstable chest wall, although its occurrence is unusual due to the elasticity of the thoracic cage and the high proportion of cartilage present in the ribs of children.[13]

Once the diagnosis is made, several modes of therapy are available, the most important of which is to stabilize the involved portion of the thoracic cage, thus increasing the effective tidal volume and ventilatory efficiency. The most expedient means of providing initial chest wall stabilization is by external support, utilizing gentle, firm manual pressure or by applying weighted objects to the injured area. A useful approach at the scene of an accident is to place the patient with the injured side down. External traction devices, using instruments such as towel clips placed around the injured ribs, have also been employed. Surgical fixation of these multiple fractures has proved effective in certain instances.[14]

At present, the use of "internal pneumatic stabilization," employing endotracheal intubation and mechanical ventilation utilizing a volume-cycled respirator, is the treatment of choice. This procedure provides optimal pulmonary expansion and splinting of the chest wall but carries a significant morbidity in infants and young children. High inflation pressures from mechanical ventilation cause pneumothorax in 25 to 30 per cent of cases,[15, 16] 25 per cent of which require tube thoracostomy.[17, 18] The incidence of tension pneumothorax increases with elevated inflation pressures and the use of positive end-expiratory pressure (PEEP). Bronchial perforation from endotracheal suctioning has also been described.

Authors have documented their ability to manage patients with mild to moderate flail chest without utilizing ventilatory assistance, employing careful patient selection and close observation.[19] Trinkle[20] has described a method for management of these injuries without the need for mechanical respiratory support, relying on vigorous treatment of the underlying lung contusion, pulmonary physiotherapy, and chest pain relief using intercostal nerve blocks.

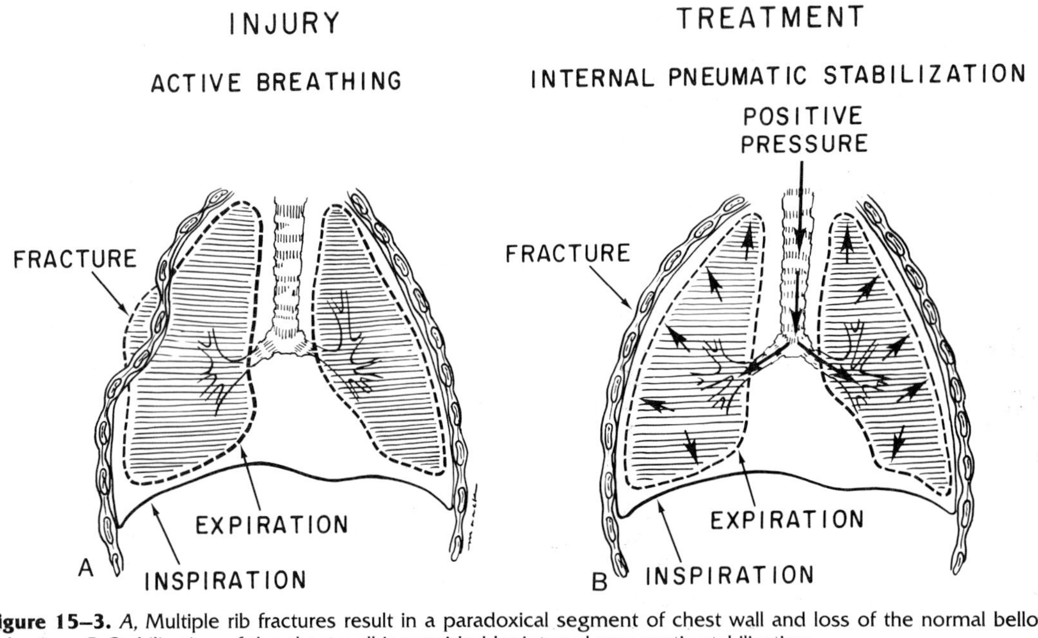

Figure 15–3. *A*, Multiple rib fractures result in a paradoxical segment of chest wall and loss of the normal bellows mechanism. *B*, Stabilization of the chest wall is provided by internal pneumatic stabilization.

Sternal Fractures

Fracture of the sternum in children is very uncommon, again owing to the marked compliance of the chest wall. However, when present it is frequently associated with other severe intrathoracic injuries.

Reduction and fixation of the fracture may be required, especially if it is displaced or contributing to the child's respiratory insufficiency. Impacted or partially displaced fractures causing no ventilatory impairment require only observation and analgesics.

Open Pneumothorax

An open or sucking wound of the chest results in acute ventilatory embarrassment from rapid equilibration of atmospheric and intrapleural pressures through the open defect. This condition thus interferes with the normal mechanical function of the thoracic "bellows" of providing the necessary pressure gradient for air exchange. Collapse of the ipsilateral lung, mediastinal shift, and decrease in venous return to the heart from loss of negative intrathoracic pressure all contribute to the cardiorespiratory insufficiency caused by the injury (Fig. 15–4).

An open chest wound should be covered immediately with any material or object readily available, thus converting the condition from an acute emergency to that of a closed pneumothorax. A definitive sterile occlusive dressing should then be applied as soon as possible. Once the child reaches a medical care facility, a chest tube can be inserted and connected to water-seal drainage. Following thorough evaluation and resuscitation, surgical debridement and closure are carried out. Mobilization and utilization of a flap of adjacent muscle is occasionally necessary to provide airtight closure.

Traumatic Asphyxia

This potentially fatal entity occurs exclusively in children, again because of their flexible thorax and the absence of valves in the superior and inferior vena cava.[21] Direct sudden compression of the compliant thoracic cage against a closed glottis causes a sudden, dramatic increase in intratracheal and intrapulmonary pressure, with concomitant temporary vena caval obstruction. This, in turn, causes a marked increase in venous pressure, resulting in capillary extravasation and hemorrhage from the brain and other organs.

Children with this condition become acutely disoriented and may lose consciousness and have seizures. Respiratory compromise with tachypnea and hemoptysis can occur. Other presenting symptoms include cervicofacial cyanosis; vascular engorgement with petechiae of the face, head, chest and neck; subconjunctival hemorrhage; and acute hepatomegaly.

Treatment initially consists of removing the causative agent. Any resultant complications, such as pneumothorax or lung contusion, are then treated in the usual manner.

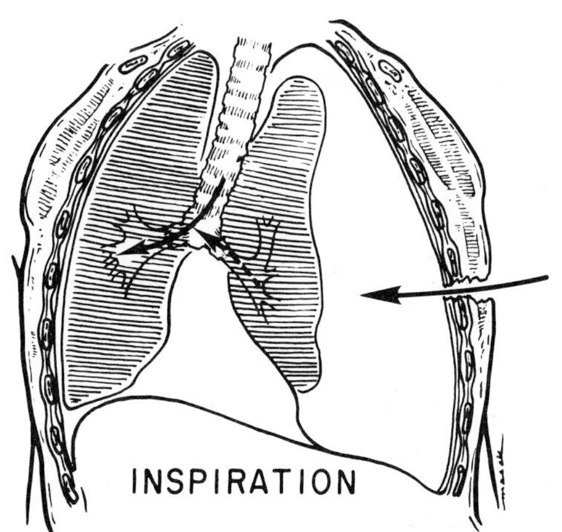

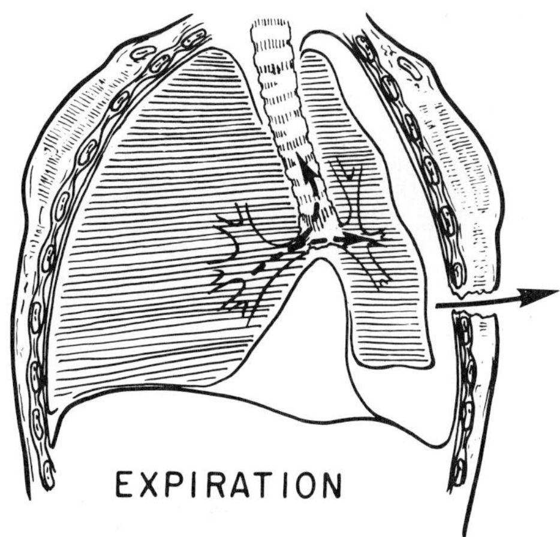

Figure 15–4. Open pneumothorax results in ipsilateral lung collapse, mediastinal shift, and impaired ventilation of the opposite lung.

Pleural Space

Closed Pneumothorax

Pneumothorax is the most commonly encountered entity in pediatric chest trauma and may result from a blunt or penetrating injury. Again, the elasticity of the child's thorax results in its occurrence in the absence, many times, of associated rib fractures.

Collapse of the lung is caused by loss of the normally occurring negative pressure within the pleural space, which can result from (1) penetration of the chest wall, (2) disruption of the lung parenchyma, (3) tear of the tracheobronchial tree, or (4) esophageal perforation.

The physical signs of a closed pneumothorax include diminished breath sounds, hyperresonance to percussion, a poorly moving hemithorax, subcutaneous emphysema, and deviation of the trachea to the side of the injury. A chest roentgenogram usually confirms the diagnosis. If closed pneumothorax is not initially present, evidence of chest trauma with findings of subcutaneous emphysema or other physical signs, as outlined previously, should alert the examiner to the possibility of the patient exhibiting the lesion on subsequent evaluations.

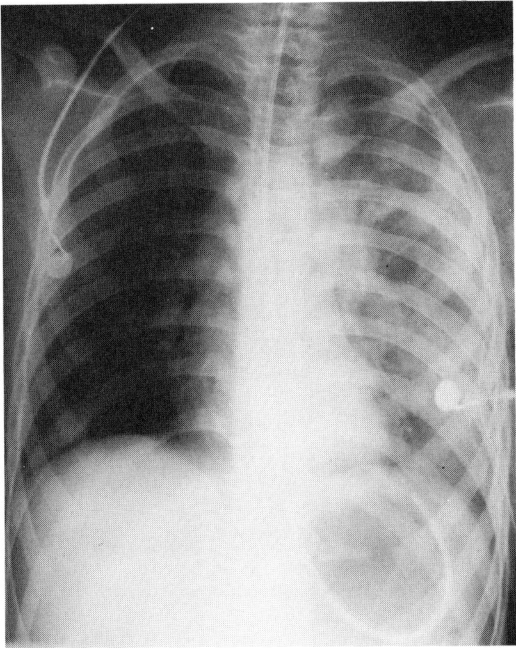

Figure 15–5. Chest roentgenogram following left tube thoracostomy for treatment of hemopneumothorax results from blunt trauma. Pulmonary contusion and pneumomediastinum are also present.

Treatment of a significant closed pneumothorax (greater than 15 per cent or in a symptomatic patient) is best provided by tube thoracostomy drainage. The optimal anatomic site of chest tube insertion is at the anterior axillary line, lateral to the pectoralis major muscle, in the fourth intercostal space. The tube is connected to underwater-seal drainage and is left in place until pleural drainage subsides, and for at least 24 hours after any air leak subsides. A persistent air leak may signify a laceration of the tracheobronchial tree, which, in turn, may require further diagnostic procedures and surgical intervention for control. Any child sustaining chest trauma who requires general anesthesia for another remote injury should have a prophylactic chest tube placed prior to anesthetic induction. The major potential complication of the procedure in infants and children is lung perforation, occurring in as many as 25 per cent of cases.[17, 18] Insertion requires experience and judicious technique. If a trocar is used, it should never be inserted beyond the rib margin (Fig. 15–5).[6]

Tension Pneumothorax

A condition that allows progressive accumulation of air under pressure in the pleural space may lead to rapid cardiorespiratory collapse and prove fatal if not promptly detected and treated. An injury to the lung parenchyma or a bronchial tear may permit air to enter the pleural space under pressure, the lesion acting as a one-way valve. Rarely, oblique wounds in the chest wall may allow movement of air into the pleural space from the outside atmosphere. The increased use of endotracheal intubation; ventilator support, especially employing PEEP; and endotracheal suctioning has increased the incidence of this disorder in infants and children.

The progressive accumulation of air under pressure within the pleural space causes not only a collapse of the lung on the side of the injury but also a progressive shift of the mediastinum to the opposite side, with compression of the contralateral lung. Impairment of ventilation and venous return ensues, leading to severe cardiorespiratory collapse (Fig. 15–6).

This condition requires prompt recognition and immediate treatment. The involved hemithorax is prominent and hyperresonant and transmits breath sounds poorly. There may be a shift of the trachea to the contralateral side, with neck vein distention and subcuta-

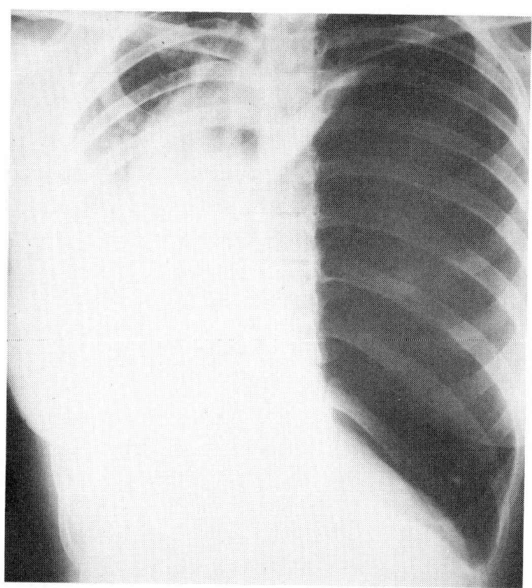

Figure 15–6. Chest roentgenogram demonstrating severe tension pneumothorax.

neous emphysema. Clinical evidence of shock, with hypotension, tachycardia, and peripheral vascular vasoconstriction, is also apparent.

The initial treatment of this disorder involves equilibration of the pleural space with atmospheric pressure, utilizing percutaneous needle puncture of the involved hemithorax. This procedure converts the injury to a simple pneumothorax, which can be treated with tube thoracostomy and underwater-seal drainage.

HEMOTHORAX

Hemothorax is one of the most common problems following major chest trauma. It results from either penetrating or blunt injuries. Thirty to forty per cent of the total blood volume may be rapidly lost into one pleural space, with little resistance being offered by the compliant lung. This amount of hemorrhage usually heralds an injury to the heart, great vessels, or major systemic artery. However, this is unusual in children as a result of their low incidence of penetrating chest injuries. Lung parenchymal injuries seldom result in this extent of blood loss, because of the low perfusion pressure and the abundance of thromboplastins within the parenchyma.[8]

A major hemothorax will result in shock and should rarely be missed in the rapid initial evaluation of a trauma victim. Ventilatory embarrassment from compression of the ipsilateral lung and shift of the mediastinal structures compound the cardiovascular collapse. Decreased breath sounds are present over the involved hemithorax, and tracheal shift may be detected. An upright chest film is essential in establishing the diagnosis, since loss of a major volume of blood within the pleural space may produce only a slight increase in density over the involved hemithorax on a supine film. Aspiration of blood by thoracentesis confirms the diagnosis.

Treatment of a major hemothorax requires early aggressive ventilatory support and adequate pleural evacuation. Oxygenation may require endotracheal intubation, and intravascular volume should be restored with blood or crystalloids. Pleural drainage is best achieved by tube thoracostomy; the chest tube is placed laterally in the fourth or fifth intercostal space, and the tip is advanced to the apex of the pleural space. Difficulty has been encountered in managing even small hemothoraces utilizing observation or thoracentesis.[22] Tube thoracostomy not only provides evacuation of the hemothorax and reexpansion of the compressed lung but also reduces further bleeding by coaptation of the pleural space and serves as a monitor for any continuing blood loss. A method of chest tube drainage of blood and its return by autotransfusion after appropriate micron filtration has been described; it provides a readily available source for transfusion without ill-effects.[23]

The vast majority of patients sustaining acute traumatic hemothorax can be managed without thoracotomy.[22, 24] However, surgical intervention is indicated if (1) bleeding continues, (2) the rate of bleeding increases, or (3) it is impossible to adequately evacuate the retained blood within the pleural space. Blood left undrained within the pleural space may chronically lead to fibrothorax, a trapped lung, and scoliosis in the growing child.[22] If thoracotomy is required, the incision is made anterolaterally through the fourth intercostal space and extended trans-sternally if necessary. This approach provides ready access to the heart, lung, and great vessels, and cardiac massage can easily be performed. Median sternotomy is contraindicated owing to the extra time and instruments involved and the poor access it provides to the hilum of the lung and the posterior mediastinal structures.

Chylothorax

The thoracic duct enters the venous system at the confluence of the left subclavian and left internal jugular veins. Its disruption leads to the accumulation of chyle within the mediastinum and its subsequent leak into the pleural space. The injury most commonly is iatrogenic, occurring at the time of patent ductus ligation or with mobilization of the trachea in tracheoesophageal fistula repair. It can occur with trauma, most commonly from a penetrating wound or hyperextension injury to the spine.

Diagnosis is confirmed by aspiration of white, milky fluid containing fat that layers out in a test tube containing ether.[25] Since chyle is bacteriostatic, chylothorax infrequently is associated with empyema. Treatment initially consists of tube thoracostomy drainage. Concomitant oral feedings of medium chain triglycerides[26] or total parenteral nutrition, or both, is also utilized to decrease thoracic duct flow. If nonsurgical therapy is unsuccessful after 1 month, thoracic duct ligation is indicated.[6]

Lungs

Intrathoracic Foreign Bodies

Problems with intrathoracic foreign bodies have most commonly been associated with penetrating chest injuries suffered in military action. Although their presence is uncommon in the pediatric population, the recent widespread use of firearms and weapons and the increased incidence of motor vehicular accidents have made it necessary for physicians to become adept in their treatment.

In general, foreign bodies involving the pulmomary parenchyma and pleura are best left alone until they produce symptoms. Only approximately 20 per cent develop complications requiring subsequent removal. On the other hand, objects in or near the tracheobronchial tree, the heart, or the great vessels warrant surgical removal. Large (> 2.5 cm), sharply contoured or grossly contaminated foreign bodies also require early surgical retrieval. Those objects not in themselves requiring surgical removal should, when possible, be removed if thoracotomy is required for other indications.

Pulmonary Contusion

Pulmonary contusion is frequently encountered in infants and children sustaining chest trauma: it occurred in 61.7 per cent of cases in Smyth's series.[1] The lesion most commonly results from a rapid non-penetrating deceleration injury and may initially be overlooked if there is no severe trauma to the chest wall or when multiple other injuries, especially those to the head or abdomen, demand urgent attention. Three basic phenomena appear to be important to its etiology: (1) the *spalling* effect, in which the liquid-gas interface is disrupted by a shock wave moving in the liquid, resulting in pulmonary hemorrhage and edema; (2) the *implosion* effect, the pressure wave producing alveolar overexpansion by moving from a more dense medium to that of air; and (3) the *inertial* effect, as low-density alveolar tissue is stripped from heavier hilar structures.[27]

The injury differs both clinically and pathologically from respiratory distress syndrome with which it is often confused. Pulmonary contusions occur within minutes of the injury, are localized to a segment or lobe of the lung, can usually be seen on the initial chest x-ray, and, if they do not become infected, tend to resolve in 2 to 6 days.[28]

The diagnosis of a pulmonary contusion can usually be made from the history and chest x-ray. Especially in children, many of the worst contusions occur without accompanying rib fractures, although they are many times associated with other serious injuries resulting from blunt trauma (Fig. 15–7).

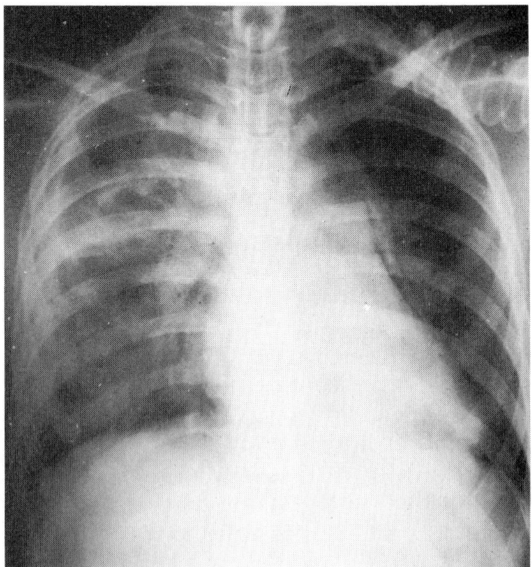

Figure 15–7. Chest roentgenogram showing significant pulmonary contusion with pneumatoceles of right lung following blunt chest injury.

Patients sustaining pulmonary contusion should be carefully monitored in an intensive care unit. Thorough evaluation for any other associated injuries must be made, and any complicating thoracic disorders (e.g., hemothorax, pneumothorax) corrected. Adequate ventilation must be maintained to all parts of the lung. Mechanical ventilation utilizing positive end-expiratory pressure (PEEP) has been shown to have a protective effect on the pulmonary parenchyma, especially if the patient's Po_2 is less than 60.[28] Judicious fluid restriction, monitored by a Swan-Ganz catheter, is mandatory. The use of diuretics and plasma or albumin to maintain a serum osmolarity of 290 to 300 mOsm and prophylactic antibiotics have also been advocated. However, the use of steroids is controversial, except when there is accompanying smoke inhalation, fat embolism, aspiration of gastric contents, or severe, progressive pulmonary insufficiency.

Pulmonary contusion can result in serious complications, the most common being infection. The extravasation of fluid and blood into the alveolar and interstitial spaces provides an excellent culture medium, especially in debilitated patients. Fifty to seventy per cent of those sustaining a pulmonary contusion will develop pneumonia in the contused segment of lung, and 35 per cent will go on to pulmonary abscess or empyema, or both.[28] Chronic pulmonary insufficiency and pneumothorax, especially in those requiring mechanical ventilation and PEEP, are other complications of this disorder.

Pulmonary Hematoma

Pulmonary hematomas result from accumulation of extravasated blood in a space created by parenchymal disruption. They appear as fuzzy outlines on the initial chest film but sharpen in definition over the next few days as the surrounding suffusion of blood resorbs, leaving a typical "coin lesion" of the lung. Most resolve spontaneously over 2 to 4 weeks.

Initial management of this injury is still somewhat controversial, although most surgeons favor a conservative approach, reserving thoracotomy and removal of traumatized lung tissue for cases of continued hemorrhage, air leak, or infection. However, if thoracotomy is required for an associated injury, most believe that resection of the involved lung tissue is indicated at that time.

Pulmonary Laceration

Pulmonary lacerations most commonly result from penetrating chest trauma. In cases of blunt trauma, they usually result from the temporary inward protrusion of a fractured rib or avulsion of previous pleural adhesions. They most commonly produce a hemothorax, a pneumothorax or a hemopneumothorax, the latter usually resulting from a penetrating injury (Fig. 15–8).

The majority of these injuries can be handled by careful observation and serial chest x-rays or by simple tube thoracostomy. Major life-threatening lacerations are uncommon,

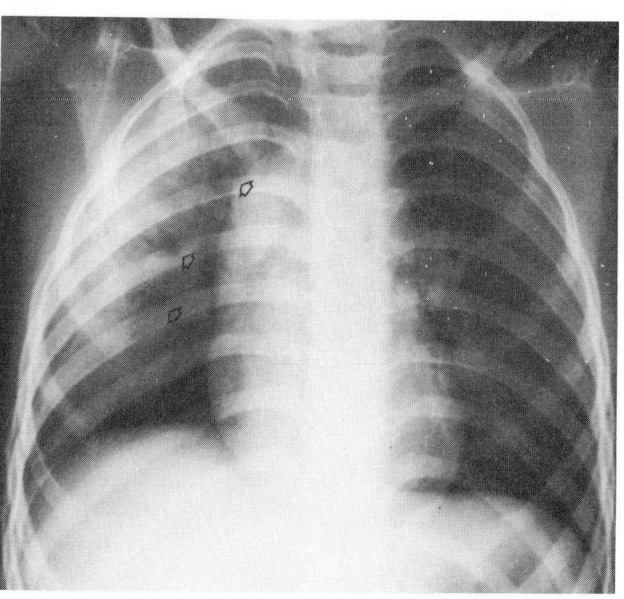

Figure 15–8. Three traumatic pulmonary lacerations with focal air collections *(arrows)* resulting from blunt chest trauma and rib fractures.

representing approximately 4 per cent of thoracic trauma, and are usually accompanied by hemoptysis, multiple rib fractures, or a hemopneumothorax with parenchymal hematoma. Children with these injuries require thoracotomy with associated segmental resection, lobectomy, or pneumonectomy to control the bleeding and air leaks.

TRACHEOBRONCHIAL INJURIES

Injury to the tracheobronchial tree is rare in the pediatric population because of the elasticity of the thoracic cage and the mobility of the mediastinal structures. In a series of 94 children, Smyth[1] found two patients with tracheal rupture and an additional 3 with a bronchial tear, one of whom died. All injuries resulted from severe blunt chest trauma.

An interruption of the tracheobronchial tree can result from either blunt or penetrating chest injuries. Blunt injuries result from (1) shearing forces, tearing the distal mobile bronchus from the fixed proximal segment; (2) compression of the trachea against the vertebrae; (3) airway distention against a closed glottis; or (4) a sudden vertical stretch. The injury most frequently occurs at the takeoff of a main or upper lobe bronchus, particularly on the right side near the carina. Kirsh and associates[29] found that 80 per cent occurred within 2.5 cm. of the carina. There is usually no accompanying injury to the pulmonary vessels.

The presence of a tracheobronchial disruption should be considered in any instance in which significant chest trauma has occurred. The diagnostic signs leading to its eventual diagnosis will differ, depending upon whether there is free communication between the tear and the pleural space. Findings requiring further investigation include (1) massive hemoptysis, commonly occurring from disruption of a bronchial artery; (2) airway obstruction; (3) progressive mediastinal or subcutaneous emphysema; (4) tension pneumothorax; (5) persistent air leak and pneumothorax; (6) massive atelectasis of one lobe or an entire lung, which does not respond to treatment; and (7) chronic bronchiectasis resulting from bronchial obstruction. The most reliable means of establishing the site, nature, and extent of the lesion is by bronchoscopy. Bronchography has occasionally been helpful in establishing the diagnosis.

Direct repair of the injury as soon as the patient's condition permits is indicated, since the morbidity and mortality are significantly increased by delay. High tracheal injuries are repaired by employing a distal tracheostomy. Lower tracheal and bronchial injuries require thoracotomy for direct repair. The torn ends are debrided and closed with nonabsorbable atraumatic sutures, with the knots tied on the outside of the lumen. Lesions in the distal tracheobronchial tree may require resection of the involved segment if an air leak persists following tube thoracostomy or if the disruption is too severe to accommodate repair. Assessment of the repair should be made bronchoscopically 3 months postoperatively and at regular intervals thereafter.

Traumatic tracheoesophageal fistula is an uncommon injury resulting from concomitant laceration of the trachea and necrosis of the adjacent esophagus by their compression between the sternum and vertebrae. The lesion usually develops 3 to 5 days following the injury, and the diagnosis is confirmed by esophagoscopy, bronchoscopy, and esophagography. Early surgical transection of the fistula and primary repair of both the trachea and esophagus is the treatment of choice.

Diaphragm

DIAPHRAGMATIC RUPTURE

Diaphragmatic rupture was first described in the 16th century by Ambrose Paré, who noted that following diaphragmatic injury, "the stomach and intestines are sometimes drawn into the thoracic cavity."[30]

This lesion most commonly follows blunt trauma resulting from a vehicular accident or a fall, the crushing force producing a sudden increase in the intrathoracic or intra-abdominal pressure against the fixed diaphragm. Penetrating lesions can also result in diaphragmatic disruption. The diagnosis can easily be missed because symptoms and signs of diaphragmatic hernia are absent. Solheim[31] reviewed 13 children with traumatic diaphragmatic rupture, 6 of whom had the diagnosis missed initially. Ninety per cent of traumatic tears occur on the left side, predominantly from the buttressing of the liver on the right.

The commonest presenting symptoms include shortness of breath and chest pain. Since 60 to 80 per cent of normal ventilation depends upon proper diaphragmatic function, unilateral dysfunction accompanied by compression of the lung and mediastinum from the herniated intra-abdominal contents may severely restrict respiration. Physical findings include decreased breath sounds on the side of herniation, a contralateral shift of the mediastinum, a markedly scaphoid abdomen (Gibson's sign), and the presence of bowel sounds in the thorax. Cardiac insufficiency may result from obstruction to venous return, myocardial contusion, or intrapericardial placement of intra-abdominal contents through the diaphragm, causing cardiac tamponade.[31]

The chest roentgenogram usually confirms the suspected diagnosis, demonstrating abnormal shadows (many times containing gas bubbles) in the lower lung field, an unclear or elevated diaphragmatic outline, and a shift of the mediastinum. Confirmation can also be made by placement of a nasogastric tube into the supradiaphragmatic stomach or by contrast studies demonstrating the stomach or loops of bowel within the thorax. The creation of a pneumoperitoneum is the best nonsurgical diagnostic procedure. Injection of air into the peritoneal cavity with subsequent demonstration of a pneumothorax confirms a communication between the pleura and peritoneum (Fig. 15–9).

Immediate surgical repair is indicated unless precluded by other more serious injuries. Although the surgical approach is somewhat controversial, most recommend transabdominal repair in acute injuries if other injuries to intra-abdominal viscera are suspected. These additional injuries are present in 75 per cent of cases. The transthoracic approach provides the best exposure, and intra-abdom-

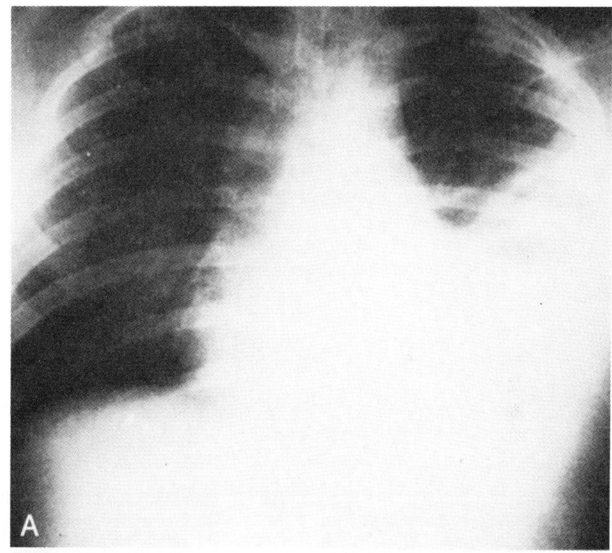

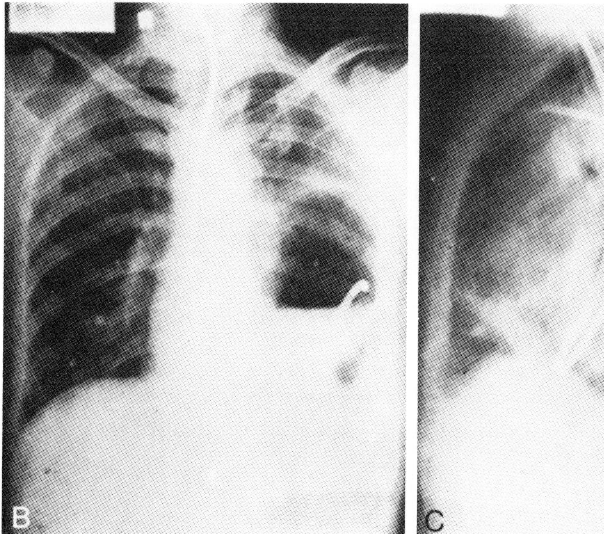

Figure 15–9. *A*, Chest roentgenogram demonstrating air-filled loops of bowel in the left hemithorax through a ruptured diaphragm. *B* and *C*, A nasogastric tube has been inserted into the supradiaphragmatic stomach.

inal injuries may be repaired through the diaphragmatic rupture. It is also recommended for repair of right-sided and chronic injuries.

Esophagus

Esophageal Perforation

Injuries to the esophagus in children are a consequence of their unique behavior or exposure to iatrogenic injury. Children tend to explore the environment and place many objects in their mouth, subjecting themselves to esophageal perforation or corrosive injury. The most common iatrogenic injury is perforation at the thoracic inlet, crossing the aortic arch or the diaphragmatic hiatus, from nasogastric tube insertion.[33] Blowout from major chest compression can occur and has been described following sudden, rapid pneumatic pressure from a child biting into an inner tube.[34–36]

Esophageal perforation represents a rather benign injury when localized to the neck, causing only localized swelling, pain, and dysphagia. However, leakage of gastric contents into the mediastinum results in severe systemic toxicity, which often results in death. Fever, tachycardia, shock, and severe chest pain accompany mediastinal inflammation. Subcutaneous emphysema may dissect up into the neck, and a "mediastinal crunch" may be noted on chest auscultation because of air within the mediastinum. Mediastinal air, widening of the mediastinum, or a reactive pleural effusion on chest x-ray tends to confirm the diagnosis. Large perforations with pleural communication are usually associated with a pneumothorax. Further confirmation of the injury and outline of the surgical approach can be attained by having the patient swallow absorbable contrast material under roentgenographic observation (Fig. 15–10).

All esophageal tears should initially be treated with vigorous intravenous (IV) fluid administration, parenteral antibiotics, and restriction of oral intake. Many times cervical perforations resolve using this regimen, although occasional open drainage is necessary. Intrathoracic injuries, on the other hand, require early thoracotomy, primary closure of the perforation, and chest tube drainage. If possible, closure should be performed in two layers, and the tips of the chest tubes placed near but not on the suture line to provide maximal drainage should the repair break down. Esophagography should be performed 1 week postoperatively to confirm closure of the perforation prior to removing the chest tubes or beginning oral feedings.

The outcome of esophageal rupture depends upon the mechanism of injury, the site of perforation, the degree of contamination, and the delay in treatment. Instrumental perforations carry the best prognosis, whereas the highest mortality follows blunt traumatic rupture.

Esophageal Corrosive Injury

Ingestion of caustic substances, most commonly lye, causes esophageal burn, which may result in full-thickness injury. Diagnosis and assessment of the extent of the injury are initially made by esophagoscopy to the proximal level of the burn. The child is given nothing by mouth and is treated with antibiotics and steroids. An upper gastrointestinal (GI) series is performed 3 weeks after ingestion to document the extent of injury and presence of stricture. If stricture is present, gastrostomy followed by serial retrograde esophageal dilatation is undertaken. If chronic stricture persists, surgery is indicated, with (1) resection and end-to-end anastomosis, (2) colon interposition, or (3) construction of a gastric tube.[36] Resection of the involved esophagus is also accomplished, since carcinoma may develop in the injured tissue.[37]

Heart

Non-Penetrating Injuries

Blunt cardiac trauma is estimated to represent the most common unsuspected visceral injury responsible for death in fatally injured accident victims. It often initially goes unnoticed because of attention to other severe injuries, lack of evidence of thoracic injury (especially in children), or lack of evidence of cardiac injury on the initial examination. Rapid deceleration resulting from high-speed vehicular impact accounts for the overwhelming majority of these injuries.

A spectrum of cardiac injuries may result from non-penetrating thoracic trauma, including (1) myocardial contusion, (2) myocardial rupture, (3) septal rupture, (4) valvar injury, and (5) disruption and thrombosis of the coronary arteries.

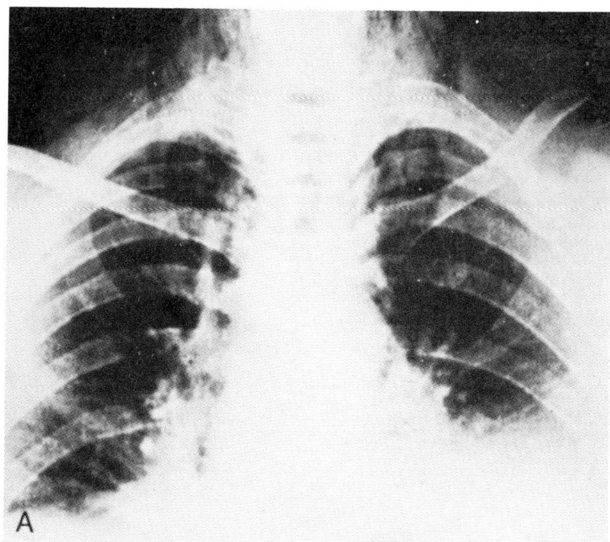

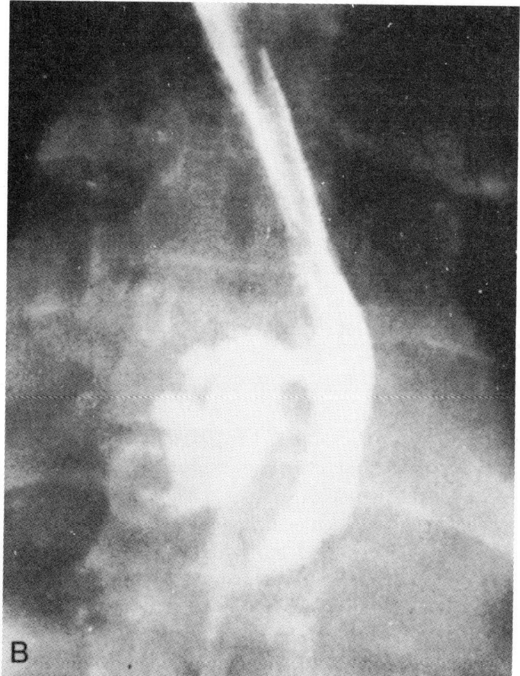

Figure 15–10. *A*, Left pleural effusion and mediastinal emphysema resulting from esophageal perforation. *B*, Contrast study demonstrates a leak in the distal esophagus.

Myocardial Contusion. Cardiac contusion represents the most common injury resulting from non-penetrating trauma to the heart. Many of the signs and symptoms of myocardial contusion are similar to those of acute myocardial infarction or pericarditis, the common presenting complaint being chest pain. The simplest method of establishing the diagnosis is by serial electrocardiography. ST- and T-wave changes similar to those of myocardial ischemia or infarction are observed, although they may not become apparent for 24 to 48 hours following injury. These changes are generally reversible, but take weeks to resolve. Serum enzymes (serum glutamic-oxaloacetic transaminase [SGOT], lactate dehydrogenase [LDH], creatine phosphokinase [CPK]) are of little value in the presence of multisystem injury, although the CPK isoenzyme CPK-MB may be more specific of myocardial injury. Early diagnosis may be aided using radionuclide imaging with technetium polyphosphate.[38]

Treatment of myocardial contusion follows the same guidelines as that of acute myocardial infarction in the adult population. Complete bed rest and oxygen therapy are instituted until electrocardiographic changes revert to normal or stabilize. Careful monitoring is essential, including the use of a Swan-Ganz catheter to monitor left-sided filling pressure. Congestive heart failure or arrhythmias are treated with appropriate pharmacologic agents. Pomerantz and associates[39] found a 50 per cent drop in cardiac output in 11 of 17 patients having sustained blunt cardiac trauma. Hypovolemia from associated injuries and, conversely, fluid overload should be avoided. Anticoagulation should be avoided because of the associated injuries involved.

Myocardial and Septal Rupture. Cardiac rupture is the most common cause of death in patients sustaining closed thoracic trauma. The anatomic location of the right ventricle directly beneath the sternum makes it the cardiac chamber most commonly ruptured, followed by the left ventricle, right atrium, and left atrium.

Intracardiac septal rupture can also occur, its prognosis being related to the size of the defect and the resultant left-to-right shunt. Pharmacologic afterload reduction can initially be employed until the diagnosis is confirmed by emergency cardiac catheterization. Surgical repair of all but the smallest defects should follow immediately.

Valvar Injury. Although relatively rare, acute cardiac valvar injury results in significant regurgitation and heart failure.[40] The valves on the left side of the heart, particularly the aortic valve, are most often involved, and previously diseased valves are more susceptible to injury. Repair requires cardiopulmonary bypass and valve repair, if possible.

Coronary Artery Injury. This condition, although rare, should be considered in children demonstrating persistent electrocardiographic changes following blunt chest injury. Because of its anatomic location, the left anterior descending coronary artery is most frequently involved, an intimal tear leading to occlusion. Conservative management, as with an acute myocardial infarction, is employed.

PENETRATING INJURIES

Penetrating injury to the heart and great vessels is uncommon in children.[33] Patients surviving long enough to reach a hospital following penetrating cardiac injuries usually do so because of some degree of pericardial tamponade. A large defect in the pericardium leads to exsanguinating hemorrhage into the pleural space. Other less common injuries resulting from penetrating cardiac trauma include (1) damage to the conduction system, resulting in various degrees of atrioventricular dissociation; (2) atrial and ventricular septal defects; (3) valvar injury; (4) coronary artery injury; and (5) intracardiac foreign bodies.

CARDIAC TAMPONADE

Tamponade results from the accumulation of blood in the tough, fibrous, nondistensible pericardium when the pericardial injury is too small to allow egress of blood or is sealed by thrombus.

Acute tamponade presents a characteristic clinical picture. Diastolic filling of the heart is impaired from external compression, accounting for the distant heart sounds, low blood pressure, narrow pulse pressure, and elevated venous pressure. The degree of shock is out of proportion to the noted blood loss. A paradoxical pulse may be noted, the blood pressure falling more than 10 mm Hg during inspiration. Peripheral vasoconstriction and tachycardia manifest the low cardiac output.

The diagnosis of cardiac tamponade must be made on the basis of rapid, thorough evaluation. Chest x-ray and other diagnostic procedures prove to be of little help and require time not available. If the diagnosis is in question, diagnostic pericardiocentesis is indicated (see Fig. 1–9, page 73).

Initial patient management requires control of the airway and intravascular volume restoration. For many years, pericardiocentesis provided the primary therapeutic approach; thoracotomy was reserved for patients who failed to respond to pericardial aspiration or who demonstrated recurrence of the tamponade.[41] Reports from major trauma centers now advocate thoracotomy as the treatment of choice for all penetrating cardiac injuries, with pericardiocentesis used only as an interim measure to stabilize the patient for surgery.[42–46]

The entire chest should be prepared. The initial incision is made in the left fourth intercostal space and is extended across the sternum, if necessary. Initial control is best achieved by digital compression, followed by suture repair. Lacerations on the diaphragmatic surface, large tangential wounds, and coronary artery injuries may require employment of cardiopulmonary bypass.

Great Vessels

Non-Penetrating Injuries

Aortic transection and rupture is very uncommon in the pediatric population, again because of children's marked tissue elasticity.

The common anatomic sites of aortic transection are at (1) the ligamentum arteriosum, just distal to the origin of the left subclavian artery; (2) the root of the aorta; and (3) the aortic hiatus in the diaphragm. Shearing forces of the otherwise mobile aorta against these fixed anatomic sites and the marked instantaneous rise in intraluminal aortic pressure are both believed to contribute to aortic rupture (Fig. 15–11).

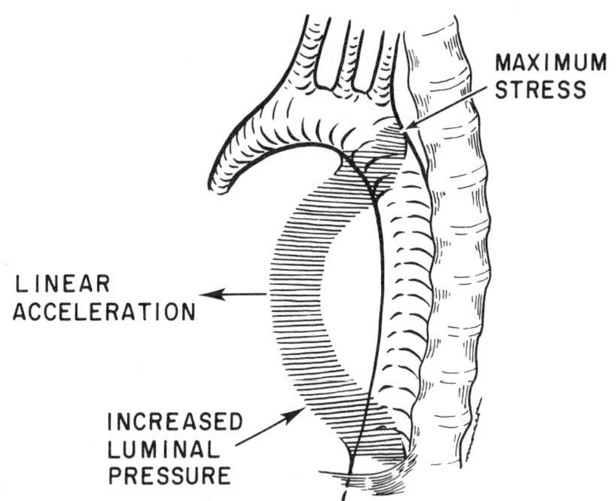

Figure 15–11. An instantaneous rise in intra-aortic pressure and abrupt shearing forces against points of fixation result in aortic transection.

An index of suspicion of this injury should be maintained in any child having sustained a high speed decelerating injury, whether or not there is external evidence of trauma. Commonly occurring coexisting injuries may mask or divert the physician's attention away from the more lethal aortic rupture. Clinical findings of importance include the acute onset of upper extremity hypertension, difference in pulse amplitude between the upper and lower extremities, and a harsh systolic murmur over the precordium or posterior interscapular area.

The most consistent sign of a ruptured aorta is a widened mediastinum on chest roentgenogram. Any suggestion clinically or roentgenographically of an aortic injury warrants immediate performance of aortography, not only to establish the diagnosis but also to specifically identify the location and magnitude of the injury. Surgical repair is indicated following diagnosis.

Penetrating Injuries

Penetrating injuries to the thoracic aorta and intrathoracic great vessels are also very rare in children. The initial management of patients with penetrating great vessel injury depends on the presentation but usually consists of maintenance of an airway and an attempt to restore intravascular volume. Cardiac tamponade is managed as discussed previously. Severe hemorrhage requires emergency submammary anterolateral thoracotomy. Injuries at the thoracic outlet may require conversion to a "book" incision by extension into an upper median sternotomy and a parallel incision above the ipsilateral clavicle. Extension of the submammary incision anteriorly across the sternum provides access to the right hilum and the ascending aorta and its branches. When time permits, localization of the injury angiographically greatly simplifies surgical exposure and repair.

The principles of vascular surgery should always be maintained. Whenever possible, proximal and distal control of the injured vessel should be achieved, or the defect excluded with a partial occlusion clamp. Small lacerations may be controlled with digital pressure and closed with interrupted or continuous vascular sutures. More extensive injuries may require vessel debridement and end-to-end repair.

MORTALITY

The mortality in pediatric chest trauma varies with the age of the victim and associated injury to other organ systems. Smyth[1] found an overall mortality of 13.8 per cent in 94 children following chest injury, with an age variability of (1) 0 to 5 years of 23 per cent, (2) 6 to 10 years of 11.3 per cent, and (3) 11 to 15 years of 8.3 per cent. Concomitant injury to the chest and two other major extrathoracic systems carried a mortality of 58.3 per cent, and 100 per cent of the patients died when three other systems were involved.

The relatively low mortality associated with thoracic trauma in children is a consequence of their usually not having pre-existing cardiopulmonary, renal, or hepatic disease. Further reduction in the incidence and mortality of chest trauma in the pediatric patient will best be achieved through avenues of accident prevention.

REFERENCES

1. Smyth BT: Chest trauma in children. J Pediatr Surg 14:41, 1979.
2. Kilman JW, Charnock E: Thoracic trauma in infancy and childhood. J Trauma 9:863, 1969.
3. Baxt WA, Moody P: The impact of a rotorcraft aeromedical emergency care service on trauma mortality. JAMA 249:3047, 1983.
4. Black RE, Mayer T, Walker ML, et al.: Air transport of pediatric emergency cases. New Engl J Med 307:1465, 1982.
5. Van Wagoner FH: Died in hospital: A three year study of deaths following trauma. Trauma 1:401, 1961.
6. Eichelberger MR, Randolph Jg: Thoracic trauma in children. Surg Clin North Am 61:1181, 1981.
7. Reul GJ Jr, Mattox KL, Beall AC Jr, et al.: Recent advances in the operative management of massive chest trauma. Ann Thorac Surg 16:52, 1973.
8. Jones KW: Thoracic trauma. Surg Clin North Am 60:957, 1980.
9. Levy JL Jr: Management of crushing chest injuries in children. South Med J 65:1040, 1972.
10. Thomas PS: Rib fractures in infancy. Ann Radiol 20:115, 1977.
11. Richardson JD, McElvein RB, Trinkle JK: First rib fracture: A hallmark of severe trauma. Ann Surg 181:251, 1975.
12. Wilson RF, Murray C, Antonenko DR: Non-penetrating thoracic injuries. Surg Clin North Am 57:17, 1977.
13. Relihan M, Litwin MS: Morbidity and mortality associated with flail chest injury. Trauma 13:663, 1973.
14. McCoy JA, Ayium E: The management of acute thoracic injuries. Anesthesia 31:532, 1976.
15. Grosfield JL, Lemons JL, Ballantine TVN, et al.: Emergency thoracotomy for acquired bronchopleural fistula in the premature infant with respiratory distress. Pediatr Surg 15:416, 1980.
16. Hall RT, Rhodes PG: Pneumothorax and pneumomediastinum in infants with idiopathic respiratory distress syndrome receiving continuous positive airway pressure. Pediatrics 55:493, 1975.
17. Ganitano ES, Pomerance JJ, Gans SL: Successful surgical repair of iatrogenic lung perforation in the neonate. Pediatr Surg 16:70, 1981.
18. Moessinger AC, Driscol JM, Wigger HJ: High incidence of lung perforation by chest tube in neonatal pneumothorax. J Pediatr 92:635, 1978.
19. Shackford SR, Smith De, Zarins CK, et al.: The management of flail chest: A comparison of ventilatory and non-ventilatory treatment. Am J Surg 132:749, 1976.
20. Trinkle JK, Richardson JD, Franz JL, et al.: Management of flail chest without mechanical ventilation. Ann Thorac Surg 19:355, 1975.
21. Haller JA, Donahoo JS: Traumatic asphyxia in children. J Trauma 11:453, 1971.
22. Griffith GL, Todd EP, McMillan RD, et al.: Acute traumatic hemothorax. Ann Thorac Surg 26:204, 1978.
23. Symbas PN: Autotransfusion for hemothorax: Experimental and clinical studies. J Trauma 12:689, 1972.
24. Kish G, Kozloff L, Joseph WL, et al.: Indications for early thoracotomy in the management of chest trauma. Ann Thorac Surg 22:23, 1976.
25. Randolph JG, Gross R: Congenital chylothorax. Arch Surg 74:405, 1957.
26. Haskin SA, Raholt HB, Babyan V, et al.: Treatment of chyleria and chylothorax with medium chain triglyceride. N Engl J Med 270:756, 1964.
27. Ratcliffe JL: Pulmonary contusion: A continuing management problem. J Thorac Cardiovasc Surg 62:638, 1971.
28. Trinkle JK, Furman RW, Hinshaw MA, et al.: Pulmonary contusion: Pathogenesis and effect of various resuscitative measures. Ann Thorac Surg 16:568, 1973.
29. Kirsh MM, Orringer MB, Behrendt DM, et al.: Management of tracheobronchial disruption secondary to non-penetrating trauma. Ann Thorac Surg 22:93, 1976.
30. Lindskog GE: Some historical aspects of thoracic trauma. J Thorac Cardiovasc Surg 42:1, 1961.
31. Solheim K: Closed thoracic injuries. Acta Chir Scand 126:549, 1963.
32. Beddingfield GW: Cardiac tamponade due to traumatic hernia of the diaphragm and pericardium. Ann Thorac Surg 6:178, 1968.
33. Welch KJ: Thoracic injuries. *In* Randolph JG, et al. (eds.): The Injured Child. Chicago, Yearbook Medical Publishers, 1980, pp. 215–231.
34. Cole DS, Burcher SK: Accidential pneumatic rupture of esophagus and stomach. Lancet 1:24, 1961.
35. Kerr HH, Sloan H, O'Brien CE: Rupture of the

esophagus by compressed air. Surgery 33:417, 1953.
36. Randolph H, Melick DW, Grant AR: Perforation of the esophagus from external trauma or blast injures. Dis Chest 51:121, 1967.
37. Applequist P, Salmo M: Lye corrosion carcinoma of the esophagus. Cancer 45:2655, 1980.
38. Doty DB, Anderson AE, Rose EF, et al.: Cardiac trauma: Clinical and experimental correlations of myocardial contusion. Ann Surg 180:452, 1974.
39. Pomerantz M, Delgado F, Eiseman B: Unsuspected depressed cardiac output following blunt thoracic and abdominal trauma. Surgery 70:865, 1971.
40. Rowland TW: Traumatic aortic insufficiency in children: Case report and review of the literature. Pediatrics 60:893, 1977.
41. Blalock A, Ravitch MM: Consideration of nonoperative treatment of cardiac tamponade resulting from wounds of the heart. Surgery 14:157, 1943.
42. Beall AC Jr, Patrick TA, Okies JE, et al.: Penetrating wounds of the heart: Changing patterns of surgical management. J Trauma 12:468, 1972.
43. Bolonowski PJP, Saminathan AP, Neville WE: Aggressive surgical management of penetrating cardiac injuries. J Thorac Cardiovasc Surg 66:52, 1973.
44. Bricker DL, Beall AC Jr: Trauma to the heart. *In* Daugherty DC (ed.): Thoracic Trauma. Boston, Little, Brown and Company 1980, pp. 141–149.
45. Evans J, Gray LA, Rayner AC, et al.: Principles for the management of penetrating cardiac wounds. Ann Surg 189:777, 1979.
46. Symbas PN, Kourias E, Tyres DH, et al.: Penetrating wounds of the great vessels. Ann Surg 179:757, 1974.

CHAPTER

16 Head Injuries

MARION L. WALKER
BRUCE B. STORRS
THOM A. MAYER

Head injury is an extremely common type of trauma in children as well as a leading cause of morbidity and mortality. Up to 75 per cent of all children suffering multiple trauma suffer head injury, and nearly 80 per cent of all trauma deaths in children are associated with significant neurologic injury.[1-2] Conversely, a high percentage of children with head injuries sustain trauma to at least one other body area. The care of children with head injuries requires rapid diagnosis and treatment but can be extremely rewarding. Aggressive recognition and appropriate therapy of such children can save lives and preserve long-term function. Of significant importance is early treatment of hypoxia, hypercarbia, and hypovolemia, since these factors adversely effect outcome.[3-4]

Head injury has three phases: the primary impact injury, the secondary injury produced by the brain's response to trauma, and the secondary injury resulting from the systemic response to trauma. Depending upon individual circumstances, primary brain injury may involve laceration of brain tissue, vascular damage with intracranial hemorrhage, and/or axon stretching and shearing. The secondary injury produced by the brain's response to trauma is a dynamic process, evolving over a period of hours to days and generally peaking at 3 to 5 days after injury. It involves loss of cerebral autoregulation, development of both extracellular and intracellular edema, breakdown of the blood-brain barrier, and, in some cases, coalescence of intracranial hemorrhage. To compound the problem, secondary systemic injury—largely cardiovascular and pulmonary in nature—may contribute to this deterioration. Hypertension, hypotension, hypoxia, hypercarbia, and diminished cardiac output may all be present, and all have the potential for further increasing the likelihood of brain damage. Emergency treatment of pediatric patients with head injury is largely directed towards preventing the secondary injury to the brain. This includes treatment of hypoxia, hypercarbia, hypotension, and increased intracranial pressure.

There are several significant differences between adult and pediatric patients with head injuries. First, as mentioned above, head injuries are much more common in children than in adults. While 80 per cent of children dying of multiple trauma have severe head injury, only approximately 50 per cent of similar adult series of trauma patients die as a result of brain injury.[5] Several reasons predispose the pediatric patient to head injury, including the fact that the head makes up an overall higher percentage of both body area and body weight in a child. In addition, the types of trauma that children suffer (motor vehicle accidents without seat-belt restraint, auto-pedestrian collisions, child abuse, falls) are also a factor in the increased prevalance of head injury in children. Second, the child's brain has significant anatomic differences from that of an adult. Particularly in infancy and early childhood, the brain is less myelinated and is much more easily injured than in an adult. Further, the protection afforded by the cranium differs from that in adults, inasmuch as the cranial bones are thinner and less developed.

Third, the child's response to brain injury differs significantly from that in an adult. Children have a much lower incidence of intracranial mass lesions following head trauma. In adult series, 40 to 50 per cent of all patients have significant mass lesions[6, 7] versus only 30 per cent in children.[8, 9] On the other hand, intracranial hypertension is much more common in children than in adults. Only 40 to 50 per cent of adult patients suffer significant intracranial hypertension following their head injury,[10-12] while significantly increased intracranial pressure is seen in 80 per cent of children.[13, 14] Children also suffer from a unique form of brain injury, previously known as "malignant brain edema." Nearly 50 per cent of children develop this entity, which actually consists not of brain edema but of significant cerebral hyperemia in the immediate phase after head injury (see below).[15]

Because mass lesions are uncommon in children and because of the fact that increased intracranial pressure and cerebral hyperemia occur frequently, children are in general more susceptible to secondary versus primary brain injury. For this reason, it is critical that the physician responsible for the initial care of the pediatric patient with a head injury be aware of these differences and the impact they may have on outcome. Finally, because the secondary head injury is in part more treatable than the primary impact injury, outcome in pediatric patients is significantly better than in adults. In children with severe head injuries (defined as unconsciousness greater than 6 hours duration with inability to utter recognizable words or follow commands) mortality is 6 to 10 per cent.[16, 17] In adults with severe head injuries mortality is 30 to 50 per cent.[6, 7, 18, 19]

INITIAL THERAPY AND ASSESSMENT

In a child with a head injury, initial assessment is directed at treatment of the secondary head injury. Therefore, the cardiorespiratory system is assessed prior to detailed neurologic examination. Because of the significant impact that hypoxia, hypercarbia, and hypotension may have on the injured brain, it is essential to provide cardiopulmonary support immediately. Initiation of preliminary therapeutic measures include the following: (1) establishment of an adequate airway; (2) assurance of adequate oxygenation; (3) initiation of hyperventilation; and (4) correction of hypovolemic shock. The most common mistakes in initial management of the severely injured child center around the failure to accomplish these important tasks. These measures are described in detail in Chapters 1 and 2.

Once an adequate airway has been assured, all patients with severe head injury should be given supplemental oxygen until it can be proved that adequate blood gases are present, since the injured brain requires a rich supply of oxygen. Arterial blood Po_2 levels should be in the range of 80 to 90 torr. If tests for blood gases are available, it is a good idea to draw blood for them as early as possible following the arrival of the patient in the emergency department.

With the establishment of an adequate airway, care should also be taken to hyperventilate the patient to provide a Pco_2 in the range of 25 to 35 torr. Changes in Pco_2 are the most important determinant of cerebral blood flow, since a reduction of 10 torr in Pco_2 can reduce cerebral blood flow severalfold.[20] Because the cranial vault is a fixed space containing brain matter, cerebral spinal fluid, and blood, changes in the volume of this space may result in clinically significant changes in intracranial pressure. The fastest means of reducing intracranial volume and pressure is by controlled hyperventilation. Astute students often question whether aggressive reduction in cerebral blood flow via hyperventilation might result in cerebral ischemia. Controlled studies in animals clearly show that cerebral ischemia is not produced until the Pco_2 drops to 15 to 20 torr.[21] Thus, a Pco_2 of 25 to 30 torr does not compromise cerebral blood flow in patients with head injuries.

The technique of hyperventilation is the same regardless of age and consists of providing adequate total volume to produce symmetrically full chest wall rise and an increase in the respiratory rate sufficient to result in a Pco_2 of 25 to 30 torr. Familiarity with the normal age-dependent respiratory rates of children is important (Table 16–1). In most cases, providing an assisted respiratory rate of approximately five to seven breaths per minute above these normal values results in an appropriate level of Pco_2 for patients with head injuries. However, arterial blood gases should be obtained early and monitored throughout the initial resuscitation. Because hypercarbia in the head-injured patient can dramatically increase the intracranial pressure, airway obstruction and hypoventilation need to be treated early.

Hypovolemic shock is rarely attributable to a head injury alone. If the child is in shock, it must be assumed that the hypotension is due to some cause other than the head injury. Exceptions to this include patients with large scalp lacerations or open skull fractures with dural sinus tears or patients with hydrocephalus, in which major bleeding into the ventricles may occur. Always look for evidence of other injuries when shock is present. However, in a small child even small scalp lacerations may produce sufficient blood loss to account for hypotension. If scalp bleeding is uncontrolled, profound shock may result, particularly in infants. Thus, control of bleeding is critically impor-

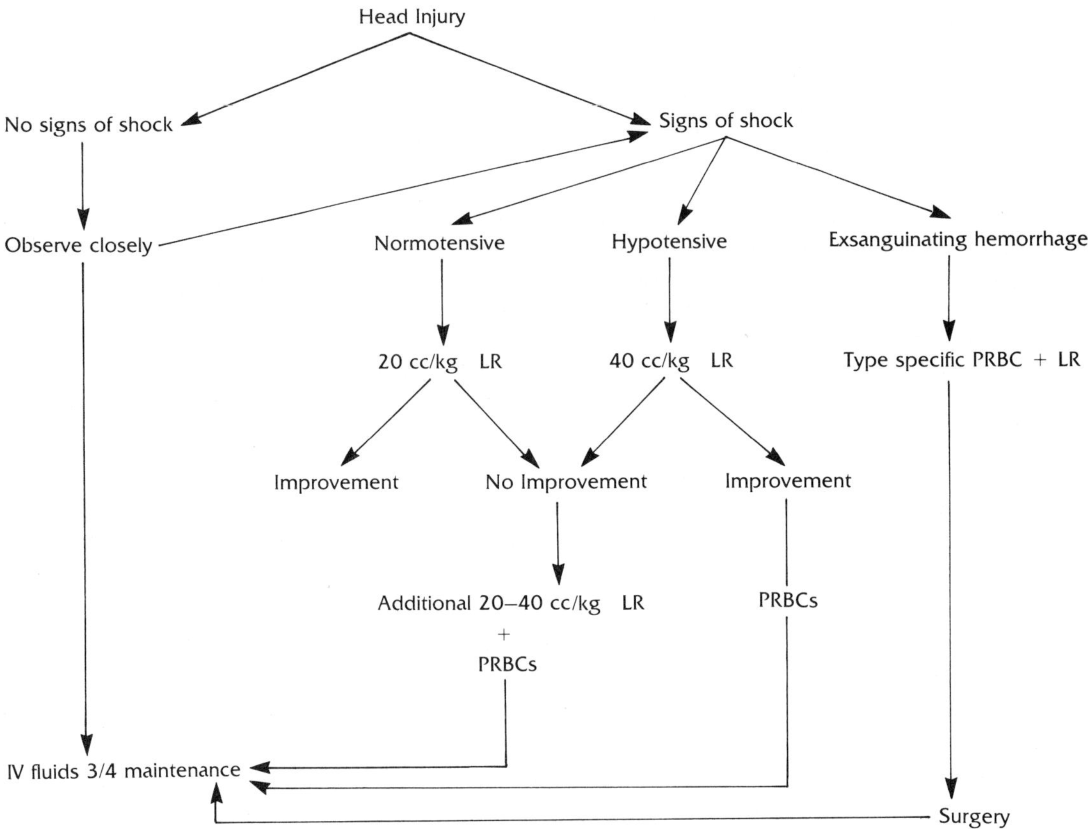

LR = Lactated Ringer's
PRBC = Packed Red Blood Cells

Figure 16–1. Fluid therapy in patients with head injury. Because of its profound effect on patients with head injury, shock should be aggressively treated. Once the effective circulatory volume has been restored and transfusion completed (when necessary), intravenous fluids should be decreased to 75 per cent of maintenance levels to limit cerebral edema.

tant to the initial care of the head-injured patient. Associated injuries may also cause bleeding, which also requires aggressive treatment. Fractures are common in children, especially in the femoral and pelvic regions, and can be the site of significant bleeding.

The importance of rapidly providing an adequate circulatory volume for the pediatric victim of multiple traumas cannot be overstated. The total blood volume of the child is considerably less than an adult but also constitutes a larger overall portion of body weight.[22] Loss of a relatively small amount of blood may be enough to produce shock and seriously compromise an already critical head injury.

Initial fluid resuscitation for all patients in shock is provided with balanced salt solution.[23, 24] It is important to maintain an adequate blood pressure (blood pressure > 80 + 2 times the age in years) in order to maintain brain perfusion. While this may seem obvious, the omission of fluid resuscitation is one of the most common errors seen in the initial management of the head-injured patient. In a child with early signs of shock (decreased pulse pressure, tachycardia, tachypnea), 20 ml/kg of lactated Ringer's solution should be infused. If hypotension is present, 20 to 40 ml/kg of balanced salt solution will be necessary. In cases of severe hemorrage, 10 to 15 cc/kg of packed red blood cells should also be transfused. There is usually time to provide type-specific packed red blood cells, but in cases of exsanguinating hemorrhage, O-negative red blood cells should be transfused (Fig. 16–1).

However, once the cardiovascular system has been stabilized, shock has been adequately treated, and bleeding has been controlled, maintenance intravenous fluids should be given at two thirds to three fourths the normal maintenance levels of 1500 $ml/m^2/24$ hours.

In patients who suffer head injury and who present in shock with an altered level of consciousness, it is important to realize that the depressed level of consciousness cannot be fully and appropriately evaluated until hypotension is reversed, since shock may produce altered mental status. Therefore, any head-injured patient with signs of shock should be aggressively resuscitated and the level of consciousness reassessed as clinical improvement in shock occurs.

Even for experienced professionals it is disturbing to see a child with a serious head injury. There is a natural tendency to rush the child to the nearest neurosurgeon. However, this is appropriate only when it does not compromise the child's overall care. During the initial phase of resuscitation, attention should be focused on controlling the airway, providing adequate oxygenation and ventilation, initiating hyperventilation, and aggressively treating hypovolemic shock. In the majority of head-injured pediatric patients, these measures are more critical than simply rushing the child to the nearest neurosurgeon.

THE EMERGENCY DEPARTMENT MINI-NEUROLOGIC EXAMINATION

A decision regarding the urgency of neurosurgical care can often be made during the first moments of the emergency department evaluation. This decision is arrived at by using the mini-neurological examination. This important and simple examination serves as a baseline for comparing future examinations and helps sort out the priorities of neurosurgical treatment. It consists of the following seven components: (1) history, (2) level of consciousness, (3) pupils and fundi, (4) movement of extremities, (5) plantar responses, (6) cerebrospinal fluid (CSF) otorrhea/rhinorrhea, and (7) vital signs. The mini-neurologic exam is described in Chapter 1.

History

Information obtained from the history is vitally important. An effort should be made to talk with those who were present at the scene of the accident. Paramedics or EMTs can often give valuable information regarding the patient's level of consciousness at the scene of the injury and whether or not it has changed since that time. Documentation of any neurologic changes, especially deterioration, is of the utmost importance. Early clues to increasing intracranial pressure (i.e., decreasing level of consciousness, pupillary changes, respiratory abnormalities, developing paresis, and so on) are important in making decisions regarding the urgency of neurosurgical intervention. These changes, of course, are best appreciated in comparison with the historical findings of the patient. We make it a point of never letting the paramedics or EMTs leave the emergency department without describing for us the neurologic findings at the scene of the accident. The patient's status is thus documented from the time of the initial impact.

Rapid deterioration in the patient's level of consciousness is a signal for urgent neurosurgical intervention.[25, 26] Early in the patient's care, this deterioration often represents an expanding intracranial hematoma, which requires immediate neurosurgical consultation.[27, 28] Other cases of rapid deterioration include refractory seizures,[29] the syndrome of malignant brain edema of childhood,[15] or the development of hypovolemic shock. The first two of these diagnoses are best differentiated through a history and a CT scan, and the later should be monitored carefully by vital signs and clinical assessment of response to therapy.

Level of Consciousness

Evaluation of the level of consciousness following head injury is the single most important factor influencing both treatment and outcome in these patients[30-36] and is best accomplished with the Glasgow Coma Scale (Table 1–4, p. 25). All patients with a score of 10 or lower on the Glasgow Coma Scale (GCS) should be considered to have a serious head injury. In addition, the GCS score is extremely accurate in evaluating changes in the level of consciousness. For example, a drop in the GCS score of 3 or more is an indication for immediate neurosurgical intervention, assuming shock has not intervened to cause the decreased level of consciousness. All physicians caring for patients with head injuries or altered level of consciousness should be familiar with the use of GCS score. Use of this score also aids in communication between nurses, prehospital care personnel, and physicians as they communicate the patient's neurologic status.

One potential problem with the use of the GSC score occurs in children under 2 years of age, in whom verbal skills are variably developed. While additional scales have been proposed and tested for this age group, we simply score such children with a full verbal score if they are able to cry after stimulation.[37] Additional factors that can influence the level of consciousness, and thus the GCS score, are hypoxia, hypotension, the presence of intoxicants, and a postictal state.[38]

Table 16–1. NORMAL RESPIRATORY RATES IN CHILDREN

Age	Breaths/Minute
Infant	25–30
Preschool	20
School-age	15
Adolescent	12–15

Pupils and Fundi

This is a simple but nonetheless important part of the examination. The pupils should be described according to size, reactivity to light and accommodation, and irregularities. Always check the pupils individually, not by shining a light in both eyes at once. This gives an assessment of the status of each pupil and avoids confusion with an intact consensual reflex when an optic nerve may have been severed. The simplest means of describing pupillary size and reactivity is by stating their size in millimeters before and after light stimulation or accommodation. All physicians should be familiar with estimating pupillary size in millimeters.

The presence of a dilated and unreactive pupil immediately following trauma may be due to traumatic iridoplegia, direct nerve damage, increased intracranial pressure, or cerebral ischemia. It is important to distinguish the first two from the latter, since only cerebral ischemia and increased intracranial pressure are of prognostic significance for long-term neurologic outcome. Dilated and unreactive pupils immediately following direct head or facial trauma in an otherwise alert and neurologically intact patient are usually secondary to traumatic iridoplegia. However, if decreased level of consciousness or other neurologic findings are present, increased intracranial pressure or ischemia may be present.

The fundi frequently yield positive information in the first few hours post trauma and should always be examined. Some of the findings in the fundi have specific implications as to the cause and type of trauma and have some prognostic value as well. Fresh retinal hemorrhages after head injury usually signify a significant degree of trauma[39] and often imply the presence of a subarachnoid hemorrhage or an acute subdural hematoma. It is a peculiar trait of children that retinal hemorrhage is notably absent in all but the most severe of head injury cases. It has been noted that the presence of retinal hemorrhages in a child less than one year of age usually represents child abuse.[40]

It usually takes 12 to 24 hours for significant papilledema to develop following trauma. Acute papilledema (present within 2 hours of the head injury) is a very serious prognostic sign. It is invariably caused by dramatically increased intracranial pressure and is usually fatal.[41]

Movement of the Extremities

Any impairment of movement that may be present should be described. Whether there is monoparesis, hemiparesis, diplegia, or other specific disorder should be noted. In assigning scores to the Glasgow Coma Scale, the best movement of the patient is used for scoring (see Table 1–4, p. 25), but the response on both sides should be recorded.

Plantar Responses

The response of the toes to a Babinski stimulation should be recorded as downgoing, upgoing, or equivocal.

Cerebrospinal Fluid Otorrhea/Rhinorrhea

This is usually easy to document but should always be looked for during the examination. Otorrhea will almost always stop within 7 days of the injury. Rhinorrhea may stop but may also continue indefinitely, requiring surgical repair.

Vital Signs

The vital signs may give important clues to the level as well as the type of injury present. In addition to the importance of the vital signs in the assessment of the general status of the multiple trauma victim, the vital signs can have special meaning for the patient with a head injury.

Temperature

A rise in the patient's temperature may cause increased cerebral blood flow, increased intracranial volume and, therefore, increased intracranial pressure. It is advisable to keep the temperature as close to normal as possible. It should always be remembered that children are very sensitive to the ambient temperature and their body temperature can drop quickly, a response that is magnified in head-injured patients.[42] Care should be taken to keep the child in a neutral thermal environment. In most emergency departments this will require heating lamps or blankets, particularly for infants and small children.

Pulse

A rapid pulse most often represents blood loss, and a search for the site of hemorrhage should be undertaken. Bradycardia in the presence of increasing blood pressure (the Cushing response) may indicate increasing intracranial pressure and should alert the examiner to seek neurosurgical consultation immediately. However, the Cushing response is usually a late response to the injury (after the intracranial pressure is quite high). One should not rely on this response as an early sign of deterioration.

Blood Pressure

Comments on the Cushing response have been made in the preceding section. As stated at the beginning of this chapter, hypotension should never be assumed to be the direct result of the head injury.

Respirations

Several patterns of respiration may have clinical significance for the location and importance of the injury.

Cheyne-Stokes Respirations. This pattern of breathing is a waxing and waning, crescendo and decrescendo pattern with a short period of apnea in between. It indicates diffuse diencephalic or upper midbrain involvement.[43] Development of this pattern of breathing after a previously normal respiratory pattern is evidence of neurologic deterioration.

Apnea. While apnea may represent a grave prognostic finding in head-injured patients, initial resuscitation should still be provided. Hypovolemic shock or cervical spine injury may be the cause of apnea. However, up to 15 per cent of pediatric patients with apnea caused by head injury survive.[37]

Central Neurogenic Hyperventilation. This respiratory pattern is characterized by a deep repetitive breath. It is seen with injuries to the brain stem at the level of the pons.[43]

EVALUATION OF THE PATIENT WITH A "MILD" HEAD INJURY

One of the most frequently encountered and challenging problems confronting emergency physicians and pediatricians is the appropriate evaluation and therapy of children with minor to moderate head injury. In most cases, these children have not suffered major multiple trauma or serious head injury. Quite often, a child has simply fallen from a chair, kitchen counter, grocery cart, swing, or some other piece of furniture or equipment. Following the injury the child develops drowsiness and vomiting and is taken to the physician for evaluation. In many cases, the parent will state, "I'd like some x-rays taken to see if it's a concussion or if anything is broken." Should all such patients be x-rayed? Should all such patients be admitted to the hospital for evaluation? If not, which patients require radiographic evaluation? Which patients can be safely observed at home and which require hospitalization?

Numerous detailed clinical studies have been performed to evaluate the efficiency of skull x-rays in such patients. A number of high-yield criteria have been proposed as screening protocols for identifying patients requiring skull films. Classic studies by Bell and Loop,[44] as well as others,[45-51] have proposed that routine skull radiographs in all patients with mild head injury are not cost effective. However, there is no unanimity of opinion on the precise criteria that should be utilized in all circumstances as an indication for skull radiographs. We utilize a general approach, integrating history, neurologic examination, and additional physical findings to identify patients who are likely to benefit from skull radiographs (Table 16–2).

For patients with mild head injuries, regardless of whether or not a skull fracture is present, the single most important treatment is careful observation in the period following the injury.[52] This observation is necessary to identify neurologic deterioration. Whether this observation is best delivered at home or in the hospital is based largely upon the patient's clinical status. Patients with a decreasing level of consciousness or findings that are not explained by the history, physical examination, or radiographs should be carefully observed in the hospital. If a linear, basilar, or occipital fracture is demonstrated on x-ray, the patient should usually be observed in the hospital for 24 to 48 hours.[53] Finally, when the physician is unsure if close neurologic observation can be given at home, the patient should be admitted to the hospital for observation.

Table 16–2. INDICATIONS FOR SKULL RADIOGRAPHS

History
Documented loss of consciousness
High-speed deceleration injury with head trauma
Significant injuries to temporal or occipital areas
"Lucid interval" documented
Previous craniotomy with shunt tube
Physical Examination
Infant < 1 year of age
Glasgow Coma Scale score ≤ 10
Focal neurologic findings
Findings suggesting basilar skull fracture (Hemotympanum, Battle's sign, "raccoon eyes")
Occipital swelling or hematoma
Depressed areas by palpation
Open skull injury
Penetrating injury

EVALUATION OF PATIENTS WITH MODERATE TO SEVERE HEAD INJURY

As indicated above, patients with more serious head injury are most easily identified by their level of consciousness, as indicated by a GCS score of 10 or lower. In addition to the level of consciousness, patients with serious head injury may be identified by other factors, including open skull fractures, depressed skull fractures, penetrating injuries to the brain, focal neurologic findings or rapid deterioration of consciousness (indicated by a decrease in the GCS of 2 to 3 points). The initial priorities of airway, ventilation, and treatment of shock are paramount, followed by the neurologic examination. Once a patient has been identified as having a severe head injury, additional evaluation is intended to clarify both the type and extent of injury. This evaluation includes laboratory tests, skull radiographs, and CT scans, when indicated.

Laboratory Tests

Although laboratory tests have a limited role in the evaluation of neurologic injury per se, they assist in identifying the extent of hemorrhage, the presence of pre-existing disease, and the extent of additional injuries, and they prepare patients for transfusion. A blood specimen should be drawn during the initial assessment. We usually draw a standard set of lab tests on all serious trauma victims. This includes a CBC, electrolytes, glucose, amylase, prothrombin time, partial thromboplastin time, platelets, and type and cross-match. A urinalysis is also done. This can be done without interfering with the examination of the patient and allows the laboratory to get started on these important tests.

Skull X-Rays

While the previous section details appropriate radiographic work-up of patients with mild head injury, skull x-rays also serve in the evaluations of patients with moderate to severe head injury. There is an understandable tendency to rely heavily on skull x-rays to assess the degree of damage in the patient with head injury. However, the degree of brain injury does not correlate well with the presence of skull fractures,[54, 55] except in certain specific instances (e.g., fractures crossing the middle meningeal artery, depressed skull fractures, occipital skull fractures).[56] Many patients with severe brain injury have no skull fractures, while other patients with linear fractures of the skull may show little or no neurologic damage. It is critical to note that skull x-rays do not replace or obviate the need for a careful history and neurologic examination. Instead, radiologic studies simply *enhance* the care of the patient, by identifying specific areas of injury. However, skull x-rays may be important because they help in deciding which patients may need admission or special observation.

Many of the x-ray examinations on a trauma patient can be done by portable equipment in the emergency department. However, if the patient's condition is stable, higher quality films can usually be obtained in the radiology department or by fixed radiographic equipment in a trauma resuscitation area. Appropriate x-rays should always be guided by a careful history and physical examination and include all areas of suspected trauma. Prime consideration should be given to the chest, cervical spine, abdomen, pelvis, and extremities (see Chapter 8).

Classification of Skull Fractures

Skull fractures may be divided into several important groups, according to type, location, and patient's age.

Type of Skull Fracture. Skull fractures are generally classified as linear or depressed. The primary importance of linear fractures is related to their location (see below). Depressed fractures are classified as open or closed according to the presence or absence of an overlying scalp laceration. Depressed fractures generally will require surgical repair, particularly if the fragment is depressed to a depth greater than the thickness of the calvarium.[57] Any open fractures should be covered with sterile saline-soaked sponges. Patients with open depressed skull fractures should be started on intravenous antibiotics early. We recommend methicillin and ampicillin (200 mg/kg/day). If brain tissue is seen through the fracture site, then anticonvulsant medication (phenytoin 10 mg/kg) should also be given.

Location of Skull Fracture. The location of the skull fracture can have very important implications. Fractures across vascular grooves (e.g., middle meningeal artery) or dural venous sinuses should be observed closely. The potential for deterioration exists because bleeding into the subdural or epidural spaces may cause elevated intracranial pressure. Occipital fractures and basilar fractures have a higher than usual incidence of complicating factors (e.g., CSF leak, meningitis, cranial nerve palsies, intracranial hematomas) than other skull fractures.[56] Hence, patients with such fractures need to be admitted to the hospital for neurosurgical observation no matter how alert and normal they may appear. While linear and depressed skull fractures are usually easily seen on plain skull films, basilar skull fractures are not usually clearly apparent on skull films.[58] The diagnosis of a basilar fracture is made on the clinical examination of the patient. There will be CSF or blood coming from the ear or nose or the typical "raccoon eye" appearance with the hematoma limited to the upper eyelid.

Age of the Patient. Infants are especially prone to complications from skull fractures. Small children dropped from infant seats or similar heights may sustain a severely lacerated brain from bony fragments pushed deep into the hemispheres of the brain. The bony fragments in such cases usually realign themselves immediately following the injury. The clue on the skull x-ray that this may have happened is the presence of a wide diastatic fracture line. These babies look surprisingly good on examination but may go on to have cerebral edema, bleeding, or seizures. If the skull film shows a wide diastasis to the linear fracture line, the infant should be admitted for close observation.

CT Scans

Computerized tomography (CT) scanning provides a rapid, safe, and noninvasive means of assessing brain injury and yields important information, including identification of intracranial hematomas, extent of subsequent mass effect, presence of cerebral edema or hyperemia, and extent of depression of skull fractures.[59, 60] In order to assure maximum benefit from utilization of the CT scan in pediatric head injury patients, pediatricians and emergency physicians should seek input from the neurosurgeons responsible for the care of such trauma patients. It is preferable to obtain necessary input on each patient individually; however, in some cases time constraints do not allow neurosurgical consultation prior to obtaining CT scans. In these instances, the emergency department will be well served by planning for such circumstances in advance by discussing the general indications for CT scans with the neurosurgical group serving the hospital. Recent data indicate that major mortality reductions may result if certain intracranial lesions are evacuated within 4 hours of injury.[61, 62] Thus, following provision of an airway, controlled hyperventilation, and therapy of shock, expeditious evaluation of head injury patients is mandatory, including obtaining CT scans when indicated.

In general, a CT scan should be obtained on all patients who are unconscious and cannot be aroused, or who undergo rapid deterioration of the level of consciousness.[63, 64] We also suggest scans on patients with penetrating brain injuries, basilar or occipital skull fractures, depressed skull fractures, or focal neurologic deficits, and on those whose degree of neurologic deficit is persistent or unexplained by coexistent findings.

TYPES OF INTRACRANIAL INJURY

Intracranial Hematomas

Expanding intracranial hematomas can cause dramatic deterioration in the patient's neurologic status and often require immediate surgical intervention. Some of the more common symptoms and signs associated with these lesions are discussed below.

Extradural Hematomas

An extradural hematoma is most commonly caused by a tear in one of the *arteries* of the dura and is almost always associated with a skull fracture. Since this bleeding is under arterial pressure, there can be a rapid increase in intracranial pressure and a rapid change in the neurologic status. The typical injury producing an extradural hematoma is a low-velocity injury (fall, object striking the head, bicycle accident, and so on). This results in a typical clinical picture of initial loss of consciousness and brief recovery, followed by deterioration in the level of consciousness.[65] It is important to recognize that the reason that a lucid interval occurs is that the brain is recovering from the concussive effects of the injury. The deterioration is due to the rapidly rising intracranial pressure. Therefore, if the patient is brought to surgery for treatment of the hematoma before irreversible brain damage is sustained, there is an excellent chance of a good recovery.[66, 67]

Extradural hematomas typically occur in the temporal region and are associated with fractures that cross and tear the middle meningeal artery (Fig. 16–2). These hematomas may occur anywhere, however. Rapid deterioration in the level of consciousness following a head injury is a sign to call for urgent neurosurgical consultation. A CT scan is indicated if rapidly available. The judicious use of mannitol in this situation may prove quite helpful (see discussion under Treatment of Severe Head Injury) until neurosurgical intervention can be provided. In general, extradural hematomas present on CT scan as dense lesions that are convex relative to the brain surface.

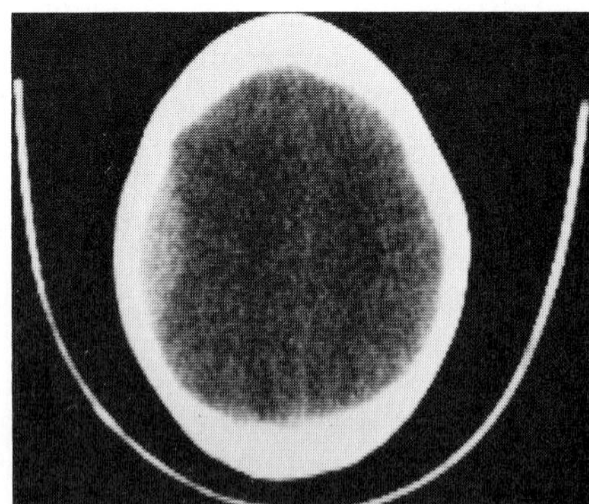

Figure 16–2. This CT scan shows an area of increased density in the temporal region, representing an extradural hematoma caused by a middle meningeal artery tear. Extradural hematomas typically present on CT scan as dense lesions convex to the brain surface. When recognized and treated early, there is virtually no mortality in children with such lesions.

Subdural Hematomas

Subdural hematomas are associated with tearing of the bridging veins between the cerebral cortex and the dura (Fig. 16–3). In young children these hematomas are more common than extradural hematomas. They often occur from high-speed injuries (automobile accidents, motorcycle accidents, auto-pedestrian accidents, violent shaking as seen in child abuse, etc.). Even though subdural hematomas are generally due to venous bleeding, they are associated with serious brain injuries (high-speed injuries) and the outcome is much worse than with extradural hematomas.[68, 69] There is rarely a lucid interval because the brain is so severely injured that a return to consciousness is not possible. The patient who has a subdural hematoma may deteriorate rapidly, but rarely has there been an intervening improvement. Any sign of worsening should alert the physician to the possibility of an expanding hematoma, and a neurosurgeon must be consulted. On CT scan, subdural hematomas present as mass lesions that are concave relative to the brain surface (Fig. 16–3). Outcome with subdural hematoma is significantly worse than with extradural hematoma.

Intracerebral Hematomas

These lesions are associated with bruising of the parenchyma of the brain. They are often not well visualized on CT scans in the first few hours post injury (Fig. 16–4). They are best seen 1 or 2 days following the injury. These hematomas rarely require surgical intervention in children. They do, however, require intensive neurologic management and are most often seen in the frontal and temporal regions.

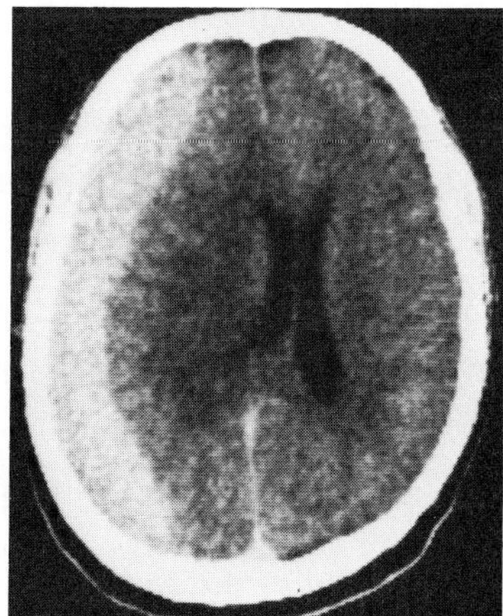

Figure 16–3. This CT scan shows a huge subdural hematoma, caused by a motor-vehicle accident. Such injuries result from tearing of the bridging veins between the cerebral cortex and the dura, presenting on CT scans as dense areas concave relative to the brain surface. Outcome is significantly worse with subdural hematomas than with extradural hematomas.

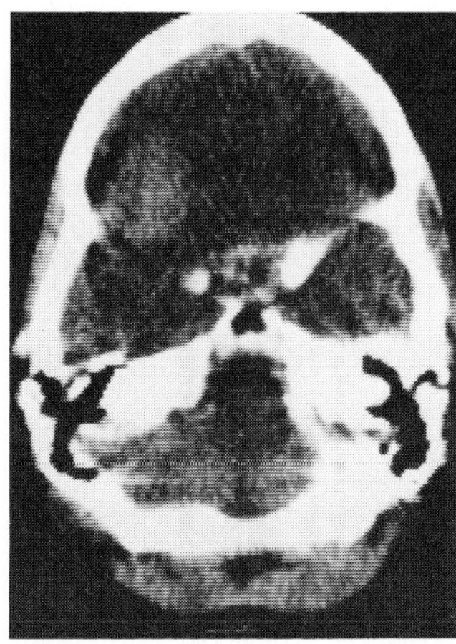

Figure 16–4. This CT scan was taken 24 hours after an auto-pedestrian accident produced deep coma. It shows an intracerebral hematoma in the frontotemporal region. Such lesions represent bruising of the brain and rarely require surgical treatment. However, intensive neurologic care and monitoring are required.

Pneumocephalus

Although pneumocephalus is relatively uncommon, it is presented here to remind the reader that it may present as an expanding intracranial mass (Fig. 16–5). If there is a

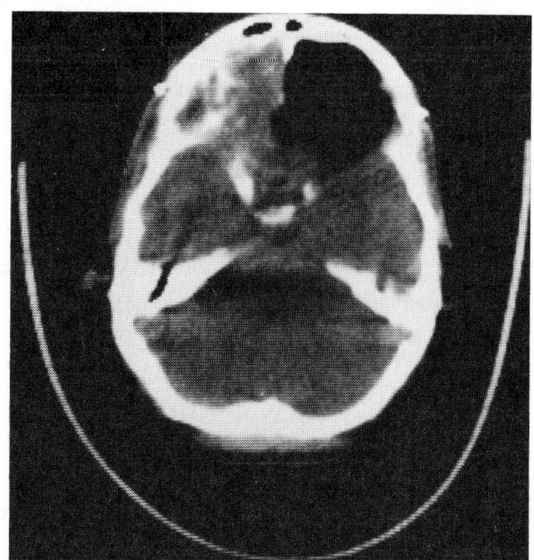

Figure 16–5. This CT scan demonstrates a large area of pneumocephalus in the frontal area, presenting as a mass lesion. When decreasing level of consciousness is present, surgical intervention may be required.

tear of the dura at the base of the skull associated with a fracture, air may get into the intracranial space. If this air is increased with each breath and is not exiting well (a ball-valve effect), the air may expand into a large mass and compress surrounding brain tissue. Pneumocephalus can usually be seen easily on plain skull films as well as on a CT scan. If a head-injured patient is found to have pneumocephalus, the patient must be admitted to the hospital for observation. We recommend antibiotics for this condition.

Cerebral Edema

Cerebral edema may present quickly following a head injury but usually takes 24 to 48 hours to develop.[70] Early treatment of the head injury, including the management of hypoxia, hypotension, and hyperventilation as soon as possible following the injury, is stressed in the first portion of this chapter. Prevention of progression of cerebral edema needs to be given a high priority, hence the emphasis on early management, which is designed to minimize the development of edema. Hypoxia is the worst complicating factor, hence the importance of the airway and supplemental oxygen in head-injured children.

Cerebral edema may be either focal or diffuse. It seems to be easier for children than for adults to develop a diffuse edema following head injury. On CT scan diffuse edema often presents as bilateral, symmetrical compression of the ventricles. Areas of focal cerebral edema may be more difficult to evaluate, since areas of true focal edema may be difficult to distinguish from areas of focal increased blood flow. If mannitol is given to these patients, further increased blood flow may result, resulting in a further increase in the intracranial pressure (see Treatment of Severe Head Injury).

Cerebral Hyperemia—The Syndrome of "Malignant Brain Edema"

There is a syndrome of malignant edema following head injury in children that may present as a rapid deterioration of the neurologic status and truly represents a neurosurgical emergency. It may be confused with an expanding intracranial hematoma, but this form of edema is actually more commonly the cause of deterioration in the pediatric age group, occurring in up to 50 per cent of all severely head-injured patients.[15] This is almost always an increased vascular response to the injury, resulting in cerebral hyperemia rather than true edema.[71, 72] A CT scan is necessary to rule out the presence of a surgical mass lesion. It is best treated by measures designed to decrease intracranial pressure (hyperventilation, oxygenation, head positioning, diuretic therapy, and so on).

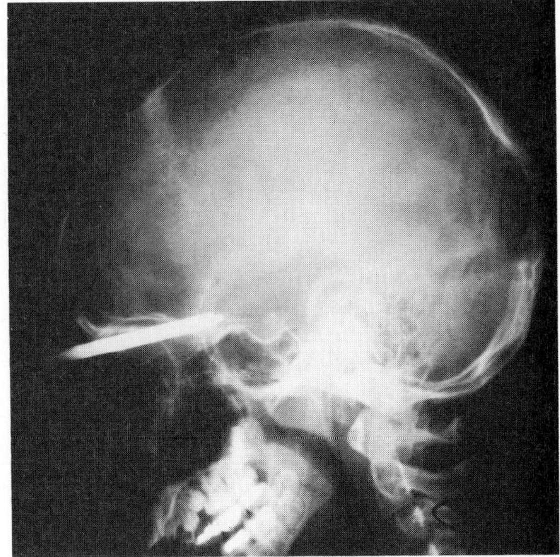

Figure 16–6. This lateral skull x-ray was taken minutes after a child had been in a motor-vehicle accident in which the car antenna was driven into the frontal lobe. Paramedics at the scene appropriately stabilized the fragment and shortened but did not remove it. Such fragments should only be removed in the operating room, since profuse hemorrhage often follows removal. This child survived without significant sequelae and is attending the appropriate grade in school.

Foreign Bodies

Foreign bodies protruding from the brain and skull should not be removed! Because of the lush vascularity of the brain, there will almost always be tamponading of blood vessels by the foreign body. The foreign body must be removed only by the surgical team when the patient is ready for the surgical procedure. To do otherwise invites disaster (Fig. 16–6).

TREATMENT OF SEVERE HEAD INJURY

Management of the Initial Head Injury and Increased Intracranial Pressure

The comments made at the beginning of this chapter regarding airway, breathing, blood pressure, and hyperventilation remain the most important parts of initial head injury management. Initiation of this optimal environment as soon as possible following the head injury will greatly decrease the development of secondary complications to the head injury (Table 16–3). The emphasis on provision of an adequate airway, hyperventilation, and treatment of shock were listed in some detail at the beginning of the chapter and will not be repeated here.

Raise the Head of the Bed. This simple maneuver can significantly affect the intracranial pressure. It should be a matter of routine unless the circulatory status is too unstable.

Position the Neck. The neck should be kept straight and in the midline position if at all possible. Turning the neck too far to one side may occlude the jugular venous drainage on that side.[73] This may then lead to a very significant increase in the intracranial pressure.

Treat Pain. A reasonable attempt should be made to minimize the patient's pain. Pain may cause muscle tension and increased intracranial pressure. Remember, however, that the head-injured patient should not be *heavily* sedated, especially if the patient is to be transported to another facility. We usually use acetaminophen (1 grain/year of age) for initial pain control.

Suction. The patient's airway must be kept clear, and this will necessitate the suctioning of the airway occasionally. If the suctioning is done through an endotracheal tube, there is great danger that this may increase the intracranial pressure. Suction the patient only as necessary.

Table 16–3. INITIAL TREATMENT OF HEAD INJURY

1. Provision of airway (PA_{O_2} = 80–90 torr)
2. Controlled hyperventilation (PA_{CO_2} = 25–28 torr)
3. Maintain blood pressure (BP $\geq$ 80 + 2 $\times$ age in years)
4. Elevate head 30–45 degrees
5. Head and neck in midline position
6. Minimize stimuli (pain, suctioning, movement, and so on)
7. Treat seizures
   Dilantin (delayed or persistent seizures) 10 mg/kg
   Diazepam (status epilepticus) 0.1–0.3 mg/kg
8. Antibiotics (penetrating injuries, open fractures, pneumocephalus)
   Ampicillin 200 mg/kg
   Methicillin 200 mg/kg
9. Diuretics (for documented deterioration)
   Mannitol (mass lesions) 1 g/kg
   Furosemide (hyperemia) 1–2 mg/kg
10. Burr holes (rarely necessary)

Stabilize Other Injuries. Other areas of injury must also be stabilized in order to provide the best possible environment for the head-injured child. This includes stopping bleeding, splinting fractures, and stabilizing the neck.

Seizures

A seizure that occurs at impact or within a few minutes thereof does not require treatment with anticonvulsant medications. If a seizure occurs more than 30 minutes beyond the time of impact, we like to start the patient on medication as soon as possible thereafter. We prefer the use of phenytoin (Dilantin) in this situation. A leading dose of 10 mg/kg is given intravenously, followed by a second IV dose of 10 mg/kg in 3 hours, or sooner if seizures persist. We then continue the phenytoin at a dose of 5 mg/kg/day IV divided in two doses. Drug levels are checked to assure adequate serum concentrations.

If the patient is in status epilepticus at the time of initial evaluation, diazepam (Valium) may be used intravenously in a dose of 0.1 to 0.3 mg/kg. Great care should be used in giving this medication, and the physician should always be prepared to manage the airway (including intubation) when diazepam is used. We would use it only for true status epilepticus, never for ongoing seizure control.

Phenobarbital is occasionally used to control seizures in the head trauma victim. We prefer not to use it unless the other medications have failed because of the sedating effects and slower onset of action.

Antibiotic Therapy

We recommend antibiotics only for penetrating brain injuries, open depressed skull fractures, and pneumocephalus. If antibiotics are used, they should be given intravenously. Some form of broad-spectrum coverage is needed in most of these circumstances. We prefer ampicillin 200 mg/kg/day and methicillin 200 mg/kg/day IV.

Evidence now suggests that there is no benefit from prophylactic antibiotics in the patient with routine basilar skull fractures.[74] If antibiotics are given in these circumstances, any meningitis that develops may be resistant to many of the commonly used antibiotics.

Additional Drug Therapy

The use of drugs in the management of the seriously head-injured patient has a very important place. However, great care must be used in the selection of which drugs are to be used and which dosages are to be given.

Steroids. There is now good evidence to suggest that steroids have no beneficial effect on the head-injured patient.[75, 76] Despite the fact that we have used these drugs for years, it now seems that they do not benefit head-injured patients and we no longer recommend their use.

Diuretics. Mannitol has a very effective dehydrating effect on the brain owing to its powerful osmotic action. This can obviously be of great benefit under the proper circumstances (such as deterioration from a rapidly expanding intracranial hematoma). However, mannitol also increases the cerebral blood flow dramatically.[77] If the increased intracranial pressure is due to hyperemia (a very common finding in the pediatric age group), then mannitol may actually be harmful to the patient. A decision regarding the administration of mannitol should be made by the consulting neurosurgeon. Mannitol should not be given as a "reflex" response to the child who has a serious head injury but who shows no evidence of neurologic deterioration.

Lasix also has an effective dehydrating action on the brain and can be used under the same circumstances as mannitol, without increasing cerebral blood flow.[78]

Burr Holes

The use of burr holes in the emergency department is rarely, if ever, necessary under current standards of emergency department care for two reasons. CT scanning is available to identify hematomas and neurosurgeons are available to evacuate such mass lesions in a timely fashion. In addition, when life-threatening deterioration manifests itself (decreasing level of consciousness, pupil deviated down and out, contralateral or ipsilateral hemiparesis, and so on) the use of mannitol or furosemide (or both) produces temporary but dramatic neurologic improvement. The use of diuretic therapy merely succeeds in buying enough time to allow neurosurgical intervention. When burr holes are necessary, the site should be planned carefully and careful technique observed (see Chapter 1, page 26).

Table 16–4. MODIFIED INJURY SEVERITY SCALE FOR HEAD INJURY*

Grade 5 (critical, survival uncertain)	
Glasgow Coma Scale (GCS) 3–4	
GCS 5–8 plus:	Presence of surgical mass lesion; or impaired or absent pupillary light reflex; or altered oculocephalic/oculovestibular reflex
Grade 4 (critical, survival probable)	
GCS 5–8	
GCS 9–12 plus:	Presence of a surgical mass lesion; or impaired or absent pupillary light reflex; or altered oculocephalic/oculovestibular reflex
Grade 3 (serious)	
GCS 9–12	
Grade 2 (moderate)	
GCS 13–14	
Grade 1 (minor)	
GCS 15	

*All other body areas use the AIS–80 classification (American Institute of Automotive Medicine, Morton Grove, Illinois).

TRAUMA SCORING

Following completion of the general physical and mini-neurologic examinations, the patient can be scored with one of the many available trauma scoring tests. The Glasgow Coma Score is the most widely used neurologic score. It is easy to score the patient using the GCS, and this information has value for prognosis as well as helping to establish the seriousness of the head injury. The emergency department should keep a wall chart of the GCS clearly visible in the trauma room so that those involved in the trauma care can have easy access to it.

There has been much work done in the past 10 years on the development of multiple trauma scales.[79-81] We have modified the Injury Severity Scale to more appropriately reflect the importance of head injury in the pediatric patient.[82] The Modified Injury Severity Scale (MISS) was first published by Mayer and associates from the Primary Children's Medical Center in 1980[1] and has been modified several times. We strongly recommend its use, since it grades the seriousness of the injury and has a very direct relationship to outcome (Table 16–4).

REFERENCES

1. Mayer T, Matlak ME, Johnson DG, Walker ML: The modified injury severity scale in pediatric multiple trauma patients. J Pediatric Surg 15:719, 1980.
2. Mayer T, Walker ML, Matlak ME, Johnson DG: Causes of morbidity and mortality in severe pediatric trauma. JAMA 245:719, 1981.
3. Grossman RG: Treatment of patients with intracranial hematomas. N Engl J Med 304:1540, 1981.
4. Miller JD, Sweet RC, Narayan R, Becker DP: Early insults to the injured brain. JAMA 240:439, 1978.
5. Baker CC, Oppenheimer L, Stephens B, et al.: Epidemiology of trauma deaths. Am J Surg 140:144, 1980.
6. Miller JD, Butterworth JF, Gudeman SK, et al.: Further experience in the management of severe head injury. J Neurosurg 54:289, 1981.
7. Pazzaglin P, Frank G, Frank F, et al.: Clinical course and prognosis of acute post-traumatic coma. J Neurol Neurosurg Psychiatry 38:149, 1975.
8. Mayer T, Walker ML, Shasha I, et al.: Effect of multiple trauma on outcome of pediatric patients with neurologic injuries. Child's Brain 8:189, 1981.
9. Bruce DA, Raphaely RC, Goldberg AI, et al.: Pathophysiology, treatment and outcome following severe head injury in children. Child's Brain 5:174, 1979.
10. Marshall LF, Smith RW, Shapiro HM: The outcome with aggressive treatment in severe head injuries. Part 1: The significance of intracranial pressure monitoring. J Neurosurg 50:20, 1979.
11. Miller JD, Becker DP, Ward JD, et al.: Significance of intracranial hypertension in severe head injury. J Neurosurg 47:503, 1977.
12. Marshall LF, Bowers SA: Medical management of intracranial pressure. *In* Cooper PR (ed.): Head Injury. Baltimore, Williams and Wilkins, 1982, p. 129.
13. Mayer T, Walker ML: Emergency intracranial pressure monitoring in pediatrics: Management of the acute coma of brain insult. Clin Pediatr 21:391, 1982.
14. Bruce DA, Raphaely RA, Swedlow D, Schut L: The effectiveness of iatrogenic barbiturate coma in controlling increased ICP in children. *In*: Schulman K, Maramou A, Miller JD, et al. (eds.): Intracranial Pressure IV. Berlin, Springer-Verlag, 1980, pp. 630–632.
15. Bruce DA, Alavi A, Bilaniuk L, et al.: Diffuse cerebral swelling following head injuries in children: The syndrome of "malignant brain edema." J Neurosurg 54:170, 1981.
16. Bruce DA, Schut L, Bruno LA, et al.: Outcome following severe head injuries in children. J Neurosurg 48:679, 1978.
17. Walker ML, Storrs B, Mayer T: Factors effecting outcome in the pediatric patient with multiple trauma. Conc Pediatr Neurosurg 4:243, 1983.
18. Gennarelli TA, Spielman GM, Langfitt TW, et al.: Influence of the type of intracranial lesion on outcome from severe head injury. J Neurosurg 56:26, 1982.
19. Becker DP, Miller JD, Ward JD, et al.: The outcome from severe head injury with early diagnosis and intensive management. J Neurosurg 47:680, 1977.
20. Wollman H, Smith TC, Stephen GW, et al.: Effects of extremes of respiratory and metabolic alkalosis on cerebral blood flow in man. J Appl Physiol 24:60, 1976.
21. Overgaard J, Tweed WA: Cerebral circulation after head injury. I. Cerebral blood flow and its regulation after closed head injury with emphasis on clinical correlation. J Neurosurg 41:531, 1974.
22. Steele MW: Plasma volume changes in the neonate. Am J Dis Child 103:10, 1962.
23. Shires GT: Pathophysiology and fluid replacement in hypovolemic shock. Ann Clin Res 9:144, 1977.
24. Committee on Trauma, American College of Surgeons: Advanced Trauma Life Support Course. Chicago, American College of Surgeons, 1981.
25. Becker DP: Severe closed head injury. Neurosurgery 4:277, 1979.
26. Tabaddor K: Emergency care: Initial evaluation. *In* Cooper PR (ed.): Head Injury. Baltimore, Williams and Wilkins, 1982, p. 15.
27. Becker DP, Miller JD, Sweet RC, et al.: Head injury management. *In* Neural Trauma (Seminars in Neurological Surgery). New York, Raven Press, 1978, p. 313.
28. Cooper PR: Post-traumatic intracranial mass lesions. *In* Cooper PR (ed.): Head Injury. Baltimore, Williams and Wilkins, 1982, p. 185.
29. Caveness WF, Meirowsky PM, Rish BL, et al.: The nature of post-traumatic epilepsy. J Neurosurg 54:300, 1981.
30. Young B, Rapp RP, Norton JA, et al.: Early prediction of outcome in head injured patients. J Neurosurg 54:300, 1981.
31. Jennett B, Teasdale G, Braakman R, et al.: Prognosis of patients with severe head injury. Neurosurgery 4:283, 1979.
32. Narayan RK, Greenburg RP, Miller JD, et al.: Improved confidence of outcome prediction in severe head injury. J Neurosurg 54:75, 1981.
33. Jennett B, Teasdale G, Golbraith S, et al.: Severe head injury in three countries. J Neurol Neurosurg Psychiatry 40:291, 1977.
34. Bowers SA, Marshall LF: Outcome in 200 consecutive cases of severe head injury treated in San Diego County: A prospective analysis. Neurosurgery 6:362, 1980.
35. Jennett B, Teasdale G, Braakman R, et al.: Predicting outcome in individual patients after severe head injury. Lancet 1:1031, 1976.
36. Stablein DM, Miller JD, Choi SC, et al.: Statistical methods for determining prognosis in severe head injury. Neurosurgery 6:243, 1980.
37. Bruce DA: Pediatric neurologic injury. Presented as part of a symposium "Pediatric Trauma," at the American College of Surgeons Clinical Congress, San Francisco, 1981.
38. Bruce DA: Special considerations of the pediatric age group. *In* Cooper PR (ed.): Head Injury. Baltimore, Williams and Wilkins, 1982, p. 315.
39. McClelland CQ, Rekate H, Kaufman B, Persse L: Cerebral injury in child abuse: A changing profile. Child's Brain 7:225, 1980.
40. Caffey J: The whiplash-shaken infant syndrome: Manual shaking by the extremities with whiplash-induced intracranial and intraocular bleeding. Pediatrics 34:396, 1974.
41. Schut L, Bruce DA: Recent advancements in the treatment of head injuries. Pediatr Ann 5:80, 1976.
42. Gregory GA: Pediatric anesthesia. *In* Miller RD (ed.): Anesthesia. New York, Churchill-Livingstone, 1981.
43. Plum F, Posner JB: Diagnosis of Stupor and Coma. 3rd ed. Philadelphia, F.A. Davis Co., 1980.
44. Bell RS, Loop JW: The utility and futility of radio-

graphic skull examinations for trauma. N Engl J Med 284:236, 1971.
45. Harwood-Hash DC, Hendrick EB, Hudson AR: The significance of skull fracture in children. Radiology 101:151, 1971.
46. Cummins RO: Clinician's reasons for overuse of skull radiographs. Am J Nat Radiol 1:339, 1980.
47. Leonidas JC, Ting W, Binkiewicz A, et al.: Mild head trauma in children: When is a roentgenogram necessary? Pediatrics 69:139, 1982.
48. Eyes B, Evans AF: Post-traumatic skull radiographs: Time for a reappraisal. Lancet 2:85, 1978.
49. DeSmet AA, Fryback DG, Thornburg JR: A second look at the utility of radiographic skull examination for trauma. AJR 132:95, 1979.
50. Roberts F, Shopfner CE: Plain skull roentgenograms in children with head trauma. AJR 114:230, 1972.
51. Boulis ZF, Dick R, Barnes NR: Head injuries in children: Aetiology, symptoms, physical findings and x-ray wastage. Br J Radiol 51:851, 1978.
52. Ransohoff J, Fleischer A: Head injuries. JAMA 234:861, 1975.
53. Fischer RP, Carlson J, Perry JF: Post-concussive hospital observation of alert patients in a primary trauma center. J Trauma 21:920, 1981.
54. Phillips LA: Emergency services utilization and skull radiography. Neurosurgery 4:580, 1979.
55. Totten J, Buxton R: Were you knocked out? Lancet 1:369, 1979.
56. Young HA, Schmidek HH: Complications accompanying occipital skull fracture. J Trauma 22:914, 1982.
57. Jennett B, Miller JD: Infection after depressed fracture of skull. Implications for management of nonmissile injuries. J Neurosurg 36:333, 1972.
58. Ghoshhaira K: CT in trauma of the base of the skull and its complications. J Computed Tomog 4:271, 1980.
59. Peyster RG, Hoover ED: CT in head trauma. J Trauma 22:25, 1982.
60. Lee BCP, Kazam E, Newman AD: Computed tomography of the spine and spinal cord. Radiology 128:95, 1978.
61. Seelig JM, Becker DP, Miller JD, et al.: Traumatic acute subdural hematoma: Major mortality reduction in comatose patients treated within four hours. N Engl J Med 304:1511, 1981.
62. Mayer T, Walker ML: Traumatic acute subdural hematoma. N Engl J Med 306:355, 1982.
63. Kishore PRS: Radiographic evaluation. *In* Cooper PR (eds): Head Injury. Baltimore, Williams and Wilkins, 1982, p. 43.
64. Clifton GL, Grossman RG, Makels ME, et al.: Neurological course and correlated computerized tomography after severe closed head injury. J Neurosurg. 52:611, 1980.
65. Cooper PR: Post-traumatic intracranial mass lesions. *In* Cooper PR (ed.): Head Injury. Baltimore, Williams and Wilkins, 1982, p. 210.
66. Phonphrasert C, Suwanwela C, Hongsaprabhas C, et al.: Extradural hematoma: Analysis of 138 cases. J Trauma 20:679, 1980.
67. Jamieson KG, Yelland JDN: Extradural hematoma: Report of 167 cases. J Neurosurg 37:137, 1968.
68. Langfitt TW, Gennarelli TA: Can the outcome from head injury be improved? J Neurosurg 56:19, 1982.
69. Fell DA, Fitzgerald S, Moiel RH, et al.: Acute subdural hematomas: Review of 144 cases. J Neurosurg 42:37, 1975.
70. Kobrine AI, Timmins E, Rajjoub RR, et al.: Demonstration of massive traumatic brain swelling within 20 minutes after injury. J Neurosurg 46:256, 1977.
71. Kuhl DE, Alavi A, Hoffman EJ, et al.: Local cerebral blood volume in head-injured patients. Determination by emission computed tomography of ^{99m}Tc-labeled red cells. J Neurosurg 52:309, 1980.
72. Obrist WD, Thompson HK Jr, Wans HS, et al.: Regional cerebral blood flow estimated by 133 xenon inhalation. Stroke 6:245, 1975.
73. Hulme A, Cooper R: Cerebral blood flow during sleep in patients with raised intracranial pressure. Prog Brain Res 30:77, 1968.
74. Ingelzi RJ, VanderArk GD: Analysis of the treatment of basilar skull fractures with and without antibiotics. J Neurosurg 43:721, 1975.
75. Saul TG, Ducker TB, Saloman M, et al.: Steroids in severe head injury: a prospective randomized trial. J Neurosurg 54:596, 1981.
76. Cooper PR, Moody S, Clark WK, et al.: Dexamethasone and severe head injury. J Neurosurg 51:307, 1979.
77. Bruce DA, Langfitt TW, Miller JD, et al.: Regional cerebral blood flow; intracranial pressure and brain metabolism in comatose patients. J Neurosurg 38:131, 1973.
78. Bourke RS, Kimelberg HK, Daze MA, Popp AJ: Studies on the formation of astrological swelling and its inhibition by clinically useful agents. *In* Popp AJ, Bourke RS, Nelson HK (eds.): Neural Trauma. New York, Raven Press, 1979, p. 95.
79. Baker SP, O'Neill B, Haddon W Jr., et al.: The Injury Severity Score: A method for describing patients with multiple injuries and evaluating emergency care. J Trauma 14:187, 1974.
80. Champion H, Sacco W, Lepper R, et al.: An anatomic index of injury severity. J Trauma 20:197, 1980.
81. Kirkpatrick JR, Youmans RL: Trauma index: An aid in the evaluation of injured victims. J Trauma 12:711, 1971.
82. Mayer T, Walker ML, Clark P: Further experience sith the modified abbreviated injury severity scale. J Trauma 24:31, 1984.

CHAPTER

17 Facial and Soft Tissue Trauma in Childhood

T. E. SPICER

Children are exposed to the same facial injuries as adults, but major facial trauma is less common in children, owing to a number of factors. First of all, children, particularly young children, lead a relatively protected life under the watchful eyes of their parents. Second, their proximity to the ground and their smaller weights mean that less energy is dissipated on impact with the ground. Third, the soft and hard tissues of the young face are more resilient and elastic. As a result, any injuries that occur are less severe than those in the older population.

Despite these facts, there is ample opportunity in a child's life for significant injury. Like adults, children are exposed to sudden deceleration in automobile crashes. The small child is exposed to the wrath of canine pets; and the older child, to a bicycle mishap. Athletics become a significant cause of injury during teenage years. Considering the vast opportunity for injury, it is most impressive that there are not more major facial injuries in childhood.

In some ways treatment of facial injuries in children differs only slightly from the care rendered in the adult. Soft tissues need to be reapproximated after thorough debridement. Requirements for atraumatic tissue handling as well as precise suture placement are the same. Fractures of the bony structures of the face require similar concern for adequate reduction and immobilization until union is secure. There are, however, many factors that make treatment of injuries in the child unique and worthy of discussion as a separate topic.

First of all, anesthetic considerations in children are more complicated. The injured child has been subjected to the pain of his initial injury, and subsequently his care is entrusted to a stranger. The initial poking and probing in the wound by that stranger does little to encourage confidence and trust. Despite this antagonistic situation, accurate anatomic repair is required for optimal results. Special techniques of local anesthesia, with or without sedation, are warranted for accurate repair. In situations in which local anesthesia will compromise the repair, a general anesthetic is indicated. General anesthesia for children requires special expertise and techniques. See Chapter 3.

Second, severe facial injuries, whether of the soft or the hard tissue, may result in significant initial deformity in both adults and children. In children, such deformity is frequently accentuated by growth. Injury to bony growth centers, which arrests growth, may result in deformity that worsens as the remainder of the face grows normally. A constricting soft tissue scar may have identical implications. Of course, the younger child has greater growth potential and therefore has greater potential for deformity.

Third, the patterns of facial bony injury are different in children. In children the facial bones are relatively hidden beneath the large cranium. Those bones are more resilient, are stronger because of the lack of sinus aeration, and are covered by tougher periosteum. As a result, facial bone fractures are rarer in children. When they occur, they are frequently accompanied by multisystem injury, particularly intracranial injury. Thus, an injury that results in a LeFort III fracture in a child often results in death because of injury to adjacent structures. The presence of deciduous or mixed dentition alters considerations for type of intermaxillary fixation as well as considerations for open reduction and internal fixation of facial fractures.

Finally, the healing potential of children is so much more exaggerated that early repair is indicated. Injuries that are left without adequate realignment for only a few days become difficult to repair without recreating the entire wound. Such exuberant healing also results in a greater tendency for hypertrophic surface scarring. Therefore proper scar management requires more careful observation during the initial 2- to 8-week wound maturation period when measures to interrupt excessive scarring can be undertaken.

INITIAL ASSESSMENT OF INJURY

Following initial stabilization of the severely injured child, an orderly approach is indicated. During the *physical examination* one must avoid focusing on an obvious deformity and overlooking the more serious associated injury. Any significant injury to the face results in the dissipation of energy by both the cranium and cervical spine, and careful assessment of neurologic function is indicated. Precise examination of the facial injury must await definitive care of life-threatening injuries.

Evaluation of the facial injury should include the extent and the nature of the injury. Often it is helpful to sketch the precise injury, for that will draw attention to facial landmarks that are crossed by the injury. As one considers the course of a facial laceration, consideration must always be given to adjacent structures that may also be injured. Those structures include the facial nerve, the parotid duct, and the lacrimal system at the medial canthus. *Assessment of nerve function must precede local anesthetic infiltration.* Precise anatomic repair is required for lacerations that cross natural landmarks such as the vermilion border of the lip, the nasal alae, and eyelid structures.

In assessing injuries of children one must compare the extent of the injury to the history that was provided. Injuries that are in excess of or in a pattern that is different from that expected from the history suggest the possibility of child abuse and indicate further investigation. That includes x-rays to document areas of previous trauma, photo documentation of the current trauma, and reporting the injury to child welfare agencies. While it is often most comfortable to ignore such discrepancies, the child's welfare is best served by exploring them fully.

X-Ray Examination

Good x-ray documentation of facial injuries in children is difficult to achieve. Children resist precise positioning. Paranasal sinuses are often incompletely developed and the presence of developing dentition may add to confusion in interpreting the x-ray. In the severely injured face, a Waters view and an x-ray of the mandible are indicated for initial assessment. The Waters view is useful in demonstrating fractures of the maxilla and maxillary sinuses, the orbit (particularly the orbital floor), and the zygomatic bone (Table 17–1). Other views may be indicated to examine specific structures: the Caldwell view is excellent for defining fractures of the frontal skull, the orbital margins (zygomaticofrontal suture area), and the lateral walls of the maxillary sinus. The submentovertex view shows the zygomatic arches.

Fractures of the nasal bones are difficult to display for the reasons cited above, and frequently clinical examination is more rewarding.

Most often children in whom a diagnosis of facial fracture is suspected have sustained significant trauma requiring hospital admission, and definitive films can await 24 hours of stabilization and observation. The recent emergence of computerized axial tomography has added a new dimension to the diagnosis of facial fractures. Such an examina

Table 17–1. COMMON FACIAL X-RAY VIEWS

View	Figures*	Areas Well Visualized
Caldwell	14.1	Frontal bone, orbital margins, zygomaticofrontal sutures, lateral walls of maxillary sinuses
Waters	14.2	Maxilla and maxillary sinuses, orbital floor and inferior orbital rim, zygomatic bones, and zygomatic arches
Oblique Orbital-optic Foramen	14.5	Optic foramen
Submentovertex	14.6	Zygomatic arches
Nasal Views		
lateral	14.8	Nasal bones, anterior nasal spine, nasal process of maxilla
superoinferior projection	14.9	Nasal bones
Mandibular Views		
oblique lateral	14.18	Fracture of body, symphysis, angle, and ramus
TM joints	14.23	TM joints
panoramic (Panorex)	14.26	Entire mandible

*Figures from Zizmor J: Roentgen examination of the facial bones. *In* Converse JM: Surgical Treatment of Facial Injuries. Baltimore, Williams and Wilkins Company, 1974, Ch. 14.

tion in children may require general anesthesia.

ANESTHESIA

General Anesthesia

General anesthesia is indicated for the more significant facial injuries in children. Simple lacerations of the face can be repaired in the emergency room with local infiltration anesthesia, with or without sedation. The choice of anesthetic is influenced by the patient's age and his ability to cooperate, the individual laceration and the precision required for repair, the need for specialized equipment, and the availability of an anesthetist skilled in pediatric anesthesiology. Thus, with an anesthesiologist well-versed in the techniques of pediatric anesthesia, one can opt for repair in the operating room more often than if such expertise were not available. Every effort should be taken to optimize the initial repair.

Local Anesthesia

Most simple lacerations of the face can be repaired in the emergency room. Children older than 4 to 5 years of age are encouraged by a forthright and honest approach to their injury. Frequently they will accept an initial ice pack over the injury. Within a few minutes, it will provide enough local anesthesia for the injection of an infiltration anesthetic. With infiltration of the edges of the laceration, pain disappears and most children will respond in a cooperative manner, allowing cleansing, debridement, and suturing of their wounds.

The choice of local anesthetic has some importance in the care of facial injuries. Because of the rich vascularity of the face, the addition of a vasoconstrictor to the local anesthetic has a great benefit for wound exploration and hemostasis. One per cent lidocaine which contains 1:100,000 epinephrine is available in most emergency rooms and is recommended. Following infiltration of the wound edges, a period of 7 to 10 minutes provides maximum vasoconstricting effect. Debridement and exploration of the wound may then be undertaken with anticipation of minimal bleeding. Significant bleeding encountered in that situation usually comes from vessels large enough to require a ligature.

Sedation

Children younger than 5 years of age and all those who are hopelessly agitated or uncontrollable can undergo repair of their injury with intramuscular sedation. When children are sedated, constant medical supervision is necessary for the time course of that sedation, including attendance of medical personnel during radiologic procedures. "Pediatric cocktails" that work well for parenteral sedation in this situation include combinations of Demerol (meperidine), Thorazine (chlorpromazine) and Phenergan (promethazine) (See Table 34–3, p. 533). Either cocktail given intramuscularly results in adequate sedation for most children within 20 to 30 minutes. Following injection, it becomes most important to allow the child to sit with parents in as quiet and unstimulating an environment as possible for best effect. As sedation takes effect, the local anesthetic can be injected with only a minimal "start." Following the establishment of local infiltration anesthesia, the child will sleep through the remainder of the repair.

Restraint

Forcible manual restraint of an unsedated child for examination and infiltration of anesthesia should be avoided whenever possible. Such restraint may make an already frightening experience terrifying. Following sedation, however, initial restraint during the period of local infiltration is useful and, if left in place during the subsequent repair, prevents the lethargic, sleepy rolling of a sedated child.

SURGICAL CARE OF LACERATIONS

The principles of wound closure are few. All skin wounds heal by producing a scar. A good wound closure serves to minimize that scar and then to camouflage what remains.

Scars are visible because they interrupt the natural hemogeneity of contour, color, and texture of the skin. A scar that is depressed or elevated relative to the surrounding tissue will produce a give-away shadow. A more deeply pigmented scar is visible in any light. A wide scar can be detected because of differences in surface texture, even if it is flat and of the same color. Realizing the potential for these imperfections, it is important to develop techniques to avoid them.

One has little control over the direction or the extent of the traumatically induced wound. It is well known that incisions or lacerations produce a minimal scar if their orientation is parallel to the natural skin creases. That orientation provides optimal local tension factors, resulting in a minimal scar. Lacerations that follow those directions can be expected to heal best. That situation is uncommon, however. Very short lacerations or lacerations whose orientation is very near natural skin creases can be re-excised to provide a wound that follows those directions. Wounds that are larger or deviate more radically from those relaxed tension lines should be repaired without extensive local manipulation in anticipation of secondary scar revision.

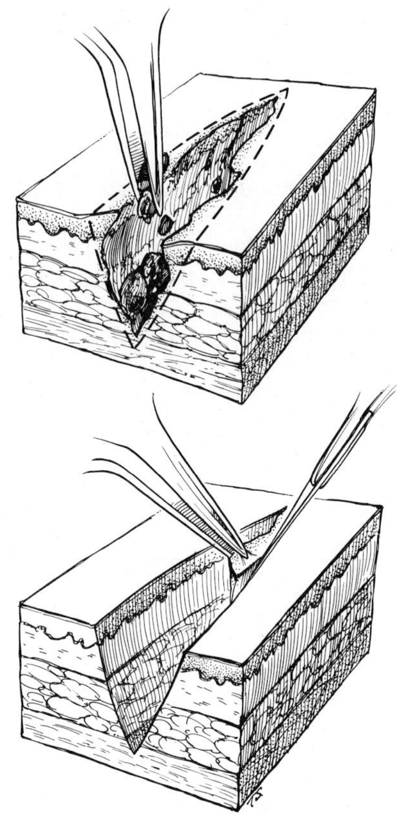

Figure 17–1. Adequate debridement of the traumatic wound leaves a clean, "healthy tissue" surface.

Wound Debridement

Soft tissue injuries result in contamination of subsurface tissues with extraneous debris. In addition, a "crush" element to the injury devitalizes wound edges. Primary uncomplicated wound healing requires debridement of devitalized tissue and extraneous material from the wound. Following local infiltration anesthesia, debridement begins with a wound antiseptic wash and irrigation. Most often irrigation is done with an antiseptic solution, though normal saline is as effective. Its purpose is less to kill bacteria than to irrigate loose foreign debris and devitalized tissue fragments from the wound.

Further debridement requires careful inspection of all of the wound surfaces, with manual removal of attached but devitalized tissue elements (Fig. 17–1). In general, any small ecchymotic tag of tissue adherent within the wound should be removed to reveal a clean surface of "healthy-tissue." While such debridement is tedious, it is as important and perhaps even more important than the manner in which a wound is finally sutured. *As a general rule, as much time should be spent preparing the wound for closure as is spent in actual closure.* Compromising this step results in prolonged inflammation in the wound and increases the possibility of wound infection and/or disruption. *The optimal scar results from minimal inflammation.*

Wound Closure

The exact technique of wound closure is important to the final result. If local infiltration anesthesia is achieved with the use of an epinephrine-containing anesthetic, *hemostasis* is usually not a problem. Any persistent bleeding points should be carefully identified and the bleeding controlled either with small ligatures or with the use of an electrocautery unit. Failure of hemostasis within a wound produces a wound hematoma, which has the same implication as leaving other devitalized tissue within the wound. Prolongation of the inflammatory mechanisms is required for its resorption, and excess scarring results.

Suturing of the wound entails distribution of any *tension* on skin edges throughout the whole wound; therefore deep as well as surface sutures are required. Fibrous tissue with strength occurs at tissue interfaces such as fat-muscle and skin-fat planes. Suture layers should be placed at each of those interfaces.

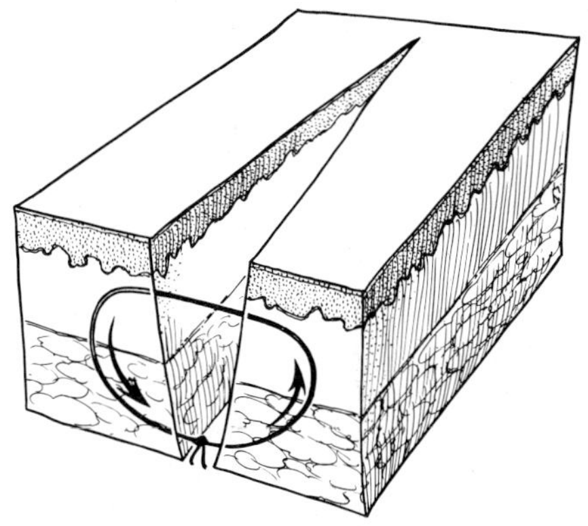

Figure 17–2. Tension on wound edges should be relieved with suture layers at each tissue interface. Place sutures with knots buried.

Those sutures are typically of the absorbable type (chromic catgut, plain catgut, Vicryl, or Dexon). They need to be of a caliber strong enough to support the tension on wound edges yet as small as possible to avoid excessive contamination of the wound with nonvital material. In facial wounds, No. 4-0 and No. 5-0 sizes are most appropriate. Such sutures can be tied with their knots buried deep (Fig. 17–2). As all sutures, they should be tied only tight enough to allow apposition of tissue interfaces. The most common error in all closures is excessively tight sutures, which result in strangulation of tissue. All sutures, whether deep or surface, should be tied securely enough to approximate edges but not strangulate encompassed tissue.

After closing the deep layers, the skin edges should be apposed. Sutures at the subdermal level should take all remaining tension if possible. Exact alignment and eversion of skin edges is completed by the final surface closure. That allows skin sutures to be of fine caliber (No. 5-0 or No. 6-0) and to be removed early to prevent the excessive inflammatory response that is activated by prolonged skin penetration. Sutures at the skin surface should be removed as soon as possible. Careful alignment of edges and removal of tension on edges by subsurface sutures will allow removal of surface sutures within the first week. If left in place too long, they result in inflammation due to ingrowth of epidermal cells along suture tracts and serve as ports of entry for infection.

The importance of *everting the wound edges* should be emphasized. As scars mature over a period of 4 to 6 months, they will lose bulk. A suture line that is perfectly level with the surrounding tissue at the completion of closure will gradually become depressed, producing a noticeable shadow. On the other hand, everting the skin edges to create a small ridge will result in a scar that will ultimately heal perfectly flat. In either event, the skin edges must be exactly approximated (Fig. 17–3).

Eversion of the skin edges may be accomplished in a number of ways. Dushoff recommends sutures that are deeper than they are wide and that include a wider bite of dermis than of epidermis (Fig. 17–4). Despite such advice, it is most difficult to evert the skin with simple sutures. Horizontal mattress sutures (Fig. 17–5) will accomplish eversion but require extra attention to avoid tissue strangulation. Overly tight sutures will result in significant suture marks. Skin eversion with either method requires conscientious practice.

The ideal *number of sutures* should be the minimum required to hold the wound edges exactly opposed. Taking fewer sutures results in small gaps that must heal secondarily, with increased scarring. An excess of

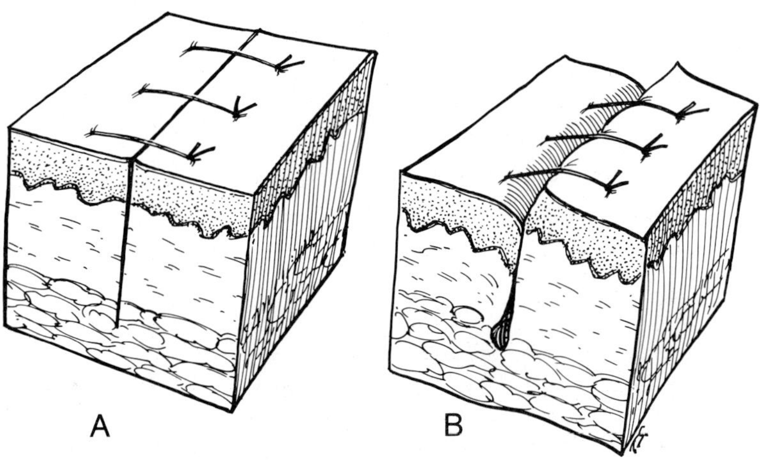

Figure 17–3. *A*, Skin edges should be exactly approximated. *B*, Avoid rolling edges.

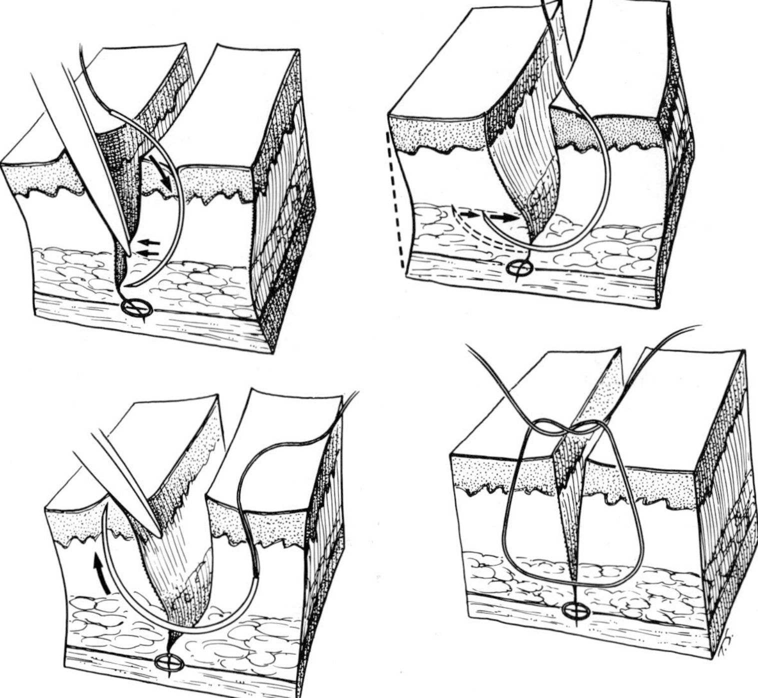

Figure 17–4. Skin eversion is accomplished with simple sutures that are deeper than they are wide and that include a wider bite of dermis than epidermis.

sutures will destroy tissue unnecessarily through the added trauma to the skin, compromising the final result. *Most facial lacerations are adequately approximated when sutures are placed 3 to 5 mm apart.*

Following final suturing of wounds, *dressings* are appropriate to splint wound edges, to absorb the exudate from the wound, and to cover the injury from view. Such dressings should have a nonadherent quality, which can be provided either by medication-impregnated gauze (Xeroform, Adaptic) or by the use of plastic films (Telfa). A properly applied dressing absorbs all of the exudate, controls edema and bleeding, and, most of all, immobilizes the injured area.

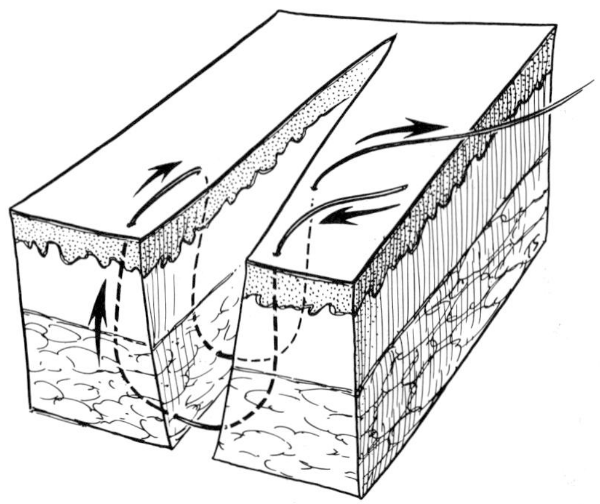

Figure 17–5. Horizontal mattress sutures guarantee eversion. Special care is required to avoid tight sutures with tissue strangulation.

The process of wound healing requires an extended period of time, with final *scar maturation* requiring a period of from 4 to 12 months, depending on the specific wound, its orientation, the age of the patient, and his genetic predisposition for wound healing. The process of scar maturation may be manipulated during that period to provide the most acceptable appearing scar. During the first few weeks following injury, splinting of wound edges using small wound tapes (Steri-strips) is advantageous. Following that period, application of pressure to wounds will produce flatter scars. Frequently a single layer of paper tape is sufficient to accomplish this. To be effective, however, pressure must be constant and must be applied for the entire maturation period. That period is complete when the scar no longer blanches on pressure, no longer is pruritic, and no longer is indurated, having assumed the normal texture of the surrounding skin.

Wounds with Tissue Loss

Wounds with minor skin loss that leave exposed fat or muscle may be effectively closed by undermining the adjacent wound

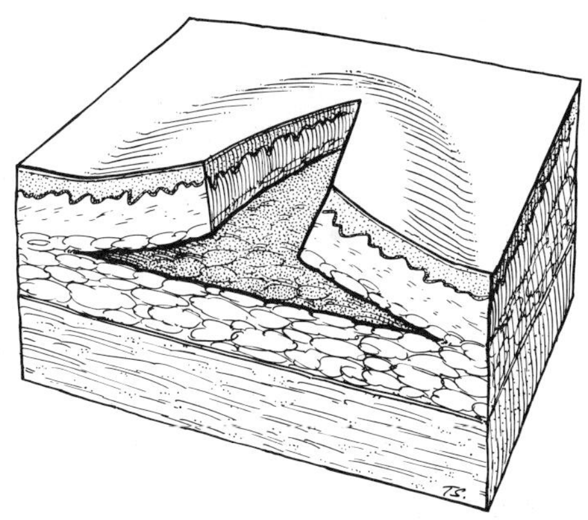

Figure 17–6. Wounds with tissue loss require undermining of wound edges to allow approximation of wound edges without excessive tension.

edges (Fig. 17–6), allowing them to be approximated with minimal tension. When such losses become extensive, or when local tissue laxity will not allow approximation of wound edges, considerations for skin grafting or for closure through local flap techniques become important.

Wounds in which there is an extensive amount of traumatic undermining or in which a small flap is elevated and attached along only one border (Fig. 17–7) represent special problems. In those wounds, distance from blood supply may leave edges devitalized. Their care requires the same considerations for debridement and irrigation. Following debridement *it is generally safe to suture a small flap that is wider than it is long.* Flaps that are very narrow may have an inadequate blood supply to support the tip. Suturing of such a flap requires careful judgment of its viability. When viability is doubtful, alternate means of wound closure (excision with primary closure, skin grafts, and so on) can be employed. More severe injuries or those in which secondary healing will result in distortion of important facial landmarks may require repair in the operating room under general anesthesia.

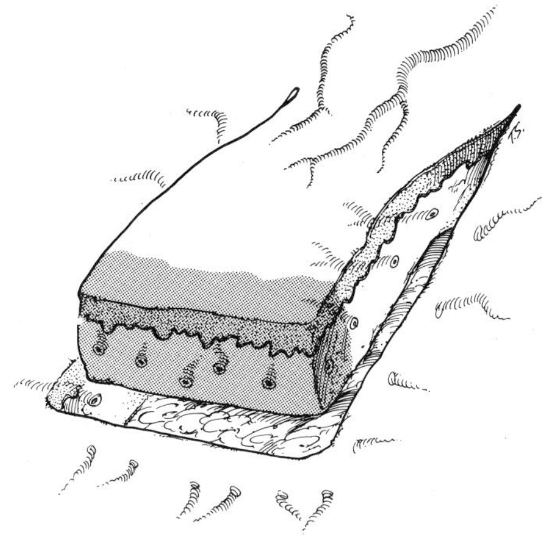

Figure 17–7. Injuries that elevate a flap of tissue may devitalize a portion of that flap by interrupting its blood supply.

Penentrating Wounds

Wounds that are caused by skin puncture by fragments of wood, glass, nails, and other materials are always more serious than they appear. Such wounds carry outside contamination deep into a subsurface location, hidden from view, where local tissue injury increases the chances of significant infection. The degree of local tissue injury is often not apparent from the observation of the surface injury. Local contamination combined with tissue devitalization provides a fertile bed for morbid infections. Fragments of the penetrating object may be left deep within the wound and increase the chances of infection.

Puncture wounds are often deeper than they appear and cause injury to deeper structures: the lacrimal apparatus within the medial canthus, the facial nerves as they course across the cheek, or the parotid duct. Appropriate care requires careful evaluation. A soft tissue x-ray of the area can be obtained in an attempt to demonstrate retained foreign body fragments. Wood and glass splinters can often be outlined against adjacent radiolucent fat. An x-ray that fails to demonstrate a retained foreign body is not absolute proof that one does not exist.

Another trick sometimes useful in locating foreign bodies is *transillumination.* Pressing a flashlight against the skin in a dark room can reveal the foreign body as a shadow in the normally pink transilluminating background. Even if such tests for retained foreign bodies are negative, all puncture wounds require careful exploration, not only to ensure that a foreign body is not present but to debride and clean the depths of the wound. As in other wounds, hemostasis is important. Final wound closure can be completed as described previously.

Bites

Human bites may result from an intentional act by smaller children as a means of aggression or defense. They more commonly occur in older teenagers during fistfights, when a clenched fist strikes an opponent's teeth. Regardless of their origin, human bites inoculate a particularly virulent combination of organisms beneath the skin surface. Bites are puncture wounds, with the attendant local tissue injury into which is injected saliva with its flora of anaerobic streptococci, spirochetes, fusiform bacilli, and other organisms. That combination may produce a rapidly progressive synergistic infection. Because of the severity of such infections, primary closure may not be attempted except in the most optimal of wound debridement situations. Human bites are best treated by aggressive debridement and irrigation and left open to insure adequate drainage. Broad-spectrum antibiotics, including penicillin, are appropriate for infection prophylaxis and should be continued for the first 5 to 7 days during the period of greatest wound infection risk. Smaller wounds may be allowed to heal by secondary intention. With larger wounds, good local wound care for the first 3 to 4 days will allow delayed primary closure at that time.

Dog bites are a common emergency problem. They may be superficial lacerations or abrasions and may result from overly aggressive play with the family pet. They may also be very extensive, ragged, deep, contaminated wounds caused by an agitated animal. The more superficial tooth abrasions require only surface cleaning and dressing with a nonadherent gauze; more extensive contaminated wounds require extensive cleansing and debridement as described previously.

Wounds from dog bites tend to be contaminated with a less virulent combination of organisms than human bites. Primary closure can be attempted, provided extensive wound debridement is completed, including excision of 1 to 2 mm of skin edge and careful removal of all wound surface to the depth of the wound. The decision to close a bite wound implies a commitment to early wound observation to provide the earliest possible intervention for wound complications.

Other bites by household pets and wild carnivores require essentially the same care. The safest course is to allow healing by secondary intention rather than wound closure.

Bites from wild animals carry a significant threat of rabies. Although the incidence of rabies in household pets has dropped considerably in the last 30 years, skunks, foxes, raccoons, bats, wild dogs, and coyotes maintain a substantial reservoir of rabies within this country. Bites from wild animals are at higher risk of transmitting rabies if the disease is known to be present within the region and if the attack that culminated in a bite was unprovoked. The likelihood of rabies is also greater if the bite results in multiple or deep puncture wounds, particularly around the hands or the face. If possible, the biting animal should be confined by a veterinarian for 7 to 10 days so that development of disease within the animal will be appreciated. A dead animal may be examined for rabies by shipping the head to a qualified laboratory.

Immunotherapy of the potential rabid wound is summarized in Table 17–2.

Injuries to Specific Structures

EYELID

In a child, only the most superficial of skin lacerations to an eyelid should be repaired under local anesthesia in the emergency room. The complex and detailed anatomy of the eyelids and the functional requirement for exact anatomic restoration dictate a general anesthetic and repair under magnification. In general, each severed structure within the eyelid should be precisely repaired separately for an optimal result. A laceration

Table 17–2. TREATMENT OF POTENTIALLY RABID WOUND

Animal Type	Disease Status	Treatment
Domestic Cat or Dog	Healthy	none*
	Unknown or escaped	RIG† and HDCV‡
	Rabid or suspected rabid	RIG and HDCV
Wild Skunk Fox Coyote Raccoon Bat	Regard as rabid	RIG and HDCV

*Animal should be observed for 10 days. Begin RIG and HDCV at first sign of rabies in observed animal.

†RIG = rabies immune globulin (passive immunization), 20 IU/kg.

‡HDCV = human diploid cell vaccine (active immunization) 1 ml IM doses on days 0, 3, 7, 14, 28. Vaccine may be discontinued if fluorescent antibody test of biting animal is negative.

of the upper lid involving tarsus, levator aponeurosis, and skin requires separate repair of each of those structures. Debridement in such complicated wounds is conservative but complete (see Chapter 18).

Injuries near the medial canthus may lacerate the fine canaliculi of the lacrimal system. All such injuries require careful exploration under general anesthesia. Repair can be completed with magnification, but prolonged intubation with a small tubular stent is necessary for eventual function. A lacerated medial canthal tendon requires repair to prevent lateral migration of the medial canthus.

EYEBROWS

Lacerations through eyebrows are frequently noticeable because the injury destroys hair follicles, leaving a hairless line through the brow (Fig. 17–8). That situation can be avoided at the time of the initial injury if the wound edges are debrided to be exactly parallel to the hair shafts. Such debridement removes the injured follicles from the wound and allows approximation of skin edges that contain productive follicles.

NOSE

Most lacerations of the nose can be handled with the same techniques noted above. Across the lower one third of the nose the skin is much thicker; healing in this area has a greater tendency to produce a depressed scar. That can be prevented by careful eversion of skin edges.

Lacerations across the alar rims frequently produce a notch in the rim as they heal. At the time of the injury, initial closure must be completed with minimal debridement in a precisely anatomic manner. Cartilages lacerated at the time of the injury should be anatomically repositioned and sutured to their mates. All layers, intranasal lining, cartilage structure, and surface skin covering should be repaired accurately and separately. Despite initial care, a notch at the alar rim frequently develops during healing but can be improved secondarily.

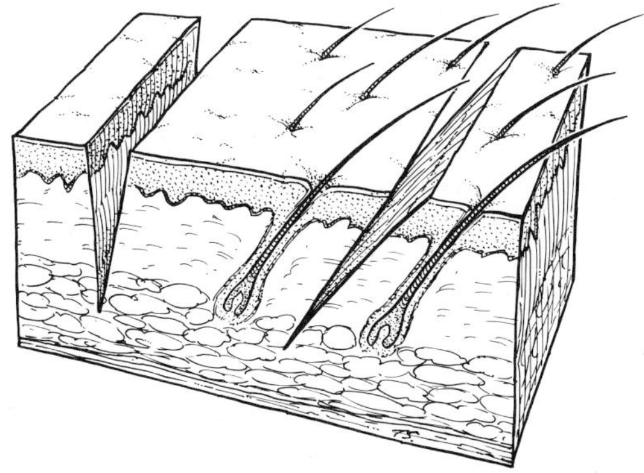

Figure 17–8. Lacerations through hair-bearing areas require debridement parallel to hair shafts to avoid the subsequent appearance of a non-hair-bearing scar. This is especially important in eyebrow lacerations.

LIPS

Lacerations that extend across the vermilion border of lips require precise realignment of that vermilion border to avoid a step deformity. A malalignment of even half a millimeter at the vermilion border is obvious from a distance. Lacerations that extend into the commissure may produce a small web on healing. Like lacerations that produce a notch on the alar rim, they must be as precisely approximated as possible at the time of the initial injury. The subsequent development of a web is best revised secondarily.

Lacerations that include the full thickness of a lip require repair of each layer involved. A full-thickness laceration would thus require repair of the intraoral mucosa, separate repair of the orbicularis muscle, and finally realignment of skin edges, again taking care to see that vermilion borders are precisely aligned.

CHEEKS

Any deep laceration across the cheeks requires assessment of facial nerve function as well as parotid duct continuity. The *location of the parotid duct* in reference to surface landmarks may be established as follows: if a line is drawn from the tragus of the ear to the ipsilateral oral commissure, the parotid duct courses along the middle third of that line. Any laceration crossing that area, and particularly one that seems to drain clear fluid, requires exploration of the parotid duct. Intraoral parotid duct cannulation with a small soft catheter will define the duct course in reference to the wound. Injuries to the parotid duct can be repaired over a stent, or may be drained directly into the mouth. Both require precise surgical techniques under general anesthesia.

Injuries to *facial nerve branches* can be repaired with the expectation of excellent recovery of function, particularly in children.

Any laceration across the lateral face should be considered a potential facial nerve injury. Examination for loss of facial motion must be completed prior to the infiltration of local anesthetic, and is best done by region. Intact innervation to the frontalis muscle is demonstrated with elevation of the eyebrows on looking up. Even the most uncooperative child will frequently follow a light. Intact orbicularis oculi function is demonstrated by ability to close the eyes. Forced eyelid closure accompanies touching the eyelid. Intact facial muscle function across the cheek presents a symmetrical facial appearance. Such children are frequently crying or grimacing, and loss of significant facial nerve function will be indicated by asymmetry, particularly involving the mouth. Small facial nerve branches coursing to the center third of the face have a great deal of interchanging nerve branches, and injury to only a few will not result in a noticeable motor deficit.

Most apparent facial muscular weakness occurs with injury to the temporal or marginal mandibular branches of the facial nerve. The surface anatomy for identifying the course of the *temporal branch* of the facial nerve is as follows: it follows a course from the tragus of the ear to 2 cm above the lateral extent of the eyebrow. Lacerations across that line may injure the temporal branch of the facial nerve, paralyzing the frontalis muscle. The *marginal mandibular branch* of the facial nerve courses within 1 cm and parallel to the lower border of the mandible. Injuries to the marginal mandibular branch paralyze the depressors to the corner of the mouth, allowing asymmetrical elevation of the ipsilateral oral commissure.

Repair of lacerated nerves is best accomplished under a general anesthetic. Adequate neurorrhaphies are completed with operative magnification. Excellent return of function is expected but requires 6 to 12 months following repair.

Ears

Lacerations across the ears require anatomic realignment of severed structures. When lacerations extend across the edge of an ear, healing with production of a notch is common, and this should be explained to the parents. Normal contours can frequently be restored secondarily. Small lacerations through the cartilage of the ear need to be repaired when there is an inherent tendency for those edges to remain out of alignment. Cartilage edges can be held in alignment using a small permanent suture such as No. 5-0 clear nylon or No. 5-0 clear prolene.

Because of its exposed position, the ear can be involved in amputation or near-amputation situations. The entire ear is often adequately vascularized by only a small remaining vascular or skin attachment. Anatomic repair of the injured structures (cartilage, skin) and careful protection from further challenge (tension, pressure, infection, hematoma, and so on) are needed.

When the ear is obviously devitalized, either by complete amputation or by a skin bridge that is too small to allow vitality, special techniques are required to allow survival of the cartilage that provides the important shape to the ear. Such techniques involve dermabrading and burying of the ear in the postauricular skin and are best done with the environmental and anesthetic control of an operating room. With a cleanly severed total ear amputation, consideration for microvascular replantation should be entertained.

Scalp

Lacerations to the scalp are of importance primarily because of their potential for significant blood loss. The scalp has a very vascular network with large vessels in the subcutaneous tissue. Because the tendency for scarring in the scalp is minimal and most scars are hidden by hair, the prime consideration in suturing is to arrest hemorrhage. Hemostasis can be provided by horizontal mattress stitches placed through the entire thickness of the scalp and tied somewhat tighter than recommended previously. They can be removed in 7 to 10 days.

SECONDARY REPAIR OF FACIAL SCARS

At the time of the original trauma, the crush injury to adjacent soft tissue makes primary uncomplicated healing questionable. Because of the risk of local infection as well as the uncertainty of the degree of local tissue injury, rearrangement of scars with local flap and Z-plasty procedures is not warranted at the time of the injury. All scars, including those that result from traumatic wounds, look their worst between 3 and 8 weeks following the time of closure. From 8 weeks until the time of final wound maturation, there will be progressive improvement in the quality of the scar. A scar is mature when it is no longer red and pruritic and has assumed normal skin texture.

At the time of wound maturation, secondary scar revision may improve scar appearance. Revision is undertaken in an attempt to resuture the wound without the local factors of contamination and local tissue injury, to realign scars better in lines of skin tension, to break up long scars into smaller segments that are less obvious, and to level skin planes where healing has produced contour differences. A variety of local tissue techniques can be used to achieve these aims, with the eventual result of a less noticeable scar.

PEDIATRIC FACIAL FRACTURES

Fractures to the facial bones of young children are less common than in adolescents or adults for a combination of reasons. First of all, children live in a more protected environment. Second, the facial bones are sheltered under a relatively larger cranium. Third, children's bones tend to be much more compact, less aerated, and more resilient. Forces great enough to produce a fracture in an adult are rarely of enough energy to do the same to a child. As a result, the occurrence of facial fractures in the child is an indication of significant injury, which should not be taken lightly. They are frequently accompanied by major multisystem injuries.

Because of the thick periosteum with great osteogenic potential, the rich vascularity and the increased metabolic rate, children's facial fractures heal very rapidly. *Early reduction is required* to avoid malunion.

The other significant concern in childhood facial fractures is their sequelae. Fractures of facial bones may injure growth centers, resulting in loss of growth potential. Those injuries result in functional derangement as well as obvious deformity. Such implications for growth are particularly significant for injuries to the mandibular condyle and the nasal septum.

There are multiple other considerations that slightly alter the approach to pediatric facial fractures. Immobilization following reduction is more difficult. Developing teeth occupy space within the mandible and maxilla. Injuries to either may alter the growth potential for such teeth.

The presence of teeth within the jaws should be considered during application of internal fixation. Should internal fixation be elected for stabilization of a pediatric facial fracture, techniques must be employed to avoid dental injury. Thus, wiring of a mandibular fracture in a child can only be employed at the most inferior border of the mandible where it will not injure developing teeth.

Most methods of immobilizing facial fractures of the maxilla or mandible are achieved through placement of the teeth in occlusion and maintaining that occlusion during the period of healing. In the adult, such methods are dependent upon interdental wiring. In children, because of the peculiar shape of deciduous teeth, interdental wiring becomes more difficult to maintain. Special wiring methods for maintaining occlusion are required.

Because of the tremendous growth potential, precise *anatomic reduction* is not required for all of these injuries. Fractures across the condylar neck can be treated conservatively despite less than anatomic reduction, with expectations of full recovery of function through the processes of bony remodeling.

As in the treatment of facial soft tissue injuries, treatment of pediatric bony injuries requires a general anesthetic. Procedures that can be completed under a local anesthesia in adults, such as placement of arch bars and interdental wiring, will require a general anesthetic in children. The same is true for removal of such appliances.

Examination and Diagnosis

Physical examination can provide helpful clues to the lines of fracture. *Conjunctival ecchymosis* is found adjacent to fractures in the inferior or lateral orbital wall. *Buccal ecchymosis* can be seen adjacent to posterior teeth in conjunction with maxillary fractures. Areas of *tenderness*, regional *bony instability*, and *crepitus* provide clues to fracture lines. In addition, *diplopia* suggests injury to orbital walls adjacent to extraocular muscles. An area of *anesthesia* across the anterior cheek and upper lip confirms injury to the infraorbital nerve in its passage beneath the orbital globe, a finding frequently observed with bony injury to that area. Lastly, it is always helpful to note the *dental occlusion*. With significant fractures to either mandible or maxilla, it is unusual to have the teeth fit together in their normal way. Malocclusion can be determined either by observation in the younger child or by questioning in the older child.

Interpretation of the x-ray examination of the pediatric face is difficult. In young children, bony structures of the face are less calcified and sutures remain open. Beginning with the second year of life, an acceleration in the rate of growth of the face occurs. It begins to overtake the cranium in terms of relative size, but the face does not entirely emerge from beneath the cranium until the end of the first decade of life. The bones of the pediatric face are less pneumatized in the areas of future paranasal sinuses. Precise positioning for x-rays is prevented by the basic uncooperativeness of injured young children. Despite the fact that facial x-rays of children are less than ideal, it is worthwhile to make an attempt to complete a Waters view and a standard mandibular view. In confusing situations, it is sometimes helpful to sedate the child for those radiographs. Because of the severe multisystem injuries that occur concomitantly with pediatric facial fractures, sedation for facial radiographs is rarely warranted on the day of injury.

Treatment

Treatment of facial fractures is rarely an emergency. Emergencies occur only when the airway is compromised or when exsanguinating hemorrhage is occurring. After establishment of an airway with endotracheal intubation and control of bleeding, attention can and should be directed to the evaluation and treatment of multisystem injuries, which are commonly present. The diagnosis and treatment of the facial injury can easily await the diagnosis and treatment of more life-threatening injuries as well as the emergency care that is required for optimal outcome of orthopedic injuries. Following completion of these more pressing needs, orderly evaluation and treatment of facial fractures may commence.

Specific Fractures

Nasal Fractures

Nasal fractures are more common than other fractures of the pediatric facial skeleton. The nasal bones in childhood retain a midline suture, which closes later in development. The presence of that suture provides a weak point at which local trauma results in disruption, causing over-riding of both lateral nasal bones (Fig. 17–9). A direct blow produces depression and widening of the root of the nose. It is recognized by the accompanying local swelling and ecchymosis and a general anesthetic will frequently be required for proper reduction. Local trauma to the root of the nose may depress or displace one or both nasal bones. Proper treatment requires repositioning to normal alignment, which can then be maintained with nasal packing and/or external nasal splint.

Many significant intranasal fractures are overlooked in childhood. Trauma to the lower two-thirds of the nose may result in internal *nasal septal injury*, which is unappreciated unless specifically investigated. Those injuries rarely have devastating early complications but more commonly result in delayed nasal deformity.

Any local nasal trauma in childhood that results in a "bloody nose" deserves a thorough nasal examination. Both nasal vaults should be inspected and attention directed to the following:

1. Identifying the position of the septum throughout its length and height. Normally, the nasal septum is flat and vertical and travels down the vomerine groove in the midsagittal plane of the nasal floor. Septal fractures can be identified when displaced by local mucosal injury and irregular contour. When displaced out of the vomerine groove, the septum presents in the floor of one nostril.

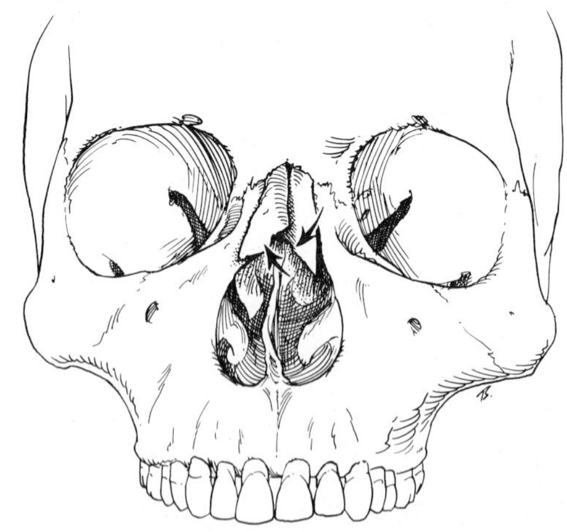

Figure 17–9. Nasal fractures in children commonly depress the side ipsilateral to the trauma and elevate the contralateral side.

2. Examination of septal mucosal surfaces for underlying hematoma. A septal hematoma appears as a *bluish* soft tissue bulge. Drainage of the hematoma via an inferior caudal incision is indicated to prevent infection with cartilage dissolution. Reapplication of septal mucosa to cartilage is accomplished with petrolatum-lubricated nasal packing.

Fractures of the Middle Third of the Face

Fractures of the middle third of the face include fractures to the naso-orbital-ethmoid region, fractures of the zygoma and zygomatic arch, fractures of the orbital floor, and fractures of the maxilla (Fig. 17–10). In general, such fractures occur in patterns similar to those in the adult, with the exception that zygomatic arch fractures are exceedingly uncommon in children. The pattern of the fracture can be demonstrated with a standard Waters x-ray view. Their treatment involves the same considerations as in adults, with anatomic reduction for displaced fractures. Occlusion provides a means of identifying adequate reduction in maxillary and mandibular fractures. Immobilizing teeth in occlusion during the early healing process guards against malunion.

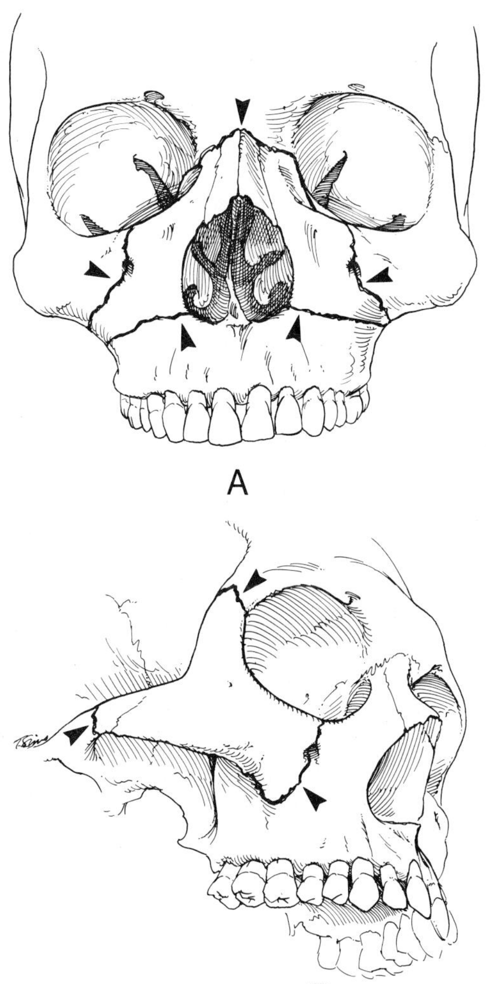

Figure 17–10. Fractures of the middle third of the face may involve the naso-orbital-ethmoid region *(A)*, the maxilla *(A)*, or the zygoma *(B)*.

Mandibular Fractures (Fig. 17–11)

Greenstick fractures of the pediatric mandible are relatively common in the condylar region; fractures with dislocation are more common in the body of the mandible. Adequate treatment requires recapturing preinjury dental occlusion, avoiding further injury to regions with growth potential, and maintaining full potential for mandibular excursion.

The *mandibular condyle* is the major growth center for the mandible. Growth occurs in a downward and forward direction by apposition of bone in the region beneath the articular cartilage. Particularly during the first 3 years of life, the condyle is composed of delicate vascular spongy tissue with a very thin covering of cortical bone. During this early pediatric development, an injury providing longitudinal stress to the region of the apex of the chin can result in compression and crushing of this important growth center. Intracapsular temporomandibular hemorrhage with hemarthrosis may cause growth disturbance as well as ankylosis of the joint. These intracapsular fractures should not be treated by immobilization but rather by early active motion. Aspiration of the joint and injection of steroids may also be indicated.

Fractures somewhat more inferiorly through the *condylar neck* are more common. They are typically of the greenstick variety,

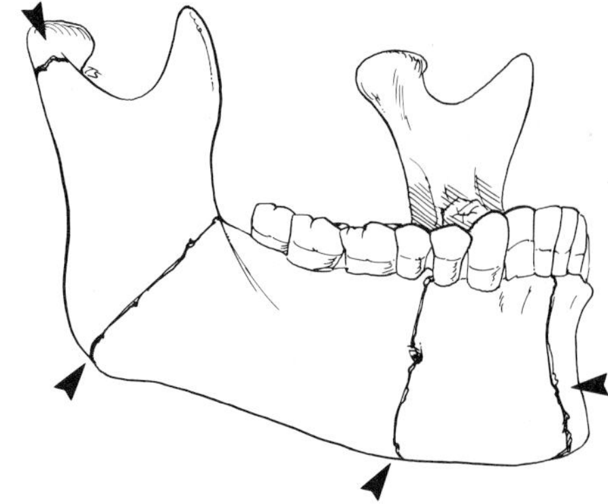

Figure 17–11. Common areas of mandibular fractures.

are displaced medially, and result in a temporary lateral crossbite. When present unilaterally, such fractures can be treated conservatively with a soft diet. Even when bilateral, they require only a closed reduction with intermaxillary fixation. An operative approach with anatomic reduction is not indicated and may further compromise growth potential. An open reduction is indicated only for the most severe injuries in which occlusion is otherwise not obtainable.

Fractures through the *body of the mandible* in children are complicated by the presence of a mixed or deciduous dentition. Because of the presence of developing dentition within the mandibular body and their influence on the strength of the bone, fractures tend to follow the enclosed teeth. Unerupted teeth in the line of fracture may be injured and subsequently undergo maleruption or be lost.

One should be aware that fractures of the body of the mandible, particularly those in the parasymphyseal position, are associated with fractures of the opposite mandibular condyle, for that injury is occasionally overlooked. Treatment of fractures of the mandibular body involves reduction of displaced fragments with maintenance of occlusion by interdental wiring.

When the injuring force is directed precisely at the teeth, the *fracture may involve the tooth* itself or the immediately subjacent bone. When those fractures do not interrupt the normal maxillary or mandibular arch, they result only in disruption of bone from the alveolar ridge. The bone may be separated from its adjacent soft tissues and may or may not be devitalized. Regardless, it should be carefully wired into its anatomic position, where it becomes a spacer. The rich collateral gingival blood supply and intact dental root canals will provide a high rate of successful healing. Definitive care of devitalized teeth requires a dental or oral surgical specialist (see Chapter 19).

Selected Readings

Bales CR, Randall P, Lehr HB: Fractures of the facial bones in children. J Trauma 12:56, 1972.

Berry T, Burg FD, Kravitz H: The toddler as a bicycle passenger. Pediatrics 49:443, 1972.

Callaham M: Dog bite wounds. JAMA 244:2327, 1980.

Dushoff IM: A stitch in time. Emerg Med 5:21, 1973.

Dushoff IM: About face. Emerg Med 6:25, 1974.

Georgiade NG, Pickrell KL: Treatment of maxillofacial injuries in children. J Int Coll Surg 27:640, 1957.

Graham WP III: Soft tissue injuries in childhood. *In* Kernahan DA, Thomson HG (eds.): Symposium on Pediatric Plastic Surgery. Vol. 21. St. Louis, C. V. Mosby, 1982, Ch. 19.

Halazonetis JA: The "weak" regions of the mandible. Br J Oral Surg 6:37, 1968.

Kaban LB, Mulliken JB, Murray JE: Facial fractures in children. An analysis of 122 fractures in 109 patients. Plast Reconstr Surg 59:15, 1977.

Karwacki JJ Jr, Baker SP: Children in motor vehicles. Never too young to die. JAMA 242:2848, 1979.

Leake D, Doykos J III, Habal MB, et al.: Long-term follow-up of fractures of the mandibular condyle in children. Plast Reconstr Surg 47:127, 1971.

Lehman JA, Saddawi ND: Fractures of the mandible in children. J. Trauma 16:773, 1976.

Linder CW: Automobile injuries to children. Curr Conc Trauma Care 16, Winter 1981.

McCoy FJ, Chandler RA, Crow ML: Facial fractures in children. Plast Reconstr Surg 37:209, 1966.

Perry AW, McShane RH: Fine tuning of the skin edges in the closure of surgical wounds. Controlling inversion and eversion with the path of the needle—the right stitch at the right time. J Dermatol Surg Oncol 7:471, 1981.

Rowe NL: Fractures of the facial skeleton in children. J Oral Surg 26:505, 1968.

Rowe NL: Fractures of the jaws in children. J Oral Surg 27:497, 1969.

Schultz RC, McMaster WC: The treatment of dog bite injuries, especially those of the face. Plast Reconstr Surg 49:494, 1972.

Schultz RC: Frontal sinus and supraorbital fractures from vehicle accidents. Clin Plast Surg 2:93, 1975.

Schultz RC, Tremolet de Villers Y: Nasal fractures. J Trauma 15:319, 1975.

Schultz RC, Oldham RJ: An overview of facial injuries. Surg Clin North Am 57:987, 1977.

Schultz RC: Pediatric facial fractures. *In* Kernahan DA, Thomson HG (eds.): Symposium on Pediatric Plastic Surgery. Vol. 21. St. Louis, C. V. Mosby, 1982, Ch. 20.

Spicer TE: Techniques of facial lesion excision and closure. J Dermatol Surg Oncol 8:551, 1982.

Tate RJ: Facial injuries associated with the battered child syndrome. Br J Oral Surg 9:41, 1972.

Waite DE: Pediatric fractures of jaw and facial bones. Pediatrics 51:551, 1973.

Waldron CW, Balkin SG, Peterson RG: Fractures of the facial bones in children. J Oral Surg 1:215, 1943.

Whitaker LA, Schaffer DB: Severe traumatic oculo-orbital displacement: Diagnosis and secondary treatment. Plast Reconstr Surg 59:352, 1977.

Zizmor, J.: Roentgen examination of the facial bones. *In* Converse JM: Surgical Treatment of Facial Injuries. Baltimore, Williams & Wilkins, 1974, Ch. 14.

CHAPTER

18 Eye Injuries

LEONARD B. NELSON

Ocular trauma may be a much more common cause of visual loss than is generally recognized. More than 2 million eye injuries severe enough to require medical care of one or more days of restricted activity occur annually in the United States.[1] The National Society to Prevent Blindness estimates that 55 per cent of eye injuries occur prior to age 25,[2] and that one-third of eye loss in the first decade of life is due to traumatic injury.[3] Clearly, eye injuries in the young have a significant impact in terms of morbidity and thus are a matter of major socioeconomic importance.

GENERAL PRINCIPLES

Eye injuries in the pediatric age group pose several diagnostic and management challenges. Confirmation of an ocular injury in a child may be difficult and occasionally may require sedation, even general anesthesia. The fibrotic component of healing in the child can be particularly exuberant, often with disastrous consequences.[4] Finally, one must consider the amblyogenic effect of patching an eye of a child after injury, even for a few days.[5]

Chemical burns of the eye and occlusion (or impending occlusion) of the central retinal artery are the only true ocular emergencies; occlusion is rare in the pediatric age group. Ocular injuries that require medical attention in hours, not minutes, include lacerations of the globe, severe lid lacerations, hyphemas (blood in the anterior chamber), and intraocular foreign bodies. In this latter group of injuries there is ample time for thorough diagnostic evaluation and management procedures.

In the evaluation of eye injuries in the pediatric age group, the examiner must always retain a high index of suspicion that an occult injury may be present. A patient with a conjunctival hemorrhage may have an occult perforation of the globe that may be missed unless the conjunctiva is carefully scrutinized for defects. A superficial lid laceration may be repaired and an unsuspected intraocular foreign body left undetected.

Finally, a thorough ocular examination is vital in the early recognition of associated intracranial damage. The pupils of both eyes should be evaluated carefully. The swinging-flashlight test is useful in the detection of afferent pupillary defects, especially from optic nerve lesions (Marcus-Gunn pupil).[6] However, the evaluation of the pupils must be interpreted within the knowledge of the possible causes of asymmetry of the pupils (Table 18–1, Fig. 18–1).

EXAMINATION

The examination of eye injuries in the pediatric age group requires considerable patience on the part of the examiner. The papoose board may be a useful adjunct, especially in the very young child. Occasionally, mild sedation or even general anesthesia may be required to evaluate the eye injuries of the child adequately.

In evaluating eye injuries the following steps are crucial:

1. Take a detailed history, to obtain an exact picture of the circumstances and the instrument or chemical involved. It is important to establish the visual status of both eyes prior to the accident.

2. Measure the visual acuity of each eye separately, using the patient's corrective lens if available. If glasses have been shattered, try to take a pinhole acuity. If massive conjunctival or lid edema prevents adequate measurement of visual acuity, record a statement to that effect in the patient's chart.

3. Determine visual fields by confrontation with an object; this may uncover an unsuspected intracranial process or retinal detachment.

4. Examine the lids and adnexa, carefully determining the extent and depth as well as the possible involvement of the canalicular apparatus. A small wound in the lid may provide a clue to an occult perforation of the globe. Eversion of the lid and swabbing with

Table 18–1. CAUSES OF ASYMMETRY OF PUPILS

A. Mydriasis (dilated pupil)
 1. Simple anisocoria
 2. Third nerve lesion
 3. Drugs
 4. Traumatic mydriasis from injury to eye
 5. Aniridia
 6. Iridodialysis or iridal-sphincter rupture
 7. Lesion of ciliary ganglion
B. Miosis (small pupil)
 1. Horner's syndrome
 2. Drugs
 3. Argyll Robertson pupil
 4. Acute pontine angle lesion
 5. Posterior synechiae

a cotton-tipped applicator after instillation of a topical anesthetic may uncover a foreign body.

5. Palpate the orbital rim, feeling for crepitus through the lids; look for an orbital or nasal fracture. Appraise the real or apparent displacement of the globe with respect to the lateral orbital rim, using either an exophthalmometer or clinical inspection from the patient's side or from above.

6. Examine the pupils and record their size, shape, and reaction to light.

7. Examine the cornea under magnification (if possible with loupes or slit lamp). Use fluorescein paper to stain the cornea and a Wood's lamp or slit lamp to delineate an abrasion.

8. Carefully examine the conjunctiva to detect lacerations, foreign bodies, and underlying scleral perforation.

9. Evaluate the anterior chamber for pus (hypopyon), blood (hyphema), and tremulousness of the iris (iridodonesis) associated with a dislocated lens.

10. Once the visual acuity and pupils have been evaluated and the general health of the patient has been determined to be without neurologic complications, dilate the pupils for adequate examination of the retina with an ophthalmoscope.

11. After the possibility of a perforation has been eliminated, evaluate the ocular motility of both eyes.

12. Obtain x-rays whenever there exists the possibility of an orbital fracture or a retained foreign body in the globe or orbit.

13. Photograph all injuries.

SPECIFIC INJURIES

Lid and Canalicular Trauma

The eyelids serve as a protective system for the eyes. They help lubricate the anterior part of the eye through the accessory tear glands located in the back surface of the lids. The normal motion of the eyelids produces a "pumping action." This moves the tears from the lacrimal gland under the upper outer lid, across the eyes, and toward the tear duct system located medially on the eyelid margin. The eyelids also prevent small foreign bodies from striking the eye with a blink mechanism that occurs in a fraction of a second.

In any trauma to the lid a careful evaluation of the full extent of the injury must be made early in the examination (Fig. 18–2). A thorough search should be performed for trauma to the canalicular system, foreign bodies, and occult perforations of the globe. The physician should consider prophylactic antibiotics and tetanus immunization in all lid lacerations, and prophylaxis against rabies in the situation of a dog bite causing a lid laceration. The proper evaluation and repair of a lid laceration in the pediatric age group may require sedation or general anesthesia.

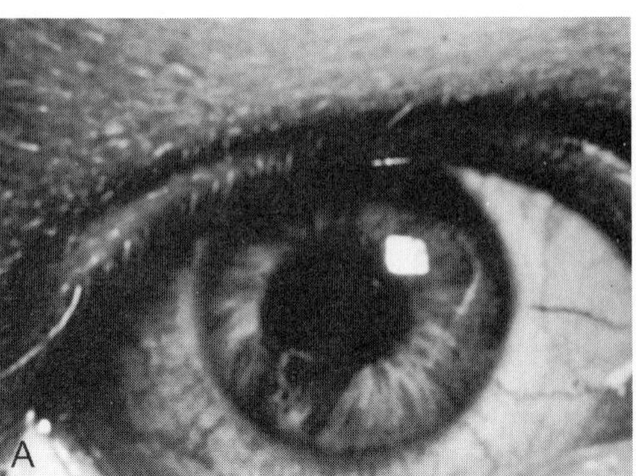

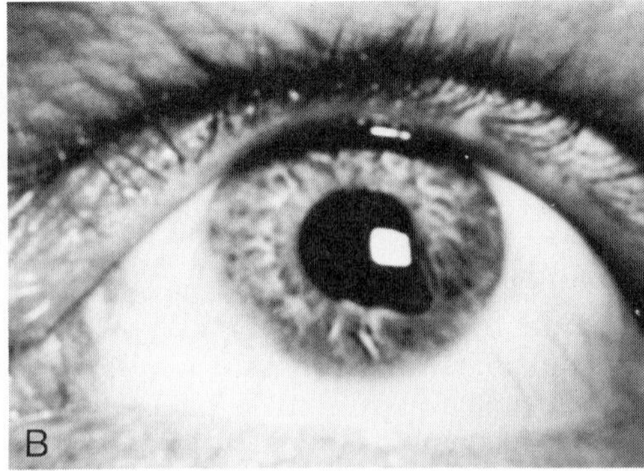

Figure 18–1. *A*, Iris atrophy inferiorly, with an irregular pupil, from a contusion injury. The lens is dislocated into the vitreous. *B*, Irregular shape of the pupil caused by a rupture of the pupillary sphincter in the inferotemporal quadrant. (Courtesy of Drs. Philip P. Ellis and James R. Cerasoli, Ocular Injuries Med-Com Inc., New York.)

Simple Lid Lacerations

Lid lacerations with startling disfigurement may present to the emergency room physician (Fig. 18–2*B*, *C*, and *D*). Careless and poorly planned repairs in the emergency room may prove to be disfiguring on a long-term basis. Once the extent of the laceration is determined, a meticulous, layer-by-layer repair should be performed. Special attention should be made in apposing the grey line (area at which conjunctiva and skin meet) so that squamification of the conjunctiva does not occur. A logical plan of repair may be performed even 24 hours after the injury, but it should be executed in a well-equipped emergency or operating room.

Traumatic Loss of the Lids

Occasionally lid trauma may result in almost complete loss of the eyelids. After a careful examination and a thorough search for a ruptured globe and foreign bodies, an effective means of protecting the eye should be employed. One good method for short-term maintenance of the exposed but uninjured globe is the use of plastic film (Saran Wrap). This material can be placed over the orbit with ophthalmic ointment at points of skin contact. Plastic film preserves the moisture necessary to the eye until a more definitive procedure can be performed. Alternative methods of protecting the uninjured globe utilize the laxity of the conjunctiva of the upper and lower fornix. Only a well-trained ophthalmologist should perform the procedure for using the conjunctiva as a protective covering over the globe.

Canalicular Lacerations

Lacerations involving the medial fourth of the lid may impair tear drainage to the nose (Fig. 18–3). Lacerations to the puncta, canaliculi, lacrimal sac, or nasolacrimal duct may not be recognized initially and may be inadequately repaired. Therefore, in any lid laceration to the medial canthal area, one must have a high index of suspicion of possible

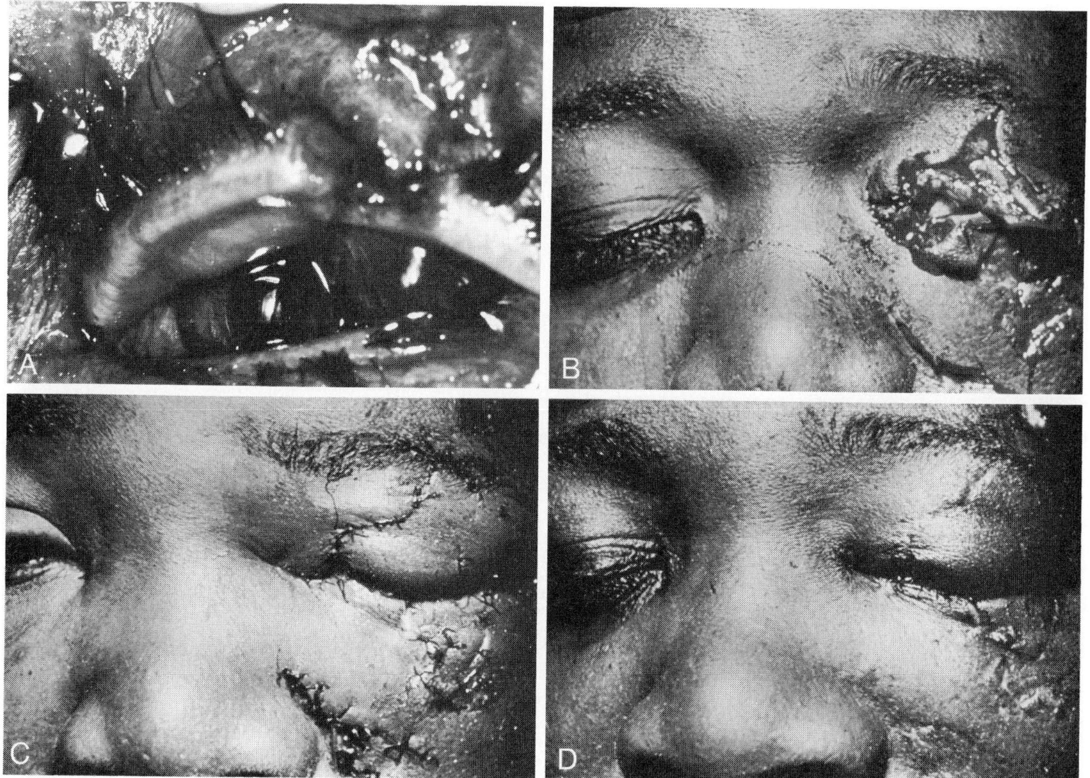

Figure 18–2. *A*, Laceration of the lid margin, with an underlying perforation of the globe. (Courtesy of Dr. Robison D. Harley.)

B, Multiple and extensive lacerations of the face and left upper and lower eyelids. *C*, Immediate postoperative appearance of the same patient in Figure 2*B* after a layer-by-layer repair of the lacerations. *D*, Three months following repair. (Figures 2*B*, *C*, and *D* courtesy of Dr. Mark Ruchman.)

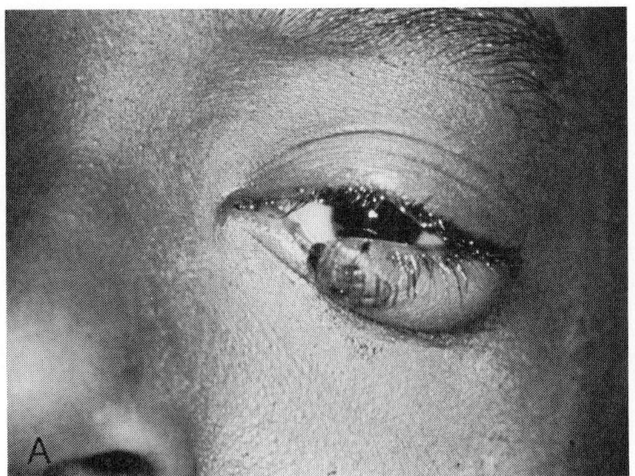

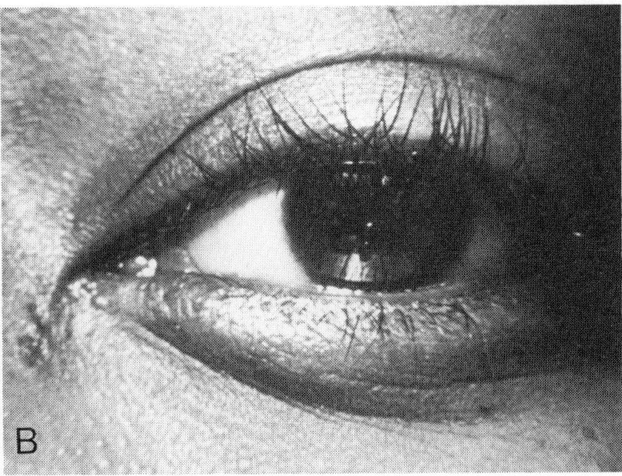

Figure 18–3. *A*, Laceration of the medial fourth of the lower eyelid, with involvement of the canaliculus. *B*, Two months following a carefully planned canaliculus anastomosis. (Courtesy of Dr. Mark Ruchman.)

trauma to the canalicular system or lacrimal sac. An experienced ophthalmic surgeon should perform a canalicular anastomosis under direct visualization with the use of a microscope or loupe. The anastomosis should be combined with the insertion of appropriate material into the lacrimal system for adequate stabilization.

Injuries of the Orbit

Orbital trauma has particular ophthalmologic importance because of the likelihood of associated ocular complications.[8] The blood vessels, extraocular muscles, and nerves lie in close proximity to the orbital bones and may be damaged from orbital fractures. Profound visual loss may occur from secondary compression of the optic nerve or from compromise of its blood supply. Lateral wall fractures are more commonly involved in optic nerve damage than other types of orbital fracture.[9] Medial wall fractures may cause restriction of horizontal motility[10] or subcutaneous emphysema, which is often visible radiographically. Finally, the possibility of intraocular injury must always be suspected and investigated.

Blowout Fractures

Blowout fractures are produced when a blunt object (such as a baseball or fist) strikes the orbital rim and causes a sudden increase in intraorbital pressure (Fig. 18–4). The force applied to the relatively incompressible soft tissues of the orbit is indirectly transferred to the bony orbital walls. The medial wall (lamina papyracea) and the orbital floor (roof of the maxillary antrum) are the weakest bones of the orbit and are most frequently damaged.[11]

Orbital floor fractures may result in incarceration of orbital fat, the inferior rectus, the

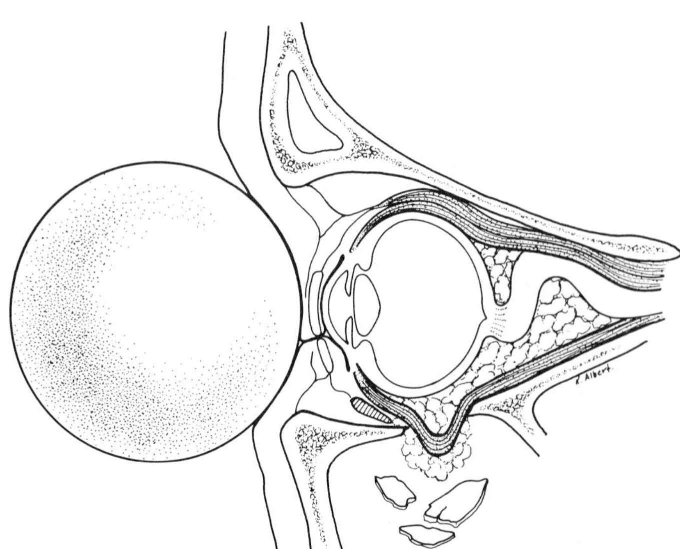

Figure 18–4. Blunt trauma applied to anterior orbit results in blow-out fracture, with incarceration of the inferior rectus and orbital fat. (Courtesy of Ms. Karen Albert.)

inferior oblique, or a combination of these. The involvement of these two muscles helps explain the restriction of extraocular motility, especially on vertical ocular movement attempts and a positive forced duction test. If the vertical movements of the eyes are generally compromised when the eye is in a abducted position, the inferior rectus muscle is probably the primary muscle involved in the floor fracture. If vertical position is affected in both the abducted and adducted positions, the inferior oblique muscle is probably involved as well (Fig. 18–5).

Ecchymosis of the lids and congestion of the orbital contents may be present, depending on the extent of soft tissue damage. Hemorrhage or edema within the orbit may also produce a positive forced duction test or possibly early exophthalmus.

Enophthalmus may occur immediately after the injury or may be delayed for several weeks or months. Causes of early enophthalmus may include protrusion of orbital fat into the maxillary antrum or redistribution of orbital contents with displacement of the globe secondary to orbital cavity enlargement following a blowout fracture. Infraorbital hypoanesthesia or anesthesia suggests a fracture in the central floor of the orbit close to the infraorbital groove.

Following a careful history and examination, the physician should obtain x-ray studies of the orbit. Radiologic evaluation demands meticulous positioning and exposure, which may be difficult in the pediatric age group. It is mandatory that the history and the presumptive diagnosis be explained to the radiology team. Frequently, x-rays of suspected blowout fractures are negative or equivocal, even when an obvious floor fracture is diagnosed clinically. Therefore, repeat x-ray studies with additional views and polytomography may be necessary to localize the precise fracture site.

A blowout fracture should never be considered an emergency. Once intraocular injury has been investigated, a conservative approach, directed toward reducing the possi-

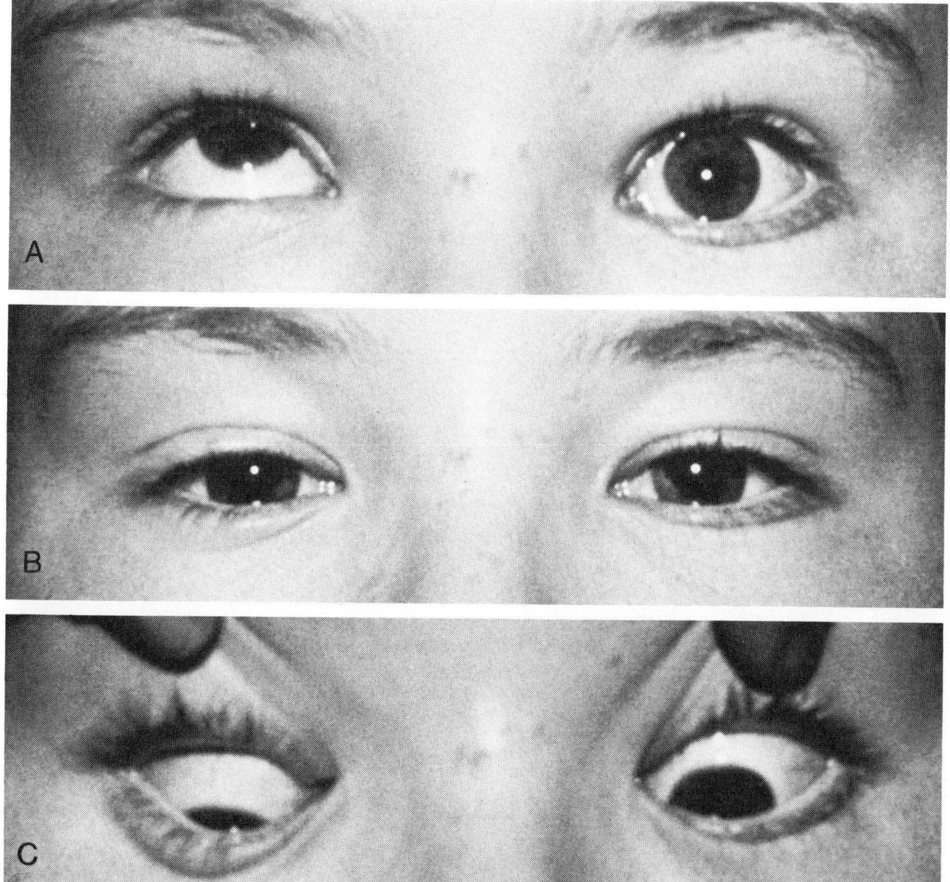

Figure 18–5. *A*, Entrapment of the inferior rectus prevented elevation of the left eye. *B*, Vertical alignment is normal in primary gaze. *C*, Contusion injury to the inferior rectus also prevents full depression of the left eye.

ble ecchymosis and edema, is initiated for 7 to 10 days. Because the surgical management of blowout fractures is controversial, no one consistent form of treatment prevails. However, since post-traumatic and postsurgical complications are ophthalmologic, it is imperative that the ophthalmologist be directly involved in the management of all patients with blowout fractures.

Chemical Burns of the Eye and Adnexa

Chemical burns are one of the few true ocular emergencies. The effects of alkalies and acids on ocular tissue are often severe, bilateral, and frequent in young people; they may result in significant visual loss or even loss of an eye (Fig. 18–6). Common household agents may cause chemical injuries to the eye (Table 18–2);[12] therefore, children are in a very vulnerable position.

Alkali burns are usually more damaging to ocular structures than acid burns. Acids quickly precipitate tissue proteins and result in an injury that is usually more superficial and slower to penetrate the cornea. Alkali burns, instead, increase the hydroxyl ion concentration beyond the limits of tissue protein stability. They react with fats to form soaps that damage all membranes, allowing rapid penetration into tissues.

Hughes' original classification of the severity of ocular chemical burns was based on the evaluation of tissue damage during the acute phase.[13, 14]

1. Mild
   a. Erosion of corneal epithelium
   b. Faint haziness
   c. No ischemic necrosis of conjunctiva or sclera
2. Moderately severe
   a. Corneal opacity blurring iris details
   b. Minimal ischemic necrosis of conjunctiva and sclera
3. Very severe
   a. Blurring of pupillary outline
   b. Blanching of conjunctival and scleral vessels

Table 18–2. COMMON HOUSEHOLD AGENTS CAPABLE OF CAUSING EYE BURNS

1. Household ammonia (ammonium hydroxide 7 per cent)
2. Other ammonia-containing agents, e.g., window cleaner and jewelry cleaner
3. Scouring cleaners
4. Deodorizing cleaners
5. Disinfectants
6. Toilet bowl cleaners
7. Lye-sodium hydroxide and other drain cleaners
8. Automotive cleaners and degreasers
9. Whitewall tire cleaners
10. Electric dishwasher detergents
11. Lime (calcium hydroxide) and plaster
12. Chlorine for swimming pools
13. Swimming pool tile cleaners
14. Bleaches

The initial treatment for chemical burns of the eye is copious irrigation with water from the nearest available source (i.e., drinking fountain, shower, or faucet). Irrigation should be repeated once the patient arrives at the hospital emergency room. For adequate benefit from irrigation, the lids should be held apart manually or with a lid retractor. Irrigation should continue for 20 to 30 min-

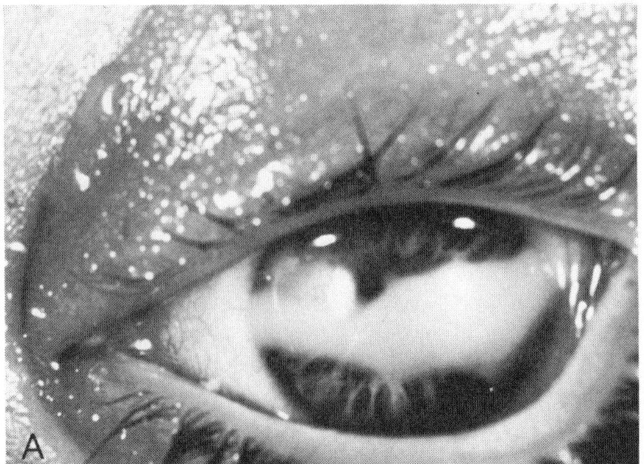

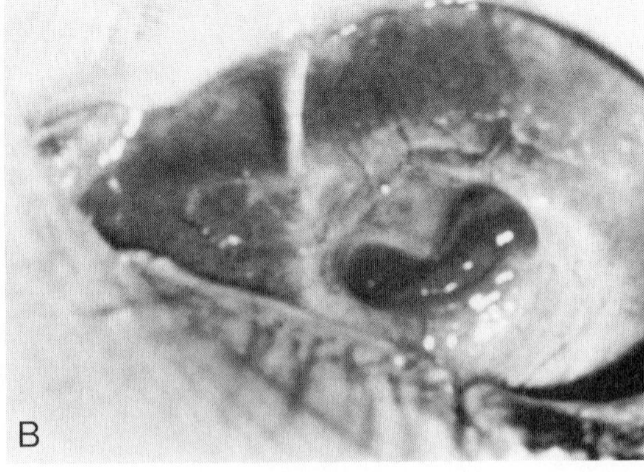

Figure 18–6. *A*, Dense corneal scar caused by ammonia splashed in the eye. (Courtesy of Dr. Robison D. Harley.) *B*, End result of an alkali burn. The upper eyelid has developed an adhesion on its margin to the bulbar conjunctiva (symblepharon). The cornea is covered by thick granulation tissue in its central position, and a dense vascularized membrane is present inferiorly. (Courtesy of Drs. Philip P. Ellis and James R. Cerasoli, Ocular Injuries Med-Com Inc., New York.)

utes with normal saline (at least 1000 to 2000 ml) connected to an intravenous tubing set. To determine neutrality, pH paper (pH of tears is between 7.3 and 7.7) can assist the emergency room physician in treating acidic or basic chemical burns.[15]

Effective irrigation may be facilitated by instillation of a topical anesthetic to ease the patient's discomfort. Avoid repetitive use of a topical anesthetic, as it will retard wound healing of the corneal epithelium. In the pediatric age group, systemic analgesics and sedation may be necessary to accomplish effective irrigation.

Once irrigation has been initiated, perform a careful investigation of the fornices to detect and remove excess debris. Double-lid eversion and swabbing of the conjunctival recesses with a cotton-tipped applicator should be performed in a careful search for caustic material that could cause additional ocular damage.

After irrigation and debridement, a cycloplegic agent is instilled. (Atropine is an excellent choice because of its prolonged cycloplegic effect.) This reduces the possibility of posterior synechiae (iridal adhesions to the lens) and ciliary spasm. Infection from an inflamed eye with surface defects and necrotic avascular conjunctiva is a constant threat. Therefore, topical antibiotics, especially against gram-negative organisms, should begin as soon as irrigation and debridement are completed. An ophthalmologist's involvement early in the care of patients with chemical burns to the eye is advantageous.

Injuries of the Conjunctiva

The conjunctiva, a mucous membrane, forms the inner surface of the eyelids and covers the anterior part of the globe up to the cornea. In any trauma to the conjunctiva, one must carefully search for occult perforations of the globe as well as for the possibility of a foreign body. A thorough investigation of the conjunctiva is accomplished most successfully with the aid of high magnification of a slit lamp or loupes.

Conjunctival Hemorrhage

Conjunctival hemorrhage in the pediatric age group is rarely spontaneous except in hematologic disorders. However, in a setting of ocular trauma, it is quite frequent. Subconjunctival hemorrhage occurs when a small conjunctival blood vessel breaks. The resulting hemorrhage usually spreads between the conjunctiva and sclera.

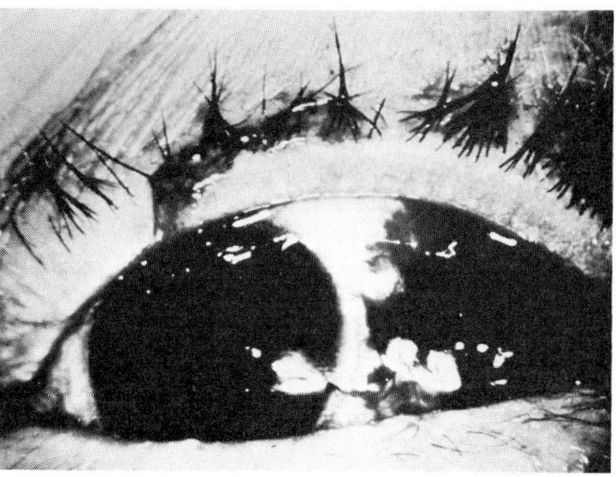

Figure 18–7. Subconjunctival hemorrhage obscuring a small perforation of the globe. (Courtesy of Dr. Robison D. Harley.)

In itself the hemorrhage is of no consequence, except that it may obscure an associated foreign body or a small perforation of the globe (Fig. 18–7). Subconjunctival hemorrhage, which generally appears darker than more superficial hemorrhage, may cause swelling of the conjunctiva between the lids. This can lead to corneal exposure, requiring lubrication with an ointment. Ice compresses applied during the first 24 hours may hasten the regression of the swelling. Subconjunctival hemorrhages usually clear without treatment in about 2 weeks. They go through the usual stages of resolution from dark red through yellow until they finally clear.

Chemosis (Conjunctival Edema)

After ocular trauma, chemosis of the conjunctiva, with or without hemorrhage, may have serious implications. Marked conjunctival chemosis may indicate a scleral rupture, especially when it is disproportionate to other indications of injury. Although chemosis is usually generalized, it may be localized to an area of scleral rupture (Fig. 18–8).

Conjunctival Crepitus

Air beneath the conjunctiva producing conjunctival crepitus occurs in association with fractures of the paranasal sinuses, par-

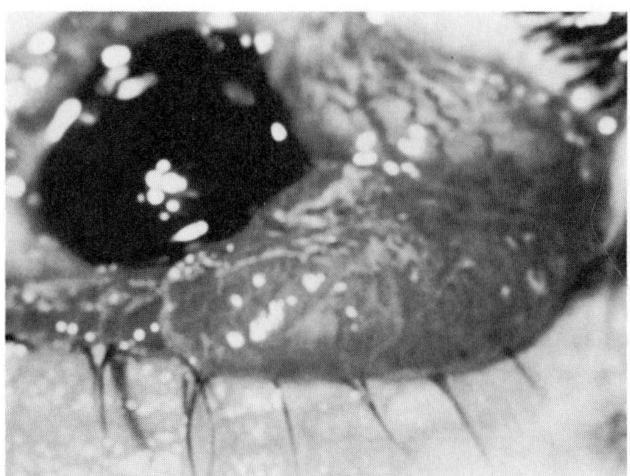

Figure 18–8. Severe conjunctival edema (chemosis) as a result of a contusion injury to the globe. (Courtesy of Drs. Philip P. Ellis and James R. Cerasoli, Ocular Injuries Med-Com Inc., New York.)

ticularly the lamina papyracea of the ethmoid. The air that causes conjunctival depths is absorbed and is of no consequence. However, its presence is an indication for prophylactic systemic antibiotics to prevent the development of orbital cellulitis from bacteria from the sinuses.[16]

TRAUMA TO THE EXTRAOCULAR MUSCLES

Intramuscular Hemorrhage

There are six muscles that rotate the eyeball. Blunt orbital trauma or direct trauma to these extraocular muscles may result in hematomas. The intramuscular hemorrhage and swelling may prevent normal function of a muscle (i.e., contraction and relaxation). Therefore, the normal movement of the eye in the direction of the involved muscle may be severely limited and difficult to differentiate clinically from neurogenic paresis.

Traumatic Muscle Disinsertion

Intraorbital trauma, especially by a sharp object, may occasionally result in a disinsertion of an extraocular muscle. The trauma may be limited to the muscle itself or may be associated with an injury to other ocular structures. The motility findings in a traumatic muscle disinsertion may be similar to those found in intramuscular hemorrhage. Therefore, a definitive diagnosis of a muscle disinsertion may not be possible clinically but would be based on the findings at the time of surgical exploration.

INJURIES TO THE GLOBE

Corneal Abrasion and Foreign Bodies

The cornea forms the window of the eye. It is composed of six distinct layers: (1) tear film, (2) epithelium, (3) Bowman's membrane, (4) stroma, (5) Descemet's membrane, and (6) endothelium. It is transparent under normal conditions because of the special arrangement of cells and collagenous fibrils and the absence of a vascular bed.

Corneal epithelial defects are extremely common in the pediatric age group. They may be caused by a foreign body caught under the upper lid (Fig. 18–9*A*) or by a scratch from a toy or a fingernail. Corneal abrasions can be quite painful because of exposure of the sensory nerve endings. The child may present with lacrimation, photophobia, severe blepharospasm, and blurring of vision.

For adequate examination of a patient with a possible corneal abrasion, a topical anesthetic is applied to relieve the ocular discomfort. Since corneal abrasions are commonly caused by a foreign body, a careful search should be undertaken. Eversion of the upper lid is a technique that every emergency room physician should know how to perform. The upper lid is grasped by the central lashes and is pulled downward; the patient is instructed to look down as well. The examiner's finger or a cotton-tipped applicator is then placed with slight pressure at the upper end of the tarsus, and the lid margin is flipped into an everted position (Fig. 18–9*B* and *C*).

If a foreign body is identified either under the upper or lower lid or on the cornea itself, it can usually be removed by forceful irrigation from a plastic squeeze bottle containing balanced salt solution or by a cotton-tipped applicator (Fig. 18–9*D*). Occasionally a foreign body is deeply embedded in the cornea, and removal requires high magnification and the use of a fine needle. In a child, it may require hospitalization and use of an operating room microscope. This latter procedure should be performed by an ophthalmologist.

If no foreign body is found, fluorescein staining can delineate diffuse punctate or focal epithelial defects (Fig. 18–10). A drop of sterile saline is placed on a fluorescein strip and touched to the palpebral conjunctiva. A Wood's lamp is a valuable instrument in inspecting the cornea for defects. It demonstrates a corneal abrasion by showing a

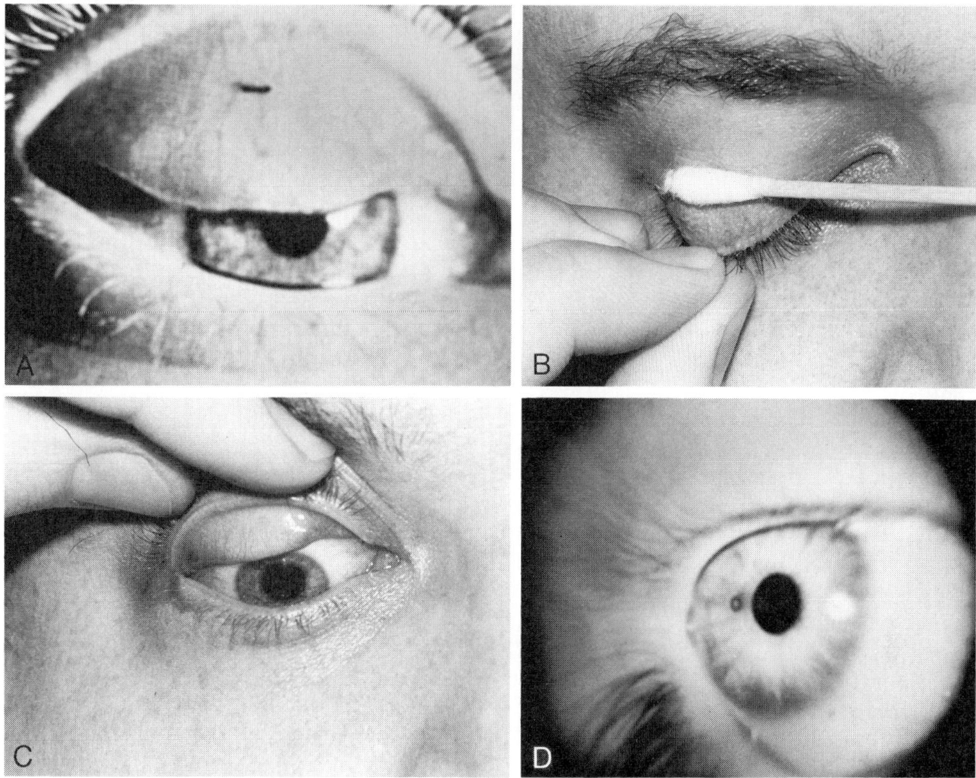

Figure 18–9. *A*, Typical location for a small foreign body located on the under surface of the upper eyelid. This foreign body can abrade the cornea with each blink. (Courtesy of Drs. Philip P. Ellis and James R. Cerasoli.)

B, The upper eyelid is everted by grasping and pulling down the lashes. A cotton-tipped applicator presses on the eyelid. *C*, The eyelid in the everted position. (Figures 9*B* and *C* courtesy of Ms. Karen Albert.)

D, A foreign body was removed from the cornea, leaving a rust ring. Removal of rust rings should be performed by an ophthalmologist. (Courtesy of Drs. Philip P. Ellis and James R. Cerasoli, Ocular Injuries Med-Com Inc., New York.)

green stain wherever an epithelial defect is present.

Corneal abrasions are treated with a short-acting cycloplegic, such as 1 per cent tropicamide (Mydriacyl) or 1 per cent cyclopentolate hydrochloride (Cyclogyl). This will alleviate the discomfort from ciliary spasm. A broad-spectrum antibiotic ointment is used to prevent potential infections. A pressure patch is applied to the forehead and cheek on the affected side to relieve the discomfort and allow the epithelial defect to heal. Corneal abrasions heal relatively quickly, usually within 1 to 3 days. However, the patient should be referred to an ophthalmologist for follow-up care the day after the injury. Under no circumstances should the patient be maintained on topical anesthetic, because it retards epithelial healing and aggravates the already present keratitis.[17]

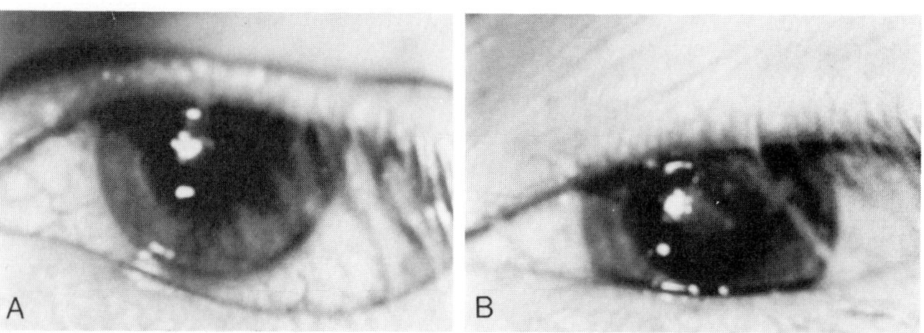

Figure 18–10. *A*, A chemical was splashed into the eye. *B*, Fluorescein was inserted into the eye and demonstrated a central corneal abrasion. (Courtesy of Drs. Philip P. Ellis and James R. Cerasoli, Ocular Injuries Med-Com Inc., New York.)

Corneal and Scleral Lacerations

All cases of ocular trauma must be evaluated carefully for possible penetrating or perforating injuries to the globe (Fig. 18–11). Penetrating injury refers to partial tissue damage to the cornea or sclera. For example, a foreign body may be trapped in the lamellae of the sclera, or a corneal laceration may cut through two-thirds of its thickness. Penetrating injuries do not involve the entire thickness of these structures. A perforating injury, however, is a complete, through and through wound of the sclera or cornea.

When the physician has determined that an eye is lacerated, pressure on the globe must be avoided. To examine the ruptured globe, the upper lid is retracted gently by pulling the superior orbital rim with a cotton-tipped applicator or with a finger. If this maneuver is inadequate, carefully placed lid retractors and the instillation of a topical anesthetic may help separate the lids and permit adequate visualization of the globe.

Corneal lacerations may be accompanied by a flat anterior chamber, and the iridal tissue may either be incarcerated in the wound or prolapsed through it (Fig. 18–12). Hemorrhage into the anterior chamber (hyphema) may prevent a satisfactory examination of the lens and retina.

Following an adequate evaluation of a ruptured globe, the eye is protected with a shield (Fig. 18–13). The patient should have orbital x-rays to establish the presence or absence of an intraocular or orbital foreign body. Tetanus immunization, broad-spectrum systemic antibiotics, and patient preparation for general anesthesia are initiated promptly.[18]

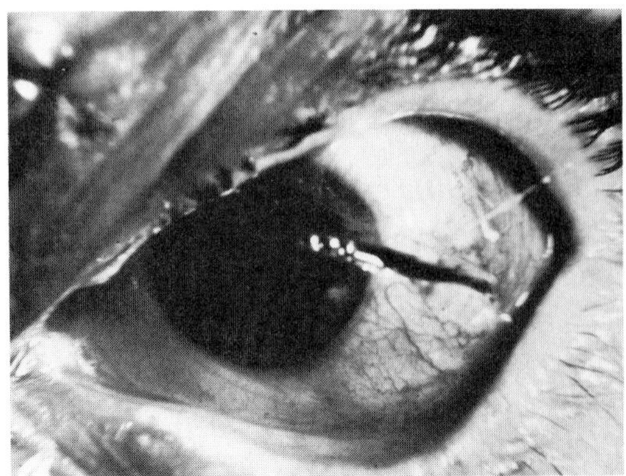

Figure 18–11. Corneoscleral laceration caused by the shattering of a spectacle lens. (Courtesy of Dr. Robison D. Harley.)

ANTERIOR SEGMENT TRAUMA

Traumatic Hyphema

The accumulation of free blood in the anterior chamber is referred to as hyphema (Fig. 18–14*A*). It is most frequently encountered in the pediatric age group and is caused by a variety of objects, including the human fist. This hemorrhage is caused by a rupture of the blood vessels of the iris or the ciliary body. The majority of hyphemas fill less than one-third of the anterior chamber; they usually last 5 to 6 days.[19] The presence of blood in the anterior chamber, especially in children, may result in marked somnolence; the mechanisms for this reaction are poorly understood. However, if a child with a hyphema presents with marked drowsiness, the possibility of head trauma should not be overlooked.

Visual acuity is evaluated with the best optical correction. The level of the hyphema is determined and recorded. Particular attention should be given to the possibility of a ruptured globe and lenticular or retinal damage.

The patient with a hyphema is hospitalized so that the ophthalmologist can perform careful daily examinations. Several different treatment regimens have been advocated to reduce the incidence of recurrent bleeding. There is, however, inconclusive evidence to support the benefit of strict bed rest[20] and binocular patching.[21] Certainly, these forms of therapy can be difficult to enforce in children. The dilemma of whether to treat with cycloplegic or miotic agents or topical or systemic steroids is also unresolved.

The patient with a hyphema may be ambulatory, with patching of the involved eye only. Elevating the head of the bed may facilitate setting of the hyphema to the inferior anterior chamber. In the absence of definitive guidelines, the use of topical or systemic medications remains arbitrary (Fig. 18–14*B*).

Trauma to the Lens

Following ocular trauma the presence of a cataract ultimately may deny the patient a good visual outcome. A traumatic cataract, which is usually unilateral, is considered the most common lens opacity in the young (Fig. 18–15).[22] There is almost always evidence of injury to related ocular structures. Clinically

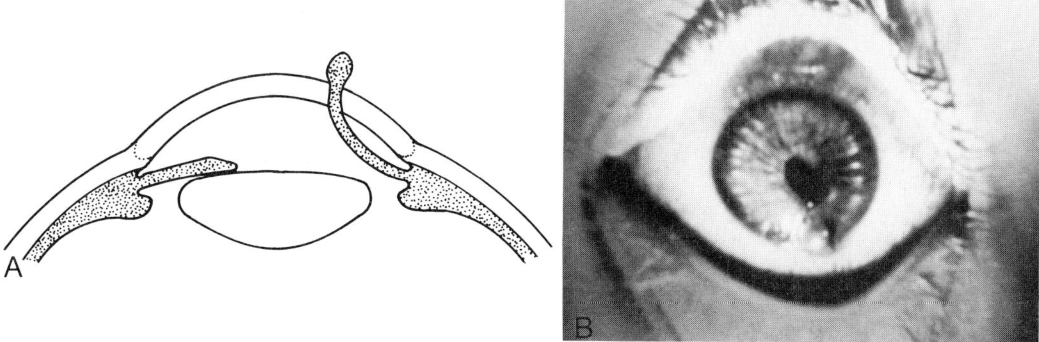

Figure 18–12. *A*, Corneal perforation with iris prolapsed externally. (Courtesy of Ms. Karen Albert.)
B, Perforating injury of the cornea with iris prolapse. (Courtesy of Drs. Philip P. Ellis and James R. Cerasoli, Ocular Injuries Med-Com Inc., New York.)

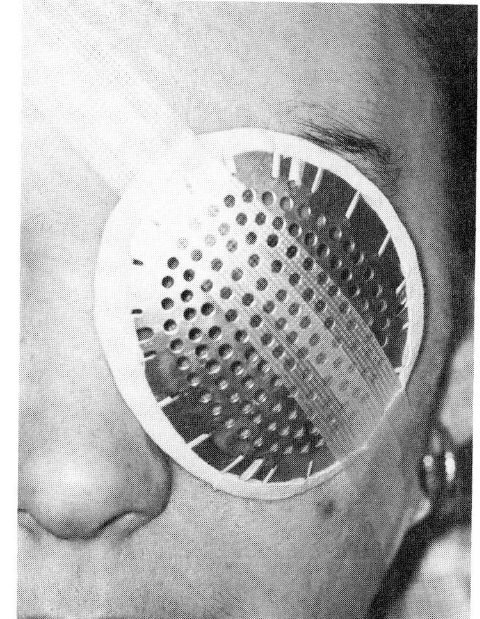

Figure 18–13. The eye is protected by a shield, following a scleral rupture.

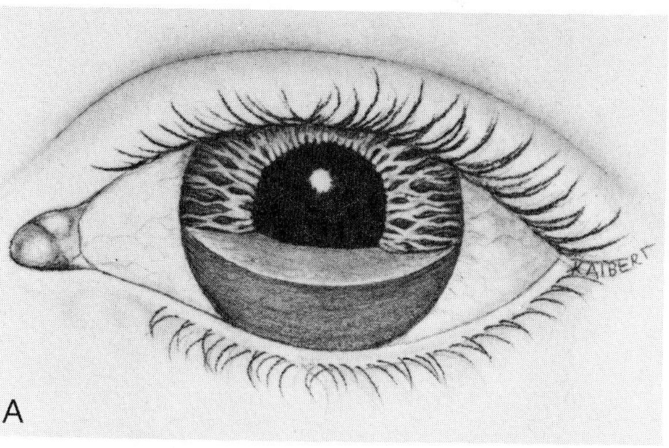

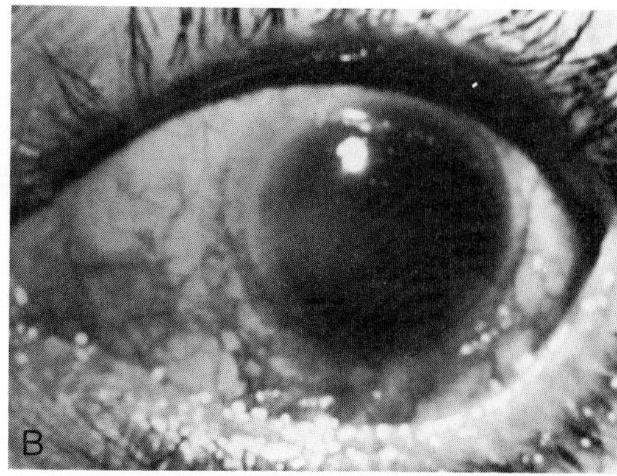

Figure 18–14. *A*, Blood in the anterior chamber (hyphema) obscures iris detail below. (Courtesy of Ms. Karen Albert.)
B, Blood staining of the cornea from a long-standing hyphema. The cornea has lost its normal transparency. (Figure 14*B* courtesy of Drs. Philip P. Ellis and James R. Cerasoli, Ocular Injuries Med-Com Inc., New York.)

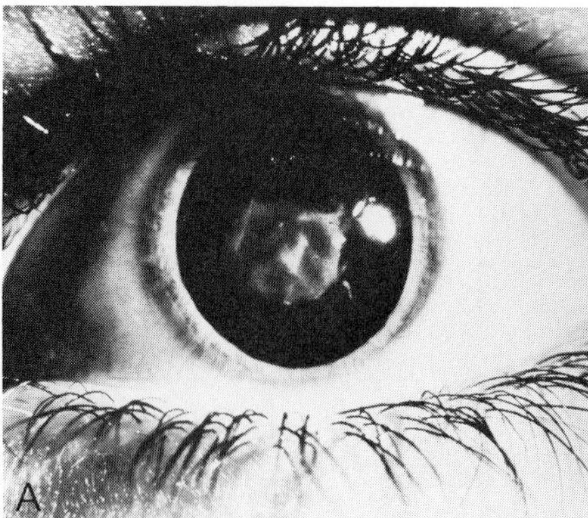

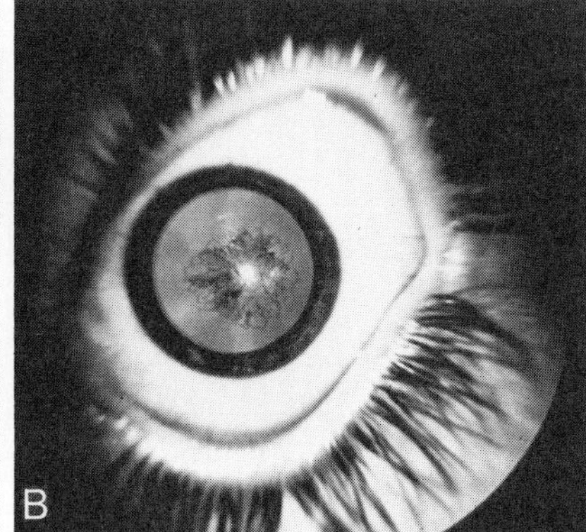

Figure 18–15. *A*, Several months following a contusion injury to the eye, a white lens opacity developed. *B*, Moderate lens opacity from blunt trauma. (Courtesy of Dr. Robison D. Harley.)

it is useful to distinguish between two types of lens opacities from trauma: a stellate posterior subcapsular opacity and an opacity at the site of lens capsule rupture. The latter opacity usually progresses rapidly to complete lens opacification.

Ocular trauma may also break the zonular fibers that encircle the lens radially and attach to the ciliary body. This may result in a subluxation of the lens when enough zonular fibers are destroyed. Lens subluxation can cause distressing visual symptoms of diplopia and distortion. Trembling of the iris (iridodonesis) is frequently observed following lens subluxation. It can be demonstrated with a hand-held flashlight while the patient moves the eyes quickly in different positions of gaze.

POSTERIOR SEGMENT TRAUMA

Vitreous Hemorrhage

Following ocular trauma, vitreous hemorrhage may result from damage to a retinal vessel. The chief symptom is usually a sudden and profound loss of vision. The hemorrhage may obscure fundus detail on ophthalmoscopic evaluation. If the hemorrhage is dense enough, the red reflex may be absent when using a hand-held light or ophthalmoscope. A careful examination of the retinal periphery should be performed by an ophthalmologist. This is extremely important, because a retinal dialysis (a break along the posterior border of the vitreous base in the periphery of the retina) may accompany a vitreous hemorrhage. In recent years, microsurgical equipment and techniques have been developed to dissect and remove large amounts of abnormal vitreous.

Commotio Retinae

Commotio retinae (Berlin's edema, concussion or contusion edema of the retina) is a common retinal injury resulting from blunt trauma to the globe (Fig. 18–16). It is thought to be caused by a paralytic vasodilation that results in edema of the retina. Visual acuity is commonly decreased. On ophthalmoscopic evaluation, a milky white edema of the retina is often found in association with a variable amount of retinal hemorrhage. The posterior pole is most often involved, with the macula standing out as a red (cherry-red) spot.

The prognosis for visual recovery from commotio retinae depends on the degree of retinal damage. There is no specific treatment, although systemic steroids have been tried but without proof of beneficial effect. Rarely, chronic cyst formation or a full-thickness macular hole may develop; these prevent full visual recovery (Fig. 18–17).

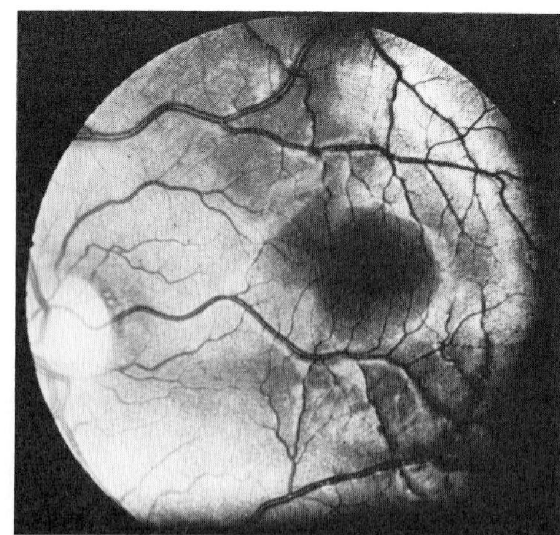

Figure 18–16. Retinal edema (commotio retinae) surrounds the macula in an eye that had sustained blunt trauma. (Courtesy of Dr. Robison D. Harley.)

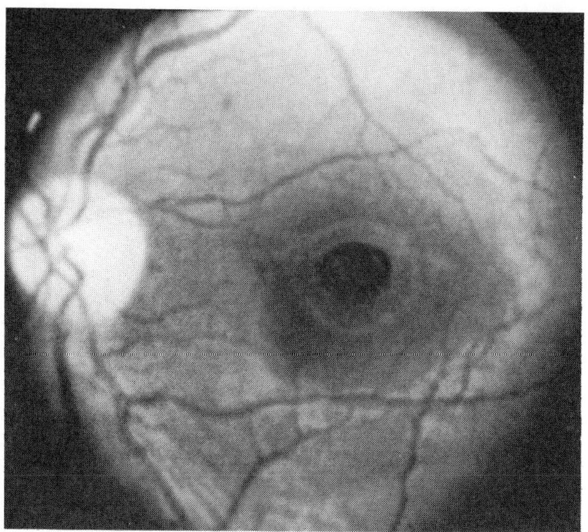

Figure 18–17. Macula hole that developed after a contusion injury to the retina. (Courtesy of Drs. Philip P. Ellis and James R. Cerasoli, Ocular Injuries Med-Com Inc., New York.)

Chorioretinal Rupture

As a result of a high-velocity missile (such as a bullet) striking the globe without penetration, a chorioretinal rupture (retinitis sclopetaria) may occur (Fig. 18–18). It is a simultaneous rupture of the retina and choroid and is usually associated with profound visual loss at initial presentation. On ophthalmoscopic evaluation, there may be severe retinal edema and hemorrhage, often breaking through into the vitreous. After clearing of this hemorrhage, a white proliferative glial scar with widespread pigmentary disturbance may be observed (Fig. 18–19). The visual outcome depends on whether the scarring and rupture are favorably located and whether the vitreous remains clear.

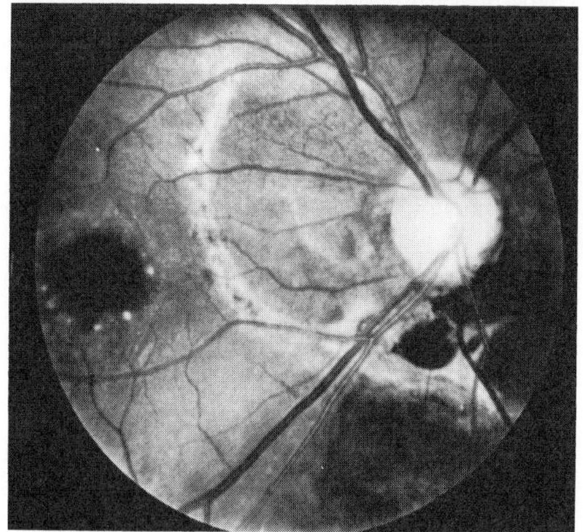

Figure 18–18. A long linear scar parallel to the optic disc is a typical residue of a choroidal rupture. (Courtesy of Dr. Robison D. Harley.)

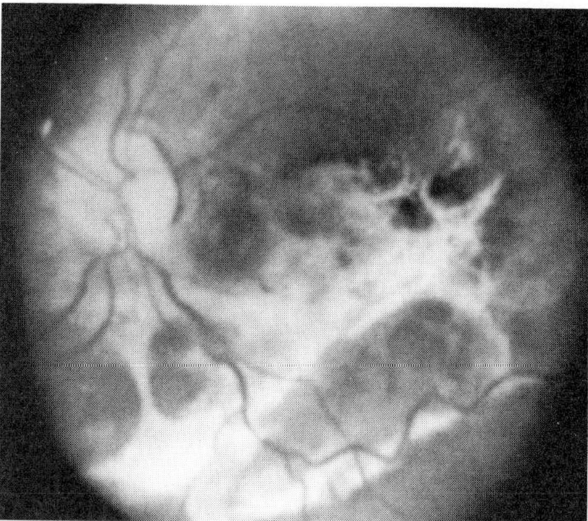

Figure 18–19. This eye suffered severe intraocular damage with hemorrhage. The end result is scarring, pigment migration, and a choroidal rupture inferiorly. (Courtesy of Drs. Philip P. Ellis and James R. Cerasoli, Ocular Injuries Med-Com Inc., New York.)

Traumatic Retinal Detachment

Ocular trauma is the most common cause of retinal detachment in children. The median age is approximately 15 years, with a statistically significant prevalence of males (84.6 per cent).[23] A dialysis (a tear at the ora serrata on the most peripheral area of the retina) is the most common cause of traumatic retinal detachment. Since many of these detachments originate in the retinal periphery, they may cause few ocular symptoms. A unique characteristic of this type of detachment is the latency period that often occurs between the time of initial trauma and the detection of the detachment (17.3 months).[28] Animal experimentation suggests that the majority of retinal breaks occur at the time of ocular trauma.[24] Since there is a high incidence of concomitant vitreous hemorrhage, which may obscure part of the retinal periphery, the ophthalmologist is required to examine the injured eye at periodic intervals.

Intraocular and Intraorbital Foreign Bodies

Whenever ocular trauma results in the possibility of a laceration of the lids or penetrating injury to the globe, the presence of a foreign body must be excluded. An intraocular foreign body may react in various ways, depending on its composition. Some foreign bodies are inert; others may react chemically with the ocular tissues. Also, small, high-velocity foreign bodies may enter the eye through the sclera and cause almost no symptoms. Therefore, a painstaking post-trauma examination must be performed to detect the location of a foreign body and the associated ocular damage.

An intraocular or intraorbital foreign body may be localized in several ways. An ophthalmoscopic examination may detect an intraocular foreign body and should be performed as soon as possible after the injury (Fig. 18–20). In many cases, an x-ray examination is necessary, especially if the ocular media is hazy, as would be expected with a traumatic cataract or intraocular hemorrhage.

Plain and soft tissue orbital x-rays may help verify the presence of a radiopaque foreign body. If a foreign body is demonstrated, a localizing x-ray may help determine whether or not it is within the globe. One method uses a Comberg contact lens. Another method, the Sweet technique, is based on mathematical calculations from x-rays of the eye at different angles. Using one of these methods, the radiologist is able to plot the approximate position of the foreign body within the eye or orbit. Ophthalmic ultrasound may be a useful ancillary method of localizing intraocular foreign bodies. Once the presence and location of a foreign body are established, it is the ophthalmologist's obligation to decide whether a conservative or surgical approach is necessary (Fig. 18–21).

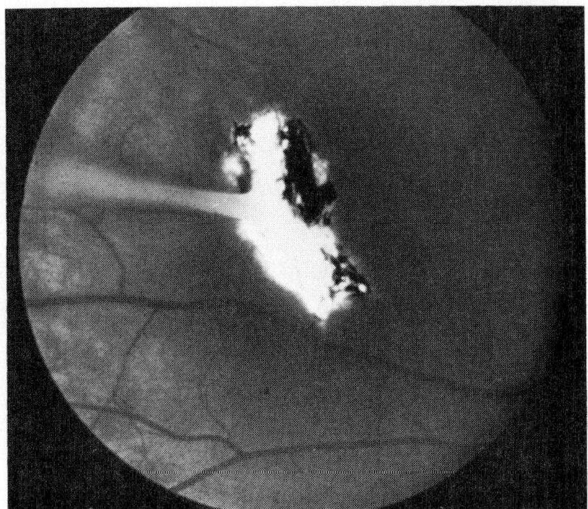

Figure 18–21. An intraocular foreign body has been removed surgically, leaving behind a chorioretinal scar with pigmentation. (Courtesy of Dr. Robison D. Harley.)

Ocular Trauma in Sports

During 1976, approximately 165,000 traumatic eye injuries occurred in school children between the ages of 5 and 17.[25] Many of these injuries resulted in time lost from school and, in some cases, in permanent total disability of an eye. Analysis of eye injuries in school children has shown that approximately two-thirds of accidents occurred during play or sports activities.[26]

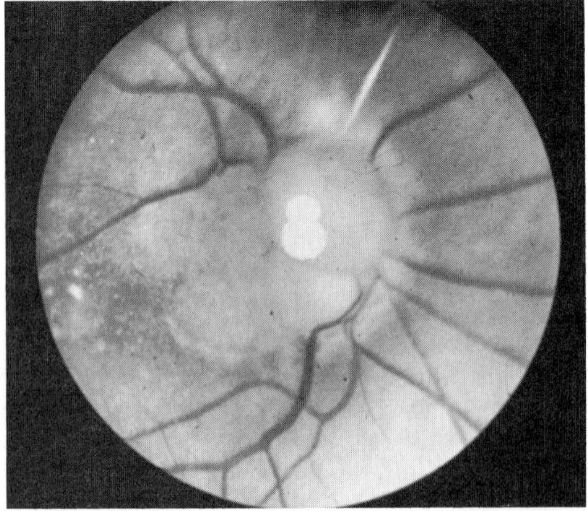

Figure 18–20. In this eye an intraocular metallic foreign body was retained for more than 10 years. It is encapsulated by a dense fibrous tissue coating. (Courtesy of Dr. Robison D. Harley.)

A review of 147 eye injuries referred for specialized treatment from general ophthalmologic practices indicated that the following sports involve severe eye injuries, in decreasing order:[27] hockey, archery, darts, and BB guns. Other sports-related injuries resulted from bicycling and motorcycling, racquet sports, baseball, boxing, and basketball. Injuries included macular edema, choroidal rupture, retinal detachment, vitreous hemorrhage, hyphema, traumatic cataracts, and perforations of the globe.

Many of these sports-related eye injuries are preventable. For instance, the mandatory use of a face mask and a rule to keep the stick below the shoulder would eliminate most of the disabling eye injuries in hockey. Public education and adequate legislation could reduce the incidence in children of eye injuries caused by the use of bows and arrows, darts, and BB guns.

Ocular Manifestations of Child Abuse

The battered child syndrome has received increasing attention as a major pediatric problem. In 1966, estimates indicated that between 10,000 and 15,000 children in the United States suffered nonaccidental injuries;[28] presently this estimate is between

75,000 and 100,000 cases annually.[29] Approximately 40 per cent of affected children have associated ocular findings, with 6 per cent initially evaluated by an ophthalmologist.[30]

Intraocular hemorrhage, often associated with intracranial bleeding, is the most common ocular finding in the battered child syndrome. Although many cases of intraocular hemorrhage clear without complications, some may lead to optic atrophy, macular scarring, or traction retinal detachment. Periorbital swelling and ecchymoses, hyphemas, cataracts, subluxated lenses, and traumatic mydriasis may also result from direct ocular trauma.

The spectrum of ocular findings in child abuse includes virtually every type of eye injury. The emergency room physician should be suspicious whenever an ocular injury cannot be explained adequately or when the parents' history is incompatible with the degree of eye damage. The finding of fractures and soft tissue injuries in various stages of healing, cigarette burns, or human bites to the skin should help confirm the diagnosis.

Acknowledgment

This work was made possible in part by grants from Fight for Sight, Inc., New York, New York, to the Fight for Sight Children's Eye Center of Wills Eye Hospital and from the Children's Eye Care Foundation, Washington, D.C. This was also supported in part by the Wills Eye Hospital Research Department.

Selected Readings

Paton D, Goldberg MF: Management of Ocular Injuries. Philadelphia, W.B. Saunders Co., 1976.

Gombos GM: Handbook of Ophthalmologic Emergency. Medical Examination Publishing Co., Inc. New York, 1977. *These two books describe the authors' extensive experience with ophthalmic injuries. They present current and specific guidelines for the management of ocular traumas. Both books are well illustrated and written for readers of all levels of training.*

Epstein DC, Paton D: Keratitis from misuse of corneal anesthetics. N Engl J Med 279:396, 1968. *This paper emphasizes the fact that chronic use of topical anesthetics on the eye can lead to severe keratitis and even permanent reduction in visual acuity. Topical anesthetics should be used to obtain transient loss of corneal sensitivity for examination purposes. It should never be used as part of a prolonged medical regimen.*

Smith B, Regan WF Jr.: Blowout fracture of the orbit: Mechanism and correction of internal orbit fracture. Am J Ophthalmol 44:733, 1957. *Classic article on the mechanism, diagnosis, and management of patients with blowout fractures of the orbit.*

Hughes WF, Jr.: Alkali burns of the eye. I. Review of the literature and summary of present knowledge. Arch Ophthalmol 35:423, 1946.

Hughes WF, Jr.: Alkali burns of the eye. II. Clinical and pathologic course. Arch Ophthalmol 36:189, 1946. *Two papers on the original classification of the severity of ocular chemical burns which is still used today. Both are well written reviews and carefully point out the many factors that may result in significant visual loss.*

REFERENCES

1. Kupfer C: Foreword. *In* Freeman HN (ed.): Ocular Trauma. New York, Prentice Hall, 1979, p. xv.
2. National Society to Prevent Blindness: Vision Problems in the U.S. New York, 1980, pp. 32–33.
3. Slusher MM, Keeney AH: Monocular blindness: Analysis of etiology and preventive needs in 424 patients. Sight Sav Rev 35:207, 1965.
4. Coles HW: Ocular surgery for traumatic injury in children. South Med J 67:930, 1974.
5. Personal communication. David S. Friendly, M.D., 1980.
6. Paton D, Goldberg MF: Management of Ocular Injuries. Philadelphia, W.B. Saunders Co., 1976, p. 10.
7. Paton D, Goldberg MF: Management of Ocular Injuries. Philadelphia, W.B. Saunders Co., 1976, p. 51.
8. Greenwald MS, Keeney AH, Shannon GM: A review of 128 patients with orbital fractures. Am J Ophthalmol 78:655, 1974.
9. Paton D, Goldberg MF: Management of Ocular Injuries. Philadelphia, W.B. Saunders Co. 1976, p. 59.
10. Rumelt MB, Ernest JT: Isolated blowout fracture of the medial orbital wall with medial rectus muscle entrapment. Am J Ophthalmol 73:451, 1972.
11. Smith B, Regan WF Jr: Blowout fracture of the orbit: Mechanism and correction of internal orbital fracture. Am J Ophthalmol 44:733, 1957.
12. Ralph RA: Chemical burns of the eye. *In* Duane TD, Jaeger EA (eds.): Clinical Ophthalmology. Vol. 4. Hagerstown, Maryland, Harper & Row, 1980, p. 1.
13. Hughes WF Jr: Alkali burns of the eye. I. Review of the literature and summary of present knowledge. Arch Ophthalmol 35:423, 1946.
14. Hughes WF Jr: Alkali burns of the eye. II. Clinical and pathologic course. Arch Ophthalmol 36:189, 1946.
15. Tenzel RR: Trauma and burns. Int Ophthalmol Clin 10:55, 1970.
16. Paton D, Goldberg MF: Management of Ocular Injuries. Philadelphia, W.B. Saunders Co., 1976, p. 186.
17. Epstein DC, Paton D: Keratitis from misuse of corneal anesthetics. N Engl J Med 279:396, 1968.
18. Gombos GM: Handbook of Ophthalmologic Emergency. New York, Medical Examination Publishing Co., 1977, pp. 123–124.
19. Read JE: Trauma: Ruptures and bleeding. *In* Duane TD, Jaeger EA (eds.): Clinical Ophthalmology. Vol. 4. Hagerstown, Maryland, Harper & Row, 1980, p. 6.

20. Read J, Goldberg MF: Comparison of medical treatment for traumatic hyphema. Tr Am Acad Ophthalmol Otolaryngol 78:799, 1974.
21. Edwards WC, Layden WE: Monocular versus binocular patching in traumatic hyphema. Am J Ophthalmol 76:359, 1973.
22. Luntz MH: *In* Duane TD, Jaeger EA (eds.): Clinical Ophthalmology. Vol. 1. Hagerstown, Maryland, Harper & Row, 1980, p. 17.
23. Tasman W: Retinal dialysis following blunt trauma. *In* Freeman HM (ed.): Ocular Trauma. New York, Appleton-Century-Crofts, 1979, pp. 295–296.
24. Weidenthol DT, Schepans CL: Peripheral fundus changes associated with ocular contusion. Am J Ophthalmol 62:465, 1966.
25. Vinger PF: The prevention of ocular trauma. *In* Freeman HM (ed.): Ocular Trauma. New York, Appleton-Century-Crofts, 1979, p. 369.
26. Kerby CE: Eye accidents to school children. Sight Sav Rev 20:11, 1950.
27. Rousseau AP: Ocular trauma in sports. *In* Freeman HM (ed.): Ocular Trauma. New York, Appleton-Century-Crofts, 1979, pp. 353–361.
28. Helfer R, Pollack C: The battered child syndrome. Adv Pediatr 15:9, 1968.
29. Harley RD: Ocular manifestations of child abuse. J Pediatr Ophthalmol 17:5, 1980.
30. Friendly DS: Ocular manifestations of physical child abuse. Trans Am Acad Ophthalmol Otolaryngol 75:318, 1971.

CHAPTER

19 Dental Injuries

CHARLES L. BRORING

The initial diagnosis and emergency care of dental injuries are often significant in assuring the survival of injured teeth. The evaluation of the degree of injury will aid in immediate treatment and provide the basis for later referral of the patient for more permanent treatment. Familiarity with types of dental injuries, effective diagnosis, and appropriate treatment are important to the emergency physician and pediatrician. Complications from dental injuries include color changes of teeth, infection, abscess formation, ankylosis, resorption of roots, loss of space in the dental arch, abnormal root development, and loss of teeth. Attention to detail in the early stages of diagnosis and management can largely prevent these complications.

Emergency care to an injured child's teeth requires prompt and efficient treatment. It is important to provide consolation and encouragement to parents and the child at this time. This chapter provides a basis for the initial evaluation, general principles of trauma management, and general prognosis for dental injuries. Definitive operative techniques for management will be described but not emphasized.

CAUSES OF DENTAL INJURIES

The teeth may be injured in a number of ways, and the cause of injury is often dependent on the child's age. Because the incisor teeth are usually not fully present until 6 months of age and because the child's ability to move about on his own is limited, dental injuries are uncommon during the first 6 to 9 months of life. Thus, most of the dental injuries sustained by infants are caused by falls. School-age children often have dental injuries related to their physical activities, including fights and sports injuries. Children of any age can be injured in automobile accidents.

Automobile accidents often cause the driver to sustain penetrating injuries of the lower lip and fractures of the lower incisors and alveolar bone. Debris is often contained in the lip wound. When the child is a passenger in the automobile, he may receive an injury from striking the dashboard, sustaining fractures of the upper teeth, alveolar process, or jaw. Tooth fragments may be found in the lacerated lip.

Fights and sports injuries often result in trauma when the lip covers the teeth at the time of impact and cushions the blow. The softened blow often causes the whole tooth to be displaced out of its socket, and the displaced tooth may carry a portion of the fractured alveolar bone with it. The anterior teeth are most often affected in this type of injury.

Falls from bicycles, stairs, or other heights may result in impact on the chin, which can injure the front teeth. According to Andreason,[1] they frequently cause other injuries, including brain concussion; fracture or contusion of the mandibular condyle; midline mandible fracture; fracture of the posterior teeth crowns, possibly involving the roots; and a bite laceration of the tongue.

Most dental injuries in small children involve falls, often causing displacement of the primary teeth. The infant's alveolar bone is a thin parchment-like structure that is soft and resilient. The bone absorbs the blow and rather than fracturing the tooth, the entire tooth is displaced, intruded within the bone, or broken out altogether.

A fall on permanent anterior teeth usually results in a fracture of the crown or root. This occurs because the stronger, harder, inelastic mature bone will not absorb the force of the blow but holds the tooth in place, causing a fracture of the tooth itself and sometimes the bone as well.

DIAGNOSIS OF DENTAL INJURIES

Dental injuries endanger the teeth both from the initial shock and trauma of the injury as well as from the possibility of deterioration by inflammation, infection, or pulpal necrosis long after the injury occurs. Dental diagnosis and treatment are therefore concerned with the initial stabilization and

Table 19–1. CLASSIFICATION OF INJURY TO TEETH AND SUPPORTING BONE

Tooth
Crack of tooth crown (infraction)
Fracture of tooth involving the following:
enamel
enamel and dentin
enamel, dentin, and pulp
Crown-root fracture
Root fracture
Mobility of tooth (subluxation)
Displacement of tooth
Supporting Bone
Compression fracture of alveolar socket
Alveolar wall fracture
Alveolar process fracture
Maxillary fracture
Mandibular fracture

Adapted from Johnson R: Traumatic injuries to the teeth and supporting structures. *In* Stewart R, Barber T, Troutman K, Wei S (eds.): Pediatric Dentistry. St. Louis, C. V. Mosby Co., 1982.

retention of the tooth and its supporting structures and preservation of the nerve central to each tooth. Table 19–1 lists the types of injuries that may affect the teeth and their supporting bones. This classification of dental injuries will be referred to throughout the course of this discussion.

The first step in diagnosis of dental injuries is determining the nature of the trauma causing the injury. Severe blows (automobile accidents or bicycle falls) frequently result in fracture of bones as well as teeth and require special attention. Injuries causing loss of consciousness should be carefully evaluated for possible head trauma. In addition, when loss of consciousness has occurred, the dentition and facial bones should be carefully assessed, since the response to pain may be decreased.

After a history of the injury has been taken, a visual examination should be performed and bleeding should be arrested before progressing with other stages of diagnosis. The ability to close the mouth in a centric bite may reveal displacement or damage to the occlusion. All teeth should be palpated for mobility and possibility of bone fracture. After each tooth has been examined by visual diagnosis and palpation, x-rays should be taken of areas involved in trauma.

Clinical Examination

The clinical examination of the patient is performed initially by careful visual examination, to determine the seriousness and extent of the injury. The following features are evaluated:

a. Bleeding: if present, it should be stopped after determining its source.

b. Swelling: if present early, it may indicate bone injury as well as laceration.

c. Laceration of tissues: should be examined for a clue to the direction and force of trauma.

d. Visible fractures of crown: gross loss of tooth structure is easily seen, but cracking is better detected with an indirect light source.

e. Pulp exposure: this is indicated by bleeding from the center of the tooth itself.

f. Loss of a tooth: a freshly traumatized space without a tooth may indicate the tooth is knocked out or that it may have been driven into the gums and bone.

g. Displacement of tooth: is the noticeable movement of a tooth out of its normal position backward, forward, or sideways?

The presence or absence of pain is noted. Local anesthesia may be indicated to facilitate treatment. Manipulation of the injured structures to determine mobility, tooth firmness, and bone fracture is performed. Radiographic evaluation is performed by taking an adequate number of films to completely cover the full extent of injury. If bone fractures are suspected, large lateral and occlusal films are needed. The following features are evaluated: (a) fractures of roots and crowns; (b) size and proximity of pulp to fractures; and (c) stage of root development.

Note: A wide immature apex has a good blood supply, which may facilitate healing, but it provides a poor field for endodontic closure. A closed apex may result in strangulation of engorged vessels following trauma but makes a good root canal prospect.

INJURIES TO THE TOOTH

Crack or Crazing (Infraction)

Infraction injuries are incomplete fractures of the enamel of the crown, without loss of tooth structure (Fig. 19–1). These injuries present as small vertical or horizontal lines or crazes. Use of an indirect light source facilitates detection of this injury. While therapy is not usually indicated, additional injuries may be present, and the child should have follow-up care arranged with the dentist.

Fractures of the Tooth

Fractures of the tooth may involve only the enamel or enamel and dentin, but more serious fractures may involve the enamel,

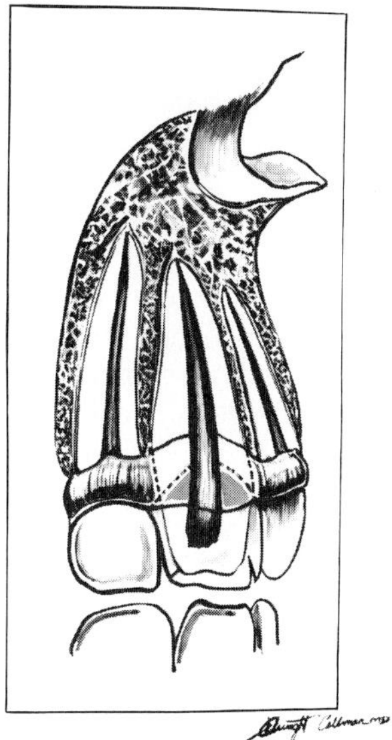

Figure 19–1. Infraction injuries are incomplete fractures of the enamel of the crown, without loss of tooth structure. These are often most easily detected using an indirect light source.

dentin, and pulp. This latter injury may involve nerve and vascular damage as well. Each injury has a different prognosis and requires different treatment. Cracks of the *enamel* appear as normal teeth with a variable portion of the tooth missing (Fig. 19–2).

If there is a question of whether a tooth has had an enamel fracture or is simply malformed, comparison with adjacent teeth or the antimere may aid the diagnosis. Fractures involving only the enamel require no immediate therapy, but instructions for later dental observation should be given.

Teeth that are fractured into the *enamel and dentin* often appear similar to enamel fractures, but they have more loss of tooth structure and often show the yellowish color of dentin in the central area of the injury. In addition, injuries of the dentin and pulp often exhibit sensitivity to air, temperature, and direct pressure (Fig. 19–3).[3] Therapy for enamel and dentin fractures is directed toward preservation of the pulp, and early consultation with the dentist should be sought.

Fractures involving enamel, dentin, and pulp usually have a red or pink area of bleeding in the center of the tooth (Fig. 19–4). Because the pulp has been exposed, bacterial contamination is common and may affect prognosis. Fractures involving enamel, dentin, and pulp require immediate dental treatment to preserve the vitality of the tooth. Delay often results in root canal or other nerve treatments, which threaten tooth vitality. The dentist may cap the nerve or perform a pulpotomy or a root canal. The earlier treatment is initiated, the better the chances of successful preservation of the tooth and its nerve.

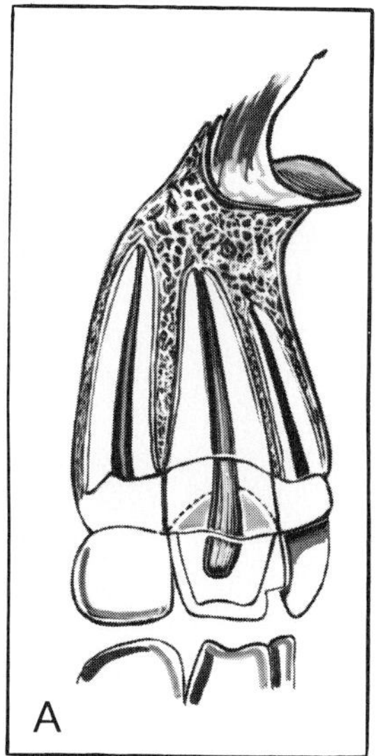

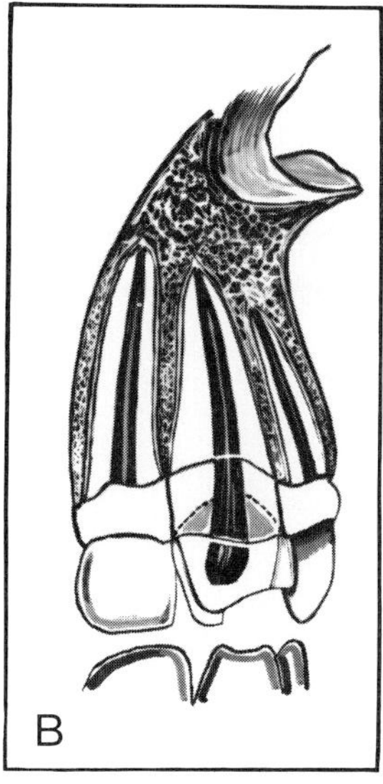

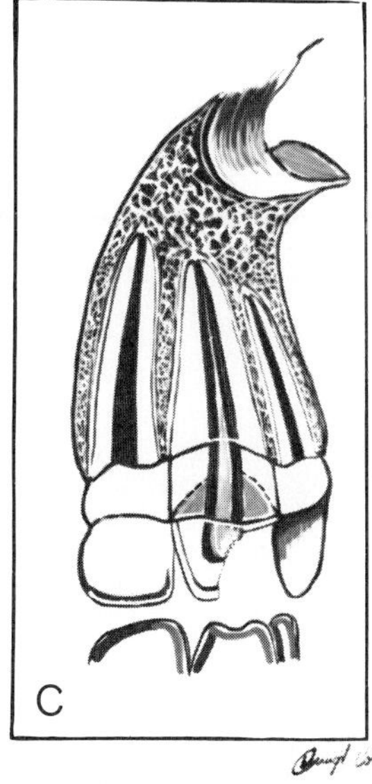

Figure 19–2. Fractures of the tooth may involve the enamel only, enamel and dentin, or enamel, dentin, and pulp. *A*, A tooth with cracks of the enamel may look like a normal tooth with a variable portion of the tooth missing. *B*, When the enamel and dentin are fractured, there is more loss of tooth structure and the yellowish color of dentin may be seen in the central area. *C*, Fractures involving enamel, dentin, and pulp usually result in a red or pink area of bleeding in the center of the tooth. These fractures require immediate dental attention to preserve the tooth.

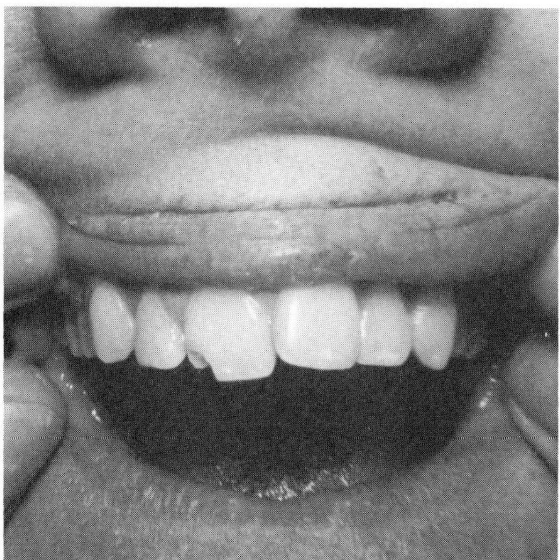

Figure 19–3. A fracture involving the enamel and dentin, without pulp involvement. This condition should receive early attention by a dentist to assure preservation of nerve tissues.

Crown-Root Fractures

A fracture extending vertically from the crown into the root of the tooth is a serious injury. In this injury, the fracture line begins above the level of the gingiva and continues through the tooth and into the root at the alveolar bone. The tooth fracture itself may involve enamel, enamel and dentin, or enamel, dentin, and pulp. When such fractures occur in primary teeth, they are usually treated by extraction of all tooth fragments. This surgery can be delayed until an opportune time after initial evaluation, especially if other tissue damage is involved. Pain is frequently absent, but when it is present, it is an indication for a rapid surgical procedure.

A crown-root fracture in the permanent dentition deserves a dental evaluation to determine if there is a salvageable amount of intact root. If there is, root canal and build up of the stump may be possible. Referral for a dental consultation is necessary.

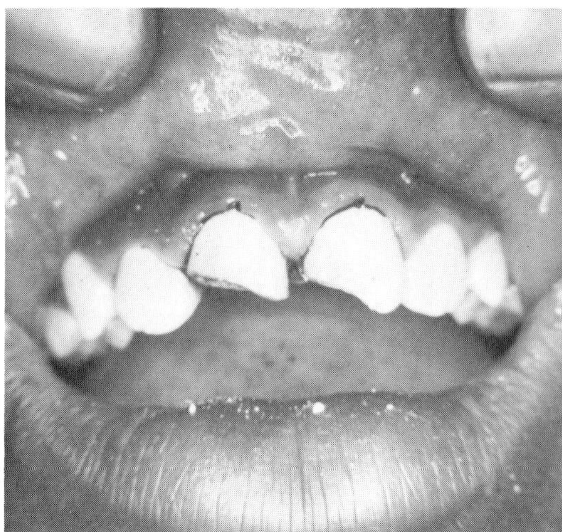

Figure 19–4. Severe crown fractures such as these often involve the pulpal tissue and require early dental attention. The pulp is visible to the examiner as a bloody spot in the middle of the tooth.

Root Fracture

Fracture of a root may be difficult to detect clinically. Looseness of the tooth and abnormal position in the dental arch are clues, and the diagnosis is confirmed by radiographs (Fig. 19–5). Root fractures can often be successfully treated by appropriate positioning and splinting of the tooth. This is done in cases in which a substantial part of the root (more than one third) remains as a unit with the crown. This provides an opportunity for reattachment and stabilization of the tooth.

Healing of the two root fragments may occur as a consequence of calcified tissue, interposition of connective tissue, interposition of bone and connective tissue, or interposition of granulation tissue. The observant dentist can determine the need for root canal treatment as the case progresses. If the root fracture occurs close to the crown or in the coronal one-third of the root, referral for extraction of the unstable tooth is advised.

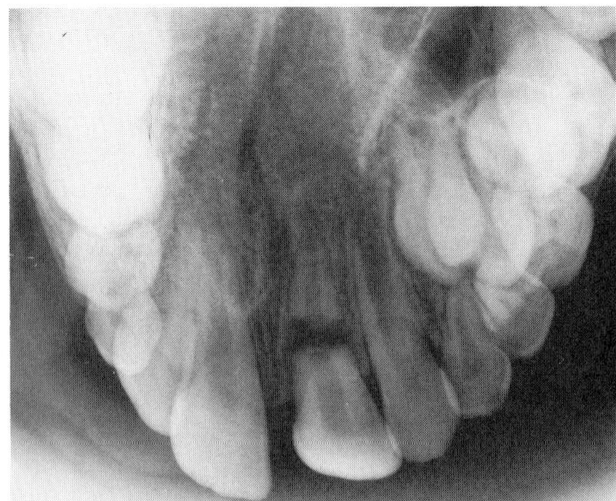

Figure 19–5. A root fracture of a permanent incisor requires a dental x-ray for diagnosis. Since a major portion of the root is attached to the crown, splinting is indicated. Stabilization with orthodontic bands promotes healing.

Sensitivity of the Tooth (Concussion)

Often the patient's complaint is one of soreness or sensitivity of the tooth after an injury. The tooth may be very sensitive to a percussion (tapping) test with a tongue blade or scalpel handle. If the tooth has no mobility or looseness, this indicates damage or irritation to the periodontal ligaments of the root. Little immediate treatment other than an x-ray is indicated. Occasionally light grinding on the occlusal part of the tooth is necessary to take the tooth out of occlusion. Teeth that have undergone concussion injuries are susceptible to pulpal necrosis. For this reason future observation by a dentist and pulp vitality testing are important to determine possible need of future root canal therapy.

Immediately after an accident, involved teeth may not be sensitive at all. These teeth may have no response to an electrical pulp test by the dentist. This is a result of the "stun" effect of the injury, resulting in a mild neuropraxia. If the nerve survives, the tooth will regain its response over a period of weeks to months. If the response to the electrical pulp test remains negative, the vitality of the nerve is in serious question.

Mobility (Subluxation)

Teeth that are mobile to the touch but have not lost their proper place in the arch must be considered for splinting to permit firming up in the bone. Mobility can be described using a scale of 1 to 10. Mobility of 1 is only slight (barely detectable movement when examined by digital pressure), while mobility of 10 describes a tooth that can be easily removed from the socket by digital pressure. To examine for mobility the thin edge of a tongue blade is placed in contact behind the tooth while one finger of the examiner presses lightly on the front of the tooth. A mobility of 1 usually represents a tooth that will stabilize of its own accord during the period of post-trauma local edema, and it does not require a splint. Teeth with a mobility of 10 usually require placement of some type of splinting (see below).

Displacement or Loosening of Teeth

Complete or partial displacement of the teeth is a common injury in children. Treatment is aimed at preserving the life of the tooth and providing patients with comfortable bite positioning during the healing process. When teeth are displaced or lost altogether, the decision of whether to try to retain the tooth is made. Removing the tooth is sometimes necessary, but this precludes survival of the tooth in the dental arch. Repositioning the tooth permits future efforts to save the tooth by orthodontic treatment or prosthetic replacement. If patient and parent cooperation permits, every reasonable effort should be made to immediately retain all lost or displaced teeth.

The Intruded Tooth

The intruded tooth is driven like a spike into the alveolar bone and presents unique problems. These teeth are usually whole, intact teeth that absorb a direct blow on the vertical axis, driving them into the alveolar bone, which fractures by compression (Fig. 19–6). An important factor in treatment is whether the tooth is primary or permanent.

The intruded primary tooth is treated by observation alone and is allowed to re-erupt of its own initiative. Most primary teeth will re-erupt, guided by lip action, tongue action, and chewing forces, to a reasonable approximation of the original position in the arch. No active treatment is indicated. Sometimes a severely traumatized primary tooth will not only re-erupt but may continue to be extruded and will be lost like a foreign body.

The intruded permanent tooth is not so likely to re-erupt but should be allowed to do so during a careful observation period.

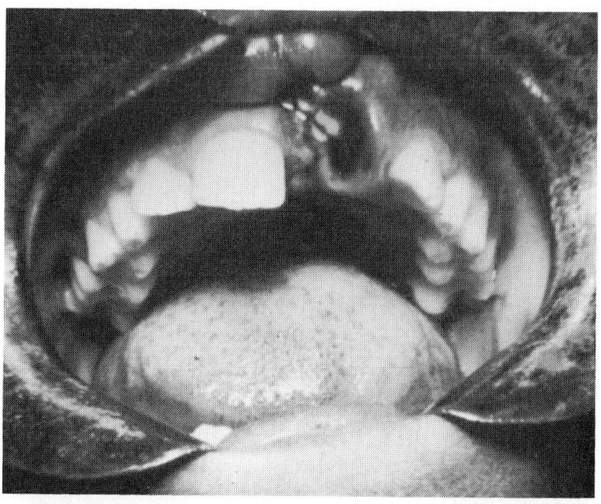

Figure 19–6. An intruded primary central incisor has been pushed up into the alveolar bone. It was diagnosed by x-ray. The primary tooth should be left undisturbed, since it will probably re-erupt. It should be observed by a dentist.

The incidence of pulp necrosis is very high in this type of injury, and root canal is often needed. A dentist should be involved in this treatment as early as possible, since newer techniques of calcium hydroxide root canal therapy may guard against ankylosis of the roots in the intruded portion. Ankylosis of the tooth will firm it into a poor arch position and will complicate orthodontic repositioning at a later date. In cases in which re-eruption and reposition do not occur, a malformed dental arch will result. The intruded tooth that is badly fractured should be carefully removed by oral surgery.

Teeth Partially Extruded From the Socket

A tooth only partially knocked from the socket provides an excellent prognosis if it is wholly intact and the alveolar socket has not been fractured. (Figs. 19–7 and 19–8). Because this tooth does not leave the oral cavity, it retains its moisture and sometimes its blood supply (Fig. 19–9). Appropriate treatment for partially extruded teeth is gentle repositioning of the tooth by finger pressure after x-ray, visual, and manual examinations for other mouth injuries. Occlusion should be checked by having the patient close his mouth in the regular way. A splint may be necessary to stabilize the teeth (see below).

Displacement Within the Tooth Socket

The tooth displaced from its upright position labially, lingually, or in a lateral direction should be gently repositioned for splinting.

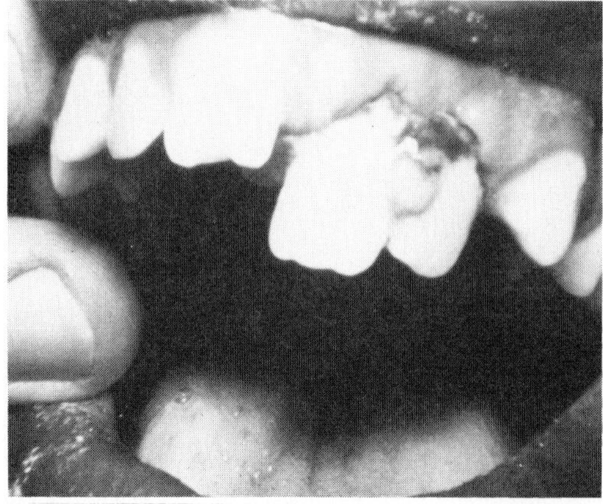

Figure 19–7. Displacement of anterior permanent teeth out of socket due to a fist fight. Since the teeth did not leave the mouth, the chances of maintaining vitality are good.

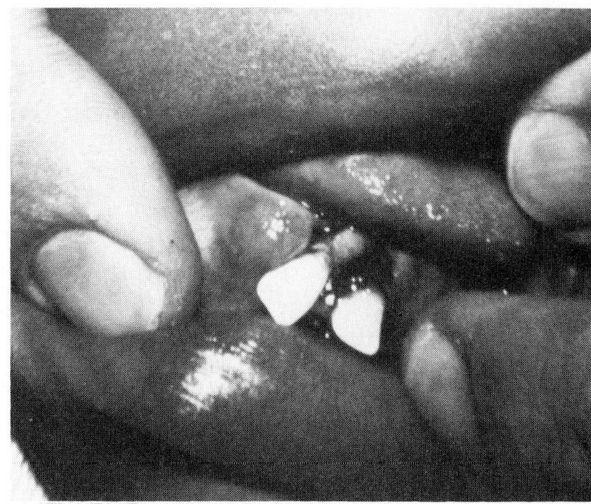

Figure 19–8. Two new primary teeth that were pulled out by yanking a blanket from an infant's mouth. There is no way to splint such teeth but an effort to reposition, followed by observation, is appropriate. If repositioning results in a very loose tooth, the operator's judgment determines if extraction is a better treatment.

This follows complete oral and x-ray examinations. Such teeth have a good chance of re-attachment, but vitality is sometimes lost due to trauma to nerve tissue (Fig. 19–10).

Evulsed Teeth

Complete evulsion of the tooth from the socket is a dramatic injury and requires a decision on whether or not the tooth should be replaced. If the tooth is not recovered at the accident scene, it is possible that instead of being knocked out the tooth has been intruded out of sight into the alveolar bone. It should be carefully sought on the x-ray.

The x-ray evaluation phase of the clinical examination becomes paramount in determining if the tooth or fragment remains in the bone. Radiographs should be taken from several angles to evaluate the alveolar area. X-rays should also be taken of the lips if any lacerations are present to determine if fragments of the tooth or the tooth itself are lodged in the lip. Occasionally patients suffer multiple injuries from a single accident (Fig. 19–11).

Permanent teeth are usually replanted if they are recovered as a whole tooth. The most commonly involved teeth are the upper incisors. The prognosis for long-term retention of a replanted tooth is variable, but replantation should be attempted, since newer techniques of follow-up care are improving the results (Figs. 19–11*B* and *C*).

The survival of the replanted tooth depends upon re-establishment of a normal

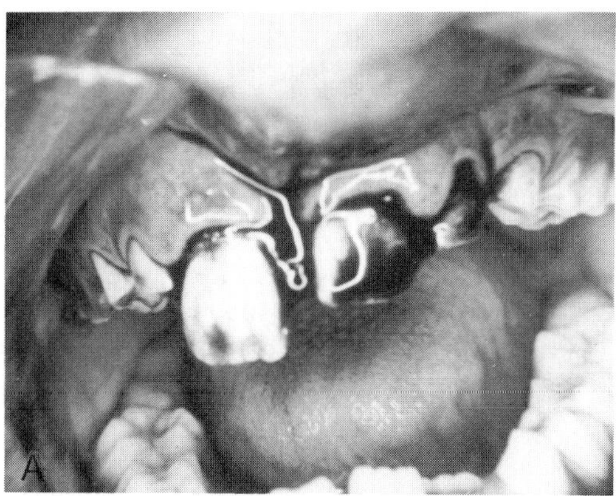
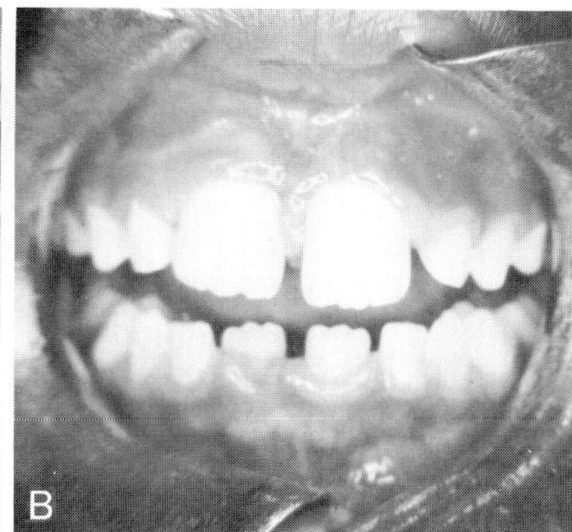

Figure 19–9. *A*, Displacement of permanent central incisors as a result of a bicycle accident. *B*, After repositioning and splinting, the teeth shown in Figure *A* have healed and stabilized in normal occlusion. Follow-up by the dentist is advised, since occlusion varies greatly in young, growing patients.

periodontal ligament attachment. This in turn requires the survival of the ligament and the management of the pulpal tissues to avoid resorption or abscess of the root.

The most critical factor in survival of the periodontal ligament is the length of time the tooth is out of the mouth. If the tooth is knocked from the socket and remains somewhere within the mouth, the prognosis is excellent. A tooth that is out of the mouth 30 minutes or less will satisfactorily replant 90 per cent of the time without root resorption.[1-2] Teeth replanted after 90 minutes or more usually show root resorption and will be less successfully replanted.[3,4]

The period of time the tooth is out of the socket is a critical factor in the survival of replanted teeth because the cells of the periodontal ligament dry out, contact foreign materials, and are traumatized by handling and exposure. Animal studies show that cell damage becomes irreversible after 60 minutes, owing to dehydration.[5, 6]

Since drying out is such a serious concern, the lost tooth should be preserved in a moist medium during transportation to the physician. The patient may carry the tooth under the tongue or in a cup of water, saline, or warm milk. Since time is of such importance in replanting teeth, the first contact with the patient by telephone should involve advising the patient to replace the tooth if possible. The best course of action is to suggest that the patient or parent wash the tooth in tap water and push it gently into the socket.

Many evulsed teeth have been treated successfully after replacement by the parents at the scene of accident or injury.[2, 3] In one case, a tooth was replaced backward by a proud, enterprising mother, who was most upset to see her error.[3] The tooth was turned, refitted, and survived, since the periodontal tissues had been protected.

The patient should be promptly brought to the emergency room for an evaluation. Replacement of the tooth by the parent or doctor should be preceded by a gentle washing of the tooth under lukewarm water. *The tooth should be gripped only by the crown to prevent further damage to the periodontal liga-*

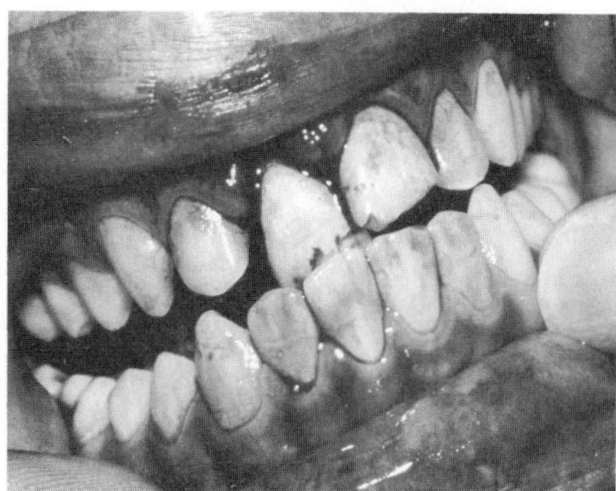

Figure 19–10. Loss of the patient's occlusion occurs in this instance of lingual displacement of upper teeth incisors. Repositioning and splinting are indicated, since the teeth are only partially knocked out. Healing is usually rapid in these circumstances.

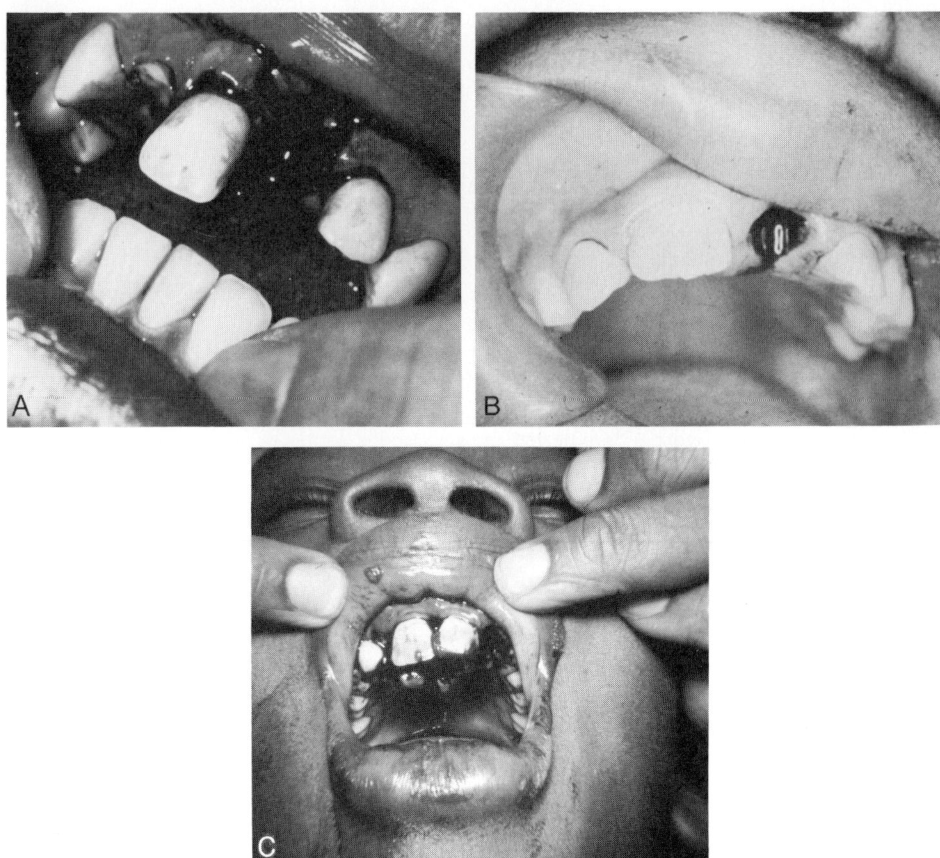

Figure 19–11. *A,* This wound involved the displacement of several teeth, loss from the mouth of one tooth, and crown fracture of another tooth. The palatal tissue is peeled back and occlusion is mangled. *B,* A tooth totally lost from the socket. If a tooth is recoverable, it may be replanted and splinted. X-rays should be used to evaluate the integrity of the socket. *C,* A fall from a tree displaced two teeth and knocked out two that were not recovered. The displaced alveolar bone was reduced, the teeth were repositioned and splinted, and the palate was repositioned and sutured.

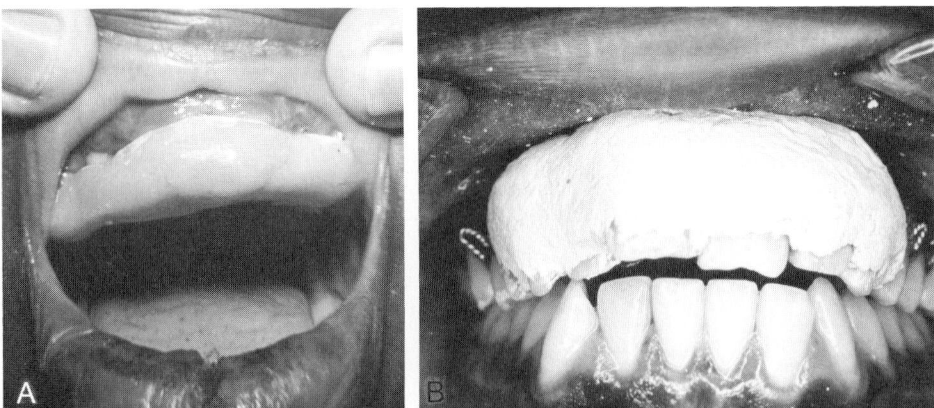

Figure 19–12. *A,* A form of splint utilized to stabilize teeth with the use of Quick-Cure dental acrylic material. This splint is easy to fabricate, but does not allow for good oral hygiene of the affected area. *B,* A serviceable temporary splint can be made of dental surgical pack. It performs well and is manipulated relatively easily for placement.

ments of the root. Before replacing the tooth, a examination and appropriate x-rays should be undertaken to evaluate other injuries. If only the tooth is involved, it may then be gently pushed into the socket, concave side on the back. If the tooth was replaced before arrival at the emergency room, the doctor should gently remove it for examination. Any foreign matter can be wiped away with a moist saline gauze.

Holding the tooth in two fingers, the physician should gently press the tooth all the way into the socket. If a clot presents an obstruction to the tooth, the socket should be cleaned by suction or gentle curettage. The tooth should be fully planted and the bite checked by having the patient gently close down. The tooth should then be splinted in place. Do not pierce the alveolus or cut the tooth apex for a better fit.

Splinting Procedures. To allow periodontal reattachment, the tooth should be securely splinted by any one of a number of procedures. A simple splint can be made of orthodontic bands cemented on the tooth and adjacent teeth and tied together by ligature wire. Another splint can be easily fabricated by assembling orthodontic bands one at a time on the tooth and adjacent teeth. As bands are fitted, they are removed and spot-welded together into a splint that grows to the approximate length needed. This complete splint is cemented in place and gives ideal splinting with some slight movement possible. This is desirable for more natural healing in the socket. Other splints, such as the Eric Arch Bar, the Essig Wire Technique, a doughy mass of quick curing acrylic (Fig. 19–12*A*), or even a surgical pack, can be temporarily applied until a better splint can be constructed (Fig. 19–12*B*). New composite materials can be acid etched on the enamel and joined with wires to give an excellent new type of splint. The important feature of the splint is maintenance of the tooth in the mouth so that healing will occur at the roots. Endodontic treatment will be decided upon within days of splinting and may be done through the splint if necessary.

Follow-up Dental Treatment. The most frequent follow-up dental treatment involves endodontic procedures to remove affected pulpal tissues and replace them with an appropriate filling material. Current endodontic practice indicates the removal of the pulp and placement of calcium hydroxide material. This material may stop inflammatory root resorption.

This material is prepared and placed no earlier than 2 weeks after the initial trauma. If inflammatory root resorption is noted on periodic follow-up x-rays, calcium hydroxide treatment should be repeated. A 1-year period without root resorption would indicate a need for replacement or gutta-percha root canal. Another result of tooth replantation is replacement resorption of the root by ingrowth of bone. This results in ankylosis of the tooth in whatever position it was placed (Fig. 19–13). The tooth may require extraction, but prognosis improves with each succeeding year.

Replanting the Primary Tooth

A primary tooth is generally not replanted because of the many difficulties in management and the danger to the developing permanent tooth bud. If the child is 2 years old or younger, quick replantation may be attempted because the immaturity of the primary roots aids in reattachment. This should be done only very soon after the accident because success decreases rapidly with time. The replanted tooth may be stabilized for a few days with a surgical pack or with wiring or suture materials. The person calling to report such an accident should be instructed to replant the tooth if possible or to keep the tooth in a moist gauze or cloth or cup of fresh milk.

Instructions should include the following:

1. Wash the tooth in tap water or saline solution.
2. Place the tooth gently into the socket as far as it will go, holding it by the crown only.
3. If the tooth cannot be replanted, place it in milk or moist gauze for transportation.

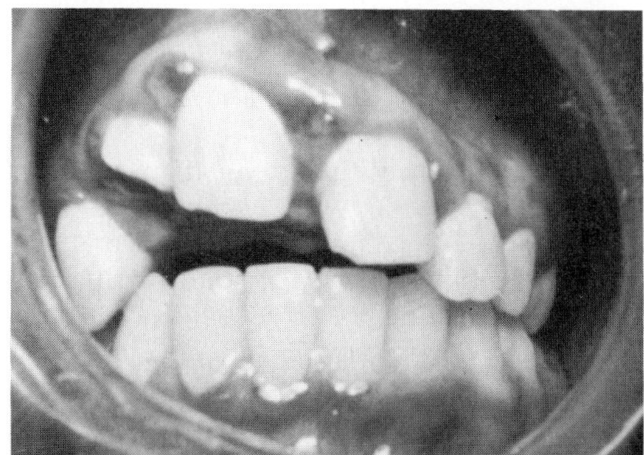

Figure 19–13. The teeth shown here were displaced by trauma and not repositioned. They have ankylosed into severe malocclusion. The dentist should be given the opportunity to reposition teeth as soon as possible.

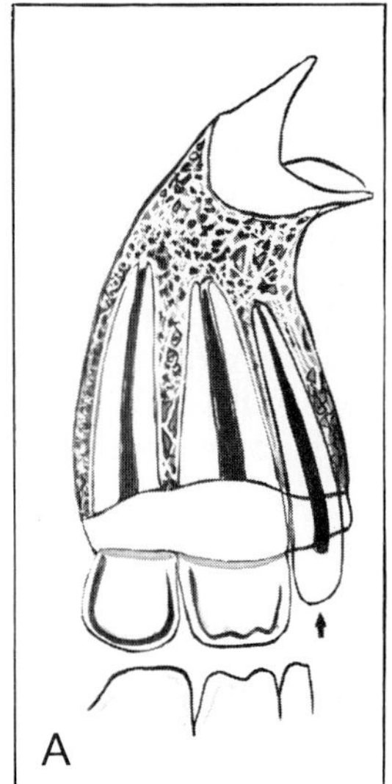

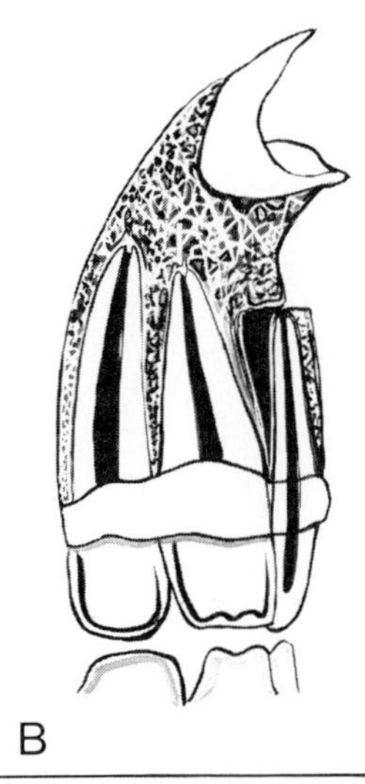

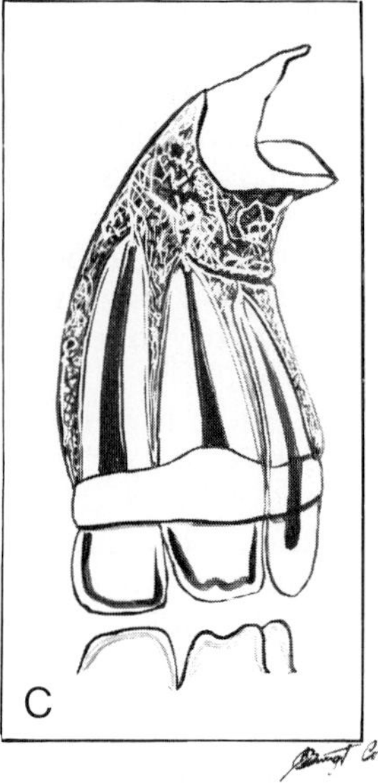

Figure 19–14. Fractures of the alveolar bone. *A*, Compression fracture of the alveolar socket due to intrusion injury. Recognition of the injury is important, and patients with this condition have more pain on palpation or percussion than those with simple intrusion injuries. *B*, Alveolar wall fracture. Palpation of the alveolar area usually reveals the fracture site. *C*, Fracture of the alveolar process. Findings vary from gross instability to minor displacement and swelling.

The injury should be followed closely by a dentist, since necrosis, abscess, root resorption, or ankylosis may occur.

Injuries to Supporting Bones

Supporting bone injuries may be classified as follows: (1) compression fractures of the alveolar socket; (2) alveolar wall fractures; (3) alveolar process fractures; (4) maxillary bone fractures; and (5) mandibular bone fractures. While these injuries are relatively less common in children than in adults, they nonetheless require astute clinical judgment to document the extent of injury.

Intrusion injuries to the teeth may cause compression fractures of the alveolar socket (Fig. 19–14*A*). Recognition of the injury is important, and these patients have more pain to palpation or percussion than those with simple intrusion injuries.

Injuries resulting in tooth displacement often cause alveolar wall fractures, particularly in the maxillary incisor area (Fig. 19–14*B*). Mobility of the tooth and palpation of the alveolar area often reveal the fracture site, and x-rays confirm the diagnosis.

Fracture of the alveolar process (Fig. 19–14*C*) may present with gross instability of the tooth and alveolar fragment but may also show simply mild displacement, hemorrhage, gingival laceration, swelling, or tenderness. These fractures are usually reduced by finger pressure and can be stabilized by splinting the teeth involved in the fractured area. Sutures placed in soft tissue lacerations associated with these wounds also help stabilize these areas.

Fractures in the maxillary or mandibular bones are less common in children and are discussed in detail in Chapter 17 (p. 299–300).

INFECTION

Penetrating wounds of soft tissues by soil-contaminated objects should be protected against tetanus. A child with no previous primary immunization requires appropriate initial passive immunity by use of tetanus antitoxin. Children who do have previous primary immunization but in whom gross contamination is present may require the use of tetanus immune globulin. Antibiotics are indicated in dental injuries when compound fractures are present or severe lacerations occur to the anterior teeth of young children. When the child is seen after the initial injury, fever and obvious infection are also indications for the use of antibiotics. In general, penicillin and ampicillin provide adequate antibiotic coverage; erythromycin may be used in cases in which penicillin allergy is present.

Patients with congenital heart disease or other problems that usually necessitate antibiotic prophylaxis prior to dental manipulation should be provided with this therapy. In some cases, patients with other chronic diseases require specific therapy (Chapters 9, 10, and 11).

REFERENCES

1. Andreason JO: Luxation of permanent teeth due to trauma. A clinical and radiographic follow-up study of 189 injured teeth. Scand J Dent Res 78:273, 1970.
2. Andreason JO: Traumatic Injuries of the Teeth. St. Louis, C.V. Mosby Co., 1972.
3. Broring C: Emergency care of fractured incisors of children. The Journal, District of Columbia Dental Society, Summer 1976.
4. Hargreaves JA: The traumatized tooth. Oral Surg 34:502, 1972.
5. Hargreaves JA, Craig J, Needleman H; The Management of Traumatized Anterior Teeth of Children. 2nd ed. Edinburgh, Churchill Livingstone, 1981.
6. Johnson R: Traumatic injuries to the teeth and supporting structures. *In* Stewart R, Barber T, Troutman K, Wei S (eds.): Pediatric Dentistry. St. Louis, C.V. Mosby Co., 1982.
7. Report of the Committee on Infectious Diseases. 18 ed. American Academy of Pediatrics, 1977, p. 3.
8. Ripa LW, Finn SB: The care of injuries to the anterior teeth of children. *In* Finn SB (ed.): Clinical Pedodontics. 4th ed. Philadelphia, W.B. Saunders Co., 1973.
9. Roberts MW: Traumatic injuries to the primary and immature permanent dentition. *In* Braham RL, Morris ME (eds.): Textbook of Pediatric Dentistry. Baltimore, Williams & Wilkins, 1980.
10. Sanders B: Pediatric Oral and Maxillofacial Surgery. St. Louis, C.V. Mosby Co., 1979.

CHAPTER

20 Abdominal Injuries

MICHAEL E. MATLAK

Trauma, specifically neurologic injury, is the number one killer of children and young adults.[1,2] Although intra-abdominal injuries account for a small percentage of total pediatric trauma deaths, failure to diagnose promptly and manage successfully these injuries accounts for the majority of *preventable* deaths following multiple trauma.[3] Generally, serious injury to the head, chest, or limbs is easy to diagnose. Serious abdominal injury tends to be quite subtle. Isolated abdominal injuries are relatively easy to assess and manage; however, confusion, needless delay, and improper establishment of priorities are not uncommon when evaluating a child with polytrauma and possible abdominal trauma.[4–5]

In this chapter, our basic premise is that improved outcome demands that the focal point of emergency management be directed at cardiopulmonary and brain resuscitation.[6] The remainder of the chapter will discuss the specifics of assessment and management of abdominal trauma.[7–9]

ASSESSMENT OF ABDOMINAL INJURIES

Abdominal injuries are usually assessed as part of the secondary survey following the resuscitative phase of management (see Chapter 1). The exception is the child with exsanguinating intra-abdominal hemorrhage.

After the *immediate* life- and limb-threatening problems are treated, attention is directed to the evaluation of regional trauma. The objective of this phase is the recognition and treatment of *potential* life-threatening problems.

History

The assessment starts with a careful history of the events surrounding the accident. Often this information is obtained from witnesses, relatives, or transport personnel. Important data include mechanism of injury, time of injury, clinical status at the scene and during transport, level of consciousness, past illnesses, medications used, allergies, bleeding tendency, and time of last meal. The history is usually obtained while the child is being examined.

Mechanism of Injury

An understanding of the mechanism of injury is essential to the assessment of the child. There are two basic types of injury to the abdomen, i.e., blunt and penetrating trauma. Trauma to the lower six ribs, whether blunt or penetrating, may result in serious injury to the upper abdominal organs. In most pediatric medical centers, blunt trauma accounts for 80 to 90 per cent of abdominal injuries.[4,10,11] Most commonly these injuries are due to motor vehicle accidents (pedestrian or occupant), in which multiple injuries are the rule rather than the exception. Falls from heights or against objects and physical abuse account for most of the other blunt injuries. Penetrating injuries are encountered infrequently in children except in some medical centers located near inner-city populations, where the use of small handguns and knives is more widespread.[12]

BLUNT TRAUMA

Blunt trauma is far more difficult to evaluate than penetrating trauma. Physical findings may be minimal despite serious injury.

Blunt trauma produces injury by compression against the spine, direct transfer of energy to an organ, or by rapid deceleration with subsequent tearing of structures. The solid organs are injured more frequently than the hollow viscera. Laceration of the spleen is the most common injury in children; other frequent sites of injury include the liver, pancreas, small bowel mesentery, duodenum, and proximal jejunum. Associated injury to the kidneys, ureter, and bladder must be identified even in the absence of

Table 20–1. PHYSICAL FINDINGS SUGGESTING GENITOURINARY INJURY

1. Fractured lower ribs
2. Flank mass, contusion, or wound
3. Lower abdominal mass or tenderness
4. Pelvic fracture
5. Genital swelling or discoloration
6. Inability to void
7. Blood at urethral meatus
8. High-riding prostrate
9. Hematuria

hematuria. Genitourinary injury is likely with a direct blow to the lower chest, flank, or pelvis. Physical signs suggesting urologic injury are shown in Table 20–1. Certain injuries occur concomitantly: fracture of the ribs or femur on the right side with liver injury; fracture of the ribs or femur on the left side with splenic laceration; pelvic fractures and bladder or rectal injury; pelvic fracture and dislocated hips; and fractures of lumbar spine with duodenal, jejunal, or pancreatic transection.

Penetrating Trauma

Penetrating wounds are usually caused by stabs or gunshot wounds.[12–14] A penetrating weapon may lacerate none, any, many or all the abdominal viscera or vessels and damage other regions. Hollow viscus injury is very common with penetrating trauma. The onset of peritonitis may be immediate if a segment of intestine full of food or stool evacuates into the peritoneal cavity. Symptoms may be delayed if peritoneal contamination is minimal or located in the retroperitoneum.

Major vascular injury with the risk of life-threatening hemorrhage is more common with penetrating trauma than with blunt injury. Patients with this injury may require immediate surgery if they survive the trip to the hospital.

In general, gunshot wounds inflict more serious injury and have a higher mortality rate than knife wounds.[13] Most surgeons will explore a gunshot wound of the abdomen immediately because of the high likelihood of visceral injury. Most centers treat stab wounds selectively, since one third of the injuries never violate the peritoneal lining, and even when the lining is penetrated, only one half of the patients have associated visceral injuries requiring repair.[15, 16] A selective approach demands repeated observation for early detection of signs of peritonitis.[17]

Penetrating wounds may also result in evisceration. The abdominal contents should be covered temporarily with moist, clean (sterile) dressings. The organs should not be replaced into the abdomen, and they should not be allowed to twist or kink. Acceptable dressing materials are clean sheets and towels covered with plastic wrap. One should not use any material that clings or loses its structure when wet, such as absorbent cotton, paper towels, or facial tissue.

Physical Diagnosis

While obtaining the history and considering the mechanism of injury, an abbreviated physical examination is performed.[18] The priorities in the assessment of the child with serious injury should follow this sequence: (1) airway, (2) cardiovascular system, (3) central nervous system, (4) gastrointestinal (GI) and genitourinary systems, and (5) injuries requiring orthopedic and plastic surgery.[9] This list stresses the initial recognition of the most life-threatening problems.

Most deaths related to intra-abdominal injuries are caused by early hemorrhage or later peritonitis.[19–21] Thus, during the abdominal examination, top priority is given to the question of whether intra-abdominal hemorrhage is the most immediate threat to life. The onset of symptoms and signs will be rapid, with major hemorrhage from splenic or liver lacerations; but occasionally, symptoms may be more subtle and occur more gradually, and the clinical findings may not accurately reflect the seriousness of the injury for several hours or days.

The physical examination of an acute abdomen in children is not significantly different from that in adults, but objective findings are often subtle, masked, or misinterpreted. This is particularly true in young children who are apprehensive, uncooperative, unconscious, or unable to communicate. Usually, the key to accurate diagnosis of serious abdominal injury is careful, repeated, and unhurried examinations coupled with selected diagnostic studies. On occasion, the child needs immediate resuscitation and exploratory laparotomy because time is not available for peritoneal lavage or other diagnostic studies.

Inspection

Inspection involves examination of the entire abdominal wall, chest, pelvis, and perineum, as well as assessment of the respiratory pattern and abdominal girth. All clothing is removed so that the child can be inspected from head to toe and from front to back. The body wall is examined for the presence of contusions, abrasions, lacerations, and penetrating wounds, which suggest underlying injury. Several hours may be required for some of the injuries to become evident.

Children breathe primarily with their diaphragms, so-called "belly-breathing." Peritoneal irritation from blood or intestinal contents, especially with irritation of the upper abdomen, changes the breathing pattern dramatically. The child will now breathe with his chest and avoid deep inspiration and expiration because it causes severe pain. Similarly, if the child is conscious, he will lie still and avoid crying loudly. These are very reliable signs, and they should not be overlooked because they alert the physician that peritonitis may be present.

The breathing pattern is also changed with chest wall injury. Respirations are rapid and shallow. The child is unwilling to breathe deeply and splints with respiration. Because of the elastic nature of their chest wall, children rarely fracture their ribs. A careful history of the mechanism of injury and close inspection of the chest wall may suggest thoracic injury although the chest radiograph is normal. Remember that blunt and penetrating trauma of the lower six ribs implies the possibility of abdominal injury. It also implies the danger of misleading abdominal physical findings.

Measurement of Abdominal Girth

The abdominal girth is serially measured at the level of the umbilicus. A distended or distending abdomen may indicate significant injury requiring exploration. The abdomen may distend because of accumulated gas or liquid, or both. Percussion of the abdomen and abdominal radiographs help differentiate air from fluid. Gas or air may collect intraluminally or extraluminally. Extraluminal air requires exploration whether the gas exited from a perforated viscus or entered from a penetrating injury. Large quantities of intraluminal gas are very common, since most children swallow significant amounts of air even with minor trauma. Acute dilation of the stomach is a specific disease process that may develop from swallowed air or esophageal intubation with an endotracheal tube (Fig. 20–1). This condition may fool the unwary clinician. Not only is the abdomen distended, but in extreme cases, respiration is embarrassed, and the child appears to be in shock. A properly positioned nasogastric tube establishes the diagnosis, offers definitive treatment, and reduces the likelihood of aspiration. Gas will pass out the nasogastric tube under pressure, and the abnormal physical findings will quickly resolve.

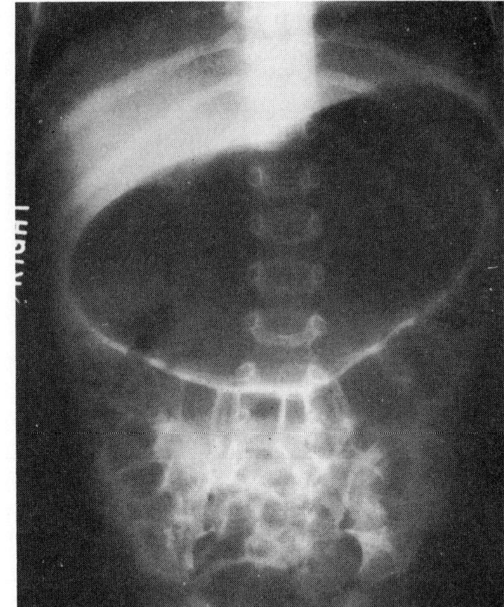

Figure 20–1. Gastric dilation frequently accompanies childhood trauma. Occasionally it may mimic a shocklike state with respiratory embarrasment. Diagnosis, treatment, and prevention are rendered by a nasogastric tube.

The most common cause for abdominal distention, besides swallowed air, is adynamic ileus. Any abdominal injury, whether minor or major, may result in this physiologic response manifested by air-fluid levels in the large and small intestine, absent or diminished bowel sounds, and gastric retention.

Abdominal distention also results from accumulation of liquids: blood, bile, pancreatic juice, urine, or intestinal contents. Serum and pus may also accumulate later as a result of inflammation, ischemia, bacterial contamination, and so on. The fluid may collect slowly or rapidly, and it may be hidden or obvious. The fluid may be inside a hollow viscus or its wall, in a solid organ, free in the peritoneal cavity, or loculated in the retroperitoneum, pelvis, or abdominal wall. Almost all these fluids result in the same physical findings, peritoneal irritation and abdominal distention. Peritoneal lavage is invaluable in detecting the presence and nature of these fluids.

Auscultation

Auscultation is the most uninformative maneuver in examination of the abdomen. Absence of bowel sounds may be normal or indicative of an ileus secondary to leakage of blood, bacteria, or chemical irritants. A bruit may indicate a significant arterial injury and suggests the need for an arteriogram.

Palpation

Palpation of the abdomen is the most difficult part of the examination to interpret in children. Frequently, children are so frightened that they are unable to cooperate. Crying and voluntary guarding challenge and frustrate the examiner. Despite these problems, detection of localized involuntary guarding and rebound tenderness is essential, since these are reliable signs of peritonitis. Palpation should include a separate evaluation of the anterior and posterior abdominal wall and intra-abdominal contents. Involuntary muscle spasm may result from injury to the abdominal wall or the underlying abdominal organs. Peritoneal irritation from intra-abdominal disease elicits more tenderness when the body wall is relaxed. Body wall injury is equally painful whether the muscle is relaxed or tightened.

The upper abdominal contents are protected by the bony thorax, making accurate examination of this area by palpation difficult. Remember that the chest wall in children is quite pliable and difficult to fracture and does not offer great protection to the underlying organs. Direct blows to the lower chest wall or compression injuries of the lower abdomen with upward transfer of destructive forces may rupture the liver, spleen, diaphragm, or stomach. Peritoneal lavage or radiographic studies may be needed to identify these injuries.

Light palpation is performed first, checking for areas of increased muscle tone. Deep palpation is used to check for masses, guarding, tenderness, and rebound pain. Rebound tenderness may be difficult to interpret because it elicits pain and results in voluntary guarding, crying, and loss of rapport. For these reasons, this physical sign should be checked last. Rebound tenderness can be reliably elicited by percussion, gentle shaking, and asking the child to cough rather than by rapid release of manual pressure. The voluntary muscle spasm associated with this sign may be misread as progression of the intra-abdominal injury. This point again stresses the need for repeated evaluations by the same observer.

Examination of Pelvis, Perineum, and Rectum

The last part of the abdominal examination is evaluation of the bony pelvis, perineum, and anorectum. A pelvic fracture is suspected if pain is elicited during compression of the wings of the ilium or symphysis pubis or with abduction of the legs. A radiograph of the abdomen and pelvis is much more accurate in establishing the diagnosis of a pelvic fracture. A pelvic fracture must not be overlooked because it may result in significant morbidity and occasional mortality. Massive pelvic and retroperitoneal hemorrhage may occur. First aid for this problem is application of the pneumatic anti-shock trousers and blood replacement. Embolization may be required for control of massive bleeding.[22–24]

Rupture of the bladder frequently accompanies pelvic fracture, although a distended bladder may rupture in the absence of a pelvic fracture. This injury is suspected when lower abdominal pain and tenderness are associated with hematuria and an inability to void. A cystogram is indicated. Urethral injuries are frequently overlooked whether they are caused by a pelvic fracture or straddle injury. The hallmarks of these injuries are perineal swelling, blood at meatus, floating prostate, distended bladder, and inability to void. Use of a urethral catheter is contraindicated, since it may convert an incomplete urethral tear into a complete urethral disruption. A urethrogram is indicated. Specific management of urinary injuries is discussed in Chapter 21. Besides causing rupture of the bladder and urethra, pelvic fracture may also penetrate the vagina and rectum, with the danger of mixed aerobic and anaerobic infection.

The rectal examination evaluates tone of the anal sphincter, position of the prostate, and integrity of the bony pelvis and bowel wall. Blood strongly suggests perforation of the colon or rectum. Proctoscopy and/or barium enema study may be indicated. The rectal examination may uncover significant abnormality as listed in Table 20–2.

Table 20–2. FINDINGS ON RECTAL EXAMINATION AND ASSOCIATED INJURIES

Physical Sign	Injury
Absent sphincter tone	Spinal cord injury
Floating prostate	Urethral disruption
Disrupted pelvic wall	Pelvic fracture
Disrupted bowel wall	Perforated rectum
Blood	Colon or rectal injury
Fullness	Retroperitoneal hemorrhage

Diagnostic Studies

Following the physical examination, appropriate laboratory studies are initiated (see Table 20–3). The number and types of studies are dictated by the clinical status of the patient and the mechanism of injury. In the seriously injured but hemodynamically stable child, minimal laboratory studies include type and crossmatch of blood, complete blood count, urinalysis, measurement of serum amylase, and chest radiograph in the upright position if possible. A lateral radiograph of the cervical spine is indicated in every child who is unconscious or who has head injury or trauma above the clavicles.

A urinalysis demonstrating hematuria demands radiologic assessment. This may include a urethrogram, cystogram, intravenous pyelogram (IVP), or the most accurate tool, contrast enhanced computerized tomography (CT). Approximately 10 to 15 per cent of severe renal injuries present with normal or minimally abnormal urinalysis. If the mechanism of injury or physical signs suggest renal trauma, a rapid infusion pyelogram is warranted. However, some clinicians prefer to observe patients with microscopic hematuria and no other findings suggestive of renal trauma.

Table 20–3. DIAGNOSTIC STUDIES USEFUL IN THE EVALUATION OF ABDOMINAL, PELVIC, AND RETROPERITONEAL TRAUMA

1. History, physical examination, vital signs
2. Hematologic tests
   a. Type and crossmatch
   b. Complete blood count
   c. Blood gases
   d. Prothrombin time, partial thromboplastin time, platelet count
   e. Serum amylase
3. Urinalysis
4. Peritoneal lavage
5. Radiologic tests
   a. Plain films
      1. Chest (upright, lateral)
      2. Abdomen (upright, supine, left lateral decubitus)
   b. Infusion pyelogram, cystogram, urethrogram
   c. Gastrografin (meglumine diatrizoate) upper gastrointestinal series
   d. Computerized axial tomography
   e. Ultrasonography
   f. Radionuclide scan
   g. Angiography

An elevated serum amylase level may indicate pancreatic injury, ischemic bowel, or more likely, transection of the proximal intestine.[25]

If major bleeding is suspected, a platelet count, prothrombin time, and partial thromboplastin time are obtained. Arterial blood gases are routinely drawn when there are signs of shock, hypoxemia, hypoventilation, or respiratory distress.

Although abdominal injuries may be evaluated by plain films of the abdomen in various positions, these studies are seldom helpful.[26] The specific radiologic signs of abdominal injury are presented in Chapter 8. An upper gastrointestinal (GI) series using water-soluble contrast medium is the most accurate test to diagnose injuries of the duodenum and proximal jejunum. Radionuclide scans accurately diagnose most splenic and liver injuries,[27, 28] but ultrasonography is not a very helpful tool.

Angiography is occasionally required to evaluate a child with a unilateral nonfunctioning kidney, hepatic or splenic hematoma, hemobilia, or retroperitoneal or pelvic hemorrhage. With crushing injuries to the pelvis associated with severe diastasis of the symphysis pubis, angiography is used for diagnosis and transcatheter control of bleeding. Remember, if angiography is required, it should be performed before other contrast studies.

The three most accurate diagnostic tools for assessing abdominal injuries are serial physical examination, peritoneal lavage, and CT with contrast enhancement. The importance of serial abdominal examinations is stressed in the section on management. CT is very helpful in children with blunt trauma.[29–31] The youngster must be hemodynamically stable because this study takes approximately 30 minutes. Indications include the following: equivocal physical findings, unexplained blood loss, need for extra-abdominal surgery, suspected retroperitoneal injury, positive or indeterminate peritoneal lavage, and contraindications to performing peritoneal lavage.

Peritoneal lavage is not performed as frequently in children as in adults primarily because it interferes with serial abdominal examinations and because post-traumatic intra-abdominal bleeding by itself is not necessarily an indication for surgery in pediatric patients.[32, 33] In children with isolated abdominal trauma, most pediatric surgeons consider clinical criteria (physical findings, deteriorating vital signs, and falling hematocrit) the main determinants of surgical intervention. Since lavage or paracentesis irritates the peritoneum for 24 to 48 hours, it is not performed early in this clinical setting.

In the setting of polytrauma, especially with head injury or bleeding from extra-abdominal sites, clinical criteria may not accurately reflect the degree of intra-abdominal bleeding. Under these circumstances, peritoneal lavage may be an appropriate diagnostic maneuver. Other indications for lavage are listed in Table 20–4. Lavage is helpful in children with altered pain response for obvious reasons. If equivocal abdominal findings or hemodynamic instability are due to occult bleeding or peritoneal contamination from bile[34] or intestinal content, peritoneal lavage may be helpful in establishing the need for surgical intervention. Negative information is also helpful, especially in children with serious head injury or those undergoing general anesthesia for repair of nonabdominal injuries. Finally, lavage is useful in reducing the number of negative laparotomies in children with stab wounds but no other evidence of peritonitis.[35, 36]

Before peritoneal lavage is performed, plain films of the abdomen in the upright, supine, and left lateral decubitus position are taken. If free air is detected, lavage is not necessary.

The site and technique for paracentesis and peritoneal lavage is depicted in Figures 20–2 and 20–3. A disposable Lazarus-Nelson kit* is used.[37] Figure 20–2 shows that the bladder in children is located in the lower abdomen and is subject to catheter trauma. Thus, the bladder should be empty and the needle inserted just below the umbilicus. After preparing the skin with povidine-iodine, a small stab wound is made in the skin to help facilitate insertion of the plastic dialysis catheter. The long 18-gauge needle is then advanced into the peritoneal cavity. The cavity is then aspirated, but usually no material returns to the syringe. A thin guide wire is threaded through the needle, and the needle is removed. Next, a plastic catheter with multiple side holes is advanced over the wire into the peritoneal cavity. After the guide wire is removed, 10 to 20 ml/kg body weight of 1.5 per cent dialysate or buffered Ringer's lactate solution is rapidly instilled into the abdomen. The buffered Ringer's lactate solution is made by adding one 50 ml ampule (50 mEq) of sodium bicarbonate to 1 L of Ringer's solution. These solutions have a physiologic pH and cause much less chemical peritonitis than acidic solutions, such as normal saline or straight Ringer's lactate solution. The abdomen is gently agitated for several minutes before dependent drainage is used to evacuate the lavage fluid. Occasionally, little, if any, fluid is retrieved because the side holes are small on the dialysis catheter. In this situation, the guide wire can

Table 20–4. INDICATIONS FOR PERITONEAL LAVAGE

1. Altered pain response
   a. Head injury
   b. Alcohol or drug ingestion
   c. Fractures of ribs, pelvis, lumbar spine
   d. Chest wall injury
2. Equivocal abdominal findings
3. Hemodynamic instability
4. General anesthesia
5. Stab wound with no peritonitis

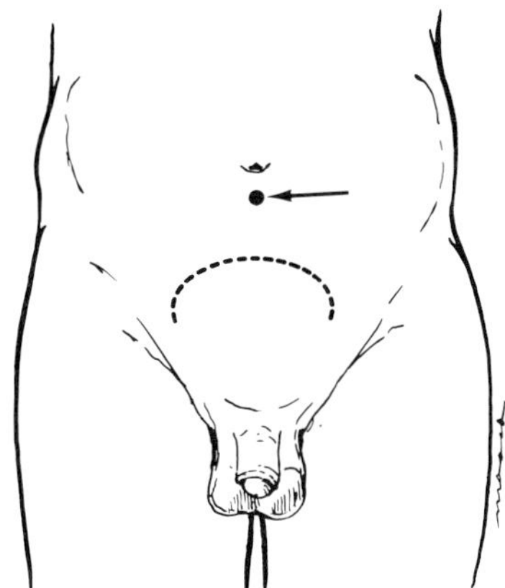

Figure 20–2. Our preferred site for paracentesis in children is below the umbilicus. Since the bladder is located intra-abdominally in young children, it should be empty before needle insertion is attempted.

*Lazarus-Nelson Peritoneal Lavage Tray. Kormed, Subsidiary of American Hospital Supply, Saint Paul, Minnesota 55120.

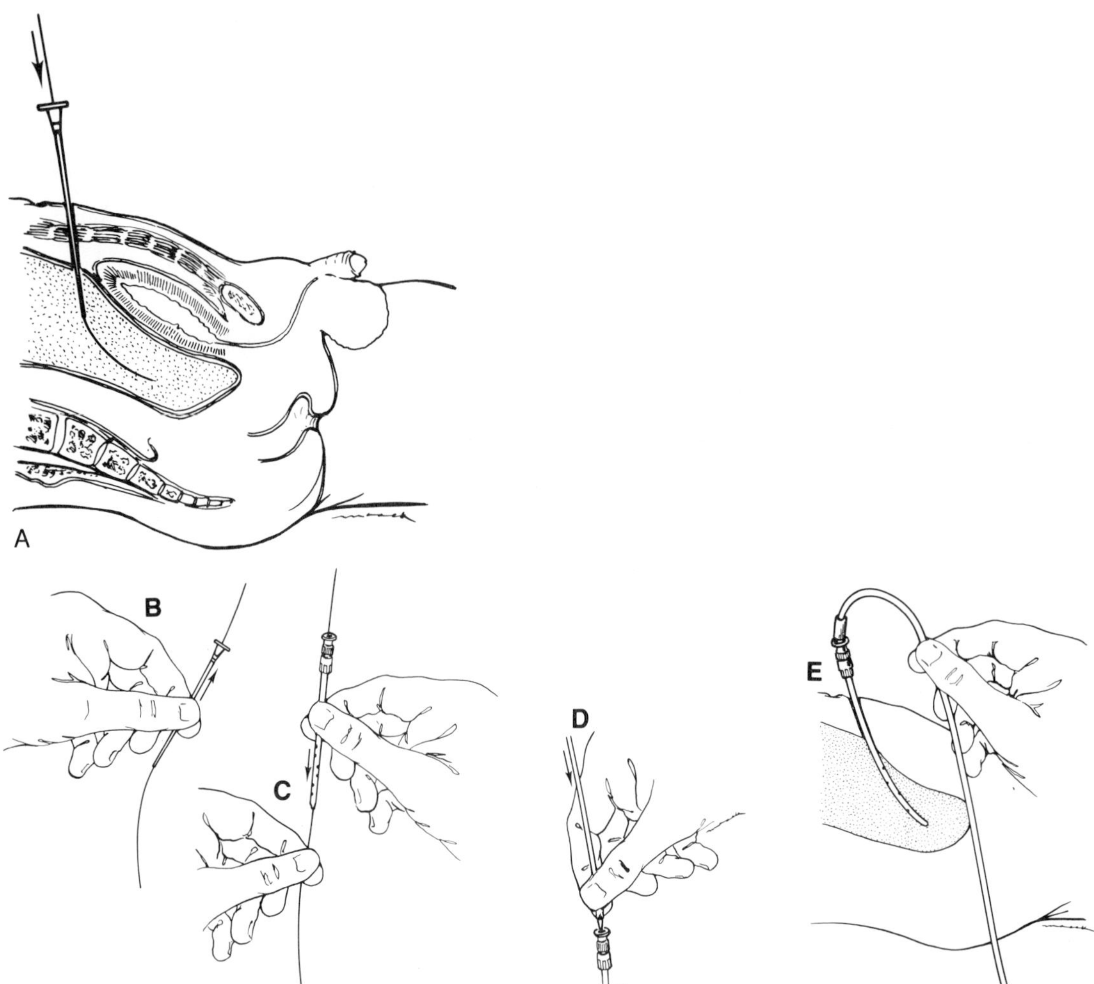

Figure 20–3. The Lazarus-Nelson technique for peritoneal lavage is demonstrated in the following figures. After the urinary bladder is emptied, the skin is sterilely prepped with povidine-iodine and infiltrated with local anesthesia. A puncture site is made with a No. 11 scalpel blade. The 18-gauge needle is advanced into the peritoneal cavity, and then a 9 French floppy guidewire is passed through the needle into the abdominal cavity (*A*). The needle is withdrawn leaving the guidewire in place (*B*). The Teflon multifenestrated catheter is advanced over the guidewire and twisted through the abdominal wall (*C*). After the guidewire is removed, the dialysis catheter is aspirated. If gross blood is not returned, then 10 to 20 ml per kg body weight of 1.5 per cent dialysis solution or buffered Ringer's lactate is instilled (*D*). Gentle agitation of the abdomen is performed for several minutes before gravity drainage is used to siphon off the peritoneal fluid (*E*).

be reinserted, and a 14 or 16 gauge angiocatheter advanced over the wire for more efficient removal of the fluid.

We do not recommend incision of the linea alba for peritoneal lavage in children because of the danger of evisceration. One child eviscerated a loop of small intestine and omentum through the small needle tract.

The findings of a diagnostic paracentesis or peritoneal lavage are as follows: A bloody or a blood-tinged aspirate that does not allow the reading of newsprint through the intravenous (IV) tubing is considered a positive lavage. Although these findings indicate intra-abdominal bleeding, the need for laparotomy is based on clinical grounds. Laboratory criteria for a diagnostic lavage are: (1) red blood cell count greater than 100,000/ml, (2) white blood cell count greater than 500/ml, and (3) the presence of bile, bacteria, or intestinal content. Rarely, lavage fluid will exit through a chest tube or urinary catheter, indicating a rupture of the diaphragm and bladder, respectively. The significance of elevated amylase levels in lavage fluid is unclear, but it may indicate a bowel perforation.

Peritoneal lavage is not reliable in detecting injury to the pancreas, duodenum, genitourinary tract, aorta, vena cava, or diaphragm. Complications of lavage include bleeding or hematoma of the abdominal wall or abdominal viscera. Transient peritonitis from the lavage fluid is common, but hollow visceral perforation is very uncommon with the technique herein described. Laceration of the bladder is avoided by evacuation prior to the procedure.

Table 20–5. ABDOMINAL INJURIES REQUIRING SURGERY

1. Massive or continued hemorrhage
2. Deterioration of vital signs
3. Gunshot wound of lower chest or abdomen
4. Stab wound of anterior abdominal wall with peritonitis
5. Gastrointestinal perforation
6. Bladder perforation
7. Evisceration

MANAGEMENT

The successful management of the child with abdominal injuries depends upon serial monitoring of vital signs, repeated physical examinations, and correct interpretation of selected diagnostic studies. Priority is often given to the establishment of a specific diagnosis, but the primary focus should be on determining the need for surgery and its appropriate timing. The key to determining when an acute surgical emergency is present is serial evaluation of the clinical course. With this in mind, children can be divided into two categories depending upon their specific therapeutic requirements: (1) the operative group and (2) the conservative or nonoperative group. Those children requiring immediate or urgent surgery are promptly resuscitated and minimal, if any, diagnostic tests are performed. The conservative group may also have potentially fatal problems, but the diagnosis may be masked for hours, days, or weeks.[38, 39] The nonoperative group is stable enough to undergo the selected diagnostic studies listed in Table 20–3.

Indications for Operation

The need for surgery may be immediate. Children in the operative group require surgery within the first few hours of injury because of a life-threatening or potentially life-threatening problem, as listed in Table 20–5. The decision for operation is largely dependent upon careful, repeated evaluation of the clinical course. Minimal laboratory or radiologic tests are required for identification of these children.

Massive Hemorrhage

The initial triage of the severely injured child may reveal that the major threat to life is profound shock from massive, uncontrolled intra-abdominal hemorrhage. The extremities are cool, mottled, and pale; the pulse is rapid and weak, and the blood pressure is below 70 mm Hg. These vital signs suggest a blood loss of more than 30 to 40 per cent of the estimated blood volume (85 ml/kg). The abdomen is distended or distending, and there are obvious signs of peritonitis.

Prehospital treatment consists of the use of pneumatic anti-shock trousers, with inflation of both leg and abdominal compartments. These trousers are not available for children less than 4 years of age, but elastic bandages can be wrapped around the lower extremities and abdomen to accomplish the same physiologic response of increasing total peripheral resistance. The trousers or elastic bandages also suppress intra-abdominal, retroperitoneal, and pelvic bleeding and help conserve body heat. The trousers usually cause transient venous dilation, which facilitates insertion of IV catheters. Two large-bore peripheral IV catheters are inserted, preferably in the upper extremities or neck. The saphenous vein at the ankle can be used for volume replacement with the anti-shock trousers, but an infusion pump is required. Fluid administered in the lower extremities may not reach the central circulation if major pelvic or retroperitoneal trauma is present. Boluses of Ringer's lactate solution (20 ml/kg) are rapidly infused.[40] Vital signs are checked before and after volume replacement to ascertain the physiologic response to therapy. If the child remains in shock after three boluses of crystalloid solution, then type-specific blood is transfused in boluses of 20 ml/kg. A nasogastric tube and urinary catheter are inserted.

A frequent error in the management of a patient with massive hemorrhage is ill-timed removal of the pneumatic trousers by inexperienced personnel. Under the circumstances described previously, the trousers should not be removed until the patient is in the operating room, anesthetized, and exploration is imminent. If the patient is stabilized, the abdominal compartment can be slowly deflated in stages while blood pressure and pulse are carefully monitored. A small amount of air is removed from the abdominal compartment, and then the valve is closed. A 5 to 10 mm Hg drop in blood pressure indicates the need for further volume expansion. The deflation process may take 30 minutes. Deflation should not be attempted before adequate resuscitation is administered. Premature removal may result in a precipitous fall in cardiac output because of redistribution of blood to the pelvis and lower extremities, rebleeding, and release of large quantities of lactic acid. The garment can be inflated for approximately 2 hours without detrimental effect.

If the child remains hemodynamically unstable, preparation is made for immediate exploration of the abdomen. Before this decision is finalized, a checklist of other causes of refractory shock is quickly reviewed (Table 20–6). Hypoxia demands immediate correction. Airway management and recognition and treatment of lethal chest injuries take precedence over abdominal injuries. Coexistant major cardiac and intra-abdominal injuries can be managed by a two-team approach, utilizing a median sternotomy and midline abdominal incision. Concommitant thoracic aortic transection or massive pulmonary hemorrhage and intra-abdominal hemorrhage present the surgeon with a major dilemma.[41] Fortunately, aortic transection is extremely uncommon in children, but if this diagnosis is a serious consideration, then aortography and expeditious repair would be required before other injuries are definitively treated.[42] It should also be noted that major intracranial and intra-abdominal operations are simultaneously performed to facilitate early management and brain preservation.

Table 20–6. ASSESSMENT OF REFRACTORY SHOCK

1. Airway patency and oxygenation
2. Ventilation
3. Lethal chest injuries
4. Unrecognized blood loss (hypovolemia)
5. Gastric dilation
6. Diabetic ketoacidosis
7. Hypoadrenalism
8. Neurogenic shock

It is not uncommon to underestimate the amount of blood or fluid lost following multiple injuries. Large volumes of blood may be sequestered in the pelvis, the thigh, the retroperitoneal space, or even the abdominal cavity and escape detection. Unrecognized blood loss may result in inadequate fluid resuscitation, unnecessary operation, persistence or worsening of the shock state, and establishment of a vicious cycle that may result in multiple organ failure. Unfortunately, the central nervous system suffers greatly from inadequate resuscitation.

Immediate celiotomy is required for control of bleeding in children who remain in hypovolemic shock after aggressive volume replacement, use of external compression trousers, and an unrevealing search for other causes of bleeding or refractory shock. A midline incision from xiphoid to symphysis pubis is employed, and most often the bleeding is from massive injury to the liver, spleen, hepatic veins, or vena cava. It is beyond the scope of this text to discuss the definitive surgical management of these complex injuries.[43–54]

Penetrating Injuries

Immediate operation is also indicated for conditions other than massive bleeding. Penetrating injuries account for 10 to 20 per cent of abdominal trauma in children,[12, 14] but many require immediate surgical care because of the high incidence of lacerations of the hollow viscera, solid organs, or major vessels. Penetrating trauma may lacerate a major vessel, requiring immediate celiotomy, as described in the previous section. Gunshot wounds of the lower chest and abdomen are associated with significant intra-abdominal injury in over 90 per cent of patients. The safest policy is to explore all these children.

Stab wounds of the anterior abdominal wall or chest wall below the sixth rib are explored when associated with signs of peritoneal irritation.[15, 16, 43] This policy results in a negative laparotomy rate of approximately 20 per cent. The major difficulty in this group of children is distinguishing those stab wounds involving only the abdominal wall from those with fascial penetration.[16, 17] Unlike adults, most children will not cooperate with exploration of the wound under local anesthesia. If signs of peritoneal irritation are present, it is safest to explore the abdomen rather than overlook a subtle, but potentially dangerous injury. The morbidity and mortality associated with a negative finding at laparotomy is negligible.[55] Another option is to perform peritoneal lavage.[35, 36] If this study is negative, observation of the clinical course can be continued. Stab wounds of the flank and lateral abdominal wall are initially treated conservatively. The development of localized peritonitis, fever, and leukocytosis may indicate perforation of the retroperitoneal colon. Exploration is again the safest option.[79] These children also require an infusion pyelogram and other radiologic examinations if urologic injury is possible. Obviously, penetrating wounds resulting in pneumoperitoneum or evisceration require expeditious operation.

Blunt Injuries

Blunt trauma accounts for the vast majority of abdominal injuries in children, but the indications for operation are far more subtle than those for penetrating trauma. Although the injury is present upon arrival at the hospital, clinical manifestations may not become evident for several hours. Despite these difficulties, the goal of the clinician is to recognize a surgical emergency as soon as possible. Basically this means recognition of continued intra-abdominal bleeding, progressive peritonitis, or deterioration of vital signs. Perforation of a hollow viscus should be recognized and repaired within the "golden period." This is the time before bacterial contamination becomes bacterial invasion, usually within the first 8 hours following perforation. Waiting longer increases the risk of septic complications.

Blunt trauma commonly results in three types of injuries to the abdominal viscera requiring surgical repair: (1) solid organ injury, (2) perforation of the small intestine, and (3) rupture of the bladder.

The most commonly injured organs are solid organs. Since the primary manifestation of this injury is bleeding, serial evaluation for continued hemorrhage is essential for diagnosis. This includes physical examination, monitoring of vital signs, urine output, peripheral perfusion, sensorium, and abdominal girth, and serial hematocrit determinations. Ordinarily, blood is very irritating to the peritoneum, resulting in involuntary guarding, abdominal distention, and ileus. Although uncommon, intraperitoneal bleeding sometimes may not cause significant peritonitis or ileus. The abdomen remains soft despite the presence of a large volume of blood. Often this problem accompanies head trauma with unconsciousness.

In children with isolated blunt abdominal trauma, continued intra-abdominal bleeding is usually easy to recognize on clinical grounds. Initially, most children receive nonoperative therapy, but if they become hemodynamically unstable, or if bleeding continues, exploratory lapartomy is required. In children with polytrauma, deterioration in clinical criteria does not necessarily signal continued abdominal bleeding. These children are difficult to evaluate.[38, 56] Early in their assessment they require peritoneal lavage or tomography CT (or both). Celiotomy is performed earlier in the group with multiple trauma because of the likelihood of identifying multiple abdominal injuries, and these children cannot afford delays in therapy.

The spleen is the most commonly injured solid organ, followed by the liver.[47, 59] Currently, most pediatric surgeons initially treat intra-abdominal bleeding by nonsurgical therapy. This approach is based on the following assumptions: (1) most injuries to solid organs heal spontaneously, (2) risk of surgery outweighs risk of conservative therapy, and (3) risk of postsplenectomy sepsis is minimized. The cost of this approach is considerable because most children require intensive care observation, blood transfusions, serial body scanning,[58] and lengthy hospitalization. Postsplenectomy sepsis is rare following post-traumatic asplenia.[59] However, this complication is so feared that it has caused the pendulum of therapy to swing far in favor of nonoperative management.[60, 61]

I favor a conservative approach in children with isolated splenic trauma or children with polytrauma who are easily resuscitated and remain stable.[62–64] I favor exploratory laparotomy in children with any evidence of continued intraperitoneal bleeding, especially that which occurs within the first few hours of injury or in the setting of possible multisystem injury.[65] Splenic repair or partial splenectomy are accomplished easily,[66, 67] associated injuries are repaired,[68] and the risk for further bleeding is virtually eliminated. Whenever possible, 50 per cent of the splenic mass is preserved for immunologic function. It is very comforting to know that the bleeding sites have been securely controlled by surgical intervention. When a splenectomy is required, children under 6 years of age are placed on penicillin prophylaxis. Regardless of age, all children with splenectomy receive pneumococcal vaccine, and parents are given instructions regarding the need for prompt medical evaluation should sepsis become a possibility.

Only a minority of liver injuries require definitive surgical care. The indications for operation are continued blood loss or deterioration in vital signs.

Perforation of the small intestine may result from compression of this structure against the spine by a narrow, rigid object, such as a handlebar, fence post, broom handle, fist, helmet, and so on. Seat belts can cause this injury, but since they are infrequently worn by children, this is an uncommon etiology. Physical findings may be minimal, and plain films of the abdomen may be normal despite a gaping hole in the intestine. Sometimes ileus, spasm of the bowel proximal to the injury, the retroperitoneal location of the injury, or partial sealing of the perforation by adjacent structures minimizes peritoneal soilage, thus accounting for the paucity of signs. In this clinical setting, a knowledge of the mechanism of injury may be more indicative of a serious injury than the physical findings.[29] Abdominal films are obtained to detect intraperitoneal air or retroperitoneal emphysema. These studies are usually normal, and a upper gastrointestinal series using water soluble contrast medium is required to establish the diagnosis. Surprisingly, the proximal jejunum is perforated more frequently than the duodenum in its fixed retroperitoneal location. Bowel perforation demands prompt exploration. Débridement and two-layer closure usually suffice for these injuries, but occasionally a segmental resection and anastamosis are required. Duodenal injuries require more extensive repair and diversion.[69, 70]

The upper GI series is also helpful in demonstrating the "coiled spring" sign of intramural hematomas of the proximal small bowel.[71, 72] Intramural hematomas usually resolve spontaneously. Therapy consists of prolonged nasogastric decompression and IV alimentation. Surgery is indicated for persistent obstruction, continued bleeding, or increasing amylase levels.

Injuries to the pancreaticoduodenal complex are infrequent because of protected position of these organs in the upper abdomen. The child may complain of severe upper abdominal and back pain with or without clear indications of peritonitis. A combination of peritoneal lavage and contrast enhanced CT are usually required for diagnosis. Injury to this area is usually devastating because of extensive hemorrhage and tissue damage from pancreatic and biliary secretions. Review articles discussing the definite operative management of duodenal and pancreatic injuries are listed in the references.[73–78]

Finally, rupture of the bladder is not difficult to diagnose, but it is frequently overlooked. Fifteen to twenty per cent of pelvic fractures have a concomitant bladder injury, but a distended bladder may tear without a pelvic fracture. Clinical findings are lower abdominal mass and tenderness, pelvic fracture, inability to void, and hematuria. If an associated urethral injury is suspected, a urethrogram should proceed the cystogram. These injuries are discussed more fully in Chapter 21.

Conservative Therapy

Most children with blunt abdominal trauma, and some with penetrating trauma, are managed nonoperatively. Often the initial evaluation is confusing because the child is apprehensive and crying. During hospital observation, the child is given IV fluids and the GI tract is decompressed with a nasogastric tube. Sedation and analgesics are avoided. The importance of serial evaluation of the clinical course has already been stressed in the section on surgical therapy.

Post-traumatic intra-abdominal bleeding by itself is not necessarily an indication for surgery in pediatric patients.[62, 64, 65] This philosophy and its problems have already been discussed. Weekly radionuclide scans or CT is used to document healing of splenic and liver trauma.[58, 63] Once the ileus is resolved, oral feedings are administered. Most children require 7 days of hospitalization and 6 weeks of restricted physical activity. Rebleeding is uncommon.

Children who do not gradually improve with nonoperative therapy may have an undiagnosed retroperitoneal injury or continued bleeding.[38, 39] Diagnostic body imaging is mandatory, and celiotomy may be required.[26–30]

REFERENCES

1. Haller JA: Pediatric trauma: The no. 1 killer of children. JAMA 249:47, 1983.

2. Karwacki JJ Jr, Baker SP: Children in motor vehicles: Never too young to die. JAMA 242:2848, 1979.
3. Trunkey DD: Overview of trauma. Surg Clin North Am 62:3, 1982.
4. Touloukian RJ: Abdominal trauma in childhood. Surg Gynecol Obstet 127:561, 1968.
5. Matlak ME, Johnson DG, Walker ML, et al.: Initial Management of the Injured Child. Salt Lake City, Zondervan Press, 1980.
6. Seelig JM, Becker DP, Miller JD, et al.: Traumatic acute subdural hematoma. N Engl J Med 304:1511, 1981.
7. Randolph JG, Ravitch MM, et al.: The Injured Child, Surgical Management. Chicago, Year Book Medical Publishers, 1979.
8. Touloukian RJ; Pediatric Trauma. New York, John Wiley and Sons, 1978.
9. Walt AJ: Early Care of the Injured Patient. Philadelphia, WB Saunders Company, 1982.
10. Philippart AI: Blunt abdominal trauma in childhood. Surg Clin North Am 57:151, 1977.
11. Tank E, Eraklis AJ, Gross RE; Blunt abdominal trauma in infancy and childhood. J Trauma 8:439, 1968.
12. Barlow B, Niemirska M, Gandhi RP: Ten years' experience with pediatric gunshot wounds. J Pediatr Surg 17:927, 1982.
13. Freeark RJ; Penetrating wounds of the abdomen. N Engl J Med 291:185, 1974.
14. Sinclair MC, Moore TC, Asch MJ: Penetrating abdominal injuries in children and adolescents. Am Surg 41:342, 1975.
15. Thompson JS, Moore EE, Van Duzer-Moore S, et al.: The evolution of abdominal stab wound management. J Trauma 20:478, 1980.
16. Wilder JR, Kudchadkar A: Stab wounds of the abdomen: Observe or explore? JAMA 243:2503, 1980.
17. Nance FC, Wennar MH, Johnson LW, et al.: Surgical judgment in the management of penetrating wounds of the abdomen: Experience with 2212 patients. Ann Surg 179:639, 1974.
18. Committee on Trauma, American College of Surgeons: Advanced Trauma Life Support Course. Chicago, American College of Surgeons, 1981.
19. Foley RW, Harris LS, Pilcher DB: Abdominal injuries in automobile accidents: Review of care of fatally injured patients. J Trauma 17:611, 1977.
20. Polk HC, Flint LM: Intra-abdominal injuries in polytrauma. World J Surg 7:56, 1983.
21. Van Wagoner FH: Died in hospital: A three-year study of deaths following trauma. J Trauma 1:401, 1961.
22. Flint LM, Brown A, Richardson JD, Polk HC: Definitive control of bleeding from severe pelvic fractures. Ann Surg 189:709, 1979.
23. Margolies MN, Ring EJ, Waltman AC, et al.: Arteriography and the management of hemorrhage from pelvic fractures. N Engl J Med 287:317, 1972.
24. Reichard SA, Helikson MA, Shorter N, et al.: Pelvic fractures in children. Review of 120 patients with a new look at general management. J Pediatr Surg 15:727, 1980.
25. Olsen WR: Serum amylase in blunt abdominal trauma. J Trauma 13:200, 1973.
26. Franken EA, Jr, Smith JA: Roentgenographic evaluation of infant and childhood trauma. Pediatr Clin North 22:303, 1975.
27. Lutzker LG, Chun KJ: Radionuclide imaging in the nonsurgical treatment of liver and spleen trauma. J Trauma 21:382, 1981.
28. McConnell BJ, McConnell RW, Guiberteau, MJ: Radionuclide imaging in blunt trauma. Radiol Clin North 19:37, 1981.
29. Federle MP: Abdominal trauma: The role and impact of computed tomography. Invest Radio 16:260, 1981.
30. Karp MP, Cooney DR, Berger PE, et al.: Role of computed tomography in the evaluation of blunt abdominal trauma in children. J Pediatr Surg 16:316, 1981.
31. Kuhn JP, Berger PE: Computed tomography in the evaluation of blunt abdominal trauma in children. Radiol Clin North 19:503, 1981.
32. Fischer RP, Beverlin BC, Engrav LH, et al.: Diagnostic peritoneal lavage: Fourteen years and 2,586 patients later. Am J Surg 136:701, 1978.
33. Powell DC, Bivins BA, Bell RM: Diagnostic peritoneal lavage. Surg Gynecol Obstet 155:257, 1982.
34. Yadav K, Pathak IC: Biliary peritonitis following blunt abdominal trauma in children. Am Gastroenterol 72:444, 1979.
35. Galbraith TA, Oreskovich MR, Heimbach DM: Role of peritoneal lavage in the management of stab wounds of the abdomen. Am J Surg 140:59, 1980.
36. Thompson JS, Moore EE: Peritoneal lavage in the evaluation of penetrating abdominal trauma. Surg Gynecol Obstet 153:861, 1981.
37. Lazarus HM, Nelson JA: A technique for peritoneal lavage without risk or complications. Surg Gynecol Obstet 149:889, 1979.
38. Ben-Menachem Y, Fisher RG, Ward RE: Are "occult" intra-abdominal and extraperitoneal injuries really occult? Radiol Clin North 19:125, 1981.
39. Flint LM, McCog M, Richardson JD, Polk HC Jr: Duodenal injury: Analysis of common misconceptions in diagnosis and treatment. Ann Surg 191:697, 1980.
40. Grosfeld JL: Symposium on childhood trauma. Pediatr Clin North Am 22:269, 1975.
41. Borman KR, Aurbakken CM, Weigelt JA: Treatment priorities in combined blunt abdominal and aortic trauma. Am J Surg 144:728, 1982.
42. Bodai BI, Smith JP, Ward RE, et al.: Emergency thoracotomy in the management of trauma: A review. JAMA 249:1891, 1983.
43. Blaisdell FN, Trunkey DD: Trauma management. Volume 1. Abdominal Trauma. New York, Thieme-Stratton, 1982.
44. Coln D, Crighton J, Schorn L: Successful management of hepatic vein injury from blunt trauma in children. Am J Surg 140:858, 1980.
45. Dickerman RM, Dunn EL: Splenic, pancreatic, and hepatic injuries. Surg Clin North 61:3, 1981.
46. Geis WP, Schulz, KA, Giacchino JL, Freeark RJ: Fate of unruptured intrahepatic hematomas. Surgery 90:689, 1981.
47. Hendren WH, Kim SH: Trauma of the spleen and liver in children. Pediatr Clin North Am 22:349, 1975.
48. Madding GF, Kennedy PA: Trauma to the liver. 2nd ed. Philadelphia, WB Saunders Company, 1971.
49. Madding GF, Lim RC, Kennedy PA: Hepatic and vena caval injuries. Surg Clin North 57:275, 1977.
50. Sandblom P: Hemobilia. Surg Clin North Am 53:1191, 1973.
51. Stone HH, Ansley JD: Management of liver trauma in children. J Pediatr Surg 12:3, 1977.
52. Suson EM, Klotz D, Kottmeier PK: Liver trauma in children. J Pediatr Surg 10:411, 1975.
53. Trunkey DD, Shires GT, McClelland R: Management of liver trauma in 811 consecutive patients. Ann Surg 179:722, 1974.

54. Walt AJ: The mythology of hepatic trauma—or Babel revisited. Am J Surg 135:12, 1978.
55. Petersen SR, Sheldon GF: Morbidity of a negative finding at laparotomy in abdominal trauma. Surg Gynecol Obstet 148:23, 1979.
56. Feins NR: Multiple trauma. Pediatr Clin North Am 26:759, 1979.
57. Oakes DD: Splenic trauma. Curr Prob Surg 6:346, 1981.
58. Fischer KC, Eraklis A, Rossello P, Treves S: Scintigraphy in the follow-up of pediatric splenic trauma treated without surgery. J Nucl Med 19:3, 1978.
59. Condon RE: Editorial. Post-splenectomy sepsis in traumatized adults. J Trauma 22:169, 1982.
60. Leonard AS, Giebink GS, Baesl TJ, Krivit W: The overwhelming post-splenectomy sepsis problem. World J Surg 4:423, 1980.
61. Sherman R: Perspectives in management of trauma to the spleen: 1979 Presidential Address, American Association for the Surgery of Trauma. J Trauma 20:1, 1980.
62. Douglas GJ, Simpson JS: The conservative management of splenic trauma. J Pediatr Surg 6:565, 1971.
63. Howman-Giles R, Gilday DL, Venogopal S, et al.: Splenic trauma—Non-operative management and long-term follow-up by scintiscan. J Pediatr Surg 13:121, 1978.
64. King DR, Lobe TE, Haase GM, Boles, ET: Selective management of injured spleen. Surgery 90:677, 1981.
65. Wesson DE, Filler RM, Ein SB, et al.: Ruptured spleen—when to operate? J Pediatr Surg 16:324, 1981.
66. Morgenstern L, Shapiro SJ: Techniques of splenic conservation. Arch Surg 114:449, 1979.
67. Pachter HL, Hofstetter SR, Spencer FC: Evolving concepts in splenic surgery: Splenorrhaphy versus splenectomy and postsplenectomy drainage: Experience in 105 patients. Ann Surg 194:262, 1981.
68. Traub AC, Perry JF: Injuries associated with splenic trauma. J Trauma 21:840, 1981.
69. Berne CJ, Donovan AJ, White EJ, Yellin AE: Duodenal "diverticulization" for duodenal and pancreatic injury. Am J Surg 127:503, 1974.
70. Snyder WH, Weigelt JA, Watkins WL, Bietz DS: Surgical management of duodenal trauma. Arch Surg 115:422, 1980.
71. Fullen WD, Selle JG, Whitely DH, et al.: Intramural duodenal hematoma. Ann Surg 179:549, 1974.
72. Stewart DR, Byrd CL, Schuster SR: Intramural hemaltomas of the alimentary tract in children. Surgery 68:550, 1970.
73. Graham JM, Pokorny WJ, Mattox KL, Jordan GL, Jr: Surgical management of acute pancreatic injuries in children. J Pediatr Surg 13:693, 1978.
74. Grosfeld JL, Cooney DR: Pancreatic and gastrointestinal trauma in children. Pediatr Clin North Am 22:365, 1975.
75. Heitsch RC, Knutson CO, Fulton RL, Jones CE: Delineation of critical factors in the treatment of pancreatic trauma. Surgery 80:523, 1976.
76. Northrup WF III, Simmons RL: Pancreatic trauma: A review. Surgery 71:27, 1972.
77. Otherson HB, Moore FT, Boles ET, Jr: Traumatic Pancreatitis and pseudocyst in childhood. J Trauma 8:535, 1968.
78. Stone HH: Pancreatic and duodenal trauma in children. J Pediatr Surg 7:670, 1972.
79. Lo Cicero J, Tajima T, Drapanas T: A half-century of experience in the management of colon injuries: Changing concepts. J Trauma 15:575, 1975.

CHAPTER

21 Genitourinary Injuries in Children

RICHARD G. MIDDLETON
MICHAEL E. MATLAK
GEORGE W. NIXON
THOM A. MAYER

Genitourinary injuries occur quite frequently in children and should be considered whenever there is trauma to the flank, abdomen, lower chest, pelvis, or perineal regions. They are especially frequent with blunt multisystem trauma, which has a higher incidence than penetrating injury in the pediatric age group. Recently, the diagnostic work-up and appropriate therapeutic intervention for genitourinary injuries have undergone important changes. Indeed, significant controversy surrounds the initial evaluation of genitourinary trauma in relation to the appropriate use of intravenous pyelography and, more recently, computed tomographic (CT) scan for patients with microscopic hematuria. Further, operative versus conservative therapy of certain renal injuries has also been greatly debated.

Because genitourinary injuries are quite common and frequently present to the practicing pediatrician or emergency physician, the significant points of each of these controversies will be presented, both with regard to diagnosis and therapy. In most cases, emergency physicians and pediatricians will be well served by consulting with appropriate urologic, pediatric, or general surgeons, as well as radiologists concerning their preferences with regard to these controversies.

RENAL TRAUMA

Injury to the kidney accounts for approximately 5 per cent of all childhood trauma.[1] The kidney is more vulnerable to injury in the pediatric age group because perinephric fat is scanty, the overlying musculature and skeletal structures are less well developed, and the kidney is relatively larger in the child as compared with the adult.

Approximately 10 per cent of children who sustain renal injuries have a pre-existing renal abnormality.[2] Hydronephrosis is the most common predisposing abnormality, although an ectopic location and horseshoe kidney are other conditions in which there is a predilection for renal injury. Relatively minor trauma may result in major renal damage when there is pre-existing hydronephrosis.

The majority of children with isolated renal trauma recover full function without requiring operation. With timely application of appropriate diagnostic testing, including computed tomography, the precise extent of genitourinary injury can usually be delineated.[3-5] Because of this, emergency exploratory surgery is rarely needed. However, the frequency of injury, the subtlety with which it may present, and the fact that early diagnosis may prevent subsequent nephrectomy require that the diagnosis of renal trauma should be considered in all children with significant trauma. Familiarity with the types of injury, clinical presentation, diagnostic work-up, and appropriate therapeutic intervention are essential to physicians caring for pediatric trauma victims.

Cause

Renal injury is much more commonly caused by blunt trauma than by penetrating injury in the pediatric age group. Falls, motor vehicle accidents, auto–pedestrian collisions, sport injuries, and child abuse are the most common mechanisms of injury.[6-7] However, any form of high-energy trauma may result in renal injury. Gunshot and stab wounds occasionally occur, usually in urban settings.[8] In general, males sustain renal trauma more commonly than females, probably owing to the fact that they engage in more strenuous play and athletic activities.[9] With changing societal roles, the sex ratio of renal injury may change.

Approximately 40 per cent of patients sustaining renal injuries have additional injured body systems. The most frequently injured body areas are the head, spleen, liver, and long bones.[10] Twenty-five per cent of patients with injuries to the left kidney also have splenic trauma. Liver injuries associated with right renal trauma are less common but are equally as serious.

Diagnosis

The diagnostic work-up of an injured child with possible renal injury is intended to adequately evaluate the following factors: (1) the overall condition of the child; (2) the type, location, and extent of injury; and (3) the status of the contralateral kidney. The overall status of the child is the most important factor. Other injuries, such as a ruptured liver or intracranial injury, may be life threatening and require immediate therapy, which occasionally results in a delay in the diagnosis and treatment of renal injuries. Knowledge of the type, location, and extent of renal injury is necessary to determine appropriate therapy. The status of the contralateral kidney is important in numerous management decisions. For example, congenital absence of a kidney greatly affects decisions regarding salvage of the opposite kidney when severe injury is present.

History

Renal injury should be suspected in any patient with a history or physical evidence

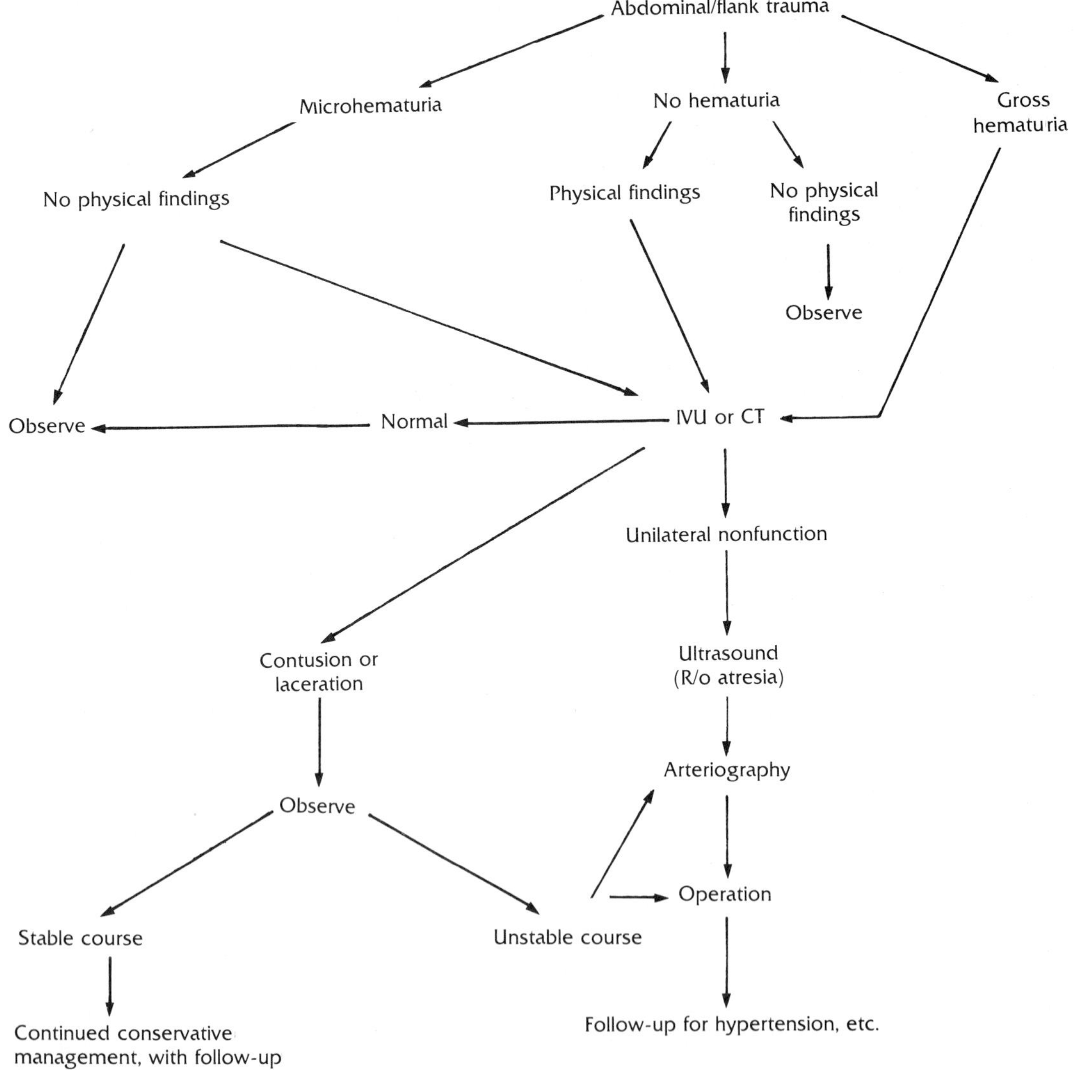

Figure 21–1. Management of renal trauma.

of trauma to the flank, back, lower chest, or abdomen (Fig. 21–1). Further, any patient with a significant head injury should be evaluated for the possibility of renal and abdominal injury. Details of the method of injury should be elicited from the patient, bystanders, and family.

Physical Examination

The signs and symptoms of renal trauma vary depending upon the type and extent of renal injury, presence of associated injuries, and the general condition of the child (Table 21–1). Hematuria and flank or abdominal pain and tenderness are usually present. Superficial abrasions, contusion, or ecchymoses may be present but are seldom the only signs of renal injury. Abdominal rigidity or a palpable flank mass may be present. Although signs and symptoms of blood loss may occasionally occur, children rarely exsanguinate from renal injuries, and patients who present with profound shock usually have associated injuries.[11] Paralytic ileus may accompany renal injuries if intraperitoneal damage is also present.[12]

Urinalysis

Virtually every child who suffers significant trauma should have urinalysis performed *early* in the evaluation. Hematuria is the hallmark of renal trauma and occurs in 80 to 90 per cent of patients with kidney injury,[13-15] although the degree of hematuria does not correlate with the severity of the injury. For example, it is not infrequent that hematuria will be absent in a patient with complete occlusion or disruption of the renal artery.[16-18] The absence of hematuria, therefore, does not exclude renal injury if other findings strongly suggest its possibility. Thus, if the history or physical examination suggests renal injury, further diagnostic work-up is indicated, even if the urinalysis is normal. It is most important that all patients with suspected renal injury be fully evaluated within 3 to 4 hours.

Table 21–1. PHYSICAL SIGNS OF GENITOURINARY INJURY

Renal
Hematuria
Flank or abdominal pain
Flank abrasion, contusion, or ecchymosis
Flank mass
Previous renal abnormality
Bladder
Hematuria
Abdominal pain
Inability to void
Pelvic fracture
Renal injury
Ureteral
Deceleration injury with hyperextension
Flank pain
Flank mass
Penetrating injuries
Hematuria
Urethral
Blood at urethra
Inability to void
Lower abdominal/pelvic pain
Scrotal hematoma/perineal swelling
High-riding prostate
Hematuria

Radiographic Studies

A plain radiograph of the abdomen may show scoliosis with the curve concave toward the injured side, fragments of penetrating foreign bodies, or associated bony fractures. Fractures of ribs or the transverse processes of thoracolumbar vertebrae are much less common in children with renal trauma as compared with adults because of increased resiliency of their bony structures. Fractures of the pelvic bones occasionally occur. Because of the small amount of retroperitoneal fat in children, failure to clearly visualize the renal and psoas margins is a much less reliable radiographic sign than in adults.

The role of radiologic evaluation of renal trauma is currently a subject of great controversy. In the past, intravenous urography was usually recommended in all patients with trauma when *any* degree of hematuria was present.[19] The major arguments supporting this approach have been the avoidance of misdiagnosing renal pedicle injury and the efficacy of surgical therapy for moderate renal injury identified by radiographic means.[20, 21] However, other urologists argue that while renal pedicle injury may occur in the absence of hematuria, children with this injury invariably show additional physical signs and symptoms suggestive of renal artery occlusion. In addition, many surgeons have argued that conservative therapy results in a lower overall nephrectomy rate for moderate renal injury.[22, 23] Thus, while pyelography clearly demonstrates the varying types of renal injury, the findings on excretory urography often do not alter the clinical management of these patients. Rather than expose all children with renal trauma to the risk of a potentially serious reaction to contrast medium, unnecessary radiation exposure and expense, and the possibility of delay in diagnosis of other injuries, many authorities recommend that intravenous urography be utilized only in children with physical findings of renal injury, an unstable clinical course with evidence of significant blood loss, or gross hematuria, or when renal artery injury is suspected.[22-26] Nonetheless, there are many urologists and general surgeons who still prefer to perform intravenous pyelography in all patients with trauma and microscopic hematuria.[19-21]

Computed tomography (CT) has become more widely utilized,[27] and many now feel that it is the procedure of choice in the evaluation of abdominal and renal trauma. Its major benefit is that all organs in the upper abdominal and retroperitoneal areas are evaluated simultaneously. This study requires the intravenous administration of radiographic contrast media to evaluate renal function. Contrast enhancement also provides for the demonstration of parenchymal injuries of kidneys, liver, and spleen as well as urinary extravasation.

The most significant justification for either intravenous urography or CT examination in the evaluation of renal trauma is to screen for renal artery occlusion. Therefore, if renal pedicle injury is suspected and either IVP or CT is indicated, it should be done as soon as possible after the patient arrives at the emergency department. Renal artery occlusion requires immediate recognition and operation within 4 to 6 hours if renal salvage is to be achieved. Aortography and renal angiography have been advocated to more clearly define the nature and extent of renal contusion, renal laceration, and areas of hematoma. Nonetheless, use of this procedure should be limited to cases in which the results will specifically alter management. Immediate arteriography is indicated to evaluate for renal artery occlusion when there is unilateral nonfunction on intravenous urography or CT. Many surgeons also think this study is indicated in cases in which continued bleeding necessitates operative intervention. In these cases, arteriography defines the renal artery anatomy for the operating surgeon. While radionuclide scanning and ultrasonography are utilized in a few institutions to evaluate renal trauma, intravenous urography or CT examination is usually more helpful in the initial assessment of genitourinary injuries.

Children with suspected renal trauma should be observed carefully. If additional findings of renal injury develop, hematuria progresses, or an unstable clinical course with evidence of blood loss ensues, further radiographic evaluation may be required. In order to provide consistent care to pediatric trauma victims, emergency physicians and pediatricians are encouraged to consult urologists or pediatric surgeons regarding their preferences with regard to the appropriate diagnostic work-up of patients with hematuria and the possibility of genitourinary disease. Figure 21–1 summarizes one approach to the diagnostic work-up of renal injuries.

Conservative Versus Surgical Therapy

As indicated previously, there is a significant controversy between surgeons who advocate early operative intervention for moderate to severe renal injuries and those who propose that conservative therapy is preferable.* Regardless of the approach to care of genitourinary injuries, all urologists and general surgeons agree that the patient must be aggressively resuscitated and treated for all life-threatening injuries, including shock, cardiopulmonary compromise, and exsanguinating hemorrhage. Each of these entities compromises renal function significantly and must be treated before definitive diagnosis and therapy of genitourinary problems are undertaken.

Surgeons who advocate early operative intervention for renal injuries point out that fewer delayed complications and better salvage rate of functioning renal tissue are accomplished through such intervention.[28, 30] Further, they argue that the majority of *serious* complications arise from conservative therapy. However, surgeons favoring conservative therapy for intermediate renal injuries note that nephrectomy rates in patients treated with early surgical intervention are nearly 50 per cent versus only 1 to 6 per cent in conservatively treated patients.[31-34] Conservative treatment of injuries, such as extravasation of sterile urine has not caused significant morbidity, and these injuries usually resolve spontaneously within a few days.[31-34] However, there are definite indications for

---

*Although there is a consensus that minor renal injuries (contusions, minor lacerations) are best managed conservatively, the divergence of opinion relates primarily to more severe injuries (urinary extravasation, ruptured kidney, and so on).

surgery, including: (1) renal arterial obstruction, indicating either avulsion of the renal pedicle or thrombosis of the artery; (2) a rapidly expanding flank mass; (3) a severely shattered, nonfunctioning kidney demonstrated on IV pyelography or CT scan; (4) lacerations of the renal pelvis that include the ureter; (5) avulsion of major renal segments that are nonfunctional; and (6) development of septic complications.

Again, the emergency physician or pediatrician will be well served by consultation with the appropriate urologic, pediatric, or general surgeon who will be responsible for the long-term care of the patient, inasmuch as controversy concerning conservative versus surgical therapy continues.

CLASSIFICATION OF RENAL INJURIES

Understanding the types of renal injuries children may sustain is helpful in understanding the clinical findings, diagnostic work-up, and rational management of such patients. Numerous classifications have been used. A simplified classification consisting of renal contusion, renal laceration of varying forms, and renal vascular injury is utilized in this chapter (Fig. 21–2).

Renal Contusion

Renal contusion is by far the most common form of renal injury, but it is also the least serious. This injury consists of localized hemorrhage into the renal parenchyma with sparing of the capsule, collecting structures, and renal blood vessels. Renal contusion results in swelling of the renal parenchyma and, since the capsule is intact, the blood vessels and collecting system are compressed, resulting in decreased urine flow from the affected kidney. Red blood cells are released into the urine, but the degree of hematuria varies depending upon the degree of diminished urine output by the affected kidney. Thus, more severe contusions may present with microscopic hematuria, while minor injuries may present with gross hematuria. Because swelling is limited by the capsule, a flank mass does not occur with simple contusion, although flank pain is often present.[35] Since the vasculature and collecting system are intact, excretion is usually sufficient for visualization on intravenous urography. In cases of mild renal contusion, the intravenous urogram will be normal. More serious contusions will demonstrate delayed excretion, incomplete visualization of collecting structures, enlargement of the kidney, or generalized compression of the collecting structures in the region of the contusion (Fig. 21–3).

This condition does not require either extended hospitalization or operative intervention. Management consists of symptomatic care and observation. Gross or microscopic hematuria may persist for up to 1 month, but there is no need for prolonged restricted activity. The major architecture of the kidney remains intact, healing proceeds rapidly with minimal scarring, and significant delayed sequelae are rare.[36, 37]

Renal Laceration

Renal lacerations are parenchymal disruptions that occur in varying degrees. There may be disruption of the pyelocalyceal system or the renal capsule. The mildest form of renal laceration is confined to the kidney parenchyma, with the capsule and pyelocalyceal structures remaining intact (Figs. 21–2 and 21–4). Signs and symptoms and treatment and prognosis are the same as with renal contusion. The laceration appears as a radiolucent fissure on intravenous urography or CT examination.

If the renal laceration extends through the capsule, bleeding into the perinephric space occurs with the formation of a perirenal hematoma. Depending upon the amount of hemorrhage, a flank mass may or may not be palpable. Flank pain and tenderness and hematuria are usually noted. If bleeding is severe, signs of blood loss (tachycardia, decreased pulse pressure, or hypotension) may be present. The hematoma is usually contained by Gerota's fascia, and exsanguination is rare. Abdominal radiographs may show scoliosis related to ipsilateral muscle spasm. Intravenous urography may demonstrate a localized radiolucent area at the site of the renal laceration and extrinsic compression of the renal parenchyma by the extrarenal hematoma. CT scanning with contrast enhancement will readily demonstrate the renal laceration and the perirenal hematoma (Figs. 21–2 and 21–5). Renal laceration with capsular disruption and perirenal hematoma will heal rapidly, since the general architecture of

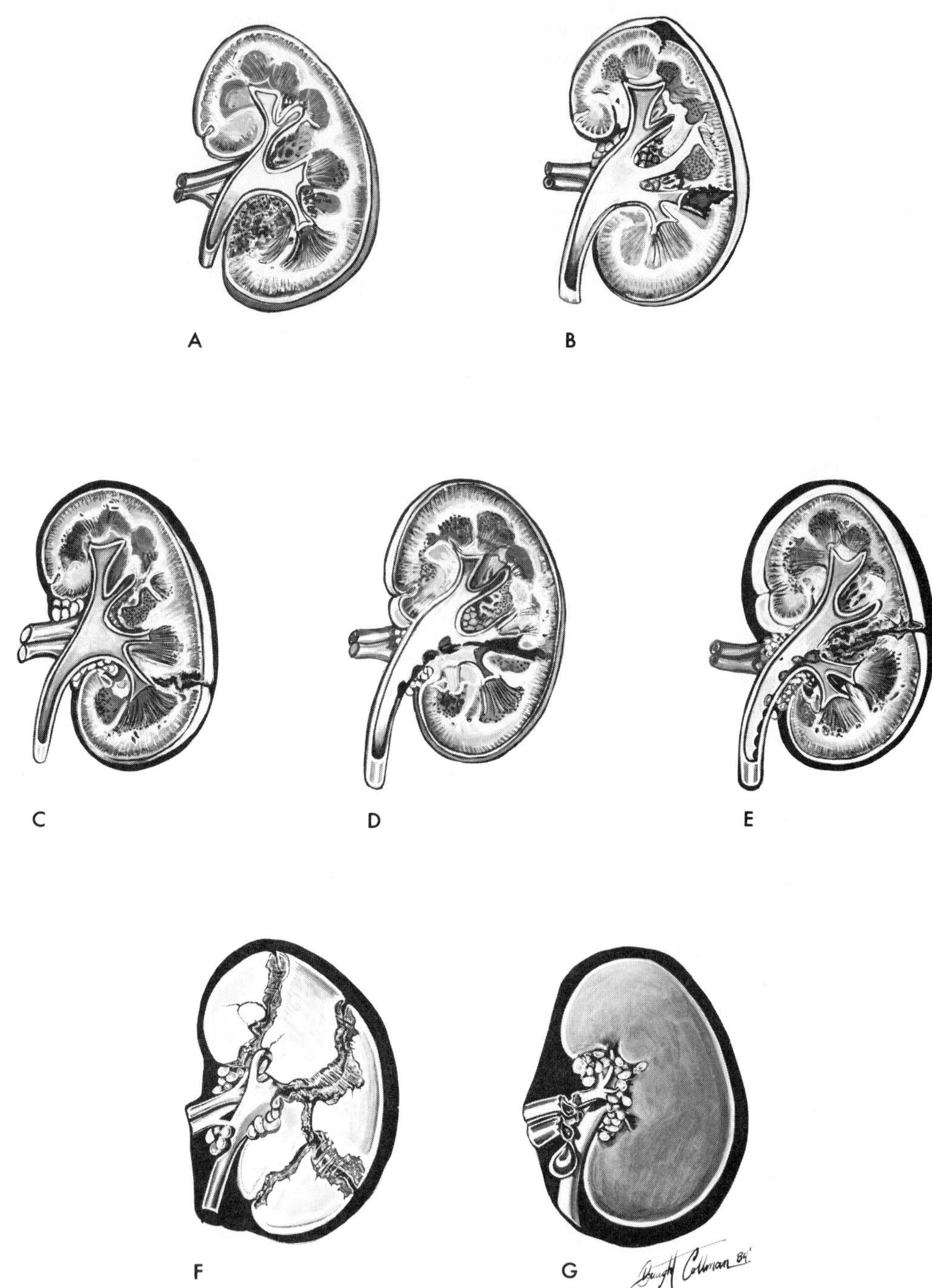

Figure 21–2. These drawings illustrate the varying forms of renal injury that may occur in children. *A,* Hemorrhage into the renal parenchyma, with the capsule and collecting structures remaining intact. This is the most common form of renal injury and usually requires simple observation. *B,* A mild renal laceration in which the collecting structures and renal capsule remain intact. Because the areas of laceration are confined to a small space a flank mass is usually not present. *C,* A mild renal laceration with extension through the renal capsule. Because the laceration extends through the capsule, a perirenal hematoma is formed. *D,* The laceration extends from the parenchyma into the collecting system. *E,* A renal laceration with extension through the capsule and into the collecting system. Because there is extrarenal extravasation, patients with this condition usually present with pain, tenderness to palpation, and possibly a flank mass. *F,* A "shattered" or "burst" kidney, in which the injury causes multiple fragments of the renal parenchyma to separate. This is an uncommon injury in pediatric patients, but partial or complete nephrectomy is generally required. *G,* This figure illustrates a renal vascular pedicle injury, which may be present as complete interruption or a renal artery intimal tear. Early diagnosis and therapy are necessary if renal salvage is to be attained.

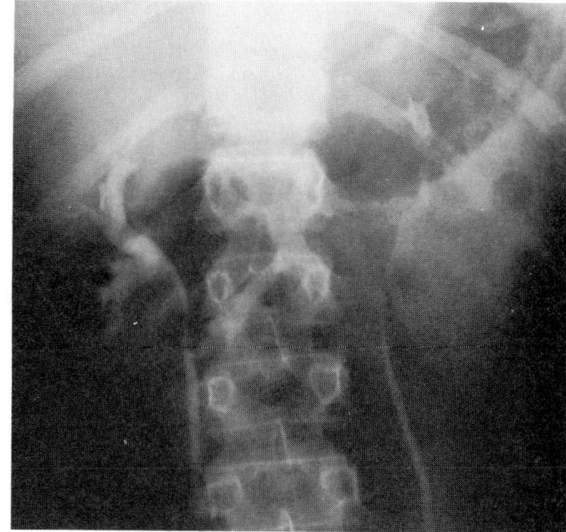

Figure 21–3. Radiograph of renal contusion in a 12-year-old boy involved in an automobile-pedestrian accident. Intravenous urography demonstrates poor visualization of the renal collecting structures in the mid and lower pole portions of the left kidney, related to compression of these structures in the region of the contusion.

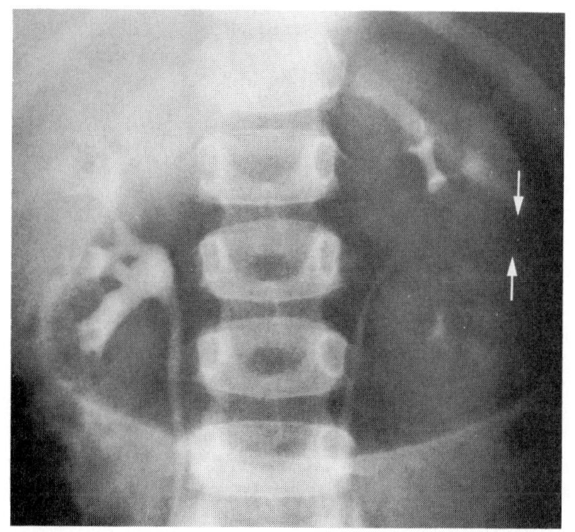

Figure 21–4. Radiograph of renal laceration in a 5-year-old child involved in an auto-pedestrian accident. Intravenous urography shows an area of diminished density in the midportion of the left kidney (*arrows*), which represents the renal laceration. No extravasation from the collecting structures is demonstrated. The patient was treated conservatively and a follow-up intravenous pyelogram 3 months later was normal.

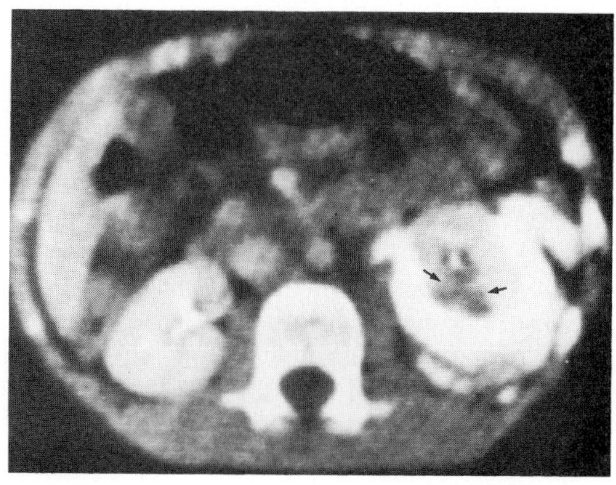

Figure 21–5. X-ray of renal laceration with disruption of the renal collectng structures on the left in a 7-year-old boy involved in an automobile-bicycle accident. Computerized tomography examination after injection of intravenous contrast material shows a renal laceration involving the posterior portion of the kidney (*arrows*) and extensive extravasation of the contrast material. The right kidney appears normal. The patient's condition remained stable and was managed conservatively.

the kidney is preserved and the bleeding contained by Gerota's fascia. Operative intervention is rarely necessary, and significant sequelae are rare.

Renal laceration may also extend from the parenchyma into the pyelocalyceal system, but with the capsule remaining intact. This is an uncommon form of renal laceration. Physical findings consist of flank pain, tenderness, and hematuria. A mass will not be palpable. Intravenous urography or CT scanning will reveal the intrarenal extravasation. This form of renal laceration usually resolves without significant sequelae.

A more severe form of renal laceration involves the capsule, parenchyma, and collecting system, resulting in extrarenal extravasation of blood and urine. Children with this injury present with flank pain, tenderness, a flank mass, and hematuria, and signs of blood loss may be present. Intravenous urography or CT scanning will demonstrate the renal laceration and extravasation into the surrounding perirenal region. Previously, the majority of patients with these injuries were managed with operative intervention, although recent reports have demonstrated favorable experience with nonoperative management.[31-34] Although the trend is toward conservative management in these cases, a urologic or pediatric surgical consultation is suggested for assistance in management decisions.

Careful management of these patients has resulted in kidney salvage in over 90 per cent of cases.[32] Although conservative care will suffice in the majority of these patients, close clinical observation and decreased physical activity are necessary in the early post-traumatic period. Patients are kept at bed rest for the first several days after injury; followed by progressive ambulation in the hospital. If clinical deterioration with evidence of progressive blood loss occurs, surgical intervention may be necessary. If the child remains stable, decreased physical activity is maintained at home. The use of antibiotics in this setting is controversial. Also, long-term follow-up is indicated to determine if hypertension develops. A difference in the incidence of hypertension, hydronephrosis, parenchymal atrophy, and infection has not yet been reported between operative and conservative forms of management.

The most severe form of renal laceration is the so-called "burst" or "shattered" type of injury, consisting of fragmentation of the kidney (Fig. 21–2). This is a rare form of injury in the pediatric age group. Persistent blood loss may necessitate operative intervention, and a partial or complete nephrectomy may be required.

Penetrating injuries to the kidney are very uncommon in childhood. Hematuria is a virtual certainty, although other physical findings will depend on the extent of damage to other organs. Intravenous urography or CT examination will demonstrate the extent of renal damage. Surgical exploration is usually necessary because of the likelihood of injuries to adjacent structures, and the initial intraoperative focus should be directed to the extrarenal structures.

Renal Vascular Injury

Renal vascular pedicle injuries are uncommon in children but require immediate recognition and appropriate surgical intervention if the affected kidney is to be salvaged. The majority of these injuries are due to blunt trauma that results in a rapid lateral acceleration of the kidney. Renal artery occlusion usually occurs secondary to intimal disruption and subsequent arterial thrombosis, although total renal artery avulsion can occur. Complete renal artery disruption is infrequent, and when it occurs, there is usually a severe intense vasospasm that prevents exsanguination. Renal artery intimal tear is the most common cause of renal artery occlusion. These injuries usually occur approximately 2 cm from the origin of the renal artery.[38] In this condition, the blood flow immediately decreases and a thrombus forms at the injury site, further decreasing perfusion. Survival of the affected kidney is a function of time, and operation is required within 4 to 6 hours.

Clinically, these children have pain and may exhibit tenderness and signs of bleeding (tachycardia, increased respiratory rate, decreased pulse pressure, and possibly hypotension). Hematuria may be present but is absent in approximately one-third of cases. Intravenous urography or CT examination demonstrates nonfunction of the kidney (Fig. 21–6). If nonvisualization was demonstrated by intravenous urography, ultrasound examination can be performed to exclude the rare instance of congenital absence of a kidney. Unilateral nonfunction is an indication for either immediate arteriography or explor-

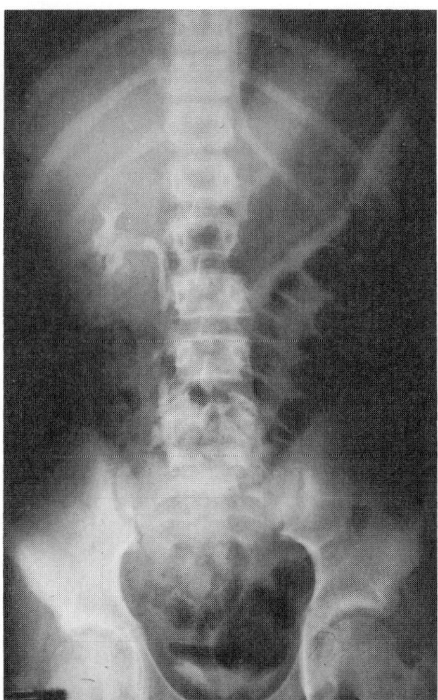

Figure 21–6. Radiograph of renal pedicle injury. Intravenous urography showing nonvisualization on the left. Angiography showed occlusion of the renal artery. At operation, the renal artery was thrombosed and nephrectomy was necessary.

atory surgery to confirm the presence of renal artery occlusion, to determine the anatomy of the renal artery or renal arteries, and to define other forms of severe renal injuries. (If a patient presents several hours after injury and renal pedicle damage is suspected, he may be taken directly for exploratory surgery in order to avoid the delay in obtaining an arteriogram.) Early operative intervention is required if the kidney is to be salvaged. Although a kidney has been saved as late as 18 hours after injury with intimal laceration and thrombus formation,[39] this is very unusual. Unless operative treatment is instituted within 4 to 6 hours of the injury, the possibility of renal salvage is unlikely.

Ureteral Injuries

The incidence of ureteral injuries is much lower in children compared with adults. This is, at least in part, related to the lower incidence of penetrating trauma in the pediatric age group.[40] Blunt trauma or sudden acceleration or deceleration with hyperextension of the spine will occasionally result in ureteral disruption in a child. In children, the level of disruption is usually at or near the ureteropelvic junction.[41] In adults with blunt trauma, this injury is often associated with a fracture of a transverse process of a lumbar vertebra, but this is a very unusual fracture in a child.

Signs of this injury are flank pain and an enlarging flank mass. This injury should specifically be considered when an enlarging flank mass is present in the absence of signs of retroperitoneal bleeding, as this implies extensive urinary extravasation. Intravenous urography usually demonstrates extravasation of contrast medium at the level of the disruption, although retrograde pyelography may be necessary to demonstrate this condition. All cases require operative repair. If recognized early and treated appropriately, ureteral injuries usually heal well without significant sequelae.

Bladder Injuries

Most bladder injuries in children are secondary to severe blunt trauma to the pelvis or lower abdomen. Occasionally penetrating injuries in the suprapubic area may lacerate the bladder. Bladder injury occurs in about 15 per cent of children with a pelvic fracture[42] and occasionally in association with renal injuries.[43] Because of associated injuries and the sometimes subtle physical findings, bladder injuries are frequently overlooked.

The bladder may rupture intraperitoneally

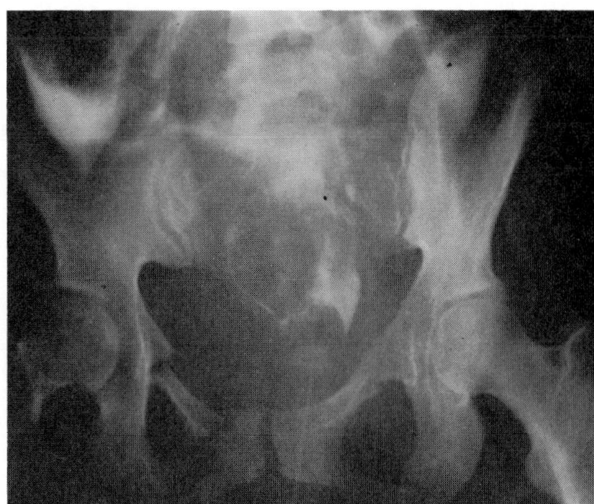

Figure 21–7. X-ray of intraperitoneal bladder perforation. There are multiple pelvic fractures. A cystogram reveals marked displacement of the bladder from perivesical hemorrhage, filling defects in the bladder (blood clots), and contrast material in the peritoneal cavity related to intraperitoneal laceration of the bladder.

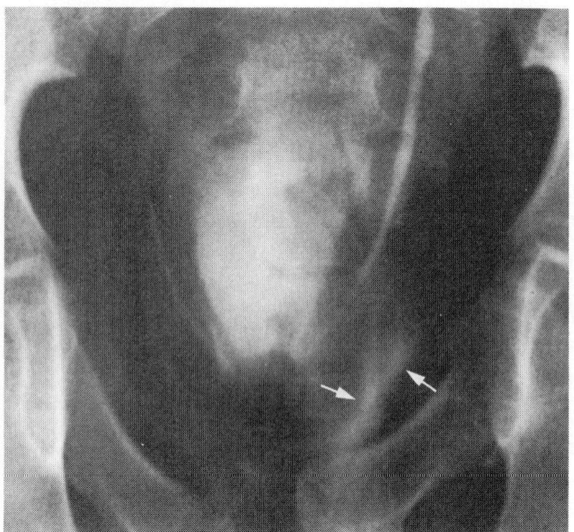

Figure 21–8. X-ray of extraperitoneal bladder perforation in an 8-year-old boy who was run over by an automobile. There are multiple pelvic fractures and separation of the pubic bones. There is extensive perivesical hemorrhage, with displacement of the bladder and ureters medially and superiorly. There is a laceration of the bladder, which results in extraperitoneal extravasation of contrast material (*arrows*).

or extraperitoneally (Figs. 21–7 and 21–8). Intraperitoneal rupture usually occurs when the bladder is full at the time of trauma and the perforation occurs in the bladder dome. This results in signs of peritonitis. Extraperitoneal extravasation of urine results in more subtle physical findings. Signs and symptoms of bladder injury include lower abdominal pain, suprapubic tenderness, hematuria, dysuria, and inability to void.

A plain film of the abdomen may show pelvic fractures or evidence of intraperitoneal fluid. A cystogram will demonstrate extravasation from the bladder and determine the location of the perforation. This study is best done with fluoroscopic control and with sufficient dye to adequately distend the bladder. In the male, a retrograde urethrogram should be done before the catheter is advanced into the bladder.

Urethral catheter drainage has been successfully used in mild bladder tears, but prompt surgical repair is usually indicated. Postoperatively, the bladder should be drained with an indwelling urethral or suprapubic catheter. Once repaired, bladder perforation heals readily without significant sequelae.

Urethral Injuries

The vast majority of urethral injuries occur in the male, in whom the urethra is longer and less well protected. Trauma to the urethra distal to the urogenital diaphragm is almost always secondary to straddle injury to the perineum. Blunt trauma to the lower abdomen or pubic area, especially when there is a resultant fracture involving the lower bony pelvis, may cause a shearing stress, which typically disrupts the urethra at the level of the urogenital diaphragm.

Signs and symptoms of urethral injury include blood at the urethral meatus, inability to void, lower abdominal or pelvic pain, and external evidence of lower abdominal or perineal trauma, and on rectal examination, the prostate may be superiorly positioned.

Patients with suspected urethral injury should not be urged to void. It is important that a urethral catheter should not be inserted until the status of the urethra has been determined by urethrography. Catheterization could result in conversion of an incomplete urethral laceration to a complete disruption. Retrograde urethrography should be performed under fluoroscopic control using aseptic technique to determine if there is a urethral laceration and to determine the location and extent of damage (Fig. 21–9). If urethral disruption is demonstrated, suprapubic drainage of the bladder should be performed. Subsequent operative repair is delayed for a few months when the proximal urethra is disrupted and for a few days if the injury involves the bulbar or penile urethra.

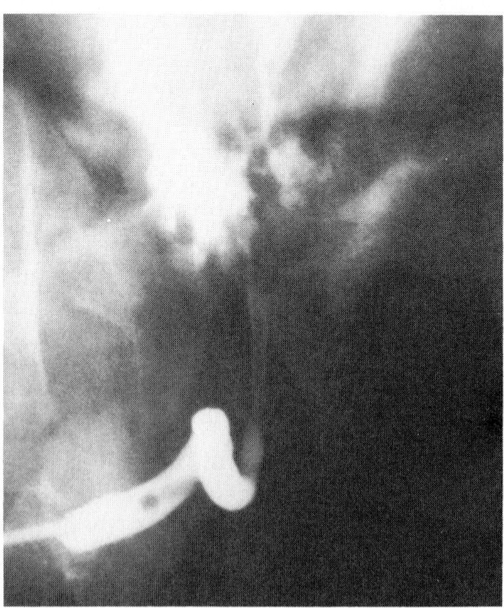

Figure 21–9. Radiograph of urethral laceration in a young boy who was run over by an automobile. A retrograde urethrogram shows extravasation of contrast material, indicating laceration of the urethra.

Injury to the Male External Genitalia

Penetrating injuries to the penis and scrotum are fairly common and are often due to falls onto sharp objects (broken glass, wire fences, wood sticks, gravel). Uncircumcised children may lacerate the redundant foreskin by catching it in the zipper of their pants. Zipper injuries entrapping the skin are best treated by placing two towel clips directly opposite each other and between the metal fasteners of the zipper. Gently twisting the clips will cause the zipper to open. This procedure is painless and does not require local anesthesia.

All lacerations should be carefully cleaned and débrided of all foreign material. Abundant irrigation with sterile saline is required. Local anesthesia may suffice in the older and more cooperative child, but general anesthesia is often necessary in younger patients. In all cases of penetrating injury to the penis, damage to the urethra should be excluded by physical exam and, if necessary, urethrogram.

Lacerations should be closed with interrupted absorbable sutures. It is often helpful to apply a bulky compression dressing to minimize subsequent swelling and ecchymosis. Because all such wounds are contaminated, antibiotic therapy may be helpful.

The penis is at times strangulated by string, wire, or hair, often in an attempt to attain urinary control. Such injuries require prompt therapy to minimize sequelae. Strangulation can result in urethral fistula or even gangrene of the glans. The strangulating material should be removed promptly. A small Foley catheter is inserted if the urethra has been traumatized. In most cases, a linear incision may be made on the dorsum to release all constricting bands. Depilatory creams may be used to remove hair, although surgical release occurs much more rapidly. Amputated fragments of penis should be retained in saline and replaced as soon as possible with fine absorbable sutures.

Blunt trauma to the external genitalia can occur from falls, kicks, or other trauma. Swelling, ecchymosis, and hematoma are common, and the injury may be very painful. Scrotal hematomas may be separate from the testicle or may be closely adherent. Small scrotal hematomas can be treated conservatively, while large hematomas that are adherent to the testicle should be explored surgically. Fracture of the corpus cavernosum is rare in the child but leads to penile deviation, marked swelling, and considerable hematoma. Surgical repair is mandatory.

Vulvar and Vaginal Injuries

Injuries to the perineum of young females occur frequently. These injuries may occur as a result of falls on sharp or blunt objects, straddle injuries, or penetrating trauma from glass, knives, and so on. If a careful history of the injury is not consistent with the type or degree of injury, sexual abuse should be considered a possible cause of the trauma. However, self-inflicted trauma also occasionally occurs. Foreign bodies may be placed in the vagina by young girls, resulting in a foul-smelling discharge and variable degrees of pain. In all injuries to the vulva or vagina, the possibility of urethral or rectal injuries must also be considered. Vesicovaginal and rectovaginal fistulas are commonly overlooked injuries, particularly with penetrating wounds of the vagina. In cases in which rectovaginal injuries have occurred, a diverting sigmoid loop colostomy is usually performed.

In cases in which perineal injury has occurred, a careful inspection of both the external and internal structures should be undertaken. Either a small speculum or endoscope may be used to assess injuries to the vagina.

In children, small vaginal lacerations that have stopped bleeding may not require suturing. When bleeding is present or lacerations are large, interrupted absorbable sutures should be used to control bleeding sites and reapproximate tissue. Strict attention to anatomic reconstruction is essential. When large vaginal hematomas are present, the hematoma should be carefully observed for possible continued expansion. In most cases the hematoma will be limited by a tamponade effect and is best left to resolve spontaneously. Attempts to incise and evacuate hematomas often result in continued hemorrhage from unidentified bleeding sites.

REFERENCES

1. Morse TS, Harris BH: Nonpenetrating renal vascular injuries. J Trauma 13:497, 1973.
2. Morse TS: Renal injuries. *In* Touloukian RJ (ed.): Pediatric Trauma. New York, John Wiley & Sons, 1978.
3. Peterson NE: Apparent exceptions to the usual patterns in renal trauma. J Urol 121:489, 1979.
4. Cockett ATK, Frank IN, Davis RS, Linke CA: Recent advances in the diagnosis and management of blunt renal trauma. J Urol 113:750, 1975.

5. Peters PC, Bright TC, III: Blunt renal injuries. Urol Clin North Am 4:17, 1977.
6. Javalpour N, Guinam P, Bush IM: Renal trauma in children. Surg Gynecol Obstetr 136:237, 1973.
7. Linke CA, Frank IN, Young LW, et al.: Renal trauma in children. New York State Med J 72:2414, 1972.
8. Sagalowsky AI, McConnel JD, Peters PC: Renal trauma requiring surgery: An analysis of 185 cases. J Trauma 23:128, 1983.
9. Emanuel B, Weiss H, Gollin P: Renal trauma in children. J Trauma 17:275, 1977.
10. Morse TS, Smith JP, Howard WHR, Rowe MI: Kidney injuries in children. J Urol 98:539, 1967.
11. Morse TS: Evaluation and initial management. *In* Touloukian (ed.): Pediatric Trauma. New York, John Wiley & Sons, 1978.
12. Uson AC, Lattimer J: Genitourinary tract injuries. *In* Randolph JG, Ravitch MM, Welch KJ, et al. (eds.): The Injured Child: Surgical Management. Chicago, Year Book Medical Publishers, 1979.
13. Glenn JF, Harvard BM: The injured kidney. JAMA 173:1189, 1960.
14. Smith JM, O'Flynn JD: Closed renal trauma. Br J Surg 64:753, 1977.
15. Banowsky LH, Wolfel DA, Lackner CH: Considerations in diagnosis and management of renal trauma. J Trauma 10:587, 1970.
16. Caponegro PJ, Leadbetter GW Jr: Traumatic renal artery thrombosis. J Urol 109:769, 1973.
17. Lang EK; Arteriography in the assessment of renal trauma. J Trauma 15:1045, 1975.
18. Persky L, Hoch WH: Genitourinary tract trauma. Curr Prob Surg, Sept., 1977.
19. Griffen WO, Belin RP, Ernst CB: Intravenous pyelography in abdominal trauma. J Trauma 18:387, 1978.
20. Editorial: Hematuria after closed trauma. Br Med J 1:841, 1979.
21. Bergquist D, Hedelin H, Lindblad B: Blunt renal trauma. Scand J Urol Nephrol 14:177, 1980.
22. Wein RJ, Murphy JJ, Mulholland SG, et al.: A conservative approach to the management of blunt trauma. J Urol 117:425, 1977.
23. Mogensen P, Agger P, Ostergaard AH: A conservative approach to the management of blunt renal trauma: Results of a follow-up study. Br J Urol 52:338, 1980.
24. Cass AS: Blunt renal trauma in children. J Trauma 23:123, 1983.
25. Peters PC, Bright TC: Blunt renal injuries. Urol Clin North Am 4:17, 1977.
26. Guice K, Oldham K, Eide B, Johanson K: Hematuria after blunt trauma: When is pyelography useful? J Trauma 23:305, 1983.
27. McAninch JW, Federle MP: Evaluation of renal injuries with computerized tomography. J Urol 128:456, 1982.
28. Cass AS: Renal trauma in the multiply injured patient. J Urol 114:495, 1975.
29. Kuzmarov IW, Morehouse DD, Gibson S: Blunt renal trauma in the pediatric population: A retrospective study. J Urol 126:648, 1981.
30. Lucey DT, Smith MJV, Koontz WW Jr: Modern trends in the management of urologic trauma. J Urol 107:641, 1972.
31. Thompson IM, Latowette H, Montie JE, et al.: Results of nonoperative management of blunt renal trauma. J Urol 118:522, 1977.
32. Evins SC, Thompson WB, Rosenblum R: Nonoperative management of severe renal lacerations. J Urol 123:247, 1980.
33. Ceccarelli FE: Expectant treatment in the management of blunt renal trauma. *In* Scott R Jr (ed.): Current Controversies in Urologic Management. Philadelphia, W.B. Saunders Co., 1972.
34. Osias MB, Hale SD, Lytton B: The management of renal injuries. J Trauma 116:954, 1977.
35. Persky L, Forsyth WE: Renal trauma in childhood. JAMA 182:709, 1962.
36. Seruca H, DeBock J, Guttman FM: Renal trauma in children. Canad J Surg 22:24, 1979.
37. Schiller M, Barris BH, Samuels LD, et al.: Diagnosis of experimental renal trauma. J Pediatr Surg 7:187, 1972.
38. Maggio AJ Jr, Brosman S: Renal artery trauma. Urology 11:125, 1978.
39. Karini SA, Yourn JD, Soderstrom C: Classification of renal injuries as a guide to therapy. Surg Gynecol Obstet 148:161, 1979.
40. Hendren WH, Hensle TW: Lower urinary tract and perineal injuries. *In* Touloukian RJ (ed.): Pediatric Trauma. New York, John Wiley & Sons, 1978.
41. Boston VE, Smyth BT: Bilateral pelvi-ureteric avulsion following closed trauma. Br J Urol 47:149, 1975.
42. Cass AS: Bladder trauma in the multiply injured patient. J Urol 115:667, 1976.
43. Mertz JH, Wishard WN Jr, Nowse MH, et al.: Injury of the kidney in children. JAMA 183:730, 1963.

CHAPTER

22 *Musculoskeletal Injuries**

ROBERT B. SALTER

Before considering specific injuries in children, it would be wise to consider some of the *special features* of fractures and dislocations in the growing years. Just as in all other clinical fields of medicine and surgery, so also in the field of fractures, children cannot be considered simply as "little adults." Fractures in children and the reaction of children's tissues to these fractures differ greatly from those in adults. Blount deserves special credit for emphasizing the fact that *fractures in children are different.*

SPECIAL FEATURES OF FRACTURES AND DISLOCATIONS IN CHILDREN

The special features of fractures and dislocations are first listed and then discussed individually. These differences are most striking in the infant and young child and become progressively less striking as the child approaches adulthood. Comparative terms, such as "more" and "less," refer to a comparison between fractures and dislocations in children and those in adults.

1. Fractures more common.
2. Stronger and more active periosteum.
3. More rapid fracture healing.
4. Special problems of diagnosis.
5. Spontaneous correction of certain residual deformities.
6. Differences in complications.
7. Different emphasis on methods of treatment.
8. Torn ligaments and dislocations less common.
9. Less tolerance of major blood loss.

Fractures More Common

The higher incidence of fractures in children is explained by the combination of their relatively slender bones and their carefree capers. Some of these injuries, such as crack or hairline fractures, buckle fractures, and greenstick fractures, are not serious, whereas others, such as intra-articular fractures and epiphyseal plate fractures, are very serious indeed.

Stronger and More Active Periosteum

The stronger periosteum in children is less readily torn across at the time of fracture, and consequently there is more often an intact periosteal hinge that can be utilized during closed reduction of the fracture. Furthermore, the periosteum is much more osteogenic in children than it is in adults (Fig. 22–1).

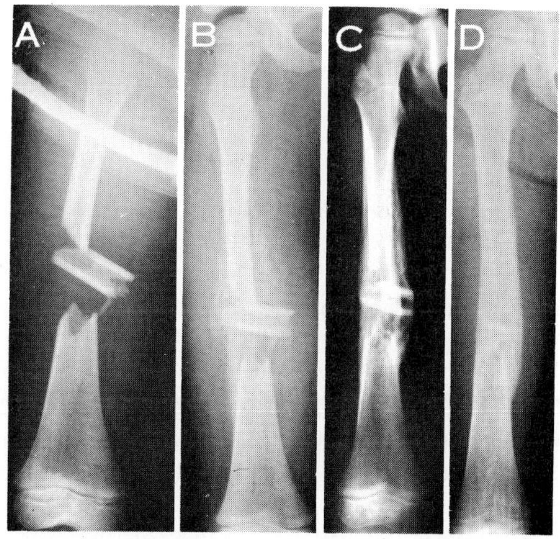

Figure 22–1. The importance of the strong and actively osteogenic periosteum in the healing process of children's fractures is demonstrated in this series of radiographs of a fractured femoral shaft in a 4-year-old child. *A*, The day of injury; a double fracture with the middle segment lying almost transversely. The strong periosteal sleeve, however, would not be completely torn across. Note the metal ring of the Thomas splint. *B*, Three weeks after injury, abundant callus is forming from the actively osteogenic periosteum; at this stage traction was replaced by a hip spica cast. *C*, Ten weeks after injury, the middle segment is well incorporated in the callus and is being resorbed; the fracture was clinically united at this stage, and the child was allowed to walk. *D*, Six months after injury, the contour of the femur is returning to normal through the process of remodeling.

*Courtesy of the Williams & Wilkins Co., Baltimore, Md. *From:* Salter, R. B.: Textbook of Disorders and Injuries of the Musculoskeletal System, 1970.

More Rapid Fracture Healing

Age is a much more important factor in the rate of healing in bone than in any other tissue in the body, particularly during childhood. This is closely related to the osteogenic activity of the periosteum and endosteum, a process that is remarkably active at birth, becomes progressively less active with each year of childhood, and remains relatively constant from early adult life to old age.

Fracture of the shaft of the femur serves as an example of this phenomenon. A femoral shaft fracture occurring at birth will be united in 3 weeks; a comparable fracture at the age of 8 years will be united in 8 weeks; at the age of 12 years it will be united at 12 weeks; and from the age of 20 years to old age it will be united in approximately 20 weeks.

Nonunion of children's fractures is rare, unless an unnecessary open operation has damaged the blood supply to the fracture fragments or has introduced the complication of infection.

Special Problems of Diagnosis

The varying radiographic appearance of a given epiphysis, both before and after the development of a secondary center of ossification, can be quite confusing; although the various secondary centers of ossification appear at relatively constant ages, these are not easy to remember. Likewise, the radiographic appearance of the various epiphyseal plates may be puzzling to the inexperienced and may be mistaken for fracture lines. These radiographic problems of diagnosis, however, can be readily overcome in limb injuries. Just as an injured limb should be compared with its normal uninjured mate during the clinical examination, so too should they be compared during the radiographic examination (see Chapter 8).

Spontaneous Correction of Certain Residual Deformities

In adults the deformity of a malunited fracture is permanent. In children, however, certain residual deformities tend to correct spontaneously, either by extensive remodeling or by epiphyseal plate growth, or sometimes by a combination of both. Just how much spontaneous correction of the healed fracture deformity can be anticipated depends upon the age of the child (and the number of years of skeletal growth remaining) and the type of deformity (angulation, incomplete apposition, shortening, rotation). This phenomenon is therefore best considered in relation to specific deformities.

Angulation. Residual angulation near an epiphyseal plate will tend to correct spontaneously with subsequent growth *provided* that the plane of the deformity is the same as the plane of motion in the nearest joint. For example, residual anterior angulation at the site of a healed fracture in the distal end of the radius is in the same plane as the flexion and extension motion in the wrist joint; thus, in a young child it can be expected to correct to a large extent (Fig. 22–2). By contrast, residual angulation at right angles to the plane of motion of the nearest joint (for example, a lateral angulation or varus deformity in the supracondylar region of the humerus, which is at right angles to the flexion and extension motion of the elbow) cannot be expected to correct (Fig. 22–3). Furthermore, angulation in the middle third of a long bone, being well away from an epiphyseal plate, cannot be expected to correct spontaneously (Fig. 22–4).

Incomplete Apposition. With incomplete apposition of the fracture fragments or even side-to-side (bayonet) apposition in children, the contour of the healed fracture improves greatly through the active process of remodeling–an example of Wolff's law (Fig. 22–5).

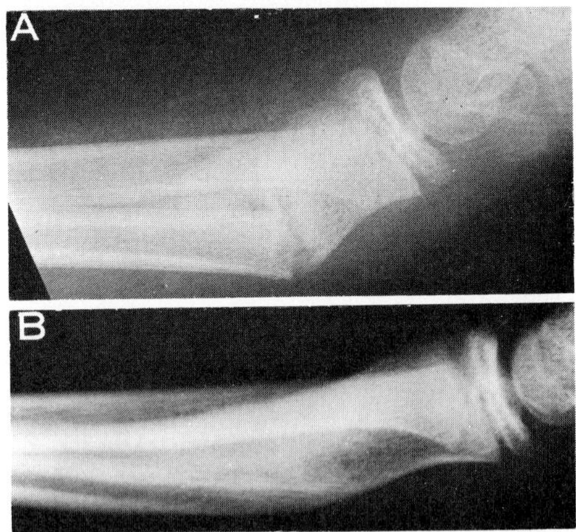

Figure 22–2. Spontaneous improvement in a residual fracture deformity with subsequent growth. *A*, Lateral projection of the distal end of the radius of a 10-year-old boy 6 weeks after injury. Unfortunately, the metaphyseal fracture had been allowed to unite with 35 degrees of anterior angulation. *B*, Six months later there is only 15 degrees of anterior angulation and the corners of the angulation deformity have remodeled. Note that the epiphysis has grown away from the fracture site during these 6 months.

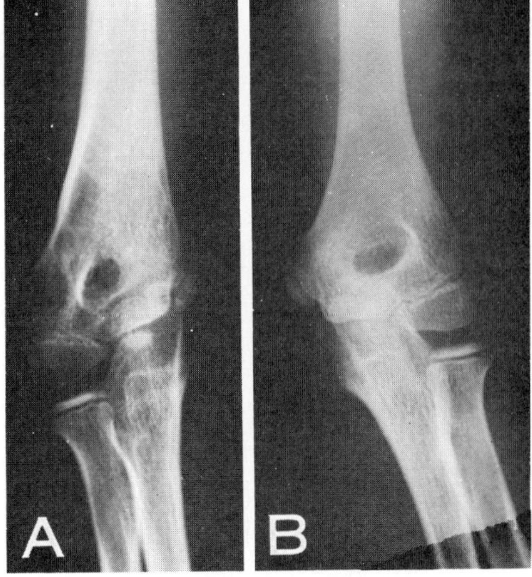

Figure 22–3. Failure of spontaneous correction of a residual fracture deformity. *A,* A supracondylar fracture of the humerus in a 9-year-old girl had been allowed to unite with 20 degrees of lateral angulation 2 years previously. *B,* The opposite elbow has a normal carrying angle of 15 degrees. Thus, on the injured side the normal carrying angle has not only been lost but also been reversed so that there is 5 degrees of varus deformity, which is permanent.

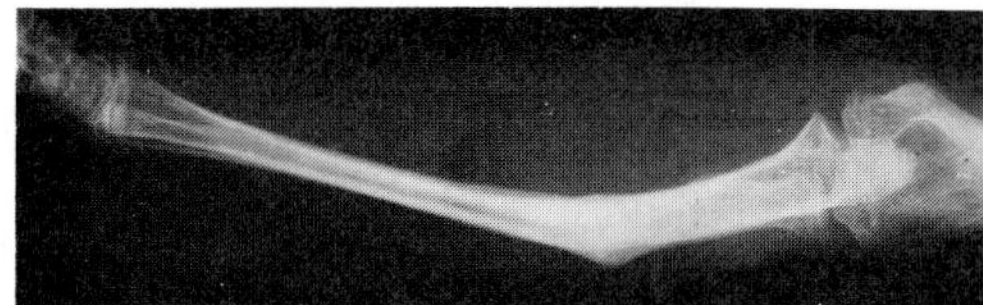

Figure 22–4. Failure of spontaneous correction of a residual fracture deformity. The fractures of the middle third of the radius and ulna of an 8-year-old girl had been allowed to unite in the unsatisfactory position of 35 degrees of posterior angulation 1 year previously. This deformity of malunion is permanent.

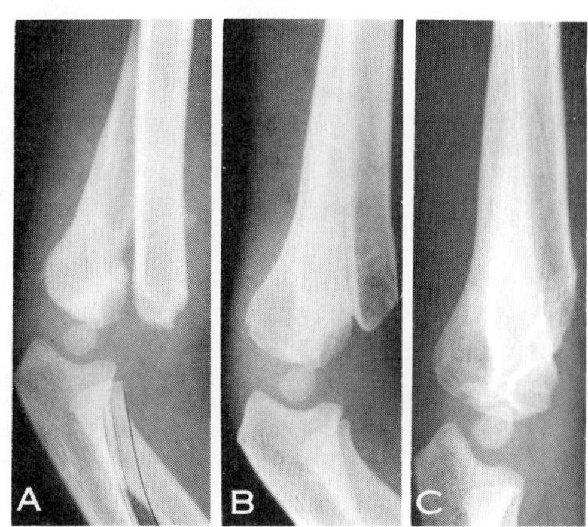

Figure 22–5. Spontaneous correction of incomplete apposition through remodeling. *A,* An unreduced supracondylar fracture of the humerus in a 4-year-old child 3 weeks after injury; note the new bone formation in the periosteal tube through which the proximal fragment is protruding. *B,* Five months after injury the periosteal tube has formed a new shaft and the original shaft is becoming resorbed. *C,* One year after injury the contour of the fracture site has been markedly improved by the process of remodeling. Note that the epiphysis has grown away from the fracture site.

Shortening. Following a displaced fracture of a long bone in a growing child, the associated disruption in the nutrient artery results in a compensatory increase in the blood flow at the epiphyseal ends of the bone. This phenomenon produces a temporary acceleration of longitudinal growth in the bone for as long as 1 year after the fracture (Fig. 22–6). This is most striking after displaced femoral shaft fractures. Therefore, overriding is a desirable aim in the treatment of such fractures, since the shortening will be corrected spontaneously by temporary overgrowth, and the two femora will become almost the same length (Fig. 22–7).

Rotation. Residual rotational deformity at the site of a healed fracture in a long bone does not correct spontaneously regardless of the child's age or the site of the deformity.

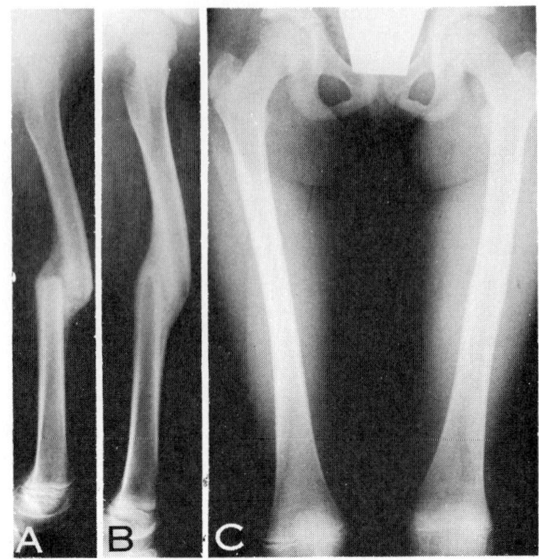

Figure 22–7. Overgrowth of the left femur after a displaced fracture of the shaft in a 9-year-old girl. *A*, Lateral projection 8 weeks after injury; the fracture had been allowed to unite with 1 cm of overriding intentionally. *B*, Six months after injury the united fracture is becoming remodeled. *C*, Eighteen months after injury the femora are virtually equal in length as a result of overgrowth of the left femur. If the fracture had been allowed to unite end-to-end, the femur would have been 1 cm too long 18 months later and the leg length discrepancy would have been permanent.

Differences in Complications

Growth disturbances after epiphyseal plate injuries occur, of course, only in children. Osteomyelitis secondary to either an open fracture or an open reduction of a closed fracture tends to be more extensive in a child, and the infection may even destroy an epiphyseal plate, with resultant growth disturbance. Volkmann's ischemia of nerves and muscles is much more common in children as are post-traumatic myositis ossificans and refracture.

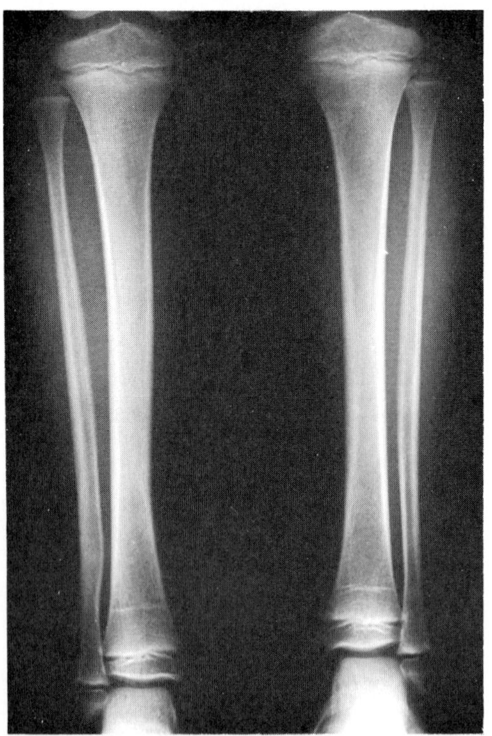

Figure 22–6. Overgrowth of a long bone after a displaced fracture. One year previously the right tibia of this 8-year-old boy had been fractured, and during the ensuing year, it had overgrown 1 cm. The transverse radiopaque lines in the distal tibial metaphyses represent the site of the epiphyseal plate at the time of injury; note that there has been more growth from the epiphyseal plate of the right tibia than from that of the left. The resultant leg length discrepancy will be permanent.

By contrast, persistent joint stiffness after fracture is relatively uncommon in children unless the fracture has involved the joint surface; consequently, physiotherapy and occupational therapy are seldom required in the aftercare of children with fractures. Likewise, fat embolism, pulmonary embolism, and accident neurosis are rare in childhood.

Different Emphasis on Methods of Treatment

Although the *principles* of fracture treatment are equally applicable to children and adults, there is a different emphasis on the *methods* of treatment in the two age groups. Virtually *all* fractures of the long bones in children can and indeed should be treated by means of closed reduction, either manipulation or continuous traction. Of course, the emotional exuberance and physical vigor of children recovering from fractures demand that their plaster of Paris casts be particularly strong.

Certain fractures in children do, however, necessitate open reduction and internal skeletal fixation, such as displaced intra-articular fractures, femoral neck fractures, and certain types of epiphyseal plate injuries, which are described in a subsequent section. There is no indication for excision of a fracture fragment and replacement by a prosthesis in children.

Torn Ligaments and Dislocations Less Common

Children's ligaments are strong and resilient. Since they are stronger than the associated epiphyseal plates, sudden extension on a ligament at the time of injury results in a separation of the epiphyseal plate rather than a tear in the ligament (Fig. 22–8). This is also true to a lesser extent of fibrous joint capsules. For example, the type of injury that would produce a traumatic dislocation of the shoulder in an adult will produce a fracture-separation of the proximal humeral epiphysis in a child.

Less Tolerance of Major Blood Loss

Although the total blood volume is proportionately smaller in a child than in an adult, the percentage of blood volume as compared with body weight is actually higher in children. A formula for estimating the average blood volume in a child is 85 ml/kg of body weight. Thus, the average blood volume of a child who weighs 20 kg (44 lb) is 1700 ml. Consequently, external hemorrhage of 500 ml/s in such a child represents nearly 30 per cent of the total blood volume, whereas a similar hemorrhage in an adult would represent only 10 per cent of the total blood volume of 5000 ml.

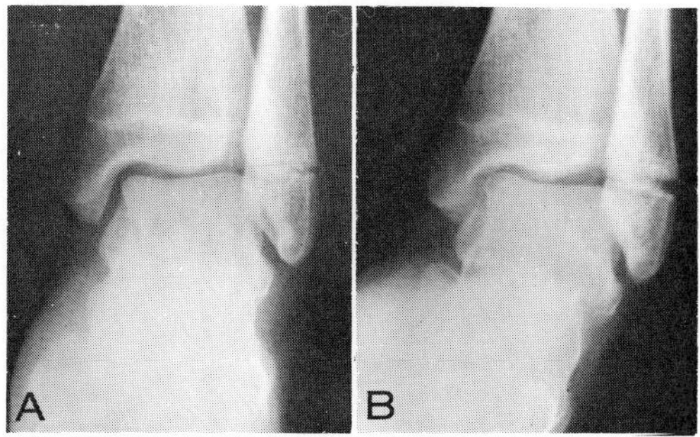

Figure 22–8. Traumatic separation of the distal fibular epiphysis in a 14-year-old boy. *A*, This radiograph appears normal because after the injury, the fibular epiphysis had returned to its normal position. *B*, In this stress radiograph (taken while a varus stress is being applied to the ankle joint with the child under anesthetic), there is a tilt of the talus and the separation of the fibular epiphysis is apparent.

SPECIAL TYPES OF FRACTURES IN CHILDREN

In addition to *stress fractures* and *pathologic fractures,* which occur in both children and adults, there are two special types of fractures that are limited to childhood, namely, *fractures that involve the epiphyseal plate and birth fractures.*

Fractures of The Epiphyseal Plate

Epiphyseal plate fractures present special problems in both diagnosis and treatment. Furthermore, they carry the risk of becoming complicated by a serious disturbance of local growth and the consequent development of progressive bony deformity during the remaining years of skeletal growth.

Anatomy, Histology, and Physiology

The types of epiphyses are shown in Figure 22–9. The weakest area of the epiphyseal

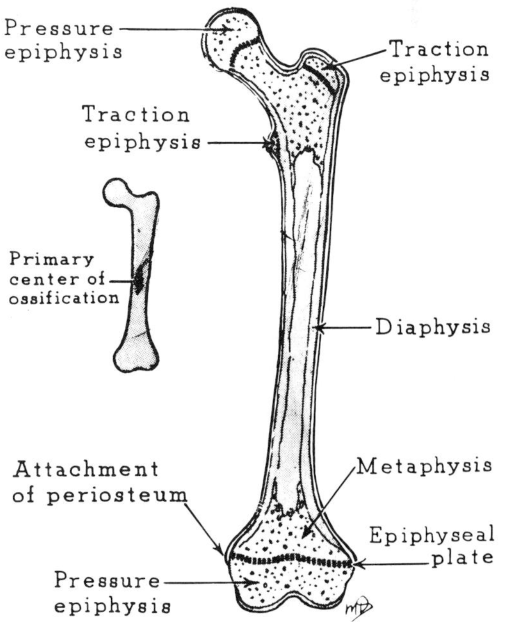

Figure 22–9. Types of epiphyses (secondary centers of ossification) in the femur. Note the attachment of the periosteum to the epiphysis.

plate is the zone of calcifying cartilage; when the epiphysis is separated by injury, the line of separation is through this zone (Fig. 22–10). Thus, the epiphyseal plate, which is radiolucent and therefore not radiographically visible, always remains attached to the epiphysis.

The blood supply of the epiphyseal plate enters from its epiphyseal surface. If the epiphysis loses its blood supply and becomes necrotic, the plate likewise becomes necrotic and growth ceases. In most sites the blood supply to the epiphysis is not damaged at the time of injury, but in the proximal femoral epiphysis and the proximal radial epiphysis, the blood vessels course along the neck of the bone and cross the epiphyseal plate peripherally. Consequently, in these sites epiphyseal separation frequently damages the blood supply and leads to avascular necrosis of the epiphysis as well as of the epiphyseal plate.

The cartilaginous epiphyseal plate is weaker than bone, and yet epiphyseal injuries account for only 15 per cent of all fractures in childhood. The explanation for this apparent paradox is that the epiphysis is firmly attached to its metaphysis peripherally by the union of perichondrium and periosteum (see Fig. 9–9). Nevertheless, as mentioned previously, epiphyseal plates are weaker than their associated ligaments and joint capsule. For this reason injuries that would result in a torn ligament or a dislocation in an adult usually produce a traumatic separation of the epiphysis in a child (see Fig. 9–8).

In the lower limb, more longitudinal growth takes place at the epiphyseal plates in the region of the knee than in the region of the hip or ankle. By contrast, in the upper limb, more growth takes place in the region of the shoulder and wrist than in the region of the elbow.

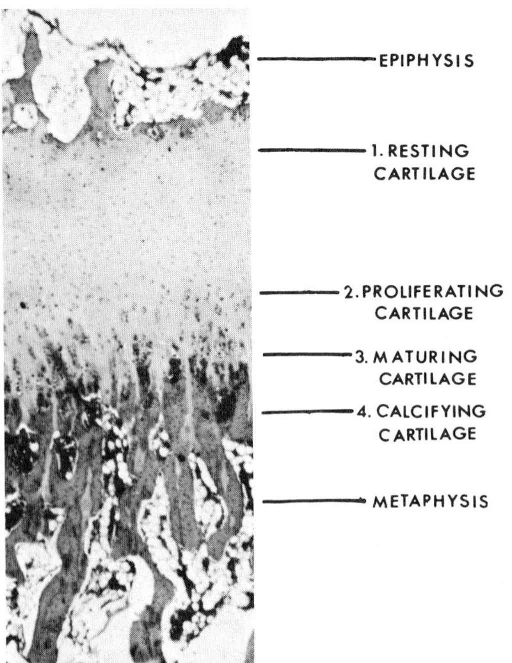

Figure 22–10. Low-power photomicrograph of an epiphyseal plate from the proximal end of the tibia of a child.

Diagnosis of Epiphyseal Plate Injuries

An epiphyseal plate fracture should be suspected in any injured child who exhibits signs suggestive of a fracture near the end of a long bone, a dislocation, or a ligamentous injury (including a sprain). However, precise diagnosis depends upon radiographic examination; at least two projections at right angles to each other are essential and comparable projections of the same region of the opposite uninjured limb should also be obtained.

Classification of Epiphyseal Plate Injuries

The following classification is based on the mechanism of injury as well as on the relationship of the fracture line to the growing cells of the epiphyseal plate. It is also correlated with the method of treatment and the prognosis of the injury concerning growth disturbance.

Type 1 (Fig. 22–11). There is complete separation of the epiphysis without any fracture through bone; the growing cells of the

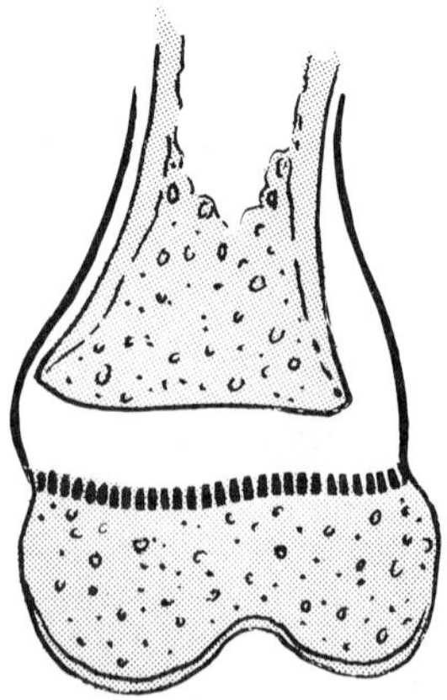

Figure 22–11. Type 1 epiphyseal plate injury. Separation of epiphysis.

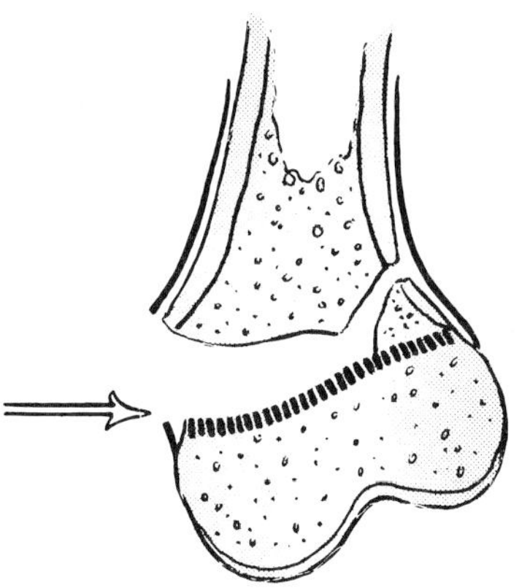

Figure 22–12. Type 2 epiphyseal plate injury. Fracture-separation of epiphysis.

epiphyseal plate remain with the epiphysis. This type of injury, the result of a shearing force, is more common in newborns (from birth injury) and in young children in whom the epiphyseal plate is relatively thick.

Closed reduction is not difficult because the periosteal attachment is intact around most of its circumference. The prognosis for future growth is excellent, provided that the blood supply to the epiphysis is intact, which it usually is in sites other than the proximal femoral epiphysis and the proximal radial epiphysis.

Type 2 (Fig. 22–12). In this, the commonest type, the line of fracture-separation extends along the epiphyseal plate to a variable distance and then out through a portion of the metaphysis, producing a triangular-shaped metaphyseal fragment. The growing cells of the plate remain with the epiphysis. This type of injury, the result of shearing and bending forces, usually occurs in the older child in whom the epiphyseal plate is relatively thin. The periosteum is torn on the convex side of the angulation but is intact on the concave side. Thus, the intact periosteal hinge is always on the side of the metaphyseal fragment.

Closed reduction is relatively easy to obtain as well as to maintain; the intact periosteal hinge and the metaphyseal fragment both prevent over-reduction. The prognosis for growth is excellent provided that the blood supply to the epiphysis is intact, which it nearly always is at sites of type 2 injuries.

Type 3 (Fig. 22–13). The fracture is intra-articular and extends from the joint surface to the deep zone of the epiphyseal plate and then along the plate to its periphery. This uncommon type of injury is caused by an intra-articular shearing force and is usually limited to the distal tibial epiphysis.

Open reduction is usually necessary to restore a perfectly normal joint surface. The prognosis for growth is good provided that the blood supply to the separated portion of the epiphysis has not been disrupted.

Type 4 (Fig. 22–14). The fracture, which is intra-articular, extends from the joint surface through the epiphysis, across the entire thickness of the epiphyseal plate, and through a portion of the metaphysis. The commonest example of a type 4 injury is the fracture of the lateral condyle of the humerus.

Open reduction and internal skeletal fixation are necessary not only to restore a normal joint surface but also to obtain perfect apposition of the epiphyseal plate. Indeed, unless the fractured surfaces of the epiphyseal plate are kept perfectly reduced, fracture healing occurs across the plate and renders further longitudinal growth impossible. Thus the prognosis for growth after a type 4 injury is very poor unless perfect reduction is achieved and maintained.

Type 5 (Fig. 22–15). This relatively uncommon injury results from a severe crushing force applied through the epiphysis to one

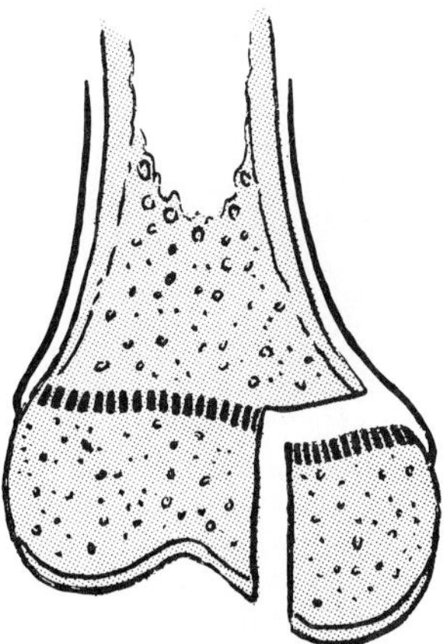

Figure 22–13. Type 3 epiphyseal plate injury. Fracture of part of epiphysis.

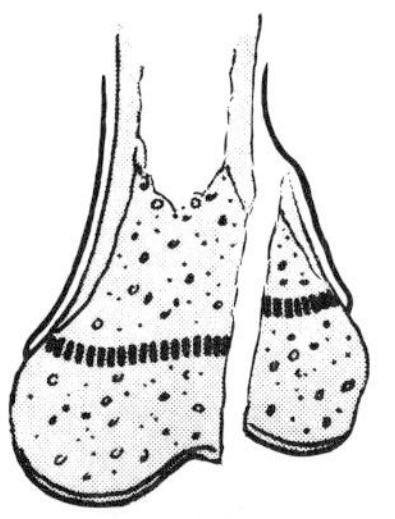

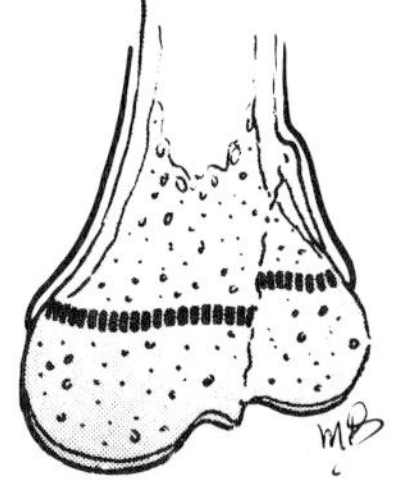

Figure 22–14. Type 4 epiphyseal plate injury. *A*, Fracture of epiphysis and epiphyseal plate. *B*, Bony union will cause premature closure of the plate.

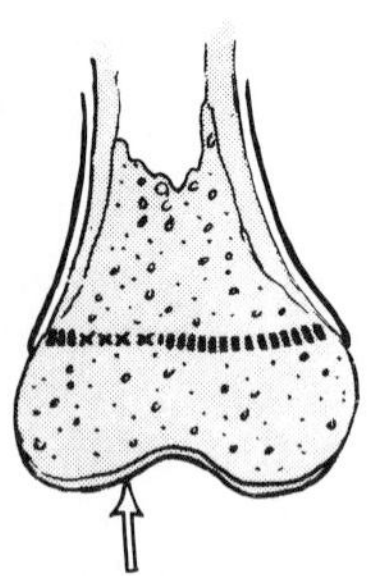
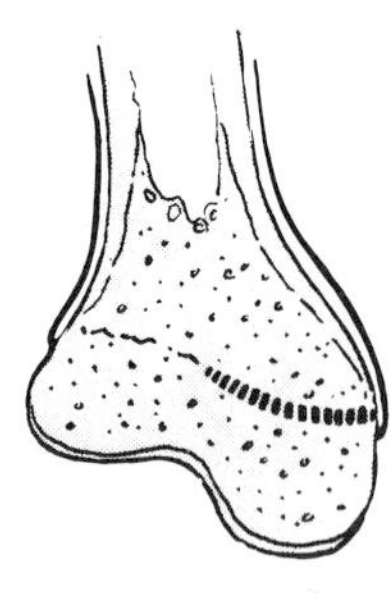

Figure 22–15. Type 5 epiphyseal plate injury. Crushing of epiphyseal plate *(left)*. Premature closure of the plate on one side, with a resultant angulatory deformity *(right)*.

area of the epiphyseal plate. It is most likely to occur in the region of the knee and ankle.

Because the epiphysis is not usually displaced, the diagnosis of a type 5 injury is difficult. Weight bearing must be avoided for at least 3 weeks in the hope of preventing further compression of the epiphyseal plate. The prognosis of type 5 injuries is decidedly poor, since premature cessation of growth is almost inevitable.

Healing of Epiphyseal Plate Injuries

After reduction of a separated epiphysis, of type 1, 2, or 3, endochondral ossification on the metaphyseal side of the epiphyseal plate is only temporarily disturbed. Thus, within 2 to 3 weeks of replacement of the epiphysis, endochondral ossification has resumed and has united the epiphyseal plate to the metaphysis. This special type of fracture healing accounts for the clinical observation that these three types of epiphyseal separations heal in only half the time required for union of a fracture through the metaphysis of the same bone in a child of the same age. Type 4 and type 5 injuries, by contrast, must heal through cancellous bone, in the same manner as any other fracture.

Prognosis Concerning Growth Disturbance

The following factors will help in estimating the prognosis of a given epiphyseal plate injury in a child.

Type of Injury. The prognosis for each of the five classified types of epiphyseal plate injury has been discussed earlier.

Age of the Child. This is really an indication of the amount of growth normally expected in the particular epiphyseal plate; obviously, the younger the child at the time of injury, the more serious any growth disturbance will be.

Blood Supply to the Epiphysis. Disruption of the blood supply to the epiphysis is associated with a poor prognosis for reasons already discussed.

Method of Reduction. Unduly forceful manipulation of a displaced epiphysis may crush the epiphyseal plate and increase the likelihood of growth disturbance.

Open or Closed Injury. Open injuries of the epiphyseal plate carry the risk of infection, which in turn is likely to destroy the plate and result in premature cessation of growth.

Possible Effects of Growth Disturbance

Fortunately, 85 per cent of epiphyseal plate injuries are uncomplicated by growth disturbance. In the remaining 15 per cent, however, the clinical problem associated with the dreaded complication of premature cessation of growth depends on several factors, including the bone involved, the extent of the disturbance in the epiphyseal plate, and the amount of growth normally expected from that particular epiphyseal plate.

If the entire epiphyseal plate ceases to grow in a single bone, the result is a progressive limb length discrepancy (Fig. 22–16). If, however, the involved bone is one of a parallel pair (such as tibia and fibula, or radius and ulna), progressive length discrepancy between the two bones will produce a progressive angulatory deformity in the neighboring joint (Fig. 22–17). If growth

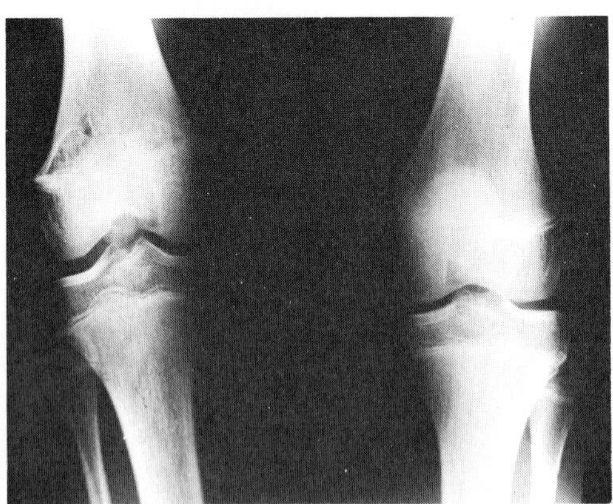

Figure 22–16. Progressive leg length discrepancy secondary to premature cessation of growth in the entire distal femoral epiphyseal plate. A type 4 epiphyseal plate injury had occurred 2 years previously in this 11-year-old boy; the discrepancy will continue to increase during the remaining years of growth.

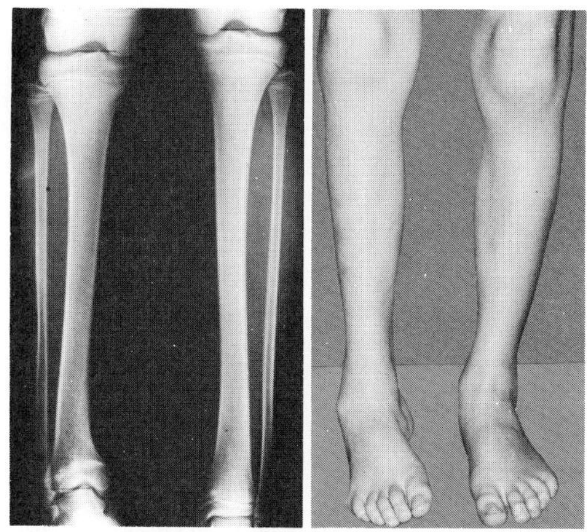

Figure 22–17. Progressive leg length discrepancy and progressive angulatory deformity in a 9-year-old girl 18 months after a type 4 epiphyseal plate injury of the right medial malleolus. Growth has ceased in the medial part of the tibial epiphyseal plate and has continued in the lateral part, as well as in the epiphyseal plate of the fibula. The result is a varus deformity of the ankle. Note also that the right tibia is shorter than the left.

ceases in only one part of the plate (for example, on the medial side) but continues in other parts, the result will be a progressive angulatory deformity (Fig. 22–18).

Premature cessation of growth does not necessarily occur immediately after an injury to the epiphyseal plate; indeed, growth may be only retarded for a period of 6 months or even longer before it ceases completely.

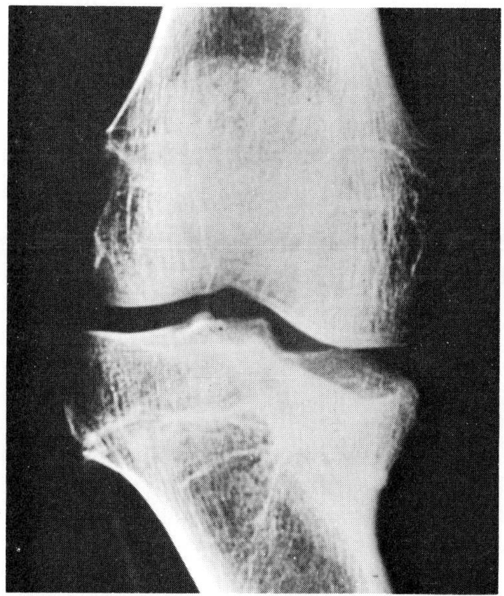

Figure 22–18. Progressive angulatory deformity of the knee in a 15-year-old boy 3 years after a type 5 injury involving the medial part of the upper tibial epiphyseal plate. Growth has ceased on the medial side but has continued on the lateral side, with a resultant progressive varus deformity of the knee.

Special Considerations in the Treatment of Epiphyseal Plate Injuries

Injuries involving the epiphyseal plate must be treated gently and as soon after injury as possible. Type 1 and 2 injuries can nearly always be treated by closed reduction. Type 3 injuries frequently require open reduction, and type 4 injuries always require open reduction and internal fixation. The period of immobilization required for types 1, 2, and 3 injuries is only half that required for a metaphyseal fracture of the same bone in a child of the same age.

It is advisable to give the parents of a child who has sustained an epiphyseal plate injury some indication of the prognosis concerning future growth without causing them undue anxiety. The child should be carefully examined both clinically and radiographically at regular intervals for at least 1 year and often longer to detect any growth disturbance.

Specific epiphyseal plate injuries are discussed on a regional basis along with specific fractures and dislocations in a subsequent section of this chapter.

Avulsion of Traction Epiphyses

A sudden traction force applied through either a ligament or a tendon to a traction epiphysis (apophysis) may result in an avulsion of the epiphysis through its epiphyseal plate. Examples of such injuries are avulsion of the medial epicondyle of the humerus and the lesser trochanter of the femur. Since the epiphyseal plates of these traction epiphyses do not contribute to the longitudinal growth of the bone, such injuries are not complicated by a growth disturbance.

Birth Fractures

During the difficult delivery of a large baby (especially a breech presentation) when the threat of fetal anoxia may necessitate rapid extraction of the baby, one limb may be difficult to disengage from the birth canal, and a bone may be inadvertently fractured or an epiphysis separated. Only rarely is a previously normal joint dislocated by a birth injury. This usually unavoidable mishap is uncommon, but when it does occur it is usually the proximal bones of the limbs that are injured.

Multiple birth fractures are nearly always pathologic and the commonest cause is osteogenesis imperfecta. Birth fracture of the tibia is rare, and when it does occur it is nearly always a pathologic fracture—congenital pseudarthrosis of the tibia.

When either the humerus or the femur is fractured during delivery, the obstetrician feels and usually hears the bone break. When an epiphysis is separated, however, it tends to slide off the metaphysis, and the obstetrician may neither feel nor hear it. Thus, the diagnosis of epiphyseal separations necessitates careful and repeated physical examination of the newborn.

Parents are understandably distressed when their new baby has sustained a birth fracture-and so is the obstetrician. However, the physician or surgeon who treats the newborn infant's injury should gently inform the parents not only that such an injury is unavoidable under the circumstances but also that is it much less serious than fetal anoxia, which the obstetrician had undoubtedly prevented by rapid extraction of the baby.

Specific birth injuries are discussed below in order of decreasing incidence.

Specific Birth Fractures

Clavicle. The slender newborn clavicle is the bone most susceptible to fracture during delivery, particularly in a broad-shouldered baby. The infant tends not to move the affected limb during the first week; this "pseudoparalysis" can be differentiated from the true paralysis of a brachial plexus injury by clinical examination (although, of course, the two may coexist). Radiographic examination confirms the presence of a fractured clavicle.

The fracture unites with remarkable rapidity, a strikingly large callus becoming apparent both clinically and radiographically within 10 days. Simple protection with a sling and bandage is the only treatment required.

Humerus. The humeral shaft is particularly susceptible to a birth fracture during a difficult breech delivery. The complete fracture is in the shaft and is frequently associated with a radial nerve injury; the latter, being only a neuropraxia, recovers completely. The newborn infant's fractured arm is obviously floppy, and the diagnosis is readily confirmed radiographically (Fig. 22–19).

The infant's arm should be bandaged to the chest for a period of 2 weeks, by which time the fracture is always clinically united. Mild residual angulatory deformities improve with subsequent growth, but rotational deformities are permanent.

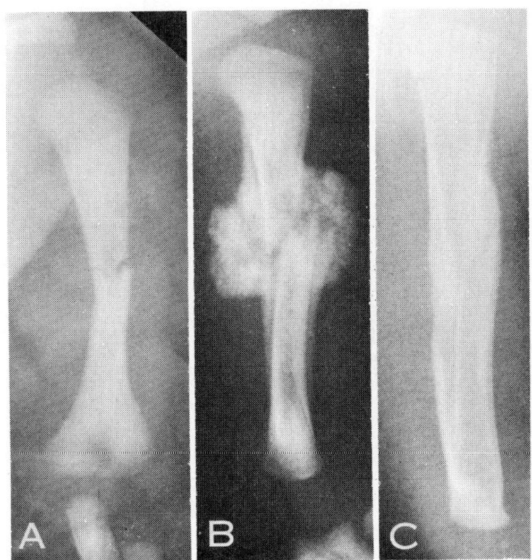

Figure 22–19. Birth fracture of the humerus. *A,* The day of birth. *B,* Ten days later there is profuse callus formation; the fracture at this stage was clinically united. *C,* Ten weeks later a remarkable amount of remodeling has occurred.

Rarely, the proximal humeral epiphysis is separated by a birth injury.

Femur. Birth fractures of the femur are most likely to occur during the delivery of a baby who has presented as a frank breech. The clinical deformity and floppiness of the lower limb are apparent, and radiographic examination confirms the diagnosis of a fracture, usually in the midshaft. Overhead (Bryant's) skin traction on both lower limbs provides adequate alignment of the fracture, which is clinically united within 3 weeks.

Traumatic separation of the distal femoral epiphysis is more difficult to recognize clinically and may escape detection until the knee becomes enlarged by extensive new bone formation (Fig. 22–20). Overhead (Bryant's) skin traction is required for 2 weeks. Since it is a type 1 epiphyseal plate injury in an epiphysis that has a good blood supply, it has an excellent prognosis for subsequent growth.

Traumatic separation of the proximal femoral epiphysis is difficult to differentiate clinically from dislocation of the hip, but the latter is rare as a birth injury. The differentiation may also be difficult radiographically, since at birth the head, neck, and greater trochanter are completely unossified; indeed, at birth the radiographic differentiation from a congenitally dislocated hip may require an arthrogram. Within 3 weeks, however, radiographic examination reveals evidence of new

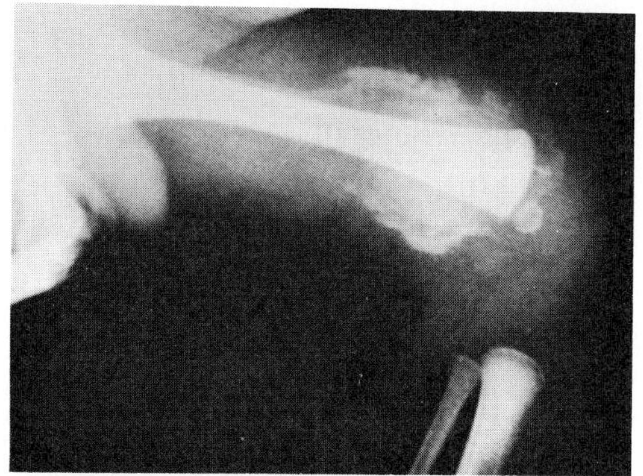

Figure 22–20. Birth injury of the distal femoral epiphysis. In this radiograph taken 10 days after birth, the center of ossification of the distal femoral epiphysis is seen to be displaced posteriorly (normally it is in line with the central axis of the femoral shaft). The marked new bone formation from the elevated periosteum would have taken approximately 10 days to develop, and therefore, by deduction, this Type 1 epiphyseal plate injury probably occurred at birth. The injury had been unsuspected at the time of the difficult breech delivery, but the radiograph was taken 10 days later because of the gross clinical swelling of the infant's knee.

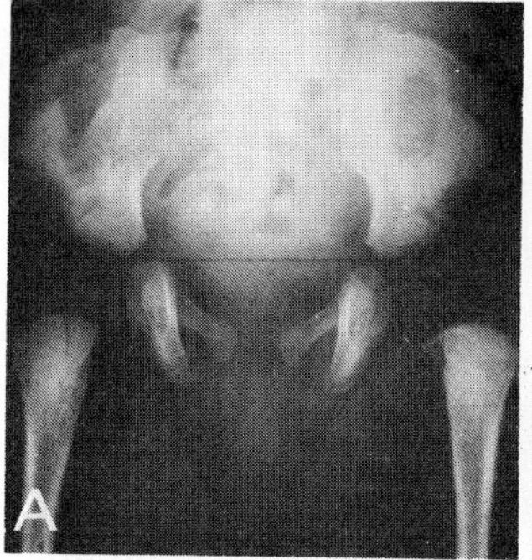

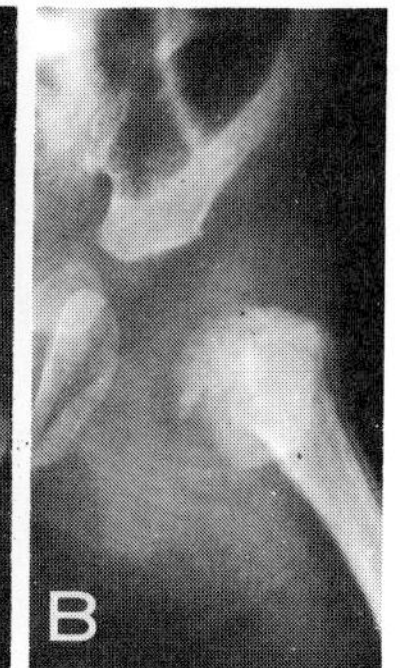

Figure 22–21. Birth injury of the proximal femoral epiphysis. *A*, Six days after birth there is obvious lateral displacement of the metaphysis of the left femur in relation to the acetabulum (the normal hip serves as a helpful comparison). Clinically, the infant was thought to have congenital dislocation of the left hip. The center of ossification does not appear until approximately six months of age. Note the slight new bone formation, however, around the metaphysis; this differentiates an epiphyseal plate injury from a dislocation of the hip. *B*, Eight weeks later there is further new bone formation and early remodeling.

bone formation in the metaphyseal region, indicating a traumatic epiphyseal separation (Fig. 22–21). Treatment consists of immobilization of the hip in abduction and flexion in a spica cast for 2 weeks. The prognosis for subsequent growth is good, since at birth the proximal femoral epiphysis consists of the head, neck, and greater trochanter, and therefore, at this stage, separation of the entire epiphysis does not jeopardize its blood supply.

Spine. Fortunately, birth injuries of the spine are rare, but they are extremely serious, since they may be complicated by complete paraplegia.

SPECIFIC FRACTURES AND DISLOCATIONS*

The Wrist and Forearm

Fractures in the region of the wrist and forearm are extremely common in childhood because of frequent falls in which the forces are transmitted from the hand to the radius and ulna.

Distal Radial Epiphysis

Fracture-separation is by far the commonest epiphyseal plate injury in the body, accounting for approximately half of the total. This injury occurs frequently in older children and may be accompanied by a greenstick fracture of the ulna. It is a type 2 injury, as indicated by the separation of the entire epiphysis with a small triangular-shaped metaphyseal fragment (Fig. 22–22). Since this fracture-separation results from a forced hyperextension and supination injury, it can be reduced by a combination of flexion and pronation. The reduced fracture-separation should be immobilized in an above-elbow cast, with the forearm in pronation for a period of 3 weeks (epiphyseal separations heal twice as rapidly as fractures through the cancellous area of the same bone in the same

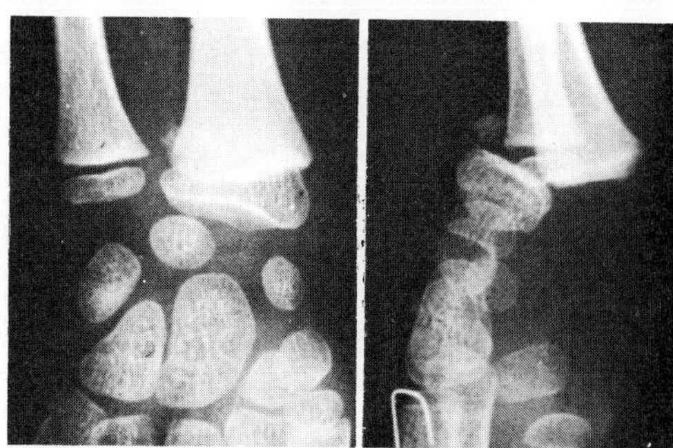

Figure 22–22. Type 2 fracture-separation of the distal radial epiphysis. In the anteroposterior projection the epiphyseal plate of the radius is not apparent because the epiphysis is displaced and angulated. In the lateral projection the backward displacement and angulation of the epiphysis are apparent. Note the small triangular metaphyseal fragment that is attached to the epiphysis and its epiphyseal plate.

*Management of hand injuries is covered in Chapter 23.

child). Because it is a type 2 injury, the prognosis for subsequent growth is excellent.

Distal Third of Radius and Ulna

Incomplete Fractures. In young children the most frequent fracture in this region is the *buckle type* (Fig. 22–23), which requires protection alone for 3 weeks.

Greenstick fractures of the distal metaphyseal region of the radius and ulna require closed reduction by manipulation if the angulation is significant. The angulation is gradually corrected to the point at which the remaining intact part of the cortex is heard and felt to crack through (Fig. 22–24). Indeed, if this is not done, the angulatory deformity will not be completely corrected and may even recur during the period of immobilization.

Complete Fractures. *Displaced fractures of the distal metaphyseal region of the radius and ulna* are particularly common in childhood (Fig. 22–25). They may be difficult to reduce unless the significance of the intact periosteal hinge is appreciated. When the radius alone is fractured, the injury has been one of supination; consequently, the reduction is most stable in pronation. When both the radius and ulna are fractured, the reduction may be more stable with the forearm in the neutral position. In either case, a well-molded, above-elbow plaster cast is required for 6 weeks.

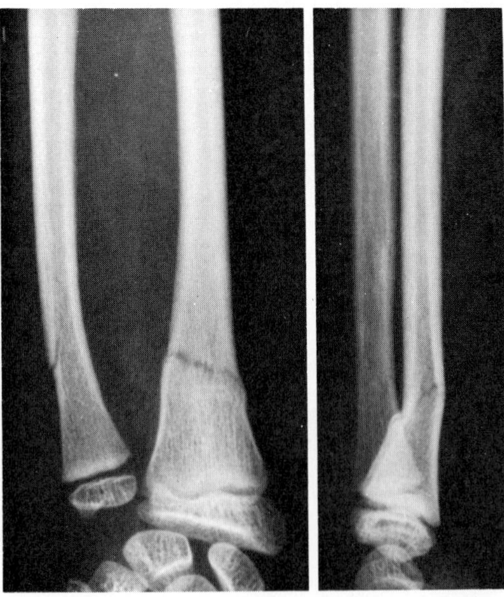

Figure 22–23. Buckle fracture of the distal metaphysis of the radius and a crack fracture of the ulna in a child. The angulation deformity with buckling or crumpling of the thin dorsal cortex is apparent in the lateral projection. This is sometimes referred to as a "torus" fracture because of the ridge on the cortex (torus, L means ridge or protuberance).

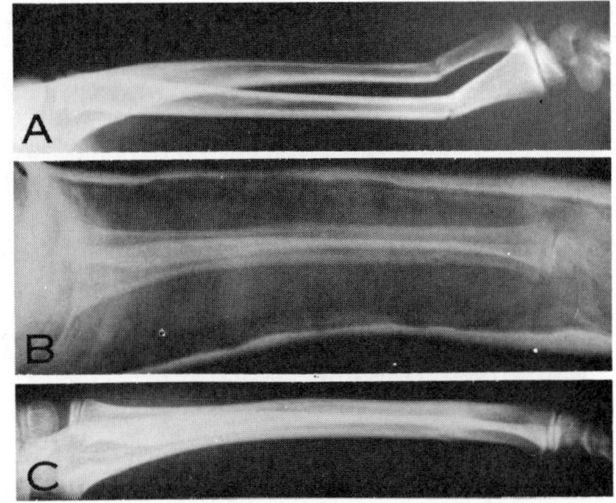

Figure 22–24. Greenstick fractures of the distal third of the radius and ulna, with anterior angulation, in a 7-year-old boy. *B*, Reduced position of the fractures in a plaster cast; the remaining intact portion of the cortex of each bone was deliberately cracked through at the time of reduction. *C*, Six weeks later both fractures have united in a satisfactory position.

Moderate residual angulation, either anterior or posterior, though not desirable, is acceptable, since it tends to correct spontaneously with subsequent growth, mentioned earlier (Fig. 22–2).

Middle Third of Radius and Ulna

Greenstick fractures of the middle third of the radius and ulna can be completely reduced by

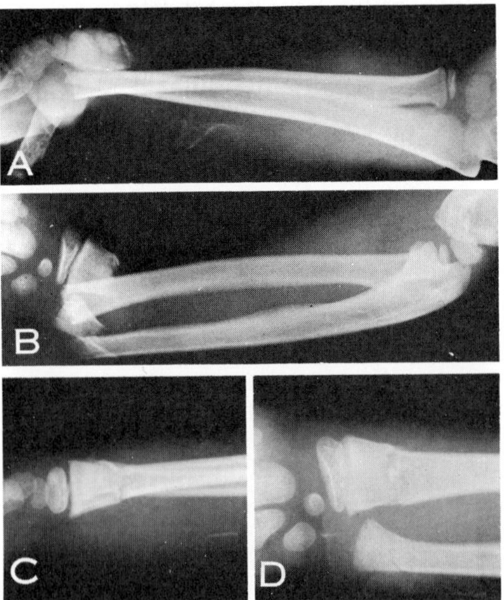

Figure 22–25. Displaced fractures of the distal metaphysis of the radius and ulna, with marked overriding. *A* and *B*, Before reduction. *C* and *D*, Immediately after closed reduction, utilizing the intact periosteal hinge.

a closed manipulation provided that the practice of cracking through the remaining intact part of the cortex is utilized (Fig. 22–26). Indeed, unless the angulatory deformity is well corrected, the normal rotation of the radius around the ulna during supination and pronation will be permanently restricted.

Displaced fractures of the middle third of the radius and ulna are unstable and may be difficult to reduce and to keep reduced. Just how much of the fracture deformity is due to angulation and how much is due to rotation is often better assessed by looking at the child's two forearms than by looking at the radiographs.

Both angulation and rotation at the fracture site must be corrected, but side-to-side (bayonet) apposition of both fractures is acceptable. Nevertheless, it is usually possible to obtain end-to-end apposition first of one fracture and then of the other, after which the most stable position of the reductions can be assessed. It is usually, but not invariably, the midposition between supination and pronation. Immobilization in a well-molded, above-elbow cast, with the forearm in the most stable position, should be maintained for 8 weeks (healing through cortical bone is slower than through cancellous bone).

Unstable fractures of both bones of the forearm should be examined radiographically each week for at least 4 weeks in order to detect any deterioration in the position of the fragments (Fig. 22–27). If angulation recurs during the period of immobilization, remanipulation is best performed about 2 weeks after the injury, at which time the fracture sites have become "sticky" and the reduction is likely to be more stable. Loss of apposition with resultant overriding should be corrected by remanipulation as soon as it is recognized.

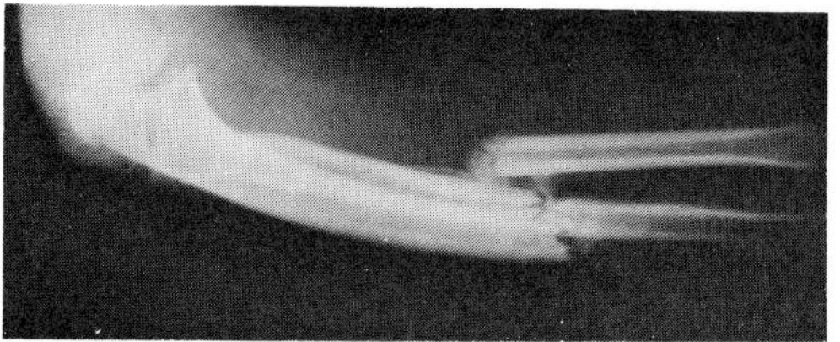

Figure 22–27. Displaced fractures of the middle third of the radius and ulna of a 15-year-old child. Six weeks after injury, the position of the fragments is obviously unsatisfactory; the ulna is out to length but there is marked overriding of the radial fracture and a rotational deformity at both fracures. At this time (after 6 weeks of healing), the fractures could not be reduced by closed manipulation, and consequently, open reduction and intenal fixation were required. Closed reduction would have been possible at an earlier stage had the loss of position of the fragments been detected by repeated radiographic examinations during the first few weeks.

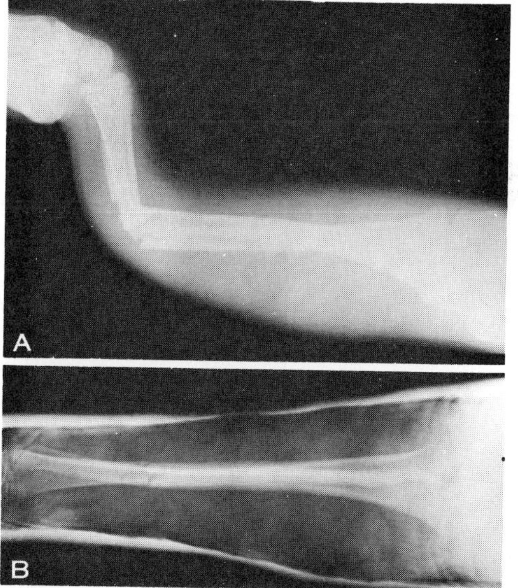

Figure 22–26. Greenstick fractures of the middle third of the radius and ulna of a 14-year-old boy. *A*, Note the gross angulation. *B*, Reduced position of the fractures in a plaster cast; the remaining intact portion of the cortex of each bone was deliberately cracked through at the time of reduction.

Fractures of both bones of the forearm in children may be difficult to treat and often are not treated well. There is virtually no indication for open reduction of these fractures in children. Some of the pitfalls of treatment are depicted as examples in order to show how to avoid them (Figs. 22–28 and 22–29).

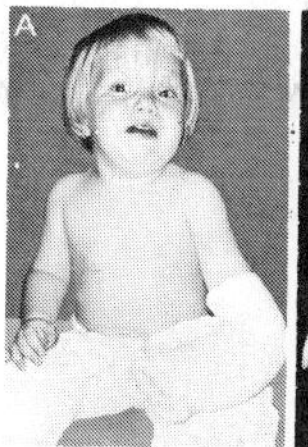

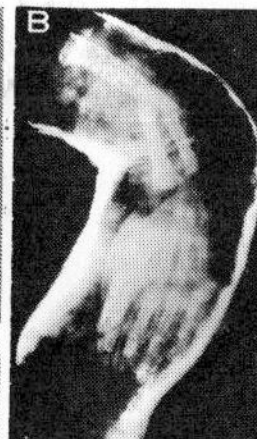

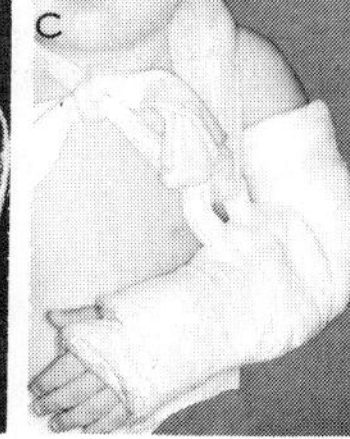

Figure 22–28. Avoidable pitfall in the treatment of fractures of both bones of the forearm in a child. *A*, This 2-year-old child has reason to cry. The incorrectly applied above-elbow cast for her fractured forearm had been gradually slipping off during the preceding three days. Note that the fingers have disappeared into the cast and that the elbow of the cast is no longer at the level of the child's elbow. It is on the way to becoming a "shopping bag cast," one that the mother brings back in her shopping bag. *B*, The child's fractures have become angulated, since they are now at the level of the elbow of the cast. A second reduction was required. *C*, After the second reduction a well-molded cast was applied and was suspended from the child's neck; these precautions prevent the cast from slipping off.

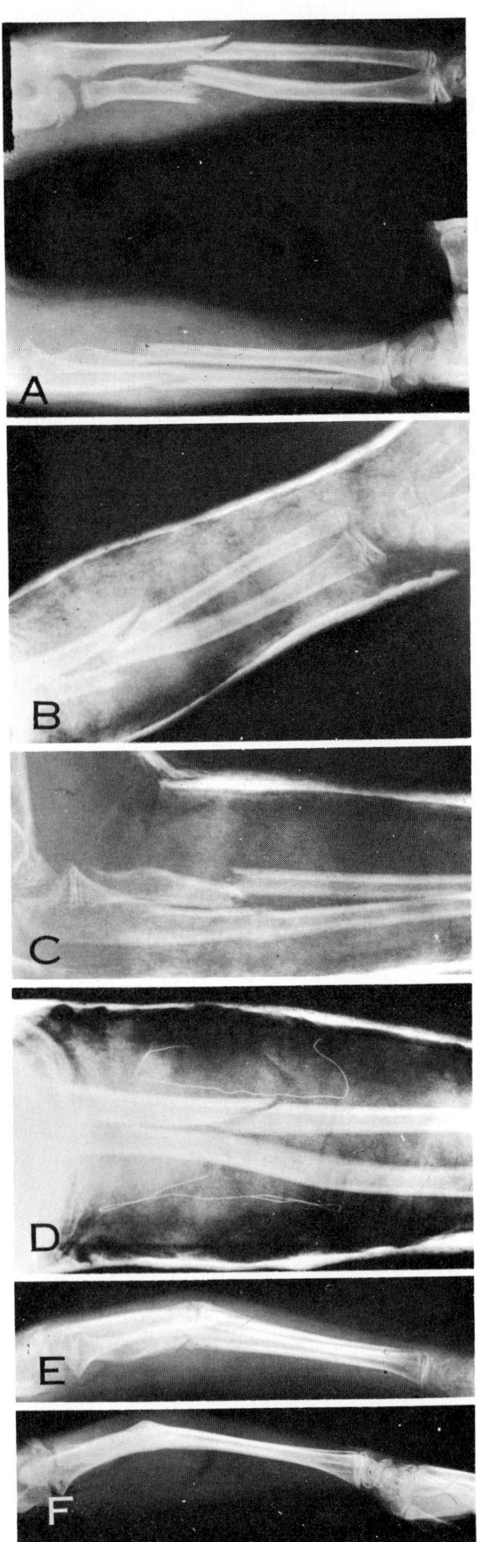

Figure 22–29. Avoidable pitfalls in the treatment of unstable fractures of both bones of the forearm in an 8-year-old girl. *A*, Initial radiographs. *B* and *C*, The position obtained by closed reduction was unsatisfactory. The surgeon did not appreciate the rotational deformity at the fracture sites. *D*, The surgeon then performed an open reduction of both fractures but failed to secure the reduction by means of internal fixation. *E*, Six weeks after injury the fractures have united with an unacceptable amount of angulation (malunion). The surgeon apparently believed this would correct spontaneously with subsequent growth. *F*, One year later the angulation remains unchanged. In addition to an ugly clinical deformity, there was gross restriction of pronation and supination of the forearm.

Proximal Third of Radius and Ulna

Fracture of the shaft of the ulna combined with dislocation of the radiohumeral joint (Monteggia's fracture-dislocation) is a serious injury not only because it is a fracture-dislocation but also because the dislocation component of the injury so often goes unrecognized and consequently remains untreated (Fig. 22–30). Because of the firm attachment of the radius of the ulna through the fibrous interosseous membrane, a fracture of the middle or proximal third of the ulna cannot become angulated unless its attached mate, the radius, either fractures or dislocates at its proximal end. Thus, the radiographic examination of a child with an angulated fracture of the ulna must include the full length of the forearm.

In children, closed reduction of a Monteggia fracture-dislocation can usually be obtained by correcting the angulation of the ulnar fracture and placing the radial head in proper relationship with the capitellum (Fig. 22–31). Immobilization of the limb in a cast, with the elbow in acute flexion, is necessary for 6 weeks to maintain the reduction. Active exercises may be required to help regain elbow motion after removal of the cast.

Neglected residual dislocation of the radiohumeral joint is difficult to treat even a few months after the injury and necessitates an extensive reconstructive operation (Fig. 22–30). If 6 months or more have elapsed since the time of injury, the dislocation is better left unreduced, since elbow stiffness after surgical correction may be more troublesome than the joint instability associated with the residual dislocation.

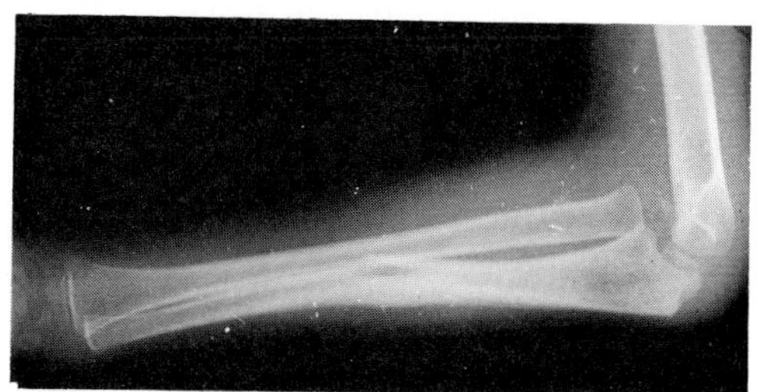

Figure 22–30. Healed fracture of the shaft of the ulna combined with dislocation of the radial head (Monteggia fracture-dislocation). The radial head should always be opposite the capitellum. The child had been treated for the fractured ulna 3 months previously, but the dislocated radial head had not been recognized. Unfortunately, at this stage, reconstructive surgery on the ulna and radiohumeral joint is required.

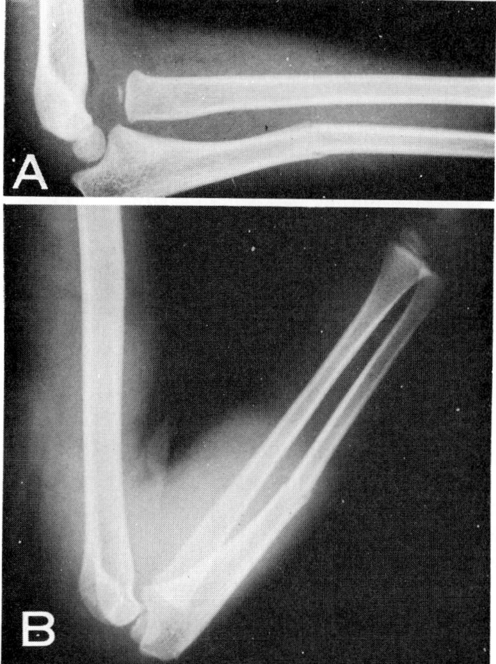

Figure 22–31. Fresh fracture of the shaft of the ulna combined with dislocation of the radial head. *A*, Before reduction. *B*, After closed reduction of the angulated ulna and the dislocated radial head.

The Elbow and Arm

Fractures and dislocations of the elbow in children are common injuries. They are also serious, not only because of inherent difficulties in obtaining adequate reduction but also because of the high incidence of complications.

One very common but minor injury, "pulled elbow," merits discussion here.

Pulled Elbow

Children of preschool age are particularly vulnerable to a sudden pull or jerk on their arms and frequently sustain the common minor injury well known to family physicians and pediatricians as *pulled elbow*.

Clinical Features. The history is characteristic; a parent, nursemaid, or older sibling, while lifting the small child up a step by the hand or pulling the child away from potential danger, exerts a strong pull on the extended elbow. The resulting injury of pulled elbow is sometimes referred to as nursemaid's elbow; although the nursemaid may cause the injury, it is the child who suffers it.

The child begins to cry and refuses to use the arm, protecting it by holding it with the elbow flexed and the forearm pronated. Understandably, the parent fears that "something must be broken" and seeks medical attention.

Diagnosis. Physical examination reveals a crying or fretful child, but the only significant local finding is painful limitation of forearm supination. Radiographic examination is consistently negative.

Pathologic Anatomy. Pulled elbow is essentially a *transient subluxation of the radial head.* For years it was assumed that in children under the age of 5 years, the diameter of the cartilaginous radial head was no larger than that of the radial neck, and that consequently the radial head could easily be pulled through the annular ligament. This assumption, however, is incorrect. Anatomic studies post mortem reveal that in children of all ages, the diameter of the radial head is always larger than that of the neck. In young children, however, the distal attachment of the annular ligament to the radial neck is thin and weak.

Post mortem studies conducted with the elbow joint exposed demonstrated that in young children a sudden pull on the extended elbow while the forearm is pronated produces a tear in the distal attachment of the annular ligament to the radial neck. The radial head penetrates part way through this tear as it is distracted from the capitellum. Then the proximal part of the annular ligament slips into the radiohumeral joint, where it becomes trapped between the joint surfaces when the pull is released (Fig. 22–32). The subluxation, therefore, is transient, and this explains the normal radiographic appearance of the elbow. The source of pain is the pinched annular ligament. The post mortem studies also revealed that with the elbow flexed, sudden supination of the forearm frees the incarcerated part of the annular ligament, which then resumes its normal position.

Treatment. On the basis of the pathologic anatomy of pulled elbow, its treatment consists simply of a deft supination of the child's forearm while the elbow is flexed. A slight click can usually be felt over the anterolateral aspect of the radial head as the annular ligament is freed from the joint. Within moments the pain is relieved and the child begins to use the arm again.

If the child has been sent to the radiology department prior to treatment, the radiographic technician frequently and unwittingly "treats" the pulled elbow while the forearm is being passively supinated to obtain the anteroposterior projection.

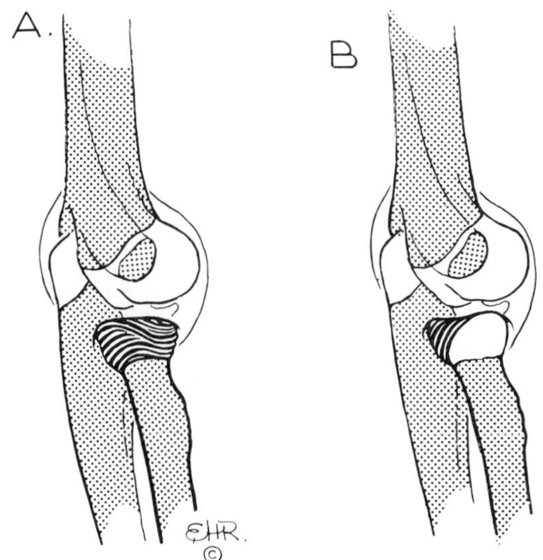

Figure 22–32. Schematic representation of the pathologic anatomy of a "pulled elbow." *A*, Normal arrangement of the annular ligament. *B*, In the "pulled elbow" there is a tear in the distal attachment of the annular ligament through which the radial head has protruded slightly; the proximal portion of the annular ligament has slipped into the radiohumeral joint, where it has become trapped.

Aftertreatment consists of use of a sling for 2 weeks to allow the tear in the attachment of the annular ligament to heal. In addition, parents are advised of the harmful effects of pulling or lifting their small child by the hand.

Proximal Radial Epiphysis

Fracture-separation of the proximal radial epiphysis is produced by a fall that exerts a compression and abduction force on the elbow joint. It is a type 2 epiphyseal plate injury with a characteristic metaphyseal fragment, and the radial head becomes tilted on the neck (Fig. 22–33).

Treatment. Satisfactory closed reduction can usually be obtained by pressing upwards and medially on the tilted radial head while an assistant holds the arm with the elbow extended and adducted.

Residual angulation of less than 40 degrees is compatible with acceptable function. Occasionally, open reduction is necessary to restore congruity between the joint surfaces of the radial head and the capitellum. Internal fixation is not necessary. Even if it has lost all soft tissue attachments, the radial

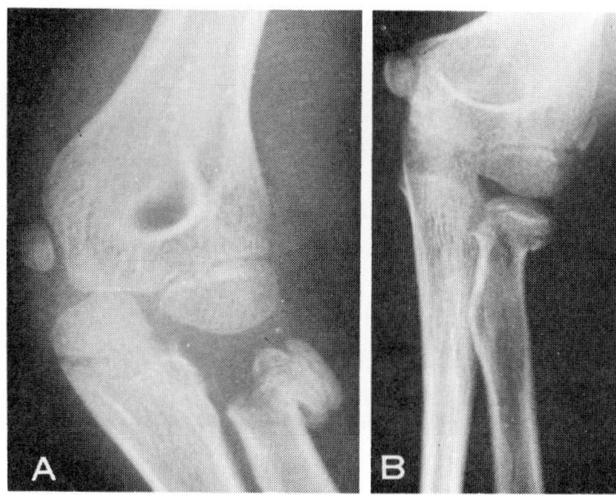

Figure 22–33. Type 2 fracture-separation of the proximal radial epiphysis in a child. *A,* Note the valgus deformity of the elbow, the angulation at the fracture site, and the loss of contact of the radiohumeral joint surfaces. *B,* The position of the fragments after closed reduction is satisfactory.

head should *never* be excised during childhood. Indeed, removal of the radial head also includes its epiphyseal plate from the proximal end of the radius. This produces a progressive discrepancy in length between the radius and ulna owing to relatively less growth in the radius. Consequently, the hand becomes progressively deviated toward the radial side. After reduction (either closed or open), the child's elbow should be immobilized for 3 weeks at a right angle with the forearm supinated, since this is the most stable position.

Complications. Since the blood supply to the intra-articular radial head is precarious, displaced fracture-separations through the epiphyseal plate may be complicated by avascular necrosis of the epiphysis. The small volume of the radial epiphysis, however, permits fairly rapid revascularization and regeneration. Little deformity of the replaced radial head ensues, but necrosis of the epiphyseal plate results in premature cessation of growth at this site and a discrepancy in length between the radius and ulna. Nevertheless, this is far superior to the results of removing the radial head in children.

Dislocation of the Elbow

Posterior dislocation of the elbow joint occurs relatively frequently in young children as a result of a fall on the hand with the elbow flexed. The distal end of the humerus is driven through the anterior capsule as the radius and ulna dislocate posteriorly.

Treatment. Closed reduction is readily accomplished by reversing the mechanism of injury; traction is applied to the flexed elbow through the forearm which is then brought forward. The reduced elbow should be maintained in the stable position of flexion above a right angle in a plaster cast for a period of 3 weeks, after which gentle active exercises are begun. *Post-traumatic myositis ossificans* may develop after dislocation of the elbow.

Fracture-dislocations of the elbow are discussed in relation to the specific fractures of the medial epicondyle and lateral condyle of the humerus.

Medial Epicondyle

Avulsion of the medial epicondyle (a traction epiphysis) results from sudden traction through the attached medial ligament in association with two types of injuries. In one type the medial epicondyle is avulsed at the time of a posterior dislocation of the elbow and is therefore carried posteriorly; as the dislocation is reduced, so also is the separation of the medial epicondyle.

More frequently, however, the injury that avulses the medial epicondyle is severe abduction of the extended elbow with or without a transient lateral dislocation of the joint; the medial epicondyle is carried distally. There is marked local swelling and tenderness. In the absence of a permanent lateral dislocation of the elbow, radiographic examination reveals only moderate separation of the medial epicondyle from the distal end of the humerus (Fig. 22–34). If there is doubt about the diagnosis, comparable radiographic projections of the opposite elbow are helpful.

Treatment. Stability of the elbow joint is the most important aspect of this second type of avulsion injury. It should always be assessed while the patient is under general anesthesia to determine the optimum form of treatment. If the elbow is stable when subjected to an abduction force, the relatively slight separation of the medial epicondyle requires only immobilization with the elbow in flexion for 3 weeks. Under these circumstances, even if the epicondyle heals by fibrous union, there is no growth disturbance, and the long-term result will be satisfactory. If, however, the elbow is grossly unstable when subjected to an abduction force, open reduction and internal fixation are indicated to restore stability of the joint (Fig. 22–35).

Complications. *A traction injury of the ulnar nerve* is a frequent complication of the abduc-

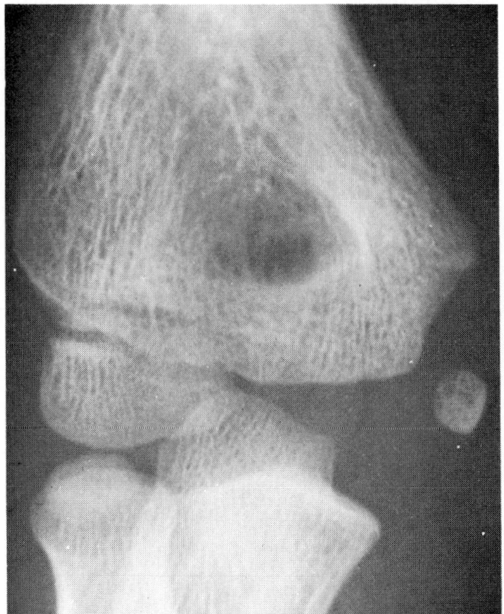

Figure 22–34. Avulsion of the medial epicondyle (a traction epiphysis) from the distal end of the humerus in a 6-year-old child. The medial epicondyle has shifted distally approximately 1 cm to reach the level of the joint line of the elbow.

tion type of avulsion of the medial epicondyle. The prognosis for recovery of the nerve lesion is excellent, and the presence of such a lesion is in itself not an indication for open reduction.

Occasionally, at the moment of spontaneous reduction of a lateral dislocation, the avulsed medial epicondyle is trapped in the elbow joint. Under these circumstances, the medial epicondyle can be freed from the joint by closed manipulation. However, since open reduction and internal fixation are indicated to restore stability to the elbow, the trapped medial epicondyle is best freed at the time of operation.

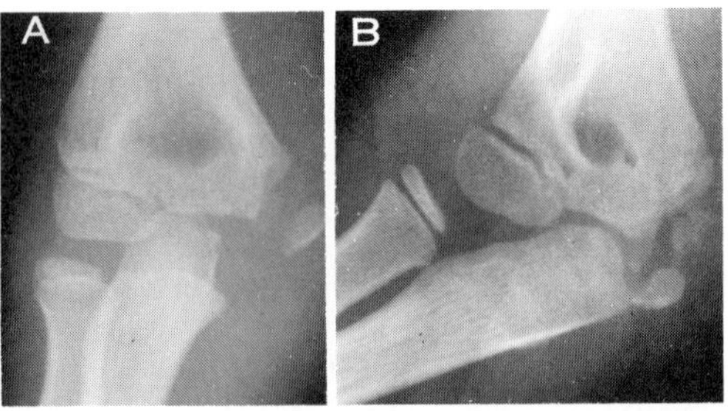

Figure 22–35. Instability of the right elbow joint of a 7-year-old boy in association with avulsion of the medial epicondyle. *A*, Anteroposterior projection of the elbow showing moderate separation of the medial epicondyle. *B*, This stress radiograph taken with the boy under anesthetic and with an abduction force being applied to the elbow reveals gross instability of the joint; the medial epicondyle has been pulled further distally.

Lateral Condyle

Fractures of the lateral condyle of the humerus in children are relatively common, frequently complicated, and regrettably often inadequately treated. The fracture line begins at the joint surface, passes through the cartilaginous portion of the epiphysis medial to the capitellum, crosses the epiphyseal plate, and extends into the metaphysis. Thus, a fracture of the lateral condyle represents a type 4 epiphyseal plate injury, the seriousness of which was discussed earlier (Fig. 22–14).

These fractures are inherently unstable, since they are predominantly intra-articular. The only periosteal covering is on the metaphyseal fragment, and this is frequently completely disrupted. Consequently, even when the fracture appears undisplaced initially, it has a tendency to become displaced subsequently with serious sequelae.

Radiographically, an undisplaced fracture of the lateral condyle may escape detection unless comparable projections of the opposite elbow are obtained. The lateral condyle (which includes the capitellum and the lateral portion of the metaphysis) may be relatively undisplaced, moderately angulated, or even completely distracted and rotated (Fig. 22–36). With severe injuries, there even may be an associated dislocation of the elbow and hence a fracture-dislocation.

Treatment. Even undisplaced fractures of the lateral condyle are potentially serious because of their instability. They may be treated initially by immobilization of the arm in a plaster cast with the elbow at a right angle. During the first 2 weeks, repeated radiographic examinations are essential, since even during immobilization the fracture may become displaced, in which case immediate open reduction and internal fixation are indicated.

Displaced fractures of the lateral condyle represent one of the relatively few absolute indications for open reduction and internal fixation in children. Since these fractures are type 4 epiphyseal plate injuries, even relatively minor displacement must be perfectly reduced, and the reduction must be constantly maintained by internal fixation to avoid an otherwise inevitable growth disturbance (Fig. 22–36*D*). After operation, the arm should be immobilized in a plaster cast, with the elbow at a right angle, for 3 weeks. The

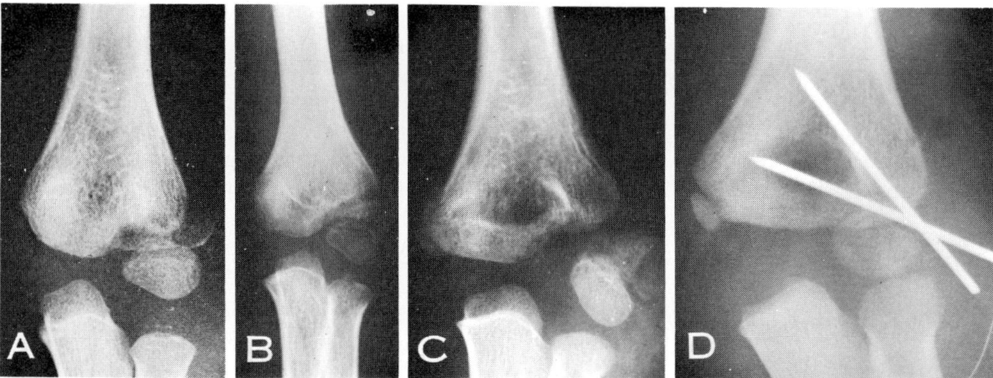

Figure 22–36. Fractures of the lateral condyle of the humerus in children, a Type 4 epiphyseal plate injury. *A*, Relatively undisplaced. *B*, Moderately angulated. *C*, Completely distracted and rotated. *D*, After open reduction and internal fixation of the fracture with Kirschner wires.

metallic internal fixation (usually Kirschner wires) should then be removed, and gentle active exercises should be started.

Complications. If the union is delayed because of inadequate fixation, the associated hyperemia may cause an overgrowth on the lateral side of the elbow, with resultant cubitus varus (loss of carrying angle) (Fig. 22–37*A*). Failure to obtain and maintain perfect reduction of a fractured lateral condyle of the humerus leads to serious growth disturbance at the epiphyseal plate (Fig. 22–37*B*). If the fracture is complicated by avascular necrosis of the capitellum, there is not only a growth disturbance and deformity but also a marked secondary enlargement of the radial head (Fig. 22–38). Inadequate treatment of a fractured lateral condyle may even result in a complete nonunion, one of the few examples of this complication in childhood (Fig. 22–39). The resultant cubitus valgus (increased carrying angle) is eventually further complicated by the gradual development of a tardy ulnar palsy.

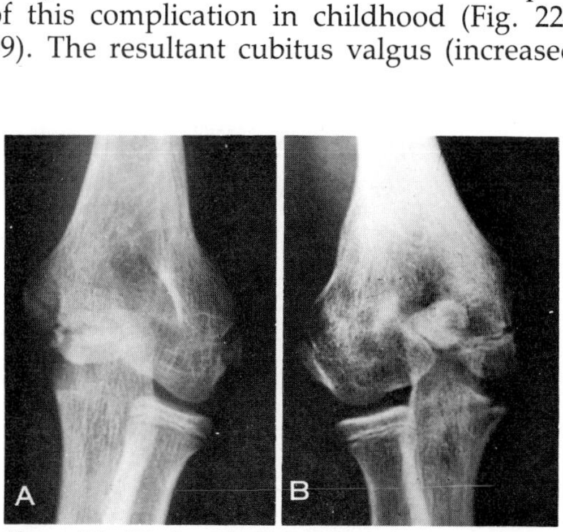

Figure 22–37. Growth disturbances complicating fractures of the lateral condyle of the humerus. *A*, Cubitus varus 1 year after a fracture of the lateral condyle due to overgrowth of the lateral part of the epiphyseal plate. *B*, Notch in the distal end of the humerus 2 years after a fracture of the lateral condyle (due to premature cessation of local epiphyseal plate growth).

Supracondylar Fracture of the Humerus

Of the significant injuries about the elbow, displaced supracondylar fractures of the humerus are the most common and certainly the most serious. They are associated not only with a high incidence of malunion with residual deformity but also with the serious risk of Volkmann's ischemia of nerves and muscles of the forearm with resultant contracture.

The following discussion refers to the extension type of supracondylar fracture, which constitutes 99 per cent of the total.

Pathologic Anatomy. The flared but flat distal metaphysis of the humerus is indented posteriorly (the olecranon fossa) and anteriorly (the coronoid fossa). Consequently, it is a relatively weak site in the upper limb. As a result of either a hyperextension injury

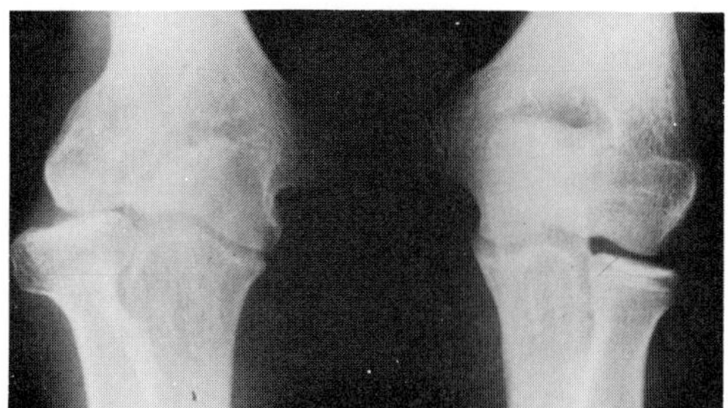

Figure 22–38. The late effects of avascular necrosis of the right capitellum, which occurred five years previously as a complication of a fracture of the lateral condyle of the humerus. Note the growth disturbance of the distal end of the humerus, the deformity of the capitellum, and the secondary enlargement of the radial head.

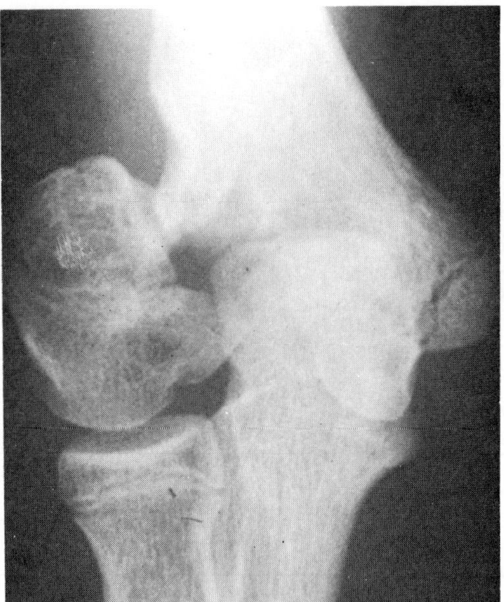

Figure 22–39. Nonunion of a fracture of the lateral condyle in a 12-year-old boy six years after an injury that had been thought to be a "sprained elbow." The boy's elbow was deformed and unstable but had a reasonable range of motion. Reconstructive surgery at this stage would be unlikely to improve the unfortunate situation.

or a fall on the hand with the elbow flexed, the forces of injury are transmitted through the elbow joint, which grips the distal end of the humerus like a right-angled wrench. Thus, the resultant fracture is consistently immediately proximal to the elbow joint. When the injury is severe, there is considerable follow-through of the fragments at the moment of fracture. The jagged end of the proximal fragment is driven through the anterior periosteum and the overlying brachialis muscle into the plane of the brachial artery and median nerve, coming to rest in the subcutaneous fat of the antecubital fossa. It may even penetrate the skin from within, thereby creating an open fracture (Fig. 22–40).

Diagnosis. Clinically, there is an obvious deformity in the elbow region, which soon becomes grossly swollen and tense as a result of extensive internal hemorrhage. The state of the peripheral circulation and the function of the peripheral nerves should be assessed immediately; impairment of the circulation demands urgent reduction of the fracture. Radiographic examination provides striking evidence of the displacement of the fragments but little evidence of the severe soft tissue damage (Fig. 22–41). The distal fragment lies posteriorly, and hence there is an intact posterior hinge of periosteum. In addition, the distal fragment is displaced either medially or laterally, but more often the former. When it is displaced medially, there is an intact medial hinge of periosteum, whereas when it is displaced laterally, there is an intact lateral hinge; these facts are important in relation to treatment.

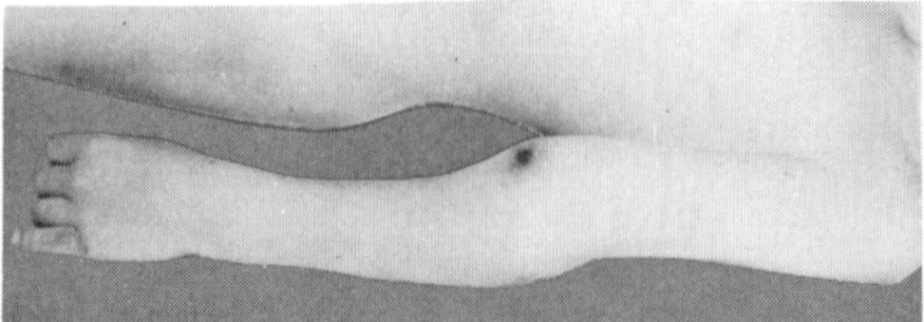

Figure 22–40. Clinical appearance of a child's arm with an open supracondylar fracture of the humerus. Note the wound in the antecubital fossa (the fracture was open from within), the gross swelling, and the striking extension deformity just proximal to the elbow joint.

Treatment. Undisplaced supracondylar fractures require only immobilization of the arm, with the elbow flexed, for 3 weeks. Most displaced supracondylar fractures of the humerus can be treated by closed reduction, which is made possible by utilizing the intact periosteal hinge. Thus, gentle traction on the forearm (with the elbow slightly flexed to avoid traction on the brachial artery) brings the fragments into general alignment, after which any rotational deformity and any medial or lateral displacement are corrected. At this stage—and not before—the elbow is flexed beyond a right angle. This maneuver tightens the posterior hinge of periosteum and helps to maintain the reduction. If the

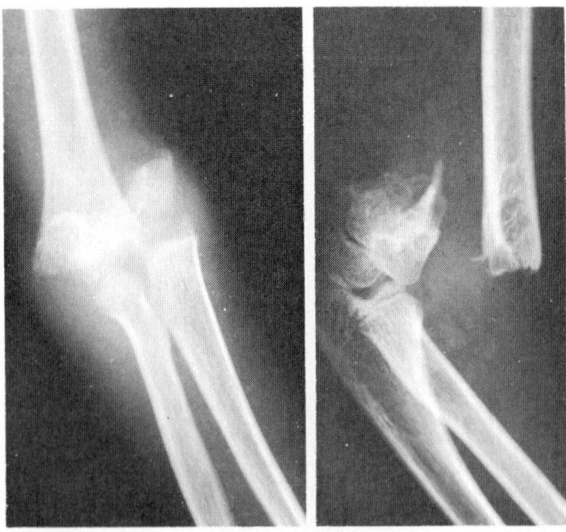

Figure 22–41. Displaced supracondylar fracture of the right humerus in a 7-year-old girl. *A*, In the anteroposterior projection the distal fragment of the humerus is displaced medially and proximally. *B*, In the lateral projection the distal fragment is displaced posteriorly and proximally. The jagged end of the proximal fragment is lying in the soft tissue of the antecubital fossa.

distal fragment was originally displaced medially, the forearm is pronated, since this tightens the medial hinge and closes the fracture line on the lateral side, thereby preventing any varus deformity at the fracture site. If, however, the distal fragment was displaced laterally, the forearm is supinated, since this tightens the lateral hinge and closes the fracture on the medial side, thereby preventing any valgus deformity at the fracture site.

After reduction of the fracture, anteroposterior (AP) and lateral radiographs are obtained by rotating the tube of the x-ray machine (rather than by rotating the child's arm) so that the reduction is not lost (Fig. 22–42). The peripheral circulation is again assessed, and if it is inadequate, the elbow must be allowed to extend slightly. The child's arm is then immobilized in a special type of cast that does not constrict the area of maximal swelling (Fig. 22–43).

Children who require closed reduction of a supracondylar fracture of the humerus should be admitted to the hospital for at least a few days of observation, with particular reference to peripheral circulation in the limb. A well-reduced fracture is stable and hence comfortable; persistent pain may be a warning signal of ischemia and should not be masked by sedation. Repeated radiographic examinations are required during the first 10 days to assess the position of the fracture fragments within the cast.

Healing of supracondylar fractures is rapid, and consequently, the cast should always be removed after 3 weeks. Immobilization for a more prolonged period is nearly always followed by prolonged elbow joint stiffness, even in children, because of the extensive soft tissue damage.

After removal of the cast, the child's elbow always lacks extension. Active exercises are

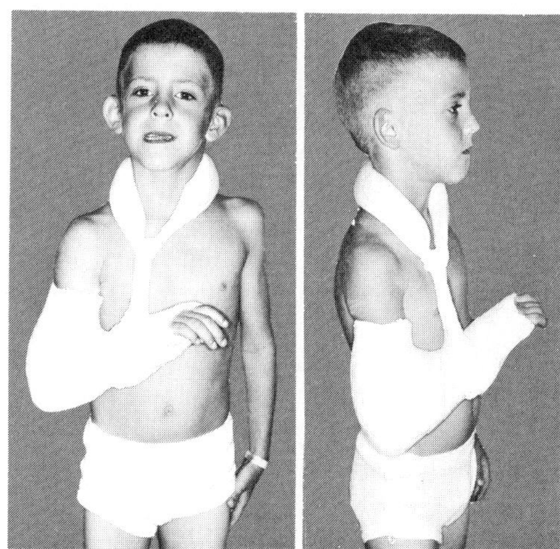

Figure 22–43. Above-elbow cast with neck sling attached for immobilization of a reduced supracondylar fracture of the humerus. The cast maintains the elbow in flexion and the forearm in pronation. Note that it does not extend into the antecubital fossa and therefore does not constrict the soft tissue in the region of the elbow.

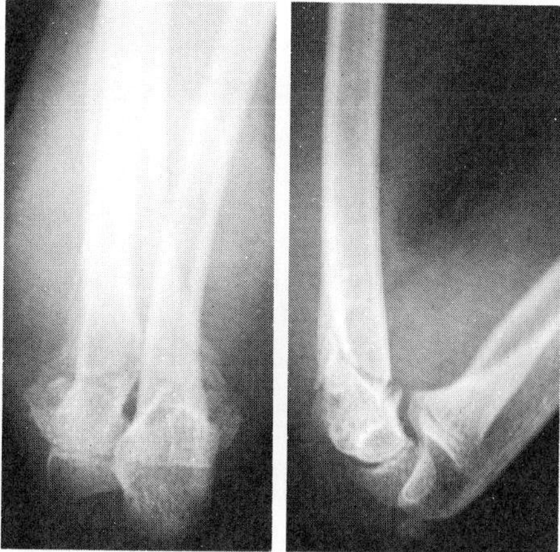

Figure 22–42. After closed reduction of the supracondylar fracture shown in Figure 22–41, the position of the fragments is satisfactory. *A*, The anteroposterior projection is taken with the elbow flexed. *B*, The position of the arm has not been altered for the lateral projection. Flexion of the elbow helps to maintain the reduction.

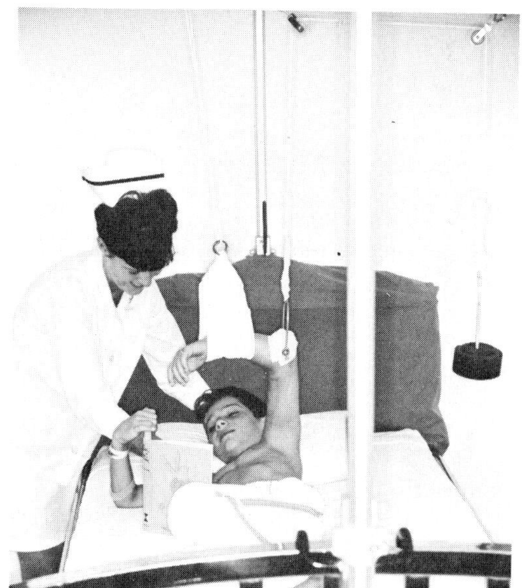

Figure 22–44. Continuous skeletal traction through a pin in the olecranon for a grossly unstable supracondylar fracture of the humerus. The position of the fragments must be monitored every few days by radiographic examination during the first 2 weeks so that the line and amount of traction may be adjusted as necessary to prevent malunion.

the only safe way of regaining joint motion and may have to be carried out for several months or even longer before a full range of motion is regained. Passive stretching of the joint is decidedly deleterious and should always be avoided.

Supracondylar fractures in which the reduction is grossly unstable as well as those with excessive soft tissue swelling or impairment of circulation are best treated by continuous skeletal traction through a pin in the olecranon (Fig. 22–44).

The rare flexion type of supracondylar fracture in which the distal fragment is displaced anteriorly is not serious. It requires closed reduction and immobilization of the elbow in extension.

Complications

Volkmann's Ischemia. The most serious complication of displaced supracondylar fractures of the humerus in children is Volkmann's ischemia of nerves and muscles of the forearm. The brachial artery may be caught and kinked in the fracture site, a complication that can be relieved only by reduction of the fracture. Moreover, the brachial artery, often contused at the moment of fracture is likely to develop severe arterial spasm, particularly if the subsequent manipulation of the fracture has been forceful or if there is rapidly progressive swelling within the unyielding fascial compartment of the arm. Excessive flexion of the elbow aggravates the tightness of the deep fascia in the antecubital fossa and may compress the brachial artery. A tight encircling cast may have the same effect.

Peripheral Nerve Injury. Although the median nerve and, less commonly, the radial and ulnar nerve may be injured at the moment of fracture, they are not divided, and consequently the prognosis for recovery is excellent.

Malunion. A common complication of displaced supracondylar fractures of the humerus is malunion, particularly residual *cubitus varus* (Fig. 22–45). Once thought to be the result of an epiphyseal growth disturbance, this unsightly deformity is now known to be the result of fracture healing in an unsatisfactory position (malunion). It can and should be *prevented* by accurate reduction of the fracture.

Malunion, if sufficiently severe, necessitates a supracondylar osteotomy of the humerus after the child has regained a full range of elbow motion.

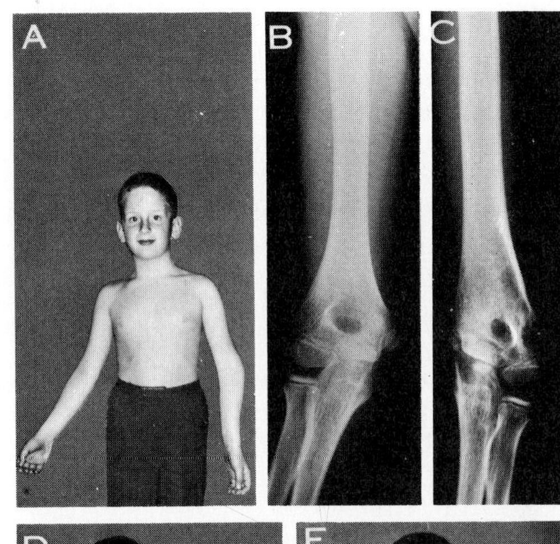

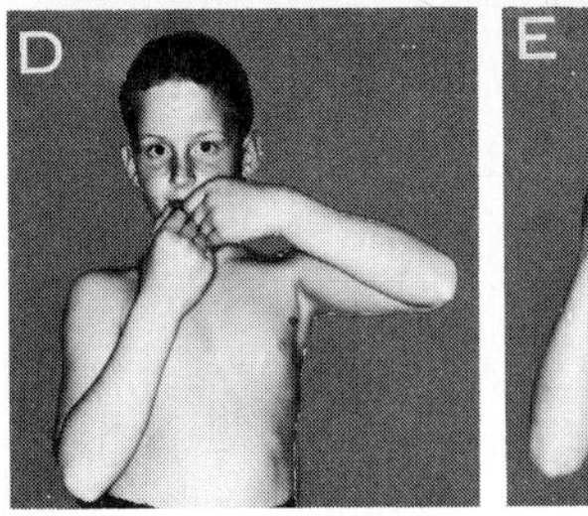

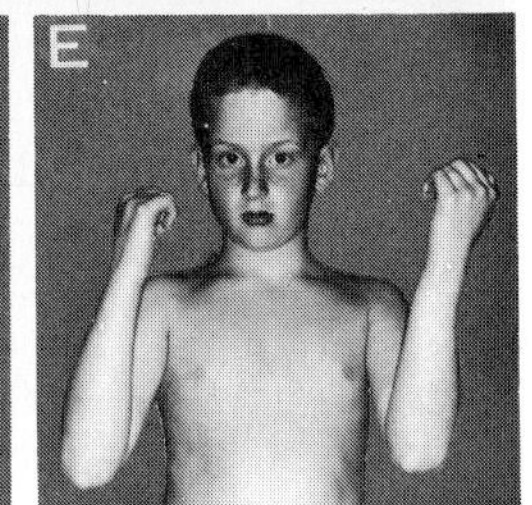

Figure 22–45. Cubitus varus (reversal of the carrying angle) of the left elbow of a 9-year-old boy due to malunion of a supracondylar fracture of the humerus one year previously. *A,* Note the unsightly deformity (sometimes referred to as a gun stock deformity). *B* and *C,* Radiographs of this boy's upper limbs. Unfortunately the supracondylar fracture of the left humerus had been allowed to unite in a varus position. *D,* Because of the altered plane of the elbow joint, the boy cannot put the left hand to his mouth without abducting his shoulder. *E,* For the same reason, his hand and forearm are deviated laterally when he keeps his elbow to his side (this could create problems for a dinner partner seated on his left side). The appearance and function of this boy's arm can be improved by a supracondylar osteotomy of the humerus.

Shaft of the Humerus

Fractures of the humeral shaft are not common in childhood, and when they do occur they are the result of a fairly severe injury. The fracture is usually in the midshaft, less commonly in the proximal metaphysis, and tends to be unstable (Fig. 22–46).

Relatively undisplaced stable fractures of the humeral shaft or proximal metaphysis can be adequately treated by a sling and a thoracobrachial bandage that binds the arm to the chest. Most displaced fractures can be managed by closed reduction followed by a shoulder spica cast for 6 weeks (Fig. 22–47). Markedly unstable fractures, particularly those in older children, may require continuous skeletal traction (Fig. 22–44) for a few weeks to maintain alignment and correct ro-

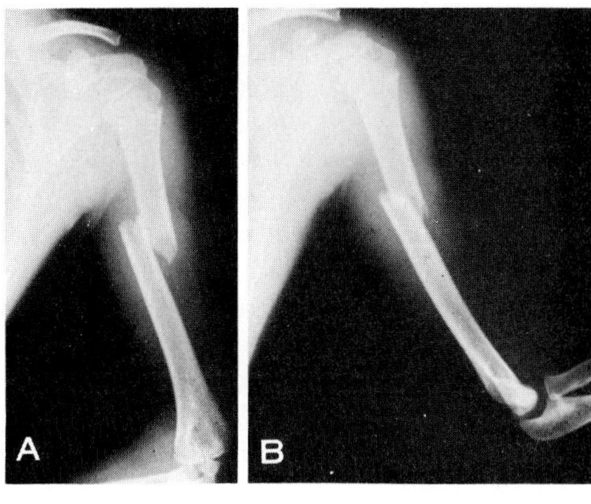

Figure 22–46. Unstable fracture of the midshaft of the left humerus in a 7-year-old boy. Prior to the radiographic examination, this boy's arm should have been splinted so that it could not be moved through the fracture site. *A,* An anteroposterior projection of both the proximal and the distal fragments. *B,* This is a lateral projection of the distal fragment but almost an anteroposterior projection of the proximal fragment. Obviously, between the two exposures the child's arm has been rotated approximately 90 degrees through the unstable fracture site by the technician. The child would have experienced much pain at this time and might even have sustained further injury to the related soft tissues.

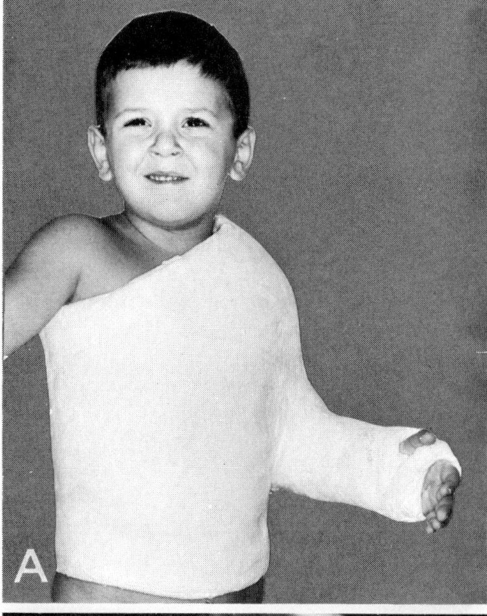

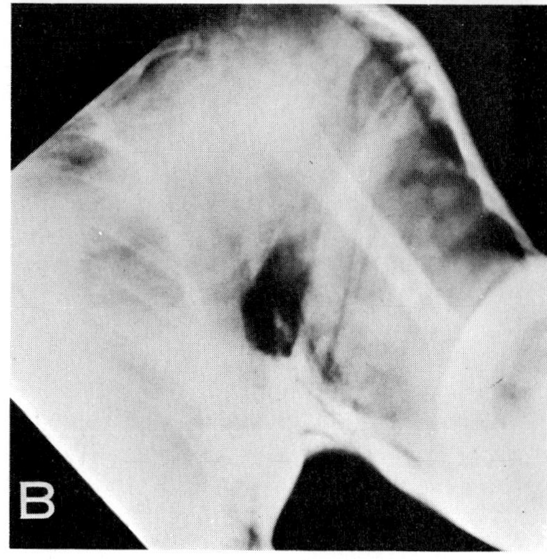

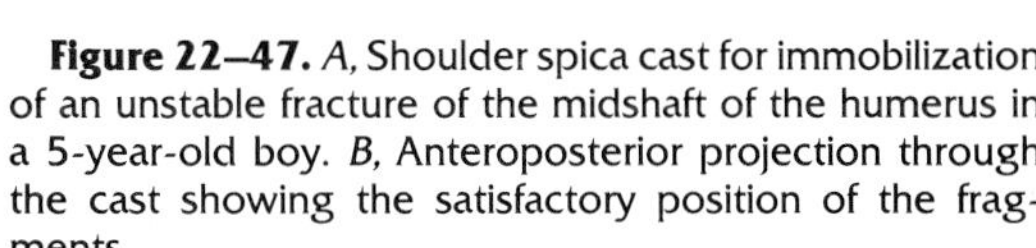

Figure 22–47. *A,* Shoulder spica cast for immobilization of an unstable fracture of the midshaft of the humerus in a 5-year-old boy. *B,* Anteroposterior projection through the cast showing the satisfactory position of the fragments.

tation, after which the fracture is sufficiently "sticky" for the traction to be replaced by a shoulder spica cast. An above-elbow cast suspended by a loop around the neck ("hanging cast") is an inefficient method of providing traction during the first few weeks, especially during sleep, and is uncomfortable for a child.

The most common complication of a fracture of the midshaft of the humerus is an associated injury of the radial nerve, which winds around the humerus at this level; the prognosis for spontaneous recovery, however, is good.

The Shoulder

Proximal Humeral Epiphysis

The type of injury that in an adult would produce a dislocation of the shoulder produces a type 2 *fracture-separation of the proximal humeral epiphysis* in a child, since the joint capsule is stronger than the epiphyseal plate (Fig. 22–48).

If the displacement is slight, closed reduction can usually be obtained, after which a sling and thoracobrachial bandage are used to immobilize the shoulder for 3 weeks.

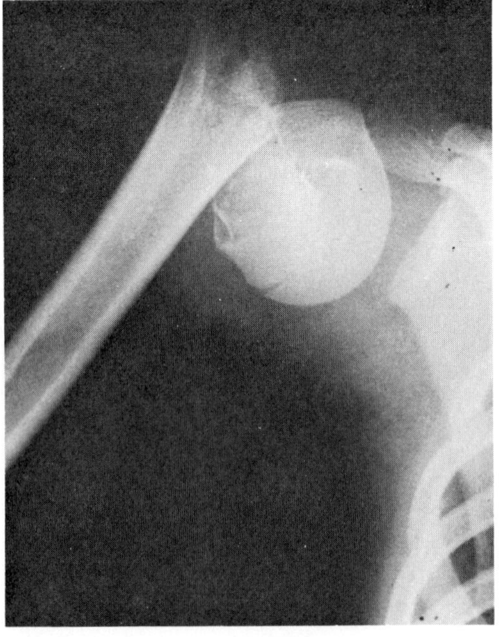

Figure 22–48. Type 2 fracture-separation of the right humeral epiphysis in a 14-year-old boy. Note the large metaphyseal fragment and the marked displacement of the fracture. The humeral head has retained its normal relationship with the glenoid cavity of the scapula.

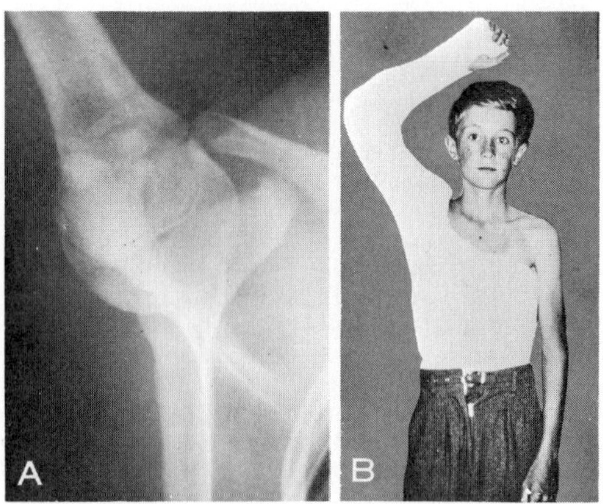

Figure 22–49. *A*, Reduced Type 2 fracture-separation of the right proximal humeral epiphysis in the boy whose initial radiograph is shown in Figure 22–48. Note that the arm is in the overhead position. *B*, Shoulder spica cast for immobilization of this boy's arm in the overhead position.

If the displacement is marked, closed reduction can be difficult unless the intact periosteal hinge is utilized. This necessitates applying traction to the arm while it is held directly over the child's head in line with the trunk, a maneuver that pulls the distal fragment into line with the epiphysis. The reduction is frequently most stable in this position. In this case, the shoulder is immobilized in the overhead position in a shoulder spica cast for 2 weeks, after which the spica cast can be replaced by a sling for an additional week (Fig. 22–49).

Even with imperfect reduction of the separated epiphysis, union occurs through the intact portion of the periosteal tube. Spontaneous correction of deformity and remodeling of the proximal end of the humerus usually produce a satisfactory result. There is virtually no indication for open reduction of these type 2 epiphyseal injuries.

The Clavicle

Fractures of the clavicle are the most common but the least serious of all childhood fractures. Preschool children, in particular, tumble almost daily, and when they land on their hands, elbows, or shoulders, their slender clavicles are subjected to indirect forces that may produce a fracture. These common fractures are not serious, however, since virtually all of them unite rapidly, and there are almost never any permanent sequelae (Fig. 22–50).

Greenstick fractures of the clavicle require only a sling for 3 weeks to provide protection

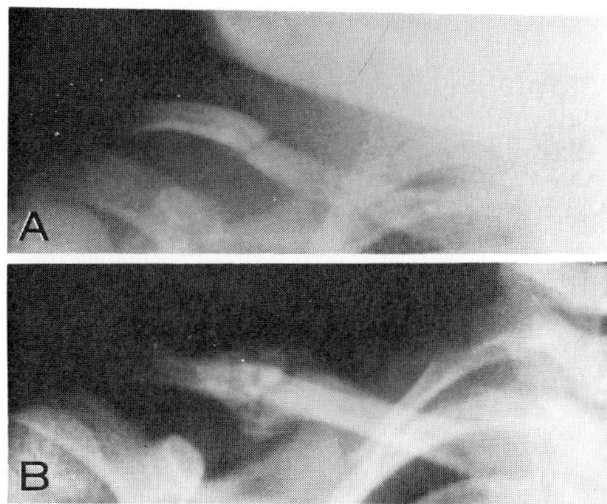

Figure 22–50. *A*, Undisplaced fracture of the right clavicle in a 2-year-old boy. *B*, Three weeks after injury there is abundant callus formation; the fracture callus was both visible and palpable as a lump.

from further injury. Displaced fractures of the clavicle in young children (under the age of 10 years) usually do not require reduction; they are best treated by a snug figure-of-eight bandage, not so much to hold the fragments in perfect position as to hold them relatively still and thereby make the child comfortable (Fig. 22–51). The parents are instructed to tighten the bandage each day as it stretches. Within 2 weeks, fracture callus is abundant in young children. The callus is even apparent clinically as a lump, but remodeling of the healed clavicle is remarkably complete within 6 months.

In children over the age of 10 years, fractures of the clavicle are more often displaced. With this age group, an attempt should be made to align the fracture fragments by pulling the shoulders up and back before applying the figure-of-eight bandage (Fig. 22–52). For older children, particularly those who are very active, the addition of plaster of Paris over the figure-of-eight bandage provides additional stability of the fracture. Even in older children the clinical results are consistently

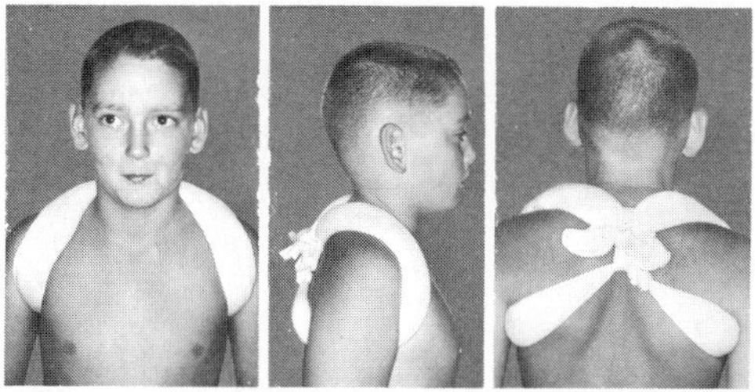

Figure 22–51. Figure-of-eight bandage for treatment of a fractured clavicle in a child; the bandage, which consists of stockinette filled with cotton wool, is adjustable so that the parent can tighten it each day.

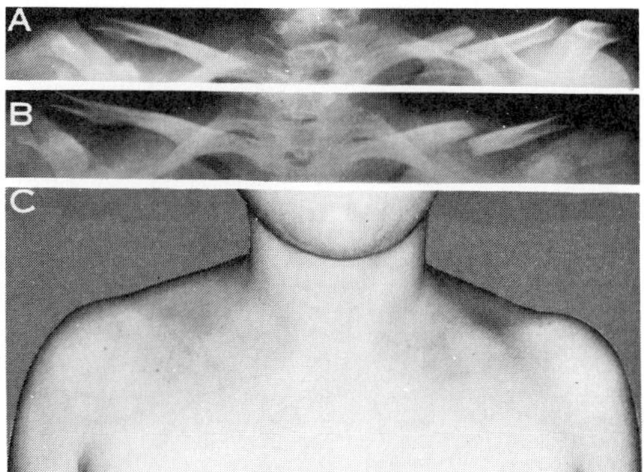

Figure 22–52. *A*, Displaced fracture of the left clavicle in a 15-year-old girl. Note the marked overriding of the fracture fragments. *B*, Three weeks after closed reduction and application of a snug figure-of-eight bandage, the clavicle is almost out to normal length; the side-to-side (bayonet) apposition of the fragments is satisfactory, callus formation is apparent, and at this stage the fracture was clinically united. *C*, The same girl 3 weeks after injury showing a lump over the left clavicle. This became inconspicuous over the ensuing 6 months.

good, and any residual deformity corrects spontaneously by growth and remodeling during the ensuing years.

There is absolutely no justification for open reduction and internal fixation in closed uncomplicated fractures of the clavicle in children.

The Foot

Fractures of the Metatarsals

An isolated fracture of a single metatarsal is not common in childhood. More common are fractures of several metatarsals, usually the result of a crushing injury, such as a heavy object dropping on the child's foot; the local arteries and veins are usually injured also. Realignment of the metatarsals by manipulation is important, but even more important is elevation of the foot to minimize soft tissue swelling, which tends to be excessive. Tight encircling bandages and casts are contraindicated because of the associated vascular injury and the risk of ischemia. Furthermore, the child should avoid weight bearing for at least 3 weeks, after which a walking cast should be applied and retained for an additional 3 weeks.

Avulsion Fracture of the Base of the Fifth Metatarsal. Occasionally, in an older child a sudden inversion injury of the foot causes an avulsion of the bony insertion of the peroneus brevis tendon into the base of the fifth metatarsal, an insertion that may be into a separate center of ossification. Local tenderness and comparable radiographic projections of the opposite foot are helpful in assessing the injury. A walking cast applied with the foot in a position of eversion provides comfort for the child during the 4 weeks required for healing.

Fracture of the Os Calcis. In children the cancellous bone of the os calcis is relatively resistant to fracture. Nevertheless, a crush or compression type of fracture may occur when a child falls from a considerable height and lands on the heels. Under these circumstances, the child's spine should also be examined both clinically and radiographically because of the high incidence of a coexistent compression fracture of a vertebral body.

After a few days of bed rest with the foot elevated, the child may be allowed up on crutches, without bearing weight on the injured foot for several weeks. Active exercises during this period help to regain a normal range of motion in the subtalar joint. In older children, as in adults, an intra-articular fracture of the os calcis may require open reduction.

The Ankle and Leg

During childhood all significant fractures about the ankle involve an epiphyseal plate and therefore should be considered in relation to the particular type of epiphyseal plate injury, as classified earlier.

Type 1 Injury of the Distal Fibular Epiphysis

Avulsion of the distal fibular epiphysis may be caused by a sudden inversion injury of the ankle. If the epiphysis returns immediately to its normal position, the child may seem to have merely sprained the ankle, since results from radiographic examination will be negative. Marked local tenderness at the site of the epiphyseal plate is an indication to obtain stress radiographs, which may reveal evidence of occult joint instability due to separation of the epiphysis, as previously described (Fig. 22–8).

Treatment consists of a below-knee walking cast for 3 weeks. The prognosis for subsequent growth is excellent.

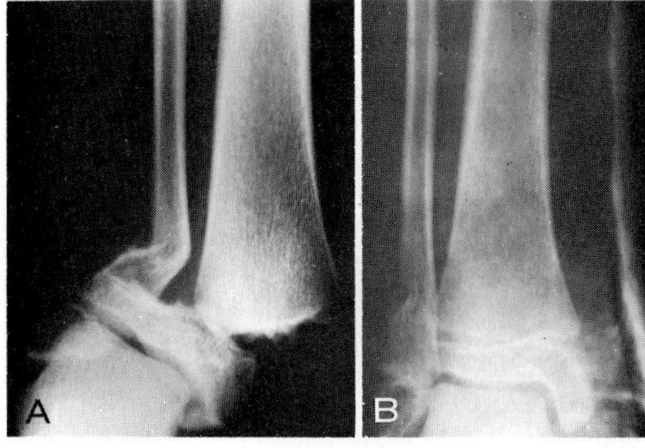

Figure 22–53. *A*, Severely displaced Type 2 fracture-separation of the distal tibial epiphysis combined with a greenstick fracture of the distal third of the fibula in a 13-year-old boy. The intact periosteal hinge is on the lateral aspect of the tibia. *B*, After closed reduction the fragments are in satisfactory position, and the reduction is maintained by a well-molded plaster cast.

Type 2 Injury of the Distal Tibial Epiphysis

Even severely displaced type 2 epiphyseal plate injuries around the ankle can be readily reduced by closed means. Furthermore, the reduction can be well maintained provided there is appropriate molding of the plaster cast (Fig. 22–53). Healing is usually complete within 3 weeks, and the prognosis for subsequent growth is excellent.

Type 3 Injury of the Distal Tibial Epiphysis

In older children who are almost fully grown, a severe ankle injury may fracture the anterolateral corner of the distal tibial epiphysis—the last part of the epiphysis to become fused to the metaphysis.

This injury is more readily detected in the lateral radiographic projection than in the AP projection (Fig. 22–54). Since the fracture is

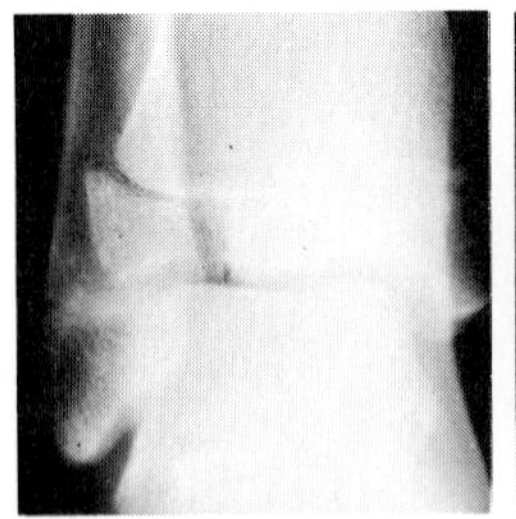

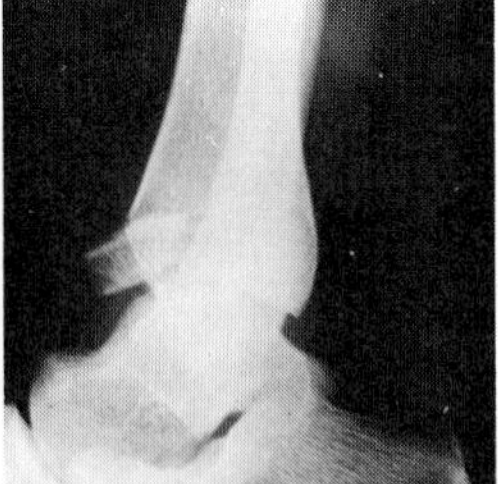

Figure 22–54. Type 3 injury of the distal tibial epiphysis in a 14-year-old boy. Note that the displacement of the anterolateral corner of the epiphysis is more obvious in the lateral projection than in the anteroposterior projection.

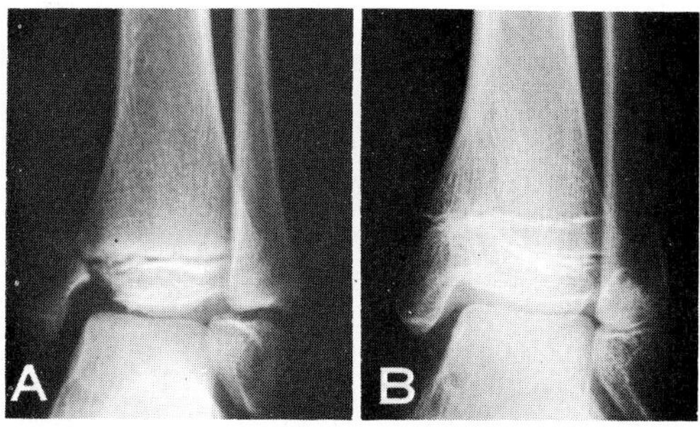

Figure 22–55. Type 4 injury of the distal tibial epiphysis. *A*, Note that the fracture line begins at the joint surface, crosses the epiphyseal plate, and extends into the metaphysis. The entire medial malleolus is shifted medially and proximally. This fracture should have been treated by open reduction and internal fixation. Also notice the Type 1 injury of the distal fibular epiphysis. *B*, One year after injury a growth disturbance is apparent; the medial part of the distal tibial epiphysis has ceased growing while the lateral part has continued to grow. The varus deformity of the ankle will be progressive.

intra-articular, open reduction is indicated to obtain perfect restoration of the joint surfaces.

Type 4 Injury of the Distal Tibial Epiphysis

A severe inversion injury of the ankle may produce a type 4 fracture through the medial portion of the distal tibial epiphyseal plate. The fracture line, which begins at the ankle joint surface, crosses the epiphyseal plate and extends into the metaphysis. Like type 4 injuries elsewhere, the fracture is unstable.

This is a treacherous injury, which requires open reduction and internal fixation to obtain and maintain perfect apposition of the fracture fragments. Indeed, even a slight residual disparity at the level of the fractured surfaces of the epiphyseal plate leads inevitably to a serious growth disturbance (Fig. 22–55).

Type 5 Injury of the Distal Tibial Epiphysis

When a child gets one foot caught, for example, between the pickets of a fence and then falls, the severe angulation of the ankle produces a tremendous compression force on the distal tibial epiphysis and epiphyseal plate. The result may be a type 5 epiphyseal plate injury.

Despite the paucity of clinical and radiographic evidence of the injury, the prognosis for subsequent growth is very poor indeed (Fig. 22–56). When a type 5 injury is suspected, the child should be kept from bearing weight on the ankle for at least 3 weeks in an attempt to prevent further compression of the epiphyseal plate. Regardless of treatment, however, subsequent growth disturbance is almost inevitable.

Fracture of the Tibia

The majority of tibial shaft fractures in children are relatively undisplaced, and this may be explained in part by the strong periosteal sleeve, which is not readily torn across. Consequently, such fractures are relatively stable and can be adequately treated by closed reduction. Widely displaced open fractures of the tibia and fibula, however, can result from major trauma, such as an automobile accident (Fig. 22–57).

Closed reduction of a fractured tibial shaft must correct both angulatory and rotational deformities. The reduction is best maintained by the application of a long leg cast, with the knee flexed to a right angle, not only to control rotation but also to prevent the child from bearing weight. After 4 weeks in such a cast, the fracture is usually sufficiently healed that a long leg walking cast can be applied and retained for an additional 4 weeks. There is virtually no indication for

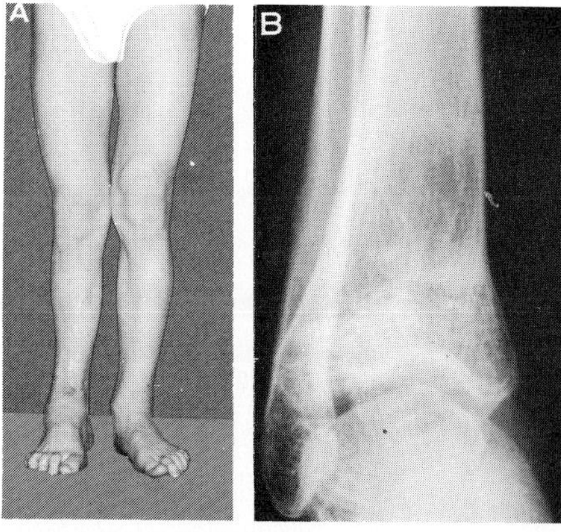

Figure 22–56. Type 5 injury of the distal tibial epiphysis. *A*, Clinical varus deformity of the ankle in a 9-year-old boy 5 years after a fall from a considerable height. He landed on his right foot and was thought to have sustained "only a sprained ankle." One year later he began to develop a progressive deformity of his ankle. Note also the shortening of the right leg. *B*, A radiograph of the ankle reveals a growth disturbance of the distal tibial epiphysis. Growth had ceased in the medial part of the epiphyseal plate because of a Type 5 crushing injury but had continued in the lateral part and also in the fibular epiphysis, with a resultant varus deformity and shortening.

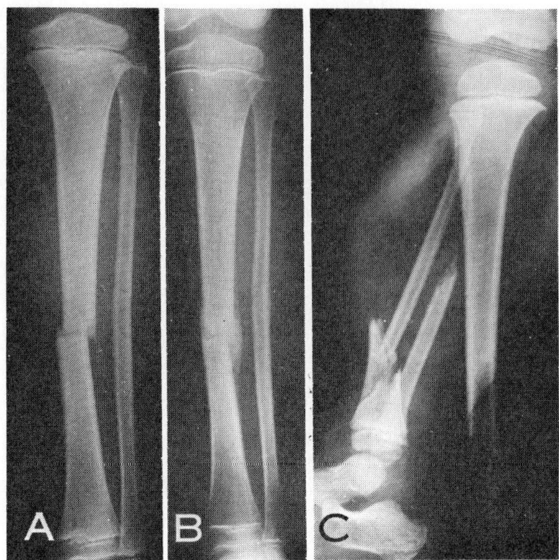

Figure 22–57. Fractures of the tibial shaft. *A*, Relatively undisplaced and stable fracture of the tibial shaft in a 6-year-old girl. No reduction was required. *B*, Six weeks later the fracture is clinically united. *C*, Widely displaced open fracture of the tibia and fibula of a 5-year-old boy who was run over by a truck. The skin was split open from the ankle to the knee, and there was extensive soft-tissue damage. Note the marked overriding and external rotation at the fracture site. After thorough debridement, the fractures were reduced and the soft tissues were repaired. Both bones and soft tissues healed without infection.

open reduction of an uncomplicated fracture of the tibial shaft in children.

Correction of alignment is particularly important when the fracture is in the proximal metaphysis of the tibia, since neither valgus nor varus deformities can be expected to correct spontaneously with subsequent growth (Fig. 22–58).

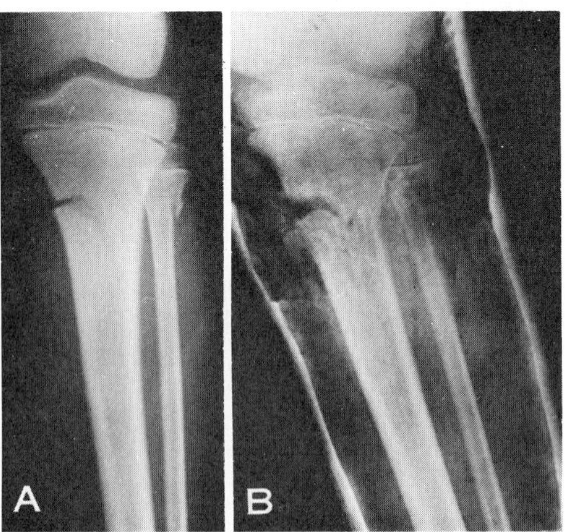

Figure 22–58. *A*, Slightly angulated fracture in the metaphyseal region of the upper end of the left tibia of a 9-year-old boy. Even this slight angulation should be corrected by manipulation, and no weight bearing should be allowed in the early stages of healing. Regrettably, the boy was treated with a long-leg walking cast. *B*, With weight bearing, the angulation increased over the ensuing 6 weeks. This angulatory deformity cannot be expected to correct spontaneously.

Fractures of the proximal third of the tibia and fibula are potentially serious because of the risk of injury to the anterior and posterior tibial arteries at the upper border of the interosseous membrane.

The Knee and Thigh

The most significant injuries about the knee in children involve the epiphyseal plate of either the proximal tibial epiphysis or the distal femoral epiphysis.

Type 2 Injury of the Proximal Tibial Epiphysis

The attachment of the proximal tibial epiphysis to the metaphysis is particularly strong because of its irregular contour; consequently, a severe injury is required to separate it. A severe hyperextension injury of the knee may produce a type 2 fracture-separation of the proximal tibial epiphysis which, though not common, is serious because of the risk of injury to the popliteal artery (Fig. 22–59).

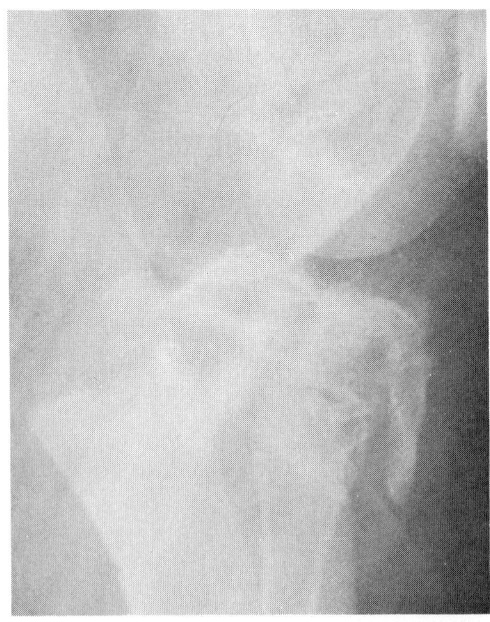

Figure 22–59. Type 2 injury of the proximal tibial epiphysis in a 14-year-old boy who was hit on the anterior aspect of the tibia by an automobile. This injury was complicated by severe damage to the popliteal artery, which necessitated local resection of the damaged portion of the artery and replacement by a vein graft.

TYPE 2 INJURY OF THE DISTAL FEMORAL EPIPHYSIS

The distal femoral epiphysis is more often separated from its metaphysis than is the proximal tibial epiphysis. A hyperextension injury may produce a type 2 fracture-separation of the epiphysis. The metaphysis of the femur tears the posterior periosteum and is driven posteriorly into the soft tissues of the popliteal fossa, where it may injure the popliteral artery as well as the medial or lateral popliteral nerves.

Clinical examination reveals a grossly swollen knee because of the associated hemarthrosis; radiographic examination reveals a striking displacement of the epiphysis (Fig. 22–60).

This fracture-separation may be difficult to reduce unless the child is lying face down. Reduction then becomes comparable to that for a supracondylar fracture of the humerus. Traction is applied to the leg with the knee slightly flexed, after which the epiphysis can be pushed into its normal position. The reduction is maintained by completely flexing the knee, since this tightens the intact anterior hinge of periosteum. The lower limb is immobilized in a cast in this position for only 3 weeks, after which active exercises are begun. Since this is a type 2 injury, the prognosis concerning subsequent growth is excellent.

TYPE 4 INJURY OF THE DISTAL FEMORAL EPIPHYSIS

Fortunately, this serious type of epiphyseal plate injury is uncommon at the knee. Because it is a type 4 fracture that traverses the joint surface as well as the epiphyseal plate, the prognosis for subsequent growth is very poor unless the reduction is perfect (Fig. 22–61).

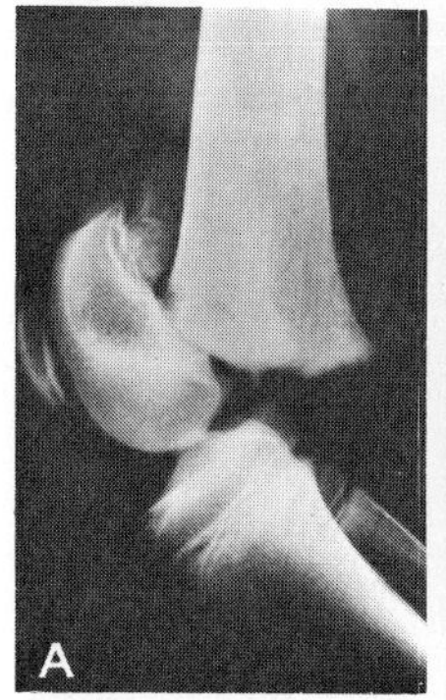

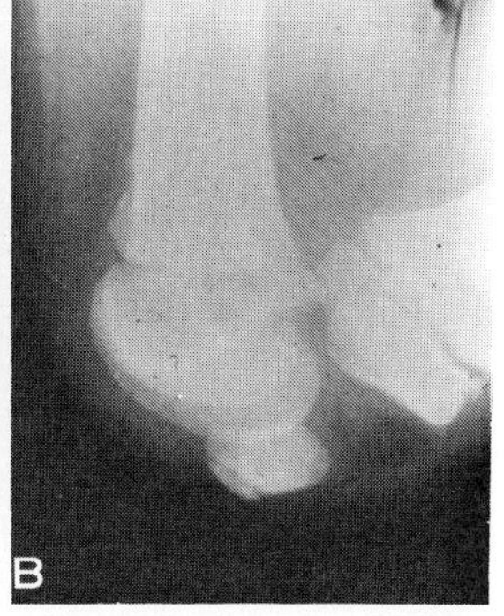

Figure 22–60. *A*, Type 2 injury of the distal femoral epiphysis in a 13-year-old boy as the result of a hyperextension injury of the knee. Note the large triangular fragment anteriorly, the side of the intact periosteal hinge. *B*, After reduction, the epiphysis is in good position and the reduction is maintained by the flexed position of the knee.

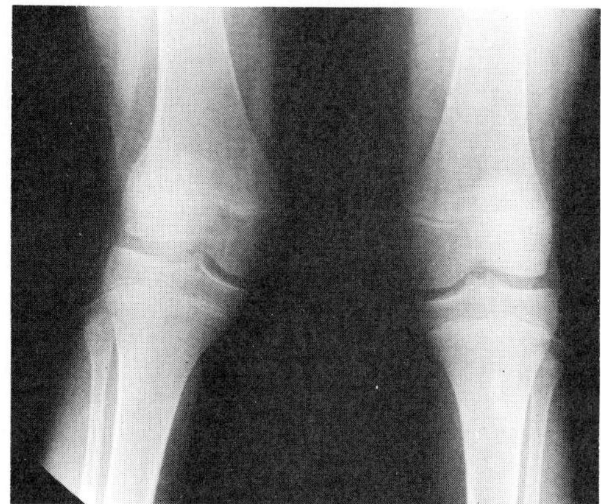

Figure 22–61. Type 4 injury of the right distal femoral epiphysis of a 12-year-old boy 1 year after injury. The fracture began at the joint surface of the lateral femoral condyle, crossed the epiphyseal plate, and extended into the metaphysis. The lateral condyle was displaced proximally and should have been treated by open reduction and internal fixation, but unfortunately it was not. One year after injury, growth has ceased in the lateral part of the epiphyseal plate but has continued in the medial part, with a resultant progessive valgus deformity.

This type of injury is extremely important to recognize because with accurate open reduction and secure internal fixation the otherwise inevitable growth disturbance can be prevented.

TRAUMATIC DISLOCATION OF THE PATELLA

Older children and adolescents, particularly girls who have some degree of genu valgum and generalized ligamentous laxity, may sustain a lateral dislocation of the patella owing to an abduction, external rotation injury to the knee. The patient experiences sharp pain, her knee gives way completely, and she falls.

Diagnosis. Physical examination reveals a grossly swollen knee as a result of a gross hemarthrosis. The patella can be felt lying on the lateral aspect of the knee. Sometimes, however, the patella has already slid back spontaneously into its normal position before the patient is seen.

Radiographic examination must include a tangential superoinferior (skyline) projection to detect the presence of an associated osteochondral fracture of either the medial edge of the patella or the lateral lip of the patellar

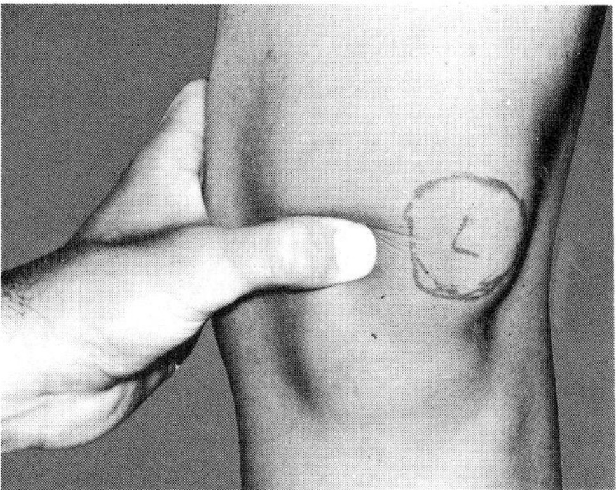

Figure 22–62. Recurring dislocation of the left patella in a 14-year-old girl who exhibited generalized ligamentous laxity. The patella could almost be dislocated by simply pushing it laterally with the thumb.

groove, the site of impact as the patella dislocates laterally.

Treatment. If there is no osteochondral fracture, the dislocated patella can be reduced by closed manipulation with the knee in the extended position. The knee is then immobilized in a cylinder cast (ankle to groin) in extension for 6 weeks. The presence of an osteochondral fracture is an indication for open operation, with removal of the fragment and repair of the torn soft tissues. During and after the period of immobilization, quadriceps exercises are important in attempting to prevent recurrence of the dislocation.

Complications. Recurring dislocation of the patella is a troublesome complication of this injury (Fig. 22–62). Moreover, with each dislocation the articular cartilage of the patella is injured, and this leads to the development of chrondromalacia of the patella and eventually to degenerative joint disease of the knee. Thus, recurring dislocation of the patella is an indication for a reconstructive operation that involves the release of tight structures on the lateral side of the joint, repair of the fibrous joint capsule on the medial side, and redirection of the line of pull of the patellar tendon by means of a tenodesis (using the semitendinosus tendon). In a growing child this type of operation is safer than that in which the tibial tubercle is transplanted, since interference with the tibial tubercle (which includes part of the proximal tibial epiphyseal plate) may cause a serious growth disturbance.

Internal Derangements of the Knee

The semilunar cartilages (menisci) of the knee in children are resilient and relatively resistant to disruption. For this reason torn menisci are uncommon in young children. Nevertheless, they may occur in older children and adolescents as a result of injuries incurred in such sports as skiing, football, and hockey.

Fractures of the Femoral Shaft

Displaced fractures of the femoral shaft are common in childhood and merit special consideration. Usually involving the middle third of the femur, the fracture may be transverse, oblique, spiral, or even comminuted, depending on the mechanism of injury. Even with marked displacement of the fragments, however, at least part of the strong periosteal sleeve remains intact, a point of considerable importance in relation to treatment and healing of the fracture.

Diagnosis. The diagnosis is obvious from clinical examination alone because of the typical deformity (Fig. 22–63). Since these fractures are extremely unstable, it is essential to apply a temporary splint before radiographic

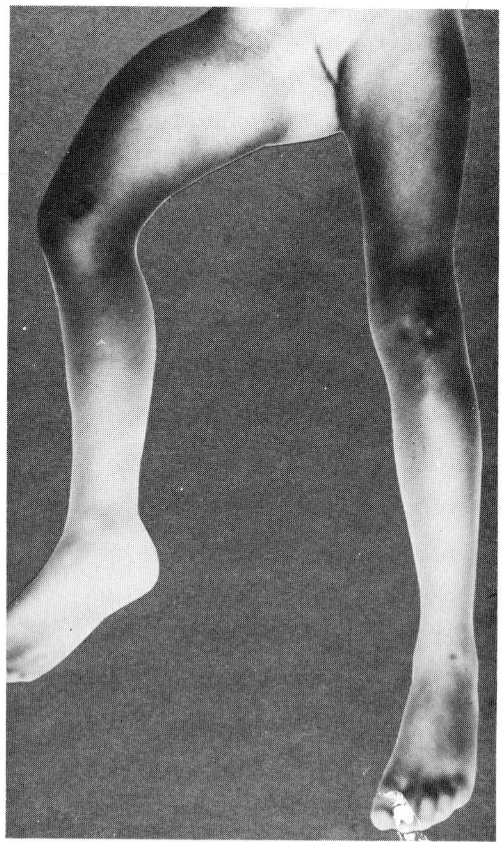

Figure 22–63. Clinical deformity in the thigh of a child with a displaced fracture of the right femoral shaft. Note the angulation, external rotation, and shortening.

examination is undertaken, not only to spare the child unnecessary pain but also to prevent further injury to the femoral artery.

Treatment. The basis of treatment for unstable fractures of the femoral shaft in children is continuous traction until the fracture is "sticky" (partially healed and hence relatively stable and painless), after which the healing femur is immobilized in a hip spica cast until it is clinically united. There is virtually no indication for open reduction of an uncomplicated femoral shaft fracture in a child. The type and duration of traction depend on the age of the child.

Children under the age of 2 years can be treated by overhead (Bryant's) skin traction, which is applied to both lower limbs (Fig. 22–64). In children over the age of 2 years, however, overhead traction is potentially dangerous because of the risk of femoral arterial spasm and consequent Volkmann's ischemia of nerves and muscles (comparable to that seen in the upper limb as a complication of supracondylar fractures of the humerus).

Thus, in children over the age of 2 years, fractures of the femoral shaft are best treated by continuous traction of the fixed type in a Thomas splint, which is slightly bent at the knee with the child lying on an inclined frame (Fig. 22–65).

Reduction of femoral shaft fractures in children is achieved gradually by the traction apparatus rather than by manipulation. Angulatory and rotational deformities must be completely corrected, since these deformities do not correct spontaneously. For reasons discussed at the beginning of this chapter, temporary overgrowth always occurs after displaced fractures of the femoral shaft. The average amount of overgrowth is 1 cm, and any residual discrepancy in length 1 year after the fracture is permanent (Fig. 22–66). It is obvious that the ideal position in which to allow the fragments to unite is side-to-side (bayonet) apposition with approximately 1 cm of overriding. This intentional shortening is compensated within 1 year by the overgrowth, as discussed earlier (Fig. 22–7).

Remodeling of the healed femoral shaft fracture is remarkable during the growing years. Although residual angulation and rotation at the fracture site do not correct spon-

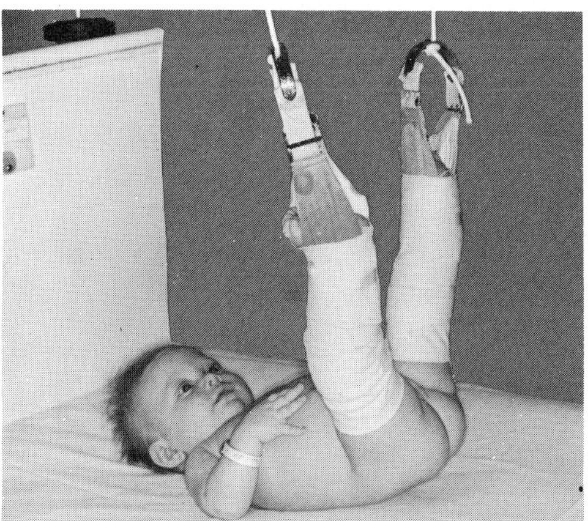

Figure 22–64. Continuous overhead (Bryant's) skin traction in the treatment of a fracture of the shaft of the left femur in a 6-month-old baby girl. Note that both lower limbs are included in the traction and that the baby's buttocks are just clear of the bed.

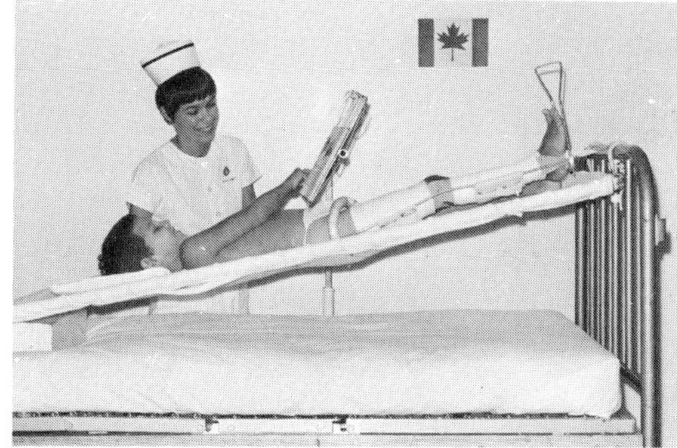

Figure 22–65. Continuous skin traction combined with a Thomas splint slightly bent at the knee for the treatment of an unstable fracture of the midshaft of the right femur in an 8-year-old boy.

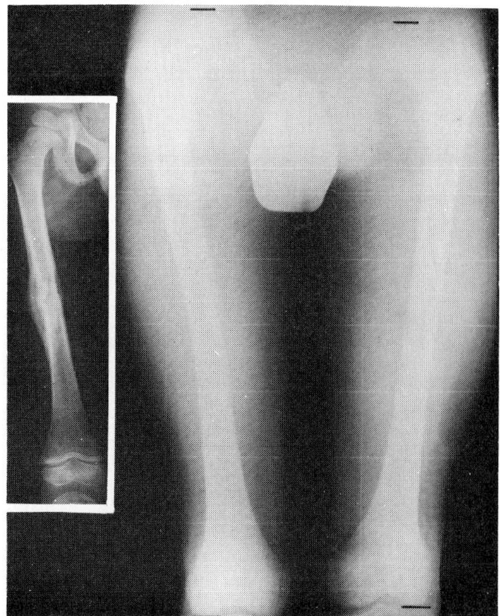

Figure 22–66. Overgrowth of the right femur after a perfectly reduced fracture of the midshaft at age 5 years *(inset)*. Eight years later the right femur is 1.2 cm longer than the left.

taneously, side-to-side apposition is beautifully remodeled over a period of years (Fig. 22–67).

Complications. The most serious complication of femoral shaft fractures in children is Volkmann's ischemia of nerves and muscles due to femoral arterial spasm. The spasm, which in turn may be secondary to a tear of the intima, is further aggravated by excessive traction on the fractured limb. The clinical manifestations of impending Volkmann's ischemia in the lower limb are the same as those in the upper limb—pain, pallor, puffiness, pulselessness, paresthesia, and paralysis. Thus, children being treated for a fracture of the femoral shaft should not be given analgesics. A well-controlled fracture should not be a source of pain, and therefore if the child has severe and constant pain—especially pain in the calf—the most likely cause is impending ischemia. Analgesics may mask this important warning signal and for this reason are contraindicated.

The moment impending Volkmann's ischemia is suspected, all encircling bandages should be removed immediately. The skin traction should be replaced by skeletal traction through the distal metaphysis of the femur, with the hip and knee flexed. If the peripheral circulation has not been re-established within half an hour, exploration of the artery is indicated. The permanent effects of Volkmann's ischemia and subsequent Volkmann's ischemic contracture are tragic (Fig. 22–68).

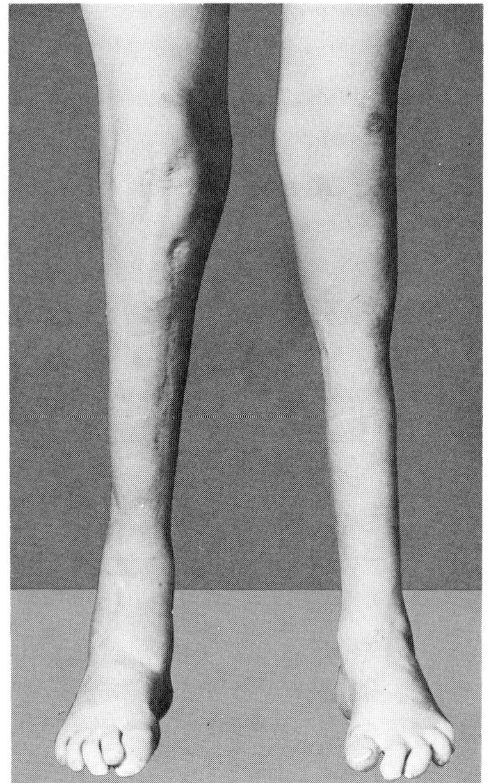

Figure 22–68. Residual Volkmann's ischemic contracture of both lower limbs in a 7-year-old boy who had been treated in overhead (Bryant's) traction for bilateral fractured femora at age 5 years, much beyond the age when overhead traction is safe. During the first 2 days of traction, the boy had complained of severe pain in both legs. The ill-advised use of analgesics relieved the pain somewhat and this masked the relentless development of severe Volkmann's ischemia until the nerve and muscle damage was irreversible. This is a preventable tragedy.

Fractures of the Subtrochanteric Region of the Femur

When the femoral fracture is just distal to the trochanters, the muscles inserted into the proximal fragment, particularly the iliopsoas and the glutei, pull it into a position of acute flexion, external rotation, and abduction (Fig. 22–69). Therefore, in order to obtain correct alignment of the fracture fragments, continuous traction must be so arranged as to bring the distal fragment up to and in line with the proximal fragment. This is best accomplished by continuous skeletal traction through the distal metaphysis of the femur, with the thigh flexed, externally rotated, and abducted (Fig. 22–70). The remainder of the treatment is comparable to that for a fracture of the midshaft of the femur in a child of the same age.

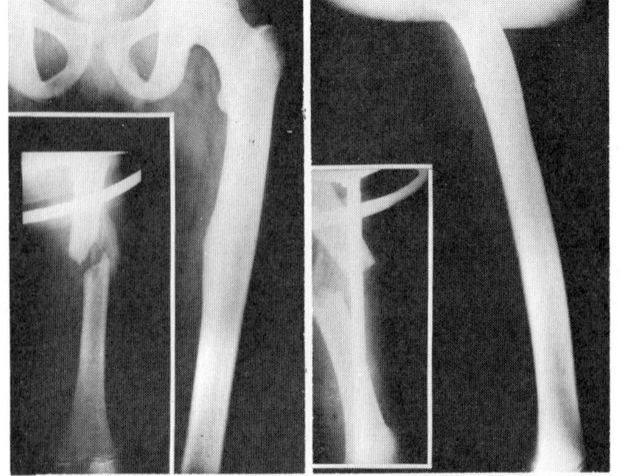

Figure 22–67. Remodeling after a displaced fracture of the femoral shaft at age 6 years *(inset).* Seven years later the fracture deformity has been beautifully remodeled.

The Hip and Pelvis

Fractures of the Femoral Neck

The femoral neck in the child, unlike that in the elderly adult, is extremely strong, and

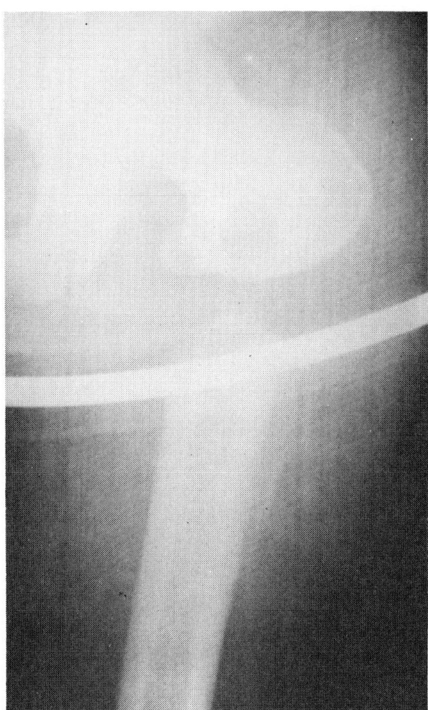

Figure 22–69. Subtrochanteric fracture of the left femur in a 14-year-old girl. Note the ring of the Thomas splint. In this anteroposterior projection the proximal fragment is flexed to 90 degrees; you are looking into its medullary cavity, which is represented by the round radiolucent area.

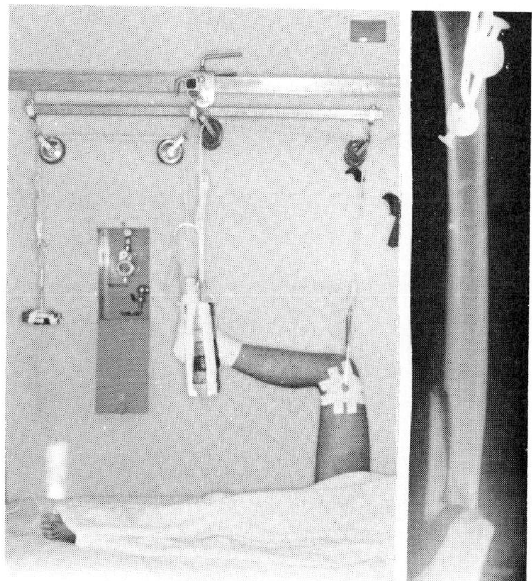

Figure 22–70. *A*, Continuous skeletal traction through a pin in the distal metaphysis for treatment of a subtrochanteric fracture of the femur. The distal fragment is thereby brought into line with the flexed proximal fragment. *B*, Lateral projection of the same fractured femur. Note the metal pin and stirrup in the region of the distal end of the femur. The distal fragment has been brought into line with the flexed proximal fragment. The comminution was not apparent in the anteroposterior projection.

consequently a severe injury is required to fracture it. Fractures of the femoral neck, therefore, are not common in childhood, but they are serious. The combination of the severe injury and the precarious blood supply to the femoral head lead to a high incidence of post-traumatic avascular necrosis. Moreover, as with femoral neck fractures in adults, they are extremely unstable and cannot be adequately treated either by closed reduction and external immobilization or by continuous traction.

Treatment. Displaced femoral neck fractures in children represent an absolute indication for internal skeletal fixation (Fig. 22–71). Since a child cannot be expected to refrain from weight bearing during the healing phase of the fracture, it is necessary to supplement the internal fixation with a hip spica cast until the fracture is clinically united; this usually requires 3 months.

Complications. If internal skeletal fixation has not been used or if it has been inadequate, fractures of the femoral neck in children are likely to be complicated by nonunion and a progressive coxa vara deformity (Fig. 22–72).

When the femoral head has lost its blood supply by disruption of its vessels at the time of a fracture, the result is post-traumatic avascular necrosis, a complication that occurs in approximately 30 per cent of children with this injury. There is little radiographic evidence of this complication until several months have elapsed. The ossific nucleus stops growing for at least 6 months after injury and at first appears *relatively* radioopaque (relative to the post-traumatic osteo-

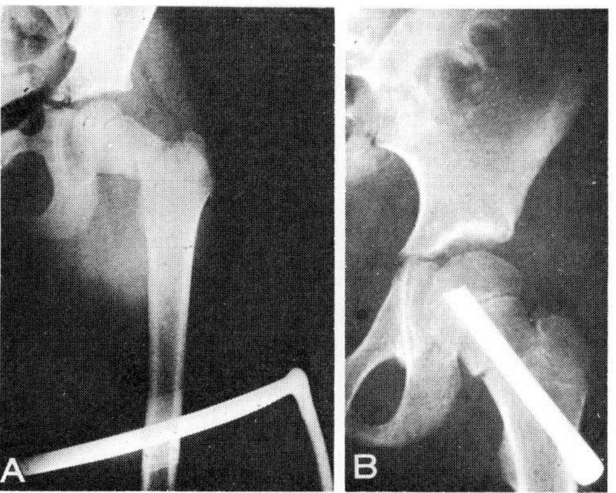

Figure 22–71. *A*, Fractured neck of femur in a 10-year-old boy. Note the ring of the Thomas splint. *B*, After closed reduction and percutaneous nailing, the fragments are in satisfactory position. Three threaded pins would have been equally satisfactory for internal fixation of this fracture.

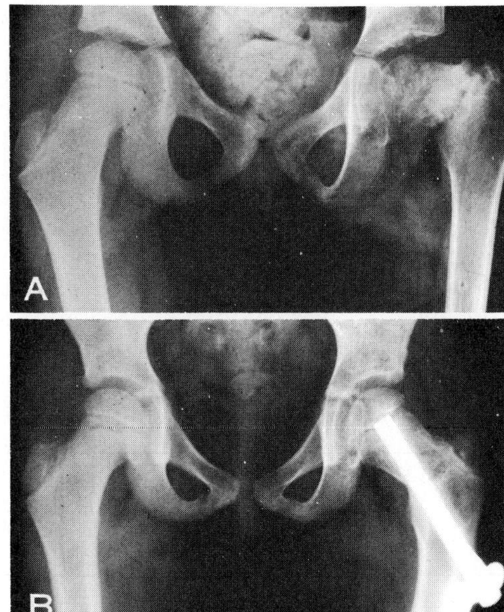

Figure 22–72. *A*, Nonunion of a fracture of the left femoral neck in a 9-year-old boy. Note the sclerosis at the fracture site and the coxa vara deformity, with resultant shortening of the limb. This fracture should have been treated by internal skeletal fixation. *B*, Correction of the deformity and union of the fracture were obtained by means of an operation that included bone grafting and the use of a nail and plate.

porosis of the living bone in the acetabulum and femoral shaft). Later, when the ossific nucleus is being revascularized and reossified, it appears *absolutely* radio-opaque as new bone is laid down on dead trabeculae. Subsequently, the femoral head may become deformed. The treatment of the complication of post-traumatic avascular necrosis of the femoral head in children is the same as that for Legg-Perthes' disease.

Type 1 Injury of the Proximal Femoral Epiphysis

This uncommon but serious injury carries the same risk of avascular necrosis of the femoral head as do fractures of the femoral neck and for the same reasons (Fig. 22–73). Like the femoral neck fracture, a type 1 injury of the proximal femoral epiphysis should be treated by internal skeletal fixation, usually with two or more threaded wires. After the injury has healed, the threaded wires should be removed to avoid a growth disturbance.

Traumatic Dislocation of the Hip

The normal hip joint is most vulnerable to dislocation when it is in a position of flexion and adduction. In this position, a force transmitted along the shaft of the femur (as may occur from a dashboard injury or a fall on the flexed knee) may drive the femoral head posteriorly over the labrum, or lip, of the acetabulum to produce a posterior dislocation. Since the femoral head escapes through a rent in the capsule, it is an extracapsular type of dislocation.

Diagnosis. The clinical deformity of a posterior dislocation of the hip—flexion, adduction, and internal rotation—is characteristic (Fig. 22–74). Traumatic anterior dislocation of the hip is rare in childhood, but when it does occur, the hip is held in the opposite position—extension, abduction, and external rotation. Posterior dislocation is obvious radiographically (Fig. 22–75).

Treatment. As long as the hip is dislocated, the torn capsule and surrounding structures constrict the femoral neck vessels, thereby jeopardizing the blood supply to the femoral

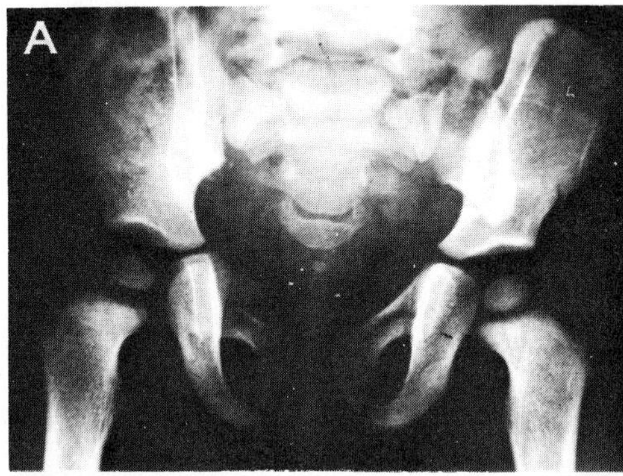

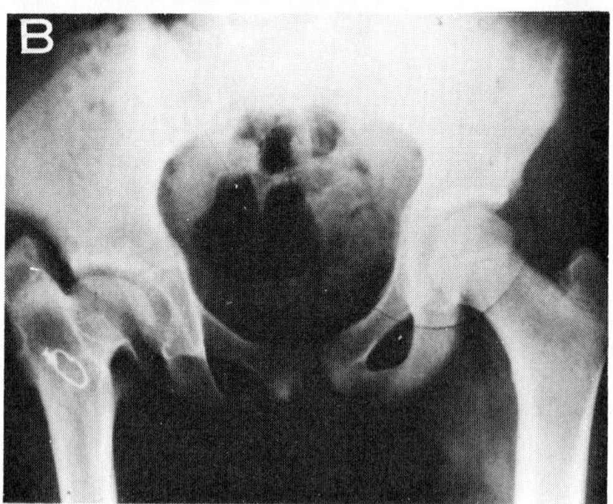

Figure 22–73. Type 1 injury of the proximal femoral epiphysis in a 1-year-old child who had been struck by a truck. *A*, Note the obvious fractures of the pelvis. Less obvious is the increased distance between the proximal femoral epiphysis and metaphysis on the right side indicating a Type 1 epiphyseal separation. *B*, Ten years later there is deformity of the femoral head (coxa plana), marked shortening of the femoral neck, and coxa vara. (The wire loop is at the site of a previous osteotomy of the femur.)

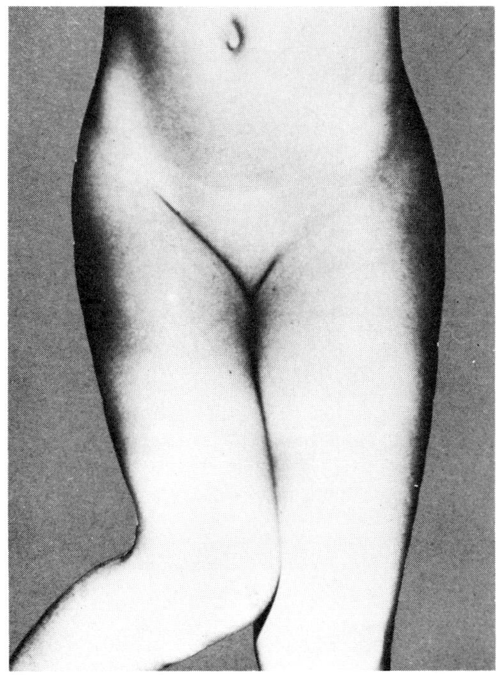

Figure 22–74. The typical clinical deformity of a child with traumatic posterior dislocation of the right hip—flexion, adduction, internal rotation, and apparent shortening.

head. For this reason, traumatic dislocation of the hip represents an emergency. The dislocation should be reduced as soon as possible in an attempt to prevent the serious complication of avascular necrosis of the femoral head. Indeed, in children whose hips are reduced within 8 hours of the time of injury, the incidence of avascular necrosis is low. However, in those whose hips have remained unreduced for longer than 8 hours, the incidence of this complication is high (approximately 40 per cent).

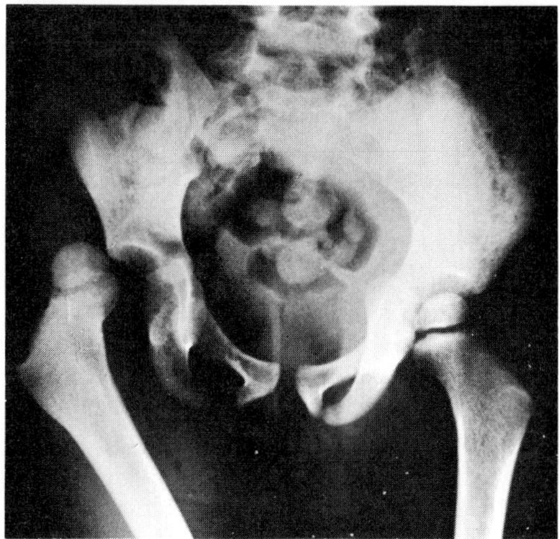

Figure 22–75. Traumatic posterior dislocation of the right hip suffered by the patient shown in Figure 22–74.

Closed reduction is accomplished by applying upward traction on the flexed thigh and by forward pressure on the femoral head from behind. After reduction, which must be perfect both clinically and radiographically, a hip spica cast is applied with the hip in its most stable position—extension, abduction, and external rotation. Immobilization of the reduced hip is maintained for 8 weeks to allow strong healing of the torn capsule.

Complications. The acetabular margin, being largely cartilaginous in children, is seldom fractured, and the sciatic nerve is seldom injured. The complication of post-traumatic avascular necrosis of the femoral head has been described earlier in relation to fractures of the femoral neck.

Pelvis

The pelvis of a child is more flexible and hence more yielding than that of an adult because of the cartilaginous components at the sacroiliac joints, triradiate cartilages, and symphysis pubis. Consequently, serious fractures of the pelvis are not common in childhood, although they do occur as the result of a severe injury, such as an automobile accident.

The most important aspects of fractures of the pelvis in children are not the fractures themselves but rather the associated complications—especially extensive internal hemorrhage from torn vessels and extravasation of urine from rupture of the bladder or urethra.

Diagnosis. Physical examination reveals local swelling and tenderness. In unstable fractures there may also be deformity of the hips as well as instability of the pelvic ring. Special radiographic projections are required to assess the precise nature of a pelvic fracture, since the AP projection provides only a two-dimensional image of the injury. The lateral projection, which would normally provide the third dimension, is unsatisfactory because of overlap of the two innominate bones. Thus, in order to obtain a three-dimensional view of the disturbed anatomy of the injury, it is necessary to obtain (1) an AP projection, (2) a tangential projection in the plane of the pelvic ring (with the tube directed upward 50 degrees) and, (3) an inlet projection looking down into the pelvic ring with the tube directed downwards 60 degrees.

Treatment. The *emergency care* of a child with a fractured pelvis centers on the two major complications.

The pelvis is a particularly vascular area, and displaced fractures of the pelvis may tear vessels (such as the large superior gluteal artery), with resultant major hemorrhage. A child may lose as much as 60 per cent of circulating blood volume into the peripelvic and retroperitoneal tissues and develop severe hemorrhagic shock.

While the child is being treated for shock, a catheter should be inserted into the bladder to investigate the possibility of associated injury to the bladder or urethra. If there is blood in the urethra and a catheter cannot be passed, the urethra is almost certainly torn. Hence, a suprapubic cystotomy must be performed pending surgical repair of the urethra. If the catheter can be passed into the bladder and the urine contains blood, cystography should be carried out immediately to determine if the bladder has been ruptured, in which case it should be repaired as soon as possible.

Since the bone of the pelvis is principally cancellous and since its blood supply is abundant, fractures of the pelvis unite rapidly. Treatment of the various types of fractures is aimed at correcting significant fracture deformities in order to prevent malunion and resultant disturbance of function.

Stable Fractures of the Pelvis

Fractures that do not transgress the pelvic ring do not interfere with stability of the pelvis in relation to weight bearing and do not require reduction.

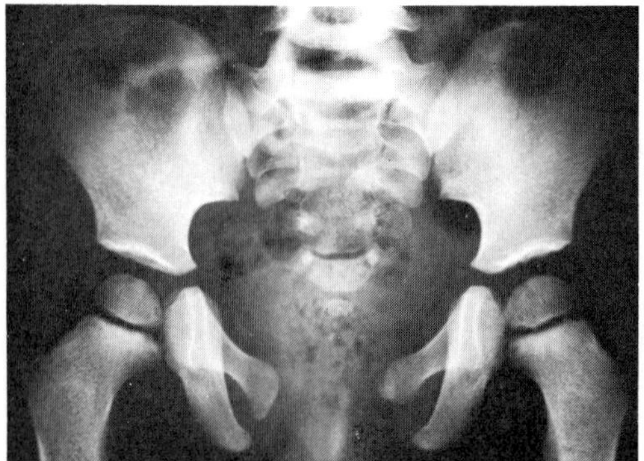

Figure 22–76. Traumatic separation of the symphysis pubis in a 2-year-old child. Both sacroiliac joints have been spread open also. The separation was reduced by internal rotation of both hips, and the open internal rotation was maintained in a hip spica cast.

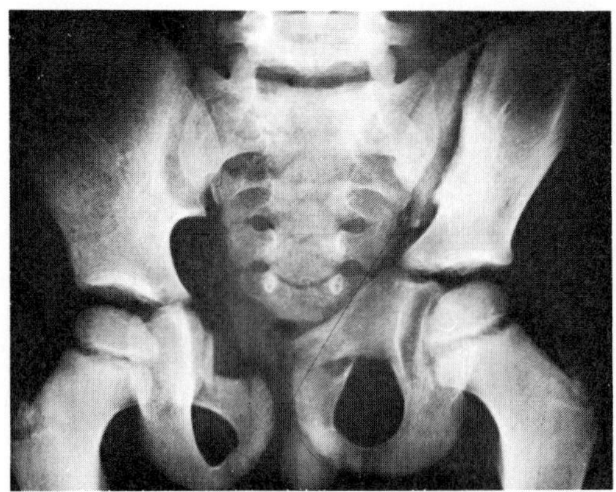

Figure 22–77. "Bucket-handle" type of unstable fracture of the pelvis of a 9-year-old boy who was run over by a truck. Note the vertical fracture just lateral to the left sacroiliac joint and the fracture of the superior pubic rami. The left half of this child's pelvis has been displaced forward and inward. The displacement was reduced by external rotation of the left hip, and the reduction was maintained in a hip spica cast.

In children, particularly in athletic boys, a sudden violent pull on the hamstring muscles may avulse their origin, the ischial apophysis. This injury usually heals well but may result in a fibrous union.

Isolated fractures of the ilium are of little significance and require only protection from weight bearing until pain subsides, within a few weeks.

A "straddle" injury of the pelvis (which may occur as a child loses his footing while walking along the top of a fence) may cause one or more fractures of the inferior pubic rami but, more important, is likely to produce a tear of the urethra.

Unstable Fractures of the Pelvis

Complete separation of the symphysis pubis and opening out of the pelvic ring is best reduced by internally rotating both hips, the reduction is maintained in a well-molded hip spica cast (Fig. 22–76).

Lateral compression of the pelvis may produce a "bucket handle" fracture in which the fractured half of the pelvis rolls forward and inward (Fig. 22–77). In children this type of fracture can usually be managed by externally rotating the lower limb, and the reduction can be maintained by the application of a well-molded hip spica cast.

Unstable fractures in which one half of the pelvis is driven proximally by an upward thrust require continuous skeletal traction through the femur to obtain and maintain reduction.

Selected Readings

Baker RH, Carroll N, Dewar FP, Hall JE: The semitendinosus tenodesis for recurrent dislocation of the patella. J Bone Joint Surg 54B:103, 1972.

Blount WP: Fractures In Children. Baltimore, Williams and Wilkins, 1955.

Boyd HB, Boals JC: The Monteggia lesion: A review of 159 cases. Clin Orthop 66:94, 1969.

Braunstein PW, Skudder PA McCarroll JR et al.: Concealed haemorrhage due to pelvic fracture. J Trauma, 4:832, 1964.

Bright RW: Surgical correction of partial epiphyseal plate closure in dogs by bone bridge resection and use of silicone rubber implants. J Bone Joint Surg 54a:1133, 1972.

Casey BH Hamilton HW, Bobechko WP: Reduction of acutely slipped upper femoral epiphysis. J Bone Joint Surg 54B:607, 1972.

Charnley J: The Closed Treatment of Common Fractures. 3rd ed. Edinburgh, E and S Livingstone, 1970.

Cooper R: Fractures in children: Fundamentals of management. J Iowa Med Soc 54:472, 1964.

Dale GC Harris WF: Prognosis in epiphyseal separation. An experimental study. J Bone Joint Surg 40B:116, 1958.

Devas MB: Stress fractures in children. J Bone Joint Surg 45B:528, 1963.

Engh CA, Robinson RA, Milgram J: Stress fractures in children. J Trauma, 10:532, 1970.

Evans EM: Fractures of the radius and ulna. J Bone Joint Surg 33B:548, 1951.

Fielding JW: Radio-ulnar union following displacement of the proximal radial epiphysis. J Bone Joint Surg 46A:1277, 1964.

Fraser RL, Haliburton RA, Barber JR: Displaced epiphyseal fractures of the proximal humerus. Can J Surg 10:427, 1967.

Gaul RW: Recurrent traumatic dislocation of the hip in children. Clin Orthop 90:107, 1973.

Griffin PP, Anderson M, Green WT: Fractures of the shaft of the femur. Orthop Clin North Am 3:213, 1972.

Griffiths SC: Fracture of odontoid process in children. J Pediatr Surg 7:680, 1972.

Haddad RJ, Saer, JK, Riordan DC: Percutaneous pinning of displaced supracondylar fractures of the elbow in children. Clin Orthop 71:112, 1970.

Hunter GA: Non-traumatic displacement of the atlanto-axial joint. J Bone Joint Surg 50B:44, 1968.

Irani RN, Nicholson JT, Chung SMK: Treatment of femoral fractures in children by immediate spica immobilization. J Bone Joint Surg 52A:1567, 1972.

Jackson DW, Cozen L: Genu valgum as a complication of proximal tibial metaphyseal fractures in children. J Bone Joint Surg 53A:1571, 1971.

Kay SP, Hall JE: Fracture of the femoral neck in children and its complications. Clin Orthop 80:53, 1971.

Kempe CH, Helfer RE: Helping the Battered Child and His Family. Philadelphia, J. B. Lippincott, 1972.

Kleiger B, Mankin HJ: Fracture of the lateral portion of the distal epiphysis. J Bone Joint Surg 46A:25, 1964.

Melzak J: Paraplegia among children. Lancet 2:45, 1969.

Murphy AF Stark HH: Closed dislocation of the MPJ of the index finger. J Bone Joint Surg 49A:1579, 1967.

Mustard WT, Simmons EH: Experimental arterial spasm in the lower extremity produced by traction. J Bone Joint Surg 35B:437, 1953.

Neer CS, Francis KC, Marcove RC, et al.: Treatment of unicameral bone cyst. J Bone Joint Surg 48A:731, 1966.

Patrick J: A study of supination and pronation with especial reference to the treatment of forearm fractures. J Bone Joint Surg 28:737, 1946.

Pearson DE, Mann RJ: Traumatic dislocation of the hip in children. Clin Orthop 92:189, 1973.

Pennsylvania Orthopaedic Society: Traumatic dislocation of the hip in children. J Bone Joint Surg 50A:79, 1968.

Rang M: Children's Fractures. Philadelphia, J. B. Lippincott, 1974.

Ratliff AHC: Traumatic separation of the upper femoral epiphysis in young children. J Bone Joint Surg 50B:757, 1968.

Ratliff AHC: Complications after fractures of the femoral neck in children and their treatment. J Bone Joint Surg 52B:175, 1970.

Rorabeck CH, Macnab I, Waddell JP: Anterior tibial compartment syndrome: A clinical and experimental review. Can J Surg 15:249, 1972.

Salter RB: Textbook of Disorders and Injuries of the Musculoskeletal System. Baltimore, Williams and Wilkins, 1970.

Salter RB, Best T: The pathogenesis and prevention of valgus deformity following fractures of the proximal metaphyseal region of the tibia in children. J Bone Joint Surg 55A:1324, 1973.

Salter RB, Harris WR: Injuries involving the epiphyseal plate. J Bone Joint Surg 45A:587, 1963.

Salter RB, Zaltz C: Anatomic investigations of the mechanism of injury and pathologic anatomy of "pulled elbow" in young children. Clin Orthop 77:141, 1971.

Sharrard WJW: Pediatric Orthopedics and Fractures. Oxford, Blackwell, Scientific Publications, 1971.

Siffert RS: Displacement of the distal humeral epiphysis in the newborn infant. J Bone Joint Surg 45A:165, 1963.

Tachdjian MO: Pediatric Orthopedics. 2nd ed. Philadelphia, W. B. Saunders, 1972.

Tator CH: Acute spinal cord injury: A review of recent studies of treatment and pathophysiology. Can Med Assoc J 107:143, 1972.

Thompson SA Mahoney LJ: Volkmann's ischemic contracture and its relationship to fracture of the femur. J Bone Joint Surg 33B:336, 1951.

Wortzman G, Dewar FP: Rotary fixation of the atlanto-axial joint. Radiology, 90:479, 1968.

CHAPTER

23 *Hand Injuries*

JEROME E. ADAMSON

Hand injuries occur frequently in children and are usually the result of the child's exploration of the unknown—of fire, machines, electrical sockets, and so on—or the child's attempt to use tools that he does not understand. Lacerations, contusions and abrasions, and burns constitute the majority of hand injuries. Fractures of the hand are relatively rare in children as compared with their occurrence in adults.

INITIAL EVALUATION

As with all aspects of medicine, to provide proper care for the child with a hand injury, a careful history must be obtained from a responsible individual who has specific knowledge of the accident. Unfortunately, with the present trend toward shopping center medicine, those of us who care for hand injuries are seeing an increasing number of children who have been taken to a neighborhood facility where local anesthesia has been injected into a laceration on the hand. When the person providing the care suddenly realizes he is "in over his head," he places a dressing on the wound, usually after putting in a few poorly placed sutures, and advises the family to take the patient to a "hand specialist." In reviewing this sequence of events with the parent, we often find that there have been very few attempts to obtain a satisfactory history of the mechanism of injury or to perform an appropriate clinical examination. We often note that these two extremely important functions have been relegated to an interviewing clerk or to a nurse at the front desk. Unfortunately, the same situation has occasionally occurred in hospitals with outstanding emergency room care, even when there is a "major trauma center" accessible. In all situations, ideal treatment begins with a careful history of the injury and of the patient.

Fortunately, most hand injuries can be diagnosed without touching the patient if a solid effort is made to obtain as much information as possible about the mechanism of injury, whether a foreign body is in the wound, and the type of and potential of a penetrating injury. A calm interview with the child frequently reveals new information about the injury, with the youngster providing important details about how his hand got cut or crushed or where he put it or what he put it in. When treating young children, a calm manner is especially important because it allows the family to relax. The general mood is transmitted immediately to the child, especially one in the late preschool years or primary grades.

Also at this time, a review of the child's past history aids the examiner and serves as a further opportunity for establishing a calm, professional atmosphere. Important information may be learned if the physician asks the standard questions all physicians learn in medical school. I cannot overemphasize the importance of carrying out this interview (which takes just a few minutes) not only for the information gained but also for the psychologic benefits to the patient and family. Unfortunately, some physicians will approach the wound very aggressively, without making an attempt to determine how the injury occurred or to assess the general state of the patient, and will immediately lose the cooperation of the child and increase the tension of the family.

Most hand injuries are not especially painful, with the exception of crush of the nail bed, with an underlying expanding hematoma. During the course of the initial discussion the examiner can gently remove the bandage on the child's hand and watch the hand during the question and answer period.

It is extremely helpful for those who are not hand surgeons and who are not faced with daily examinations of an injured hand to have the youngster place both hands side by side, noting that the normal hand and its normal anatomic posture are controlled by the delicate balance between the extensor and flexor tendon systems. For example, in injury to the profundus flexor tendon of one of the fingers from a laceration in the plam, the difference between the position of the injured hand compared with that of the normal one becomes readily apparent. The injured finger will be in a more extended position, with the posture being controlled only by the sublimus flexor tendon. On the extensor side of the hand, if the patient holds out both hands together, a severed extensor tendon with its dropped finger distal from the laceration also becomes dramatically apparent. For example in a hand with a flexor tendon laceration, any imbalance of position in the injured hand compared with the normal hand will immediately alert the examiner to the fact that the laceration has been deep enough to injure the tendon. If a laceration in this area has been deep enough to involve the tendon there is often an associated digital nerve injury.

Fractures can be studied in a similar fashion by comparing the normal with the injured hand and observing the balance, posture, and position of the fingers beyond the area of injury. Thus, one can determine the possibility of injuries to tendons, nerves, blood vessels, and bones without even touching the hand. Fortunately, the hand lends itself beautifully to this kind of intelligent observation—much more so than any other part of the body.

ANATOMY

Successful examination of the hand requires very good knowledge of anatomy. It is beyond the purview of this chapter to discuss details of hand anatomy. The reader is referred to standard texts that are of basic value.[1–9] In your review of anatomy, notice in a cross section of the finger that the extensor tendon mechanism is on the dorsum. The digital central circle containing the bones, tendons, nerves, and blood vessels is occupied in its upper two-thirds by the bone, which is round on the dorsum and flattened in the region of the shaft on its volar surface. This circle is completed on the volar surface by the flexor tendon system. Tucked into the same fascia encircling the flexor tendons, the extensor tendons, and bone, is the neurovascular bundle on the volar-lateral surface just adjacent to the flexor tendon sheath. There is little subcutaneous tissue in the hand, except in the very obese person and in the "pudgy" child.

A basic understanding of hand anatomy and a working knowledge of underlying structural permits more effective examination and treatment of hand injuries in the child.

INITIAL CARE

One should anticipate that the deeper structures have been injured and rule this out with an appropriate examination. Much can be learned without even touching the patient. As mentioned earlier, tendon injuries are easy to determine by studying the posture of the various digits that may be involved. Comparing the injured hand with the normal hand is valuable in making a correct diagnosis. Parental support is helpful in encouraging the youngster to move the injured hand to demonstrate an abnormal movement or to verify normal function. Nerve injuries should always be suspected early but confirmed last.

The natural impulse is to test for areas of denervated skin by sticking them with a pin. However, initially sticking a child with a sharp point is the worst thing you can do. Few patients will extend an injured finger and allow an examiner to stick it with a pin without involuntarily pulling the hand away, usually with a loud scream. The stimulus of touching, which frequently will be the first contact with the finger, will not produce involuntary withdrawal. Gently brush your fingertip over a normal area to let the patient know that this is an easy examination and nothing to be concerned about. Ask if this feels "Okay." Then examine the injured area. In my experience, the most common response of a child to a light, moving touch on a digit with a damaged nerve is, "It feels like a piece of wood." If the physician needs further evidence of digital nerve injury, he should then carefully palm a safety pin and shield the injured area with the other hand. With the blunt end of the pin he should first test the normal sensory areas and then gently examine the injured area. He should then touch the normal area gently and then the injured area with the sharp end as the last test before applying a wound dressing. The moving, light touch test is a helpful sensory examination and is almost foolproof if the examiner moves from the normal area to the injured area in this manner.

If there is a possibility of bony injury, x-rays should be obtained as promptly as possible. Do not be satisfied with a dorsal view, but request lateral and oblique views as well. If you have questions about the presence or absence of a fracture, the parents will respect your willingness to seek the counsel of others.

With ligament injuries, especially in teenagers engaged in active sports, painful swelling usually occurs in the area of injury. The posture of the finger may be completely normal or only slightly altered. Extension or flexion may produce pain. Injection of local anesthesia without adrenaline into the area of injury and abduction away from the joint to spread the area of ligament tear in order to demonstrate an abnormal posture are very helpful. These stress tests, as they are appropriately named, are impossible to perform in the very young but can be performed in the mature teenager. Be sure to use local anesthesia that does not contain a vasoconstricting agent such as adrenaline so as not to cause constriction of the vessels in the neurovascular bundle and subsequent development of gangrene distally. In a suspected ligament injury, x-rays must be obtained. Look carefully for a small chip of bone adjacent to the articular surface of the joint where the ligament attaches. If the injury is severe, frequently a small piece of bone will be avulsed at the ligament attachment site.

Injuries to the nail are usually crush injuries and should be treated very promptly. An immediate history and visual examination will usually define the problem. A subungual hematoma, if present, should be evacuated by one of several effective techniques. The simplest is to touch the affected area with a high-speed drill such as a dental burr and make a 1 mm or slightly larger opening to allow drainage. This provides immediate pain relief and allows a more detailed examination to determine if there is an underlying fracture or tendon injury. If a nail laceration has occurred, one should not be immediately concerned with draining a hematoma, since the injury itself will permit drainage.

Examination of compound injuries with multiple fractures, lacerations, or tendon and nerve injuries in children frequently must be undertaken in the operating room under general anesthesia. Once you have determined that the injury is in one of these categories, do not attempt an aggressive, detailed examination, but merely to obtain an x-ray and place the child where he can receive definitive care under general anesthesia. With a severely injured patient, do not subject the child, parent, your assistants, or yourself to the anxiety of a detailed examination. This is for the operating room under general anesthesia.

I will mention the importance of examining the child as a whole and not focus on the hand injury. Did the child fall? Why did he fall? Did he have a seizure? Did he have a fever? Make a careful review of symptoms. Find out the general state of the child's health, and try to relate any problems to the injury.

If the child has sustained multiple injuries, simple splinting of the hand will permit general care (see Chapter 1). Determine that circulation is adequate by comparing the color of the injured hand with that of the normal hand and apply simple splinting with a wrist-forearm-hand slab splint of almost any type, with appropriate padding between the splint and the hand and a soft circumferential, nonconstricting fluff-type bandage dressing. A vascular injury is the most demanding in a child. Once bleeding has been controlled by pressure and circulation to the part does not seem to be impaired, there is no urgency to treat the injured hand. Care should be obtained as soon as possible; if this can be achieved in 1 to 3 hours, that is perfectly permissible. It is not wise to spend a major effort in cleaning out an obviously contaminated hand if definitive care is not going to be given at that time by that physician. It is better to do nothing other than dress the hand in a sterile dressing with an immobilizing slab splint, place it in a high sling, and get the child to the individual who can provide definitive care. It compromises the problem significantly if the patient is seen in the physician's office or in the emergency room, local anesthesia is injected in the hand, possibly obscuring nerve injury, and a cursory examination is made prior to referral. Unfortunately, many young children we see have already undergone this initial treatment. By the time they reach us, they are so compromised psychologically we can do little except take them to the operating room and with general anesthesia learn as much as possible about the extent of the injury. It is better to communicate directly with the treating surgeon and spare the extra trauma for the child. In hand injuries especially, as in many other injuries, the person who treats the patient first has the best chance to get the best result.

When the patient is referred it is helpful to send information regarding previous immunization, history of allergies, any general disorder, and a record of treatment provided such as local anesthesia, antibiotic therapy, and antitetanus immunization. Every physician knows the value of this type of communication, but unfortunately some do not transmit this basic information.

In order to inform the patient's family as to what to expect, it is advisable to provide two options for treatment that should cover most anything the surgeon will do. First, with the patient under appropriate anesthesia, the surgeon may determine the problem and reconstruct the hand primarily. Second, in many instances it is preferable to clean and close the wound, occasionally with drainage, and at a second sitting, under more ideal circumstances, the surgeon may elect to do a delayed primary reconstruction. Informing the patient's family of the possibility of these options helps to establish rapport with the family without challenging the referring physician's position. Invariably, the family, upon being referred to a specialist who will care for the child's hand injury, will ask the referring pediatrician, "What will he do?" If one is not aware of these two basic possibilities, *primary* or *delayed primary care*, the credibility of the referring physician and hand surgeon may be compromised.

SKIN INJURY

Superficial skin lacerations are frequently overtreated by unnecessarily aggressive suturing. After being flushed with copious amounts of water under the spigot in the physician's office, many lacerations can be treated with taping. Usually well-fitting Shur-strips or Steristrips will close the wound satisfactorily. These products allow for wound drainage and are easy to apply, usually producing an ideal result. However, application of skin adhesives and supportive dressings is not enough for some wounds. An external covering and supportive dressing are needed, especially in the child, to protect the wound from further contamination.

Superficial wounds sustained in a clean environment do not require flushing with antibacterial agents (which in themselves may damage the wound and cause pain for the patient). The use of extensive wound irrigation is taxing for the patient and in most instances is probably unnecessary. For deep wounds with obvious contamination, irrigation should not be attempted in the very young child without a light general anesthetic on an outpatient basis. Such wounds should not be closed primarily but left open and treated as soon as possible in the operating room.

Animal bites of the hand are typical contaminated lacerations and should rarely, if ever, be closed primarily, even after aggressive wound toilet (see also Chapter 30). If the child is involved in a fist fight with a playmate and cuts his knuckle on his friend's front teeth, as 7- and 8-year-olds occasionally do, this injury should be treated very aggressively with wound irrigation, allowing it to stay open and heal secondarily with appropriate antibiotic prophylaxis. Oral penicillin is usually adequate, although cephalosporins are occasionally used. These wounds usually heal in 72 hours.

In deep lacerations without evidence of injury to underlying tendons, nerves, vessels, bone, or ligaments, the wound simply can be closed with a single layer of fine suture after infiltration of plain 1 per cent lidocaine (Xylocaine) or similar anesthetic into the surrounding tissue. It is unwise to inject local anesthesia into a wound through the laceration because of the possibility of implanting bacterial contaminants of the wound deep into the periwound area. If there is concern about further drainage or bacterial contamination, a small sterile rubber band type drain can be placed into the wound, bringing it out from one end or the other and attaching it so that it cannot slide out of the wound. All hand injuries should be dressed loosely, usually with a soluble grease-type dressing gauze with an absorbent layer of sterile 4 × 4 gauze dressing and a loose circumferential supportive dressing of fluff-type gauze. In the very young, the prudent physician closes lacerations on the hand with fine plain catgut, which will not have to be removed. This type of suture remains 2 to 3 weeks before it comes free. A small amount of tissue reaction may occur with catgut used in skin closure.

Sutures of 5-0 fine nylon or polypropylene are excellent, with minimal tissue reaction in the wound. Sutures should be spaced approximately 5 to 6 mm apart and tied loosely. The quality of the scar is not related to the number of sutures used. Necrosis of the wound margins and pain will occur when post-injury edema develops if sutures are tied too tightly or placed too closely. A patient who has post-suture pain should have the wound evaluated. Post-suture pain is usually the result of too tightly tied sutures, edema, hematoma or, several days after the injury, the development of infection.

Dependent hands swell. The child should be provided with a sling and the parents advised as to the importance of preventing edema that results from dependency. The common triangular sling available in most emergency rooms as a three-cornered section of coarse muslin is completely inadequate for good support of a child's injured hand. Frequently, this sling is poor fitting and not properly applied. The knot at the back of the neck serves as a focus of constant irritation and soon encourages the child to abandon the sling when out of the sight of his parents. The best slings are those with a foam cushion around the strap over the neck and a series of adjustable straps so as to raise and lower the elbow as well as adjust the height of the wrist. Elevation should be continued at night.

Care should be taken to appropriately pad any dressing of the hand and arm. Children tolerate discomfort and pain well and may not be able to communicate their concern. The development of numbness from compression caused by edema, stagnation of blood flow, and necrosis of tissue may be overlooked. Volkmann's ischemic contracture is most often seen in the child and can always be prevented by intelligent watchfulness, a properly fitting noncompressive dressing, splint, or cast and elevation. *Elevation is mandatory.*

In the very young child, the usual sling will be inadequate. It is best to encase the extremity in a bias cut stockinette tube with an opening cut in the tube for evaluation of the hand (Fig. 23–1). This slit in the circumferential supporting stockinette is taped closed to protect the wound from inquiring fingers. Children tolerate stockinette slings very well.

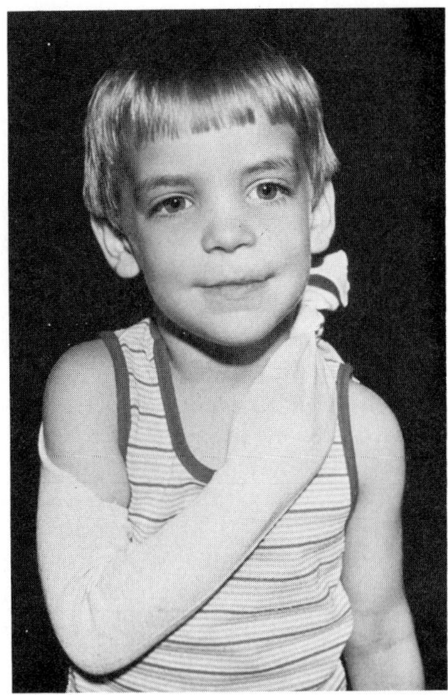

Figure 23–1. A bias cut stockinette sling comfortably elevates, protects, and effectively immobilizes the child's hand. Examination of the hand within a dressing can be accomplished by slitting the stockinette as needed.

Abrasions of the hand are frequently seen in patients who have had bicycle and other moving accidents and usually occur on the palm or the dorsal aspects of the interphalangeal and metacarpophalangeal joint regions. They are extremely painful and are often contaminated with imbedded foreign material. The treating physician should determine if there are underlying injuries and obtain x-rays to rule out suspected fractures. Abrasion wounds are best cleaned by irrigation with water from the tap. Occasionally, foreign material can be removed gently by forceps. A magnifying hand lens or loupes are of great help. Abrasions are best treated by antibiotic-impregnated gauze dressings. The most useful one in our practice has been Silvadene, which has a very low incidence of drug sensitivity. Other antibiotic ointments may produce allergic reactions, especially upon repeated use. Antibacterial dressings should be water soluble to allow the exudate from the abrasion to flow through the antibiotic dressing into the overlying absorbent layer of gauze. As for lacerations, this layer of 4 × 4 gauze dressings is held in place with loosely applied fluff roll gauze. Foreign material not removed initially may be removed by further dressings being loosened with the wound exudate. With deeply imbedded foreign material in severe abrasions, secondary cleaning with the patient under anesthesia may be necessary within 72 hours.

Dressings should always be applied with the hand in a relaxed position. This is determined by supinating the hand and allowing the fingers and thumb to fall into a natural position. Exceptions to this general rule will be reviewed when appropriate. In an extensive laceration or abrasion injury, dress the entire hand and involve all digits in the dressing. If the child realizes that he cannot use any part of his hand, he will accept total immobilization. If he finds he can use a part, he will diligently begin to find ways to use all of it. Wounds need rest.

BURN INJURY

Burns of the hand are extremely serious injuries in children.[3, 7, 9–12] Improper care produces significant problems that may result in deformities that compromise function and appearance forever. A history is absolutely essential as the first step in planning treatment. The extent of burn is related to the type of injury, the length of time the injury occurred, and the temperature of the causative agent. For example, a high voltage electrical burn that lasts for only milliseconds can produce extensive damage because of the high energy involved.[12] This may be contrasted with the hot grease burn, which involves a temperature only a fraction of that of the electrical burn, but because of the child's age and the parent's inability to flush the hot grease from the burned part immediately, the extent of damage may be equally devastating. The extent of burn is a function of the amount of energy exchanged over a period of time.

In emergency care of all burns, the physician should determine whether the burn is superficial or deep. The well-established doctrine of first-, second-, third-, and fourth-degree burns has been supplanted in a practical fashion by recognition of superficial or deep burns.[2, 7] The superficial, or partial-thickness, burn involves the outer layers of the epidermis and heals primarily. Examination reveals reddened, blistered skin, which will be extremely painful to touch. The deep, or full-thickness, burn involves damage to all or almost all of the thickness of skin, with only a few islands of dermis around hair follicles remaining intact. These burns are painless to touch, which signifies total destruction of the skin. Treatment of each type of burn is significantly different; therefore, accurate determination of the depth of the burn is essential. Unfortunately, few burns are homogeneous in depth of injury. One must try to determine the major area of injury, and the major level or depth of burn and relate treatment to that information. The fourth-degree burn involves skin and underlying structures such as tendons, nerves, vessels, and bone. This type of burn, of course, requires aggressive surgical therapy.

If the burn is superficial, with proper cleaning and prevention of infection (which converts the superficial burn to a deep burn), there will be enough viable skin elements remaining to provide good healing and the development of satisfactory skin scar. A healed superficial burn results in minimal scarring and good functional result. If a burn diagnosed as superficial heals with a thick scar or infection develops, one has misjudged the depth of the burn. Superficial burns are best treated by first preparing the whole hand with an antiseptic solution to sterilize the regions surrounding the burn wound as much as possible. Using sterile technique, which should include the use of a mask, sterile gloves, and sterile instruments in a sterile field, one carefully débrides all the blister present in the superficial burned region. An antibacterial ointment is applied. It is usually advisable to postpone the second dressing for 3 days. Thereafter, often the patient's family can change the dressing daily, as outlined in the care of abrasion wounds. The total hand is included in the dressing and is immobilized in an appropriate sling during the day with elevation at night. Elevation is extremely important in the care of the burned hand, since dependency produces edema, edema produces stasis, stasis provides a fertile area for bacterial growth, and bacterial growth may convert a superficial burn to a deep burn.

The deep burn in the hand of a child is a major injury.[2, 7] Treatment requires hospitalization and prompt surgical removal of all damaged skin by reconstruction with an appropriate skin graft (Fig. 23–2). On the dorsum of the hand and digits, excision fo the damaged skin is followed by resurfacing with split-thickness skin grafts, usually 15 to 18 thousandths of an inch thick. Primary excision and grafting with the patient under general anesthesia, tourniquet control with good take of the skin graft, and early mobilization almost always produce an excellent functional and cosmetic result. Delayed treatment of the severe hand burn almost always produces a nonfunctioning, scarred, almost useless hand (Fig. 23–3). There is no reason to delay treatment of a severely burned hand beyond two to three days after injury unless there is a life-threatening primary condition. Treatment of burns of the palmar surface requires more judicious care with thicker skin grafts. Very thick split-thickness of skin grafts or full-thickness skin grafts usually are satisfactory. The severe burn of the hand in the child is a major surgical emergency and should be dealt with promptly. The basic principles of early burn wound excision and appropriate skin coverage by the skilled plas-

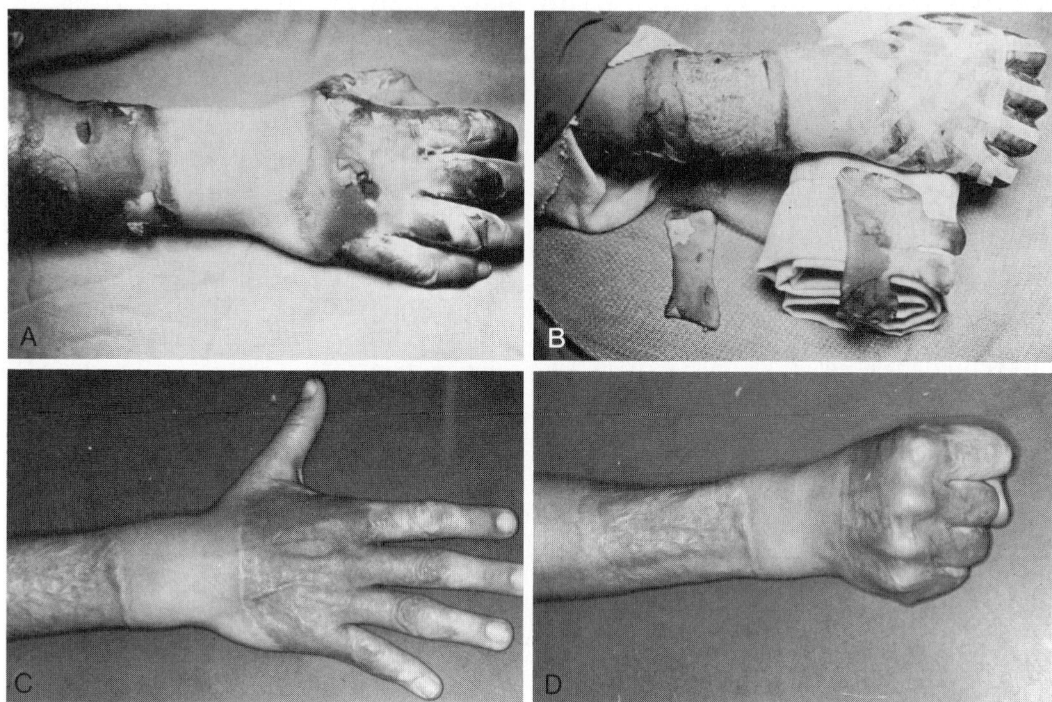

Figure 23–2. *A,* Third-degree gasoline burns of the hand and a circumferential burn of the forearm of an 8-year-old boy. *B,* After initial evaluation, the area of the third-degree burn was surgically excised, with the patient under general anesthesia. A split-thickness skin graft has been placed over the dorsum of the hand and fixed with paper adhesive. Note the marked contracture of the excised skin as opposed to the appearance of the wound following excision. *C,* Six weeks postoperatively, extension is normal. *D,* Six weeks postoperatively, flexion is normal. The patient has done well.

tic surgeon or hand surgeon usually produce excellent results.

Emergency care of severely burned hands consists of rapid cleaning with a mild antiseptic soap-type solution and application of a dressing with the metacarpophalangeal joints flexed approximately 80 degrees and the proximal and distal interphalangeal joints extended 180 degrees. The thumb web should be opened widely and the thumb placed in a position of extension. Soft gauze dressings should be applied between the fingers, and the entire hand enclosed in a supportive, fluff-type roll gauze dressing. Elevation is mandatory. Prompt transfer of the patient to a surgeon should be accomplished whenever possible. If other injuries prevent such transfer, a plastic surgeon or hand surgeon should be called in consultation for the specialized specific are that the burned hand requires. There is no place in the care of the badly burned hand for "watchful waiting." Waiting longer than 72 hours will significantly compromise the final result—the longer the wait, the worse the result.[7]

In the severely burned hand, one must be constantly aware of the problems of adequate circulation and postburn edema. The neurovascular bundles in the digits are in a vulnerable spot adjacent to the flexor tendons and contained within a fascial covering that circumscribes the extensor and flexor tendon systems. Burn edema of the digit will frequently cause secondary occlusion to the digital arteries and veins and completely obstruct blood flow. If not recognized, necrosis of the distal portion of the finger will occur. The use of anti-inflammatory agents in this area has not met with significant success. If edema is suspected, one should proceed to surgical decompression of the tight skin envelope of the digit, release of the constricting fluid, and restoration of circulation. In ideal situations, this surgical release is performed with the patient under general anesthesia, but in many instances this can be performed without anesthesia as a digit-saving emergency maneuver. The incisions are best made along the midlateral line of the finger, extending from the midportion of the distal phalanx proximally to the level of the metacarpophalangeal joint or web space. Usually the decompression needs only to be performed on one side, but patients should be watched carefully and expectantly; if indicated, decompression on the opposite side should be performed without hesitation. Because of the danger of damage to the dorsal branches of the digital nerve, which provides sensation to the dorsal aspect of the finger, decompression should first be performed in the index, middle, and ring fingers on the ulnar side. In the little finger and the thumb, decompression is best performed on the radial side. If with digital pressure on the injured finger's nail bed the blanching pulse of normal circulation cannot be seen and the patient does not perceive sensation in the fingertip, one should seriously consider prompt decompression of the compromised digit. These guidelines are important in the evaluation and care of burns involving all extremities.

In the care of the superficial burn wound, systemic antibiotics are usually not necessary. The patient should be carefully followed and if there is any indication of infection, antistreptococcal prophylaxis should be given for the first 72 hours.

In the deep burn with excision of the burn wound, prophylactic antibiotics are usually given for 72 hours.

Figure 23–3 illustrates the tragedy that may occur if burns of the hand are not appropriately treated. A teenage trumpet player, who supposedly had a brilliant career ahead of him because of his musical ability, was treated "expectantly" or "conservatively" for 3 weeks in a major hospital. He now has almost totally functionless hands with stiffened interphalangeal joints, painful scar, and grotesque-appearing fingers, which he covers from public view with gloves. Prevention of this disaster is related to very early (usually within 72 hours) removal of the burned tissue with the patient under general anesthesia and reconstruction with appropriate skin coverage. This is followed by early active motion. Immobilization of an injured hand produces stiff joints, scarred adherent tendons, and wasting of hand and forearm musculature. Rehabilitation is difficult and many times leaves an inadequate result. Early excision, skin replacement, and early active use normally produce an excellent result.

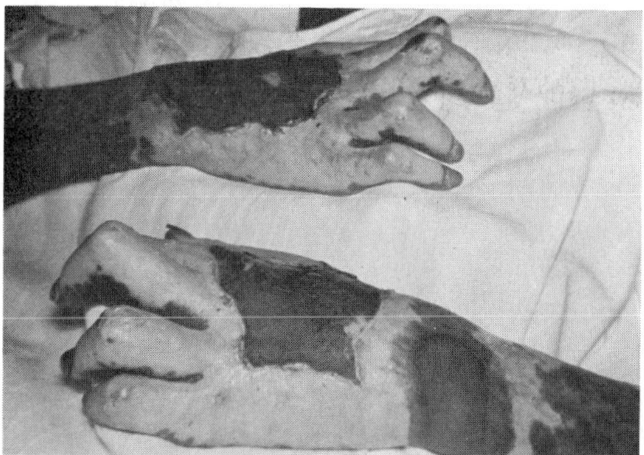

Figure 23–3. Severely deformed, badly scarred, burned hands of a 12-year-old boy. There was rupture of the extensor tendon mechanism over the proximal interphalangeal joint and severe dorsal burn scar contracture. The patient was treated for 2 months using a burn dressing prior to closure of the dorsal wound with split-thickness skin grafts. Reconstruction of this type of injury is extremely difficult, with a significantly compromised prognosis. Contrast the results of treatment in this patient with those in the patient shown in Figure 23–2, following early excision and prompt split-thickness skin grafting.

Post-Burn Reconstruction

Post-burn scarring produces many reconstructive challenges. Frequently, scarring in the web spaces on the dorsal aspect of the hand produces burn scar syndactyly. By local excision of scar tissue, utilization of the noninjured skin in the cul-de-sac of the web space, and application of heavy or thick split-thickness skin grafts, reconstruction is usually most rewarding. Dorsal burn scar contracture may prevent complete flexion of the fingers. Excision and reconstruction with split-thickness skin grafts, providing more supple skin in replacement of the constraining burn scar, is usually successful. Treatment of dorsal constraining scar contracture should be prompt because of the development of ligament shortening in the interphalangeal joint area, especially in the region of the proximal interphalangeal joint. Fortunately, children recover well from such injuries if appropriate skin coverage can be used to promptly replace either the burn wound or the post-burn scar.

Only in children with long-standing severe deformities is it necessary to proceed with extensive joint and ligament reconstruction such as capsulectomy or ligament advancement. Contractures of the web space between the thumb and index finger are frequent in post-burn hands and lend themselves very well to reconstruction. This is best achieved by a Z-plasty rearrangement of the tissues surrounding the web space. Occasionally, tissue from a distance (such as a flap of skin from the dorsal aspect of the hand overlying the second metacarpal) may be rotated into the defect of the web space to provide adequate reconstruction. Tissue from another part of the body such as the groin, dorsum of the foot, or upper medial arm, which is similar to the tissue of the web space, can be moved into this region either as a pedicle graft transfer or as a free flap vascular transfer to provide adequate replacement skin. Concomitant procedures such as muscle shifting around the thumb can be used to expand the scar-contracted web space.

EXTENSOR TENDON INJURIES

The most frequent tendon injury in the child involves the extensor tendon at its insertion on the dorsal aspect of the distal phalanx just proximal to the nail bed. This is usually damaged by a laceration or crush from getting the finger caught in a door or whatever. Often the injury will involve a portion of the bony insertion of the extensor tendon mechanism. After appropriate x-rays have been obtained, a large bony fragment is best treated with open reduction and fine Kirschner wire pinning of the fragment in position and immobilization of the distal joint in 10 to 15 degrees of hyperextension, with a second Kirschner wire placed across the joint. These pins are left in place approximately 6 weeks. In the very young, the pins are removed under light anesthesia on an outpatient basis; in an older child, Freon or similar topical sprays provide some local anesthesia of the skin overlying the pin. Results are usually satisfactory.

In children older than 6 to 7 years who are cooperative, splinting is the treatment of choice if there is no bony insertion fracture. If a hyperextension splint is applied soon after the injury, one must be cautious that postinjury edema does not constrict the circulation of the finger. After swelling has subsided, a hyperextension splint is fitted, holding the distal joint in at least 15 to 20 degrees of hyperextension. This position is maintained for a minimum of 6 weeks. One can anticipate an excellent result in at least 85 per cent of cases. However, if the patient inadvertently removes the splint and the finger is flexed or the hyperextension position is lost, secondary reconstruction with insertion of a fine Kirschner wire across the distal interphalangeal joint in the hyperextended position will be necessary. If a conservative regimen of splinting in the hyperextended position is chosen, one should inform the parents of the potential for a less than ideal result in up to 15 per cent of those treated in this manner. In the adult, such treatment may result in decreased range of motion with stiffness from either open or closed splinting, but in the child, this rarely occurs.

In infants, injuries of the proximal interphalageal joint region with a tear of the insertion of the middle slip of the extensor tendon at the base of the middle phalanx, will produce a boutonniere deformity. This is difficult to treat conservatively in the very young. Diagnosis of a tear of the middle slip always demands operative treatment with the patient under general anesthesia and suture of the avulsed tendon. A bony fragment that is avulsed at the middle slip tendon insertion must be repositioned anatomically. Immobilization of the proximal interphalangeal joint in slight hyperextension of 3 to 5 degrees above normal is maintained for 4 to 5 weeks.

In the juvenile age group, tears of the middle slip of the extensor mechanism at the level of the proximal interphalangeal joint are best treated by splinting with a safety pin splint. If this splint is maintained for 6 weeks, the ligament tear usually heals well with return of normal function. These injuries rarely produce bony avulsions at the insertion of the middle slip of the extensor mechanism, but in all cases appropriate x-rays should be obtained to be sure. If a bony deformity is noted, open reduction and repositioning of the bony fragment and repair of the tendon are the treatment of choice. Immobilization from 5 to 6 weeks with a safety pin splint is excellent therapy and almost always produces good function.

Injuries of the extensor tendon mechanism of the metacarpophalangeal joint, dorsum of the hand, or wrist from direct laceration should always be treated by operative reconstruction as soon as possible (within the first 8 hours is ideal). If the injury is not recognized initially, the skin should be closed, either with a dressing or a few sutures, and a delayed primary operative repair of the extensor tendon in 7 to 10 days should provide equally good results. In all instances, the metacarpophalangeal and wrist joints should be immobilized for 4 weeks to allow adequate time for tendon healing. The metacarpophalangeal joint should be maintained in hyperextension with the wrist in approximately 15 degrees of extension, the splint allowing normal motion of the proximal and distal interphalangeal joints of the fingers.[4]

Treatment of injuries to the extensor tendon mechanism of the thumb produces equally satisfactory results, and the same general rules may be applied.

Young children rarely require postoperative hand therapy following periods of immobilization, which permit adequate tendon healing. Removal of the splint and return to fulltime activity results in good motion. In all extensor tendon injuries of the hand in children, one should expect excellent results with the preceding modes of therapy.

FLEXOR TENDON INJURIES

Flexor tendon injuries to the fingers and hand in children do not respond well to splinting techniques (Fig. 23–4). Operative reconstruction is indicated in all instances. Because of the delicate interplay and balance between the deep (profundus) flexor tendons, which insert into the base of the distal phalanx, and the superficial (sublimus) flexor tendons, which insert into the base of the middle phalanx, both tendons whenever possible should be reconstructed following injury.[6] The sublimus tendons provide a tremendous amount of power in gross grip whereas the profundus tendons provide a major amount of power in pinch and more delicate actions. Each is equally important and repair of only one in the child should be avoided. Both tendons should be repaired. Operative reconstruction involves retrieval of the tendon if it has withdrawn in the palm, and careful coaptation of the lacerated tendon ends with a technique as delicate as possible. If possible, the flexor tendon sheath should also be reconstructed. Use of the operative microscope, which has proved effective in the treatment of nerve and vessel injuries in the hand, is becoming more common for tendon injuries. The same principles of careful attention to anatomic reapproximation and atraumatic technique give the best results.[2, 6] Treatment should be instituted as soon as possible to decrease the danger of infection. If this is not possible, equally satisfactory results can be obtained if the wound is closed and delayed primary repair is performed, usually within 7 days. If other injuries demand immediate attention, simple closure of the wound and adherence to the delayed repair principle can be followed with anticipation of a good result.

Flexor tendon injuries are usually caused by lacerations to the fingers or palm. One unique mechanism of injury involving teenagers should be noted. Rarely, we will see a teenage athlete who while playing football or some other contact sport sustains a forced hyperextension of the finger and receives an avulsion tear of the distal insertion of the profundus flexor tendon at the base of the distal phalanx on the volar surface of the finger. The patient complains of sudden pain. Upon examination, one notes that the patient has lost the ability to flex the distal interphalangeal joint region and on the volar surface of the finger there may also be tenderness over the flexor tendon sheath. Swelling and ecchymoses in the palm result from bleeding caused by rupture of the tendon

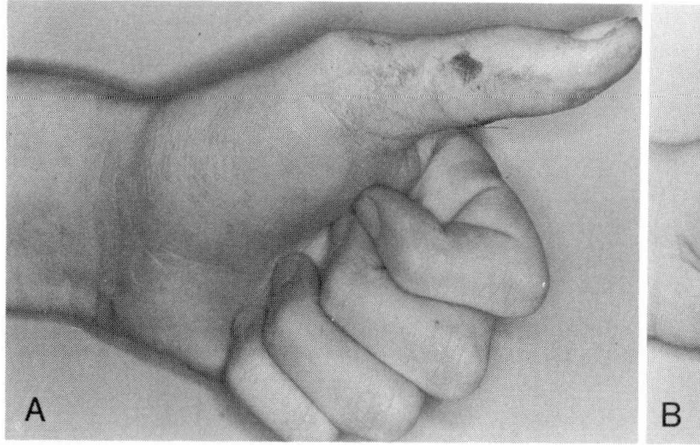

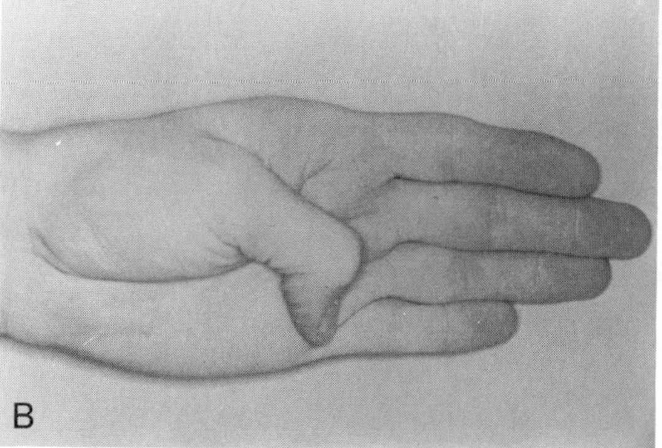

Figure 23–4. *A*, Knife tip laceration on the volar aspect of the left thumb of a 14-year-old boy. In this view, the patient is trying to flex his thumb and fingers. Flexion of the distal phalanx of the thumb is not possible and indicates an injury to the flexor pollicis longus tendon. *B*, Seven weeks after-delayed primary repair of the flexor pollicis longus tendon, there is a normal range of flexion.

insertion and the distal vinculum, which provides the blood supply to the tendon in that area. The hematoma progresses proximally through the flexor tendon sheath and presents in the palm at the level of the distal palmar crease as a painful swelling. In a few days this is noted as an ecchymosis. Occasionally, we will see this in a baseball pitcher who has thrown a fastball and felt a pain or snap upon release. It also occurs in the football quarterback when passing or in the football lineman who while attempting to clutch the jersey or pants of a fleeing runner, feels the finger painfully snap following acute flexion.

Operative treatment of the avulsion tendon injury involves retrieval of the tendon, which has frequently retracted proximally, and repositioning of the bony avulsion fragment in the distal phalanx in its anatomic position. With all flexor tendon injuries, immobilization in flexion should be carried out for at least 4 weeks.[6] Passive motion with some type of dynamic splinting prevents acute extension of the finger and allows the tendon to slide back and forth within its sheath during the healing phase, thereby preventing scar adhesions. This is usually not a problem in the very young, but even in the young teenager, dynamic tension exercises to prevent flexor tendon scar adhesions should be instituted postoperatively to achieve best results. Hand therapy is indicated to assist the child in obtaining maximum improvement. It is not often that one achieves completely normal function after flexor tendon injuries except in the very young. The older the patient, the less range of motion is achieved. This is related to the scarring that occurs in the delicate flexor tendon system during the limitation of motion necessary for adequate tendon healing.

If the flexor tendon is lacerated from the midportion of the middle phalanx to its distal insertion, tendon reconstruction in that area can usually be performed by advancement of the end of the tendon and reattachment into the normal bony insertion. This technique removes the potential of scarring within the tendon sheath from a laceration site repair. It is advisable to reconstitute the flexor tendon sheath system, most often by closing it primarily. This maintains a smooth synovial-lined, gliding surface, which enhances tendon healing and decreases the potential for scarring of surrounding, nongliding, fixed structures.

Flexor tendon injuries in the middle and proximal portion of the finger as well as in the palm or wrist should be repaired either primarily or as a delayed primary reconstruction using fine suture and magnification techniques. Splinting with the hand in a relaxed position using a supportive dorsal splint and preventing extension with some type of dynamic traction, allows the repaired tendon to slide back and forth for a short distance and prevents limiting scar adhesions.

Often in children who had sustained flexor tendon injuries many years previously, the tendon can be reconstituted either by direct repair, which may not be effective because of atrophy or forearm musculature, or by transfer of an adjacent sublimus tendon to replace the injured flexor tendon. Sublimus transfer from the adjacent finger, often the ring or the little finger, is easily performed with the patient under general anesthesia, with postoperative immobilization of 4 weeks. One should caution the family that the donor finger from whence the transfer is obtained may not function normally. The child with hyperextensile joints may develop a hyperextension bowing of the finger at the level of the proximal interphalangeal joint. This may be prevented if the surgeon is able to leave a portion of the sublimus insertion to serve as a slight check rein across the level of the proximal interphalangeal joint. Postoperative therapy is essentially the same for all flexor tendon injuries.

Flexor tendon injuries at the level of the wrist, palm, and forearm should all be treated in a similar fashion—direct repair using the most delicate techniques possible.

In the child with a compound injury of the hand involving many structures or in the child who has had a previous flexor tendon injury that has resulted in scar adherence at the repair site and a nonfunctioning digit, the possibility of secondary reconstruction is usually good. Failure to refer a patient for consideration for secondary reconstruction suggests inadequate awareness of such a potential and is certainly not ideal care.

NERVE INJURIES

Nerve injuries, whether sensory or motor, whether involving the median, radial, or ulnar nerve in the wrist or palm or their branches as digital nerves, are best treated by operative repair using microtechniques.

These techniques are well practiced by many surgeons who are skilled in microsurgery. Through the years, the attitudes regarding reconstruction of all hand injuries have been modified by the advances made in function following nerve repair. This is reflected in the adoption of more refined operative techniques. One should expect good results in repair of simple nerve lacerations treated by ideal coaptation of the nerve fasicles using microscopic techniques.

Previously, it was believed that primary repair of an injured digital nerve was the treatment of choice. However, if the wound is not ideal as with tendon injuries, it is best to close the skin, splint the hand in a protective position with elevation, and in 5 to 7 days proceed with a delayed primary nerve repair. Thus one deals effectively with the everpresent menace of infection, which would seriously compromise a nerve reconstruction. Delayed primary nerve repair, as evidenced by studies performed in our laboratory, gives better results because the time interval since injury serves as a period for the nerve cell nucleus to "gear up" its reparative capabilities and transmit this to the site of injury.[13] One should expect nerve regeneration in the pure sensory nerve of the finger, for example, to occur at a rate of approximately 1 cm or more a week. In contrast, before World War II, the rate of nerve regeneration following repair was reported to be approximately 1 mm per day after a lag period of approximately 6 weeks. These improvements are related to the development of microneural surgical techniques. Nerve injuries should always be reconstructed in children, since normal nerve function is essentially for normal development. A nonsensate finger is not used normally.

BONY INJURIES

Bony injuries are not seen as frequently in children as are the previously mentioned problems.[2, 14] Many times, simple fractures that are not displaced can be treated with splinting and a soft dressing for 3 to 4 weeks. The child can then be released to full activity, and healing usually occurs without difficulty. If fractures occur through the symphysis, located usually at the base of each phalanx, anatomic realignment is essential for satisfactory results. If there is displacement of the fractures, open reduction and anatomic repositioning of the fragments with appropriate fine wire fixation is the treatment of choice. In most, this requires general anesthesia usually on an outpatient hospital visit. These fractures require somewhat longer immobilization (4 to 5 weeks). In the mature young juvenile, immobilization of complicated fractures of the metacarpals and wrist with appropriate plaster splinting should be instituted for approximately 5 to 6 weeks. Simple fractures can be released from fracture fixation in these bones after about 4 to 5 weeks. Postimmobilization x-rays will frequently not show significant callus formation, only traces of beginning healing. Fortunately, bony healing in children occurs at an ideal rate.

Simple fractures of the phalanges, if nondisplaced, are best held in position for 3 to 4 weeks with a soft dressing and the finger slightly flexed in a position of function. In teenagers, there is a tendency toward joint stiffness and collateral ligament shortening. Fortunately, hand therapy is seldom needed in most children because of the rapid return to a full range of motion with active use. Fracture displacements should be openly reduced and held in position with appropriate internal fixation, usually Kirschner wire pins, wire loops, screws, or occasionally onlay compression plates. These more complicated fractures require immobilization for 5 to 6 weeks. If open reduction is performed, the adjacent joints should be passively moved through almost a full range of motion to prevent joint stiffness.[15]

Tuft fractures of the distal phalanges, which are frequently seen in crushed fingertips, require almost no specific treatment except protective immobilization, usually with a metal or plastic fingertip guard. They heal well and are usually pain-free after 6 to 8 weeks.

With the development of compression plate systems, the duration of immobilization necessary for satisfactory healing of a phalanx or metacarpal fracture has been reduced approximately 20 per cent. Of course, the use of a compression plate establishes the need for a second operation for plate removal. In the teenager, which is the children's group most frequently treated with compression plates for complicated fractures, plate removal utilizing peripheral nerve block anesthesia carries low morbidity.

INJURIES TO LIGAMENTS

Ligamentous injuries are complicated and need careful attention to achieve satisfactory results. One of the most frequent ligament injuries involves the extensor tendon insertion at the distal joint producing the so-called mallet finger or baseball finger deformity. This avulsion or tear of the insertion of the dorsal extensor tendon mechanism may include a chip fracture of the dorsal lip of the proximal edge of the distal interphalangeal joint. This bony chip into which the tendon inserts should be replaced anatomically. If an x-ray fails to reveal any fracture, one can safely splint the distal joint in hyperextension of at least 15 degrees for a minimum of 6 weeks.[4] Such splinting in the child has been reviewed under tendon injuries.

Collateral ligament tears of the distal interphalangeal joint are rare. They should be treated for approximately 4 weeks by conservative splinting in a plastic or metal splint with the joint held in a neutral extended position.

If a ligament injury is suspected, peripheral nerve block anesthesia in the older child is essential to determine the diagnosis with stress x-rays. After the anesthesia has been obtained, one abducts and adducts the joint to see if it can be "opened," thus revealing a torn ligament. In ligament injury in a very young child, general anesthesia is usually necessary. If x-rays reveal an avulsion fracture of the ligament insertion, open reduction and replacement of the fragment are indicated, followed by appropriate plaster immobilization for 4 to 5 weeks. Results are good in children. After immobilization, therapy rarely is needed.

If a ligament tear is demonstrated without a chip fracture and the stress x-ray maneuver suggests a marked instability of the joint such as a complete tear, open reduction and suturing of the torn ligament are indicated in the older child usually beyond age 12. In the younger child, immobilization in a plaster splint for 4 weeks will usually provide good healing. However, the parents should be apprised of the possibility of unsatisfactory healing the the need for a second reconstructive procedure. The ligament may heal in an attenuated position. Scar that has formed in the area must be removed, restoring the ligament to its more short, natural state.

NAIL INJURIES

Crush injuries to the nail often produce a painful hematoma beneath the nail, which demands evacuation for pain relief. A paper clip heated to a red hot temperature and held with an appropriate insulating clamp quickly burns through the nail, leaving an appropriately sized opening for drainage of the hematoma and relief of pain. A high-speed dental drill with a fine burr is also satisfactory in producing a drainage hole. A No. 10 scalpel blade can be used but the pressure necessary produces significant pain. A digital nerve block is indicated to perform this type of hematoma evacuation. An antibiotic-impregnated protective dressing should be placed over the drainage site to prevent subungual infection. If there is any question of underlying bony damage x-rays should be obtained.

Lacerations of the fingertip involving the nail bed demand that the nail bed be sutured anatomically.[15] Sutures of 6-0 plain catgut are ideal. A Vaseline gauze-type dressing is

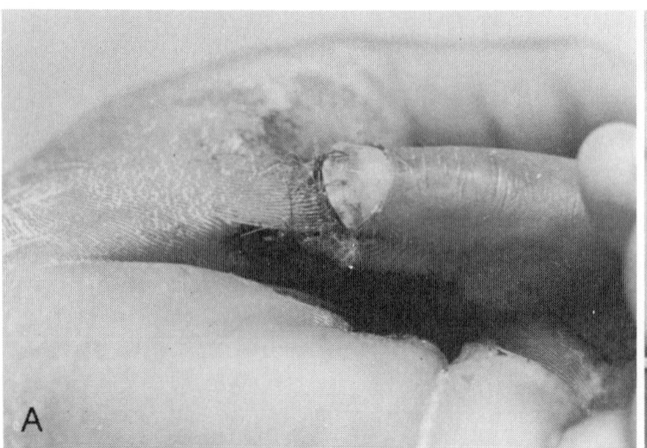

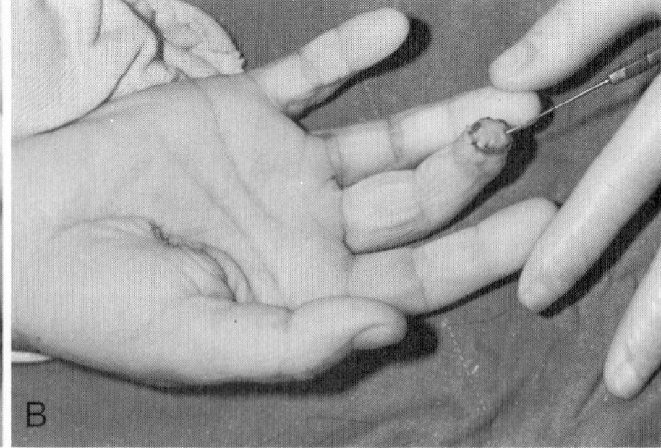

Figure 23–5. There are many techniques to correct fingertip injuries. When a significant amount of padding is needed, a thenar full-thickness flap of skin and subcutaneous tissue can be transferred to the deformed finger in two stages. *B*, The flap is detached with the patient under local anesthesia (without epinephrine) in approximately 18 days.

placed over the nail bed and held in position with a supportive dry dressing. It is not necessary to remove these sutures. The Vaseline gauze will remain adherent to the nail bed. A new nail grows out in 3 to 4 months over an intact nail bed to produce a nail without disfigurement. If the nail bed has been badly scarred and/or the laceration has not been anatomically approximated, a deformity of the nail develops. This can frequently be improved by secondary reconstruction.[15]

FINGERTIP INJURIES

Compound injuries of the tip of the finger involving nail, bone, and soft tissue are treated in a variety of ways, depending upon the extent of injury (Fig. 23–5). An effective method for primary repair of tip amputations is the development of a volar skin-pulp triangular V-flap with the apex of the V extending toward the distal flexion crease. This flap is carefully elevated and advanced to cover the amputation site. The donor area is closed as a Y. If the nail bed has been avulsed on the dorsum, the amputated part should be retrieved and the nail bed with its intact nail (if present) reattached as a free graft. Reconstitution of the nail bed is essential to obtain satisfactory correction of tip injuries. Most always the skin and soft tissue molds itself well, but lacerations within the nail bed itself are unforgiving, producing a deformed nail.

Pedicle flap reconstruction of post-traumatic deformities of the fingertip can be greatly improved by utilization of tissue from other parts of the hand. The cross-finger flap and thenar flap are examples of staged reconstructions.

Secondary reconstruction of nail bed deformities may vary from removal of the deformed nail and excision of the scar deformity within the nail bed, with careful reapproximation of the bed, to removal of the scarred deformed area of an avulsed or partially avulsed nail bed and replacement with a free nail bed graft from the second or third toe. The donor site is reconstructed most satisfactorily with a splint-thickness skin graft.

VASCULAR INJURIES

Vascular injuries of the fingers of children usually require little care if only one artery or vein has been severed. If two arteries have been severed in the finger a micro-arterial repair is indicated to restore blood flow and prevent the development of a painful, cold-intolerant digit with inadequate circulation. This is best performed as soon as possible in a hospital environment with the appropriate microreconstructive team. Trauma to the radial or ulnar arteries should also be treated as an important vascular injury. The state of the reconstructive art has progressed to the point that microreconstitution of these vessels, regardless of the age of the child, is the treatment of choice. When either the radial or ulnar artery is severed, the other will always supply the vascular demands of the hand. However, it assists prevention of cold intolerance if the radial or ulnar artery is repaired with microvascular technique.

Compound injuries involving skin, muscle, bone, tendon, and nerve should be handled in the hospital environment by an appropriately trained hand specialist with the patient under general anesthesia. The addition of the microsurgical operating capability has greatly enhanced the quality of primary and delayed reconstruction of hand injuries and has become the "standard of care" for children with these problems. The details of flap coverage resurfacing of an acute injury, free transplantation of an amputated part, or primary bone grafting for avulsed bony fragments in the acute situation are beyond the scope of this chapter. Referral to the appropriate hand surgeon after careful cleaning of the wound, dressing the wound in a sterile gauze, immobilization of the area with either a volar or dorsal slab splint, and placing the extremity in a supportive sling is the initial treatment of choice.

AMPUTATIONS

The physician who provides primary care for children should be aware of the closest surgical unit with microreconstructive capability so that, if necessary, prompt referral can be made for consideration of replantation of injured fingers or hands.*

---

*The centers nearest you can be obtained from the American Society for Surgery of the Hand, 3025 South Parker Road, Suite 65, Aurora, Colorado, 80014 (phone number 303/755-4588), and the American Society of Plastic and Reconstructive Surgery, 233 N. Michigan Avenue, Suite 1900, Chicago, Illinois (phone number 312/856-1834).

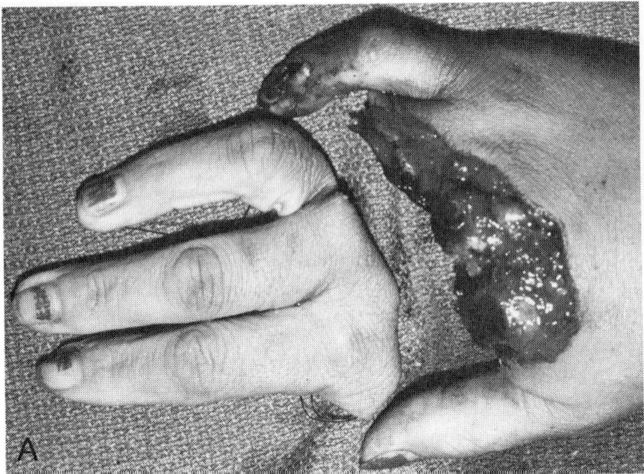

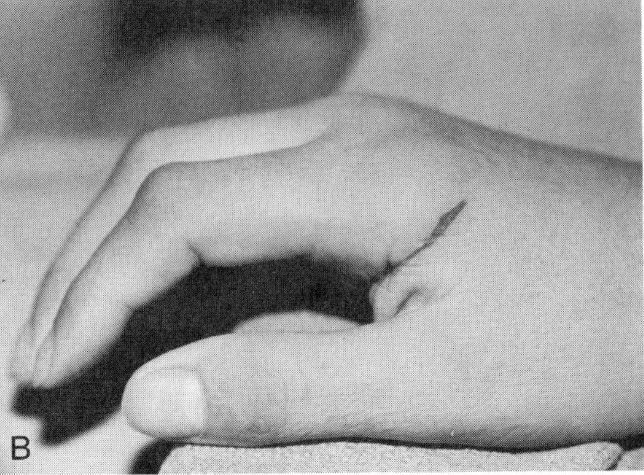

Figure 23–6. *A*, Partial or complete amputations of fingers or the hand should always be considered for possible replantation. Early transfer to a microsurgery center is essential. The amputated part should be placed in a voluminous sterile gauze supportive dressing. This should be placed in a plastic bag. The plastic bag should then be placed in an ice bag and transported with the patient as soon as possible. *B*, The hand of a 14-year-old girl who had successful replantation of the index, middle, and ring fingers after they were amputated in an automobile accident.

Total or partial amputations should be cared for with the primary purpose of getting the amputated part and the patient to a microreconstructive center as soon as possible (Fig. 23–6).

The amputated part should be retrieved and placed gently in sterile dressings. Leave the aggressive scrubbing to the treating surgeon. These dressings should be surrounded by a cotton or Dacron wool type of protective dressing approximately 3 inches thick. This should then be placed in a waterproof plastic bag, which is packed in an ice bucket. At no time should ice be allowed to come in contact with the amputated part. This will produce tissue necrosis.

The patient should be referred to the microsurgical center by telephone with as much information given to the receiving surgeon as possible. The details of the injury, the past medical history of the patient, and the care that has been provided in the initial triage are essential. If the amputated part and the patient cannot be transferred to a microvascular center before 6 to 8 hours, the chances of survival of the part decrease precipitously. If the amputation has been a clean laceration with minimal tissue destruction, the chances for survival of the part following replantation, regardless of the age of the child, are good to excellent.[11] The success of replantation is directly related to the promptness of referral as well as the extent of the original injury.

PROSTHESIS

Most young children who have one normal extremity will not use or even tolerate a partial prosthesis for the other extremity. If their handicap is severe and the prosthesis provides a significant benefit, they will use it readily, usually with consummate skill. Attempts to fit a prosthesis to replace a part of the hand are not wise in a child whose other hand is normal because of the child's ingenious ability to improvise with the intact parts.

The use of cosmetic prostheses is best postponed until after puberty when appearance becomes more important.

Any prosthesis provided to a child should be the product of a team approach developed in a center where all needed skills for designing, fitting, training, and maintenance are available.

REFERENCES

1. Pickrell KL, Georgiade N, Morris F, Adamson JE: Plastic surgical conditions in infancy and childhood. Postgrad Med 27:704, 1960.
2. Adamson JE, Horton CE, Crawford HH: The diagnosis and treatment of hand injuries in children. Va Med Mon 95:407, 1968.
3. Adamson JE: Postoperative care of the injured hand. *In* Symposium on the Hand. St. Louis, C.V. Mosby Company, 1971.
4. Adamson JE, Horton CE, Mladick RA, Carraway JH: Splinting the hand. *In* Symposium on Reconstructive Hand Surgery. St. Louis, C. V. Mosby Company, 1974.

5. Adamson JE, Fleury AF Jr: Incisions in the hand and wrist. *In* Operative Hand Surgery. New York, Churchill-Livingstone, 1982.
6. Bell JL, Mason ML, Koch SL, Stromberg WB: Injuries to flexor tendons of the hand in children. J Bone Joint Surg 40A:1220, 1958.
7. Bondoc CC, Quinby WC, Burke JF: Primary surgical management of the deeply burned hand in children. J Pediatr Surg 11:355, 1976.
8. Buncke JH, Gonzalez RI: Fingernail reconstruction. Plast Reconstr Surg 30:452, 1962.
9. Flatt AE: The Care of Minor Hand Injuries. 4th ed. St. Louis, C.V. Mosby, 1979.
10. Adamson JE, Crawford HH, Horton CE, Brown LH: Treatment of dorsal burn adduction contracture of the hand. Plast Reconstr Surg 42:355, 1968.
11. Kleinert HE, Juhala CA, Tsai TM, Van Beek A: Digital replantation—selection, technique and results. Orthop Clin North Am 8:309, 1977.
12. Peterson RA: Electrical burns of the hand: Treatment by early excision. J Bone Joint Surg 48A:407, 1966.
13. Adamson JE, Horton CE, Crawford HH: Sensory rehabilitation of the thumb. Plast Reconstr Surg 40:53, 1967.
14. Adamson JE, et al.: The treatment of acute injuries of the fingers. Norfolk General Hospital Bulletin, Vol. 2, No. 1, 1964.
15. Adamson JE: Treatment of the stiff hand. Orthop Clin North Am 1:476, 1970.

CHAPTER

24 Vascular Injuries

T. PETER DOWNING

Infants and small children present infrequently to the emergency room with injuries to significant arterial and venous vessels. In the past, vascular injuries to the trunk frequently were not diagnosed because resuscitation measures often failed when major vascular disruption was not aggressively treated. Trauma centers are now capable of resuscitating a severely injured child, and it has consequently become more important to be aware of large vessel injuries associated with diffuse trauma. Historically, peripheral vascular injuries have been treated expectantly, since infants and children have extensive collateral blood flow protecting the viability of limbs, and because surgical techniques of small vessel repair were not available. More recent publications examining long-term prognosis following major vessel disruption have disclosed serious interference with growth, however, if vessel injury is not repaired.[1–3] The use of Fogarty catheters, the success of regional and systemic heparinization, and more refined small vessel surgical techniques can be used to reinstitute perfusion to devascularized limbs. Early diagnosis can now prevent unnecessary loss of life, and expeditious aggressive treatment can prevent functional and psychologic deficits that could affect every aspect of a child's growth and development.

Truncal trauma resulting in major vessel damage is usually compounded by critical injury to other vital structures, which must be handled in sequential fashion as discussed in other sections of the book. Experience in pediatric trauma combined with present-day vascular techniques enables emergency personnel, in coordination with qualified surgeons, to provide expeditious resuscitation and repair of major vessel injury in those children fortunate enough to survive transportation to an appropriate emergency center. Although trauma sufficient to cause central vascular injury is often too severe to allow time for transport, some will survive because the pediatric population is often protected from multiple vessel injury by the elasticity of their skeletal structure, by the tendency of children to respond to physical injury without reflex muscular guarding (they relax rather than tense during blunt trauma), and by lower torso momentum because of their small weights. Frequently, in those reaching the emergency room, vessel disruption has been tamponaded or protected by spasm. In these patients, *awareness* of potential vascular injuries will direct diagnostic methods to arrive at an expeditious therapy preventing delayed morbidity or mortality.

SPECIAL CONSIDERATIONS

The ease of treatment and often of diagnosis depends upon patient age and size. Vascular injuries in children over the age of 6 or above 20 kg may be treated similarly to those in adults, although physicians must be aware of the additional problems with growth retardation following injuries that create relative vascular ischemia. Children and infants below this age and size present a difficult problem because of the increased propensity for low-flow states secondary to volume depletion to progress to distal thrombosis, whether in vessels with proximal disruption or those with spasm secondary to blunt or penetrating trauma. The smaller the vessel injured, the more likely the chance of spasm, although even aortic spasm precipitating distal thrombosis has been associated with blunt injury in small infants.

In children, fractures frequently occur in the supracondylar area of the humerus, with subsequent edema surrounding the restrictive joint space, causing vessel compromise. In these cases, early reduction of fractures or dislocations is necessary. Fortunately the abundance of collateral circulation preserves limb viability in most cases but does not preclude the necessity for reconstitution of large vessel integrity.

Invasive diagnostic procedures and therapeutic maneuvers such as the insertion of central infusion lines or monitoring catheters are themselves the most common cause of vascular injury in infants less than 2 years of age and are occasionally injurious in older children.[4] Arteriography; subclavian, internal jugular, and femoral vein cannulation; intra-arterial monitoring; intramuscular injection; femoral arterial and venous blood sample acquisition; and the more specialized use of umbilical artery or vein catheterization and hyperalimentation lines are often necessary, but physicians must remain aware of the potential risks.[5] Delayed stenosis, dissection, perivascular leak causing extrinsic compression, and central venous and arterial embolus and thrombosis are sequelae that must be avoided by applying appropriate technique and selective use, as well as recognized early when they occur.

ETIOLOGY

The mechanism of vascular injury is clearly dependent upon age and size. The majority of injuries (excluding those with iatrogenic causes) occur during the ages when children are mobile and without guidance. Because infants and small children lack the ability to protect themselves, even minor automobile accidents may have disastrous consequences. Usually, however, multisystem injuries serious enough to cause vascular damage preclude a patient's survival prior to reaching the emergency room. In the series of pediatric vascular trauma collected from the literature,[6–9] 28 per cent of the noniatrogenic injuries to major vessels were secondary to blunt trauma, 35 per cent were from gunshot wounds, and 21 per cent were from other penetrating objects.

Extremity injuries are most common, as normal childhood activities endanger limbs. Fractures, crush injuries from relatively heavy objects, penetrating injuries from glass doors, broken glass, and misuse of sharp objects and firearms are commonly associated with lack of supervision, increased mobility with age, and inability of the infant or child to recognize potential danger. Patients with abdominal injuries secondary to penetrating wounds and pelvic injuries caused by crushing trauma often survive to reach the emergency room. The latter, if associated with persistent bleeding, have a high mortality and are usually associated with motor vehicle accidents. Penetrating wounds to the thorax generally occur in older children but may be seen in young children. Children with blunt injuries to the thorax associated with major vascular damage seldom survive to the emergency room because of associated injury.

Penetrating neck injuries are uncommon in childhood but can occur secondary to gunshots or sharp objects. These patients often survive to the hospital if the injury is localized and is rapidly tamponaded. Long-term survival is dependent upon expeditious treatment. Even with a complete carotid transection, there is only a 30 per cent incidence of neurologic deficit in children. Upper thoracic trauma from blunt or penetrating injury, excluding aortic disruption, often results in survivors, and repair is dependent upon suspicion and appropriate diagnostic maneuvers.

Of particular pertinence to the infant age group is the frequency of arterial spasm, which in the presence of a hypotensive low-flow state may result in distal vessel thrombosis. In these settings, conservative treatment may be injurious by allowing progression of vessel thrombosis. Early surgical treatment is mandatory.

In addition to compromise of distal organs, physicians must be aware that virtually all identifiable arterial injuries are associated with injury to other structures, especially nerves and veins in proximity to the area of injury. Attention must also be directed toward resolution of these concomitant injuries.

DIAGNOSIS

Classic signs of vessel injury are similar to those seen in adults. Hypotension and shock with evidence of external injury often indicate blood loss but not always vessel damage. Complete evaluation by routine screening examination, comparative peripheral pulse and pressure evaluation, chest x-ray, peritoneal lavage, and thoracentesis will usually reveal potential central vascular damage. The presence of penetrating injuries in proximity to major blood vessels should limit diagnostic maneuvers and expedite transport to the operating room for exploratory surgery.

Peripheral injuries associated with a large or expanding hematoma, bruit, distal pallor and coolness, limb immobility and weakness, and loss of sensation should alert the physician. In questionable limb injuries as well as pelvic and upper thoracic trauma, bilateral blood pressure measurements and Doppler examination often reveal vascular injury. Serial Doppler ultrasound examination may also be needed to distinguish spasm from occlusion as vessels in spasm commonly allow some distal flow, which increases as volume expansion is achieved. Even in questionable cases, urgent exploration is preferable to waiting longer than 3 to 5 hours for spasm to resolve, in order to prevent further thrombosis and irreversible ischemic effects.

Arteriography should be reserved for patients not in shock with questionable damage to intra-abdominal vessels as evidenced by abdominal tenderness, negative peritoneal lavage, loss of distal pulses, or presence of a mass on examination, and to patients with cervicomediastinal trauma with clinical signs of vessel injury, for example, loss of carotid or arm pulse, hemothorax, bruit, or expanding mediastinum, widened descending aortic contour, or subpleural hematoma on chest x-ray (see Chapter 15). In these patients, arteriography is useful in delineating the operative approach as well as confirming the diagnosis. Penetrating neck injuries usually do not need arteriography unless associated with blunt trauma that may have caused reparable intracerebral damage, or if the level of injury is not clear. Blunt cervical injuries with evidence of vascular compromise often require arteriography to determine the level of transmural or intimal damage. Patients with pelvic fractures and loss of pulses or persistent retroperitoneal bleeding requiring transfusion greater than their predicted intravascular volume should undergo angiography to delineate any surgically accessible lesion. Peripheral injuries seldom require arteriography, as surgical exploration commonly reveals the significant pathology.

In the major published series, preoperative angiography was utilized from 8 to 50 per cent of the time, but it is usually unnecessary in peripheral injury. It may be useful in delineating the etiology of delayed vascular compromise or in locating lesions associated with diffuse fracture or blunt trauma. A newer approach utilizing digital contrast angiography is less invasive but may be equally as time consuming. Computed tomography (CT) may be of benefit in cases of aortic tears or pelvic or intraperitoneal bleeding.

EMERGENCY TREATMENT

Precise diagnosis and surgical intervention must be delayed until evaluation and resuscitation have been undertaken. Ventilation must be adequate, volume replacement attempted via appropriately selected central or peripheral venous access, blood cross-matched, obvious bleeding tamponaded, and unstable anatomy splinted or protected. After hemodynamic stability has been achieved, re-examination should proceed and appropriate diagnostic tests ordered. Physical examination, aided by roentgenograms, yields the diagnosis in most instances.

Penetrating injuries associated with shock or with distal pulse loss require immediate operative exploration following resuscitation. Blunt trauma or fracture often requires further evaluation and if cardiorespiratory function permits, operation can be delayed until specific diagnoses are reached. In this regard, roentgenograms, Doppler ultrasound, and, if necessary, an arteriography following a waiting period are usually indicated. Early *suspicion* of vascular injury will generally yield the correct diagnosis.

Concomitant injuries necessitate a coordinated effort to control oxygenation, relieve cardiac arrest and tamponade, and stop bleeding. Often, especially with blunt trauma, the requirement for thoracotomy, laparotomy, or fracture reduction allows a direct look at vascular anatomy that may have been disrupted and should be an integral part of any reparative operation.

Carotid Artery Injury

Penetrating or blunt trauma to the cervical region complicated by loss of carotid pulse, expanding hematoma, or persistent bleeding through the open wound warrants exploration. Only if the possibility of injury proximal to the obviously injured site exists, is there a necessity for arteriography. The presence of subcutaneous emphysema or a "hissing" sound with ventilation requires exploration for tracheal or esophageal repair and simultaneous examination of jugular vein and carotid arterial injury as well as vagus and phrenic nerve damage.

Direct compression of an expanding hematoma or bleeding during resuscitation usually suffices until the infant or child is in the operating room. Little diagnostic work-up other than cervical and chest x-rays are required while the surgical team is mobilized. In general, disruption of unilateral cerebral circulation from a common or internal carotid tear or intimal disruption is well tolerated in the child, with less than 30 per cent having any neurologic sequelae even when a ligation is necessary. Current practice, however, is to immediately restore vascular integrity through various surgical approaches.[10]

Cervicomediastinal Injuries

Blunt trauma sufficient to cause damage to the aorta, vena cava, and arch vessels rarely presents to the emergency room. A child's pliable thoracic cage and elastic fascial tissues protect from most injuries except those sufficient to cause irreparable damage. Occasionally, intimal disruption will occur or major lacerations or ligamentum tears will tamponade; and if other injuries are not severe, repair can be accomplished. Arteriography and CT will delineate the site of the tear and will assist in selecting the operative approach.

Isolated cases of penetrating injury to this region have been reported, although in the largest series in the literature, the youngest child seen in the emergency room was two.[11] The approach to children is identical to that for adults in that if the child has survived to reach the emergency room, tamponade usually exists and there is time for intravenous (IV) line insertion, control of hypotension, and appropriate diagnostic maneuvers. Evidence of a bruit, loss of extremity pulse, hemothorax, first or multiple rib fractures, thoracic spine fracture, apical subpleural hematoma, and diminished carotid pulse all imply vascular injury and in this special situation warrant arteriography prior to surgical intervention.

The surgical goal is to achieve hemostasis of major vein tributaries and to reconstitute arterial circulation. In select circumstances in young children and infants, the subclavian arteries may be sacrificed without major consequence, but attempts at complete restoration should be made prior to ligature.

Related injuries involving the pulmonary vasculature must likewise be evaluated after resuscitative maneuvers. Although most pulmonary injuries may be treated with nonsurgical conservative measures, unrelenting pulmonary hemorrhage requires bronchoscopy and possible unilateral bronchial occlusion to effect tamponade and appropriate resection.

A frequent unsuspected injury is the development of a bronchovenous fistula, which is often associated with an air embolus. Sudden unexplained cardiac arrest or a cerebral event, often precipitated by the institution of positive pressure ventilation, should alert the emergency team of the necessity for immediate thoracotomy and examination of the heart for evidence of air emboli. In the interim, the child should be placed in the head down position rotated with the injured side most anterior to protect the carotids and coronary vasculature from further emboli during resuscitative measures.[12]

Abdominal Injuries

Injuries to the trunk involving major vessel injury are usually associated with other organ injury. Penetrating injuries from sharp objects usually result in localized visceral injury and associated vessel laceration often with tamponade. Exploration of wounds in a patient not in shock is warranted, and those with peritoneal penetration deserve exploration. All major vessels and their tributaries should be examined for hematoma. A retroperitoneal hematoma will generally not need surgery, but those involving the aorta and iliac arteries as well as the vena cava and iliac veins usually require direct closure. Emergency personnel must direct attention to preparation for surgery so that tamponade aided by hypotension is not released when blood pressure is restored by the required resuscitation. Penetrating objects in a small child and injuries that appear small in the adult are nevertheless large when compared with the relative sizes of the viscera and vasculature in the child. A narrow object can easily cause complete aortic or caval disruption even though distal pulses may be present. In many cases, the vessel is tamponaded by the elastic adventitia surrounding vessels in the young age group, and pulses are maintained by collateral flow.

Patients with blunt abdominal trauma who survive to reach the emergency room seldom have major vessel injury. Hemoperitoneum is usually from visceral injury and warrants exploration with examination of vascular anatomy.

Vascular Injuries Associated with Pelvic Fractures

Because of the flexibility of the skeletal anatomy associated with reduced ossification in immature bones, shattering fractures to the pelvis are uncommon. Crush injuries, however, may cause major vascular disruption. Diagnosis can be made by the loss or diminution of femoral pulses, the presence of shock associated with the fracture, and the presence of hemoperitoneum associated with fracture. Shock requiring volume replacement greater than the estimated intravascular volume warrants angiography if time permits or immediate explorative surgery if hemoperitoneum exists. Pelvic retroperitoneal hematoma should not be explored if other cause for blood loss can be located and repaired and should rarely be explored unless a specific lesion has been identified. Children requiring pelvic exploration for continued uncontrollable hemorrhage have an 80 per cent mortality rate,[13] due not only to associated injuries but also to the inability to control hypogastric, iliac, and gluteal arterial and venous disruption. If arteriographic examination reveals a specific site of bleeding, autologous clot infusion is probably the safest method of securing hemostasis.

Emergency room treatment should be directed toward preparing vascular access for transfusion and determining the extent of other injuries while remaining aware that urologic injury is also common.

Peripheral Vascular Injuries

Although loss of blood supply to a limb is seldom life threatening, reinstitution of flow within a 3 to 6-hour period is essential to avoiding sequelae of thrombosis and later decreased limb growth.

Penetrating injuries, most commonly from glass but also from gunshot wounds, knives, and so on should be explored if an expanding hematoma exists or if distal pulses are absent. Doppler ultrasound examination will help reveal the presence of nonpalpable pulses, but even when a weak signal is present, ischemia persisting longer than 3 hours is an indication for surgical exploration without the necessity for arteriography. Emergency room care consists of proper recording of limb temperature levels, capillary filling, palpable and/or Doppler pulses, and hematoma demarcations while the wound is being tamponaded. Surgical repairs must involve repair of concomitant venous injury and, if necessary, primary or secondary nerve reanastomosis as well as compartment decompression.

Crush injuries or blunt trauma, especially in the infant, usually will inflict intimal damage without vessel wall disruption, and often no hematoma is present. Here, diagnosis is very difficult, as spasm of arteries is very common in the relatively small-caliber vessels found in infants. Sequential Doppler examination is useful. Ischemia for longer than 3 hours will have serious sequelae, and surgical exploration is indicated. Angiography may be used if the level of injury is not clear. The use of systemic heparinization to prevent thrombosis is controversial. Perhaps it is most successfully applied to those injuries without an expanding hematoma and without injury to other body structures.

Vascular compromise compounding fractures is relatively uncommon, estimated in one larger series at 1 in 300 fractures.[14] Vessels in proximity to suprachondylar fractures are particularly prone to occlusion.[15] If fracture reduction fails to return arterial flow, then open exploration is warranted. If open fixation is required, then vessel integrity should be assessed. In general, fractures should be reduced and stabilized prior to vessel repair, bearing in mind the time constraints of limb ischemia.

With blunt or fracture trauma, concomitant compartment fasciotomy is often indicated to relieve swelling secondary to hematoma and edema. Vessel repair will vary from simple suture closure to resection, mobilization, and closure, or to interposition vein or prosthesis grafting. Attempts should be made to preserve venous integrity and to identify and appropriately manage nerve damage either with primary or delayed repair. Fogarty catheters should be used to evacuate thrombus until limb back bleeding is present. Regional and systemic heparinization should be used judiciously if other injury is not present.

Although popliteal and brachial injuries are more serious than more proximal or distal injuries because collateral supply over the knee and elbow is limited and easily compromised by edema, current management requires primary repair of all axillary, brachial, radial, and ulnar arteries in the upper extremity and femoral and popliteal arteries in the lower extremity. Venous repair should be performed if possible to expedite wound healing and prevent edema. Vessels treated effectively by tamponade without surgery may later present with aneurysm formation or rupture, so they should be repaired even if distal perfusion appears adequate.

In a large well-documented series of vascŭlar injuries at a major trauma center,[7] 43 cases were in the pediatric age group. Forty-five per cent were associated with nerve injury and 18 per cent with fracture. Operative therapy brought a universally good result except for one failed popliteal repair resulting in amputation. Ligation of the radial and ulnar arteries did not compromise blood supply to the hand but is not recommended. Most importantly, however, the series disclosed that even appropriate repair had a less satisfactory result if repair was delayed 6 hours or longer.

Iatrogenic Injuries

Most commonly, iatrogenic injuries occur in neonates or in infants under the age of 2. They are associated with the insertion of monitoring lines or IV infusion sites or occur as complications of arteriography. Emergency room personnel may be called on to insert intravascular lines and must be aware of proper technique and must take care to avoid complications.[5]

In neonates, placement of umbilical artery and vein catheters and subsequent misuse may result in direct vessel injury, with dissection or stenosis if improperly placed, or with embolus and distal thrombosis related to spasm induced by the catheter or the infusion of hypertonic solution. The spasm creates a low-flow state in a vascular system that is often hypercoagulable. Prevention is the best treatment. Silastic umbilical artery catheters should be small (20 or 22 gauge) and should be localized near the L4 level as confirmed by a postinsertion abdominal roentgenogram. The catheters should be constantly infused with heparinized saline, and any evidence of distal ischemia should be treated with immediate catheter withdrawal and systemic heparinization. No other infusion should be made through the arterial line unless absolutely necessary. Aortic thrombosis as evidenced by loss of both femoral pulses should be treated with Fogarty catheter thrombectomy through an abdominal approach and unilateral loss of pulse treated with thrombectomy through a femoral cutdown site. The limb with questionable ischemia should be examined by Doppler ultrasound to ascertain if spasm or thrombosis is the etiology. Evidence of flow by a positive Doppler examination at the femoral level dictates nonoperative therapy relying on systemic heparinization only to preserve distal vessel patency. Suspected catheter dissection should be examined by arteriography and may be treated conservatively if subsequent luminal occlusion has not occurred.

Umbilical vein cutdown and line insertion are frequent causes of caval thrombosis, suppurative thrombophlebitis, hepatic vein thrombosis often related to malposition (not in the inferior vena cava) or to the infusion of hypertonic solutions. They should be used infrequently. The best sites for large-bore IV access, if peripheral insertion is impossible, include the internal jugular and subclavian veins, but placement should be performed only by those familiar with anatomy and technique. The safest sites for access are peripheral veins, utilizing as large a catheter as possible, either percutaneously or by saphenous or brachial vein cutdown. These latter two locations are frequent sites of thrombophlebitis, especially after cutdown, and removal of the catheter with early signs of inflammation is warranted to prevent these problems.

Arterial monitoring is best accomplished via the radial artery, which if necessary can be sacrificed. Again a small (20 or 22 gauge) catheter should be inserted using a guide wire if necessary. If a cutdown is required, the catheter should be inserted through a separate percutaneous puncture so that no sutures need be placed. This will decrease wound infection and optimize arterial patency following catheter removal. The femoral artery may be used for monitoring, but possible spasm and distal thrombosis creating limb ischemia make this a less desirable site. All catheters should have constant infusions of heparinized saline, should have no other IV infusion, and should be removed with evidence of distal thrombosis or ischemia, followed by systemic heparinization. Persistence of femoral thrombosis longer than 3 to 5 hours should be treated with thrombectomy.

Needle injuries to major arteries can occur with improper technique. Blood aspirated from the needle prior to injection or the development of a hematoma indicates vessel puncture. Should either of these occur, compression should be applied to avoid extrinsic compression by hematoma or intrinsic thrombosis secondary to dissection. Use of the anterolateral thigh for injection, with the avoidance (if possible) of femoral arterial punctures, is the best method for circumventing the complications of dissection, distal thrombosis, and false aneurysm formation.

Heparinized patients require compression for a minimum of 15 minutes.

Injuries associated with arteriography have been reported to be as high as 17 per cent but have been reduced to virtually zero by changes in technique, the use of smaller diameter catheters, and systemic heparinization. In a recent series, 1000 catheterizations were performed with only 10 transient episodes of spasm and no other complications.[16] The physician must be aware, however, of the possibility of femoral artery thrombosis or stricture, which may cause ischemia or subsequent growth disturbance or even partial limb loss if not repaired. Thrombosis must be identified early, but strictures usually present at a later date with diminished pulse. These should be treated surgically as soon as the diagnosis is made.

Late sequelae of these iatrogenic injuries may present to the emergency physician, and a careful history combined with physical examination will usually lead to the diagnosis of stricture, arteriovenous fistulae, or false aneurysm, which will require surgical repair.

These complications are discussed not because the emergency room personnel will see many such problems but because they are in a position to cause them. Avoidance of improper technique, selection of appropriate sites for cannulization, and assurance that a child with indwelling lines or undergoing diagnostic angiography is well hydrated will usually prevent these unfortunate sequelae.

REFERENCES

1. Bloom JD, Mozersky DS, Buckley CJ, Hagood CO: Defective limb growth as a complication of catheterization of the femoral artery. Surg Gynecol Obstet 138:524, 1974.
2. Whitehouse WM, Coram AG, Stanley JC, Kuhns LR, Weintraub WH, Fry WJ: Pediatric vascular trauma: Manifestations, management and sequelae of extremity arterial injury in patients undergoing surgical treatment. Arch Surg 111:1269, 1976.
3. Peacock JB, Procter JH: Factors limiting extremity function following vascular injury. J Trauma 17:532, 1977.
4. O'Neill JA: Traumatic vascular lesions in infants and children. *In* Dean RH, O'Neill JA (eds.): Vascular Disorders of Childhood. Philadelphia, Lea & Febiger, 1983, pp. 181–193.
5. Hughes WT: Pediatric Procedures. Philadelphia, W. B. Saunders Company, 1980.
6. Shaker IJ, White JJ, Signer RD, Golladay ES, Haller JA: Special problems of vascular injuries in children. J Trauma 16:863, 1976.
7. Stanford JR, Evans WE, Morn TS: Pediatric arterial injuries. Angiology 27:1, 1976.
8. Meagher DP, Defore WW, Mattox KL, Harberg FJ: Vascular trauma in infants and children. J Trauma 19:532, 1979.
9. Richardson JD, Fallat M, Nagaraj H, Groff DB, Flint LM: Arterial injuries in children. Arch Surg 116:685, 1981.
10. Sheeley CH, Mattox KL, Reul GJ, Beall AC, DeBakey ME: Current concepts in the management of penetrating neck trauma. J Trauma 15:895, 1975.
11. Bricker DL, Noon GP, Beall AC, DeBakey ME: Vascular injuries of the thoracic outlet. J Trauma 10:1, 1970.
12. Yee ES, Verries ED, Thomas AN: Management of air embolism in blunt and penetrating thoracic trauma. J Thoracic Cardiovasc Surg 85:661, 1983.
13. Quinby WC: Fractures of the pelvis and associated injuries in children. J Ped Surg 1:353, 1966.
14. Cole WG: Arterial injuries associated with fractures of the lower limb in childhood. Injury 12:460, 1981.
15. Rang M: Childrens' Fractures. Philadelphia, J. B. Lippincott Company, 1974.
16. Stanley P, Miller JH: Pediatric Angiography. Baltimore, Williams and Wilkins, 1982.

CHAPTER

25 Burns

GREGORY S. GEORGIADE
JOSEPH MOYLAN

Burns are the second most common cause of death in children from birth to age 4 years and are the third leading cause of death in children ages 4 to 15 years.[1] They are also an extremely common cause of morbidity in the pediatric patient, since the majority of burns are not life threatening.[2] Because of this, most pediatric patients with burns are not cared for at major burn centers but are seen by pediatricians, emergency physicians, and surgeons in the communities in which the injury took place. Furthermore, most burns occur at home and are therefore relatively preventable.[3] Examples of successful efforts to prevent burns include the recent campaign to lower water temperature in hot water heaters in homes[4] and legislation to require fire retardant materials in sleepwear for children.[5]

Thermal trauma is one of the most complex injuries sustained by pediatric patients, since it has the potential to significantly affect virtually all body systems. Although skin is the major organ affected, the cardiopulmonary, nervous, endocrine, gastrointestinal (GI), and renal systems may also be involved. Burns may cause sudden death on the basis of respiratory insufficiency, carbon monoxide poisoning, or massive fluid shifts. Thermal injury produces maximum stress for all organ systems, any or all of which may be overwhelmed by such stress, threatening the patient's survival.

INITIAL EVALUATION OF THE THERMALLY INJURED PATIENT

Physicians caring for burned children must recognize that they are not "little adults" and present a number of unique problems that must be recognized and treated rapidly. Children have a much larger total body surface area (BSA) compared with their body weights than do adults. This results in a higher metabolic turnover and water loss rate for any child with a burn injury.[6] The ability to tolerate the stress of hypothermia is diminished in children. When presented with a hypothermic insult, infants' and small children's hypothalamic regulatory mechanisms respond less efficiently and nonshivering thermogenesis is activated earlier. This is an active energy expenditure process mediated by catecholamines, resulting in heat production. Because of their smaller total blood volumes, children are less able to tolerate massive fluid loss than adults. For these reasons, children are more prone to depletion of existing energy stores, contraction of intravascular volume, and development of metabolic acidosis when they suffer a burn injury.[7] Therefore, physicians must approach all pediatric patients with burn injuries carefully, ensuring that they are evaluated and treated rapidly and efficiently.

A detailed history of the burn injury and the patient's past medical history should be obtained. If the circumstances of the history do not match the type, extent, or degree of burn, the possibility of child abuse or child neglect should be considered.[8] Current tetanus immunization status and the presence of pre-existent illness or infection should be noted.

All burn patients should receive a careful and meticulous physical examination following a protocol approach (see Chapter 1) to assess the burn and to ensure that other injuries, in addition to the burn, are not present. This examination requires removal of all clothing; therefore, it should be carried out in an appropriately prewarmed room to prevent the development of hypothermia in the patient. A detailed assessment of the total extent of the burn injury and a preliminary estimation of the depth of the burn are undertaken (see Fig. 25–1). They should be meticulously recorded on a standard burn chart depicting the representative body surface areas injured and the estimated depth of injury. Initial laboratory evaluation should include complete blood count; determination of electrolyte concentrations, arterial blood gases, and carbon monoxide level; urinalysis; chest x-ray; and electrocardiogram (EKG).

The burn wound should be cleaned with a saline solution, and a topical antibacterial agent should be applied to the injured area. The decision should be made at this time to treat the injury in an open fashion or to dress it with closed occlusive dressings. In most cases the latter technique is preferable. Prophylactic systemic antibiotic therapy is instituted only if there is a previously established infection, such as one of the respiratory tract or urinary tract or a previous history of rheumatic fever. Otherwise, prophylactic antibiotics are not used in the treatment of the burn patient.[9] The weight of the patient should be accurately determined in the emergency department before dressings are applied. The burn wound is highly prone to tetanus, and unless accurate documentation can be obtained of previous tetanus immunization, tetanus prophylaxis should be carried out.

CLASSIFICATION OF BURNS

Treatment of the pediatric burn patient depends upon the extent, depth, and type of burn, as well as the presence of coexistent injuries. The following guidelines assist in classifying minor or major burns in pediatric patients (Table 25–1). Previously, burns were classified as first, second, or third degree. First-degree burns were erythematous burns with extensive underlying edema. In this type of burn, no blisters are produced, but the edema causes extreme pain. Burns involving the epidermis and upper dermis were classified as superficial second-degree burns; those involving the epidermis, upper dermis, and deep dermis were considered deep second-degree burns. Burns in which the entire skin thickness, including the epidermis and dermis and hair follicles, nerves, and sweat glands in the underlying subcutaneous tissue, was injured were classified as third-degree burns. More recent burn classifications have used the terms partial-thickness injury (to refer to burns involving the epidermis and dermis) and full-thickness injury (to refer to complete skin destruction). Although the presence or absence of anesthesia is helpful in distinguishing partial-thickness from full-thickness injuries, it has become apparent that the exact depth of deep skin destruction often cannot be determined at the time of injury. Reassessment is often necessary to delineate the precise depth of the burn.

Table 25–1. CLASSIFICATION OF BURNS IN CHILDREN

Minor Burns
<10% BSA* partial thickness (outpatient)
10–20% BSA partial thickness (inpatient)
Major Burns
≥10% BSA full thickness
≥20% BSA partial or full thickness
Burns to hands, face, feet, or perineum
Electrical burns
Inhalation injuries
Burns complicated by other injury

*BSA = body surface area

Most burns in children are mild to moderate, involving 10 to 20 per cent of total BSA, with less than full-thickness injury. In general, patients with a burn involving 10 per cent or less of BSA are managed as outpatients, unless the burn is full thickness or there are additional injuries requiring inpatient treatment. Patients with burns involving 10 to 20 per cent of BSA usually require hospitalization and fluid resuscitation (see below). Major burns include those characterized by full-thickness involvement of more than 10 per cent of BSA; by partial-thickness involvement of greater than 20 per cent of BSA; by involvement of the hands, face, or perineum; and by complications of inhalational injury, electrical injury, or injury to additional body systems. Many patients with major burns require hospitalization in specialized burn units.

PATHOPHYSIOLOGIC BASIS FOR FLUID THERAPY

Virtually all body systems are affected to varying degrees in burn injuries. A complete discussion of the pathophysiology of burns is beyond the scope of this textbook, and the reader is referred to excellent overviews on the subject.[10,11] However, with regard to fluid therapy, the following pathophysiologic facts are pertinent. First, beginning at the time of initial injury and continuing for approximately 24 hours, water, electrolytes, and molecules with a molecular weight of up to 350,000 daltons leak from the intravascular space into the burn wound and the interstitium.[12] This rapid fluid egress is mediated by multiple mechanisms, including simple increased capillary permeability, altered ability of muscle cells to maintain the normal sodium-potassium gradient, and increased affinity of denatured collagen for sodium and water.[13,14] Approximately 24 hours after the injury, the burn wound is sealed in the vast majority of patients, and the rapid translocation of water, electrolytes, and molecules from the vascular space ends.

Fluid Resuscitation During the First 24 Hours

Because of the preceding pathophysiologic factors, the majority of burn surgeons recommend initial resuscitation of the burn patient during the first 24 hours with a balanced salt solution. Because of the increased capillary permeability during this phase, blood and colloids are not usually administered.[15] Once the burn wound has sealed and resuscitation has been completed during the first 24-hour period, colloid may be added to the crystalloid regimen for resuscitation. The goal of fluid replacement is to appropriately replace the immense body water, electrolyte, and protein losses presented by burn injuries in a timely fashion. A number of formulas have been utilized to estimate the amount and type of fluid that should be administered to burned patients. Children present with significant differences in their response to burn injuries, and therapy should therefore be managed in a protocol fashion. The following specific recommendations are utilized at our burn center.

Virtually all formulas for burn resuscitation base the amount of fluid necessary for resuscitation on the patient's weight and percentage of total body surface area that is involved with partial- or full-thickness burns. The patient's weight and total body surface area should be accurately determined at the time of primary evaluation so that the fluid requirements can be calculated. The initial burn resuscitation is managed with crystalloid replacement therapy using Ringer's lactate solution, with sodium bicarbonate added. This allows for adequate replacement of the isotonic sequestration of the intravascular fluid into the third space at a rate equal to its loss from the intravascular space. One-half ampule of sodium bicarbonate is added to each liter of Ringer's lactate solution using the Duke formula (Table 25–2). With this formula, a calculation can be made of the amount of fluid required for resuscitation by multiplying the weight in kilograms times the percentage of body surface area involved in the burn times 3 ml of the above solution:

3 ml crystalloid solution × weight in kilograms × % BSA burned

Table 25–2. FLUID RESUSCITATION FOR BURNED CHILDREN

First 24 Hours Post-Burn
- Fluid: Ringer's lactate solution + ½ ampule $NaHCO_3$/L
- Rate: 3 ml/kg body weight/ % BSA* burn/24 hr
- Method: ½ volume 1st 8 hr ¼ 2nd + 3rd 8 hr
- Monitor: Urine output (1 ml/kg/hr) + blood pressure (≥80 + [2 × age in years])

24 to 48 Hours Post-Burn
- Fluid: Ringer's lactate solution + $NaHCO_3$
  5% Albumin (3–5 g/kg + 1 g/% BSA burn)
- Rate: To maintain adequate urine output and blood pressure

>48 Hours Post-Burn
- Fluid: 5% glucose in water (D_5W) + blood (as necessary)
- Rate: 2 ml D_5W/% BSA burn/24 hr
- Monitor: Electrolytes, urine output, blood pressure, hemoglobin

*BSA = body surface area.

One half of this total volume is to be administered over the first 8-hour period following the burn, with the remainder of the total volume to be administered equally in the second and third 8-hour periods. It is extremely important that this volume is transfused over the first 24 hours after the injury. When there is a significant delay in obtaining medical care, it will be necessary to increase the amount of fluid transfused over the first 8-hour period to make up for the delay.

As indicated previously, all burn formulas are estimates of the approximate amount of fluid required for resuscitation of the burn patient. For this reason, all patients suffering burns require close monitoring to ensure that fluid resuscitation is adequate. For most patients, this involves monitoring urine output, vital signs, and mental status. These elements serve as indicators of the adequacy of the patient's cardiac output. Urine output should be maintained at 1 ml/kg/hour in children and 50 ml/hour in adults. In children, the blood pressure should be maintained at or above 80 plus twice the patient's age in years. In patients with large burns or those in whom complications develop, more invasive monitoring, including Swan-Ganz catheterization and cardiac output determination, may be necessary.[16] Regardless of whether noninvasive or invasive monitoring is required, careful record keeping with 24-hour flow sheets is essential to ensure appropriate and effective fluid resuscitation.

All children suffering burns covering more than 10 per cent of the total BSA should be admitted to the hospital to receive intravenous (IV) fluid resuscitation. An IV catheter and a Foley catheter are inserted in these patients. Crystalloid replacement therapy is the preferred method of resuscitation for the first 24-hour period following injury. During this time, patients having even moderate burns of 10 to 20 per cent of body surface area may have problems with reflex GI ileus. Any patient demonstrating decreased bowel activity and all patients with burns covering more than 20 per cent of the BSA should have nasogastric tubes inserted.

Fluid Resuscitation During the Second 24 Hours

During the second 24-hour period postburn, administration of Ringer's lactate solution with sodium bicarbonate may be required. The fluid needs for this subsequent 24-hour-period should reflect fluid loss through the burn wound plus maintenance requirements for the patient. As mentioned previously, the adequacy of replacement is monitored by assessing vital signs, urine output, and mental status and, when necessary, by using more invasive methods. Because the burn wound seals at 24 hours following injury in the majority of patients, colloid solutions may be added at this time. Protein requirements may be calculated on the basis of 3 to 5 g/kg plus 1 g/percentage BSA burn. This colloid can be provided by the use of 5 per cent albumin or fresh frozen plasma.

The burn injury always involves the induction of a hypermetabolic state, requiring increased protein and calories to meet the metabolic needs of the patient.[17] As soon as the patient's reflex ileus is gone, oral fluid intake should be started. All burn patients will have some degree of ileus, and oral intake should be slowly increased until dietary caloric and protein requirements can be met. In some cases, parenteral hyperalimentation may be added to oral alimentation to meet the protein and caloric requirements of the patient. However, the GI tract should be used whenever possible. When adequate hydration and caloric needs can be met by oral alimentation, IV infusion should be discontinued, since the IV line may act as a source of sepsis for the patient.[18]

Management of the Burn Patient after 48 hours Following Injury

After the initial resuscitation of the burn patient has been completed during the first 48 hours, the major source of fluid loss in burn patients is evaporative water loss.[19] Fluid therapy during this period is designed to maintain serum electrolytes in the normal range by replacing this water loss and to maintain an hematocrit in the 35 to 40 range. The evaporative water loss can be replaced using the following formula: 2 ml of 5 per cent dextrose and water per per cent burn per 24 hour period. To provide for maximum survival, the physician must ensure that the patient has appropriate initial resuscitation and appropriate fluid and nutritional support to minimize later burn complications and must detect associated injuries.

Acute Problems During the Period of Initial Resuscitation

Patients who do not respond to the initial resuscitation with administration of appropriate fluid volume require careful reassessment. The physician should recalculate the patient's total BSA of burn and the patient's weight. A careful reassessment of previous fluid therapy should be undertaken to ensure its accuracy. If all these measurements are correct, it is possible that the patient's burn wound has not sealed as predicted and more invasive therapy and monitoring will be required. At this time, a pulmonary artery catheter with a thermodilution cardiac output monitor should be considered. This form of monitoring provides accurate evaluations of the filling status of the left heart and myocardial performance.[20] In some children, small amounts of colloid may need to be administered by bolus therapy. In rare cases, inotropic drugs such as dopamine may be required.

PERIPHERAL VASCULAR COMPROMISE

During the initial period of fluid resuscitation, the burned child will develop marked peripheral edema. When there are third-degree burns present, the burn wound may act as a tourniquet, producing compromise of the distal circulation. This restrictive effect can also occur in the chest area, where constriction can produce secondary respiratory failure. This is a common problem in children due to the compromise of the elasticity of their chest wall. Management of this syndrome requires incision through the burn wound to the underlying subcutaneous tissues to produce adequate relief of the constrictive effects of the full-thickness burn. This improves distal circulation in the extremity and improved ventilatory dynamics in the chest wall. Escharotomy is carried out in the midmedial and midlateral lines of the extremities and in a shieldlike pattern on the chest. Care should be taken not to expose tendon sheaths, arteries, or nerves. The procedure can be carried out without anesthesia because the incisions are made through full-thickness burned areas, where the nerve endings have been coagulated and destroyed. Adequate hemostasis is usually obtained with compression, elevation and later with electrocautery if required.

ANALGESICS

All analgesics are given intravenously, and appropriate dosages are based on the weight of the individual child (morphine 0.1 mg/kg, meperidine hydrochloride [Demerol] 1 mg/kg). No analgesics should be given intramuscularly as they are poorly and variably absorbed when given by this route.

MANAGEMENT OF A MINOR BURN IN THE PEDIATRIC PATIENT

Most pediatric burns are minor in that they cover less than 10 per cent total BSA. They are in general secondary to contact with either a hot stove or hot liquids. These burns should be carefully cleaned initially and débrided, after which a determination of the depth and extent of injury should be carried out. The depth of the burn at the time of initial presentation may be deceptive, and subsequent examinations at 24 to 48 hours post-burn may reveal a deeper burn than initially suspected. In addition, infection can also deepen the initial burn wound. After the burn injuries are initially cleaned, they should be dressed with a topical agent such as silver sulfadiazine cream and wrapped occlusively. Arrangements should be made for the patient to be seen in follow-up for repeat dressing change 24 to 48 hours later. This allows for reassessment of the depth of the injury and provides for the necessary follow-up for wound care until the period of complete wound healing has been effected. It is important to remember that burns in young children are usually deeper than initially suspected and close follow-up is mandatory.

Although patients with burns covering less than 10 per cent of total BSA do not usually require hospitalization for IV fluid resuscitation, there is nonetheless a considerable degree of fluid loss from the burn wound. All patients treated on an outpatient basis should receive adequate oral fluid intake to ensure adequate hydration. In addition to assuring that no cardiovascular compromise is present, such oral fluid therapy can help prevent complications of the burn, including hyperpyrexia, pain, and infection.

SPECIALIZED BURN INJURIES

Inhalation Injury

The diagnosis of inhalational injury is suspected primarily on clinical findings. Factors that may indicate the presence of inhalation injury include the following: the burn occurred in an enclosed space; there is physical evidence of burns in or about the mouth; the face is burned; facial or nasal hairs are singed; hoarseness, wheezing, dyspnea, or a rasping cough develop; or the carbonaceous sputum is produced. A patent upper airway must be secured in patients with suspected inhalational injury, and the diagnosis can be confirmed by flexible bronchoscopy or xenon radiography.[21,22] If there are questions as to the patency of the airway, it is preferentially maintained by nasotracheal intubation. Tracheostomy should be avoided because of the problems associated with continued pulmonary sepsis from the surrounding burn wound. Patients with inhalation injury are supported as required with appropriate mechanical ventilatory assistance.

Patients with pulmonary inhalation injuries have fluid losses greatly in excess of patients with simple skin burn. Water losses through a damaged tracheobronchial tree are difficult to estimate accurately. For this reason, the patient with a pulmonary inhalation injury should be strongly considered for invasive monitoring to minimize the possibility of fluid overload and iatrogenic pulmonary compromise. Steroids should not be administered to such patients, since these drugs increase the risk of infectious complications.[23]

Electrical Injuries

Most electrical burn injuries in the pediatric population are due to open electrical sockets or cords. Many of these injuries can be prevented by covering electrical sockets with plastic prongs. Electrical injury due to contact with high voltage wires, other power sources, or lightning is unusual in children and is usually limited to the teenage group. Electrical injuries are the result of the conversion of electrical energy to thermal energy. Electrical injury disperses from the point of injury through the lowest pathway of resistance in a manner similar to all electrical current. In a patient this energy diffuses through the low resistance blood vessels in the body. Because of this, electrical injuries are frequently much more extensive and serious than may be initially suspected from examination of the skin.

Electrical injuries can produce fractures as a result of muscular tetany, vascular thrombosis leading to subsequent muscle death, and possible severe internal injuries. Third space fluid loss may be massive and muscle compartment ischemia may be produced locally or distally where the current has traveled. The subsequent muscle necrosis may produce myoglobinuria, which may lead to tubular necrosis and acute renal failure. A profound metabolic acidosis is a frequent sequelae of electrical injuries.[24]

The initial treatment of the patient with electrical injury requires evaluation of the cardiac status of the patient with an electrocardiogram (EKG), since the heart is also susceptible to muscle necrosis secondary to the electrical stimulus. A careful neurologic examination (including examination of the peripheral nerves) should be undertaken. The severity of an electrical injury is suggested by swelling, which may vary from mild to extremely severe. Pain on passive extension of the extremity, contracture, absence of pulse, distal cyanosis, and poor capillary refill also suggest the development of a compartment syndrome due to swelling from an electrical injury.

The early management of the electrical burn consists of the empircal administration of large quantities of Ringer's lactate solution to maintain urine output at or above 1.5 ml/kg of body weight/hour. The physician should carefully monitor for myoglobinuria, which presents classically as burgundy-colored urine. This complication should be treated with alkalinization of the urine with sodium bicarbonate and forced osmotic diuresis with mannitol, if necessary. Continuous cardiac monitoring is mandatory, and early fasciotomy of the extremity should be carried out when indicated. Vital structures exposed by débridement and fasciotomy should be covered with biologic dressings such as pig skin and kept moist until coverage can be effected with adjacent or distant myocutaneous flaps. The most important elements in the management of patients with electrical injuries are adequate fluid resuscitation and close monitoring for the development of possible complications.

Electrical burns about the mouth characteristically are caused by a child making contact with an open electrical source. This usually means the child has sucked on the end of a live extension cord or an open electrical socket. This injury produces a high temperature in the surrounding area and a subsequent wide area of tissue necrosis. These injuries are best treated with topical dressings and cleaning and are allowed to heal primarily. Delayed reconstruction of the area may be necessary, but many of these injuries heal well primarily. It is important to realize that a commonly encountered complication of this injury is erosion of the burn wound into the labial artery several days to 1 week following the injury. This may produce significant blood loss, but this can usually be well controlled by manual pressure. Parents should be warned of this possible complication and instructed to provide the appropriate first-aid measures until the bleeding can be controlled at the hospital.

Chemical Burns

Chemical skin burns differ from thermal burns mainly because the agents produce skin destruction by coagulation necrosis, with prolonged exposure resulting in vascular thrombosis. Chemical burns are treated by copious water lavage. The period of time required to effect return of the pH of the skin to normal with lavage varies depending on the chemical agent involved. Skin exposed to an alkali such as 50 per cent sodium hydroxide, requires a prolonged period before pH returns to normal, whereas skin subjected to acid burns requires a shorter time for return of normal skin pH. Some specialized injuries such as lye burns are affected very little by water lavage after they are 1 hour or more old. They may actually be increased in depth with lavage if it is instituted after 1 hour or later post-burn because of the facilitation of the passage of hydroxidions into the deeper layers of the dermis.

Extreme care should be given in providing for adequate copious lavage of the burned area, and a detailed history should be taken concerning the offending agent if adequate therapy is to be instituted. Chemical injuries can produce significant problems relative to the underestimation of their size because of the occult nature of the injury. This is especially true in young infants. Consideration should be given to the inhalation of toxic vapors, which could subsequently produce secondary pulmonary injury. Chest x-ray and measurement of arterial blood gases are important, and fiberoptic laryngoscopy or bronchoscopy should be considered in appropriate cases.

The calculation of requirements for fluid resuscitation of patients with chemical burns is determined in the same way as it is for patients with a thermal burn of similar BSA.

Specific chemical antidotes to chemical burns are of dubious value, and saline lavage should be carried out immediately. Undiluted chemical neutralized agents may do further damage by the production of heat by exothermic chemical reactions. Specific information concerning individual chemical injuries can be obtained from standard reference texts.[25]

The management of chemical burn wounds parallels that of thermal burns, with the use of topical antimicrobial agents, excision, and early coverage if possible.

TRANSFER CONSIDERATIONS

Thermally injured patients with partial-thickness burns of 20 per cent of BSA or third-degree burns of 10 per cent BSA should be considered for transfer to a specialty burn care unit. In addition, patients with burns of complex structures such as the hands, face, perineum, and feet should be considered for transfer if a well-trained reconstructive surgeon familiar with burn injuries is not available to manage the patient. Patients with electrical burns and burn injuries complicated by inhalation injury or associated with major soft tissue injuries, fractures, or other traumatic injuries should be considered for transport to a specialized facility. Burn patients may be transferred at any time following burn injury but often are best transferred shortly after the initial injury if the length of time required for transfer is short and resuscitation procedures have been initiated prior to transfer. Longer distance transfers require increased planning and organization if they are to be carried out without compromise to the patient. It is the responsibility of the referring physician to contact a suitable burn care facility. Most hospitals have a long-standing relationship with several burn facilities. A list of regional burn care facilities is available from the American Burn Association.

Adequate communication between the referring and receiving physicians is essential. Adequate initial steps in resuscitation should be initiated prior to transfer, and records and laboratory data on the patient should be maintained throughout the resuscitation and period of transfer. The receiving physician should provide the necessary instructions for effecting a safe transport and gather appropriate data on the initial severity of the injury to allow for appropriate preparations by the receiving unit.

It is difficult to perform a procedure during transport, and for this reason, the necessary airways and IV lines and nasogastric tubes should be inserted before the patient leaves the primary facility. Resuscitation with adequate peripheral or central IV catheters should be well underway prior to initiating transport.

OUTCOME

Burn injuries cause a significant amount of morbidity and mortality in this country, particularly among children. Perhaps no injury is more horrifying than a burn. However, it is important to realize that major strides have been made in both mortality reduction in burn patients as well as rehabilitation for patients with minor and major burn injuries. Aggressive fluid resuscitation, prevention of burn wound sepsis, and anticipation and management of additional complications have resulted in survival for many patients with major burns. Modern techniques of plastic surgical reconstruction have allowed many patients with disfiguring injuries to return to a relatively normal lifestyle. In general, morbidity and mortality from burns are related to the percentage of the BSA burned, the depth and location of the burn, the presence of respiratory failure (whether produced by respiratory distress syndrome or inhalation injury), sepsis, renal failure, and age. Because of their poorly developed immune and homeostatic regulatory mechanisms, infants with major burns have a much higher mortality than school-age children or adolescents. It is important to remember that sepsis is difficult to predict in burn patients, partially because leukocytosis and hyperthermia are extremely common in all burn patients. Burn wound biopsies and careful physiologic monitoring are necessary for the timely detection of the development of sepsis.

With adequate training, preparation, and implementation of appropriate resources, the majority of burns in pediatric patients can be successfully managed.

REFERENCES

1. Wagman ME: Annual summary of vital statistics. Pediatrics 72:755, 1983.
2. O'Neill JA: Evaluation and treatment of the burned child. Pediatr Clin North Am 22:407, 1975.
3. Raine PAM, Azmy A: A review of thermal injuries in young children. J Pediatr Surg 18:21, 1983.
4. Feldman KW, Schaller RT, Feldman JA, et al.: Tap water scald burns in children. Pediatrics 62:1, 1978.
5. McLaughlin E, Clarke N, Stahl K, Crawford JD: One pediatric burn unit's experience with sleepware-related injuries. J Pediatr 60:405, 1977.
6. Dartschi MB, Kohler TR, Finley A, Heimbach DM: Burn injury in infants and young children. Surg Gynecol Obstet 150:651, 1980.
7. Brack HM, Asch MJ, Pruitt BA: Burns in children: A 10 year experience with 412 patients. J Trauma 10:658, 1970.
8. Hight DW, Bakaler MR, Lloyd JR: Inflicted burns in children: Recognition and treatment. JAMA 242:517, 1979.
9. Larkin JM, Moylan JA: The role of prophylactic antibiotics in burn care. Ann Surg 42:247, 1976.
10. Moncrief JA: Burns. N Engl J Med 288:444, 1973.
11. O'Neill JA: Burns in children. *In* Artz CP, Moncrief DA, Pruitt BA Jr (eds.): Burns: A Team Approach. Philadelphia, W. B. Saunders Company, 1979.
12. Moylan JA, Mason AD, Rogers SP, Walder HL: Postburn shock: A critical evaluation of resuscitation. J Trauma 13:354, 1973.
13. Parks DH, Carvajal HF, Larson DL: Management of burns. Surg Clin North Am 57:875, 1977.
14. Moyer CA, Margraft HW, Monafo WW: Burn shock in association with extravascular sodium deficiency. Arch Surg 90:799, 1965.
15. Lewis VL Jr: Management of the burned patient. *In* Beal JM (ed.): Critical Care for Surgical Patients. New York, MacMillan Publishing, 1982, p. 274.
16. Baxter CR: Problems and complications of burn shock resuscitation. Surg Clin North Am 58:1313, 1978.
17. Wilmore DW: Catecholamines: Mediator of the hypermetabolic response to thermal injury. Ann Surg 180:653, 1974.
18. O'Neill JA, Pruitt BA Jr, Moncrief JA: Suppurative thrombophlebitis, a lethal complication of intravenous therapy. J Trauma 8:256.
19. Moncrief JA, Mason AD: Evaporative water loss in the burned patient. J Trauma 4:180, 1964.
20. Agarwal N, Petro J, Salisbury RE: Physiologic profile monitoring in burned patients. J Trauma 23:577, 1983.
21. Stone HH: Pulmonary burns in childhood. J Pediatr Surg 14:48, 1979.
22. Moylan JA, Wilmore OW, Mouton DE, Pruitt BA Jr: Early diagnosis of inhalation injury using ^{133}xenon lung scan. Ann Surg 176:477, 1972.
23. Clarke AM: Thermal injuries: The care of the whole child. J Trauma 20:823, 1980.
24. Hunt JL: The pathophysiology of acute electrical injuries. J Trauma 16:335, 1976.
25. Haddad LM, Winchester JF (eds.): Clinical Management of Poisonings and Drug Overdoses. Philadelphia, W. B. Saunders Company, 1983.

CHAPTER

26 Child Abuse

DAVID L. KERNS

In any emergency medical setting in which a significant number of children present with injuries, physicians will frequently face the often difficult diagnostic challenge of distinguishing accidental from inflicted trauma. A refined expert approach is essential—an inappropriate diagnosis of child abuse will initiate sociolegal interventions that can be extraordinarily disruptive and traumatic for families, and a missed diagnosis of child abuse may result in repeated and possibly fatal injuries. To accurately identify those children who are likely to have been physically abused, the physician must be skillful at interviewing parents and children, familiar with the motor development of young children, and knowledgeable regarding the physical and radiologic findings in accidental and characteristic inflicted trauma.

THE MAGNITUDE OF THE PROBLEM

For a variety of reasons, the true incidence of child abuse is unknown: (1) there is no "perfect" or uniformly accepted definition of child abuse from which data can be derived (for purposes of discussion in this chapter, *physical abuse* is used interchangeably with *child abuse* and is defined as *physical trauma that has been inflicted on a child by an adult or by a minor with caretaker responsibilities for that child*); (2) to a significant extent there are frequent failures in diagnosing physical abuse; (3) physical abuse that is identified is often not reported and therefore not entered in any data base; and (4) there is great variation in the way the data is categorized in reporting jurisdictions (states and counties).

The incidence of child abuse can be only roughly estimated from the collation of heterogenous data from various reporting jurisdictions. Because of the nature of the methodologic problems, it can be safely assumed that the derived incidence estimates are actually underestimates. From data of the 1981 National Study on Child Abuse and Neglect Reporting (see Table 26–1), several general conclusions can be made:

Table 26–1. 1981 NATIONAL STUDY ON CHILD ABUSE AND NEGLECT REPORTING*

Total case reports		850,980
Physical abuse reports (45%)		382,941
"Major" physical injury (4%)		34,039
Average age of reported children		7.2 Years
Average age of case fatalities		3.3 Years
Cases reported by medical personnel (11%)		93,608
Percentage of families with economic problems		44%
Ethnic distribution of maltreated children	White	68%
	Black	22%
	Hispanic	8%
	Other	2%

*Data from the American Humane Association: 1981 National Study on Child Neglect and Abuse Reporting. Denver, American Humane Association, 1983.

1. Hundreds of thousands of children are being physically abused in the United States each year.
2. Tens of thousands of children are suffering major inflicted physical injuries and are at risk for fatality and permanent disability in the United States each year.
3. Younger children are at greater risk for fatality than older children (Fig. 26–1).
4. Although certain ethnic/racial minorities are over-represented, the majority of families involved in child maltreatment are white.
5. Although certain families with economic stress are over-represented, the majority of families involved in child maltreatment are not experiencing economic difficulty.

THE PHYSICIAN'S RESPONSIBILITIES

In each instance of pediatric trauma in which physical abuse is suspected, the physician is responsible for:

1. Initiating a medical treatment plan for the child's injuries.
2. Providing support for patients and family members in often stressful and emotionally charged situations.
3. Through history, physical examination, radiographs, and laboratory studies, estimating the probability that an injury has been inflicted.

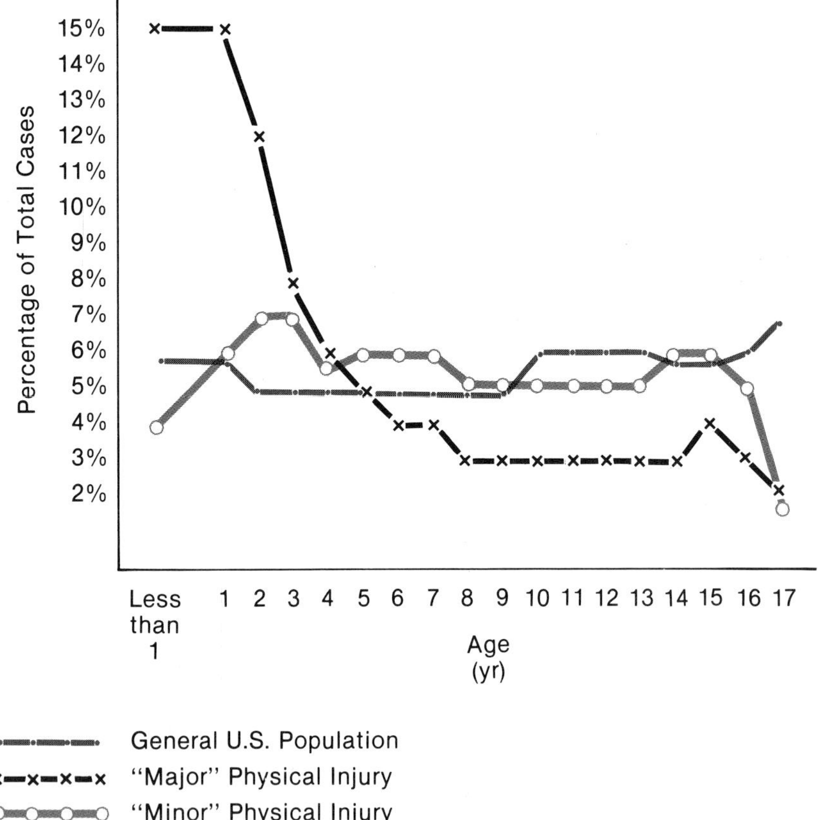

Figure 26–1. Age distribution of child abuse (American Humane Association, 1983).

4. When appropriate, initiating sociolegal interventions, i.e., reporting to child protective services and possibly to law enforcement authorities.

5. When appropriate, providing immediate child protection through hospitalization.

6. Carefully recording clinical details in the medical record, bearing in mind that these entries may become the data base for subsequent civil and criminal court testimony.

This chapter focuses on the diagnostic process in the emergency setting, the objective findings in common and characteristic cases of physical abuse, and the physician's dispositional responsibilities beyond the strictly medical and surgical aspects, which are abundantly discussed throughout this book.

THE CLINICAL HISTORY

History taking in potential child abuse cases may be particularly challenging because the parents, although concerned about the well-being of the child, may be anxious, angry, secretive, intimidating, guilt-ridden, and so on. The physician needs to explore in detail the circumstances of the trauma and at the same time convey a supportive, nonauthoritarian concern for the family. This can best be accomplished by a calm, friendly, nonaccusatory demeanor and an emphasis on the physical condition of the child. It is important to emphasize that diagnostically *it is the physician's responsibility to attempt to determine whether the trauma is accidental or inflicted; it is not the physician's responsibility to determine "who did it."*

Children who have been physically abused will present to the emergency department with one of four chief complaints: (1) accidental injury, (2) trauma without explanation, (3) unrelated nontrauma symptoms, or (4) inflicted injury. Most commonly a history of accidental trauma will be given. However, it is not unusual for parents to state that they have no explanation for injuries that they have discovered or for injuries discovered by the physician while examining the child for an unrelated complaint. The absence of an explanation, of course, does not necessarily imply that the parent is "covering up," since children may be accidentally injured without the knowledge of the parents and they may receive inflicted injuries from other adults or children. Occasionally children will present with a chief complaint of inflicted injury. The parent may directly state that he or she lost control with the child, or the child may be brought in by the police or protective services personnel for medical assessment and documentation after abuse has been identified or at least strongly suspected.

Areas of Emphasis in the Clinical History

Timing in Seeking Medical Care for the Child. When significant accidental trauma has occurred, parents will almost always seek immediate medical attention for their child. If a significant delay occurs, the parents may not understand the seriousness of the injury, they may be avoiding possible discovery of an inflicted injury, or they may be manifesting neglect of significant accidental trauma.

Reaction of the Parents. Although it is certainly expected that the parent of an injured child will be anxious, signs of parental detachment or depression and particularly inappropriate hostility and defensiveness should raise suspicion regarding the etiology of the injury. As parents of children who have been accidentally injured become aware that the possibility of child abuse is being entertained, they often seem surprised and may become slightly defensive or irritated. In general, however, they do not become blatantly hostile or intimidating as abusive parents frequently do in this situation.

Focus of Concern of the Parents. The common and expected response of a parent to a child's injury is concern for the child's physical and emotional state. If the parent is principally concerned with his or her own needs (e.g., how inconvenient this hospital visit is), this suggests at least some problem in the parent-child relationship.

Mental Status of the Parents. It is particularly important to note if the parent of an injured child is saying bizarre things, is acting "spacy," is intoxicated, or appears to be retarded. Although such a finding does not necessarily imply that an injury was inflicted, it raises concern regarding the capacity of the parent to provide a safe environment or to respond appropriately if serious accidental injury occurs.

History of Prior Trauma. A careful history of prior trauma should be elicited. A review of the medical record may reveal a pattern of multiple injuries over time and may, of course, indicate that child abuse has been suspected or diagnosed in the past. If the medical records of siblings are available, they should be reviewed. In cases in which skin bruises are the principal physical finding, questions regarding bleeding disorders should be asked, e.g., history of easy bruisability, excessive bleeding with circumcision, hemarthroses, use of aspirin, family history, and so on.

The Psychosocial History. When child abuse is suspected, a hospital social worker or, if none is available, a protective services social worker should elicit a family psychosocial history. Given the special talents of the social worker and the practical demands of the hospital emergency department, it is not reasonable for the emergency physician to attempt to perform this role.

The following areas of emphasis refer specifically to those cases in which a child's physical injury is attributed to an accident (i.e., accidental explanation).

Elicit Precise Details of the Accident. To the extent possible, determination of the exact circumstances of the accident should be made. For example, if an infant has allegedly fallen from a dressing table, the height of the table, the nature of the flooring (carpet, tile, and so on), and the position of the infant at impact should be determined. Even if the accident has not been witnessed, knowledge of the physical characteristics of the accident site may be quite helpful.

The Value of Multiple Histories. When possible, it is important to interview separately all witnesses (including the injured child and siblings if they can speak) regarding the circumstances of the injury. Gross discrepancies point toward a nonaccidental etiology, whereas consistencies are reassuring regarding the accidental explanation.

Developmental Capabilities of the Child. An estimation of the motor development of the child is important, particularly in cases of trauma to infants. If the motor activity allegedly leading to the accidental injury is well beyond the expected maturation of the infant, doubt is cast upon the accidental explanation. Table 26–2 summarizes the timing of the attainment of milestones of gross motor development for infants and toddlers. It is important to remember that there are

Table 26–2. MILESTONES IN GROSS MOTOR DEVELOPMENT IN INFANTS AND TODDLERS

Milestone	Range of Attainment
Pushing up prone to 90 degrees	1–3 months
Rolling front-to-back	2–5 months
Rolling back-to-front	4–6 months
Sitting independently	5–7 months
Creeping	7–10 months
Pulling to standing	8–10 months
Cruising	9–11 months
Walking	10–15 months
Climbing stairs*	18–30 months
Climbing stairs†	24–36 months
Running‡	Begins approximately at 27 months

*Leading with same foot.
†Alternating feet.
‡Both feet off surface simultaneously.

occasional instances of precocious gross motor performance. Observation of the actual motor activities of the individual infant can be helpful, presuming that the infant's injuries are not such that the activity in question is impeded.

Application of Experience and Common Sense. Occasionally an accidental explanation is seriously in doubt because it simply does not make sense in light of one's experience with commonplace physical events. For example, a toddler would not sustain multiple bruises and fractures from a simple fall on a carpeted floor.

All details of the elicited history should be analyzed in the context of their consistency or discrepancy with the physical findings.

COMMON AND CHARACTERISTIC OBJECTIVE FINDINGS IN CHILD ABUSE CASES

Skin Trauma

Injuries to the skin are by far the most frequent physical manifestation of child abuse. These can be principally categorized into bruises, burns, and bite marks.

Bruises

Healthy children collide with the environment regularly. In fact it is unusual to see active preschool children without their share of small and even not-so-small ecchymoses. Typically, these signs of minor accidental trauma are seen over bony prominences such as shins, knees, hands, elbows, chin, and forehead. Bruises over soft surfaces such as the facial cheeks, neck, abdomen, back, buttocks, and thighs are *somewhat* less likely to have been acquired accidentally.

The approximation of the "age" of a bruise may be helpful in determining the consistency of an accidental history. Table 26–3 reviews the color changes found in bruises of different ages. Although social workers and attorneys often expect physicians to make very accurate estimations of the age of a bruise, only relatively broad assessments can be made. In general, skin trauma great enough to rupture capillaries will produce an initial red color, which will become reddish-purple in the first 24 hours and will progress to a predominantly purple color for 5 to 7 days. Hemoglobin degradation will then yield changes to yellow, brown, and green hues. This appearance will last, with gradual fading, for 1 to 3 weeks. Therefore, it is generally possible to distinguish gross discrepancies with a given history (e.g., reddish-purple bruises alleged to have occurred 2 weeks earlier) but not fine discrepancies (e.g., bruises 3 days old versus 5 days old).

Often the configuration of a bruise will reveal its etiology. The following are examples of bruise patterns that are diagnostically helpful:

Grab Marks. These bruises are oval in shape with indistinct borders; they may be somewhat indistinguishable from random amorphous bruises or may appear in a pattern suggesting violent grabbing with fingers. In the latter, a single bruise from the thumb will be opposed by multiple bruises in linear arrangement from the fingers.

Pinch Marks. These marks will appear as linear or slightly crescentic bruises of 1 to 2 cm in length.

Slap Marks. The mechanisms of a slap with the open hand are such that the skin capillaries rupture at the edges of the perpetrator's fingers, leaving a complete or,

Table 26–3. ESTIMATING THE "AGES" OF SKIN BRUISES

Age	Color
Immediate	Red
Within first 24 hours	Red-purple
Day 1 to day 5–7	Dark purple
Day 5–7 to weeks 2–4	Green/yellow/brown
After 2–4 weeks	Returns to normal

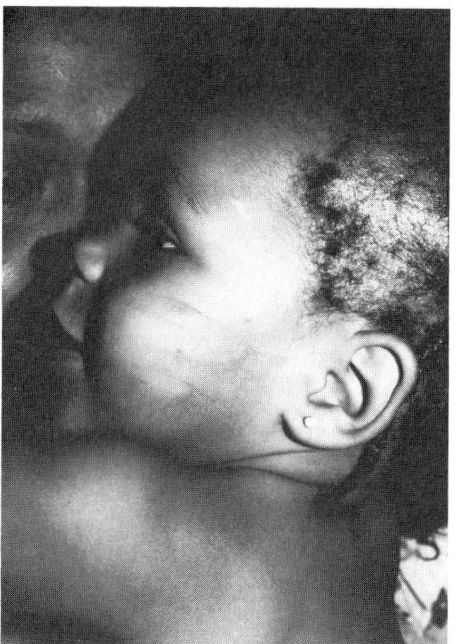

Figure 26–2. Facial slap marks caused by capillary rupture at the impact points of the edges of the fingers of the slapping hand.

more frequently, an incomplete hand print (Fig. 26–2).

Belt Marks. These broad linear bruises are usually easily identifiable; trauma from a ruler may leave a similar pattern. Occasionally, the impression of a belt buckle may be seen at one end of the linear belt mark.

Loop Marks. Elliptic bruises are usually the result of trauma inflicted with a looped electrical cord (Fig. 26–3).

Hair Brush Injuries. Trauma inflicted with the bristle side of the hair brush may leave a field of multiple punctate bruises and superficial puncture wounds (Fig. 26–4).

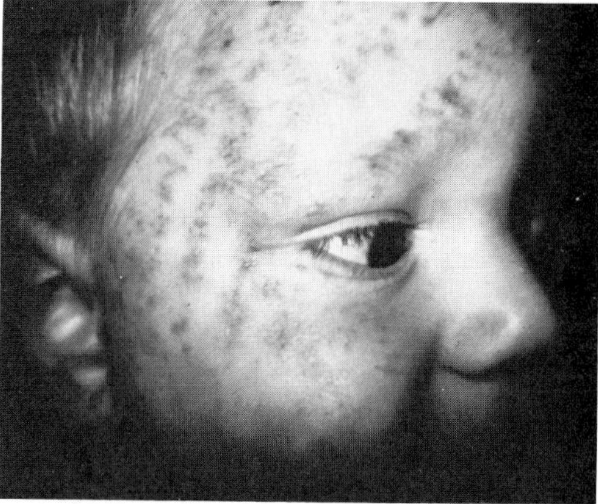

Figure 26–4. Multiple puncture wounds caused by the impact of the bristle side of a hairbrush.

Comb Marks. Multiple parallel linear abrasions and bruises are seen as a result of a comb being forcefully dragged across the skin (Fig. 26–5).

Circumferential Bruises. Bruises encircling the wrists or ankles indicate that the child has been tied or restrained with a rope or a similar object. Circumferential bruises of the neck indicate strangulation.

To resolve the issue of the possibility of underlying coagulopathy in a patient with bruises, the following studies constitute an adequate "screen": prothrombin time, partial thromboplastin time, platelet count, and bleeding time. In the absence of a suggestive history, these studies rarely uncover a previously unrecognized bleeding disorder.

Of greatest concern are inflicted bruises to the head, face, neck, chest, abdomen, and perineum. These imply the greatest loss of

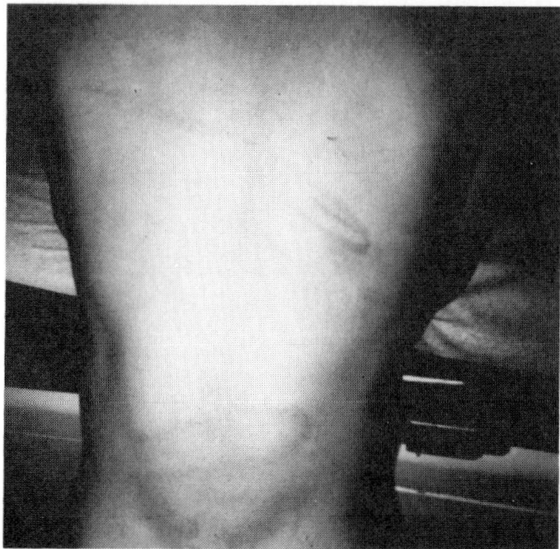

Figure 26–3. Loop marks caused by the impact of a looped electric cord.

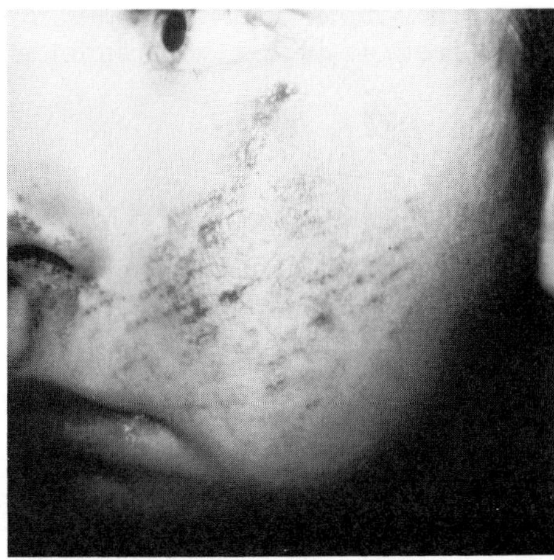

Figure 26–5. Multiple parallel linear abrasions caused by forceful scraping with a metal comb.

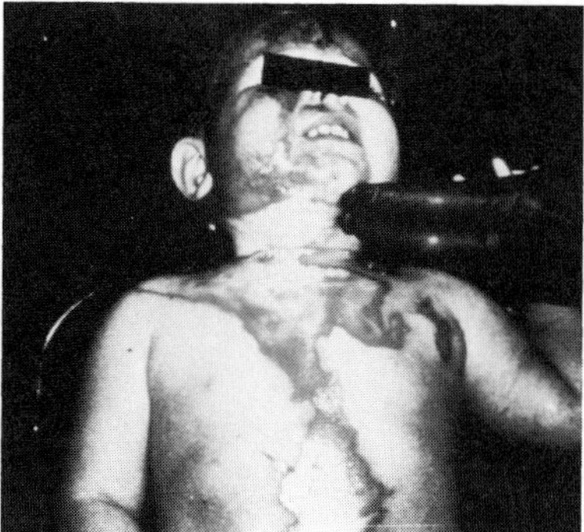

Figure 26–6. Second- and third-degree burns inflicted by a hot liquid splash.

control and impairment of judgment on the part of the perpetrator and are the most likely to result in serious and life-threatening injuries.

BURNS

Burns are present in approximately 10 per cent of physical abuse cases. There are principally three types of inflicted burns: hot liquid splash burns, hot water immersion burns, and burns with hot solid objects (branding).

Splash Burns. These burns can be caused by hot liquid (water, coffee, cooking oil, and so on) being thrown at or poured over a child. They typically result in a large confluent area of second- or third-degree burns surrounded by smaller scattered burns caused by splattering and "run-off" (Fig. 26–6). Such burns can, of course, be acquired accidentally. The physician must rely heavily on historical criteria to determine the probability of abuse in these cases.

Hot Water Immersion Burns. Children who have had parts of their bodies immersed

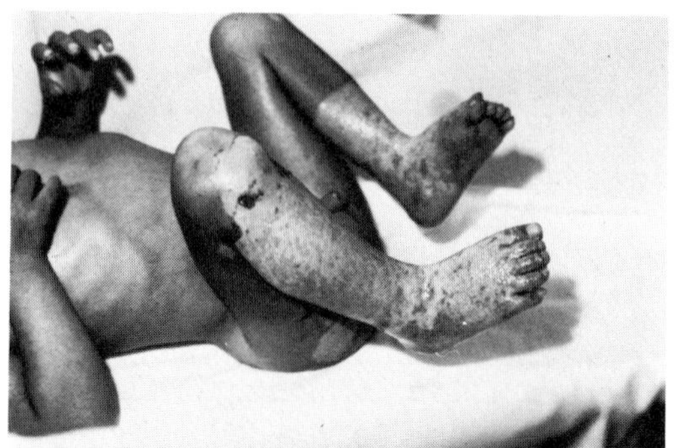

Figure 26–7. Severe hot water immersion burn in "stocking" distribution on both legs. An immersion burn of the buttocks can also be seen.

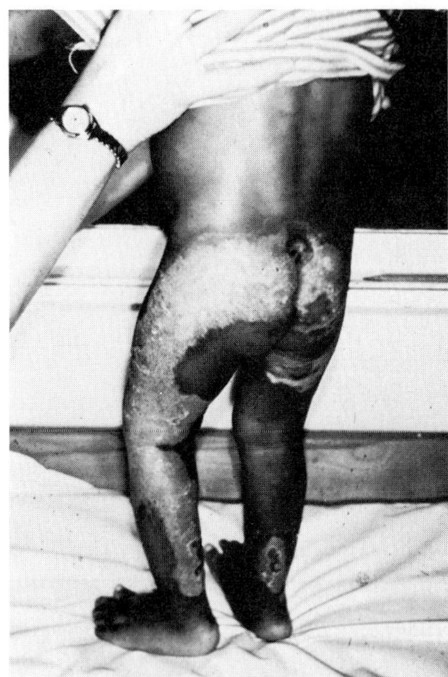

Figure 26–8. A classic hot water dunking burn after several days of healing. The central area of the buttocks was spared by direct contact with the cool surface of the bathtub.

in hot water will demonstrate typical burn patterns on physical examination. When hands or feet are immersed, confluent "stocking-glove" burns are seen (Fig. 26–7). Immersion of a child buttocks-first into a tub of very hot water can result in the *classic dunking burn.* These are most typically seen in toddlers who are being "disciplined" following a toileting accident. The burn is usually confluent on the buttocks, ending in a "water level" line near the waist. The perineum, genitalia, and parts of the lower extremities may be included, depending on the exact position of the child. Intertriginous folds are usually protected, and if the child has been in solid contact with the cooler surface of the bathtub, the central area of the buttocks may be spared, leaving a "donut" configuration to the burn (Fig. 26–8).

In assessing hot water immersion burns, the temperature of the hot water is an important consideration. A scald will develop with 60 seconds of contact at 127° F, but within 1 second if the water temperature is 158° F.[2] Knowledge of the water temperature within a household hot water heater may significantly affect the credibility of a given history in such a case.

Branding. Burns inflicted with hot solid

objects are considerably less common than hot liquid burns. These may be relatively amorphous or may take the form of the object involved, such as a waffle iron, clothes iron, heating grate, electric range heating element, and so forth. The most frequently considered burn of this type is the *cigarette burn.* An accidental "brush" with a cigarette will leave a superficial tangential burn across the skin in the fashion of an abrasion. Perpendicular forced cigarette burns will result in circular ulcerating lesions, which may blister and which will often heal with hyperpigmentation. They are most often seen on the palms and soles and generally indicate serious psychopathology on the part of the perpetrators. *It is crucial that cigarette burns be diagnosed with the utmost caution.* They are easily mimicked by infected insect bites and superficial puncture wounds.

Details of the emergency department management and follow-up care of thermal injuries are listed in Chapter 25.

BITE MARKS

Although considerably less common than bruises or burns, bite marks are seen several times each year in a busy pediatric emergency setting. They may take several forms, the most common of which are linear puncture wounds on fingers (Fig. 26–9) and characteristic curvilinear to circular bruises on any part of the body (Fig. 26–10). The latter may be vague and confluent, or the "impression" of individual teeth may be seen. Occasionally, suction petechiae (hickeys) are present, encircled by the bite marks. Most commonly, the given history will be that the child was bitten by another child, and this may indeed be true. Individual tooth characteristics, arch width, and intercanine distance can be determined by forensic odontologic techniques if photographic evidence, including a metric tape in the field, has been collected. Even with bite marks that appear to be rather vague, forensic experts can discern child from adult bites and may be able to accomplish specific perpetrator identifications.

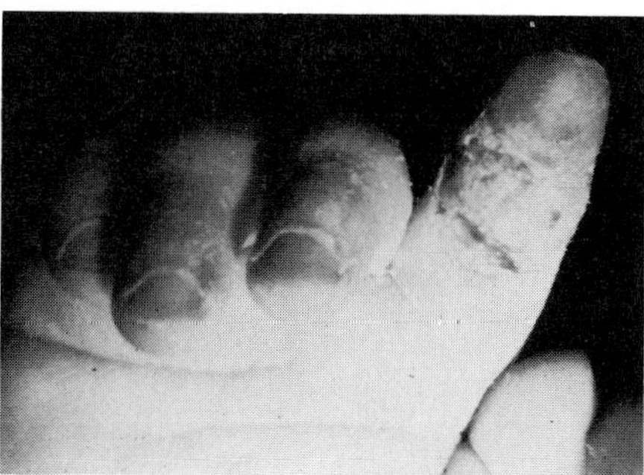

Figure 26–9. Severe linear human bite of index finger, in this instance inflicted by an angry sibling.

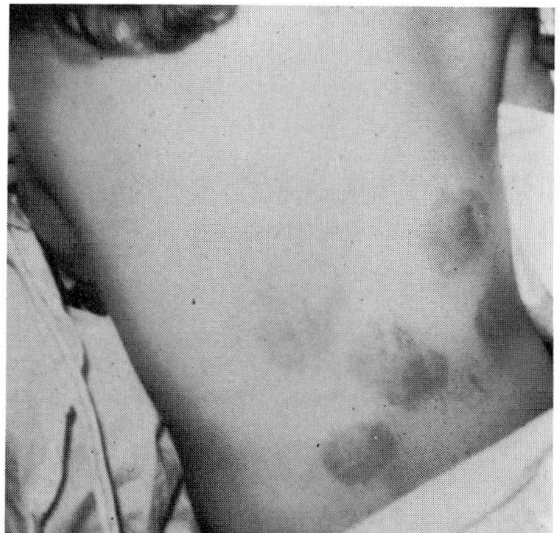

Figure 26–10. Opposed curvilinear bite marks with central suction petechiae; individual tooth marks are distinguishable.

Head and Central Nervous System Trauma

Intracranial injuries are the principal source of mortality and chronic organic morbidity in abused children. Neurodevelopmental research suggests that as many as 17 per cent of reported physically abused children demonstrate significant neurologic sequelae.[3] Early diagnosis and protective intervention are therefore particularly crucial for children sustaining inflicted head injuries.

SCALP INJURIES

Direct trauma to the head may, of course, cause a variety of scalp findings, including bruises, lacerations, abrasions, and edema. Violent hair-pulling can result in focal hair loss (traumatic alopecia) and, if forceful enough, can dissect the scalp off the skull, resulting in cephalhematoma. Although common as a neonatal birth injury, cephalhematoma rarely results from blunt trauma to the head.

SKULL FRACTURES

In general, the nature of the appearance of a skull fracture on a radiograph will not suggest whether the trauma has been accidental or inflicted. As is true with other trauma, correlation with the history given should indicate the possible cause. *Multiple skull fractures* can be caused by a single skull collision; of course if the fractures are in different stages of healing, repeated trauma to the skull has taken place. *Depressed skull fractures* are typically caused by trauma with protruding objects and not by collisions with flat surfaces, such as falls to the floor. Importantly, falls from minimal heights (less than 3 ft) rarely result in skull fractures (approximately 1 per cent of the time or less), and intracranial complications are infrequent.[4] Children with basilar skull fractures may present with ecchymoses in a periorbital distribution or over the mastoid bones. These must be distinguished from direct trauma to these areas. Occasionally, a child with neuroblastoma will present with bilateral periorbital ecchymoses.

INTRACRANIAL INJURIES

Severe inflicted trauma to the head may result in the expected gamut of serious intracranial complications: cerebral edema, epidural and subdural hematoma, subarachnoid hemorrhage, and intracerebral contusion, laceration, and hematoma. Immediate life-support, computerized tomography (CT) imaging, and neurosurgical interventions are frequently necessary in these cases (see Chapter 16).

WHIPLASH-SHAKEN–INFANT SYNDROME

In recent decades, clinical and experimental studies[5,6] have documented that violent shaking of infants, causing rapid accelerations and decelerations of the head, can lead to the development of acute subdural hematomas. These most frequently occur in the posterior parieto-occipital region between the cerebral hemispheres.[7] They are frequently accompanied by retinal hemorrhages and occasionally by metaphyseal fractures of the long bones (see below) and grab marks on the skin. The subdural hematomas are created by tearing of the bridging veins (running from arachnoid to dura) during rapid accelerations and decelerations of the head. The retinal hemorrhages are thought to be due to sudden rises in intracranial pressure, which are transmitted to the retinal vasculature, leading to small vessel ruptures. Most commonly the hemorrhages are of the large crescentic sublaminar (preretinal) variety, but flame and dot hemorrhages, indicating bleeding in the deeper retinal layers, are seen as well. Retinal hemorrhages of all three varieties occur in up to 50 per cent of normal newborn infants as a result of "normal" birth trauma. These resolve in days to weeks, with the sublaminar hemorrhages occasionally still present after several weeks.[8]

The infant who has been violently shaken but not struck will, of course, have no evidence of blunt trauma to the head. Presentation of the child to a physician will likely be triggered by the appearance of symptoms arising from increased intracranial pressure (e.g., alteration of behavior or consciousness or respiratory problems). Careful neurologic and fundoscopic examination combined with CT scanning will lead to the diagnosis. Telltale grab marks on the chest, shoulders, or head and the appearance of traction fractures on a bone survey may strengthen the diagnosis. *Importantly, there is no evidence that spontaneous subdural hematomas exist as a clinical entity. Acute subdural hematomas are traumatic in origin caused either by direct head injury or by violent shaking.*

Skeletal Injuries

Fractures are a common manifestation of child abuse and are second in frequency only to injuries of the skin. The probability that a given fracture has been inflicted will rest upon careful correlation with the clinical history. This will require estimation of the age of the fracture and recognition of patterns of bony injury that are seen in accidental and nonaccidental trauma.

ESTIMATING THE AGE OF THE FRACTURE

As is the case with the "dating" of a bruise, only a broad estimation of the age of a fracture can be made, which is often frustrating to social services, law enforcement, and court representatives who are seeking very specific "accurate" estimates of the time of injury.

Immediately following a fracture, there will usually be soft tissue swelling clinically, which may be identifiable radiologically. Fracture lines are usually, but not invariably, seen. Deformity such as angulation and displacement may be identified. For the next 7 days to 2 weeks no further radiologic changes will be seen except for a diminution in soft tissue swelling. At approximately 10 to 14 days, calcification will begin to be seen both of the developing callus at the fracture site (Fig. 26–11) as well as along the elevated periosteum of the involved bone (Fig. 26–12). This process will continue, with abundant and obvious calcification, for the next 2 to 3 months. Approximately 2 months after the initial injury, the initially observed fracture line will usually be obliterated by calcified callus (Fig. 26–13). Over the next 2 to 4 months the bone will undergo remodeling. At the end of the process there may be some permanent bony deformity or the bone may appear to be completely normal. Given this sequence, the physician will generally be able to "date" fractures within the following time intervals: (1) 0 to 10 days, (2) 10 days to 2 months, (3) 2 to 6 months or (4) older than 6 months. Therefore, gross discrepancies in historical timing will be discernible, but fine discrepancies will not. Importantly, bones that have been fractured owing to birth trauma should show callus and periosteal calcification by the time the infant is 2 weeks old. If an infant of that age or older has a noncalcified fracture, it has been acquired postnatally.

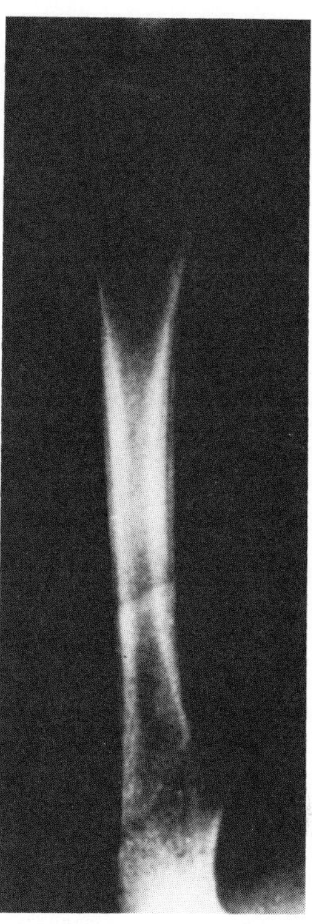

Figure 26–12. Calcification of subperiosteal hematoma, extending the length of the long bone proximal to the fracture site; the fracture is 3 weeks old.

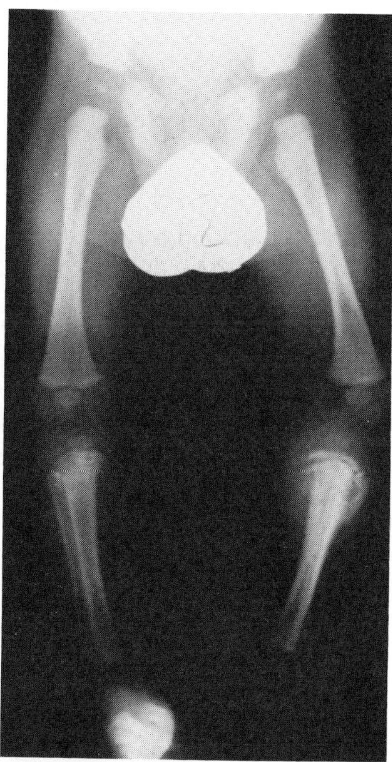

Figure 26–11. Early calcification of callus at proximal metaphyseal fracture site of the left tibia; the calcification has the configuration of the classic "bucket-handle" variety.

Fractures that Indicate a High Probability of Child Abuse

Inconsistent or Absent History of Injury. In any instance in which a fracture is unexplained by the history, the possibility of abuse should be seriously considered. This is particularly true in infants, who are less likely to suffer accidents because they are not fully ambulatory and because they are at the greatest risk for serious morbidity and mortality if they are being abused.

Multiple Fractures of Different "Ages." This finding indicates that a child is being repeatedly injured. Although there may be several accidental explanations that are plausible, such cases should be explored very carefully, particularly cases involving infants.

Metaphyseal Fractures of Long Bones. These are the "classic," and often considered pathognomonic, injuries seen in abused infants and toddlers. They are "chip" or "corner" fractures of the metaphyses of long bones (Fig. 26–14) and are caused by violent torsion or traction of the extremities. Al-

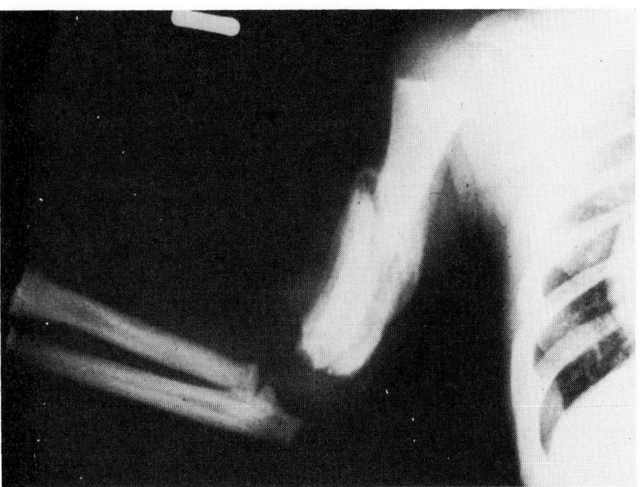

Figure 26–13. Calcified callus nearly obliterating humeral fracture site; the fracture is 2 months old.

though such fractures may occur accidentally in older children, they should be considered as strong evidence of child abuse in infants and toddlers.

Spiral Fractures. These fractures, usually of the tibia, femur, radius or humerus, are also the result of torsion injuries. Powerful twisting forces on an extremity result in a spiral fracture (Fig. 26–15). In older children and adults, these injuries are usually accidental. However, in children under 2 years of age, and particularly in infants, spiral fractures should be regarded as having been inflicted. There is no evidence that minor falls or legs entrapped in crib slats lead to these serious major injuries.

Bilateral Rib Fractures. When seen in infants and toddlers, fractures to both sides of the rib cage should be regarded as inflicted unless an extraordinary and consistent accidental history is given. These fractures occur when infants' chests are crushed between two hands. This behavior may accompany violent shaking and its resultant injuries.

Skeletal Surveys

When children under the age of 6 years have any significant evidence of physical abuse, sexual abuse, or serious neglect (e.g., nonorganic failure to thrive), a radiologic skeletal survey (bone survey) should be performed. This should include radiographic examination of the *skull, ribs,* and *extremities.* To avoid unnecessary radiation exposure, the pelvis should be excluded from the survey because of the low yield of positive findings. However, films of the pelvis are justified if there is a specific indication prompted by the

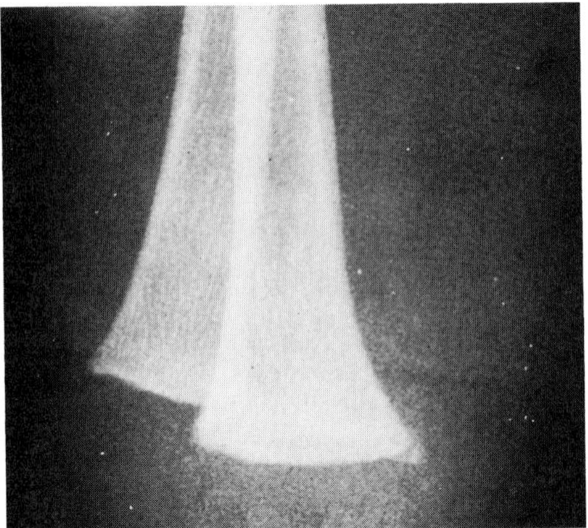

Figure 26–14. A metaphyseal "corner" fracture discovered on the skeletal survey of an infant with suspicious bruises.

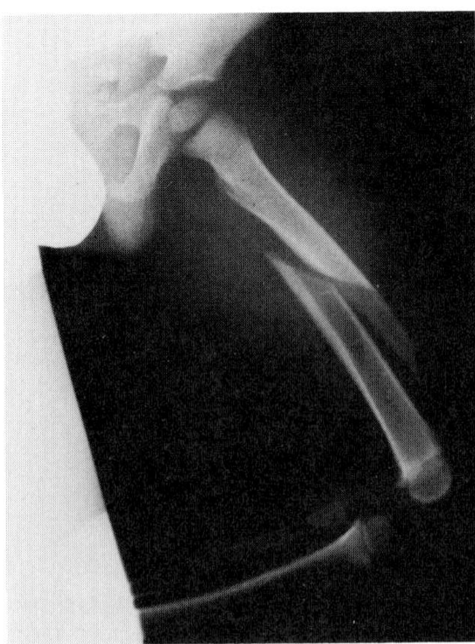

Figure 26–15. A femoral spiral fracture in an infant; this type of injury is not caused by trivial trauma but by powerful torsion forces.

history or physical examination. The most common "discoveries" from the skeletal survey are unsuspected healing metaphyseal fractures of the long bones.

Intra-Abdominal Injuries

Inflicted abdominal trauma is a major source of mortality, second only to intracranial injuries, among abused children.[9] Abused children have sustained the full spectrum of intra-abdominal injuries, including gastric and intestinal perforations; hepatic, splenic, and renal ruptures and lacerations; pancreatic injuries; major vessel lacerations; and lower urinary tract injuries.

Of particular interest diagnostically are two entities that result from blunt trauma to children and may present in a delayed and veiled fashion: intramural duodenal hematoma and acute pancreatitis, with or without pseudocyst formation.

Intramural Duodenal Hematoma

Blunt trauma to the abdomen may result in hemorrhagic injury to the wall of the fixed third portion of the duodenum as it is compressed against the vertebral column. The resulting intramural hematoma will lead to the manifestations of upper gastrointestinal obstruction. The clinical presentations are variable in severity and are usually delayed from hours to days following the initiating trauma. The classic accidental injury leading to intramural duodenal hematoma is blunt trauma from a bicycle handlebar following sudden deceleration. In child abuse cases, the patient may present with bilious vomiting and abdominal distention, with no historical or physical findings consistent with trauma. However, in many cases, the finding of multiple trauma will lead the physician to suspect that this particular duodenal injury is present. When radiologic studies are confirmatory and no reasonable accidental explanation is given, child abuse should be strongly suspected even in the absence of other traumatic findings.[10]

Pancreatic Trauma

The principal etiology of pancreatic disease in children is trauma. Blunt trauma may cause parenchymal pancreatic damage and hemorrhage leading to an "acute abdomen" and possibly to the appearance of peritonitis. Levels of pancreatic enzymes, particularly amylase, will be elevated in serum and abdominal fluid. Occasionally, pancreatic injury is more localized and less evident acutely. However, within a few weeks, an ongoing encapsulated inflammatory process can lead to the formation of a pancreatic pseudocyst, with accompanying epigastric and/or back pain, vomiting, and an upper abdominal mass. Serum amylase levels will be elevated and radiologic studies will reveal characteristic duodenal displacement. As is the case with intramural duodenal hematoma, unless a plausible accidental explanation is given, child abuse is probable.[11]

Other Inflicted Injuries

Since the original description of the "battered child syndrome,"[12] hundreds of reports of extraordinary varieties of inflicted trauma to children have been published. In addition to the principal injuries to skin, central nervous system, retina, skeleton, and abdomen that are reviewed above, case studies have described the association of child abuse with injuries to virtually every part of the anatomy.[13]

PHYSICAL FINDINGS MIMICKING CHILD ABUSE

With some regularity, children are reported to child protection agencies with physical findings that may appear to be, but are not, secondary to inflicted trauma.

Mongolian Spots

These unfortunately named hyperpigmented areas have often been confused with unexplained bruises. They are macular and dark purple-black in color and are distributed principally in the sacral area. However, it is not uncommon to see a wider distribution, with spots on the lower extremities, trunk, and/or upper extremities. Most frequently seen in black infants and toddlers, they are also common in other dark-skinned racial groups. Mongolian spots very gradually fade, disappearing as early as several months or as late as 3 to 4 years. Although there is a gross similarity between a mongolian spot and a bruise that is in its first week of evolution, generally the characteristic appearance and distribution of the mongolian spot is quite distinguishable.

Coin Rubbing

With the migration of Asian refugees to the United States in the 1970s came the awareness of a harmless folk medicine technique that was initially confused with child abuse by Westerners. Coin rubbing (CiaGio) is a technique used by the parent principally to rid the child of fever.[14] Usually, warm oil is rubbed on the skin and the edge of a coin is repeatedly rubbed across the skin in linear strokes. With capillary dilatation and repeated friction, bruising results. The process is not uncomfortable to the child but rather is experienced much like a massage. The residual appearance of a nonaccidental bruise pattern may be striking (Fig. 26–16).

Car Seat Burns

Infants may sustain burns of peculiar and suspicious configurations from contact with automobile vinyl seats or metal buckles that have been exposed to intense sunlight.[15] Most typically, these burns have a bilateral linear distribution on the back of the thighs.

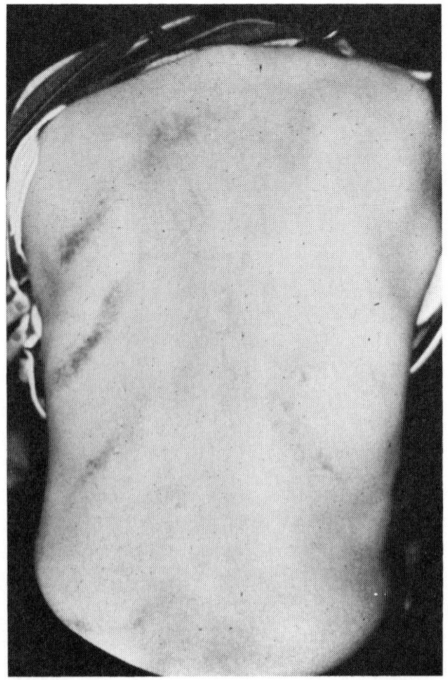

Figure 26–16. Multiple linear bruises caused by coin-rubbing (CiaGio), a Southeast Asian folk medicine remedy.

Careful history should distinguish them from inflicted burns.

Subluxation of the Radial Head

Strictly speaking, this extremely frequent injury to young children is inflicted trauma. However, it is so common and so easily caused by suddenly fully extending the elbow and pulling on the wrist or hand that the application of the term "child abuse," with its sociolegal ramifications, would grossly mislabel parents who are just in need of some straightforward education.

Caffey's Disease (Infantile Cortical Hyperostosis)

Superficially, the bones of a child with this mysterious disease may radiologically resemble those of a battered child. Areas of abundant subperiosteal calcification mimic the appearance of multiple healing fractures. However, radiologic distinctions can be made, and children with this disease often have evidence of systemic illness, such as low-grade fevers and elevated erythrocyte sedimentation rates.

UNIQUE CONSIDERATIONS FOR THE PHYSICIAN IN SUSPECTED CHILD ABUSE CASES

The strictly medical or surgical management of these cases will not vary from the therapeutic approaches described in this book. However, a number of additional important considerations arise in child abuse cases.

The Need for Immediate Child Protection

In each instance of suspected child abuse, a determination needs to be made regarding the immediate safety of the child. If hospitalization is medically indicated, then the problem of providing immediate protection is at least temporarily solved.

However, if hospitalization is not medically indicated, the physician, generally in concert with the hospital social worker or protective services worker, must determine if it is safe for the child to return home. A number of important factors need to be considered in this decision, such as the age of the child, the nature of the trauma, the past history of trauma, and the specific characteristics of the family. Each case is unique and requires an individualized assessment. In general, it is best to err on the side of child protection if the circumstances are "marginal" and the decision is difficult.

Reporting to Child Protective Services

In all counties in the United States, physicians are required to immediately report *suspected* child abuse cases to the local child protective services agency. All state child protection laws contain the following:

1. Physicians are required to report if they have *reason to suspect* inflicted injuries.
2. Physicians who report in good faith are *immune from civil and criminal liability* for having done so.
3. Various penalties (usually fines) may be levied if a physician fails to report.

In addition, nonreporting has been found to constitute medical malpractice in a number of cases.

Law Enforcement Notification and Emergency Custody

In some states, immediate notification of the local police is required in all cases of suspected abuse. In particularly volatile situations, law enforcement officials should be immediately involved even if this is not mandated by law. If there is a reasonable probability that a parent is likely to flee the emergency department or inpatient ward with an abused child, emergency custody can be obtained through police or court-ordered "holds." The logistics of obtaining these holds varies in different locales. The physician should be familiar with the details of the local child protection statutes and the mechanisms for accomplishing emergency custody. Individualized hospital protocols are particularly helpful in these situations.

The Medical Record

Because the medical record becomes a significant portion of the data base for protective services and civil and/or criminal court dispositions, the historical and physical findings must be recorded in a meticulous, thorough, and legible fashion. To the extent possible, the caretaker's explanation of the cause of the trauma should be recorded verbatim in quotation marks. All positive physical findings should be described in qualitative and quantitative detail and carefully sketched on the medical record and/or child abuse reporting form. When documenting each case, the physician must recognize that the recorded information will become the sole source of data for physician testimony in court, possibly months or years later.

Photography

Physical manifestations of child abuse should be photographed in color with high-quality equipment, preferably a single lens reflex 35-mm camera with electronic strobe. State child protection statutes and hospital legal representatives should be consulted for the development of protocols dealing with consent and confidentiality issues.

Court Testimony

It is a fair observation that most physicians—in fact, most people—are reluctant to testify in court. The physician's knowledgeable participation may be critical to the appropriate and safe disposition of a child abuse case. The following guidelines should be helpful to the physician in carrying out testimonial responsibilities:

1. *Insist on a pretrial interview with the attorney.* Either by telephone or in person, both the process and the content of the testimony should be reviewed. The attorney should clarify his expectations of the physician and should answer any questions that the physician may have.
2. *Go to court only "on call."* Delays, recesses, and unexpected cancellations and rescheduling are routine in the conduct of court cases. It is reasonable to first request a firm commitment as to the date and time of the testimony and then to request telephone notification shortly before the actual court appearance. Countless hours have been wasted waiting in anterooms prior to testimony.
3. *Know the details of the case.* Court testimony is most difficult when the witness is unclear about the facts. The medical record and photographs should be reviewed in detail. Summary notes, particularly with quan-

titative information, are most helpful on the witness stand. There is no need to commit the data to memory; this, in fact, is likely to lead to difficulties.

4. *Take your time.* Testimony should be presented calmly, clearly, and slowly. It is helpful to take a few moments to formulate a verbal response before actually speaking. One's own relaxed thoughtful pace should be maintained regardless of the style of an attorney's examination.

5. *Maintain a "neutral" position.* The physician's obligation is to testify on behalf of the truth, not in service of one side or the other. The communication of neutrality will enhance the credibility of the content of the testimony to the parties involved.

6. *Do not answer complex questions with simple answers.* Although less frequently than television drama would indicate, attorneys will occasionally ask for simple answers, e.g., "yes or no" responses, to complicated or subtle questions. In these instances, the physician should state that the question cannot be appropriately or understandably answered in that fashion. The judge will inevitably allow the witness to give a comprehensive response.

7. *Do not be intimidated.* Occasionally, cross-examining attorneys will attempt to confuse or embarrass a physician witness, particularly while reviewing credentials. It is important to keep in mind that it is the attorney's job to attempt to "win" for his client, using whatever tactics are available to do so. Therefore, do not take it personally. It is most unusual for a judge to permit any significant harrassment of a professional witness.

SUPPORTING THE PARENTS

It is indeed difficult, in the presence of injured children and often suspicious, guilty, and angry parents, to maintain a supportive, friendly, professional style. Health care professionals are often angry and suspicious themselves in these clinical situations, and the sociolegal interventions required have adversary qualities that are quite unlike traditional medical care transactions. It should be kept in mind that most abusive parents have themselves been abused as children, that they are generally quite frightened, and that despite their role in having harmed their children, they are in fact seeking help for them and, more subtly, are likely to be seeking help for themselves as well. An empathic awareness of the pain and the complexity of the lives of these parents will be most likely to lead to an approach that is medically and legally responsible and at the same time supportive of all family members.

REFERENCES

1. American Humane Association: 1981 National Study on Child Neglect and Abuse Reporting. Denver, American Humane Association, 1983.
2. Feldman KW, Schaller RT, Feldman JA, et al.: Tap water scald burns in children. Pediatrics 62:1, 1978.
3. Martin H, Beezley P, Conway E, et al.: The development of abused children. Part 1: A review of the literature. Part 2: Physical, neurologic and intellectual outcome. Adv Pediatr 21:25, 1974.
4. Helfer RE, Slovis TL, Black M: Injuries resulting when small children fall out of bed. Pediatrics 60:533, 1977.
5. Caffey J: On the theory and practice of shaking infants. Am J Dis Child 124:161, 1972.
6. Ommaya AK, Faas F, Yarnell P: Whiplash injury and brain damage. JAMA 204:285, 1968.
7. Zimmerman RA, Bilaniuk LT, Bruce D, et al.: Computed tomography of craniocerebral injury in the abused child. Radiology 130:687, 1979.
8. Barsewisch von B: Perinatal Retinal Hemorrhages. Berlin, Springer-Verlag, 1979.
9. O'Neill JA, Meacham WF, Griffin JP, et al.: Patterns of injury in the battered child syndrome. J Trauma 13:332, 1973.
10. Wooley MM: Duodenal hematoma in infancy and childhood. Changing etiology and changing treatment. Am J Surg 136:8, 1978.
11. Slovis TL: Pancreatitis and the battered child syndrome. Report of two cases with skeletal involvement. Am J Radiol 125:456, 1975.
12. Kempe CH, Silverman FN, Steele BF, et al.: The battered child syndrome. JAMA 181:17, 1962.
13. Ellerstein NS: Child Abuse and Neglect. A Medical Reference. New York, John Wiley and Sons, 1981.
14. Yeatman GW, Shaw C, Barlow MJ, et al.: Pseudobattering in Vietnamese children. Pediatrics 58:616, 1976.
15. Schmitt BD, Gray JD, Britton HL: Car seat burns in infants: Avoiding confusion with inflicted burns. Pediatrics 62:607, 1978.

CHAPTER

27 Sexual Abuse of Children

JUDITH G. CHEEK

In recent years, the problem of rape and the medical, psychologic, and legal issues involved in caring for the victim have become more apparent. In urban areas, many health care professionals and law enforcement agencies have begun to recognize the complexity of the problem and assume some responsibility for improving the quality of care and success of legal action afforded the rape victim. Despite this growing awareness, the problem of sexual abuse of children has remained relatively suppressed. There are many factors that contribute to the failure to recognize and deal effectively with the sexually abused child. This chapter will present an overview of the problem, attempting to highlight those aspects of child sexual abuse that have allowed it to remain unrecognized. The unique considerations in caring for child victims and their families will be discussed in the context of a multidisciplinary approach. The specific role of the emergency care physician in evaluating the child victim of sexual abuse will be emphasized.

It is difficult to determine the precise magnitude of the problem of childhood sexual abuse. The incidence of reported rape cases in the United States was estimated at 76,000 in 1979.[1] This represented a fourfold increase in reported cases over the previous 20 years. Most authorities agree that less than 50 per cent of sexual assaults are actually reported. Children constitute a surprisingly large proportion of the victims of reported crimes. Various studies have reported that 20 to 40 per cent of victims are under age 15, and 12 to 15 per cent are under age 9.[2–4] It is clear that these reported cases represent only a fraction of the children actually subjected to some form of sexual abuse. In order to understand the true magnitude of the problem one must consider the various types of sexual abuse and the relationships between the offender and victim.

The definition of sexual abuse varies according to state criminal codes. Most states now include the following as sexual offenses: rape, aggravated rape, incest, sodomy, and indecent liberties.[4] The definition of rape is controversial but most legal authorities consider four components essential to establish *rape*:

1. A victim (of any age or sex).
2. Lack of consent—construed as a conscious unwillingness to submit or an inability to consent because of mental impairment. (The victim does not have to show evidence of struggling.)
3. Use of force—either actual or threatened.
4. Penetration (using sexual organ or inanimate objects) into the vagina, anus, or mouth.

Aggravated rape is defined as a rape in which there is use or threatened use of a weapon or force. *Incest* is defined as sexual activity with a relative closer than first cousin or with a surrogate family member. *Indecent liberties* covers a range of offenses including physical advances, exposure, and genital fondling or manipulation.

Many cases of child sexual assault do not fit the legal definition of rape. Studies of the actual sexual activities in child abuse indicate that genital fondling in conjunction with masturbation is the most common form of abuse of prepubertal children.[5] An actual sexual relationship involving penetration is found more commonly when the victim is postpubertal.

Although female victims outnumber males in reported cases 10 to 1, one must remember that male children may be victims of fondling, anal intercourse, and other forms of abuse and, secondly, that women may also be guilty of sexual assault.[6] A form of childhood sexual abuse often overlooked by medical authorities involves the female offender who places foreign objects in the vagina or anus of a child. It should not be assumed that the child is responsible for the placement of these objects. Authorities must learn to recognize subtle presentations of sexual abuse in children. Lack of genital trauma does not rule out sexual abuse. Children with complaints involving the genitalia may be victims despite the lack of specific allegations or physical findings.

The relationship of the offender to the victim further complicates the recognition and reporting of these crimes. Offenders fall into three basic categories in relation to the victim. Parents or parent surrogates (stepparent or live-in boyfriend or girlfriend) constitute an estimated 30 to 40 per cent of offenders, with other relatives and friends constituting an additional 30 to 40 per cent. Thus 80 per cent of offenders may be known and trusted by the child. Strangers are responsible for the minority (20 per cent) of child sexual assaults.[6] The popular image of the child molester as a perverted recluse, the stranger we are all warned to avoid, is both inaccurate and naive. It is similarly unsafe to assume that sexual assault is a frightening or even an unpleasant experience for the child. Because the offender is often a loved one and the offense occurs in familiar surroundings, many children may derive some pleasure or may have at least a neutral response to the relationship. Sexual abuse of children is often a recurrent or ongoing problem within a family. The isolated assault by a stranger is in many respects handled more easily by authorities as well as the family of the victim.

The child victim of sexual abuse may be reluctant to report the problem for many reasons. If the offender is a family member, the child may fear rejection or actual retaliation by the involved relative. Furthermore, fear of precipitating a family crisis or a sense of guilt about a secretive relationship may compound the problem. Children are often warned about the consequences of revealing their relationship. Even if the offender is a stranger, children may be inhibited from reporting the incident by guilt, embarrassment, or fear of parental punishment. Similar concerns often dissuade adult victims from reporting sexual crimes. In addition, the child victim may not perceive the relationship as undesirable. Thus, the failure to recognize sexually abused children is in part a function of the nature of the crime and the characteristics of both victim and offender.

MANAGEMENT OF CHILD ABUSE VICTIMS—AN INTERDISCIPLINARY APPROACH

Unfortunately, medical and legal authorities are frequently responsible for a failure to recognize childhood sexual abuse. There is a tendency among health care and legal authorities to doubt the validity of many complaints of abuse that are reported. Several factors contribute to this attitude. Many health care personnel feel uncomfortable in these situations. Pediatricians may doubt their ability to do an adequate gynecologic evaluation. Gynecologists may be hesitant to attempt an examination of a pediatric patient. Both may feel inadequate in dealing with the psychologic complexities of the family relationship. In addition, there is often subconscious revulsion in response to this sort of crime, which may be based on personal experience or deep seated psychologic factors. As a result, physicians may consciously or subconsciously avoid becoming involved in these cases. Many emergency rooms are inadequately equipped to handle rape victims and have not established a mechanism to insure appropriate follow-up care.

The response of authorities is further limited by their inability to verify the complaint. A common scenario consists of distraught mother who presents a confused and unresponsive child to the emergency room, claiming sexual abuse by another family member. The physical findings may be unremarkable or inconclusive and the stories presented may be contradictory. Confronted with this situation, the physician may overlook or disregard serious childhood abuse.

Having acknowledged the difficulties in recognizing childhood rape, I will discuss how physicians and other authorities can improve their response.

Let us first consider the role of various authorities. One key to successful management of child victims and their families is the involvement of various professionals. Police officers, nurses, emergency care physicians, and mental health and social workers all assume important roles. Emergency care facilities must coordinate the efforts of these individuals in order to insure appropriate comprehensive care for these patients.

Role of Law Enforcement Officials

Law enforcement officials should be trained to handle these cases. Their initial responsibility includes assessment of the reported crime. If the offense occurs outside the home, there may be witnesses to interview or evidence to collect. Police may not be contacted initially in intrafamilial cases.

When contact is made, police must be sensitive to the dangers of exposure and confrontation of offending adults. Children and adolescents may be reluctant to discuss their situation unless they can be assured that their statements will not be conveyed to the family. This fear of confrontation is usually well founded. There is controversy over whether immediate separation of a child from an offending family member is the best approach. In some situations in which the offender is nonviolent and voluntarily seeking help, it may be possible to leave the child in contact with the offender. However, authorities agree that the child may be placed in serious jeopardy if a secretive sexual relationship involving a family member is exposed and the child remains in contact with the offending adult.[7] If the potential for further harm exists, no exposure or accusation should be made unless removal of either the child or the offender from the situation can be ensured. Police and social workers must cooperate in handling these situations.

Police officials should avoid detailed questioning of parents and victims. The history is a sensitive aspect of the overall evaluation. Trauma can be minimized if only one complete history is obtained. Having assessed the basic complaint, police should direct families to the appropriate medical facility. Their role then involves collection of forensic evidence from the medical personnel. Finally, police should attempt to standardize their reporting of these crimes. Incest, sodomy, and indecent liberties involving child victims should all be considered variants of child sexual abuse and filed as a single crime.

In addition to law enforcement officials, families and child victims will usually come in contact with emergency room nurses, various physicians (pediatricians, gynecologists, psychiatrists), psychologists, and social workers. Although all these individuals play an important role, they can be overwhelming to the child and family. Further psychologic trauma can be avoided by compassionate management of the situation in the emergency room.

Care in the Medical Facility

Families of abused children are often extremely upset. They may overreact to typical emergency room procedures and demand immediate attention. Immediate attention to these families should be provided. A sympathetic nurse should speak with the family in a private setting, assuring them that their child will be seen promptly and briefly describing what the evaluation will include. At the same time, an assessment is made as to whether a medical emergency exists. This initial contact should *not* be used to elicit a detailed account of the incident. Its purpose is rather to provide immediate reassurance and sympathy for the family.

Prior to beginning the actual history and physical examination, consent papers must be obtained. These must include permission to perform a genital examination. Specific permission to collect and submit specimens, and records, including photographs, for possible legal action should be obtained. This permit must be signed by a parent or guardian if the victim is a minor and witnessed by the emergency room staff.

Obtaining a History

Children are largely influenced by the reactions of adults. They are especially sensitive to the reaction of their parents. Efforts to calm hysterical parents are often crucial in obtaining the cooperation of the child victim. The influence of the parents also must be considered in obtaining the history. If possible, each parent or involved adult should be questioned privately away from the child. He or she should be told that children in general provide better information when questioned by a skilled individual without parental influence. Some young children (2 to 4 years old) may suffer separation anxiety or fear of strangers and will do better if their parents remain with them. In this situation, parents should be advised to encourage the child to answer questions but not to coach or answer for the child. In cases of intrafamily abuse, separation of the child from both the offending and accusing parent may be essential if an accurate history is to be obtained.

Obtaining a medical history from a child can be a challenge, and the history of a sexual assault is especially problematic. Children may justifiably fear the consequences of their comments. Their anxiety, fear, shame, and guilt all contribute to an unwillingness to discuss the situation. This is compounded by a general fear of strangers and a specific fear of physicians and hospitals. Children may have further concern about the upcoming examination. Confronted with so many anxieties, many children may refuse to respond.

In order to deal effectively with these children, professionals need experience and some degree of expertise. Any interested and compassionate professional can develop some techniques that are useful in dealing with these children. If possible, children should be interviewed in a comfortable private setting, an office rather than an examination room. Children should be given some form of diversion (books or toys) and allowed some time to adjust to their surroundings before an interview is attempted. The interviewer should begin with nonthreatening questions of interest to the child. The interviewer must be able to communicate on the child's level. Using appropriate vocabulary is especially important. Children may use nonanatomic terms such as "pee-pee" or "doodle" in describing genitalia. It may be useful to use an anatomically correct doll or drawing to establish the child's terminology. The interviewer must then use terms that are familiar to the child. Dolls, drawings, or puppets may also be used to "act out" or demonstrate the events. Children may be willing to project their experience in the form of play acting. Other interviews have used role reversal technique to elicit information by encouraging the child to direct the questioning:

Doctor: "Now let's play that you are the doctor and I am the one who is sick. You ask *me* how I got sick."
Child: "OK. I am the doctor. How did you get sick?"
Doctor: "Guess"
Child: "Did you get it on a bus?"
Doctor: "No"
Child: "Did you get it from your teddy bear?"
Doctor: "No"
Child: "Did you get it from your cousin?"
Doctor: "Maybe so."[6]

In this case the child had contracted gonorrhea from older cousins who were also infected.

Older children and adolescents may be too embarassed by the interview situation to discuss the actual events. An interviewer of the same sex may be of some help. The interviewer may also offer to ask direct questions to which the victim can respond with a simply yes or no.

In obtaining a history from adolescents, it is important to consider their menstrual history and other possible sexual encounters. One must specifically consider the timing of the menstrual cycle relative to sexual activity in order to assess possible pregnancy risk. The adolescent may be sexually active, and information regarding contraceptives is significant. Finally, both children and adolescents must be questioned about bathing, washing, or douching following sexual encounters.

Interviewing a child in a stressful situation can be very frustrating. There are many other techniques that trained professionals may employ. However, the most important aspect of the interview, is to remain compassionate, nonthreatening, and nonjudgmental. Child victims need to be reassured that they will not be further humiliated, punished, or hurt.

The initial contact with the patient and the way in which the interview is conducted are important in managing child abuse cases. Before discussing the details of the physical examination, the importance of an organized and efficient emergency setting will be considered.

Assignment of Medical Personnel

Hospital emergency rooms are often very busy and the staff is frequently overwhelmed by patients and families demanding their attention. The general emergency room staff may not be able to provide the special care required by sexually abused children and their families. An ideal arrangement would identify specific nurses and primary care physicians who are responsible for managing all such cases. The responsible physician may be a member of the emergency room staff, a pediatrician, a gynecologist, or a general practitioner. What is essential is that several physicians participate so that someone is always available. Ideally the involved physicians and nurses will have a special interest in providing quality care to these children and will be willing to make the commitment of time and develop the necessary skills that will enable them to manage these situations effectively.

Coordination of Medical, Legal, and Social Service Efforts

The staff of the medical facility should coordinate its efforts with those of law enforcement officials. In order to prosecute offenders successfully, the medical evaluation must conform to the legal requirements for admissible evidence. This involves appropriate release forms from witnesses, accurate labeling of evidence, legible, signed medical records, and strict adherence to the "chain of evidence." The chain of evidence insures that the specimens, clothing, and laboratory tests submitted are in fact the victim's. It protects the victim from defense attorneys' attempts to discredit the physical evidence. All specimens must be labeled and submitted immediately to the appropriate laboratory (forensic or hospital), with a standardized form indicating the date and the name of the individual who received the specimen. Facilities should have a "lock box" in which specimens are kept at night until delivery to the appropriate laboratory is possible. The system is most effective if a minimum number of people handle the specimens. If possible, only one transporter and technician should be assigned to handle these specimens.

Further cooperation with legal authorities is necessary during the trial of these cases. Unfortunately, rape trials often do not occur until many months after the actual incident. Physicians may have relocated by the time they are called to testify. Ideally, the physicians who are responsible for these cases will be practicing physicians with a commitment to the area and a willingness to participate in the legal process.

Finally, the medical facility must be able to provide appropriate psychologic counseling and social intervention for victims and families. Trained psychologists or psychiatrists must be available to provide immediate counseling as well as long-term follow-up. A social worker with the capability of providing immediate crisis intervention and placement is also a vital member of the team. Thus, the medical facility must be able to coordinate the efforts of law enforcement, medical, psychologic, and social work professionals to provide comprehensive care for the sexually abused child.

Equipment

The facility in which the abused child is evaluated may also affect the quality of care. Not all hospitals or emergency rooms are equipped to provide the range of services that these cases may require. The facility should have an appropriate private room in which to conduct interviews. The emergency room itself must have all the necessary equipment for evidence collection and physical examination. A prepackaged "rape kit" can prevent oversights and maximize efficiency in performing the examination. This kit should include

1. sealed glass slides
2. diamond point labeling pencil
3. adhesive labels
4. 6 to 12 plastic handled sterile Q-tips
5. 8 to 12 test tubes
6. saline
7. urine container
8. needle and Vacutainer
9. blood specimen tubes (VDRL, B-HOG)
10. Thayer-Martin medium bottle
11. gonorrhea culture and PAP mailers
12. comb—sterile package
13. scissors
14. fingernail scraper

For children, special equipment, including long nasal speculum or special pediatric vaginal speculum, is necessary. Children may also require some form of diversion (toys, dolls, and so forth) during both the interview and the examination. It may be necessary to provide mild sedation for the child or occasionally the parents. Access to an operating room with full anesthesia capabilities may be necessary for surgical repair of trauma or proper examination. Gynecologic and general surgical consultants should be available.

Physical Examination

Having considered many of the general problems in dealing with child sexual abuse, let us now concentrate on the physical examination of the child victim. As with the history, the physical examination should be conducted in private. Children under 6 years may be more relaxed with a parent present, whereas many older children cooperate better when seen without a parent. Again children reflect their parent's anxiety reactions. It is important to discuss the examination with the parent and enlist his or her cooperation in putting the child at ease.

The examination should begin with observation and description of the child's manner and general appearance. Judgmental comments should be avoided. For example, if a child appears calm and relaxed, this should be stated without adding "she does not appear abused" or "as if nothing has happened." Each aspect of the examination should be described to the child before it is performed.

Any evidence of physical trauma should be carefully described, illustrated, and, if possible, photographed. Particular attention should be directed to the neck, wrists, and ultimately the genital/anal areas. If restraint or force was used, these areas are likely to show ecchymoses. Fingernail scrapings from the child should be obtained if the history or examination suggests resistance by the victim. Any hairs found on the abdomen or pubic region should be submitted. In adolescent girls, pubic hair should be combed and a small clipping submitted for possible hair or secretions from the assailant. Clothing with secretions must be submitted as evidence. Similarly foreign bodies should be labeled and submitted. Wood's lamp illumination in the dark will cause fluorescence of semen and may be used to detect areas of staining on the clothing, abdomen, or genital region.

The most difficult aspect of the evaluation of the child victim is the gynecologic or genital examination. Children should be reassured that the examination will be as gentle as possible and that it is necessary to be sure that they are not injured or "sick." Very young children may be held in a frog leg position on the mother's lap. Some examiners have recommended placing young children in a lithotomy position (Fig. 27–1). This position may allow adequate visualization of the vaginal orifice. Some children may find the lithotomy position more familiar than a frog leg or modified lithotomy position (Fig. 27–2). Whatever position is used, the child should be gently placed and not forced into position. Begin with simple visualization of the perineum, anus, and external genitalia. Any erythema, abrasion, or laceration is significant and should be noted. The child should be told that you are going to touch her leg or thigh, and then slide your hand slowly down to the genitalia. Avoid abruptly touching the genital region without warning.

Whether visualization of the vagina is essential is a point of controversy. In prepubertal children with no evidence of genital trauma (i.e., no erythema, bleeding, laceration), full visualization is not necessary. This does not mean that specimens need not be collected. In adolescents or in children with trauma, visualization of the vagina can usually be accomplished with a long narrow pediatric vaginal or nasal speculum. Some

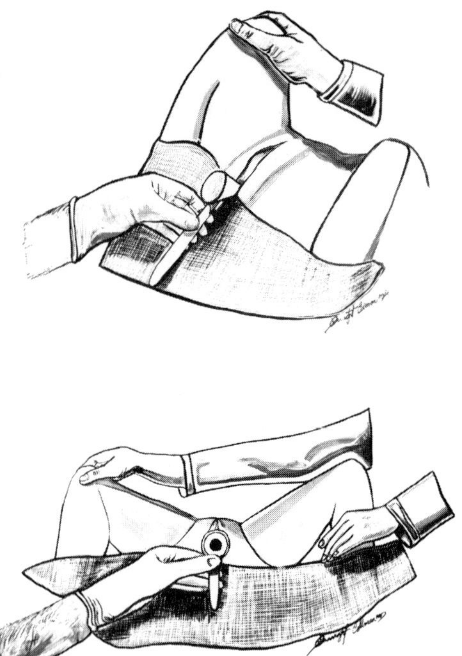

Figure 27–2. The frog leg position for pediatric genital examination allows adequate visualization of the genitalia. However, this position is usually somewhat less familiar to the patient than the lithotomy position, and as a result, the physician may have more difficulty maintaining adequate visualization.

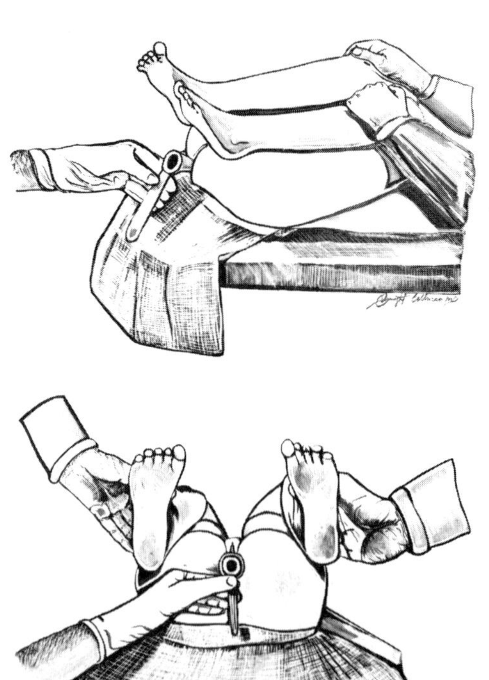

Figure 27–1. The lithotomy position for pediatric genital examination provides adequate exposure and is an easy position for most young children to maintain. It is of critical importance to carefully describe the position, as well as all procedures to be performed, to the patient.

examiners have used a hysteroscope or cystoscope for high lacerations. If there is any bleeding or significant trauma, thorough examination is essential and anesthesia may be required.

Children vary in their willingness to cooperate for a genital examination. Every attempt should be made to allay anxiety and establish rapport. This includes describing the examination in nonfrightening, understandable terms; allowing the child to feel both your fingers and the speculum on the leg or thigh; and then gradually moving towards the genital area, describing the sensations that the child will be feeling as the examination is performed. Despite these efforts, the examination may be both frightening and painful. If a child cannot be examined using these techniques, sedation or anesthesia should be employed. Forcible restraint may further traumatize a child and should never be employed in evaluating a child rape victim.

If trauma is evident, surgical repair may be required. As such, the child should be treated only by a trained gynecologic or, if appropriate, anorectal surgeon. The child should never be subjected to multiple examinations whether awake or asleep.

Unless the child is exceptionally cooperative, anesthesia should be utilized to evaluate all vaginal bleeding. Lacerations may occur on the anterior or posterior vaginal wall, which may be difficult to visualize even with a nasal or pediatric speculum. A hysteroscope may be useful for lesions high in the fornix or when used in conjunction with a test tube dilator to illuminate the vaginal vault. The glass dilator should be used only with full anesthesia, since resistance may result in further trauma.

In children, lacerations may extend into the peritoneum, resulting in intra-abdominal bleeding. Careful vaginal and rectal palpation for hematomas should be routinely performed in cases requiring anesthesia. If intra-abdominal extension of laceration or hematoma formation is suspected, children should be hospitalized and serial hematocrits followed. Laparotomy may be required in some cases.

Small lacerations that are not bleeding do not require suturing. Interrupted absorbable sutures can be used to control bleeding sites or to reapproximate tissues. Strict attention to accurate anatomic reconstruction is essential in major trauma involving the perineum or anus.

In cases of large vaginal hematomas, the area must be carefully observed for continued expansion. Generally these hematomas will be self-limited by a tamponade effect and are best left to resolve spontaneously. Attempts to incise and evacuate hematomas may result in further hemorrhage with unidentifiable bleeding sites or infection. However, if the hematoma is expanding, it may be necessary to isolate and ligate large vessels. If this effort fails, pressure packing will often control further bleeding. In cases of excessive bleeding, selective embolization of vessels utilizing angiography may be considered as an alternative to an abdominal approach with ligation of the anterior hypogastric vessels. These techniques are rarely necessary.

Even when actual visualization of the vagina and cervix is not required, specimen collection is still essential. One must remember that oral and anal penetration is common in child abuse cases. As such, specimens should be obtained from the oral pharynx, anus, and vagina. The first swab of each area should be plated on Thayer-Martin medium for gonorrhea culture. Gonorrhea infection of a child is evidence of sexual contact (oral/genital, genital/genital, or hand/genital) with an infected adult or adolescent. Children do not acquire gonorrhea from towels, bedding, or toilet seats! Children who present with vaginal discharge that proves to be gonorrhea should be considered child abuse victims, and appropriate investigations should be instituted.[8]

The oral, genital, and anal areas each should then be swabbed for secretions, which are smeared on a slide and viewed immediately for the presence of motile sperm. Motile sperm usually persist in the vagina for 2 to 3 hours and occasionally longer. A second swab from each area should be submitted for PAP smear or Gram's stain to determine the presence of nonmotile sperm, which may persist up to 72 hours in the vagina and 10 to 14 days in the endocervix.[9, 10] A third swab from each region should be submitted for an acid phosphatase determination. An elevated acid phosphatase indicates the presence of semen for up to 12 hours.[11, 12] It may be necessary to irrigate with a small amount of normal saline solution to obtain these specimens.

In cases in which ejaculation is suspected to have occurred, a specimen from the appropriate area may be submitted for blood group determination. This is only necessary if the offender is not known, as it is an aide to positive identification. Approximately 80 per cent of individuals will secrete blood-group antigens in saliva, semen, and other secretions. Secretions from the mouth or vagina can be tested for the presence of blood-group antigens. Because these antigens may be the child's, their secretor status must also be determined. This may be done by having the child spit or chew on a piece of cloth and submit this specimen. Comparison of the blood-group antigens from the specimens with the blood group of the child and the blood-group of the suspect may help identify the offender.

The examination should be individualized depending on the history and initial findings. However, it is important, to maintain a high index of suspicion despite lack of history or physical findings. Swabs for gonorrhea, sperm, and acid phosphatase are simple to obtain and should always be collected. These specimens along with clothing, pubic hair, fingernail scrapes, and a baseline VDRL blood test should be submitted to the appropriate laboratory. All specimens should be carefully labeled and initialed by the physician, and the chain of evidence procedures must be strictly observed.

Additional Considerations

Additional medical treatment may be indicated for venereal disease and pregnancy prevention. Again treatment must be individualized. If the history suggests possible exposure to venereal disease, prophylactic antibiotics should be given. For adolescents or children who weigh more than 40 kg, the standard therapy of probenecid 1 g followed in 1 hour by procaine penicillin 4.8 million units IM is appropriate coverage for both gonorrhea and syphilis. Children weighing less than 40 kg should receive probenecid 25 mg/kg po followed by procaine penicillin 100,000 units/kg IM.

Children who are allergic to penicillin may be treated with tetracycline 25 mg/kg po and then 40 to 60 mg/kg/day in 4 divided doses for 1 week. Tetracycline should *not* be used in children less than 10 years of age because of staining of dental enamel. Erythromycin 40 mg/kg/day in 4 doses for 1 week may also be used although its efficacy in treating syphilis is not established.

Follow-up for exposed children should include repeat GC culture as well as repeat VDRL and pregnancy test in 6 weeks. These follow-up examinations are especially important if antibiotic treatment is not given.

Prophylaxis against pregnancy is a controversial issue. In any postmenarchal victim, the issue should at least be considered. The timing of the assault relative to probable ovulation and use of any contraceptive measures should be determined in order to assess the risk of pregnancy. The principle side effect of pregnancy prophylaxis is nausea and vomiting. Prophylaxis is approximately 80 per cent effective in preventing implantation. If no prophylaxis is given and pregnancy does occur, many victims will consider abortion, which involves further physical risks and emotional trauma. These factors must all be considered in deciding whether to provide prophylaxis. Pregnancy prophylaxis may be given as diethylstilbesterol (DES) 25 mg po bid for 5 days or 40 to 50 mg/day for 3 days in conjunction with an antiemetic. Although exposure to DES or estrogen prior to 4 weeks gestation is not associated with fetal genital tract abnormality, medicolegal considerations demand that possible teratogenic effects be discussed. Patients must understand that prophylaxis is not 100 per cent effective and that therapeutic abortion may be indicated if pregnancy does occur. In adolescents who are sexually active with a partner other than the offender, a serum β-HCG pregnancy test should be performed to help rule out conception prior to the rape and to avoid confusion in the event of pregnancy.

Following physical examination and specimen collection, the preliminary findings should be reviewed with the family. The child and family should be reassured regarding the extent and nature of any injuries and the possibility of any permanent damage. Families may fear future problems with sexual relations or childbearing, and these issues should be discussed. Parents should be given a written sheet describing what tests were performed and the nature and purpose of any treatment rendered. This sheet should also include follow-up appointment information. Under duress, many people cannot absorb and retain information. A written information sheet is thus essential to insure patient understanding and follow-up.

A great deal has been written on the psychologic effects of sexual abuse. When the victim is a child, the psychologic effects may be extremely complex and have long-term implications. Not only the child but also various family members may require immediate counseling as well as long-term follow-up. This may require referral to individuals specially trained in child abuse therapy. The staff of the emergency care facility should be able to provide access to both crisis counseling and referral for long-term follow-up within the community. As with medical care, families should be provided with written instructions for obtaining psychologic help.

Similarly the family may require the immediate and long-term services of a social worker. Temporary placement of the child or offending adult may be an essential part of successful management. Quality care of the child victim and family must include immediate and long-term monitoring of the home situation. These services should be included in the initial evaluation of the abused child.

There are many complex issues in caring for the child victims of sexual assault and their families that exceed the scope of this chapter. The psychologic and social ramifications of these situations may be profound. Although special training may be required to deal effectively with the long-term effects of child sexual abuse, the emergency care physician should be capable of the initial evaluation of these patients.

REFERENCES

1. Sweeney J: Enlightened management of the rape victim: Part I: Definition, incidence, history. ER Reports 2:91, 1981.
2. Keefe L: Police investigation of child sexual assault. *In* Burgess AW, Groth AN, Holstrom LL, Sgroi SM (eds.): Sexual Assault of Children and Adolescents. MA, Lexington Books, 1982.
3. Schiff AF: Attending the child "rape victim." South Med J, 72:906, 1979.
4. Tilelli JA, Turek D, Jaffe AC: Sexual abuse of children. N Engl J Med 302:319, 1980.
5. Groth AN: Patterns of sexual assault against children and adolescents. *In* Burgess AW, Groth AN, Holstrom LL, Sgroi SM (eds.): Sexual Assault of Children and Adolescents. MA, Lexington Books, 1982.
6. DeVine RA; Sexual abuse of children: An overview of the problem. *In* Sexual Abuse of Children: Selected Readings. National Center of Child Abuse and Neglect. U.S. Department of Health and Human Services, DHHS Publication No. (OHDS) 78-30161, November 1980.
7. Groth AN, Guidelines for the assessment and management of the offender. *In* Burgess AW, Groth AN, Holstrom LL, Sgroi SM (eds.): Sexual Assault of Children and Adolescents. MA, Lexington Books, 1982.
8. Knasel AL: Venereal disease in children. *In* Sexual Abuse of Children: Selected Readings. National Center of Child Abuse and Neglect. U.S. Department of Health and Human Services, DHHS Publication No. (OHDS) 78-30161, November 1980.
9. Silverman EM, Silverman AG: Persistence of spermatozoa in the lower genital tracts of women. JAMA 240:1875, 1978.
10. Soules MR, Pollard AA, Brown KM, Mool V: The forensic laboratory evaluation of evidence in alleged rape. Am J Obstet Gynecol 130:142, 1978.
11. Findley TP: Quantitation of vaginal acid phosphatase and its relationship to time of coitus. Am J Clin Pathol, 68:238, 1977.
12. Gomez RR, Wunsch CD, Davis JH, Hicks DJ: Qualitative and quantitative determinations of acid phosphatase activity in vaginal washings. Am J Clin Pathol 64:423, 1975.

Selected Readings

Breen JL, Greenwald E, Gregori CA: The molested young female: Evaluation and therapy of alleged rape. Pediatr Clin North Am, 19:717, 1972.

Burgess AW, Groth AN, Holstrom LL, Sgroi SM: Sexual Assault of Children and Adolescents. MA, Lexington Books, 1982.

Greenberg NH The Epidemiology of childhood sexual abuse. Pediatr Ann 8:16, 1979.

Halbert DR, Darnell-Jones DE: Medical management of the sexually assaulted woman. J Reprod Med 20:28, 1978.

National Center of Child Abuse and Neglect: Sexual Abuse of Children: Selected Readings. Children's Bureau, U.S. Department of Health and Human Services, Publication No. (OHDS) 78-30161, November 1980.

On DP: Management of childhood sexual abuse. J Fam Pract 11:1057, 1980.

On DP, Prietto SV: Emergency management of sexually abused children: The role of the pediatric resident. Am J Dis Child 133:628, 1979.

Pascoe DJ: Management of sexually abused children. Pediatr Ann 8:44, 1979.

Paul DM: The medical examination in sexual offenses against children. Med Sci Law, 17:251, 1977.

Pepiton-Rockwell F: Patterns of rape and approaches to care. J Fam Prac 6:521, 1978.

Price JM, Valdiserri EV: Childhood sexual abuse: A recent review of the literature. J Am Med Wom Assoc 36:232, 1981.

CHAPTER

28 Poisoning

A. R. TEMPLE

Dealing with poisoning is an everyday problem for the emergency room physician. The number of poisoning episodes annually in the United States is estimated to be between 5 and 10 million, of which some 15 to 20 per cent require emergency medical evaluation. Poisonings are both accidental and intentional. Accidental poisonings account for 80 to 85 per cent of poisoning exposures, whereas intentional poisonings account for 15 to 20 per cent. However, individuals who purposefully overdose have a much higher rate of significant toxicity, have a greater need for treatment in the emergency department, and have higher rates of hospitalization, intensive care monitoring, and death. Among children aged 5 and under, essentially all poisonings are accidents related to their natural exploratory behavior, but among older children and adolescents, the physician must consider the possibility of suicide attempts (Table 28–1).

The number of toxic substances involved in poisonings is extensive, requiring a broad range of knowledge in toxicology if one is to treat poisonings adequately. Table 28–2 presents a list of substances most frequently ingested by children under age 5 years. Table 28–3 presents a list of the most common drugs involved in adolescent and adult emergency room poisoning visits. There are significant differences between the pediatric (accidental) and the adolescent and adult (purposeful) profiles. In adolescents, there is a much higher percentage of cases in which psychopharmacologic drugs (sedatives, tranquilizers, and antidepressants) are the source of the poisoning, compared with young children, in whom there is a much higher frequency of exposure to household chemicals and plants.

Table 28–1. BREAKDOWN OF POISONING CASES BY THE AGE OF THE VICTIM

Age in Years	1975 (Per Cent)*	1983 (Per Cent)†
Under 1	6.4	16.9
1	17.0	37.8
2	21.0	13.5
3	14.4	4.5
4	5.4	1.4
5	2.7	1.2
6–17	10.2	6.5
18 and over	20.5	15.6
Not recorded	2.3	2.6

*Data from the Intermountain Regional Poison Control Center, 1975.

†Data from coöperative regional poison control center pilot study, Jan.–Feb., 1983, American Association of Poison Control Centers.

Poisoning exposures can occur by ingestion, which accounts for the vast majority of occurrences, or by ocular exposure, inhalation, cutaneous or topical exposure, or envenomation (Table 28–4). Poisonings may occur from either acute or chronic exposures, but most poisonings are a result of a single, acute exposure. Nonetheless, chronic toxicity is an important issue for the clinician to consider because in such cases the source is not always obvious, the toxicity not always clear, and the toxic process not often obvious until serious clinical derangements occur. Knowing how to approach each of these various types of poisoning is an essential part of clinical medicine.

EVALUATION OF A POISONING

Exposure to Known Poisons

In most cases of known exposure, the history is the single most important factor in assessment of the severity of that poisoning. In the absence of symptoms of toxicity, the decision to institute treatment is almost always based on the history of the exposure. Therefore, an accurate history of the exposure is essential in determining appropriate treatment. When the poisoned patient is first encountered, an assessment of the potential severity of the toxic exposure must be made as rapidly as possible. Basic information to obtain (Table 28–5) should include (1) confirmation that a toxic exposure has occurred, (2) specific identification of the product and toxic agent(s), (3) the route and magnitude (dose) of the exposure, (4) the time of the exposure, and (5) the present condition of

Table 28–2. SUBSTANCES MOST FREQUENTLY INGESTED BY CHILDREN UNDER AGE FIVE*†

Substance	Cases in 1978 Number	Per Cent
Plants	11,010	11.7
Soaps, detergents, cleaners	5,836	6.2
Antihistamines, cold medications	4,003	4.3
Perfume, cologne, toilet water	3,748	4.0
Vitamins, minerals	3,677	3.9
Aspirin	3,557	3.8
Baby	2,557	0.4
Adult	380	0.4
Unspecified	640	0.7
Household disinfectants, deodorizers	2,752	2.9
Miscellaneous analgesics	2,752	2.9
Insecticides (excluding mothballs)	2,675	2.9
Miscellaneous internal medicines	2,303	2.5
Fingernail preparations	2,270	2.4
Miscellaneous external medicines	2,151	2.3
Liniments	2,016	2.2
Household bleach	1,863	2.0
Miscellaneous products	1,627	1.7
Cosmetic lotions, creams	1,625	1.7
Antiseptic medications	1,603	1.7
Psychopharmacologic agents	1,463	1.6
Cough medicines	1,443	1.5
Hormones	1,386	1.5
Glues, adhesives	1,384	1.5
Rodenticides	1,347	1.4
Internal antibiotics	1,246	1.3
Corrosive acids, alkalies	1,204	1.3
Paint	1,204	1.3

*From Temple AR: Poisoning I. Monograph 52. Kansas City, American Academy of Family Physicians, 1983. Reproduced by permission.

†Individual poison reports (phone inquiries and treated cases) submitted to the National Clearinghouse for Poison Control Centers by 326 centers in 44 states, District of Columbia, Panama and military bases abroad.

Table 28–3. TWENTY MOST COMMON DRUGS INVOLVED IN ADULT EMERGENCY ROOM POISONING EPISODES REPORTED TO DRUG ABUSE WARNING NETWORK FOR 1979*

Drug	Number of Mentions	Drug Rank in 1981	Drug Rank in 1980
Alcohol-in-combination	28,718	1	1
Diazepam	14,932	2	2
Heroin/morphine	9,666	3	3
Aspirin	6,947	4	4
Methaqualone	4,955	5	5
Cocaine	4,777	6	9
Marijuana	4,671	7	7
Acetaminophen	4,467	8	10
Flurazepam	4,432	9	6
PCP/PCP combinations	3,752	10	8
Codeine combinations	3,551	11	12
Amitriptyline	3,400	12	11
Phenobarbital	2,936	13	14
Diphenylhydantoin sodium	2,778	14	15
Pentazocine	2,606	15	22
Chlordiazepoxide	2,591	16	17
Propoxyphene	2,556	17	13
Methadone	2,522	18	18
Amphetamine	2,444	19	16
Speed	2,212	20	26

*From Temple AR: Poisoning I. Monograph 52. Kansas City, American Academy of Family Physicians, 1983. Reproduced by permission.

Table 28–4. CLASSIFICATION OF POISONING CASES BY MODE OF EXPOSURE

Mode	1975 (Per Cent)*	1983 (Per Cent)†
Ingestion	85.0	87.9
Topical	3.3	4.8
Ocular	4.6	4.5
Inhalation	3.5	2.4
Envenomation	2.9	0.1
Other	0.7	0.3

*Data from the Intermountain Regional Poison Control Center, 1975.

†Data from cooperative regional poison center pilot study, Jan.–Feb., 1983, American Association of Poison Control Centers.

the victim, including signs, symptoms, and recent changes in the patient's status. Only with an accurate history is it possible to make a sound judgment regarding the level of treatment required. During the initial assessment, consultation with a poison control center may save considerable time and, by providing necessary information, may enhance the clinicians management skills.

Whenever a serious poisoning has occurred, the victim must be seen by appropriately trained personnel. As in any medical emergency, initial assessment and management should include establishment of an airway, artificial ventilation to restore breathing, and appropriate measures to restore circulation. Specific attention should be paid to heart rate, blood pressure, central nervous system status, (deep tendon reflexes, corneal reflexes, response to verbal and painful stimuli, and pupil size and response to light), and hydration.

Table 28–5. KEY QUESTIONS IN OBTAINING A POISONING HISTORY*

To whom are you talking?
Was there an exposure?
What was the toxic agent? Exact nature or name of item?
What were the circumstances of the exposure?
To how much was the patient exposed?
What was the route of exposure?
When was the exposure?
What is the age, weight, sex and name of the patient?
What was the condition or state of mind of the patient prior to the exposure?
What is the present condition of the patient?
When did any symptoms begin?
Have the symptoms become worse?
Can you describe the symptoms?
Is the container and item of exposure available?

*From Temple AR: Poisoning I. Monograph 52. Kansas City, American Academy of Family Physicians, 1983. Reproduced by permission.

Exposure to Unknown Poisons

Obtaining a history when an exposure is suspected but the agent or reality of the exposure is unknown requires careful scrutiny. It is important to know why an exposure is suspected. In most such circumstances the patient presents with symptoms potentially referable to a toxic exposure, ranging from the chronic and vague in nature to the acute and life threatening. Immediate evaluation of severity should be made to determine if the patient is in immediate and life threatening danger, some potential danger, or no real danger at all. To do this, symptoms demonstrated by the patient are of primary diagnostic help, with laboratory confirmation also being helpful.

Diagnosis

Children who are poisoned do not always come to the physician with a clear history of exposure followed by the onset of symptoms. Often they develop signs and symptoms of illnesses that mimic other diseases and may give no history of a toxic exposure. Thus, physicians must consider the possibility of an ingestion when treating young children who have unusual behavior, sudden onset of illness, or unexplained symptoms. Other factors to suggest the possibility that poisoning may be a problem include the poison-prone age range of 1 to 3 years; past history of pica or a known accidental ingestion; evidence of substantial environmental stress, either acute (arrival of a new baby, family move, serious illness in a parent) or chronic (marital conflict, parental inadequacy); unexplained multiple organ system involvement; or significant alteration in level of consciousness. Many findings on physical examination may suggest an intoxication, including altered vital signs, neuromuscular dysfunction, unusual eye findings, skin alteration, and unusual odors on the breath.

When a patient has a poisoning exposure, it is important to determine whether or not any symptoms present are a result of the exposure. Symptoms generally occur within 2 to 4 hours after the ingestion of most poisons, except with nontoxic amounts, but symptoms may be delayed for several hours to several days. The degree of severity and type of symptoms are dependent upon the amount ingested. Symptoms of toxicity from drugs generally occur at about the same time following the overdose that pharmacologic effects would occur following the taking of a therapeutic dose. However, massive overdoses may result in earlier onset of symptoms. In addition, products in solution (alcohol, cough and cold medicines, and so on) are more rapidly absorbed and so toxic symptoms occur earlier, while enteric-coated or time-release products have a delayed onset of symptoms. Contact irritants (inhaled gases, spilled liquids, swallowed caustics) may have a variable onset of symptoms, but generally symptoms will be present within 2 to 4 hours if they are to occur at all. Not all of the symptoms associated with a poisoning will occur at the same time. Symptoms referable to local irritation generally precede systemic effects. In some cases, certain symptoms occur at one level of intoxication while others do not occur until a higher level of intoxication is reached.

The assessment of severity also depends on the degree to which a given symptom is manifest. There are varying degrees of coma as there are varying degrees of burns. For central nervous system (CNS) symptoms, which occur most commonly, various classification schemes have been devised. Table 28–6 presents classification systems that can be used to assess the severity of symptoms

Table 28–6. RATING SCALES FOR SEVERITY OF SYMPTOMS*

Classification of Depth of Coma *Physical Findings*	*Coma Stage†*				
	0	1	2	3	4
Responds to verbal stimuli	+	0	0	0	0
Responds to minimal tactile stimuli	+	0	0	0	0
Responds to maximal tactile stimuli	+	+	0	0	0
Deep tendon reflexes present	+	+	+	0	0
Pupillary light reflexes present	+	+	+	0	0
Spontaneous respirations present	+	+	+	+	0
Stable blood pressure present	+	+	+	+	0
Classification of Degree of Hyperactivity *Physical Findings*	*Stage†*				
	1	2	3	4	
Restlessness, tremors, hyperreflexia	+	+	+	+	
Sweating, mydriasis, flushing	+	+	+	+	
Confusion, hyperactivity, tachypnea	0	+	+	+	
Hypertension, hyperpyrexia	0	+	+ +	+ +	
Delirium, mania, self-injury	0	0	+	+	
Tachycardia, arrhythmias	0	0	+	+	
Convulsions, coma, circulatory collapse	0	0	0	+	
Classification of Withdrawal *Physical Findings*	*Degree‡*				
	0	1	2		
Diarrhea					
Dilated pupils					
Goose flesh					
Hyperactive bowel sounds					
Hypertension					
Insomnia					
Lacrimation					
Muscle cramps					
Tachycardia					
Yawning					
Total points					

*From Temple AR: Poisoning I. Monograph 52. Kansas City, American Academy of Family Physicians, 1983. Reproduced by permission.

† – + = present; 0 = absent; + + = severe.

‡– Score on 0, 1, 2, point basis: 0 = absent; 1 = present; 2 = severe. Severity rating (total points): 1-5 = mild; 6-10 = moderate; 11-15 = severe.

associated with coma, hyperactivity, and withdrawal.

Combinations of Symptoms. A symptom complex is often helpful in evaluating a poisoning victim. Specific combinations of toxic signs and symptoms may suggest specific types of poisonings. These "toxidromes" are often so characteristic as to provide guidance for initiating therapy even before laboratory confirmation of a specific diagnosis is available (Table 28–7). For example, if a patient is comatose, has depressed respirations, and has constricted pupils (miosis), a diagnosis of narcotic overdose would be very likely.

Table 28–7. CHARACTERISTICS OF SPECIFIC INTOXICATIONS (TOXIDROMES)*

Anticholinergics (Atropine, Tricyclic Antidepressants)
Fixed dilated pupils
Fever
Dry skin and mucous membranes
Rubor
Hallucinations, mania
Increased heart rate

Anticholinesterases (Organophosphates, Carbamates)
Constricted or pinpoint pupils
Profuse sweating and salivation
Bronchial secretions and bronchospasms
Muscle fasciculations
Coma
Bradycardia

Carbon Monoxide
Coma
Labored breathing
Cherry-red skin coloration (only rarely)
Possible involvement of multiple individuals

Cyanide
Coma
Rapid breathing
Hypotension
Odor of bitter almonds on breath

Narcotics and Other Central Nervous System Depressants
Pinpoint pupils
Decreased respiration
Coma
Hypotension
Decreased or absent reflexes

Salicylates
Vomting
Deep labored breathing
Lethargy and/or disorientation
Ringing in ears
Dehydration
Fever
Coma or convulsions

*From Temple AR: Poisoning I. Monograph 52. Kansas City, American Academy of Family Physicians, 1983. Reproduced by permission.

Diagnoses are often based on the symptom complex, but severity is best judged by whether there are symptoms or not. For example, if a patient was alleged to have taken ten 100-mg phenobarbital capsules 10 hours prior to call but has had no symptoms, the ingestion cannot be very severe, even though the alleged amount is potentially very serious.

Nontoxic Ingestion

Frequently the emergency physician will be asked about childhood ingestion of common household products, many of which are nontoxic unless taken in huge amounts. The availability of lists of such nontoxic products often allows the physician to reassure the parent and avoid unnecessary noxious therapy. Before using such a list, however, several precautions need to be borne in mind. The fact that an ingestion is nontoxic does not necessarily mean it has no medical significance. Ingestions often occur in the context of a poor social environment. Furthermore, parents may be innaccurate in their history. The child may have taken other products in addition to the non-toxic agents identified. Careful history and physical examination may assist in identifying patients who have ingested additional poisons.

GENERAL MANAGEMENT OF POISONINGS

Initial First Aid and Decontamination Procedures

A number of methods may be utilized to terminate the patient's exposure to a toxic substance or to mitigate potential toxicity. Table 28–8 summarizes basic consumer first aid recommendations. Obviously, it is necessary to identify the mode of exposure to the toxic agent, that is, whether the exposure was ocular or topical or the result of inhalation, ingestion, envenomation, or a combination of any of these. The following outlines procedures that should be instituted for each type of exposure.

Ocular Exposure

Involved eyes should be washed thoroughly, examined carefully, and then irrigated further, with additional therapy ad-

Table 28–8. FIRST AID TREATMENT FOR POISONING*

I. DO THESE THINGS BEFORE YOU CALL SOMEONE
   A. Remove poisons from contact with eyes, skin or mouth.
      1. Eyes: Gently wash eyes with plenty of water (or milk) for 10 to 15 minutes with the eyelids held open. Remove contact and again wash the eyes. Do not allow victims to rub their eyes.
      2. Skin: Wash poisons off the skin with large amounts of plain water. Then wash the skin with a detergent if it is possible. Remove and discard all contaminated clothing.
      3. Mouth: Look into victim's mouth and remove all tablets, powder, plants, or any other material that you find. Also examine for cuts, burns, or any unusual coloring. Wipe out mouth with a cloth and wash thoroughly with water.
   B. Remove victim from contact with poisonous fumes or gases.
      Get the victim into fresh air.
      Loosen all tight-fitting clothing.
      If the victim is not breathing, you should start artificial respiration immediately. Do not stop until the victim is either breathing well or help arrives. Use oxygen if available. Send someone else to call for help.
   C. If a caustic poison has been swallowed, you should dilute it by giving 1 or 2 glassfuls of milk or water.

II. CALL FOR INFORMATION ABOUT WHAT TO DO NEXT:
   A. Call your doctor, or call the poison control center.
      1. Identify yourself and your relationship to the victim.
      2. Describe the victim by name, age and sex.
      3. Have the package or poison in your hand and identify exactly (as best as you can) what the victim took and how much he took.
   B. Call for information even if you are not sure. Keep calm. You have enough time to act, but don't delay unnecessarily.

III. IF YOU ARE INSTRUCTED TO INDUCE VOMITING
   Never induce vomiting until you are instructed to do so.
   A. Have syrup of ipecac available to induce vomiting. Purchase one ounce of ipecac syrup from your pharmacist. You may do this without a prescription. It will keep stored at room temperature for several years.
   B. To use ipecac:
      In an adult give 2 tablespoons (30 ml), in a child over one year give one tablespoon (15 ml), and in a child less than one year (10 ml), of ipecac syrup followed by a glass (8 oz) of liquid (water, juices, etc.). Then give additional liquid as tolerated. If patient hasn't vomited within 15 to 20 minutes, repeat the dose of ipecac and give more water.
   C. Don't waste time trying other ways to make the victim vomit.
      Tickling the back of the throat with your fingers, a spoon, or some other object is not very effective. Do not use salt water. It is potentially dangerous.
   D. Never induce vomiting if the patient:
      Is unconscious.
      Is having convulsions (fits).
      Has swallowed strong caustics or corrosives.
      And induce vomiting only if instructed, if the patient:
      Has swallowed petroleum products, cleaning fluids, gasoline, lighter fluid, etc.

IV. IF YOU GO TO THE HOSPITAL:
   A. Take or send the poison container, poisonous plant, etc., with you.
   B. Take any vomitus you collect.
   C. Don't give substances like coffee, alcohol, stimulants, or drugs to the victim.

*From Temple AR: Poison control. *In* Osol A, Chase GD, Gennaro AR, et al. (eds.): Remmington Pharmaceutical Services. Easton, PA, Mack Publishing Company, 1980. Reproduced with permission.

ministered as necessary. First aid steps consist of (1) immediate flushing of the eye with water, (2) removal of contact lenses, if any, and then (3) further irrigation for at least 10 to 15 minutes. Irrigation of the eye(s) can be done with tap water, lactated Ringer's solution, or normal saline. In the emergency room, it may be necessary to anesthetize the eye(s) to facilitate treatment. Examination should consist of a thorough examination of all surfaces, measurement of conjunctival pH following an alkali exposure, and even slit lamp examination when potentially serious damage may have occurred.

Topical (Dermal) Exposure

For dermal exposures the affected area should be immediately flushed with water and then washed thoroughly. Soap should be used in cases of exposure to oily substances or ones that are potentially systemic toxins. Contaminated clothing should be removed and discarded if adequate cleaning is not subsequently possible. This is particularly important with pesticide exposures. Protective clothing should be worn by medical personnel involved in decontaminating the patient in cases in which contamination of treating personnel is possible, as in cases involving a pesticide. For caustic or corrosive exposures the current recommendation is not to use a neutralizing substance.

Inhalation Exposure

For respiratory exposure, removal of the victim from the toxic environment is the primary first aid step, which in most cases means moving the victim from the area of exposure into an area of fresh air. Caution should be exercised in entering a potentially contaminated environment. Protective gear may need to be worn and closed spaces adequately ventilated before entering. Clothing should be loosened and artificial respiration administered if needed. Following initial resuscitative measures, the patient should be observed for latent pulmonary symptoms, particularly following pulmonary to exposure irritant gases.

Ingestion Exposure

For ingestions, management should focus on gastrointestinal decontamination through dilution, evacuation, local detoxification, or catharsis.

Dilution. Dilution is indicated only when the toxin produces local irritancy or corrosivity. Water is the preferred diluent in most circumstances. On the other hand, for drug ingestions dilution *alone* should not be used, since it may enhance absorption by increasing dissolution rates of the tablets or capsules or promote more rapid transit into the lower gastrointestinal tract. However, administration of fluids during the induction of emesis is appropriate. Milk may add a demulcent effect and may be used to ameliorate the local irritancy of corrosive or irritating substances.

Gastric Evacuation. Gastric evacuation is most effective if done within 2 to 4 hours, but in selected circumstances may be of value up to 24 hours following ingestion. Emesis is effective in the removal of a substantial portion of ingested poisons in children and is indicated except when the patient has ingested caustics, or when the patient is comatose, experiencing seizures, or has lost the gag reflex. The drug of choice for inducing emesis under most circumstances is ipecac syrup (not fluid extract). Syrup of ipecac is safe and effective when administered properly. The dose is 30 ml for adolescents (and adults), 15 ml for children, and 10 ml for infants under 1 year of age. This should be accompanied by 100 to 200 ml (4 to 8 ounces) of fluid (water, juice) by mouth. The ipecac and fluids should be repeated if emesis does not occur in 20 to 30 minutes. Toxicity has resulted from the misuse of fluid extract of ipecac, manifest primarily as cardiovascular effects, including EKG abnormalities, and severe gastrointestinal discomfort, but toxicity has not been shown to occur with appropriate use of ipecac syrup.*

Apomorphine is an alternative drug to ipecac for inducing emesis but is used only when ipecac fails to induce emesis and lavage is contraindicated. It induces emesis somewhat more rapidly than does syrup of ipecac, but produces CNS depression and is more likely to cause protracted vomiting. Apomorphine is administered subcutaneously in a dose of 0.07 to 0.1 mg/kg. Some of the side effects of apomorphine may be terminated by the administration of naloxone hydrochloride (Narcan).

Gastric Lavage. This is also a useful method of recovering stomach contents. In children it may be less effective than emesis owing to the fact that tablets or fragments may be too large to pass through the small tubes generally used in children. However, in adolescents, when an adequate size tube may be used, it may be as effective or more effective than emesis. Gastric lavage is particularly indicated to remove stomach contents in the following situations: CNS depression or altered consciousness, failure to induce emesis with syrup of ipecac or apomorphine, and situations in which syrup of ipecac or apomorphine cannot be used. Contraindications to gastric lavage include ingestion of caustic materials, ingestion of petroleum distillates, and total or subtotal gastrectomy.

Lavage should be done using the largest tube that can reasonably be passed (usually 22 Fr in child, 36 to 50 Fr in adult). The tube should be passed and, after checking for the presence in the stomach by instilling 25 to 50 ml of air, secured at the nose. The gastric contents should be aspirated *before* introducing lavage fluid into the stomach. The aspirate should be saved for later toxicologic analysis if necessary. One particularly simple technique is to initiate a continuous flow pattern of lavage fluid with intermittent suction. To do this requires a double-lumen tube

*Because fluid extract and syrup of ipecac can be easily confused, we recommend that emergency departments stock only the syrup.

with the inflow connected to a hanging bottle of fluid and the stomach allowed to fill by gravity. The outflow is connected to intermittent suction. For adolescents, a total volume of at least 2 to 4 liters, at a rate of 1 to 2 L every 5 minutes, can be used. For children, a total volume of at least 2 L, at a rate up to 1 L every 5 minutes should be used. Lavage may be performed using either tap water or saline.

Local Detoxification. Activated charcoal is the most commonly used local adsorbent. It minimizes absorption by adsorbing drugs on its surfaces. Its use should be considered in all cases of poisoning, although a number of compounds are not well absorbed (iron, cyanide) and its use may interfere with other critical therapy (orally administered antidotes). Activated charcoal is most effective if given during the first several hours after ingestion. The usually recommended dose is 10 g of activated charcoal for each gram of drug or chemical ingested. When the amount of toxic substance ingested is unknown, a minimum of 20 g should be given to adolescents. The activated charcoal should be mixed with a sufficient amount of water to make a slurry, which can then be taken orally or administered by nasogastric tube. Added flavoring or suspending the charcoal in sorbital does not substantially interfere with its adsorptive capacity. However, charcoal should not be given with milk or ice cream.

When used in conjunction with ipecac syrup, activated charcoal should not be used until after vomiting has occurred, since it will otherwise inactivate the ipecac. It should be noted that the once-advocated "universal antidote," comprised of activated charcoal, magnesium oxide, and tannic acid, is not recommended. Similarly, burnt toast is not effective. Repeated dosing with charcoal may be beneficial for reducing absorption of drugs undergoing enterohepatic recirculation or active excretion into gastric fluids but should only be given in the presence of active bowel sounds. Enhanced clearance of several drugs with repeated charcoal dosing has recently been demonstrated even in the absence of active excretion or recirculation.

Catharsis. After emesis or lavage, catharsis may be used to hasten the elimination of remaining ingested material. Saline cathartics are preferred. Oil or stimulant cathartics are not recommended, since they may increase absorption of some poisons or cause prolonged catharsis. Saline cathartics may be given after administering activated charcoal and after gastric lavage or emesis. The usual doses for saline cathartics are sodium sulfate, 250 mg/kg, as a 20 to 50 per cent solution; magnesium sulfate, 250 mg/kg, as a 20 to 50 per cent solution, and magnesium citrate, 4 ml/kg. The cathartic dose should be repeated at regular intervals (every 1 to 2 hours) as long as bowel sounds are present. Passage of any administered charcoal can be used as a marker of successful clearing of the intestinal tract.

Antidotal Therapy

The overall number of ingestions for which a specific antidote is necessary or available is small. When a specific antidote can be used, it is vital that it be administered as early as possible and in appropriately monitored doses, which could be done by paramedic units under appropriate medical control. Those antidotes that should be available for immediate administration are listed in Table 28–9. Other antidotes usually do not require urgent administration and may be given subsequent to initiation of other management modalities. Antidotes can be put into two categories: local antidotes and systemic antidotes. Local antidotes act (usually in the stomach) against poison that is not yet absorbed. The mechanism is by inactivation, dimution of solubility, or blocking of absorption. Systemic antidotes are given to counteract the effects of poisons that have already been absorbed. Table 28–10 presents a list of

Table 28–9. EMERGENCY ANTIDOTES THAT MAY NEED TO BE GIVEN IN PRE-HOSPITAL PHASE OF CARE*

Antidote	Indications
Naloxone	Opiates Heroin Morphine Methadone and similar substances
Oxygen	Carbon monoxide
Amyl nitrite Sodium nitrite Sodium thiosulfate	Cyanide
Atropine	Anticholinesterases Organophosphates Carbamates
Methylene blue	Methemoglobinemic agents Nitrites Chlorates Nitrobenzene

*In spite of the extreme urgency in administering these antidotes, they should be given only under appropriate medical control.

Table 28–10. LOCAL AND SYSTEMIC ANTIDOTES*

Poison	Local Antidote	System Antidote
Acetaminophen	Activated charcoal (not to be used if *N*-acetylcysteine is to be given)	*N*-acetylcysteine (Mucomyst): initial dose, 140 mg/kg orally in cola, fruit soda, fruit juice or water, followed by 70 mg/kg every 4 hours for 68 hours (17 doses)
Acids, corrosive	Dilute with water or milk	
Alkali, caustic	Dilute with water or milk, followed by demulcent	
Alkaloids (coniine, quinine, strychnine, ect.)	Activated charcoal	
Amphetamines	Activated charcoal	Chlorpromazine (Thorazine), 1 mg/kg intramuscularly or intravenouysly (administer slowly if given intravenously); may be repeated in 15 minutes; reduce to 0.5 mg/kg if other central nervous system depressants involved
Anticholinergics	Activated charcoal	Physostigmine (Antilirium): adults, 2.0 mg, children, 0.5 mg given slowly intravenously: may be repeated in 15 minutes until desired effect is achieved; subsequent doses may be given every 2 to 3 hours as needed; use only for specific indications associated with severe toxicity
Anticholinesterases Organophosphates Neostigmine (Prostigmin) Physostigmine Pyridostigmine (Mestinon)	Activated charcoal	Atropine, 1 to 2 mg (for children under age two, 1.0 mg or 0.05 to 0.1 mg/kg) intravenously repeated every 10 to 15 minutes until atropinization is evident, followed by pralidoxime chloride (Protopam), 25 to 50 mg/kg (1 g in adults) intravenously; repeat in eight to 12 hours as needed
Carbamates		Atropine as above, but do not use pralidoxime
Antihistamines	*(See Anticholinergics)*	
Arsenic	*(See Heavy metals)*	
Atropine	*(See Anticholinergics)*	
Barium salts	Sodium sulfate, 300 mg/kg	Sodium or magnesium sulfate, 10 ml of 10% solution intravenously every 15 minutes until symptoms stop
Belladonna alkaloids	*(See Anticholinergics)*	
Bromides		Sodium or ammonium chloride, 6 to 12 g per day orally or the equivalent as normal saline every 6 hours intravenously
Cadmium	*(See Heavy metals)*	
Carbon monoxide		100% oxygen by inhalation for at least 4 hours (hyperbaric oxygen is a recommended alternative in comatose patients)
Cholinergic compounds	*(See Anticholinesterases)*	
Copper	*(See Heavy metals)*	
Cyanide		Adults: amyl nitrite inhalation (15 to 30 seconds every 60 seconds) pending administration of 300 mg sodium nitrite (10 ml of 3% solution) slowly intravenously (over 2 to 4 minutes): follow immediately with 12.5 g sodium thiosulfate (2.5 to 5.0 ml per minute of 25% solution) slowly intravenously (over 10 minutes)
Cyanide		Children: Dose should be adjusted based on hemoglobin level (sodium nitrite should not exceed recommended dose because fatal methemoglobinemia may result)

Hemoglobin	Initial Dose 3% Sodium Nitrite Intravenously	Initial Dose 25% Sodium Thiosulfate Intravenously
8 g	0.22 ml (6.6mg)/kg	1.10 ml/kg
10 g	0.27 ml (8.7 mg)/kg	1.35 ml/kg
12 g	0.33 ml (10.0 mg)/kg	1.65 ml/kg
14 g	0.39 ml (11.6 mg)g	1.95 ml/kg

Poison	Local Antidote	System Antidote
Ethylene glycol	*(See Methanol)*	
Fluoride	Calcium gluconate or lactate, 150 mg/kg, or milk	Calcium gluconate, 10 ml of 10% solution slowly intravenously until symptoms abate; may be repeated as needed

Table 28–10. LOCAL AND SYSTEMIC ANTIDOTES* *(Continued)*

Poison	Local Antidote	System Antidote
Gold	*(See Heavy metals)*	
Heavy metals		BAL (dimercaprol): 3 to 5 mg/kg dose deep intramuscularly every 4 hours for 2 days, every 4 to 6 hours for an additional 2 days, then every 4 to 12 hours for up to 7 additional days
		EDTA: 75 mg/kg per 24 hours deep intramuscularly or slow intravenous infusion in 3 to 6 divided doses for up to 5 days; may be repeated for a second course after a minimum of two days; each course should not exceed a total of 500 mg/kg body weight
Arsenic	Usual chelators used: BAL	
Cadmium	Satisfactory use not demonstrated	
Copper	BAL, penicillamine	Penicillamine: 100 mg/kg per day (maximum, 1 g) orally in divided doses for up to 5 days; for long-term therapy, do not exceed 40 mg/kg per day
Gold	BAL	
Lead	BAL, EDTA, penicillamine	
Mercury	BAL, penicillamine	
Silver	Satisfactory use not demonstrated	
Thallium	Prussian blue	
Hypochlorites	*(See Alkali, caustic)*	
Iron	Sodium bicarbonate, 1 to 5% solution, preferably by lavage	Deferoxamine (Desteral), 20 to 40 mg/kg intravenously as slow drip over four hours (not to exceed 15 mg/kg per hour); followed by 20 mg/kg every four to eight hours until urine color normal or iron level normal (may give 20 mg/kg intramuscularly every 4 to 12 hours if no intravenous sites available)
Isoniazid	Activated charcoal	Pyridoxine (vitamin B_6), 1 g per g of INH ingested 5 to 10% concentration in 5% dextrose in water) intravenously over 30 to 60 minutes
Lead	*(See Heavy metals)*	
Mercury	*(See Heavy metals)*	
Methanol		Ethanol: loading dose to achieve blood level of 100 mg/dl, 0.6 g/kg body weight. Maintenance doses should be 100 mg/kg per hour started at time of loading dose and adjusted according to measured blood ethanol levels
Methemoglobinemic agents Nitrites Chlorates Nitrobenzene		Methylene blue, 1 to 2 mg (0.1 to 0.2 ml/kg) of 1% solution slowly intravenously over five to 10 minutes if cyanosis is severe (or methemoglobin level is greater than 40%)
Narcotics	Activated charcoal	Naloxone (Narcan), 0.01 mg/kg (adult: 0.4 mg) intravenously; if no response, 0.1 mg/kg (adult: 4.0 mg) intravenously; alternative approach: 0.03 mg/kg intravenously up to three or four doses
Nitrites	*(See Methemoglobinemic agents)*	
Oxalate	Dilute with water or milk, followed by calcium gluconate or lactate, 150 mg/kg	Calcium gluconate, 10 ml of 10% solution slowly intravenously until symptoms abate; may be repeated as needed
Phenothiazines (neuromuscular reaction only)		Diphenhydramine (Benadryl), 0.5 to 1.0 mg/kg intramuscularly or intravenously, or benztropine (Cogentin), 2 mg intramuscularly or intravenously
Phosgene		Methenamine, 20 ml of 20% solution (4 g) intravenously; probably ineffective after full development of pulmonary edema
Physostigmine	*(See Anticholinesterases)*	
Quaternary ammonium compounds	Ordinary soap solution	
Silver	Normal saline (lavage)	
	(See Heavy metals)	
Thallium	Prussian blue (250 mg/kg per 24 hours via nasojejunal tube in two to four divided doses)	
	(See Heavy metals)	

Table continued on following page

Table 28–10. LOCAL AND SYSTEMIC ANTIDOTES* *(Continued)*

Poison	Local Antidote	System Antidote
Tricyclic antidepressants	*(See Anticholinergics)*	
Warfarin		Vitamin K_1, 0.5 to 1.0 mg/kg intramuscularly or intravenously Adults: 10 mg intramuscularly or intravenously Children: 1 to 5 mg intramuscularly or intravenously
For Envenomation†		
Animals		*Antivenin‡*
Snake, Crotalidae (all North American rattlesnakes and moccasins)		Antivenin (Crotalidae), polyvalent
Snake, coral		Antivenin *(Micrurus fulvius)*, monovalent
Spider, black widow		Antivenin *(Latrodectus mactans)*

*From Temple AR: Poisoning I. Monograph 52. Kansas City, American Academy of Family Physicians, 1983. Reproduced by permission.
†All antisera should be tested for sensitivity to horse serum.
‡See package insert for dosage and administration.

most currently available antidotes, their indicated use, and appropriate doses. Even when available, antidotes do not diminish the need for good supportive care and indiscriminant use of antidotes without other forms of management is certainly appropriate.

Hastening the Elimination of Absorbed Poison

The procedures with the greatest value for enhancing the elimination of an absorbed poison in the management of the pediatric patient are diuresis, dialysis, and hemoperfusion. Because some risk is involved, these procedures should be considered only in those cases in which the patient's recovery would be unlikely without it or in which a specific significant benefit is expected.

Diuresis

Diuresis may be useful in cases of poisoning with agents that are excreted primarily by the renal route. Fluid diuresis may increase glomerular filtration, and, if accompanied by proportionally less tubular reabsorption of the toxic agent, may result in enhanced excretion. However, administering large fluid loads alone is of limited value. The addition of an osmotic diuretic, such as mannitol, will prevent reabsorption of an ingested drug in the proximal tubule, Henle's loop, and the distal tubule, using the principle of an osmotic load, and is a preferable approach. Diuresis has been shown to be particularly effective with long-acting barbiturates and salicylates and is often combined with alkalinization.

Ionized diuresis takes advantage of the principle that excretion is favored when a drug is in its ionized state in the glomerular filtrate. Alkaline or acid diuresis involves adjustment of urine pH so that the drug will be in its ionized form and thus remain within the tubular lumen and not be reabsorbed. For drugs that are weak acids, alkalinization of the urine accomplishes this if the pH reaches 8.0 or so (Fig. 28–1). In fact, recent studies suggest that alkalinization alone may be as effective as the combination of alkalinization plus diuresis in the management of

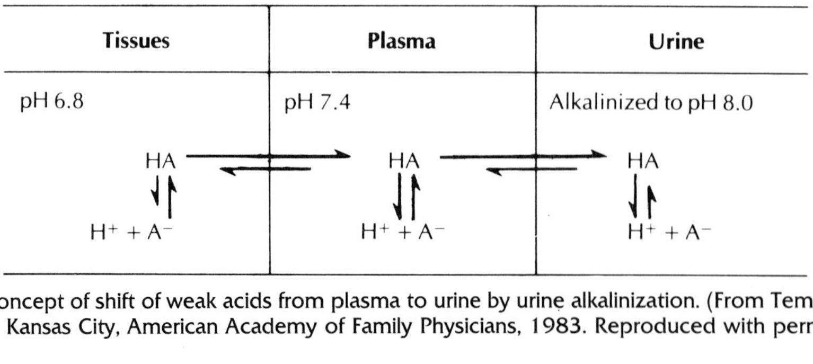

Tissues	Plasma	Urine
pH 6.8	pH 7.4	Alkalinized to pH 8.0
HA ⇄ $H^+ + A^-$	HA ⇄ $H^+ + A^-$	HA $H^+ + A^-$

Figure 28–1. Concept of shift of weak acids from plasma to urine by urine alkalinization. (From Temple AR: Poisoning I. Monograph 52. Kansas City, American Academy of Family Physicians, 1983. Reproduced with permission.)

salicylate overdose. Acid diuresis similarly may enhance the excretion of weak bases.

Criteria for initiating diuretic therapy include (1) a satisfactory systolic blood pressure, (2) clinical evidence of adequate renal function, (3) no evidence of cardiac failure, (4) no evidence of respiratory insufficiency, (5) coma of expected extended duration, or (6) drug blood level in the serious or potentially fatal range. It is obvious that the drug should be well excreted via the renal route.

The principal osmotic diuretic that has been used in treating poisoning is mannitol. A urinary catheter should always be placed when this drug is utilized. Mannitol is given as a 25 per cent solution in a loading dose of 0.5 g/kg. A satisfactory flow, once established, can be maintained using a 10 per cent mannitol solution. Urine output, fluid input, Na, K, Cl, CO_2, BUN, Ca, P, serum osmolality, urine osmolality, and central venous pressure should be monitored during diuresis. Ideally, the initial diuretic load should produce a urine output of approximately 5 ml/kg/hour. Additional doses of diuretics should be adjusted to produce a urine output of 6 to 9 ml/kg/hour. Diuresis may be discontinued when the patient regains consciousness, when serious toxic manifestations abate, or when drug blood levels are below toxic levels.

Urine alkalinization is usually accomplished by using sodium bicarbonate at a dose of 1 to 2 mEq/kg intravenously over a 1- 2-hour period. Urine pH is monitored regularly, and the infusion is continued at the same rate or modified to maintain a urine pH of 8.0 or greater. Acidification of the urine is usually initiated with ammonium chloride at a dose of 75 mg (2.75 mEq/kg/dose) orally every 6 hours via a nasogastric tube until the urine pH is equal to or less than 5.0. The urine should be maintained at this pH. As an adjunct to this therapy, ascorbic acid in a dosage range of 0.5 to 2.0 g in 500 ml of fluid can be administered intravenously at a normal infusion rate every 6 hours.

Dialysis

Dialysis is indicated for selected cases of severe poisoning or when renal failure is present. Indications for dialysis are based both on patient-related and drug-related criteria. Patient-related criteria include (1) anticipated prolonged coma with the high likelihood of attendant complications, (2) development of renal failure or impairment of normal excretory pathways, and (3) progressive clinical deterioration in spite of careful medical supervision. Drug-related criteria include (1) satisfactory membrane permeability, (2) a correlation between plasma drug concentration and drug toxicity of the agent, (3) plasma levels in the potentially fatal range or the presence of a significant quantity of an agent that is normally metabolized to a toxic substance, and (4) an expectation of significant enhancement of clearance during dialysis. Hemodialysis is the most effective means of dialysis. Because it requires highly technical skills and both a physician and a technician it is not always readily available. Peritoneal dialysis is considerably less efficient than hemodialysis and is usually not a satisfactory alternative.

Hemoperfusion

Hemoperfusion is the process of passing blood through an extracorporeal circuit over (or through) an adsorbent, such as activated charcoal or resins, to remove toxins from the blood. A number of hemoperfusion devices are now commercially available. Hemoperfusion appears to be as effective or more effective than hemodialysis for a wide range of drugs. The indications for its use include those listed for hemodialysis.

General Supportive Care

Basic Life Support

In all cases of poisoning, basic life support is essential. Basic life support for a poisoning case should be consistent with other medical emergencies and consists of recognizing respiratory and cardiac arrest and initiating the proper steps of cardiopulmonary resuscitation, including establishing an airway, restoring breathing through artificial ventilation, and attempting to restore circulation by performing external cardiac compression. Other common complications of poisonings include respiratory failure, hypotension, seizures, cerebral edema, acidosis, cardiac arrhythmias, drug abuse reactions, and drug withdrawal manifestations. General supportive measures should be instituted for each of these conditions as appropriate.

CARDIAC ARRHYTHMIAS

Many toxic substances, especially in large amounts, can produce cardiac arrhythmias. For all substances with which cardiac arrhythmias are known to occur, a cardiac monitor should be positioned on the patient. An attempt should be made to determine if the patient has a pre-existing heart condition. If the initial recording appears abnormal, a complete 12-lead EKG should be done to more fully evaluate cardiac status. Appropriate supportive and therapeutic measures should be identified for any patient with cardiac abnormalities. When appropriate, measures should be instituted to normalize the electrical pattern and output of the heart by the judicious use of drugs or other modes of therapy.

RESPIRATORY FAILURE

Certain poisoned patients may need respiratory support even though spontaneous respirations seem to be effective at the time of the initial physical examination. To establish an effective airway, the mouth and upper respiratory passages should be examined and cleared of any debris. If the patient is unresponsive to minimal tactile stimuli, a cuffed endotracheal (either nasotracheal or orotracheal) tube should be inserted and the bronchial passages gently suctioned. Appropriate inhalatory support should be instituted, including administration of humidified air, oxygen for cyanosis, and continued bronchial toilet. For patients who are deeply comatose or have evidence of hypoventilation, respiratory support using a volume respirator should be instituted. With a respirator in place, tidal volume can be measured and should be kept in the range of 10 to 15 ml/kg. Arterial blood gas determinations need to be made frequently to assess the need for altering respiratory support procedures. If a cyanotic patient with good cardiac function does not respond to the administration of oxygen, other causes for the cyanosis must be evaluated, such as various toxic agents that may alter the oxygen-carrying capacity of the blood, ventilation/perfusion mismatch, or other identificable causes. There are no indications for the use of analeptics or central nervous system stimulants. There is no evidence that analeptics are beneficial; on the contrary, they may produce adverse side effects, including convulsions, cardiac arrhythmias, hyperpyrexia, and vomiting.

HYPOTENSION

In poisoned patients, hypotension and decreased cardiac output often occur. An initial blood pressure should be obtained, and in deeply comatose patients, a central venous pressure line should be inserted, even if the patient is normotensive. Systolic blood pressure should be maintained at greater than 80 mm Hg ($80 + 2 \times$ age in years). For patients with mild hypotension, correction of respiratory status and acidosis is usually therapeutic. Nonetheless, in any hypotensive patient, the first step is elevation of the victim's feet. If no benefit follows this and respiratory support, expansion of the intravascular volume with appropriate fluids should be attempted. In almost all cases, this will be sufficient. In the rare cases when this fails to restore an adequate blood pressure, dopamine therapy may be required (see p. 8).

SEIZURES

In central nervous system stimulant poisonings, the principal problems are acute termination of seizures and prophylaxis against subsequent seizures. For terminating acute toxic seizures, diazepam or phenytoin is usually effective and relatively safe. Short-acting barbiturates are also effective. The drugs of choice for seizure prophylaxis are phenobarbital and phenytoin. The former can also be used to acutely terminate seizures; however, these drugs have a longer duration of action, which must be taken into account.

CEREBRAL EDEMA

Cerebral edema may occur in certain types of poisonings or may follow hypoxia or fluid overload. Cerebral edema can usually be managed with hyperventilation or an intravenous infusion of mannitol.

ACIDOSIS

Unless it is very severe, acidosis can be corrected by the administration of hypotonic, polyionic parenteral solutions. Severe acidosis requires the administration of sodium bicarbonate in doses of 1 to 2 mEq/kg. Correction of acidosis is very important in a number of poisoning situations, like salicylate toxicity or tricyclic antidepressant overdose.

Psychedelic Drug Reactions

In psychedelic drug poisoning, the approach is one of cautious interaction, with the avoidance of unnecessary procedures. The effects of most psychedelics are qualitatively similar. Almost all of the symptoms experienced with mild intoxications of psychedelics are of no serious medical consequences and require only reassurance of the patient. Nonetheless, careful monitoring of heart rate and blood pressure and medical evaluation of other subjective symptomatology is necessary. Close friends or acquaintances can help calm and reassure the victim during the period of intoxication. They should be supportive, positive, and concerned. Trained staff can assist in "talking down" the patient from the undesirable reaction. External sensory input (lights, sounds, movement) should be minimized. Severe agitation that may result in harm or damage can be treated with diazepam. Chlorpromazine or haloperidol can also be used.

Acute Drug Withdrawal States

Drug abuse continues to be a problem among adolescents. Drugs that produce physical dependence (opiates, barbiturates, ethanol, nonbarbiturate sedatives, minor tranquilizers) can generally be tapered gradually without too much difficulty. Drugs that produce psychological dependence (amphetamines and related stimulants, cocaine, marijuana) can produce a more difficult withdrawal picture. Dependence can recur months after discontinuance of the drug. For specific drug withdrawal regimens, the physician should contact a drug abuse treatment facility, toxicology service, or poison control center.

Temperature Alteration

For temperatures less than 97° F (36° C), simple procedures to prevent heat loss from the body and maintain appropriate environmental temperatures should be instituted. Active rewarming is required for marked hypothermia at or below 86° F (30° C). Temperatures greater than 105° F (40° C) may be controlled by using ice blankets.

Fluid Therapy

Intravenous fluids should be administered throughout the duration of any coma. If there is evidence of dehydration, appropriate replacement fluids should be administered. Maintenance fluids, using dilute electrolyte solutions, should be given at usual rates; however, additional fluids may be required for patients on respirators. Bladder catheterization should be instituted in severe intoxications when accurate fluid balance monitoring is required.

APPROPRIATE AND TIMELY REFERRAL OF SEVERELY POISONED PATIENTS

General Guidelines

Consultation should be obtained on any patient when the attending physician feels that additional clinical expertise is necessary, and in particular, when dangerous antidotal therapy or special analytical monitoring is needed, or in patients who meet the criteria for comprehensive level care. At the time of consultation, transfer versus on-site management should be considered and disposition determined jointly by the attending physician and toxicology consultant, taking into consideration the benefits of transfer of the patient over transfer of appropriate therapeutic modalities to the patient's bedside. Instituting the special procedures below should be carefully considered, and the determination to transfer a patient should always be based on physician-to-physician consultation.

Transfer Process

All procedures necessary for immediate care, including decontamination of the patient, should be completed prior to any attempt at transport. General symptomatic and supportive measures needed to stabilize the patient should also be completed. When the patient is transferred, send along a sample of the poison involved, in the original container if it is available, and samples for toxicologic analysis that are available (blood, urine, and/or vomitus). If this is a transfer to another medical care facility, one also should include facility record, physician or treating personnel notes, laboratory results, and x-rays. General symptomatic and supportive care must be provided during transport by an appropriate medical team.

EVALUATION AND REFERRAL OF THE SUICIDAL PATIENT

General Information

All cases involving adolescent overdoses must be evaluated relative to the psychiatric state of the patient and the potential suicidal intent of the incident. Even more specifically the attending physician must make an initial determination of the meaning of the suicide attempt to determine whether death was the ultimate objective or whether it was more accurately a gesture. Pertinent information relative to this determination should be gathered during the process of treating the toxic state.

Medical Clearance for Psychiatric Evaluation

All necessary initial management measures must be instituted prior to psychiatric evaluation. A complete psychiatric evaluation of the patient cannot be made until the patient is alert enough to participate in the interview. Thus, the patient cannot be drowsy or stuporous or have sufficiently disquieting feelings that he or she cannot concentrate on the content of the interview or conversation. Transfer to a psychiatric care unit from a medical care unit should not be made until the patient no longer needs respiratory support or evaluation, cardiac monitoring, intravenous fluids or alimentation, or constant nursing supervision. In addition, all need for antidotal therapy or monitoring of outcome should be terminated.

Psychiatric Evaluation or Referral

It is important that each case of intentional poisoning, whether a gesture or a genuine attempt at death, be psychiatrically evaluated. Patients should be evaluated for degree of depressive symptoms and factors making the likelihood of an additional suicide attempt greater. When a psychiatrist or crisis team is not available, the attending physician should make use of standard criteria to make an assessment. When a crisis team is available, cases should be seen before discharge from the emergency room or in-patient unit. When a crisis team is not available, cases in which further suicidal risk is estimated to be high should be admitted or detained until psychiatric consultation is obtained. When further suicidal risk is low, in the sense that the attending physician is assured that another suicide attempt is not imminent, the patient may be scheduled for subsequent psychiatric evaluation and discharged to the care and supervision of concerned and supportive family or friends.

CHAPTER

29 Near Drowning

JOEL THOMPSON

The term drowning refers to a fatal episode of submersion, whereas the term near drowning refers to submersion followed by survival for at least 24 hours.[1]

Approximately 8000 drownings occur each year in the United States, and 40 per cent of these occur in children under 4 years of age.[2] It is estimated that several times this number of children are victims of near drowning each year.[3]

Significant morbidity and mortality result from near drowning, which usually occurs in private swimming pools, lakes, rivers, canals, irrigation ditches, and bathtubs. Toddlers are particularly vulnerable to toppling into pools or ditches, while teenagers and adults are victims of overestimation of swimming skills often secondary to consumption of alcoholic beverages.

Clearly, with a problem of this magnitude, vigorous preventive measures are needed to avert episodes of submersion. Should they occur, however, a program of vigorous resuscitation and supportive therapy is vital to reducing morbidity and mortality. The following is a discussion of the pathophysiology and treatment of near drowning.

PATHOPHYSIOLOGY

Near drowning is a process involving several different organ systems. Although the damage done to the pulmonary system may result primarily from direct contact with water and debris, the damage done to other organ systems is usually the result of hypoxia and ischemia.

Pulmonary System

Most near drowning victims aspirate small quantities of water and debris, although approximately 10 to 20 per cent of the victims have no aspiration, perhaps secondary to laryngospasm early in the course of drowning.[2,4]

Freshwater drowning may result in significant surfactant washout, resulting in decreased surface tension, and progressive alveolar collapse, resulting in atelectasis.[5] Intrapulmonary shunting with ventilation-perfusion mismatching commonly occurs in this setting. Pulmonary edema may also occur secondary to circulatory overload and also from hemolysis, resulting in the breakdown of erythrocytes and platelets, which may damage pulmonary capillaries.[6]

Victims of saltwater submersion may sustain direct injury to the alveolar-capillary membrane from the hypertonic saline. A hypertonic solution also osmotically draws fluid out of the circulation and into the alveoli, further inhibiting gas exchange.[7]

In freshwater or saltwater submersion, the primary pulmonary disturbances often include (1) reduction in pulmonary compliance, (2) increase in dead space to tidal volume ratio, (3) intrapulmonary shunting with ventilation perfusion mismatching, and (4) an increase in the difference in oxygen tension between the alveoli and arterial blood.[8]

Occasionally, infection further complicates the underlying pulmonary disturbance sustained in a submersion accident. It is uncommon, however, for permanent pulmonary dysfunction to occur.[9]

Central Nervous System

Most of the morbidity or mortality associated with submersion accidents results from damage to the central nervous system (CNS). The basic injury is one of hypoxic ischemic encephalopathy, and it varies in severity depending on (1) pre-existing health in the patient, (2) age of the patient, (3) water temperature, and (4) duration of the submersion.

Hypoxic Ischemic Encephalopathy

Near drowning is just one of many causes of hypoxic ischemic encephalopathy. The basic pathology is largely the same regardless of the underlying cause, however.

The brain is dependent on a constant supply of high-energy compounds to supply the energy needed for maintenance of membrane potentials and the multitude of synthetic and catabolic processes that occur. Normally, when a sufficient quantity of oxygen is present, one molecule of glucose, which is the main energy-producing compound in the CNS, can be metabolized to carbon dioxide and water, producing 32 molecules of adenosine triphosphate (ATP). If an insufficient quantity of oxygen is present, the pyruvate produced from glycolysis cannot enter the Krebs cycle and ultimately the electron transport system. Instead, the pyruvate is converted to lactate, and the ultimate energy yield is only 2 molecules of ATP. Accumulation of lactic acid causes dilation of cerebral blood vessels and improves oxygen and glucose delivery temporarily, but ultimately this method of compensation is inadequate unless sufficient oxygen is introduced.

Ischemia further aggravates the problems caused by hypoxia. It not only further decreases the oxygen delivery to tissues but also decreases the delivery of other vital substrates such as glucose. The stasis resulting from ischemia results in accumulation of lactic acid and other toxic products, which eventually have an adverse effect on local enzymatic reactions. Studies in experimental animals suggest that if perfusion is maintained, animals may tolerate rather long periods of substantial hypoxia.[27]

If hypoxia or ischemia of sufficient duration occurs, then neuronal death or residual neuronal dysfunction may occur. Cytotoxic cerebral edema may result in increased intracranial pressure (ICP), which may further injure the nervous system, particularly if the ICP begins to exceed the mean peripheral blood pressure, resulting in a drop in cerebral perfusion pressure (mean arterial blood pressure–ICP) to critical levels below 40 torr.

Hypoxia and ischemia may also result in damage to autoregulation of cerebral circulation. Normally this system controls cerebral blood flow through a wide range of cerebral perfusion pressures. If the system of autoregulation malfunctions, however, certain areas of the brain may be overperfused, resulting in edema, and others underperfused, resulting in ischemia, despite normal perfusion pressures.

If circulatory arrest is of sufficient duration, then certain areas of the brain may not be reperfused secondary to capillary occlusions, a situation known as the no reflow phenomenon.

Posner and associates have described the delayed onset of neurologic deficit secondary to hypoxic insults.[10] Some individuals who sustain hypoxic injury from a variety of causes may have a hiatus of reasonably normal neurologic function varying from hours to a few weeks after which they develop substantial neurologic deterioration and may expire. These individuals appear to have secondary demyelination of cortical white matter, presumably the result of an initial hypoxic insult.

Factors Determining Survivable Time Of Submersion

Many factors influence the amount of elapsed time necessary to produce severe irreversible cerebral injury. Generally some degree of cerebral injury begins within 20 seconds of the onset of complete anoxia, and after 5 minutes of complete anoxia, a substantial amount of damage has usually occurred. Several factors do, however, determine the amount of damage sustained over a certain elapsed period of time.

State of Health. The pre-existing state of health may clearly influence the amount of time an individual can be submerged without substantial central nervous system injury. Complicating factors such as myocardial infarction or other chronic health problems may shorten the tolerated time of submersion. Children, for a variety of reasons, will generally tolerate a longer period of submersion than adults.[11]

Primitive Reflexes. Certain primitive reflexes such as the diving reflex or drowning reflex may help to protect the submerged individual.[12,13] The diving reflex occurs more commonly in infants and may be potentiated by fear of the water or low water temperature. The reflex is triggered by submersion of the face in cold water and results in shunting of blood flow, predominantly to the heart and brain, accompanied by profound bradycardia. The heart may continue to beat after 5 to 10 minutes of submersion, thus providing for some delivery of oxygen and necessary substrates to tissues. This reflex may clearly prolong the amount of time submersion may be tolerated.

Immersion–Hypothermia. A number of investigators have reported normal survival after periods of submersion up to 40 minutes in cold water, attributing the survival to hypothermia.[14] The metabolic demands of the brain are reduced by lowering body temperature, and the tolerance for hypoxia and ischemia increases. Immersion in cold water produces a gradual decrease in body temperature. Immersion in very cold water (≤ 5° C) results in paralysis of cutaneous capillaries, which greatly accelerates heat loss. If the patient struggles, the vasodilation in skeletal muscle further accentuates the heat loss. Infants and children may lose heat more rapidly because of their large body surface area and sparse subcutaneous fat. Swallowing and aspiration of water further accelerate the cooling of the body core temperature.

An occasional individual may develop ventricular fibrillation from sudden immersion in icy water, an event termed the "immersion syndrome." Most individuals will survive until the body core temperature drops to between 34° and 30° C, at which time unconsciousness occurs and drowning results. In individuals supported by life preservers, death does not occur until the body core temperature drops to 28° C, at which time ventricular fibrillation occurs, or 22° C, at which time asystole results.[16] The infant and child may have a survival advantage over the adult in that the diving reflex may promote circulation for a long enough time to allow adequate cooling to occur. If asphyxia and immersion hypothermia have a simultaneous onset, termed "submersion hypothermia," then the survival prognosis is less favorable. If substantial cooling occurs before the cessation of respiration, then the protective effects are more substantial.

Cardiovascular System

The effects of hypothermia and the diving reflex on cardiovascular function were described in the previous section. Most of the impact of near drowning on the cardiovascular system relates to initial hypoxic damage to the myocardium and the secondary effects of decreased arterial oxygen content, pulmonary dysfunction, and acid-base disturbances. As a general rule, substantial problems with myocardial function are not observed once resuscitation has been completed and adequate oxygenation and acid base balance have been restored. If myocardial dysfunction persists, then the amount of cerebral injury is usually very severe, since the myocardium is much more resilient to hypoxia than the brain. A wide range of electrocardiographic changes have been observed in victims of near drowning, although no dominant patterns characteristic of near drowning have been noted. The arterial blood pressure may be normal, high, or low in freshwater and saltwater drowning victims. The central venous pressure is increased immediately after aspiration of small amounts of water (fresh or salt) but rapidly returns to normal.[16] This may be related to increased pulmonary resistance and resultant right heart failure. After aspiration and ingestion of large amounts of fresh water, the central venous pressure may be elevated for an hour or more, presumably secondary to volume expansion.[17] After aspiration or ingestion of large amounts of salt water, the central venous pressure may increase briefly and then decrease to low levels secondary to volume contraction.[18] The central venous pressure may be falsely elevated despite intravascular depletion in patients with right heart failure or increased pulmonary vascular resistance secondary to hypoxia or acidosis. Severe problems in maintaining blood pressure usually reflect severe central nervous system damage with some intrinsic cardiovascular dysfunction as well.

Renal System

Renal dysfunction may be seen in freshwater or saltwater near drownings and usually reflects a substantial hypoxic ischemic injury.[19] Occasionally renal injury is seen secondary to hemolysis with hemoglobin deposition in the tubular system. Myoglobin deposition secondary to muscular trauma or anoxic muscle injury may also cause tubular injury. In these instances the degree of hypoxic injury may not be as severe.

Fluid and Electrolyte Disturbances

Studies in research animals suggest that severe fluid and electrolyte derangements might occur in victims of near drowning.[20] This is rarely observed in human drowning victims, however, in either freshwater or saltwater. It is distinctly rare for a human to aspirate or swallow fluid volumes exceeding 20 ml/kg of bodyweight.[21]

Coagulation Disorders

The hypoxia, acidosis, hypoperfusion, and occasionally sepsis associated with near drowning may result in hemolysis, coagulation defects, and disseminated intravascular coagulation.[22] Presumably the metabolic and traumatic insults result in a release of tissue thromboplastin and activation of Hageman factor and other parts of the coagulation cascade.

TREATMENT OF NEAR DROWNING

The ultimate outcome for the patient with near drowning is largely related to the amount of irreversible hypoxic ischemic brain injury sustained, since complications from involvement of other organ systems are rare and usually not chronic. All efforts should be expended to minimize the cerebral insult by providing immediate supportive care, and in some cases, a specific effort should be extended to provide "cerebral resuscitation."

At The Scene

Immediate efforts at cardiopulmonary resuscitation (CPR) should be initiated at the scene of the near drowning, since the elapsed time of hypoxia and ischemia clearly reflects on the ultimate prognosis. The airway can be cleared digitally and mouth-to-mouth resuscitation initiated in the water if the patient cannot be immediately removed. Clearing of the airway is of great importance, since attempting to resuscitate an individual with a blocked airway will result in gastric distention and vomiting, which occurs in at least 50 per cent of those individuals who are victims of near drowning. If the patient has been removed from the water, the presence or absence of spontaneous respirations and heartbeat should be determined and appropriate CPR initiated immediately. Supplemental oxygen should be given to the patient enroute to the emergency room. If an appropriate mobile rescue unit is available, then cardiotonic drugs and intravenous sodium bicarbonate can be administered at the scene.

Hospital Care

Pulmonary Support

The amount of pulmonary support required will depend on the patient's state of consciousness and the magnitude of the physiologic disturbance in pulmonary function. In the hospital setting a nasogastric tube may be placed to help evacuate water and debris from the stomach, reducing the likelihood of aspiration. Endotracheal intubation should be considered in any patient with a substantially depressed level of consciousness and poor airway protection. Inadequate respiration as determined from observation or blood gases is another indication. Most intubated patients will require mechanical ventilation.

Some conscious patients can be maintained on a mask with continuous positive airway pressure (CPAP) to open the aveoli and prevent atelectatic changes, although, in freshwater drowning, the loss of surfactant may make adequate expansion of the aveoli extremely difficult, even in the conscious patient who is expending great effort in respiration.

In the patient requiring mechanical ventilation, positive end expiratory pressure (PEEP) is added to prevent atelectasis and help overcome intrapulmonary shunting, which may account for up to 70 per cent of the cardiac output. In patients with precarious cardiac output it is important to remember that PEEP and to a lesser extent CPAP at higher pressures may decrease cardiac output.[23]

A few patients with aspiration develop bronchospasm, which can be appropriately treated with aminophylline. Pulmonary edema is best treated with either PEEP or CPAP, with titration of these modalities against the blood gases. It is important to avoid sudden removal of either of these supports; gradually taper them and allow the patient to equilibrate.

Pneumonitis may occasionally complicate aspiration of water and debris, but prophylactic antibiotics and steroids have not been of proven benefit in preventing this complication.[24] Daily complete blood counts and cultures of tracheal aspirates are advised to monitor possible development of infection in the intubated patient, particularly if hypothermia is utilized as a mode of therapy.

Cerebral Support

Ultimate cerebral function is dependent upon rapid restoration of adequate oxygenation and correction of acid-base derangements. Although carefully controlled studies of the outcome of near drowning are difficult to perform, there has been general agreement on the fact that the level of consciousness on arrival at the hospital is a good prognosticator of outcome.[25,26] Since the greatest morbidity and mortality reside in the group of children who are comatose on arrival at the hospital, much attention has been given to evaluating various therapeutic measures to improve the outcome in this group of patients.

Some investigators have confined therapy to vigorous supportive care, while others have added more extensive measures termed "cerebral resuscitation," which is aimed at restoring central nervous system function. Those utilizing cerebral resuscitation conclude that cerebral injury does not end with restoration of adequate oxygenation and acid-base balance. They specifically conclude that neuronal deterioration may be progressive and that cerebral edema may further add to the injury.[26] Measures aimed at preventing further neuronal injury presuppose that maintaining brain cells in a "hypometabolic state" for varying periods of time after the injury may prevent further neuronal loss. Hypothermia and barbiturate coma have both been utilized for this form of therapy. Some investigators have questioned the value of these measures once adequate oxygenation and acid-base balance have been restored.[25]

Cerebral edema secondary to hypoxia and ischemia has been treated with fluid restriction, head inclination, osmotic diuretics, diuretics, hyperventilation, hyperoxygenation, barbiturate coma, and hypothermia. Although these methods clearly control intracranial pressure in many patients, we are concerned that cerebral edema of sufficient magnitude to require vigorous therapy usually reflects a severe cerebral anoxic injury. Control of severe, increased intracranial pressure usually results in the preservation of individuals with only vegetative functions.

A comparison of two recent studies, one utilizing intensive supportive care and the other "cerebral resuscitation," revealed no significant differences in morbidity or mortality between the two groups.[25,26] Further well-controlled studies are clearly needed to resolve this important issue.

If the decision is made to institute cerebral resuscitation, then an intracranial pressure monitor such as the subarachnoid bolt is usually indicated. A monitor may be particularly helpful in individuals undergoing hypothermia or barbiturate coma therapy, since these therapies may alter brainstem reflexes (pupillary light reflexes, doll's eyes, respirations) utilized to assess neurologic deterioration in the patient.

Hypothermia

Conn and others have suggested that hypothermia maintained for several days after near drowning may arrest neuronal damage and aid recovery.[1] Immediate cooling of the patient to 30° ± 1° C, utilizing a cooling blanket and chlorpromazine to prevent shivering, is suggested. Continuous rectal core temperature monitoring is necessary, since ventricular fibrillation occurs at 28° C. Frequent blood cultures and complete blood counts are suggested, since sepsis is more likely in the hypothermic patient. After several days the patient is allowed to slowly and passively warm to normal temperatures.

Barbiturate Coma

Barbiturate coma has been advocated by Conn and others.[25] Animal studies have suggested that pretreatment with barbiturates will increase the normal survival of animals subjected to hypoxia.[27] The mechanism of action presumably involves reduction of the cerebral metabolic rate, thus making the patient less susceptible to hypoxia. In this respect the effect may be similar to that of hypothermia. No clear-cut benefits have been demonstrated, however, in treating individuals after a hypoxic event. Barbiturates have, however, been clearly demonstrated to help reduce increased intracranial pressure. An initial pentobarbital loading dose of 3 to 6 mg/kg of body weight is suggested, with a maintenance dosage of 1 to 3 mg/kg of body weight per hour. A continuous EEG monitor is useful for monitoring EEG patterns. A burst suppression pattern generally indicates maximum physiologic benefit from barbiturates with no further benefit to be expected by increasing the blood level. Serum levels of pentobarbital should not exceed 50 μ/ml. Side effects include hypotension and cardiac arrhythmia. An intracranial pressure monitor is essential, since barbiturate coma causes cessation of pupillary light reflexes, oculovestibular reflexes, and spontaneous movement.

Increased Intracranial Pressure

Many investigators have reported cerebral edema in association with near drowning. In most cases it is probably the result of severe hypoxic ischemic encephalopathy and only rarely due to fluid overload. Evaluation of intracranial pressure with intracranial pressure monitoring and treatment with head elevation (30 degrees), hypothermia, barbiturates, hyperventilation, fluid restriction, steroids, and osmotic diuretics in various combinations have been advocated by different investigators. Elevation of the head at a 30 degree angle from the bed will increase cerebral venous return and reduce intracranial pressure. It is important to avoid fluid overload, but severe fluid restriction in the normovolemic patient is probably of little benefit. Although frequently used, steroids are of no proven benefit in hypoxic ischemic encephalopathy.

Hyperventilation reduces intracranial pressure by lowering the P_{CO_2}, which results in cerebral vasoconstriction. This probably constitutes the safest way to reduce increased intracranial pressure in the near drowning victim, assuming that lung disease does not limit attaining a P_{CO_2} of 22 to 25 torr. Maintaining a P_{O_2} of 100 to 150 torr will also help reduce intracranial pressure by promoting cerebral vasoconstriction, but prolonged elevation of the P_{O_2} should be avoided to prevent pulmonary oxygen toxicity. Mechanical ventilation with paralysis utilizing pancuronium 0.1 mg/kg of body weight is generally necessary to achieve the necessary respiratory parameters.

Osmotic diuretics such as intravenous mannitol, 1 g/kg of body weight may also help reduce intracranial pressure. These do reduce vascular volume and, in the hypotensive patient, may be contraindicated.

The use of barbiturate coma and hypothermia for control of increased intracranial pressure has been discussed.

Cardiovascular Problems

The majority of the cardiovascular problems seen in the near drowning victim resolve with restoration of adequate oxygenation and correction of acid-base imbalances. If problems with cardiac output appear to be present and of sufficient severity, a Swan-Ganz catheter is recommended for measuring the pulmonary wedge pressure. The pulmonary wedge pressure reflects the left ventricular end diastolic pressure or preload. If the cardiac output is decreased, then slow administration of fluid until the wedge pressure reaches 15 to 18 cm of water should help in increasing the cardiac output.[7] If, despite volume loading and correction of acid-base problems and hypoxia, the patient remains hypotensive, a trial of a vasopressor such as dopamine should be considered.[28]

Renal Abnormalities

If acute tubular necrosis secondary to hypoxia and ischemia has occurred, then appropriate fluid restriction and management of acute renal failure should be instituted. If hemoglobinuria or myoglobinuria are detected, then therapy with mannitol may be indicated to improve urine production and reduce the likelihood of tubular precipitation of these substances.

Coagulation Abnormalities

A prothrombin time, partial thromboplastin time, and platelet count should be obtained routinely. If these studies are abnormal, a thrombin time, fibrinogen level, fibrin degradation products, and euglobulin lysis time are indicated. Efforts should be directed at treating the primary cause of the coagulopathy, such as cardiac or pulmonary dysfunction. Therapy with fresh frozen plasma and platelets should be considered. Therapy with heparin should also be considered, but its use is more controversial.

PROGNOSIS

The ultimate prognosis for the victim of near drowning rests heavily on the amount of hypoxic ischemic encephalopathy sustained by the patient. Factors such as preexisting health, age of the patient, the diving reflex, hypothermia, and the promptness and skill of resuscitation efforts all reflect the amount of damage done. The level of consciousness at the time of presentation in the emergency room weighs heavily on the ultimate prognosis. Those patients arriving awake have a survival rate of near 100 per cent if appropriate supportive measures are instituted. Those who have mild blunting in level of consciousness have a survival rate of 90 to 100 per cent; deaths reported in this group are largely secondary to pulmonary causes. The group of patients who arrive in the comatose state have a more variable outcome. Approximately 44 per cent of these patients will survive without major neurologic residua. Seventeen per cent will survive with incapacitating central nervous system damage, and 39 per cent will die.[25,26] Clearly, meticulous care must be directed at the comatose patient in hopes of improving survival and decreasing morbidity. A variety of therapeutic approaches such as "cerebral resuscitation" need to be carefully evaluated with controlled studies but to date have not been proved superior to vigorous supportive care. In any controlled study, patients must be carefully matched for level of consciousness when presenting for therapy.

REFERENCES

1. Conn AW, Edmonds JF, and Barker GA: Cerebral resuscitation in near-drowning. Pediatric Clin North Am 1979, pp. 691–701.
2. Giammona ST: Drowning: Pathophysiology and management. Curr Probl Pediatr 1:1, 1971.
3. Schuman SH, Rowe JR, Glazler HM, et al.: The iceberg phenomenon of near-drowning. Soc Crit Care Med 4:127, 1976.
4. Rivers JF, Orr G, Lee HA: Drowning: Its clinical sequelae and management. Br Med J 2:157, 1970.
5. Giammona ST, Modell JH: Drowning by total immersion: Effects on pulmonary surfactant of distilled water, isotonic saline and sea water. Am J Dis Child 114:612, 1967.
6. Hoff B: Multisystem failure: A review with special reference to drowning. Crit Care Med 7:310, 1979.
7. Modell JH, Moya F, Williams EJ, et al.: The effects of fluid volume in sea water drowning. Ann Intern Med 67:68, 1967.
8. Modell JH, Graves SA, Ketover A: Clinical course of 91 consecutive near-drowning victims. Chest 70:231, 1976.
9. Jenkinson SG, George DB: Serial pulmonary function studies in survivors of near-drowning. Chest 77:777, 1980.
10. Plum F, Posner JB, Hain, RF: Delayed neurological deterioration after anoxia. Arch Intern Med 110:56, 1962.
11. Orlowski JP: Prognostic factors in drowning and post-submersion syndrome. Crit Care Med 6:94, 1978.
12. Gooden BA: Drowning and the diving reflex in man. Med J Austral 2:583, 1972.
13. Hunt PK: Effect and treatment of diving reflex. Can Med Assoc J III:13330, 1974.
14. Young RSK, Zaineraitis EL, Dooling EC: Neurological outcome of cold water drowning. JAMA 244:1233, 1980.
15. Keatinge WR: Survival in cold water: The physiology and treatment of immersion hypothermia and of drowning. Oxford, Blackwell Scientific 1969, pp. 5, 42.
16. Model JH, Moya F: Effects of volume of aspirated fluid during chlorinated fresh water drowning. Anesthesiology 27:662, 1966.
17. Farthmann EH, Davidson AIG: Fresh water drowning at lower body temperature. An experimental study. Am J Surg 109:410, 1965.
18. Swann HG, Brucer M, Moore C, et al.: Fresh water and sea water drowning: A study of the terminal cardiac and biochemical events. Tex Rep Biol Med 7:604, 1949.
19. Grausz H, Amend WJC Jr, Earl LE: Acute renal failure complicating immersion in sea water. JAMA 217:207, 1971.
20. Swann HG, Brucer M: The cardiorespiratory and biochemical events during rapid anoxic death. VI. Fresh water and sea water drowning. Tex Rep Biol Med 7:604, 1949.
21. Modell JH, David JH: Electrolyte changes in human drowning victims. Anesthesia 30:414, 1969.
22. Culpepper RM: Bleeding diasthesis in fresh water drowning. Ann Intern Med 83:675, 1975.
23. Kirby R, Perry JC, Calderwood HW et al.: Cardiorespiratory effects of high positive end expiratory pressures. Anesthesiology 43:533, 1975.
24. Modell JH, Graves SA, Kefover A: Clinical course of 91 consecutive near-drowning victims. Chest 70:231, 1976.
25. Modell JH, Graves SA, Kuck EJ: Near-drowning: Correlation of level of consciousness and survival. Can Anaesth Soc J 27:213, 1980.
26. Conn AW, Montes JE, Barker GA, et al.: Cerebral salvage in near-drowning following neurological classification by triage. Can Anaesth Soc J 27:201, 1980.
27. Bleyaert AL, Nemoto EM, Safar P, et al.: Amelioration of postischemic encephalopathy by sodium thiopental after 16 minutes of global brain ischemia in monkies. Physiologist 18:145, 1975.
28. Holzer J, Karliner JS, Olrouke RA, et al.: Effectiveness of dopamine in patients with cardiogenic shock. Am J Cardiol 32:79, 1973.

CHAPTER

30 Animal, Snake, and Insect Bites

CLIFFORD C. SNYDER
THOM A. MAYER

During 1982, an average of 800 humans per day were bitten by animals in the United States; it should not be surprising to pediatricians or emergency physicians that the majority of victims were between 2 and 15 years of age. Parents often purchase "tame" monkeys, skunks, raccoons, hamsters, rats, snakes, or lizards as pets for their children. However, advice and supervision are necessary for safe and appropriate care of such animals. The privilege of maintaining pets and learning to respect and love them can be an excellent experience for children, but possible hazards may result from bites by the animals. The domestic animal population is increasing, and with the addition of wild and exotic animals as household pets, physicians must be familiar with the types of concomitant accidents and the specific therapy for such accidents, as well as the means of managing the sequelae.

DOG BITES

Dogs are responsible for 9 out of every 10 mammalian bites. Cats are the source of 5 per cent of bites, and monkeys, rats, bats, raccoons, foxes, skunks, hamsters, horses, camels, and bears are causative agents for the remaining 5 per cent. The dog breeds responsible for most of the attacks are German shepherds, collies, spaniels, and terriers. In children, facial and upper extremity wounds are the commonest injuries because the youngster usually is teasing or playing with the animal at close range. Lower extremity bites are frequently seen in postmen, parcel deliverers, milk carriers, bicyclers, and joggers.

Dog bite wounds have always been considered exorbitantly contaminated and, therefore, are seldom closed primarily. Careful débridement with secondary skin closure is advisable for acute, large, avulsive lesions or wounds of long duration with inflammatory exudate (Fig. 30–1). However, there are many dog bites that may be treated by thorough cleansing, surgical débridement, and loose closure, particularly wounds involving the face that may lead to disfigurement if secondary closure is attempted. Superficial canine lacerations may be copiously irrigated, the margins débrided, and the wound closed loosely to allow drainage (Fig. 30–2).[2]

Prevention of dog bites is the preferable course, and the following tenets may be beneficial:

1. Select family pets carefully.
2. Educate children in proper pet care.
3. Ignore dogs engaged in fighting.
4. Refrain from petting mother dogs nursing pups.
5. Do not awaken a dog abruptly.
6. Avoid a dog that is eating.
7. Restrain watchdogs.
8. Avoid strange, prowling, or ailing dogs.
9. Use leashes and muzzles on pet dogs in public.

RABIES

Epidemiology

The Centers for Disease Control (CDC) in Atlanta reported that there were 7211 documented cases of animal rabies recorded in 1981 in the United States and its territories of Guam, Puerto Rico, and the Virgin Islands, of which most were detected in wild animals. This is the highest number reported since 1954.[1] Although there is an increase of rabies in wild animals, there has been a decrease of rabies in domestic animals in recent years. Less than 10 humans contracted rabies in 1981 in the United States, yet about 30,000 people are treated annually because of contact with possible rabid animals. Of the confirmed rabies-infected animals, skunks, foxes, raccoons, coyotes, bobcats, and bats are the commonest rabies virus vectors.

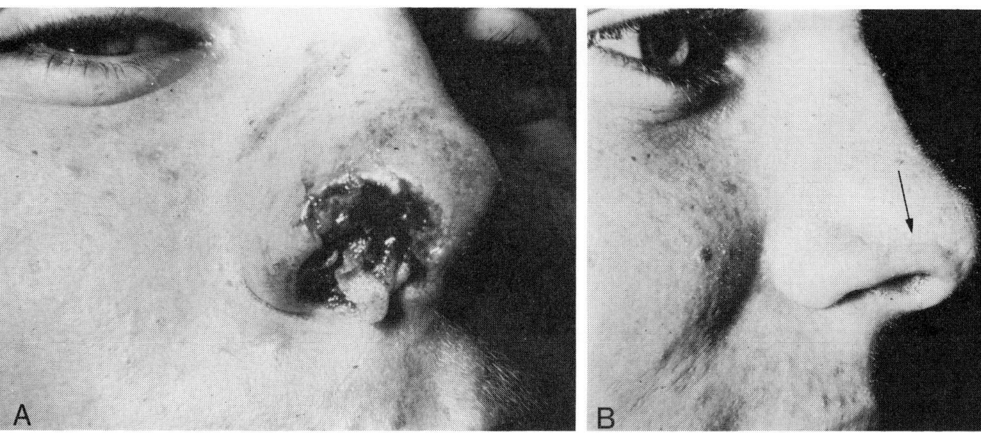

Figure 30–1. *A*, The adage "clean as a hound's tooth" is an extravagant error. Avulsive dog bite wounds are cleaned thoroughly, debrided judiciously, and treated intensively until free of sepsis. *B*, A compound loss of tissue (skin and cartilage) is corrected with a compound-free graft of identical tissue (skin and cartilage) from the auricular concha.

The responsible etiologic organism is an ultramicroscopic, filterable, neurotropic virus transmitted to man through bites, skin or mucosal contact, and inhalation. Although the usual incubation period varies from 10 days to months, the prodromal period is shortened remarkably with severe infections. The victim complains early of pain at the bite site, which disperses and becomes so intense that the patient will not tolerate the least touch or palpation. Following this generalized hyperesthesia, there ensues a dislike of light (photophobia), when the patient will squint and turn the head from the brightness due to dilated pupils. As the nervous system becomes more irritable, the least noise bothers the patient to the extent that he will jump with a knock at the door or a slap on the bed. Uncontrollable sudorific activity is promoted, which is responsible for diaphoresis, excessive lacrimation, and salivation (known erroneously as hydrophobia). As the status worsens, muscle spasms and convulsions become evident, swallowing is a problem. Cheyne-Stokes respiration develops, hyperthermia evolves, and death becomes unavoidable.

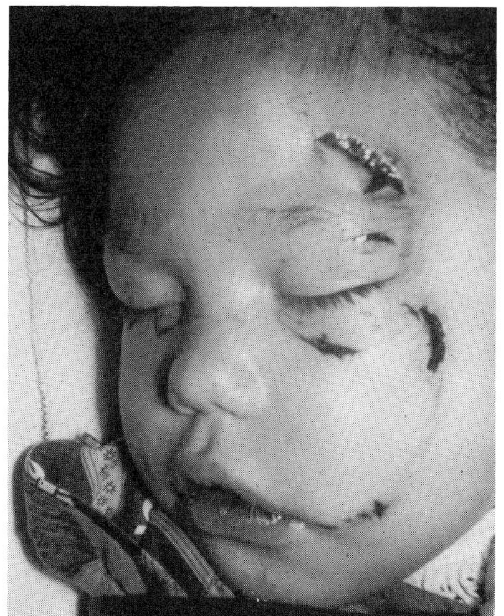

Figure 30–2. Dog bites of the face are more common in children because children play and tease animals at close range. Because of the vascular composition of facial integument and the possibility of the development of deforming cicatrices, facial dog bites are immediately washed, rinsed, and debrided, and the margins are leniently approximated.

Diagnosis

Among the various methods of diagnoses are the following:

1. The suspected rabid animal is kept under surveillance for 10 days, and if it is alive without suspicious actions, it should be considered not rabid. If it becomes ill or dies within the 10 days, it is reasonable to suspect infection and the animal must be studied.
2. Brain tissue retrieved from the animal is examined and reveals Negri bodies in the motor nerves.
3. A smear of brain tissue from the animal is bathed with rabies antibody and stained with fluorescein dye and fluoresces under a black lamp, indicating the virus tagged onto the antibody.

4. The suspected material is injected into the brain of 3-week-old mice who succumb in 3 weeks if the material is rabid.

Treatment

The epizootic incidence of rabies in animals warrants immediate concern, and possible rabies in the human patient should *always* be considered. Chemotherapy and antibiotics offer little control of this neurotrophic virus; therefore, in highly suspicious or known cases, immediate local therapy and active immunization with human diploid cell rabies vaccine (HDCV), supplemented with human rabies immune globulin (HRIG), may be the difference between life and death. HDCV has replaced duck embryo vaccine (DEV) in the treatment of rabies, because the latter entailed 23 painful injections and produced a high incidence of neurologic side effects. HDCV is composed of less foreign protein than DEV, produces higher antibody titers, promotes a prompt antibody response, and necessitates only three pre-exposure or five postexposure injections.

The therapeutic regimen begins with thorough cleansing of the wound with Betadine or Hibiclens, which is then rinsed with sterile water and débrided surgically in depth and circumferentially. The wound edges are not closed. Only 5 per cent of purposefully inflicted research animals with rabies virus whose wounds were scrubbed with soap and water developed the disease. As a comparative study, 90 per cent of the controls whose wounds were not cleansed died of rabies. The physician who is not familiar with the disease will often benefit by consulting public health doctors, who always graciously offer guidance. The most important decision for an attending physician is *when* to treat and *when not* to treat. Before treating the victim, the physician must know the following:

1. The circumstances at the time of exposure.
2. The animal species involved in the exposure.
3. The type of exposure.
4. The epidemiology of rabies in the area of exposure.
5. The vaccination status of the animal.
6. The therapeutic alternatives.

The above criteria may be employed as follows (see Table 30–1):

1. Was the victim bitten, scratched, or licked by a possibly rapid animal? If the answer is no, treatment for rabies is unnecessary. If the answer is yes, then,
2. Is rabies present in the vicinity or suspected in the animal? If the answer is no, do not treat for rabies. If the answer is yes, then,
3. Is the animal available? If the answer is no, then,
4. Is the animal a dog or cat? If the answer is no, administer HDCV and HRIG. If the answer is yes, then,
5. Was the person bitten? If the answer is no, give only HDCV. If the answer is yes, give HDCV and HRIG. If the answer to number 3 above (is the animal available?) is yes, then,
6. Is the animal's behavior normal and is it a vaccinated dog or cat? If the answer is yes, then,
7. Did the animal become ill during the next 10 days? If the answer is no, no rabies treatment is indicated. If the answer is yes, then,
8. Does the laboratory examination of the brain confirm rabies? If the answer is no, forget the treatment. If the answer is yes, then administer HDCV and HRIG.

The human diploid cell rabies vaccine (HDCV) is recommended for people with a high risk of being exposed to rabies virus (veterinarians, laboratory personnel, dog pound laborers) as a *pre-exposure vaccine* in three 1-ml deltoid muscle injections, given

Table 30–1. INSTANT TREATMENT FOR RABIES

Wound Type	Healthy Family Dog or Cat	Unidentified Nonvaccinated Domestic Animal	Rabid Domestic Animal	Wild Skunk, Fox, Raccoon, Bat
No lesion	no HDCV, no HRIG	Observation	HDCV, HRIG	Observation
Scratches	no HDCV, no HRIG	HRIG	HDCV, HRIG	HDCV, HRIG
Superficial bite	no HDCV, no HRIG	HRIG	HDCV, HRIG	HDCV, HRIG
Severe attack	HRIG	HDCV, HRIG	HDCV, HRIG	HDCV, HRIG

on days 0, 7, and 21. Those persons with a continuing risk of exposure should receive a booster dose of 1 ml intramuscularly at least every 2 years. Those *postexposure* people who have experienced a wound from a possibly rabid animal should be hastened to a physician or hospital where the wound can be briskly scrubbed and débrided and antirabies therapy instituted. Human rabies immune globulin (HRIG) should be administered in a dosage of 20 IU/kg intramuscularly. Simultaneously, 1 ml of HDCV is given intramuscularly and repeated on days 3, 7, 14, and 28. If there is great concern, a sixth dose on day 90 may be administered. Those previously immunized people with demonstrable rabies antibodies (e. g., veterinarians) who are exposed to rabies should receive 2 doses of 1 ml of HDCV, the first immediately and the second 3 days later. HRIG is not necessary for these patients. The Advisory Committee for Immunization Practices (ACIP) reviewed data on 510 individuals immunized with HDCV vaccines. The Committee reported that 100 per cent had protective levels following pre-exposure treatment, and that of 1300 postexposure HDCV-treated persons, 99.9 per cent exhibited protective antibody levels.

Physicians should be alert for any reactions to the HDCV, which include local redness, itching, and pain. Occasionally fever, nausea, abdominal pain, headache, and muscle aching occur. These reactions usually subside upon completion of the therapeutic injections, but symptomatic relief is appreciated during the episodes. If the patient encounters adverse reactions to the HDCV such as local erythema, pain, and itching, epinephrine is helpful, but cortisone should not be used because it decreases the victim's immune reaction and so releases the potency of the rabies virus. Physicians should realize that a tear or puncture in the skin is not the only portal of entry for the rabies virus. Eating, drinking, breathing, and handling infected materials may also be the cause for infection. Mucosal ulcerations are also vulnerable to rabies. Animals placed in bat-infested caves have contracted airborne rabies after 10 hours exposure, and bat urine and guano may cause infection when handled.

CAT BITES

Bites by domestic cats differ from those by dogs owing to the thin needle-like teeth of cats, which produce deep narrow puncture wounds. They rarely produce avulsions. The bacteria from the cat's oral cavity and from the victim's skin are deposited into the depths of the puncture wound, and when the wound closes, the nidus is developed for anaerobic bacteria to multiply. Because these wounds are difficult to cleanse topically with a cloth or brush, they are débrided by excision and irrigated thoroughly. If the injury is severe, it should not be closed. Most bites inflicted by household cats or kittens occur during play and need only cleansing.

Bites from pet rabbits, guinea pigs, hamsters, and rats are treated similarly to those by cats.

EQUINE BITES

Children are very vulnerable to bites by pet horses and burros, but may also be bitten by zebras and camels because of the abundance of zoos. Equines have large wide incisor teeth, which are responsible for bruises, crushes, and avulsions. It is not uncommon to see soft tissues missing in the wound (Fig. 30–3). This type of wound is painful and becomes infected early if treatment is not provided. For these reasons equine wounds are initially cleansed, débrided, and repaired when seen.

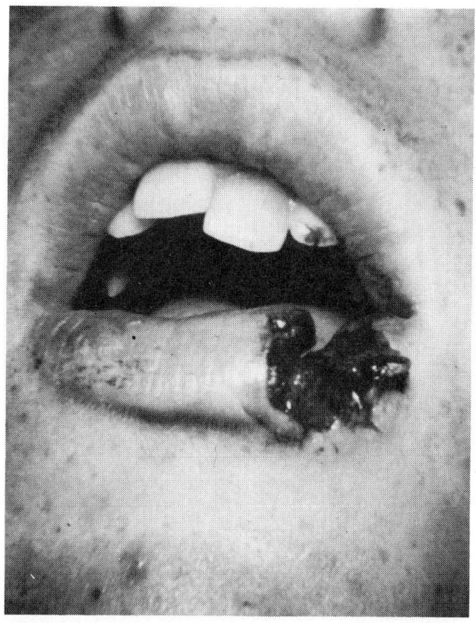

Figure 30–3. The child's face, especially the lips, is a frequent site of equine inflictions. The pony's large and wide incisors produce a crushing avulsive type of wound with loss of tissue.

REPTILE BITES

Alligators, crocodiles, caimans, and large lizards have massive heads of nearly solid bone, powerful jaws, and rows of sharp teeth. Bite wounds from these animals produce crushing and avulsive injuries with loss of a leg or an arm or a body crush occurring frequently.

The first goal of treatment of reptilian wounds is to control bleeding. Then the wound is cleansed by profusely irrigating and débriding the wound depths of foreign material and devitalized structures. The wound margins may be brought loosely together and the irrigation tubes left in position, or the wound may be left open to granulate, and a skin graft applied later.

ARTHROPOD INFLICTIONS

Almost all of the 800,000 species of arthropods are envenomous to humans, and more poisonings to man are encountered from these than from the entire remaining phyla combined. There are three times as many deaths in the United States from arthropod inflictions than from rattlesnake bites. Most of these are attributed to anaphylaxis rather than to direct effects from the venoms.

Black Widow Spider (*Latrodectus*) Bites

The pediatrician must be aware that this dangerous American arthropod (Fig. 30–4), the black widow spider, has an established envenomation mortality of 4 per cent. Although most *Latrodectus* bites are self-limiting and need only immediate treatment for pain and possible anaphylaxis, cellulitis, lymphangitis, and ulceration may ensue (Fig. 30–5). Arachnidism has been known to mimic pneumonia, myocardial infarction, appendicitis, and peritonitis. Patients may not recall being bitten or may recall a sharp pinprick incident that was forgotten. A careful search of the skin will reveal a minute red fang mark with local edema.

Cold compresses or ice packs on and about the local infliction, with adjuvant local application of an anti-inflammatory drug such as betamethasone dipropionate (Diprosone), 0.05 per cent, or flurandrenolide (Cordran), 0.05 per cent ointment, will relieve the pain

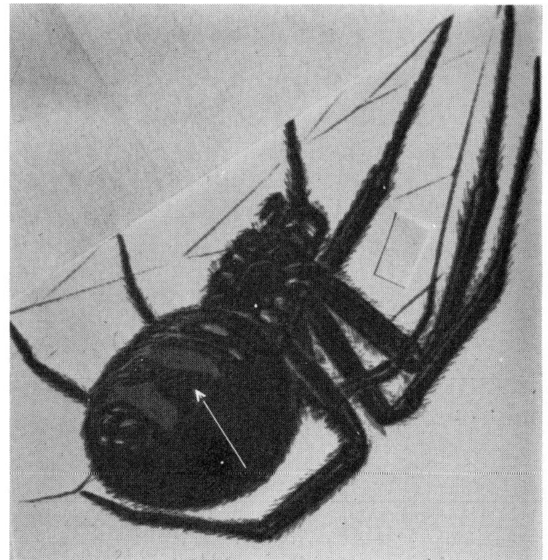

Figure 30–4. The female black widow spider *(Latrodectus)* hangs from its web in the supine position, exposing the cardinal-colored abdomen *(arrow)* by which it is notoriously identified.

immediately. If the victim has been severely envenomated, dyspnea and muscular spasms should be treated first with a slow IV infusion of 10 ml of 10 per cent calcium gluconate in children 6 months or older, repeated at 4-hour intervals as necessary. Additionally, for muscle spasm, nausea, and vomiting, give diazepam (Valium) 0.3 mg/kg by slow IV infusion, up to 5 mg in infants and toddlers, and up to 10 mg in older children. For severe pain the use of acetaminophen initially, and later meperidine (Dem-

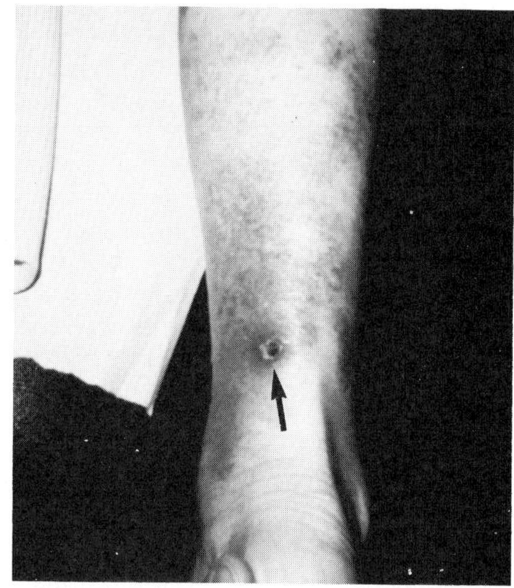

Figure 30–5. The pediatrician must be aware that arachnidism may lead to ulceration *(arrow)*, cellulitis, and lymphangitis and may mimic myocardial infarction, appendicitis, or a ruptured peptic ulcer.

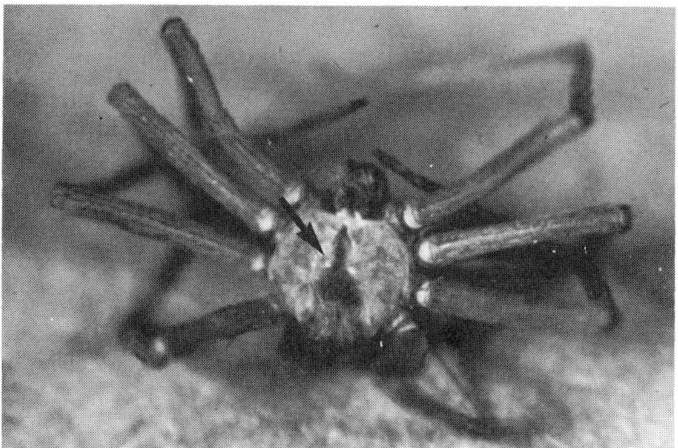

Figure 30–6. The brown recluse spider *(Loxosceles)* is commonly called the fiddler spider because of the violin-shaped figure on its back.

erol) up to 1 mg/kg or morphine (0.1 mg/kg), may be helpful.

The only specific therapy for latrodectism is antivenin, and this may be purchased under the name of Antivenin (Merck, Sharpe, and Dohme). It should be used only in severe envenomation or in highly susceptible individuals. Because it is a horse serum product, sensitivity testing must be conducted as the package flyer indicates. The dose is 2.5 ml IM and may be repeated. For allergic manifestations and urticaria, use antihistamines.

Brown Recluse Spider (*Loxosceles*) Bites

Loxosceles reclusa is tan colored with a dark brown violin-shaped figure on its back (Fig. 30–6). The "fiddler" spider bite is seldom painful initially, but within a few hours a blood-filled bleb becomes apparent at the bite site (Fig. 30–7). The bleb soon ruptures, and a small ulcer develops, with a white ischemic periphery surrounded by an erythematous halo (Fig. 30–8). This red, white, and blue pathognomonic finding soon ulcerates and becomes painful and tender. If not attended to, the ulceration continues to progress for several weeks, and many such bites are erroneously diagnosed as basal cell carcinomas (Fig. 30–9). Corticosteroids given early are effective but adequate dosage is required, beginning with 1 mg/kg of body weight of methylprednisolone (Solu-Medrol), or an equivalent IM corticosteroid, repeated at 6-

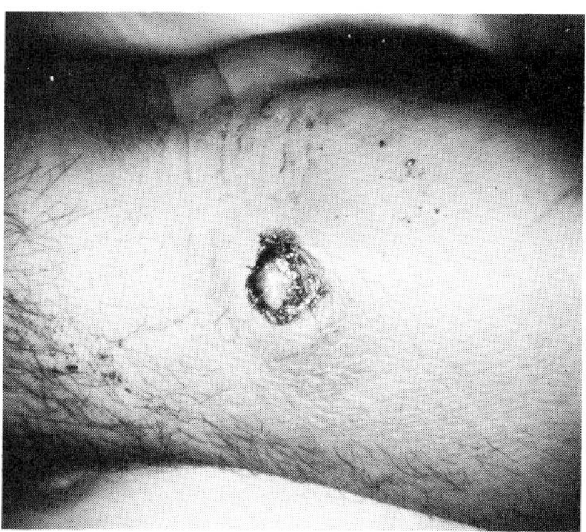

Figure 30–8. The ulceration caused by the bite of the recluse spider develops a bluish central necrosis, a white ischemic periphery, and a surrounding erythematous halo. These concentric rings are known as the red, white, and blue phenomenon.

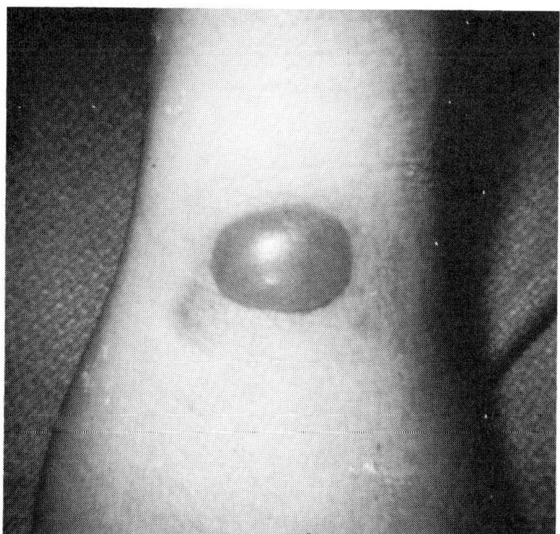

Figure 30–7. Within a few hours, on the bite site of the recluse spider appears a bulla filled with a hemorrhagic transudate, which ruptures to form an ulceration.

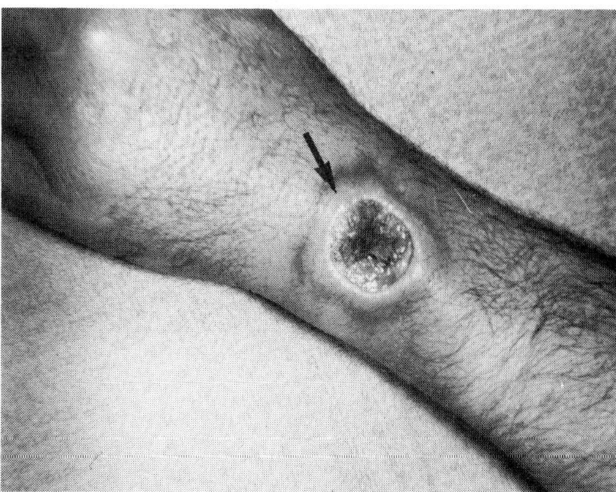

Figure 30–9. If unattended, the ulcer from the bite of the recluse spider will become indolent and resemble a basal cell carcinoma with an elevated periphery and an umbilicated center, and the pathognomonic finding of red, white, and blue coloration *(arrow)* will illuminate like a neon signal.

hour intervals. If the bite is identified as that of a brown recluse spider, immediate excision and closure of the site under local 1 per cent lidocaine (Xylocaine) is usually successful. If ulceration has developed, late excision and closure will accelerate healing and produce a more satisfactory scar. Cephalexin (Keflex) or an equivalent is used for secondary infection, in doses of 125 mg every 6 hours until the infection has subsided. Tetanus prophylaxis should be considered in nonhealing lesions.

Scorpion Stings

All scorpion infections are venomous and have diverse reactions. Stings by *Centruroides* species produce severe systemic effects and can be fatal. The stinger is designed with an ampulla, which stores the venom (Fig. 30–10). Epinephrine is synergistic to scorpion stings and must be eliminated from any treatment. To relieve the sharp pain and edema produced by the venom injection, apply local cold compresses or household ammonia to the sting as soon as possible (Fig. 30–11). For the annoying itching that accompanies the wound, 0.05 per cent betamethasone dipropionate (Diprosone) ointment applied freely to the sting site is relieving. For apprehension, nervousness, or muscle spasm, administer diazepam (Valium) intravenously, up to 5 mg in infants and toddlers and up to 10 mg in older children. Muscular fasciculations and convulsions can be treated with 5 to 10 ml of 10 per cent calcium gluconate IV, repeated at 4-hour intervals as necessary. Hypersalivation is combated with atropine sulfate in IM doses of 0.3 mg.

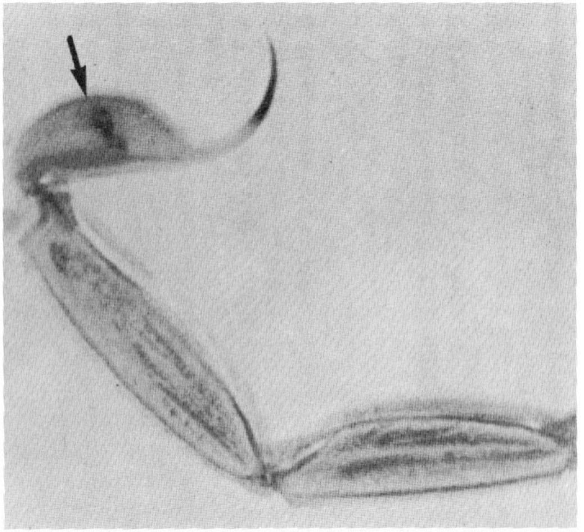

Figure 30–10. The stinging apparatus consists of a durable, curved, needle point shaft, and an ampulla *(arrow)*, which stores the venom until used by the scorpion.

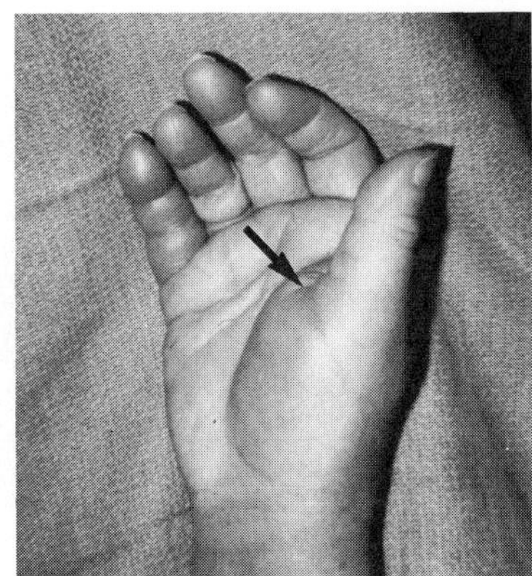

Figure 30–11. This edematous hand of a 10-year-old boy who was injected by a scorpion of the *Centruroides* species in the thumb–index finger web space *(arrow)* 1 hour previous to the photograph.

Hymenoptera Stings

This order of arthropods includes bees, wasps, hornets, ants, and other membrane-winged insects whose venomers are females. Most Hymenoptera attacks are more of an aggravation than a disaster, although there are some very envenomous species. Pediatricians should be aware that at least 25 per cent of the world population is sensitive to Hymenoptera venoms and that the high mortality from these is attributed to anaphylactic shock as a result of hypersensitivity of the victim. Female Hymenoptera are endowed with a canalized ovipositor (stinger), which has a dual purpose of depositing eggs and injecting venom. Some ovipositors are barbed, and these are detached from the insect's body, causing its death, whereas other ovipositors are smooth and the insect is able to sting repeatedly and fly away. Hymenoptera kill more people in our nation than any other venomer, so their envenomation may be an acute medical problem deserving emergency attention (Fig. 30–12).

If the ovipositor is deposited in the skin, it will appear as a black dot. Retrieve it with a sharp-pointed No. 11 scalpel blade, without squeezing the skin or using tweezers as the venom sac is attached and venom will be spread in the wound. The inflammation at the sting site is relieved by an ice pack and betamethasone dipropionate (Diprosone), 0.05 per cent, or betamethasone valerate (Val-

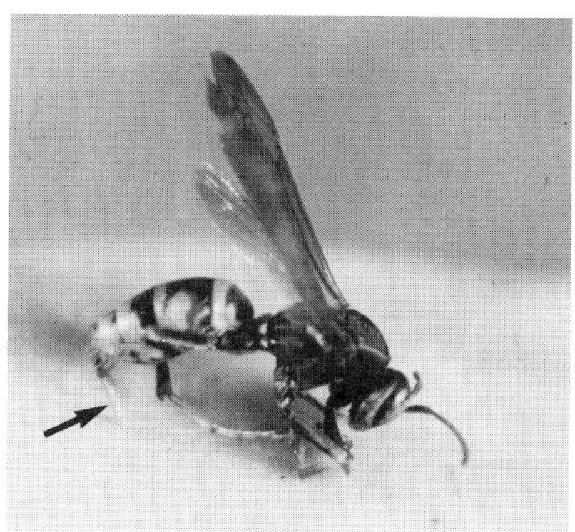

Figure 30–12. This wasp, nicknamed the Southern Belle because of the large thorax and abdomen joined by a ribbon waist, is trigger-tempered and compulsive. The ovipositor or stinger *(arrow)* is smooth without barbs and is capable of injecting many times.

isone), 0.1 per cent ointment. A paste of monosodium glutamate powder applied to the site also may be tried. If urticaria develops, administer 0.3 ml epinephrine 1:1000 subcutaneously. For progressive symptoms or dyspnea, begin an IV infusion of 1 ml epinephrine 1:1000/10 ml normal saline and titrate to the relief of symptoms. Other adjunctive therapy is diazepam (Valium), 5 to 10 mg IV for agitation and 1 mg/kg of body weight of methylprednisolone (Solu-Medrol) IV for joint pains. Occasionally a victim will have an acute generalized allergic reaction with dyspnea that necessitates immediate emergency care. Inject 0.5 ml of epinephrine 1:1000 subcutaneously and repeat in 5 minutes, with up to 2 additional doses if necessary. Start an IV lifeline with normal saline and use an epinephrine infusion as described previously. Use levarterenol (Levophed) for shock and aminophylline for bronchospasm.

For children prone to anaphylaxis, prophylaxis can be achieved with a commercial polyvalent hymenopteran antigen kit available from Center Laboratories (Port Washington, New York). These children must avoid exposure to infested areas of stinging insects, avoid floral and perfume scents, and wear white clothing and shoes when hiking or camping.

Fly Bites

The order Diptera includes such flies as the horse fly, deer fly, and sand fly. Most of these are bloodsuckers that deposit a salivary fluid into the skin that is irritating to the recipient. The immediate therapy is to clean the bite area with soap, water, and alcohol to reduce the chance of infection, and cover the local area with a corticosteroid ointment. If the patient is allergic to the bite as evidenced by migrating pain, arthralgia, and generalized urticaria, a therapy regimen identical to that for Hymenoptera is advocated.

AQUATIC ANIMAL STINGS

Jellyfish, Portuguese-man-of-war, sea anemones, hydras, and corals, who inject their toxins by a nematoid apparatus functioning through a microscopic trigger mechanism, are all agents of aquatic stings. The thousands of nematocysts in the tentacles of the attacking organism become imbedded in the skin of the victim. Erythematous streaks where the tentacles have touched the skin are extremely painful and become exaggerated when the lesions are rubbed. Emergency treatment inactivates the nematocysts by rinsing the involved area with alcohol and then treating the stings locally with household ammonia. An unguent of baking powder, papain, lidocaine 0.05 per cent, and betamethasone valerate (Valisone) 0.1 per cent is superb for relieving the symptoms.

SNAKEBITES

The care of children with snakebites is one of the most fascinating problems in pediatrics. Snakebites occur with relatively great frequency in children, since over 50 per cent of all such injuries occur in those under 19 years of age.[4] Care of the snakebite victim requires rapid assessment, specific knowledge of therapeutic needs, and preparation for delivery of intensive therapy. Because over half of all snakebites are potentially life or limb threatening, the high degree of skill required for appropriate management can be extremely gratifying, inasmuch as the physicians' skills can lead to patient salvage. This is particularly true in children, since pediatric snakebite victims react much more intensely to envenomation than do adults. The intent of this chapter is to present a balanced approach to evaluation and management of snakebite injuries in children.

Types of Snakes

In the United States, as in most countries, the vast majority of snakes are not poisonous. It is extremely important to assess whether a snakebite has come from poisonous or nonpoisonous species. Two families of snakes (the Crotalidae and Elapidae) account for most of the world's poisonous snakebites. Snakes of the Crotalidae family are pit vipers and include large rattlesnakes, several small rattlesnakes found in the western United States, copperhead or highland moccasins, and the cottonmouth snakes (or water moccasins). While detailed reference texts and charts are available for snake identification,[5] some general rules assist in the determination of whether a snake is of the Crotalidae (pit viper) family. Pit vipers are named for the presence of fangs as well as for a pair of small indentations, or "pits," located between the eye and the snout. These indentations are thermoreceptor organs and assist the snake in locating warm-blooded prey. Snakes of the pit viper family usually have a triangle-shaped head with vertical pupils, in contrast to the round pupils and heads of harmless snakes.

Rattlesnakes may be identified by the characteristic row of rattles or tail plates. However, these rows of rattles may be lost or deformed during the snake's life, so their absence should not mislead proper identification. Rattlesnakes may be found in all areas of the mainland United States. The copperhead moccasin is named for its coppery color but can also be identified by its hourglass-shaped markings. These snakes inhabit a large area, stretching from middle New England southward to north Florida and westward to an area extending from central Illinois to Texas.

The cottonmouth or water moccasin resides in semiaquatic or aquatic environments in states from Virginia to Florida and westward to the eastern part of Texas. Aside from its characteristic white buccal mucosa, the snake can also be identified by its broad, flat head and dark color.

The Elapidae family of snakes includes some of the world's deadliest, including cobras, kraits, mambas, and a variety of snakes with extremely neurotoxic venoms. The Eastern and Sonoran coral snakes are the only members of this family that occur naturally in the United States, although other Elapids may be found in zoos throughout the country. The Eastern coral snake (*Micrurus fulvius*) is by far the most common elapid in the United States and is found in southern states from the Carolinas to Texas. This snake is quite beautiful in color, with a black snout and a body encircled by bands of red, yellow, and black. While there is occasionally some difficulty in distinguishing this snake from the similarly colored scarlet king snake, the verse "Red bands on yellow can kill a fellow" assists in identifying the coral snake. The Sonoran coral snake is found in the Arizona desert and is rarely encountered by man.

Venom

The venom of poisonous snakes comprises a "witches brew" of some of the world's most powerful enzymes, proteins, and polypeptides. While venom varies in composition and amount between species and according to the size of the snake, it can generally be characterized as a protein-rich substance injected through the snake's fangs. It may contain up to 17 enzymes. In addition to a broad range of effects exerted by the enzymes, a number of proteins and polypeptides may be released, producing a number of autopharmacologic effects. Bradykinin, serotonin, and histamine also form a part of the organism's reaction to the injection of the snake venom.

The concatenation of enzymes present in the snake venom produces an extremely broad array of pharmacologic effects. L-arginine esterase results in release of bradykinin, which is thought to be responsible for the pain, reflex hypotension, nausea and vomiting, and sweating that are often initially present after the snakebite. A broad variety of proteases are present in snake venom, which combine to produce varying degrees of tissue necrosis. Phospholipase A results in hydrolysis of red blood cell membranes. Connective tissue is broken down by hyaluronidase, which allows further spread of the enzymes and toxins present in snake venom. Snake venom usually contains a variable amount of amino acid esterase, which prevents clotting by partially splitting fibrinogen to fibrin. When amino acid esterase is present in sufficient quantities, the classic syndrome of disseminated intravascular coagulation can result. Finally, cholinesterases and anticholinesterases are present in some snake venoms, primarily in members of the Elapidae family. In addition to the effects of these multivaried enzymes, nonenzymatic polypeptides and proteins present in snake venom damage endothelial cells of blood vessels and result in capillary leak syndrome with loss of serum proteins.

Several neurotoxic effects may be seen both in the action of Crotalids and Elapids. The effect of neurotoxins is particularly impressive in the Mojave and Eastern diamondback rattlesnakes as well as in the Eastern coral snake.

Clinical Symptoms

All of the enzymes, proteins, and polypeptides of venom interact to produce a complex and highly variable pathophysiologic state in snakebite victims. Patients may present with a wide array of effects, including (1) multiple effects of the venom occurring in a specific sequence; (2) the simultaneous appearance of multiple effects of the snake venom; and (3) dominance of a single set of clinical symptoms until death.

However, the early *cardinal* findings in the snakebite victim are *immediate, burning pain; rapid swelling* (within 15 minutes) with *advancing edema;* and the *appearance of soft tissue ecchymosis.* In most patients, the bite mark shows evidence of the paired fangs. In many cases, particularly in children, nausea and vomiting, profound diaphoresis, and transient hypotension may be present. Patients that have been bitten by the Eastern diamondback rattlesnake often have a bitter, metallic taste in their mouths. A variety of other neurologic symptoms may occur following snakebite, including perioral tingling, numbness, fasciculations, tremor, weakness, miosis, ptosis, and seizures.

In general, how rapidly the symptoms spread depends upon the degree of envenomation, the patient's size, and the potency of the snake's venom. Edema, pain, and ecchymosis tend to advance proximally on the extremity. In some cases, vesicles or petechiae may appear at the sight of the bite as well as proximally. As the effects of the venom continue, there can be increasing edema with an advancing border and a decrease in the circulating blood volume, with resultant hypotension. Renal problems may occur as a result of either hypotension or the effects of hydrolysis of red blood cells. As mentioned previously, specific enzymes may be responsible for coagulation changes that result in a clinical picture of disseminated intravascular coagulation.

It is important to recognize that the clinical symptoms present following snakebite are highly variable. These variations depend upon the amount of envenomation, the size of the patient, and the patient's pre-existing medical condition. In addition, envenomation with three specific snakes commonly results in a clinical picture that differs from that outlined above. Patients bitten by the Eastern diamondback or Mojave rattlesnakes have relatively less pain and swelling than is seen following bites by other Crotalids, but neurologic manifestations are increased early in the course of their illness. Appearance of these symptoms at an early stage should suggest a bite by either of these snakes. In the case of the Eastern coral snake and other Elapids, there are even less dramatic initial systemic findings or changes in the wound site. However, 6 to 12 hours after the initial bite, profound neurologic symptoms leading to paralysis and death may result. For this reason, any patient even remotely suspected of having been bitten by an Eastern coral snake or other Elapids should be observed in the hospital quite closely. In the past, deaths have resulted because patients have been discharged owing to a paucity of initial physical findings. Later, rapid advancement of neurologic symptoms has resulted in death.

In addition to variations by the type of snake, two other areas warrant concern. In cases in which the snakebite has resulted in subfascial injection of venom, the early physical findings are often very mild. However, after a variable delay, there is the onset of profound systemic symptoms resulting from release of the enzymes and proteins in the subfascial space. Second, when envenomation occurs in highly vascular areas, symptoms may progress quite rapidly, and present with profound systemic insults. Snakebites on the scalp or into large venous beds, such as popliteal or saphenous veins, may result in quite rapid progression of symptoms and serious medical emergencies.

Clinical Classification of Envenomation

Clinical experience with literally thousands of patients suffering snakebites has resulted

Table 30–2. CLASSIFICATION AND TREATMENT OF CROTALID ENVENOMATION

Degree of Envenomations	Signs and Symptoms	Antivenin Treatment*
None	No local or systemic findings	0
Minimal	Local swelling alone, no progression	1–5 vials
Moderate	Swelling, pain, ecchymosis beyond the bite site; systemic and/or laboratory changes	up to 15 vials
Severe	Marked local reaction, multiple or severe systemic findings, coagulation changes	up to 15 vials

*In small children, the antivenin dose may need to be doubled to effect cure.

in classification systems designed to allow the practioner to predict *general* therapeutic needs. Such systems depend, to a large degree, on the presence of local findings, progressing in a systematic and predictable fashion. As noted above, there may often be exceptions to this sort of clinical picture. Thus, classification schema should always be tempered by the individual circumstances of the bite, the type of snake, and the physician's clinical judgement. Tables 30–2 and 30–3 list the envenomation classifications for both the Crotalidae and Elapidae family. In any situation in which extenuating circumstances (location of bite, length of time from initial envenomation, size of the patient, subfascial or intravascular envenomation, and so on) are present, the patient should be considered to have a more serious envenomation.

GENERAL MANAGEMENT OF THE SNAKEBITE VICTIM

All snakebite victims should be considered a *top priority emergency* until it can be clearly demonstrated that either a poisonous snake was not responsible for the bite or that the patient has not received significant envenomation. The initial 15 minutes to 1 hour of care is critical in ensuring that these seriously ill patients are appropriately cared for. All emergency medical personnel should be familiar with the appropriate diagnostic and therapeutic protocols for snakebite victims.

The initial approach to the snakebite patient is designed to satisfy four specific therapeutic goals. The first goal is to determine whether the patient was bitten by a venomous snake, and if so, what specific type of snake. Second, the degree and extent of envenomation must be assessed as well as the progression of symptoms and the current status of the patient. Third, for all patients with moderate to severe envenomation, it is important to determine if the patient has horse serum allergy, either by establishing a clear history of such allergy or through skin testing. Finally, the emergency medical team should protect the patient's life and limbs with aggressive therapy. However, all such therapy should be tempered by Hippocrates's ancient dictum: *"Primum non nocere"* (First, do no harm).

In order for the physician and the emergency medical team to attain these therapeutic goals, it is usually advisable to follow a protocol approach to the diagnosis and workup of the snakebite victim. Such protocols are based on clinical experience in treating large numbers of snakebite victims. The diagnostic and therapeutic guidelines provide a general framework in which to approach the patient. Nonetheless, it is always necessary to temper one's approach to the protocol

Table 30–3. CLASSIFICATION OF ELAPID ENVENOMATION

Degree of Envenomation	Signs and Symptoms
Grade 0–none	Positive history; superficial scratches with local swelling; no neurologic symptoms
Grade 1–moderate	Grade 0 findings plus any neurologic findings or the following: euphoria, nausea, vomiting, paresthesias, ptosis, weakness, paralysis, dyspnea
Grade 2–severe	Any Grade 1 findings plus complete respiratory paralysis within first 36 hours

with the clinical judgment based on the individual patient's circumstances. Further, in pediatric patients who are victims of snakebites, the patient's age and size become a significant factor. As mentioned previously, children are much more sensitive to snake venom than adults and usually require more intensive therapy and much higher doses of antivenin. An additional factor that effects the protocol approach to the patient is the time that has elapsed from the original injury. The sooner a patient is seen by a physician and emergency medical team, the more likely it is that early intervention with aggressive therapy will decrease morbidity and mortality.[6]

The following protocols establish the general guidelines for therapy in patients with both crotalid and elapid bites. Each is listed separately, since the symptoms and treatment vary widely between the two families. In addition, the treatment is also listed according to whether it is provided in either the field or the hospital.

Crotalid Envenomation

Field Treatment

1. *Transport the victim rapidly and directly to the nearest hospital emergency department.* If it is possible to do so, the snake responsible for the bite should be killed and brought in with the patient. However, the snake should be kept in a bag and away from both the victim and other potential victims. No time should be lost in chasing or killing the snake. If retrieving the snake will cause more than 10 to 15 minutes' delay, the patient should be transported to the hospital and the snake brought in by a separate vehicle. The first priority in all snakebite injuries is to obtain medical assistance as rapidly as possible. The old adage that "car keys are the best first aid for snakebites" is a wise one.

2. A *loose venous tourniquet* should be applied proximal to the snakebite site and well above the site of injury. Most of the major morbidity from the use of tourniquets has resulted from the fact that they are applied too tightly and for too long. The application of the tourniquet is designed to occlude superficial venous and lymphatic flow *alone.* The tourniquet should not be applied so tightly that the deep venous system or arterial system is compromised. In practical terms, this means that the tourniquet should be just snug enough that the fingers will easily slide under the tourniquet. In some cases, as a result of venous congestion and advancing edema, the tourniquet needs to be replaced during transport. In such cases, a second tourniquet should be applied well proximal to the first prior to releasing the initial tourniquet.

3. *Immobilize the body area where the bite occurred.* This serves to decrease venous return and relatively incarcerates the venom in the area of deposition. The victim should be kept as calm and as quiet as possible in order to keep the heart rate and venous return at a minimal level.

4. *The victim should not be given anything to eat or drink.* Aside from the fact that a number of patients with significant snakebites suffer nausea and vomiting, it is difficult to tell at the scene of injury whether surgery will be required for snakebite victims. Therefore, all snakebite victims should be given nothing by mouth until they can be evaluated by a physician.

5. If transport time is expected to exceed 45 minutes, *a call should be placed to the hospital emergency department* to advise them that a snakebite victim is en route. In all cases in which transport time will exceed 45 minutes, it is advisable to place a loose venous tourniquet to assist in incarcerating the venom. The field use of excision and suction has been debated greatly in the literature.[6–8] Detailed studies in laboratory animals have indicated that *immediate* excision and suction of the wound can result in recovery of a significant portion of the snake venom.[9,10] However, other studies have been less conclusive, and no detailed studies exist in human beings. At the present time, we do not advise excision and suction in the field unless transport time will exceed 30 to 45 minutes.

When excision and suction are used, several specific guidelines should be kept in mind. First, this procedure should be performed by medical personnel or those with specific training. Second, the procedure should be performed as early as possible, preferably within the first 5 hours of injury. Third, the use of cruciate incisions should be avoided. Instead, elliptical incisions of the fang marks should be used to apply suction. In cases of severe envenomation, some authors have utilized elliptic incisions around the bite site and to the fascia to remove the venom from the patient.[9]

6. *Avoid prolonged application of ice packs, but*

judiciously applied cool compresses may reduce metabolic reaction at the wound site. Application of ice cold packs may further increase the tissue necrosis caused by the snake venom by increasing vasoconstriction at the site of injury.

7. *The patient should be observed closely during transport* for both progression of symptoms of the snakebite as well as systemic findings. As in all emergencies, priority should be given to the airway, breathing, and circulation should systemic symptoms progress.

Hospital Care

1. The first step in assessment of the snakebite victim is to confirm envenomation. This should be done by a rapid but careful history taken from both the patient and any companions that can confirm the bite. In cases in which the snake is present, the physician should examine it carefully to determine whether the snake is a pit viper and, if so, what type. In cases in which either the history is vague or the snake is not captured, the physical exam may document the presence of envenomation. Classic fang marks (occurring singly, in pairs, or in multiples) along with classic symptoms of burning pain, advancing edema, and ecchymosis essentially confirm the diagnosis of crotalid envenomation. An additional element that should be considered early in the course of assessment of the snakebite victim is the timing and progression of the patient's symptoms. Try to determine as precisely as possible the time at which the patient was bitten. Question the patient, companions, and emergency medical personnel regarding the progression of symptoms. Rapid progression of symptoms suggests severe envenomation, which will require rapid and aggressive therapy.

The size and species of snake should be recorded clearly on the chart. When possible, the number of bites suffered should be recorded, as well as the type of bite (brief strikes versus prolonged, squeezing contact). The general location of the bite should also be recorded carefully. Bites on the scalp, those with subfascial envenomation, and those near the popliteal or saphenous venous systems may result in more rapid progression of symptoms.

The size of the child is a critical determinant of the relative need for invasive therapy. In general, the smaller the child, the more rapid the progression of symptoms will be and therefore the more urgent the need for definitive therapy. A final concern during the initial evaluation of the snakebite victim is to clearly document and assess the results of any therapy given in the field.

2. During the process of confirming envenomation and during the history and physical examination, two large-bore intravenous lines should be started, preferably in an extremity other than the one bitten by the snake. The usual fluid infused through these lines is Ringer's lactate with dextrose. Two lines are necessary, to ensure that one is available for antivenin therapy, when needed, while the other is used for intravenous bolus fluid therapy and invasive monitoring.

3. Early in the course of the patient's care, appropriate laboratory parameters should be assessed. These should include a blood count with differential, a coagulation profile (prothrombin time, partial thromboplastin time, platelet count, fibrin split products, fibrinogen level), electrolytes, urinalysis, and blood urea nitrogen and creatinine.

4. Unless the patient has a clearly documented history of previous tetanus immunization, appropriate dosages of tetanus toxoid or diphtheria-tetanus toxoid should be given.

5. Depending upon the degree of envenomation and progression of symptoms, antivenin therapy may be indicated. The following section details the specific elements of antivenin therapy, including appropriate skin testing for horse serum allergy. It is important to remember that the physician's clinical judgement is essential in assessing the need for antivenin therapy. In patients with rapid progression of symptoms, the general guidelines listed for antivenin therapy may need to be exceeded. In general, small children may require two to three times the antivenin dose recommended for adults with similar progression of symptoms.

6. Excision of the wound and suction are sometimes indicated in emergency department management. Such treatment should be offered only if the patient is seen within the first several hours after envenomation. While excision and suction can be extremely helpful in removing the venom, they should be performed only by an experienced physician, using an elliptical incision. Whenever the snakebite occurs in close proximity to the hospital, excision and suction should be considered.

7. The patient's extremity should be assessed carefully. The size and girth of the bitten extremity should be measured care-

fully and recorded, and the opposite extremity should be measured as well. It is usually a good idea to mark the advancing border of edema and/or ecchymosis with a pen in order to document progression of symptoms. If swelling and ecchymosis are severe, particular attention should be paid to the possible development of a compartment syndrome. Pain on passive stretch is the classic initial finding of compartment syndrome, but this symptom may be confused with the advancing pain of the injury itself. Therefore, additional clinical signs or symptoms of a compartment syndrome should also be assessed.

8. The role of fasciotomy in snakebite victims has been widely and heatedly debated.[11–13] In current management of snakebite victims, fasciotomy is rarely indicated. Most authors agree that as an *initial* treatment for the snakebite victim, fasciotomy offers no therapeutic benefit. However, in patients in whom edema has advanced significantly and a compartment syndrome has developed, prompt fasciotomy can result in dramatic improvement. Thus, the use of fasciotomy for treatment for compartment syndrome remains a time-honored concept. However, the development of compartment syndrome following snakebites occurs less frequently, probably because victims are more rapidly transported to the hospital and more effectively treated with antivenin. Occasionally, patients develop symptoms of a compartment syndrome several hours after their initial treatment with antivenin. In many cases, this represents inadequate initial treatment with antivenin, which results in progression of symptoms.

9. For all snakebite victims with significant envenomation, broad-spectrum antibiotics are advised.

10. The use of corticosteroids in snakebites remains somewhat controversial. However, the inflammation from snakebites results from pathophysiologic mechanisms that may be responsive to the mechanism of action of corticosteroids. For this reason, we generally recommend the use of steroids in snakebite victims.

Elapid Bites

Field Measures

Because the identification of the coral snake can be difficult unless the snake is killed and brought to the emergency department, and because the symptoms of coral snake envenomation may be markedly delayed, the field treatment of elapid injuries differs somewhat from those of the Crotalid family. Whenever possible, the snake responsible for the bite should be killed and brought to the emergency department to allow positive identification. If this is not possible, the patient's companions should observe the snake as closely as possible for markings to allow more precise identification.

Although the local effects of the elapid venom differ markedly from those caused by venom of the Crotalid family, early use of incision and suction and tourniquet application can be beneficial. The bite should be washed gently with whatever solution is rapidly available, the extremity should be immobilized, the patient should be kept at rest, and transported to the nearest hospital emergency department immediately.

Hospital Care

Care of the child with a suspected coral snake bite can be an extremely challenging problem. If the snake can be positively identified as a coral snake, it is much simpler to offer appropriate therapy. As opposed to the bite of pit vipers, coral snake bites often result in small lines of puncture wounds that are very similar to those of nonpoisonous snakes. There is very seldom a significant amount of pain, edema, or ecchymosis following coral snake bites, so the local findings do not distinguish the elapid from nonpoisonous bites. However, the neurotoxic symptoms developing because of elapid envenomation may occur as late as 7 to 24 hours after the original bite. Such symptoms can be lethal. For this reason, no patient with suspected coral snake envenomation should be discharged from the hospital. All such patients should be admitted for 48 hours of close observation.

Grade 0—No Envenomation. These patients have a positive history of a bite by a coral snake but no evidence of envenomation. There may be superficial scratches or punctures with mild local swelling, but no systemic signs or symptoms develop within the first 24 to 48 hours following the bite. In children with this degree of injury, two therapeutic options are available. First, the patient may be observed closely for the development of neurotoxic symptoms or progression of local symptoms. At the earliest evidence of any such symptoms, antivenin therapy can be begun. However, this requires intensive and sustained monitoring of the patient with close physical examination. For this reason, many physicians choose to treat patients with *documented* grade 0 coral snake envenomation with two units of antivenin, in order to bind the circulating neurotoxins. Additional antivenin therapy is withheld until further symptoms develop.

Grade 1—Moderate Envenomation. These patients have a positive history of a bite and local findings suggestive of coral snake envenomation, with mild to moderate local swelling. In addition, nausea, vomiting, euphoria, excessive salivation, paresthesias in the extremity, weakness, abnormal reflexes, paralysis, and ptosis may be present. Appearance of any of these symptoms documents grade 1 envenomation and requires appropriate therapy (see Antivenin Therapy below), including incision, when appropriate.

Grade 2—Severe Envenomation. This degree of envenomation is present when any or all of the grade 1 symptoms are present in addition to the development of complete respiratory paralysis within the first 36 hours following envenomation. Treatment of this degree of injury requires both antivenin therapy as well as appropriate short- and long-term control of the airway. A nasogastric tube should also be placed and suction applied to assure that the stomach empties appropriately. Appropriate enteral or hyperenteral alimentation should be provided according to intensive care unit protocols. In most of these patients, a central venous line and indwelling Foley catheter should be inserted. Oxygen therapy and renal dialysis should be administered when necessary.

Antivenin Therapy

Snake antivenin was first made available in this country in 1927, when Mulford's antivenin *Nearctic Polyvalent* was introduced. Prior to this time, snakebite therapy had been limited to efforts either to incarcerate the venom (by incision and suction, excision, or poultices) or to obliterate it (by cauterization, kerosene immersion, or chemical application). While there was an early decrease in mortality with such antivenin therapy, increased use of this therapy showed a high incidence of serum sickness and an inability to prevent peripheral soft tissue destruction. As a result, antivenin therapy did not attain widespread use until 1954. At that time, Wyeth Laboratories released a more powerful and less antigenic polyvalent antivenin. This purified product resulted in decreased mortality and had a preventive effect on local tissue destruction as well.

The extensive clinical experience of Russell,[10,12,14,15] Snyder,[9,13] Wingert,[16] and others[17] has clearly indicated that antivenin therapy can be effective in combating both local and systemic effects of snake venom and in decreasing mortality from snakebite envenomation. Because of this, antivenin therapy is an essential part of effective management of a snakebite victim.

The currently marketed pit viper antivenin is Anitvenin *Crotalidae* Polyvalent, a horse serum product produced by Wyeth Laboratories. This equine serum is produced by hyperimmunization of horses with four potent crotalid venoms. Elapid antivenin (Antivenin *Micrurus fulvius*) is produced by a similar process with coral snake venom injected into the horses. The resultant hyperimmune serum is then precipitated with ammonium sulphate, producing a polyvalent serum that cross-reacts with venom from all crotalids or the coral snake, respectively.

However, the production process is unable to remove all residual horse serum and proteins. Therefore, the antivenin contains horse serum albumin, IgG, IgM, and alpha and beta-1 globulins. The presence of these equine proteins accounts for the high incidence of serum sickness reactions in patients given antivenin therapy (see below).

While antivenin therapy is clearly appropriate for patients with significant envenomation by poisonous snakes, four caveats regarding its use are necessary. First, antivenin therapy must be given early in the course of the patient's disease. Any significant delay in providing such therapy results in increased local tissue destruction and further systemic spread of the toxin, with resultant widespread autopharmacologic effects.[4,5,9,13,14–17] However, even if a patient is seen many hours after the original bite has occurred, antivenin therapy should still be offered in appropriate doses to neutralize any remaining venom. Second, antivenin should be administered by the intravenous or intra-arterial route. McCollough and associates[6] demonstrated that when dogs previously envenomated with Eastern diamondback rattlesnake venom were treated with ^{131}I-tagged antivenin, 85 per cent of the antivenin accumulated at the site within 2 hours when given by the intravenous route. The subcutaneous and intramuscular routes resulted in 5.6 and 1.43 per cent accumulation, respectively. Numerous other clinical studies have documented the effect of intravenous administration.[8,10,14–17] Snyder has shown that intra-arterial injection combined with excision of the snakebite wound resulted in excellent results with no mortality.[9] His results indicated that intra-arterial injection required a decreased dose of the antivenin. However, most authorities currently recommended the intravenous route of administration, because of the significant ease of administration and clear-cut effectiveness.

Third, when antivenin therapy is instituted, the *full neutralizing dose* must be given. Failure to give antivenin in sufficient quantities to inactivate existing venom remains the most important therapeutic failure in the management of snakebite victims.[4] Snake venom can remain in the tissue and systemic circulation for days following the original injury, resulting in prolongation of both local and systemic reactions. Thus, undertreatment with the snake antivenin represents a common and serious problem in patients suffering snakebite.

Fourth, because pediatric patients have a large amount of venom injected relative to their body mass, children frequently react much more intensely to envenomation than do adults. Consequently, the usual therapeutic recommendations for antivenin therapy (Table 30–2) may need to be doubled or even tripled in small children.

In light of the above, antivenin therapy should be guided by the clinical response to therapy, patient age, time from onset of the snakebite, and rapidity of progression of symptoms. The goal of antivenin therapy is to fully and completely inactivate the venom. This is evidenced clinically by decreased pain, decreased advancement of edema and ecchymosis, and ablation of the systemic signs and symptoms of disease. It is better to slightly overtreat patients with antivenin and have circulating antivenin remaining than to undertreat and leave circulating venom. The general guidelines for treatment are based on clinical symptoms of envenomation and have been formulated from the experience with thousands of snakebite victims. However, these guidelines should serve as a general format and should be altered according to the patient's response to therapy. If increased doses of antivenin are required, the clinician should not hesitate to administer them under appropriate circumstances.

Skin Testing

Skin testing for horse serum allergies should be instituted only after a careful history for previous allergy has been taken and *only* when antivenin therapy will be required. If the patient's symptoms are not of sufficient severity to offer clear-cut indications for antivenin therapy, skin testing should not be done. However, it should be noted that current recommendations indicate that even patients with minimal envenomation (local swelling and pain) can benefit from antivenin therapy.[10,12,15–17]

Prior to skin testing, an IV line should be established, preparation should be made for provision of an airway and other resuscitative measures, and epinephrine, diphenhydramine, and steroids should be available. Although rare, anaphylactic reactions can occur following skin testing, and they require aggressive, intensive management. We recommend that the appropriate dose (0.01 ml/kg) of epinephrine 1:1000 be drawn into a syringe prior to testing in case anaphylaxis develops.

The actual process of skin testing for horse serum allergy involves intradermal injection of 0.02 ml of normal horse serum (1:10 dilution) and a like amount of normal saline as a control. (The 1:10 dilution of horse serum is provided in the Wyeth Antivenin Kit.) If horse serum allergy is suspected, the 1:10 dilution should be further diluted to 1:100.

A positive reaction to horse serum includes erythema and wheal formation, although some patients experience additional symptoms ranging from generalized itching and urticaria to anaphylaxis.

If the patient has a negative skin test, the physician should proceed to antivenin therapy based on the general guidelines of up to five vials of antivenin for minimal envenomation with higher doses used for cases of moderate or severe envenomation (Table 30–2). As indicated previously, small children often require larger antivenin doses than those just listed. In addition, when a clear identification of envenomation by the Mojave rattlesnake is present, earlier and more aggressive antivenin therapy is indicated, since the neurologic manifestations of this snake's venom can be substantial.

In patients with Eastern coral snake envenomation, one to five vials of *Micrurus fulvius* antivenin should be given. Such treatment *must* occur early in the course of therapy for elapid envenomation. Once the neurologic manifestations of coral snake envenomation develop, they may prove extremely difficult to reverse.

Antivenin should be diluted 1:2 or 1:4 with normal saline and given over 1 to 2 hours, or at the rate of 20 ml/kg/hour. Cardiovascular parameters, physical examination, and urine output should be monitored closely during the course of antivenin therapy. In patients with severe envenomation in whom hypovolemia has developed, large volumes of colloid infusion may be necessary, and the rate of antivenin administration may need to be increased. In patients with severe coagulopathy, fresh frozen plasma and platelets may need to be administered. If antivenin therapy is given early and in appropriate dosage, such coagulation changes are never seen.[10,17] Antivenin therapy should be continued until the advancing edema and localized pain decrease and systemic signs, symptoms, and laboratory indicators show a reversal of trend or clear-cut stabilization. If stabilization develops but symptoms are not decreased, 5 to 10 vials of antivenin every 2 hours may be administered.

Treating the child with significant envenomation who also has a *positive* horse serum allergy (documented by skin testing or history) is one of the most challenging problems in pediatric emergency care. All such cases require careful consideration of the risk-benefit ratio of antivenin therapy balanced against the risk of anaphylaxis. In general, patients with no or minimal envenomation should be closely observed for progression of disease after aggressive therapy to incarcerate the venom has been undertaken. If these patients' symptoms progress to signs of moderate disease, antivenin therapy should be begun.

With moderate to severe envenomation, patients should be pretreated with diphenhydramine hydrochloride 50 to 100 ml IV. The antivenin solution should be diluted 1:4 or higher and dripped in over 2 to 4 hours. If local or systemic findings develop, the infusion should be stopped and the patient should be treated with epinephrine 1:1000 in doses of 0.01 ml/kg or higher. In all cases of antivenin therapy with positive skin test allergy, it is wise to consult an expert in snakebite care as soon as possible.

Serum Sickness

Serum sickness may manifest itself as fever, malaise, rash, arthralgias, nausea and vomiting, or diverse neurologic symptoms. Serum sickness usually occurs from 3 to 14 days following initial antivenin therapy. Some authorities have argued that the high incidence of serum sickness following antivenin therapy should preclude widespread use of this type of treatment. However, Corrigan and associates[15] clearly documented that while up to 75 per cent of all patients receiving antivenin therapy in a group of 600 developed symptoms of serum sickness, most had mild symptoms and virtually all cases of serum sickness could be adequately treated with appropriate therapy. They noted that of the 75 per cent of patients developing serum sickness, 40 per cent had insignificant symptoms or responded rapidly to diphenhydramine therapy. In 30 per cent of patients, symptoms were more severe (fever, nausea and vomiting, angioneurotic edema, arthralgis, and so on), but all responded to antihistamine or steroid therapy. In 5 per cent of patients, the serum sickness reactions were severe and required intensive therapy, but even this small group of patients did quite well.

When serum sickness is diagnosed, patients should be begun on 2 mg/kg/day of prednisone, which should be tapered over a 7 to 10 day period. More severe cases of serum sickness may require pharmacologic doses of IV steroids and intensive care management.

Subacute Phase

Once the process of envenomation has been reversed, whether by incarceration, antivenin therapy, or both, patients with snakebite still require aggressive therapy. In patients with crotalid bites, there may be large areas of necrotic tissue and/or ulceration present on the extremities and proximally. These should be soaked in Burow's solution and a consultation with a plastic surgeon should be obtained for appropriate wound care and follow-up.

One interesting diagnostic problem that occasionally develops may occur several days after snakebite envenomation and following antivenin therapy. Some patients then develop malaise, nausea and vomiting, and other constitutional symptoms. At times it may be difficult to determine whether this represents an early serum sickness reaction or continued effects of unneutralized venom. In general, if *any* signs of advancing edema, pain, increased ecchymosis, or other progressions of the local wound findings are present, inadequate venom neutralization is suggested and additional antivenin therapy is required. If the patient's wound findings are improving or other specific symptoms of serum sickness are present, steroid therapy would then be appropriate.

REFERENCES

1. Fox JE: Rabies incidence highest in years. U. S. Medicine 19:(11):3, 1983.
2. Robinson DA: Dog bites and rabies: An assessment of risk. Br Med J 1:1066, 1976.
3. Snyder CC, Hunter GR, Browne EZ: Malevolent inflictions: Bites and stings. *In* Shires TG (ed.): Care of the Trauma Patient. New York, McGraw-Hill Book Co., 1979.
4. Pitts WJ: Snakebite. *In* Randolph JG, Rovitch MM, Welch J, et al. (eds.): The Injured Child: Surgical Management. Chicago, Year Book, 1979, pp. 331–367.
5. Klauber LM: Rattlesnakes: Their Habits, Life Histories, and Influence on Mankind. Berkeley, University of California Press, 1956.
6. McCollough NC, Gennoro JF, Jr: Evaluation of venomous snakebite in the U.S. from parallel clinical and laboratory investigators. J Fla Med Assn 49:959, 1963.
7. Jackson D: First aid treatment for snakebite. Texas St J Med 23:198, 1927.
8. Russell FE: Rattlesnake bites in Southern California. Am J Med Sci 239:51, 1960.
9. Snyder CC, Pickens JE, Knowles RP, et al.: A definitive study of snakebite. J Fla Med Assn 55:330, 1968.
10. Russell FE: First aid for snake venom poisoning. Toxicon 4:215, 1967.
11. Glass TG, Jr: Early debridement in pit viper bites. JAMA 235:2513, 1976.
12. Russell FE: Snake venom poisoning in the United States. Am Rev Med 31:247, 1980.
13. Snyder CC, Knowles RP, Pickens JE, et al.: Pathogenesis and treatment of poisonous snakebites. J Am Vet Med Assn 15:1635, 1967.
14. Russell FE: Snake venom poisoning in the United States. Experiences with 550 cases. JAMA 233:341, 1975.
15. Russell FE: Snake Venom Poisoning. Great Neck, New York, Scholium International, 1983.
16. Wingert WA, Wainschel J: Diagnosis and management of envenomation by poisonous snakes. South Med J 68:1015, 1975.
17. Simon TL, Grace TG: Envenomation coagulopathy in wounds from pit vipers. New Engl J Med 305:443, 1981.
18. Corrigan P, Russell FE, Wainschel J: Clinical Reactions to Antivenin. *In* Rosenberg P (ed.): Proceedings of the Fifth International Symposium. Oxford and New York, Pergamon Press, pp. 457–465.

CHAPTER

31 Foreign Bodies

MICHAEL E. MATLAK

I have seen
A curious child, who dwelt upon a tract
Of inland ground, applying to his ear
The convolutions of a smooth-lipped shell,
To which, in silence hushed, his very soul
Listened intensely; and his countenance soon
Brightened with joy, for from within were heard
Murmurings, whereby the monitor expressed
Mysterious union with its native sea.

WILLIAM WORDSWORTH, *The Excursion (1814)*

Children are innately inquisitive, and while Wordsworth suggests this characteristic may brighten their countenance with joy, this adventuresome trait may also place them in grave danger. Small foreign objects are frequently explored, and then misplaced into a variety of body cavities. The presence of a foreign body may result in more embarrassment than harm, but in some instances an acute life-threatening emergency develops. Annually over 500 children die in the United States from accidental inhalation or ingestion,[1] a statistic underscoring the need for a plan of action in dealing with this problem.

This chapter reviews the clinical presentation and management of foreign bodies of the ear, nose, throat, airway, gastrointestinal tract, and vagina. In simpler cases, the initial evaluation and removal of a foreign object may be safely undertaken by the emergency room physician. Management requires a cooperative, immobilized child and proper equipment, including adequate illumination, suction, extraction devices, and radiographic equipment. Many foreign bodies require endoscopic removal with a general anesthetic.

FOREIGN BODIES OF THE EAR, NOSE AND THROAT

Ear

Foreign bodies of the ear are usually easy to diagnose. A typical history reveals that an object has been placed into the ear, although it may not be seen externally. Often a child presents with pain and persistent purulent drainage from one ear that has not responded to antibiotic therapy. The examination should be performed under optimal conditions. Instrumentation should not be attempted unless the child is cooperative and the head immobilized. Topical or local anesthetics may decrease the pain, but usually adequate anesthesia cannot be achieved. Mild sedation may be useful in an anxious child but may occasionally result in greater fear and trepidation. If a child cannot cooperate, evaluation under general anesthesia is safer than risking impaction against or perforation of the ear drum.

Inspection of the ear canal is performed with an otoscope or operating microscope. The foreign body is easily seen unless obscured by purulent drainage. Suctioning is done gently to avoid bleeding or deeper impaction. Removal of the object depends on size, shape, location, and nature of the object. Small alligator forceps, a cerumen curette, or angled hooks can be used for removal. Irrigation with water may deliver the foreign body, but this technique should be avoided with a history of drum perforation or in the presence of blood in the ear canal, which suggests recent perforation. Water causes vegetable matter to swell and should not be used if this type of object is present.

Live insects, especially the biting variety, should be killed before removal. The ear canal is filled for several minutes with mineral oil, alcohol, ether, or lidocaine. The dead insect can then be safely and completely removed. After the foreign body is removed, the ear is reinspected for additional foreign bodies or damage to the ear canal or drum. Lacerations of the canal respond nicely to topical antibiotic drops while perforation of the drum requires oral antibiotics. Proper healing of the ear drum should be documented by subsequent examinations. Hearing loss may necessitate audiologic testing.

Nose

Nasal foreign bodies should be suspected in children with persistent unilateral nasal discharge. Radiographic examination is usually not helpful, since most foreign bodies tend to be radiolucent. The diagnosis is made by interior rhinoscopy with a nasal speculum. Good illumination and suction are again mandatory for proper examination of the nasal cavity. Topical anesthetics (lidocaine, cocaine) and vasoconstrictors (Neo-Synephrine*) usually permit a more comfortable and complete evaluation. The foreign object is usually located beneath the middle turbinate, where it can be grasped with a forceps, hooked with a curved probe, or removed with a suction catheter. Small balloon-tipped catheters (Fogarty† or Shiley‡) are occasionally used to extract the foreign body, but the cost of these catheters limits their routine use. The object should not be pushed posteriorly into the nasopharynx, since removal from this location is more difficult and there is danger of aspiration. If the object cannot be removed easily, examination under general anesthesia is necessary.

Once the foreign body is removed, both nasal cavities should be re-examined for residual material. The nasal discharge is cultured, and the child is placed on broad-spectrum antibiotics. Sinusitis, although uncommon, is a dreaded complication of nasal foreign bodies. If there is evidence of sinus involvement on x-ray, careful follow-up evaluation is mandatory. Consultation with an otolaryngologist should be considered.

Throat

Small, sharp objects, such as fish or chicken bones, frequently become imbedded into the mucosa of the throat. They often become stuck in the tonsil, pharyngeal wall, or base of the tongue. The child complains of sore throat, dysphagia, or neck pain following a meal of fish or poultry. Direct visualization of the oral cavity and indirect mirror examination of the hypopharynx and larynx are performed. In a cooperative child, the offending object, if visualized, can be carefully removed using grasping forceps.

Some foreign bodies of the throat are difficult to visualize. In these situations radiographs of the neck utilizing high kilovoltage with filtration have been most useful.[2] Since most foreign bodies are radiolucent, multiple views, especially the lateral view, are required for proper evaluation. Some centers recommend fluoroscopic evaluation of the throat with ingestion of barium-soaked pieces of bread, cotton or marshmallows. We have seldom found this technique necessary or helpful. Furthermore, the contrast media may coat the mucosa, making direct visualization in the operating room more difficult. If the physician still suspects a foreign body but cannot demonstrate it, an examination under anesthesia is justified.

AIRWAY OBSTRUCTIVE DISEASE

Laryngeal foreign bodies, while uncommon, provide a most challenging clinical problem. Most small foreign bodies that reach the larynx are either coughed out or pass into the lower respiratory passages. Some foods and objects, however, become trapped within the glottic region, resulting in an immediate threat to life because of airway obstruction. Prompt recognition and immediate management of this emergency are necessary to prevent asphyxiation.

Infectious Airway Obstructive Disease

Foreign body aspiration must be differentiated from three common infectious pediatric diseases: laryngotracheitis (croup), epiglottitis, and bacterial tracheitis. While each condition causes airway obstruction (partial or complete), their etiology, recognition, and management are quite different, as summarized in Table 31–1. The clinical history is of paramount importance in separating these entities. With aspiration, a previously healthy child chokes while eating or playing with small toys and *immediately* develops difficulty with breathing. With infectious airway obstructive disease the child has constitutional symptoms for some time and the respiratory difficulty is *progressive*. Most children with croup, epiglottitis, and bacterial tracheitis initially present with partial airway ob-

*Neo-Synephrine, Winthrop Laboratories, New York, N.Y. 10016.

†Fogarty Catheters, Edwards Laboratory, Division of American Hospital Supply Corp., Santa Anna, CA 92711.

‡Shiley Catheters, Shiley Sales Corp., Irvine, Calif. 92714.

Table 31–1. TYPES OF AIRWAY OBSTRUCTION

	Croup	Epiglottitis	Bacterial Tracheitis	Laryngeal Foreign Body
Onset	1 to 3 days	10 to 12 hours	1 day	Seconds
Etiology	Viral	*H. influenzae*	*S. aureus*, others	Foreign object
Location	Subglottis	Supraglottis	Subglottis, trachea	Supraglottis, glottis
Mortality	Very low	High	High	Very high
Treatment	Mist, epinephrine	Intubation, antibiotics	Intubation, antibiotics, tracheal suctioning	Removal

struction. It is extremely important to remember that manipulation or instrumentation of the airway may precipitate complete airway obstruction. These maneuvers should not be performed unless proper equipment, lighting, and personnel are available for immediate establishment of an airway.

If air exchange is adequate, we prefer radiologic examination before direct visualization of the oral cavity. A physician should accompany the child to the radiology department to insure that the airway remains patent. Equipment for securing an airway should be readily available. The initial examination should be plain roentgenograms of the neck in the frontal and lateral projections. Radiographs utilizing high kilovoltage with filtration[2] or fluoroscopy may also prove helpful.

Laryngotracheitis (Croup)

Croup is a common, usually benign, self-limited viral[3] infection affecting children between 6 months and 3 years of age.[4] Upper respiratory tract symptoms and low-grade fever are typically present for 1 to 3 days before these children develop signs of respiratory distress. Inflammation of the cricoid area results in inspiratory and expiratory stridor and a barking cough, while edema of the vocal cords causes hoarseness. Usually there is no sore throat, dysphagia, drooling, or preferred posture. Neck films reveal a long tapered narrowing in the subglottic portion of the trachea.[5] The epiglottis and aryepiglottic folds appear entirely normal on radiographs but may be erythematous when visualized by laryngoscopy.

The clinical scoring system proposed by Downes[6] is quite helpful in objectively following the progress of the disease and effectiveness of therapy. The clinical croup score is presented in Table 31–2. Most children are initially treated at home with humidification of the airway and clear liquids by mouth.[7] If respiratory symptoms persist or progress, or if the croup score is 4 or more, a trial of racemic epinephrine and supplemental oxygen is administered in either the emergency room or the hospital.[8–10] Children treated in the emergency room are observed for 2 to 4 hours, since rebound edema may occur following treatment. Racemic epinephrine administered by intermittent positive pressure ventilation via a facemask is more effective than aerosolized mist. Our customary dose of racemic epinephrine ranges from 0.25 to 0.50 ml of a 2.25 per cent solution mixed with 4 to 5 ml of sterile water.

Rarely a child will develop progressive or severe airway obstruction (croup score 7 or more) despite receiving proper therapy. Some of these children may actually have

Table 31–2. CLINICAL CROUP SCORE*

Clinical Sign	0	1	2
Inspiratory breath sounds	Normal	Harsh with rhonchi	Delayed
Stridor	None	Inspiratory	Inspiratory and expiratory
Cough	None	Hoarse cry	Bark
Retractions and flaring	None	Flaring and suprasternal retractions	As under 1, plus subcostal, intercostal retractions
Cyanosis	None	In room air	In 40% oxygen

*From Downes JJ, Raphaely R: Pediatric intensive care. Anesthesiology 43:242, 1975. Reproduced with permission.

bacterial tracheitis, but they still require endotracheal intubation or tracheostomy. Intubation is also required for hypoxemia (arterial PO_2 less than 50 torr) with supplemental oxygen, hypercarbia (arterial PCO_2 greater than 50 torr), and exhaustion. If the child's condition permits, these procedures should be done in the operating room with a set-up for bronchoscopy and tracheostomy immediately available. Endotracheal intubation is challenging because of marked edema of what is already the narrowest portion of the child's airway. Because of subglottic narrowing we suggest intubation with a tube smaller than the size predicted for the child's age. Using a stylet or stiffening the tube by immersing it in ice facilitates introduction of the tube. Since intubation is generally required for only a few days, a tracheostomy can usually be avoided.[6,11] Extubation is attempted when an air leak develops around the tube and tracheal secretions are diminished and thin. Steroids and antibiotics are not routinely used for uncomplicated cases.

EPIGLOTTITIS

Epiglottitis caused by *Haemophilus influenzae*, type B,[12] is a life-threatening illness[13] characterized by an acute onset of symptoms with rapid progression to severe respiratory distress in several hours.[4] Most children afflicted are between 2 and 5 years of age. Physical findings include an acutely ill, apprehensive child with high fever (39 to 40° C), difficulty swallowing, sore throat, drooling, mild inspiratory stridor, dyspnea, and profound respiratory distress. Breathing is easier when sitting up and leaning forward. The recumbent position may obstruct the airway. Respiratory arrest secondary to exhaustion or complete airway obstruction may develop acutely, accounting for the relatively high mortality in this condition. If the child's condition permits, it is recommended that roentgen visualization replace physical examination of the epiglottis in these patients. Under no circumstances should examination of the pharynx and larynx be attempted by inexperienced staff as it could induce instantaneous airway obstruction and death. Criteria for this diagnosis is marked enlargement of the aryepiglottic folds and/or epiglottis on a lateral radiograph of the neck.[5] The subglottic area is normal.

The mainstays of therapy are endotracheal intubation, systemic antibiotics, supplemental oxygen, and airway humidification in an intensive care setting.[14,15] Generally, racemic epinephrine is not helpful. The administration of steroids is controversial, but the current trend is to avoid their use. The indications for endotracheal intubation are any child who is diagnosed as having epiglottitis because respiratory arrest may develop suddenly and without warning. It is crucial to remember that if a child becomes apneic and unconscious, it is almost always possible to ventilate the child with a bag and mask at a slow rate with high pressure.[16,17] This manuever allows time to better secure the airway. Intubation is generally quite difficult because anatomic landmarks are obscured by edema and inflammation. Nasotracheal intubation by an experienced anesthesiologist in the operating room is our preferred method of managing the airway in these children.[18,19] The surgeon is also in the operating room ready to perform a cricothyroidotomy or tracheostomy if necessary. Most often a surgical airway can be avoided.

Extubation is usually possible in 24 to 48 hours. The best indicators for decannulation are disappearance of toxemia and diminution in the size and degree of inflammation of the epiglottis.

Since epiglottitis is an uncommon condition, especially in a community hospital, a detailed interdisciplinary protocol would help assure that proper steps in management are established and followed. Several protocols have recently been published.[20–22]

BACTERIAL TRACHEITIS

Bacterial tracheitis is a distinct, life-threatening condition sharing clinical features with both epiglottitis and croup.[4,23] Most patients are less than 3 years of age and have symptoms for 24 hours or less prior to presentation. These children are toxic with high fever (39 to 40° C). The brassy cough, inspiratory stridor, and respiratory distress fail to respond to aerosolized racemic epinephrine. The respiratory status may rapidly deteriorate. Radiographs of the neck reveal subglottic narrowing, while chest films may show focal infiltrates, air-trapping, or patchy pneumonitis. Direct laryngoscopy reveals a normal epiglottis and aryepiglottic folds. Passage of a suction catheter or endotracheal tube into the trachea results in the expulsion of copious amounts of purulent secretions (Fig. 31–1). Cultures most often grow *Staph-*

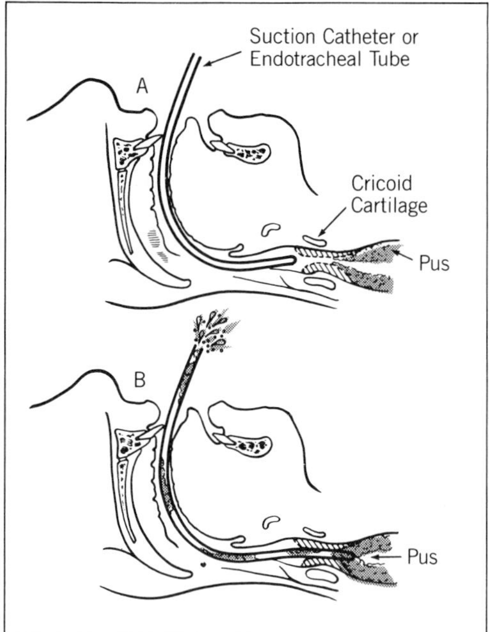

Figure 31–1. The pathophysiology of bacterial tracheitis consists of subglottic edema and copius tracheal secretions. (From Jones R, Santos J, Overall J: Bacterial tracheitis. JAMA 242:721, 1979. Copyright 1979, American Medical Association.)

ylococcus aureus, but group A *Streptococcus* and *Haemophilus influenzae* have also been isolated. In addition to broad-spectrum antibiotics, most of these children require endotracheal intubation or tracheostomy for relief of airway obstruction, and periodic tracheal suctioning.

Laryngeal Foreign Bodies

Children who aspirate foreign bodies into the glottic region generally fall into two categories depending upon whether the airway obstruction is partial or complete. While the recognition and management of each group is slightly different, both require expeditious therapy to prevent suffocation. An acute choking episode usually occurs while the child is either eating or playing with small toys. Foods most commonly reported to cause asphyxiation include hot dogs, peanuts, gum drops, chunks of apple, candy, sandwiches, potatoes, and other products; medications may also cause asphyxiation.[24] Nonfood objects at risk of causing suffocation are primarily toys or pieces of toys measuring less than 3 cm in diameter, such as pacifiers, rattles, rubber or wooden balls, marbles, wheels, balloons, screws, and nuts and bolts.

Partial Airway Obstruction

Children with partial airway obstruction may be capable of either good or poor air exchange.[25,26] With good air exchange the child is able to breathe, cough effectively, and make sounds. Hoarseness and stridor are usually present. The child should be encouraged to remain calm and breathe slowly. If the child is cooperative, he may take a deep breath and attempt to cough out the foreign body.[27] Methods that induce an artificial cough (back blows, abdominal and chest thrusts) are unnecessary and potentially dangerous unless the obstruction becomes complete.[28] Heimlich recommends the use of the abdominal thrust,[29] but most authorities prefer instrumental removal.[30] Artificial ventilation is not required, but supplemental oxygen is administered if it does not agitate the youngster. Blood sampling is usually avoided, since this may cause vigorous crying and poor air exchange.

The child is quickly prepared for the operating room, where direct laryngoscopy or tracheoscopy is performed. If time allows, radiographs of the neck may disclose the specific nature and location of the foreign body (Fig. 31–2). These films may assist in the choice of the safest anesthetic management of this problem. Options for anesthetic

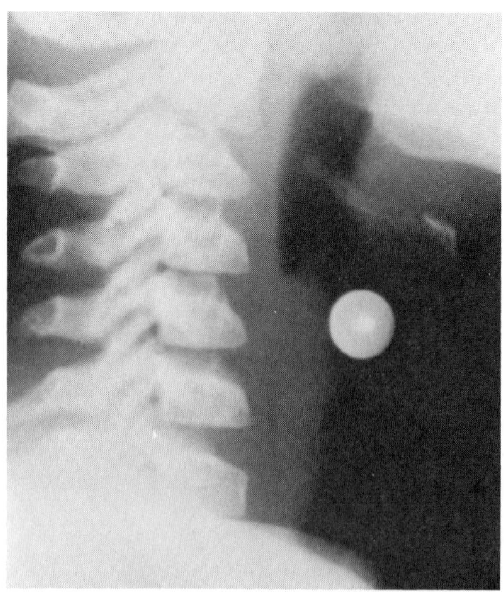

Figure 31–2. Thumbtack lodged in glottis, resulting in partial airway obstruction.

management include (1) awake oral or nasal tracheal intubation following topical anesthesia, (2) rapid-sequence induction of anesthesia using barbiturates and muscle relaxants followed by intubation of the trachea, (3) inhalation induction of anesthesia followed by intubation of the trachea, (4) intravenous barbiturate induction of anesthesia followed by insufflation of anesthesia using a nasopharyngeal tube, and (5) tracheostomy under local anesthesia.[31] Most of these methods are impractical and potentially dangerous in children because they require patient cooperation. Possible complications include loss of airway control, inability to secure the airway with intubation of the trachea, uncontrolled bleeding, and foreign body dislodgement with precipitation of complete airway obstruction.

Recently we described the induction of anesthesia by inhalation of halothane, followed by the careful placement into the trachea of a small cuffed endotracheal tube.[31] The airway was secured quickly and safely, thus negating the need for tracheostomy and its related hazards.[32,33] The possibility of airway obstruction from the foreign body during removal was also avoided. Only after the airway is secured are attempts made to extract the foreign material.

Complete Airway Obstruction

The choking child with partial airway obstruction but poor air exchange is managed

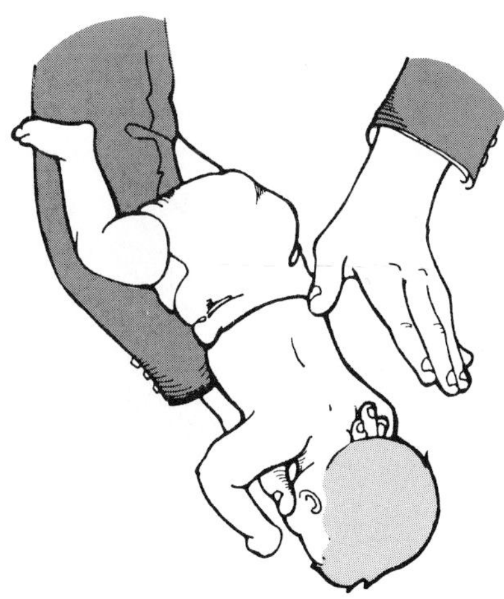

Figure 31–3. In a choking infant, back blows are delivered with the child in the head-down position. (From Lewis JA, et al.: A Manual for Instructors of Basic Cardiac Life Support. Texas, American Heart Association, 1981, pp. 145, 146. © Reproduced with permission. American Heart Association.)

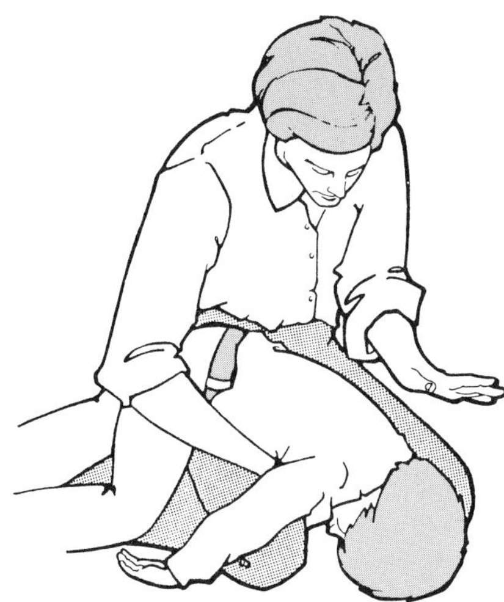

Figure 31–4. Proper way of delivering back blows to a choking child. (From Lewis JA, et al.: A Manual for Instructors of Basic Cardiac Life Support. Texas, American Heart Association, 1981, p. 146. © Reproduced with permission. American Heart Association.)

as a complete obstruction.[26,27] The child may be making vigorous respiratory efforts but ventilation is inadequate. The cough, if present, is ineffective. Inspiratory stridor may still be present but usually the child is unable to make sounds. Cyanosis of the lips, nails, and skin indicates the need for immediate therapy. Radiographs and blind finger sweeps of the mouth are not indicated.

The best treatment for the choking child with complete airway obstruction is currently the subject of considerable attention and controversy.[11,25–30,34–37] Scientific and sound clinical data are not available for review. Despite these problems, an expeditious plan of action is required to establish a patent airway. Management options include back blows, chest thrusts, abdominal thrusts, finger probing, direct laryngoscopy, and cricothyroidotomy.

Conscious Choking Child. If the victim is still conscious, we follow the guidelines of the American Heart Association, American Academy of Pediatrics, and the American Red Cross for basic life support.[25,27,28,34] The child is placed in the head-down position and four measured blows (back blows) are delivered in rapid succession between the scapulae as demonstrated in Figures 31–3 and 31–4. The child is then turned and four chest thrusts are rapidly delivered. A chest thrust is the same maneuver as an external chest compression for cardiac massage. For infants, thrusts are delivered to the midsternum, since the liver resides higher in the abdomen

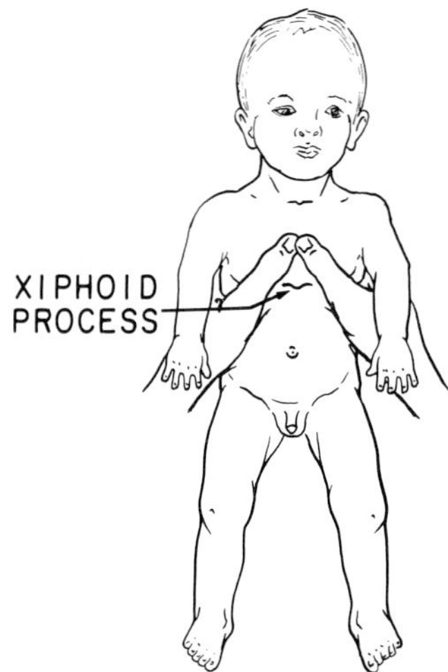

Figure 31–5. For a choking infant, chest thrusts are delivered to the mid sternum.

and is in danger of injury (Fig. 31–5). Chest thrusts are delivered to the lower sternum for children between 1 and 8 years of age. Currently, abdominal thrusts (Heimlich maneuver) are not recommended for children under 8 years of age because of the danger of lacerating the abdominal organs.[27]

Heimlich strongly disagrees with the approach of these authorities.[11,29,35–39] He suggests that back blows force the foreign body deeper into the larynx; and chest thrusts are too dangerous.[40] Thus, in his opinion the only acceptable first aid technique is an abdominal thrust. This maneuver delivers a rapid and strong force to the upper abdomen, pushing the diaphragm upward, compressing the lungs and expelling the obstructing bolus[39] (Fig. 31–6).

The American Heart Association contends there is no scientific or theoretic reason to suspect that back blows wedge a foreign object into the airway.[35,38] The procedure is easy and takes little time (3 to 5 seconds). Complications, if any, are negligible. The major value of this technique seems to be that it loosens the object from the glottis, thus facilitating further expulsion by other manuevers such as the chest or abdominal thrust. Which maneuver is safest and most effective in relieving the airway obstruction? No one knows. Despite Heimlich's arguments to the contrary,[40] complications from the chest thrust (cardiac massage) while well-documented are rare. Furthermore, this procedure may be as successful as an abdominal thrust in opening the airway.[30] The American Academy of Pediatrics contends that the abdominal thrust is more dangerous than the chest thrust, [28] but it fails to present any meaningful documentation to support this contention. Recently we cared for a toddler who had complete transection of his liver and a pancreatic injury following application of a single abdominal thrust by his anxious mother. The airway obstruction was completely relieved, but this proved to be a very expensive peanut butter sandwich.

Clearly, the abdominal thrust is very effective in relieving airway obstruction. How often in the pediatric population, however, does a Heimlich maneuver result in serious complications even when properly applied? Should a chest or abdominal thrust be tried first? Meaningful data to answer these questions are not available. Perhaps a combination of maneuvers would be preferable to a single procedure.[30] Whatever sequence or procedure is attempted, it must be applied

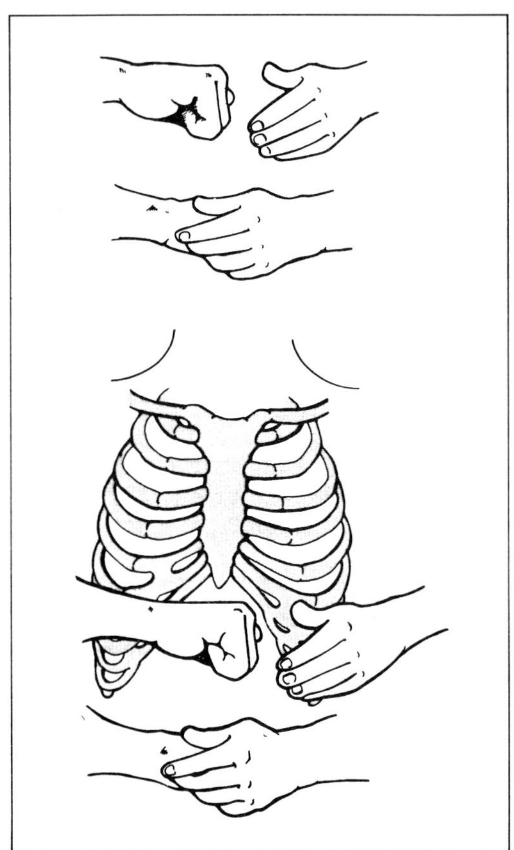

Figure 31–6. Proper hand placement for abdominal thrusts (Heimlich maneuver). (From Standards and guidelines for cardiopulmonary resuscitation [CPR] and emergency cardiac care [ECC]. JAMA 244:465, 1980. © Reproduced with permission. American Heart Association.)

Table 31–3. OPTIONS FOR MANAGEMENT OF COMPLETE LARYNGEAL OBSTRUCTION

Conscious Choking Child

1. Recognize airway obstruction
2. Artificial cough:
   a. 4 Back blows (3 to 5 seconds)
   b. 4 Chest thrusts (4 to 5 seconds)
   c. 4 Abdominal thrusts (4 to 5 seconds)
3. Repeat artificial cough until effective or unconscious

Unconscious Choking Child

1. Assess airway patency:
   a. Proper position of head and neck
   b. Open airway
   c. Remove foreign object if visualized (finger sweep)
   d. Attempt assisted ventilation (mouth-to-mouth, bag and mask)
2. For persistent, complete airway obstruction:
   a. Artificial cough (back blows, chest and abdominal thrusts)
   c. Attempt assisted ventilation again
   d. Repeat above steps
   e. Direct laryngoscopy
   f. Cricothyroidotomy

expertly and quickly because a life is in danger. The options for relief of laryngeal obstruction in the conscious child are summarized in Table 31–3. Note that finger sweeps, laryngoscopy, and cricothyroidotomy are not recommended until the child has lost consciousness from hypoxia.

Unconscious Choking Child. When a choking child becomes unconscious, the first treatment priority is reassessment of airway patency. With unconsciousness, the foreign body may become disimpacted or relief of laryngospasm may temporarily allow delivery of adequate air exchange by slow, deep positive pressure ventilation. Occasionally, the converse is true. Artificial ventilation may convert a partial into a complete obstruction.

The following sequence is recommended for the relief of laryngeal obstruction in the unconscious child (Table 31–3). The head and neck are properly positioned and the mouth opened. If the foreign body is visualized, it should be removed by the rescuer's finger or an instrument. If the object is not visualized, blind finger probing is not recommended as it may cause further impaction. Breathing is checked. If poor air exchange persists, then four slow, deep breaths are delivered by mouth-to-mouth resuscitation or ventilating bag and mask. Assisted ventilation may temporarily result in adequate air exchange and prevention of hypoxia. If the obstruction persists, the chest will not rise. Back blows, chest thrusts, and/or abdominal thrusts are rapidly, repeatedly, and persistently delivered. After each sequence, the mouth is reopened and gently checked with a finger sweep, and assisted ventilation is tried again.

If ventilation is still ineffective or impossible, direct laryngoscopy and attempted removal by suction or forceps are performed. Hopefully, the foreign body can be disimpacted, extracted, and airway patency reestablished. If these manuevers are unsuccessful, airway patency is rapidly established by either needle or surgical cricothyroidotomy. Ventilation is maintained by these means until the foreign body is removed or tracheostomy is established.

A cricothyroidotomy is indicated in any child with high-grade or complete upper airway obstruction when assisted ventilation is inadequate or when the trachea cannot be intubated.[41] In a life-threatening emergency, a standard tracheostomy is not recommended as the initial procedure to establish a patent airway, since it cannot be performed quickly enough to prevent hypoxia.

A needle cricothyroidotomy (see Fig. 1–3, p. 6) is performed by inserting a 14- or 16-gauge plastic catheter over a needle apparatus through the cricothyroid membrane. Because this membrane is soft in children, care must be taken to avoid intubation of the esophagus. After the stylet is withdrawn, an intermittent jet of oxygen is delivered to the catheter needle hub either through oxygen tubing attached to a Y connector or through a 3-mm endotracheal tube adapter attached to a ventilating bag. Oxygen must be delivered at a high flow rate. The jet of air may dislodge the foreign body into the pharynx. Exhalation occurs passively. If the upper airway remains completely obstructed, exhalation may be enhanced by gentle compression of the chest. Hypoxemia and hypercarbia develop in 30 to 45 minutes. This allows time for removal of the foreign body and establishment of a tracheostomy. The major advantage of this procedure is that it can be accomplished in several seconds. The major disadvantage is that large tidal volumes and high airway pressures may result in a tension pneumothorax, pneumomediastinum, or subcutaneous emphysema. This is particularly true if the upper airway is totally obstructed. Bleeding and esophageal perforation may also occur.

A surgical cricothyroidotomy is performed by incising the cricothyroid membrane (Fig. 31–7). We suggest using a No. 10 or 15 scalpel

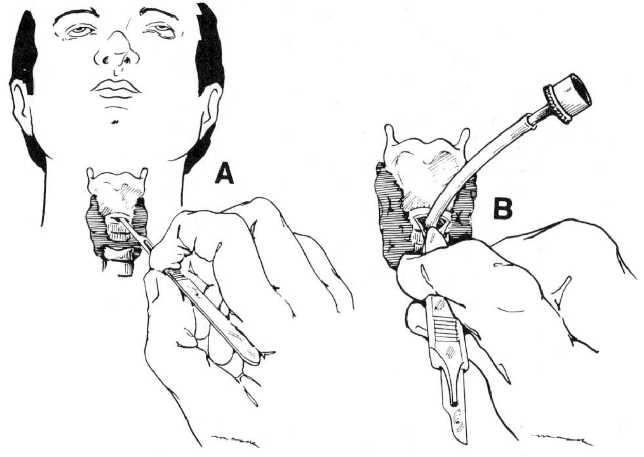

Figure 31–7. *A*, A surgical cricothyroidotomy is performed by incising the cricothyroid membrane with a No. 10 or 15 scalpel blade. *B*, A small endotracheal tube (3 or 3.5 mm) is inserted for ventilation.

blade and avoiding the pointed No. 11 blade, which may perforate the esophagus. A small endotracheal tube is then inserted for effective ventilation. This procedure allows rapid access to the airway but has a higher complication rate than needle cricothyroidotomy. Both of these procedures are temporary, and they should be converted to a standard tracheostomy as soon as possible.

Tracheobronchial Foreign Bodies

Aspiration of foreign material into the lower respiratory passages occurs frequently in children between 9 months and 3 years of age or in the retarded child.[42–46] The typical setting involves a toddler who starts choking and coughing while eating peanuts. Violent coughing, gagging, and cyanosis may occur and then the child appears to recover. Often the parents ignore this situation and medical consultation is obtained in a few days for evaluation of intermittent but persistent respiratory symptoms. The physical examination and radiographs may be normal. It must be stressed, however, that the history of initial aspiration coupled with the persistence of respiratory symptoms are the most important factors in deciding upon the need for endoscopy.[47] Foreign body aspiration should also be considered in children who suddenly develop asthma, or in those having persistent or recurrent pneumonia, hemoptysis, bronchitis, or bronchiectasis.[48]

In our society peanuts are the most common airway foreign body. Other foods commonly aspirated include fragments of carrots, potatoes, celery, peas, and seeds. Nonfood objects accidentally inhaled include toys, parts of toys, hardware products, and a long list of strange objects. The reason for the high incidence of aspiration in toddlers is unclear. First, permanent molars generally erupt at 6 years of age. The addition of these teeth greatly facilitates grinding and chewing. Furthermore, oral tactile sensation in younger children may be poorly developed, accounting for some difficulty in preventing aspiration. Whatever the reason, from a preventive standpoint we recommend that youngsters less than 6 years of age avoid peanuts, popcorn, seeds, raw carrots, and celery sticks.

Most bronchial foreign bodies are radiolucent, and initially the bronchus is either unobstructed, partially obstructed, or totally obstructed. The foreign body may be located in any bronchial segment; its location may change and the degree of obstruction may also change. It is not unusual, then, to see a youngster within 24 to 36 hours of aspiration who has a normal physical examination and a normal chest radiograph. A common error, however, is to send these children home without bronchoscopy.[47,48]

Physical findings will aid in detecting and locating the aspirated foreign body. The child may be short of breath, coughing, and febrile. Nasal flaring, chest retractions, and decreased chest excursion may be present. With partial bronchial obstruction, wheezing and decreased breath sounds will be heard over the involved lobe. With complete obstruction, no breath sounds will be heard. If atelectasis or consolidation is present, bronchial or tubular sounds may be auscultated.

The initial radiologic examination should be frontal inspiratory and expiratory films. A lateral chest film is also obtained. In an un-

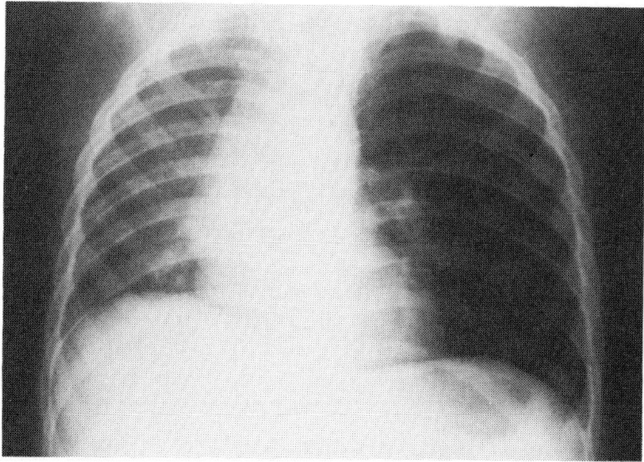
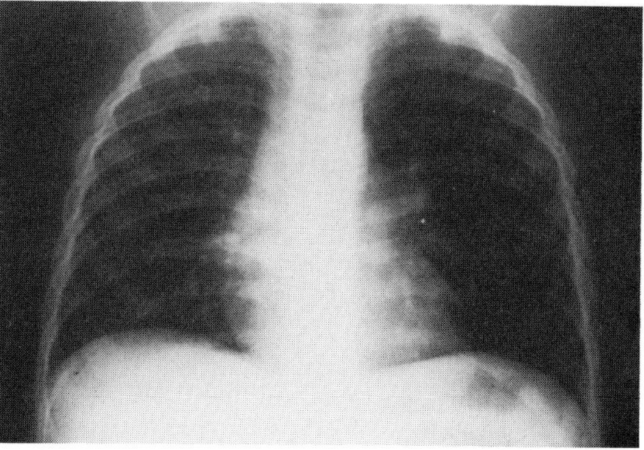

Figure 31–8. Left bronchus is partially obstructed by a peanut fragment. The expiratory film on the left demonstrates air trapping and a mediastinal shift away from the foreign body. (From Johnson DG, Matlak ME: Ambulatory pediatric surgery. *In* Wolcott MW (ed.): Ambulatory Surgery and the Basics of Emergency Surgical Care. Philadelphia, J. B. Lippincott Company, 1981, p. 477. Reproduced with permission.)

cooperative child, right and left lateral decubitus films are obtained. If these films are normal, chest fluoroscopy is warranted. The radiologic findings depend on the degree of bronchial obstruction. With partial obstruction air can enter the involved segment, but it is not completely expelled on expiration. The expiratory film will show air trapping or obstructive emphysema on the side of the foreign body with a shift of the mediastinum away from the object (Fig. 31–8). The decubitus films will also detect air trapping. In a normal child the mediastinal structures shift towards the normal dependent lung. In a child with obstructive emphysema, however, the mediastinum will not shift when the obstructive lung is dependent. If the bronchus is completely occluded, the film will show atelectasis or consolidation and a shift of the mediastinum towards the foreign body (Fig. 31–9). Usually these children have marked respiratory distress.

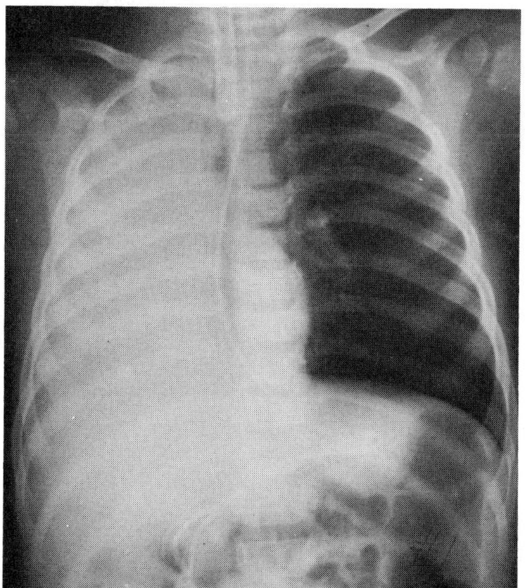

Figure 31–9. Complete obstruction of right bronchus from aspiration of a navy bean.

Bronchoscopy and foreign body removal is the treatment of choice for foreign body aspiration.[46,49] The timing of the foreign body removal is quite important. In general the earlier the extraction the better. Many children have a stomach full of food, however, which makes the anesthetic management potentially hazardous. When the respiratory status is satisfactory, we prefer waiting 4 to 6 hours before proceeding with the operation. If the respiratory status is precarious, then it may be best to proceed with early endoscopy rather than risk a respiratory emergency. Quite often supplemental oxygen is all that is required to temporarily tide these children over while the stomach is emptying. Newer infant and child-sized endoscopic equipment utilizing the Hopkins rod-lens telescope provides a magnified view with sharp resolution of even the subsegmental bronchi. Diagnostic evaluation and foreign body extraction can be done with safety and precision. Endoscopy performed by experienced personnel is also the safest procedure for avoiding retained foreign bodies and their sequelae. Most patients require a single day of hospitalization for postoperative chest physical therapy, airway humidification, and observation.

Several years ago, postural drainage with percussion and vibration was advocated as the initial treatment for youngsters seen within 24 hours of aspiration.[50,51] This method is uncertain, and only an exceptional child successfully expelled the foreign body. Furthermore, there is danger of dislodging the foreign body from the bronchus, where it is causing insignificant respiratory distress, into the larynx, where it may cause complete airway obstruction.[29] If a free-floating tracheal foreign body suddenly lodges in the larynx, subglottic edema and laryngospasm usually trap the object, preventing expulsion by methods that induce an artificial cough. The best therapy for this problem is immediate endotracheal intubation, which forces the foreign object back into the larger section of the trachea. Thus, complete airway obstruction is converted to partial obstruction, allowing time for transport to the operating room. An acceptable alternative is a cricothyroidotomy. If no equipment is available to secure an airway, back blows and abdominal and chest thrust may be given for complete tracheal obstruction, although successful expulsion is unlikely.

FOREIGN BODIES OF THE GASTROINTESTINAL TRACT

The majority of foreign bodies ingested by children pass uneventfully through the digestive tract. Some lodge at certain points, however, and require specific action. For example, esophageal foreign bodies require prompt removal because of the danger of aspiration and esophageal perforation. On the other hand, a foreign body that enters the stomach has a 95 per cent chance of spontaneous passage without the need for specific therapy. The clinician should be familiar with those foreign body ingestions that represent potential trouble, such as perforation, bleeding, or obstruction. This will help him determine the timing of serial radiographs and the need for hospitalization, endoscopy, or operative removal.

Esophagus

The most dangerous site for lodgement of an ingested foreign body is the esophagus. The child is in constant danger of aspiration, asphyxiation, and perforation until the object is removed. Thus, without exception, these children require prompt evaluation and expeditious therapy.[52]

An esophageal foreign body should be suspected when a child has a choking episode with something in his mouth. An asymptomatic interval commonly occurs, and this does not necessarily mean that the object has been coughed out or passed into the stomach. Other symptoms of esophageal obstruction include dysphagia, sore throat, a change in eating habits, excessive salivation (drooling), regurgitation of food, substernal pain, a suffocating sensation, or respiratory symptoms. A foreign body of the upper esophagus may compress or perforate the larynx or trachea. Thus, some children with esophageal foreign bodies present primarily with respiratory symptoms or symptoms of partial airway obstruction or a tracheo-esophageal fistula.[53] Occasionally a large esophageal foreign body will completely obstruct the airway, resulting in asphyxiation and death. On rare occasions a child may present with massive bleeding from erosion of the object through a major blood vessel or the heart. Thus, esophageal foreign bodies present in a variety of ways, depending upon the nature of the object, its location and longevity, and the presence or absence of complications.

Esophageal foreign bodies lodge at one of four levels of physiologic compression: (1) upper sphincter, (2) thoracic inlet, (3) aortic arch–left main stem bronchus, or (4) hiatus of diaphragm. Most objects are found in the cervical esophagus above the aortic arch. Objects may also lodge at previous operative sites or at points of congenital or acquired narrowing, such as strictures secondary to lye ingestion or gastroesophageal reflux.

Radiographic examination of a child with a foreign body of the throat or esophagus should include several projections of the neck and chest. These films may reveal the exact location and nature of the foreign body, the presence or absence of complications, and the presence of additional foreign bodies. Radiographic demonstration of a foreign body depends on its size, opacity, and site. Objects with slight radio-opacity, such as glass or bones, may be visualized if surrounded by air. Radio-opaque objects containing metal are easily demonstrated. Semiopaque or nonopaque objects may require contrast media for identification. If contrast media is used when esophageal obstruction is suspected, it should be used cautiously and in small volumes because of the danger of aspiration or interference with endoscopic identification. A limited esophagram is considered when the diagnosis is unclear or when balloon-catheter extraction is contemplated. Prior to the study a thin suction catheter is placed in the proximal esophagus for aspiration of saliva. The radiocontrast can be administered and removed carefully through this small catheter under fluoroscopic control to avoid the problems noted previously.

The nature of ingested foreign bodies, especially those of the esophagus, significantly influence recognition and management. Bones (chicken, fish, or pork) are the most commonly swallowed pointed foreign bodies. Usually they wedge into the pharynx or hypopharynx, but occasionally they imbed into the esophageal wall. Removal under direct vision or through an endoscope is clearly indicated.

Coins are the most common ingested foreign bodies in children. Most coins wedge in the cervical esophagus where they are orientated in a coronal plane. Detection may be delayed for weeks because of an initial paucity of symptoms. While complications are rare, coins can erode through the esophageal wall.

Large boluses of meat may be impacted against the cricopharyngeus, resulting in the so-called "cafe coronary." Recognition and first aid management have been discussed under Laryngeal Foreign Bodies. Meat lodged in the lower esophagus can be removed by balloon-catheter extraction, esophagoscopy, or dissolution with meat tenderizers. If the catheter technique is employed, the radiologist must be certain that the meat does not contain a fragment of bone. The use of meat tenderizers (papain, papaya juice, Adolph's, and others) is controversial because of numerous reported cases of esophageal perforation occurring with this technique. Whether these perforations are due to ischemic necrosis produced by the foreign body or digestion of the esophageal wall by the trypsinlike enzyme seems only of academic importance. As previously emphasized, esophageal foreign bodies should be removed shortly after discovery. For this reason most centers avoid the use of this mode of therapy except for isolated cases in which a general anesthetic may be hazardous.

Open safety pins are one of the greatest challenges to the endoscopist. Mishandling can result not only in perforation of the esophagus but of the heart and great vessels as well. Methods of removal include (1) bringing both ends of the safety pin into the lumen of the rigid esophagoscope, (2) endoesophageal version, (3) endogastric version, (4) straightening of the pin, and (5) the use of a pin closer. Fortunately, ingestion of safety pins is rarely seen today because of the common use of paper diapers and the use of large safety pins that are more difficult to swallow.

Fragments of commercial glass are generally difficult to detect radiographically, because the radiodensity is similar to bone. Surprisingly the incidence of complications of ingested glass is extremely low, although occasional disasters do occur. An exception to this generalization is the ingestion of fragments of a Christmas bulb.[54] The glass is very thin, brittle, razor sharp, and in multiple small fragments. Radiologic and endoscopic visualization is almost impossible. In this instance the glass tends to lodge, lacerate, and cause massive gastrointestinal hemorrhage rather than perforation. This is a serious potential health hazard to small children, and the best therapy is prevention.

Since the 1960s, aluminum pop-tops have littered our countryside.[55,56] In order to clean up America, environmentalists stressed placing the pop-top in the can, and thus, inadvertently, a new health hazard was produced. Furthermore, curious children love to place shiny objects into their mouth. A pull-tab measures 0.2 mm in thickness and 14 mm in width. They are only radio-opaque when visualized on end. For this reason, pop-tops are best visualized with a lateral radiograph of the chest (Fig. 31–10). Delays in diagnosis are still common. The foreign body may obstruct, ulcerate, or perforate the esophagus, resulting in a tracheosophageal fistula, mediastinal abscess, or massive gastrointestinal hemorrhage from erosion of a major vessel. Parents should be cautioned about this dangerous problem.

All foreign bodies in the esophagus must be removed. Watchful waiting is not indicated. The only exception would be the occasional child who has persistent esophageal symptoms despite passage of the foreign body into the stomach. If an esophagram is normal, the child may be observed, but esophagoscopy should be performed if symptoms persist for 24 to 36 hours.

Blunt, smooth, round, soft, opaque, or nonopaque foreign bodies can be safely removed with a balloon-tipped catheter by an experienced radiologist.[57] First, a small cath-

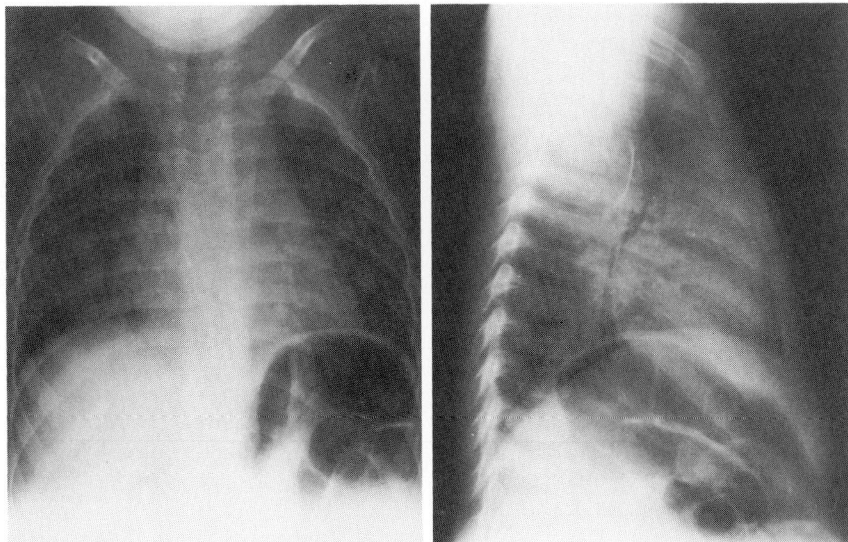

Figure 31–10. Aluminum pop-top is invisible on posteroanterior film, but it can be visualized on lateral view. The esophagus is perforated and foreign body is lodged against the aorta. (From Johnson DG, Matlak ME: Ambulatory pediatric surgery. *In* Wolcott MW (ed.): Ambulatory Surgery and the Basics of Emergency Surgical Care. Philadelphia, J. B. Lippincott Company, 1981, p. 478. Reproduced with permission.)

eter is inserted into the proximal esophagus for aspiration of retained secretions. Then a balloon-tipped catheter is passed through the nose and advanced beyond the foreign body. The balloon is filled with barium and under fluoroscopic control the object is gently disimpacted and withdrawn (Fig. 31–11). This technique has been successfully employed in

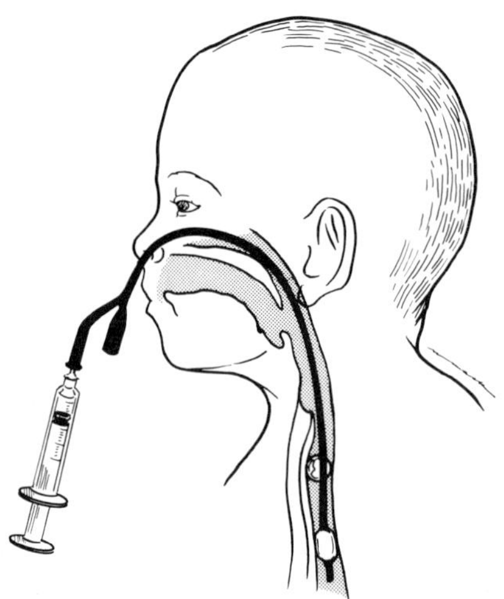

Figure 31–11. Demonstration of balloon-tipped catheter technique for removal of esophageal foreign bodies. (From Johnson DG, Matlak ME: Ambulatory pediatric surgery. *In* Wolcott MW (ed.): Ambulatory Surgery and the Basics of Emergency Surgical Care. Philadelphia, J. B. Lippincott Company, 1981, p. 479. Reproduced with permission.)

several hundred youngsters in our institution over the past 10 years. No complications have occurred except an occasional nosebleed. When performed by experienced personnel, the method of extraction is safe and inexpensive and avoids general anesthesia and hospitalization. It must be emphasized that pointed objects should not be removed by this technique, and one must be certain that a fragment of bone is not present in a piece of meat.

When the balloon-catheter extraction technique is contraindicated or unsuccessful, then a rigid open esophagoscope is usually employed for endoscopic removal of foreign material. General anesthesia is required in children, and this may be particularly hazardous because of the danger of aspiration. The complications of retained esophageal foreign bodies include asphyxia, perforation with abscess formation or mediastinitis, bleeding, hemopericardium and cardiac tamponade, endocarditis, tracheoesophageal fistula, esophageal obstruction, and chronic pulmonary disease.

Stomach and Intestines

Once in the stomach, 95 per cent of all ingested foreign bodies pass through the gastrointestinal tract without difficulty. Only rarely will a foreign body below the diaphragm cause complications such as perforation, obstruction, or bleeding. The usual treatment is watchful waiting, regular diet, and avoidance of cathartics. Most objects successfully negotiate the gut in 2 or 3 days but some require 3 to 4 weeks.

The nature of the foreign body influences management. Objects that are smooth, with no sharp edges or projections, almost never cause harm. Rarely they fail to pass or they obstruct, necessitating surgical removal. One important exception is swallowed small alkaline batteries.[58] Leakage of highly caustic potassium hydroxide produces liquefaction necrosis and perforation. Fatalities have resulted from esophageal perforation. Willis and Ho suggest that "if the battery becomes arrested in the esophagus, remains in the stomach for 24 hours or longer, or fails to negotiate the entire gastrointestinal tract in 48 hours, or if the patient exhibits signs of peritoneal irritation, surgical intervention is strongly indicated."[58] We prefer immediate removal of batteries in the esophagus or stomach. Recently, we removed a small battery from the stomach of two children by first passing a magnet into the stomach for retrograde advancement of the foreign body into the upper esophagus. A balloon-tipped catheter completed the extraction and avoided a general anesthetic and hospitalization.

Surprisingly, small, short foreign objects with sharp or pointed edges almost always pass through the gut without complications. Stools should be strained, and daily roentgenograms help monitor progressive movement of the object. Small amounts of blood in the stool may indicate a mucosal tear, but if the object is moving down the intestinal tract, nonoperative management is still warranted. Surgical removal becomes necessary when the object fails to move, or if evidence of significant bleeding or peritonitis develop.

The worrisome swallowed foreign bodies are elongated, slender objects (Fig. 31–12). Because of their length and pointed ends, these objects have difficulty negotiating the pylorus, duodenal loop, ligament of Treitz, ileocecal region, and sigmoid. As a general rule, an object 2 inches or longer in length in a 2 year old will not pass spontaneously. These patients are hospitalized because of the greater risk of complications and failure of passage. If the object is still in the stomach, removal with a flexible gastroscope is attempted.[59] If removal is unsuccessful, not possible or the object has passed through the stomach, then observation and daily radiographs are performed. Surgery is indicated if signs of complications develop or when the object fails to change position daily. Of particular concern is an object stuck in the duodenal loop or ligament of Treitz. Impingement or perforation in this area can cause thrombosis of the superior mesenteric vessels and infarction of the midgut. Frequent radiographs and early operation should prevent this dreaded complication.

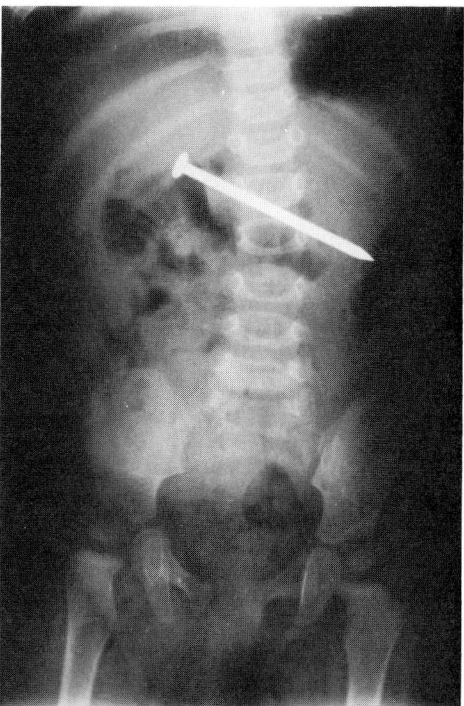

Figure 31–12. Worrisome ingested foreign bodies are long and slender like this nail lodged in the stomach. (From Johnson DG, Matlak ME: Ambulatory pediatric surgery. *In* Wolcott MW (ed.): Ambulatory Surgery and the Basics of Emergency Surgical Care. Philadelphia, J. B. Lippincott Company, 1981, p. 479. Reproduced with permission.)

VAGINAL FOREIGN BODIES

Occasionally the vagina serves as a favorite hiding place for small foreign bodies. Vaginal bleeding or a foul-smelling vaginal discharge usually bring these children to medical attention. Occasionally the foreign body can be palpated by transrectal examination, but often the foreign material is soft enough to elude detection. Instrumentation of the vagina in a small child is traumatic. A light anesthetic for examination of the vagina with an infant cystoscope or small speculum is the most satisfactory way to determine the presence of a vaginal foreign body.

REFERENCES

1. Accident Facts. Chicago, National Safety Council, 1980, p. 7.
2. Joseph PM, Berdon WE, Baker DH, et al.: Upper airway obstruction in infants and small children: Improved radiographic diagnosis by combining filtration, high kilovoltage, and magnification. Radiology 121:143, 1976.
3. Glezen WP, Denny FW: Etiology of acute lower respiratory disease in children. N Engl J Med 288:499, 1973.
4. Lockhart CH, Battaglia JD: Croup (laryngtotracheal bronchititis) and epiglotittis. Pediatr Ann 6:262, 1977.
5. Rapkin RH: The diagnosis of epiglottis: Simplicity and reliability of radiographs of the neck in the differential diagnosis of the croup syndrome. J Pediatr 80:96, 1972.
6. Downes JJ, Raphaely R: Pediatric intensive care. Anesthesiology 43:238, 1975.
7. Jones RS: Management of acute croup. Arch Dis Child 47:661, 1972.
8. Adair JC, Wallace HR, Jordan WS, et al.: Ten-year experience with IPPB in the treatment of acute laryngotracheobronchitis. Anesthes Analg 50:649, 1971.
9. Taussig L, Castro O, Beaudry P, et al.: Treatment of laryngotracheobronchitis (croup): Use of intermittent positive pressure breathing and racemic epinephrine. Am J Dis Child 129:790, 1975.
10. Westley CR, Brooks JG, Cotton EK: Nebulized racemic epinephrine by IPPB for the treatment of croup: A double-blind study. Am J Dis Child 132:484, 1978.
11. Day RL, Crelin ES, DuBois AB: Choking: Heimlich abdominal thrust vs. back blows. An approach to measurement of inertial and aerodynamic forces. Pediatrics 70:113, 1982.
12. Margolis CZ, Colletti RB, Grundy G: Hemophilus influenza, type b: The etiologic agent in epiglottitis. J Pediatr 87:322, 1975.
13. Bass JW, Steele RW, Wiebe RA: Acute epiglottitis: A surgical emergency. JAMA 229:671, 1974.
14. Adair JC, Ring W: Management of epiglottitis in children. Anesth Analg 54:622, 1975.
15. Lazoritz S, Saunders BS, Bason WM: Management of acute epiglottitis. Critical Care Med 7:285, 1979.
16. Glicklich M, Cohen RD, Jona JZ: Steroids and bag and mask ventilation in the treatment of acute epiglottitis. J Pediatr Surg 14:247, 1979.
17. Szold PD, Glicklich M: Children with epiglottitis can be bagged. Clin Pediatr 15:792, 1976.
18. Battaglia JD, Lockhart CH: Management of acute epiglottitis by nasotracheal intubation. Am J Dis Child 129:334, 1975.
19. Milko DA, Marshak G, Striker TW: Nasotracheal intubation in the treatment of acute epiglottitis. Pediatrics 53:674, 1974.
20. Hannallah RS, Rosales JK: Acute epiglottitis: Current management and review. Canad Anaseth Soc J 25:84, 1978.
21. Oh TH, and Motoyama EK: Comparisons of nasotracheal intubation and tracheostomy in management of acute epiglottitis. Anesthesiology 46:214, 1977.
22. Rayburn RL, Gatch G: Epiglottitis in pediatric patients. AORN J 36:59, 1982.
23. Jones R, Santos J, Overall J: Bacterial tracheitis. JAMA 242:721, 1979.
24. Baker SP, Fisher RS: Childhood asphyxiation by choking or suffocation. JAMA 244:1343, 1980.
25. Committee on Accident and Poison Prevention, American Academy of Pediatrics: First Aid for the Choking Child. Pediatrics 67:744, 1981.
26. Lewis JA, et al.: A Manual for Instructors of Basic Cardiac Life Support. Texas, American Heart Association, 1981, pages 145 and 146.
27. Report of National Conference on CPR and Emergency Cardiac Care held in Dallas, 1979: Standards and Guidelines for Cardiopulmonary Resuscitation (CPR) and Emergency Cardiac Care (ECC). JAMA 244:453, 1980.
28. Greensher J, Mofenson HC: Emergency treatment of the choking child. Pediatrics 70:110, 1982.
29. Heimlich HJ: First aid for choking children: Back blows and chest thrusts cause complications and death. Pediatrics 70:120, 1982.
30. Hoffman JR: Treatment of foreign body obstruction of the upper airway. West J Med 136:11, 1982.
31. Roberts LS, Rayburn RL, Matlak ME, Nixon GW: Unique method for the anesthetic management of laryngeal foreign bodies. Anesthesiology 56:480, 1982.
32. Gaudet PT, Peerless A, Sasaki CT, et al.: Pediatric tracheostomy and associated complications. Laryngoscope 88:1633, 1978.
33. Stowe DG, Kenan PD, Hudson WB: Complications of tracheostomy. Am J Surg 36:34, 1970.
34. Gann DS: Emergency management of the obstructed airway. JAMA 243:1141, 1980.
35. Gordon AS, Belton MK, Ridolpho PF: Emergency management of foreign body airway obstruction. *In* Safar P, Elam JO (eds.): Advances in Cardiopulmonary Resuscitation. New York, Springer-Verlag, Inc., 1977, pp. 39–50.
36. Hughes T: Comparative analysis of Dr. Henry J. Heimlich's data on 536 case reports of the application of the Heimlich maneuver. Submitted to National Research Council, July, 1976.
37. Patrick EA: Choking: A questionaire to find the most effective treatment. Emergency 12:59, 1980.
38. Redding JS: The choking controversy: Critique of evidence on the Heimlich maneuver. Crit Care Med 7:475, 1979.
39. Heimlich HJ: The Heimlich manuever. Clin Symp 31:3, 1979.
40. Enarson DA, Gracey DR: Complications of cardiopulmonary resuscitation. Heart Lung 5:805, 1976.
41. McIntyre KM, Lewis AJ (eds.): Textbook of Advanced Cardiac Life Support. American Heart Association, 1981.
42. Aytac A, Yurdakul Y, Ikizler C, et al.: Inhalation of Foreign Bodies in Children: Report of 500 Cases. J Thor Card Surg 74:145, 1977.
43. Blazer S, Naveh Y, Friedman A: Foreign body in the airway: A review of 200 cases. Am J Dis Child 134:68, 1980.
44. Johnson DG, Matlak ME: Ambulatory pediatric sur-

gery. *In* Wolcott MW (ed.): Ambulatory Surgery and The Basics of Emergency Surgical Care. Philadelphia, J. B. Lippincott, 1981, pp. 466–496.

45. Kim IG, Brummitt WM, Humphry A, et al.: Foreign body in the airway: A review of 202 cases. Laryngoscope 83:347, 1973.
46. Kosloske AM: Bronchoscopic extraction of aspirated foreign bodies in children. Am J Dis Child 136:924, 1982.
47. Puterman M, Gorodischer R, Leiberman A: Tracheobronchial foreign bodies: Impact of a postgraduate educational program on diagnosis, morbidity, and treatment. Pediatrics 70:96, 1982.
48. Katzenelson D: On the diagnosis of foreign bodies in the respiratory tract in children. Clin Pediatr 17:107, 1978.
49. Gans SL, Berci G: Advances in endoscopy of infants and children. J Pediatr Surg 6:199, 1971.
50. Kosloske AM: Tracheobronchial foreign bodies in children: Back to the bronchoscope and balloon. Pediatrics 66:321, 1980.
51. Law DK, Kosloske AM: Management of tracheobronchial foreign bodies in children: A reevaluation of postural drainage and bronchoscopy. Pediatrics 58:362, 1976.
52. Rosenow III EC: Foreign bodies of the esophagus. *In* Payne WS, Olsen AM (eds.): The Esophagus. Philadelphia, Lea and Febiger, 1974, pp. 159–170.
53. Newman DE: The radiolucent esophageal foreign body: An often forgotten cause of respiratory symptoms. Pediatrics 92:60, 1978.
54. Norberg HP, Reyes HM: Complications of ornamental Christmas bulb ingestion. Arch Surg 110:1494, 1975.
55. Burrington JD: Aluminum "pop tops." JAMA 235:2614, 1976.
56. Rogers LF, Igini JP: Beverage can pull-tabs. JAMA 233:345, 1975.
57. Nixon GW: Foley catheter method of esophageal foreign body removal: Extension of applications. Am J Radiol 132:441, 1979.
58. Willis GA, Ho WC: Perforation of Meckel's diverticulum by an alkaline hearing aid battery. Can Med Assn J 126:497, 1982.
59. Christie DL, Ament ME: Removal of foreign bodies from the esophagus and stomach with flexible fiberoptic panendoscopes. Pediatrics 57:931, 1976.

SECTION

IV Organization and Management of Pediatric Emergency Care

CHAPTER

32 Organization of a Regional Pediatric Trauma and Emergency Center

J. ALEX HALLER, JR.

Regional centers of excellence for specialized medical care are well-tested sources of medical care in the United States. These regional centers have developed in a number of speciality areas, including cancer, heart disease, burns, and newborn and infant care. As a result of this centralization of specialized care, significant decreases in duplication of medical services have been accomplished and individuals with specialized skills and technical know-how have been concentrated in units that provide the best care for complicated medical problems. This has been true not only in closely related disciplines such as cardiology and cardiac surgery but also in neonatal centers, where surgeons skilled in the operative care of newborn babies, neonatologists, and pediatric radiologists can work together. Another good example of regionalization has been the development of cancer centers, which include many complicated technologies under one roof or in one center, where close interplay can occur in the management of individual patients, allowing the accumulation of new clinical knowledge and the formulation of standards of care throughout the United States.

REGIONAL TRAUMA CENTERS

Following the lead of these specialized centers of excellence, regional trauma centers have gradually evolved to focus on the "disease of modern society," as trauma has been called by physicians working in the field of multiple systems injuries. One of the earliest of these regional trauma centers was the Maryland Shock Trauma Unit under the direction of Dr. R. A. Cowley. It has subsequently developed into a more complex statewide emergency system now called the Maryland Institute of Emergency Medical Services. Within a few years of the establishment of this center similar trauma centers were organized and had a very impressive impact on the management of trauma in the San Francisco area, in Chicago,[1] and in Denver, to mention but a few of the leading trauma centers in the United States. Fortunately, these centers recognized the importance of new information. One of their components was clinical research, and in a few centers, basic laboratory research was carried out on resuscitation and the metabolism and pathophysiology of major injuries. These research interests received delayed but ultimately important support from the National Institutes of Health, with the organization of trauma clinical research units in a few major centers throughout the country. The development, evolution, and future of these clinical research units have been well documented and discussed by one of their early and innovative contributors, Dr. Charles Baxter, in his presidential address to the American Association of the Surgery of Trauma (October 1981).[2] These research units have been responsible for the development of standards of care based upon solid clinical and laboratory research. In this way the acute care of patients has been improved, and to some extent the long-term care and ultimate outcome have been enhanced.

Research centers supported by these includes the contributions of Shires and associates[3] to the identification of crystalloid solutions as the appropriate replacement fluid for patients with hemorrhagic or hypovolemic shock; Peter's work[4] toward a better understanding of the pathophysiology of adult respiratory distress syndrome; and the proposals of Pruit and colleagues[5] for the initial management of the burn wound, including use of topical antibiotic and antiseptic solutions; and the eventual development of standards of initial resuscitation, emphasizing the ABCs of trauma care,[6] which have been formalized in the recent instructional courses of the American College of Surgeons, entitled Advanced Trauma Life Support Courses. All of these advances are a result of the basic concept of regional centers of excellence for specialized care of trauma.

The ultimate value of such systems will be reflected in a lower mortality and morbidity from the diseases upon which they are focused. There is now clear evidence that regional trauma centers not only improve the outcome of resuscitation in life-threating injuries, but, as a result of this focused attention, also promote better systems of transportation from the scene of the accident to the appropriate center as well as ongoing intensive care within the trauma institution.[7–9] This systems approach is still evolving,[10] but the model is there and the preliminary evidence clearly supports the value of regional centers to improved care of this complicated disease entity called *trauma*.

Although much progress has occurred in regionalized care for special problems, and trauma is one of the outstanding examples of the effectiveness of this approach to management, care of the severely injured child has not received adequate identification and emphasis. Until the last few years there had been no loud outcry for specialized care of children with major injuries.[11, 12] Only when it is recognized that more than 50 per cent of the deaths in the childhood years from 1 to 14 in the United States are a result of major trauma, as compared with approximately 1 death in 10 from injuries in the total general population, do we begin to realize the impact of trauma (Fig. 32–1). A similar situation is present in all the industrialized nations of the world, but in the United States we must focus more actively on this special problem in children. Trauma is clearly the leading cause of death by a wide margin.[13]

The death of a *normal child* is in itself a great tragedy, and most children with major injuries are normal, since they have already come through the period of early infancy without birth defects or major congenital abnormalities (or these have been corrected).[14] On the other hand, crippling injuries to a child and the resulting need for rehabilitation may have an even greater impact on our health care system.[15] The expenditure of resources and personnel as well as the economic loss from termination of work potential in a child are relatively enormous when compared with similar costs resulting from adult injuries. This is true not

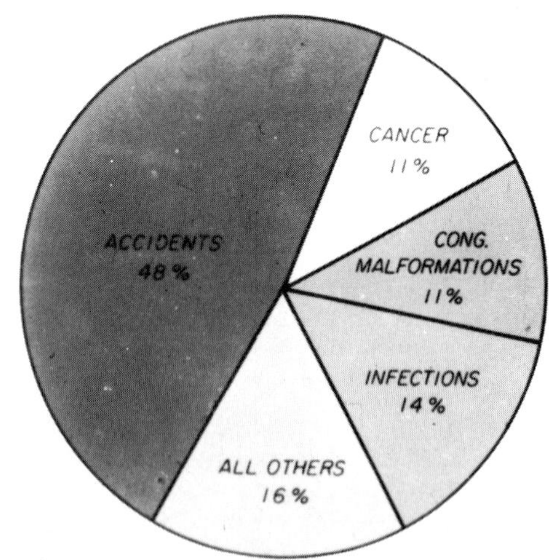

Figure 32–1. Causes of death in children, ages 1 to 14 years, in the United States, 1980. Trauma accounts for nearly half of all deaths in this age group.

only because of the long-term nature of such rehabilitation but also because of the growth and development that must take place simultaneously in an immature child. These adjustments to severe disability and a child's image of himself as an incomplete individual may be overwhelming to a young patient unless highly trained professionals participate in the process of recovery. It has been estimated that more than 100,000 children are seriously crippled each year by accidents and that more than 2 million may be temporarily incapacitated by their injuries.[16, 17] The need for emergency resuscitation as well as long-term rehabilitation will put further strains on overburdened health care systems unless we can prevent more accidents and become more aggressive in acute care management, which will decrease the need for long-term rehabilitation.

As in the case with other diseases, each region must solve its own organizational problems based upon its available facilities and potential, but perhaps no mode exists that is ideal for the management of major injuries in children. Nevertheless, the first such unit organized specifically for the management of life-threatening injuries in children in a large university hospital took place in 1973 at the Johns Hopkins Children's Center.[17] This unit will be described in detail as *one approach* to system management of major injuries in children.

A statewide emergency trauma system has existed in Maryland since 1958. Beginning early in 1960, the Division of Pediatric Surgery at Johns Hopkins was intimately involved in the overall system of the development of triage of emergency care in Maryland, and ultimately the decision was made to designate the Hopkins Children's Center as a regional pediatric trauma center for the entire state of Maryland, to which children with life-threatening injuries, except burns and isolated eye and hand injuries, would be preferentially taken both by land transport and by helicopter. Since 1973 major pediatric trauma cases have been transported to the John Hopkins Emergency Room by state police helicopter and fire department ambulance. A few children are initially evacuated from the site of injury and treated at outlying hospitals and then transferred after consultation to the Children's Regional Trauma Center. Care in the field is provided by emergency medical technicians, all of whom have been trained under the direction of the Emergency Medical Systems Training Program and have received special instruction in the handling of pediatric trauma cases.

The mother program for emergency care is the Maryland Institute of Emergency Medical Services, which is composed of five arbitrarily selected but geographically appropriate regions in the state, each with an administrative director and with physician representatives on the advisory board to the Maryland Center. It is within these regions that organization of emergency care has taken place, using guidelines locally developed and based upon facilities and available personnel. These programs are correlated and ultimately administered through the Maryland Institute of Emergency Medical Services (Fig. 32–2). The child component of this plan was developed

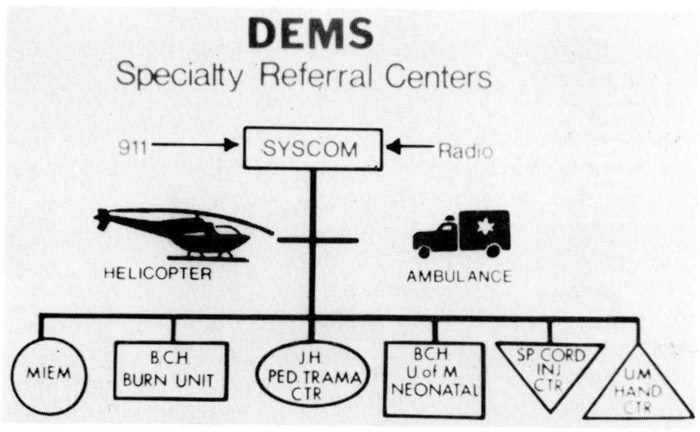

Figure 32–2. Diagram showing the components of the Division of Emergency Medical Services (DEMS).

within the general organizational structure and utilizes all the systems that were already in effect.

COMPONENTS OF THE REGIONAL PEDIATRIC TRAUMA CENTER

Communication System

The support components of the communication system include police *helicopter transport* on a radio-controlled basis, which is initiated through an *emergency medical relay center*. This center functions as a communication link for the system. Transport is arranged through the relay center for each case and the appropriate specialty facility to which the patient should be taken is also determined. *Two-way radio communication* with the emergency medical technicians at the scene of an emergency not only allows for physician communication and advice but also identifies the presence or absence of medical specialists in nearby hospitals and determines the destination of the individual patient whether a child or an adult.

Transport System

The *emergency medical technicians* receive specialized training in the care of newborn infants and children from medical specialists such as neonatologists, pediatric surgeons, and anesthesiologists. They are qualified to begin intravenous (IV) treatment for small infants and to intubate babies and young children if this is indicated. Their training is a part of the ongoing training program for emergency medical technicians within the state system. Care of pediatric emergencies is also included in the training program for fire department ambulance personnel in the Baltimore metropolitan area. Children with major life-threatening injuries within the Baltimore metropolitan area are usually transported in fire department ambulances rather than by state police helicopter. These children are also brought to the Hopkins Children's Center after consultation through the emergency medical relay center and after direct communication with both the emergency room and the pediatric intensive care unit.

Pediatric Trauma Center

The Regional Pediatric Trauma Center is an entity consisting of multiple facilities in several locations that are integrated programatically within the Johns Hopkins Hospital. The facilities are located within the Children's Center and attached emergency room buildings.

After communication from the scene of the life-threatening injury, a child is brought by appropriate transport, i.e., state-wide helicopter or city-wide fire department ambulance, to either the helicopter landing pad on top of the Children's Center or to the emergency room on the ground floor (Fig. 32–3). The child is met by a team of pediatric emergency physicians and pediatric surgery specialists who are trained in initial resuscitation and management of life-threatening injuries. The geography of the system includes a ramp that connects the helipad to a dedicated emergency elevator, which within seconds delivers the injured child to the emergency room for resuscitation or to the pediatric intensive care unit or to the pediatric operating rooms at the discretion of the resuscitating trauma team. This dedicated elevator is thus the connecting link to all components

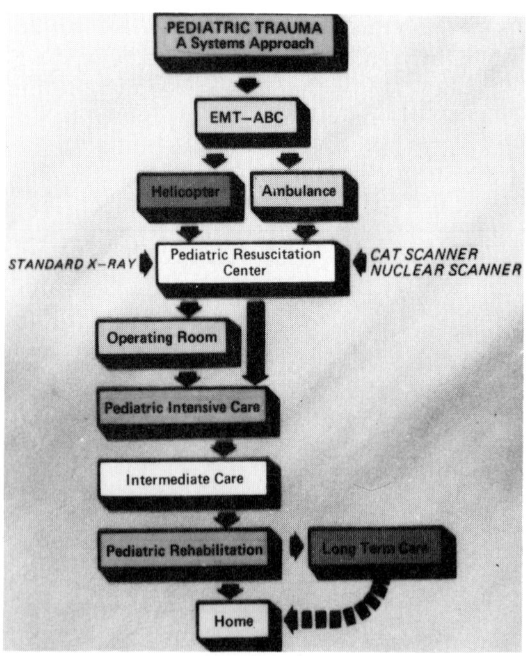

Figure 32–3. A systematic and regionalized approach to trauma care has resulted in significant reduction of morbidity and mortality.

of the trauma center and is controlled by keys maintained by the trauma center staff.

The child is managed in a resuscitation unit designed specifically for children, and it has miniature intubation equipment, including tracheostomy tubes, and other specialized equipment for children, such as central venous pressure lines. This unit is one of four for resuscitation of life-threatening conditions and is converted into a specialized pediatric resuscitation unit by a mobile unit containing all the necessary equipment.

The captain of the resuscitation team is either the senior resident in pediatric surgery or a staff pediatric surgeon working closely with the appropriate pediatric surgical specialists, such as pediatric neurosurgeons and pediatric orthopedic surgeons. X-ray equipment is immediately available in the unit for both the initial diagnostic studies and subsequent special films. It is important to emphasize that all children with injuries are resuscitated by pediatricians and pediatric surgeons, all of whom are part of the pediatric trauma team.

After resuscitation and stabilization and appropriate diagnostic tests and specialty consultations, a child may go directly to the operating room or be admitted to a 14-bed pediatric intensive care unit with a four-bed component dedicated specifically to the care of children with major injuries. Patients with multiple systems injuries are admitted on the general pediatric surgery service and are closely followed in consultation with both the pediatric intensivists and thepediatric surgical specialists who are involved in the management of different organ systems. Subsequently, the child may be transferred to a specialty service if a single organ becomes the predominant problem, such as a major head injury, with no other organ systems importantly involved.

Pediatric Intensive Care Unit

The inpatient focal point of the Pediatric Trauma Center is the 14-bed pediatric intensive care unit, which is directed by a pediatric intensive care specialist with a background in pediatric anesthesia and pediatric acute care. All the patient stations are equipped with sophisticated multiple-channel monitoring equipment and ventilators, but the four-bed trauma unit is specifically organized for the management of multiple injuries and has equipment for the immediate detection of cardiopulmonary arrest, for resuscitation, and for continuing post-trauma management. Other equipment includes a mass spectrometer, cardiac output computers, blood gas analyzers, ionized calcium analyzers, and pacard gamma camera for determination of cardiac output and similar clinical research studies. A small dedicated onsite blood gas laboratory provides immediate access to blood gas determination.

Pediatric Surgical Operating Room

Within a few hundred feet on the same floor is the general operating room suite, which includes a dedicated operating room for the management of emergencies in children. This pediatric operating room has temperature control and special lighting and anesthesia facilities, which make it appropriate for the operative management of multiple injuries. Although it is not used exclusively for trauma, it is assigned to the pediatric surgeons and may be pre-empted at any time for the management of trauma. This priority of surgical care is initiated by a communication alert to the regional trauma center that a child with life-threatening injuries is arriving. In this way there is not delay in the operative management of children who require emergency surgery.

Additional Facilities

Three important additional facilities round out the total concept of a regional center for the care of major trauma in children. These are (1) an *intermediate care unit*, which is under the direction of pediatric neurologists, (2) *a pediatric rehabilitation unit* under the direction of a pediatric physiatrist, and (3) *a long-term care facility* for children who have chronic rehabilitation and nursing needs.

The neurology-neurosurgery intermediate unit for pediatric trauma is directed by a pediatric neurosurgeon and a pediatric neurologist who both have special interests in the care of the child with head injuries. This is a direct continuation of the intensive care of those children with severe brain injuries, including continued monitoring of their neurologic recovery as soon as they no longer require constant monitoring and the use of intracranial bolt measurements.[18, 19] Within this unit, pediatric rehabilitation begins, and the work of the pediatric physiatrist becomes an increasingly important component of patient management.

Preliminary evidence from this experience strongly suggests that children with major head injuries producing coma lasting longer than 24 hours have a greatly improved recovery rate over that reported in the literature. Data suggest that only 6 per cent of the total and 9 per cent of the surviving children have any intellectual or motor residual defects, and 88 per cent of the survivors over 2 years of age have good recovery without measurable major motor or intellectual deficits. It remains to be seen whether these preliminary data predict continuing trends, but certainly they are encouraging.[20–22]

The new Pediatric Trauma Rehabilitation Unit is a component of the John F. Kennedy Rehabilitation Institute and has a high priority within that institution. A four-bed unit has been designed, and it allows for inpatient care and parent participation in ongoing rehabilitation programs and evaluation. This provides for better day-to-day patient care and also an opportunity for studying the emotional and physical responses to rehabilitation and for designing new protocols for treatment.

A pediatric trauma long-term rehabilitation and management unit is housed in an affiliated children's nursing home and has committed itself to long-term management of children with residual neurologic and physical problems following major injuries. This unit has full-time supervision by a pediatrician and also has all of the physician members of the pediatric trauma group at Johns Hopkins on its consultative staff, with frequent interdisciplinary discussions and presentations.

EVALUATION

The Regional Trauma Center for Children in the state of Maryland provides a systems approach to the management of life-threatening injuries. The success of this system is clearly reflected in better standards of patient care. Equally importantly, it is a focus for integrated interdisciplinary approaches to the management of multiple organ injuries.[23] From this regional center has come a trauma registry for children and a recent opportunity to evaluate several of the new anatomic indexes of injury severity both for adults and children.[8–10, 24] Material from the clinical evaluation of patients is available for in-service discussion and ongoing peer review in an attempt to identify better management techniques as well as to document cost effectiveness, in the overall treatment plan, of this very expensive form of emergency care.

On the basis of data from this preliminary experience, gathered over less than a decade, the operation of the Regional Pediatric Trauma Center appears to be effective, and it is hoped that this center will be a stimulus for concentrated pediatric trauma research as well. It provides for excellent initial management at the scene of the accident and rapid transport under the care of specially trained emergency medical technicians to a designated trauma center for children.

In-hospital management follows by medical personnel who are experienced in the emotional and physical care of all aspects of childhood trauma, including the social and psychologic ones. In addition, the large volume of cases (approaching 50 per month) at the Johns Hopkins Children's Center allows for development and evaluation of new techniques in trauma management and provides invaluable training for general surgery residents, pediatricians, and emergency care physicians in this important area of pediatric care. Preliminary data strongly suggest that such a system of management will decrease the morbidity and mortality associated with some, if not all, types of injuries and that it will have a significant effect on head injuries, which are the major cause of death from childhood trauma. This component of the Maryland Emergency Medical System will perhaps serve as a prototype for the establishment of regional pediatric trauma centers in other parts of the United States. These units must, of course, be modified in each region by the special characteristics of the health care system in that part of the country.

REFERENCES

1. Boyd DR: A symposium on the Illinois trauma program: A systems approach to the critically injured. J Trauma 13:275, 1973.
2. Baxter, Charles R. Personal communication.
3. Shires GT, Canizaro PC: Fluid resuscitation in the severely injured. Surg Clin North Am 53:1341, 1973.
4. Peter RM: Work of breathing following trauma. J Trauma 8:915, 1968.
5. Pruitt BA Jr, Mason AD Jr, Moncrief JA: Hemodynamic changes in the early post-burn patient. J Trauma 11:36, 1971.
6. Zuidema GD, Cameron JL, Sabatier HS Jr: Initial

evaluation and resuscitation of the injured patient. *In* Zuidema GD, Rutherford RB, Ballinger WF (eds.): The Management of Trauma. 3rd ed. Philadelphia, W. B. Saunders Co., 1979, pp. 1–27.

7. American College of Surgeons Committee on Trauma: Field categorization of trauma patients and hospital trauma index. Bull Am Cell Surg 65:28, 1980.
8. Baker SP, et al.: The injury score. A method for describing patients with multiple injuries and evaluating emergency care. J Trauma 14:187, 1974.
9. Baker SP, O'Neill B: The injury severity score: An update J Trauma 16:882, 1976.
10. Champion HR, et al.: An anatomic index of injury severity. J Trauma 20:197, 1980.
11. Gratz RR: Accidental injury in childhood: A literature review on pediatric trauma. J Trauma 19:551, 1979.
12. Haller JA Jr, Talbert James L: Trauma workshop report: trauma in children. J Trauma 10:1052, 1970.
13. Haller JA Jr: Problems in children's trauma. J Trauma 10:269, 1970.
14. Keddy JA: Accidents in childhood. Canad Med Assoc J 91:675, 1964.
15. O'Neill JA, Meacham WF, Griffin PO, Sawyers JI: Patterns of injury in the battered children syndrome. J Trauma 13:332, 1973.
16. Haller JA Jr: Newer concepts in emergency care of children with major injuries. Md St Med J 22:65, 1973.
17. Haller JA Jr: An overview of emergency care for children with major injuries. Collected Papers in Emergency Services and Traumatology, 1979.
18. Langfitt TW: Measuring the outcome from head injuries. J Neurosurg 48:673, 1978.
19. Mayer T, et al.: Causes of morbidity and mortality in severe pediatric trauma. JAMA 7:245, 1981.
20. Becker D, et al.: The outcome from severe head injury with early diagnosis and intensive management. J Neurosurg 47:491, 1977.
21. Bruce D.: Outcome following severe head injuries in children. J Neurosurg 48:697, May, 1978.
22. Mayer T, et al.: The effect of multiple trauma on morbidity and mortality in pediatric patients with neurologic injuries. Presented to the International Society for Pediatric Neurosurgery, Marseilles, France, June, 1980.
23. Mayer T, et al.: Effect of multiple trauma on outcome of pediatric patients with neurologic injuries. Child's Brain 8:189, 1981.
24. Mayer T, et al.: The modified, injury severity scale in pediatric multiple trauma patients. J Pediatric Surg 15:719, 1980.

CHAPTER

33 Transportation of the Injured Child

THOM A. MAYER

Virtually any injured child who is evaluated by a physician requires transportation at some stage in his medical care. The method of transportation ranges from the family car to sophisticated rotary or fixed-wing transportation. The majority of injured patients are transported by ambulance from the scene of an accident to a hospital. Over 1 million patients were transported by this means in 1981.[1]

The injured child has special needs and presents special problems with regard to emergency transportation. This chapter attempts to highlight both the general problems of transportation of the injured patient and care of the child, as well as detailing specific problems of pediatric transport.

Transportation may be classified as either prehospital or interhospital in nature, the former accounting for the vast majority. Prehospital transportation refers to the transfer of the patient from the scene of the accident or illness to the hospital. Interhospital transportation arises when a patient has been evaluated at a receiving hospital and requires transfer to a second hospital for definitive care. The reason for transfer to another hospital may range from patient's personal preferences in hospitals or physicians to the necessity for specialized care at regional centers (e.g., burn, head injury, spinal cord, or trauma centers).

HISTORICAL SUMMARY

Descriptions of transportation of the ill and injured can be traced to biblical times. In the Gospel According to Mark (Mark 2:1–4), a description is given of a paralytic who was lowered through the roof of a house in order to be healed. From that time until the first half of the 19th century, there was no systematic means of transporting patients to and from sources of medical care, except in cases of battlefield casualties. Litters, horse drawn sedans, and street chairs were intermittently used to transport injured patients in the 19th century.[8] An 1835 report describes a dock worker who was transported in a sedan after being trapped between a large cask and the ship from which it had been unloaded. Interestingly, he was not taken to a hospital, but to his home.[9] By 1847 at least three London hospitals had vehicles designed to transport sick patients, and in 1857, the Metropolitan Asylum Board of London encouraged provision of transportation to areas outside the city.[10]

The first known use of air transportation of the wounded occurred during the Prussian siege of Paris in 1870, when 160 wounded Frenchmen were lifted out of the city by hot air balloon.[11] An air ambulance system was proposed shortly after the first successful powered flight by the Wright brothers in 1903. In 1910 two American Army officers proposed modification of an aircraft to transport patients, but their requests for funds to develop this project were summarily denied.[12]

Although air and ground transportation of wounded soldiers was utilized during World War I, these efforts were extremely limited and did not significantly advance knowledge of transportation of injured patients. However, in World War II ground and air transportation, as well as the concepts of prehospital medical aid and triage, were increasingly well developed.[13] Mortality figures from that war attest to the success of these endeavors, since there was only a 3.3 per cent mortality among battlefield wounded who reached medical treatment facilities.[14]

Further refinements in care were effected in the period between World War II and the Korean War. In particular, the helicopter, which had previously been used to rescue pilots, was increasingly adapted for medical transports. This was of particular importance in Korea, since the terrain, lack of roads, dispersion of medical treatment facilities, and nature of the conflict made ground ambulance evacuation less feasible than it had been in Europe. Over 20 thousand serious casualties were evacuated during the Korean conflict, with a mortality of 2 per cent for those reaching medical facilities.[15, 16]

In addition to use of more rapid means of transportation, the presence of large numbers of highly skilled medical teams, availability of large quantities of whole blood, and availability and effective administration of forward-area hospitals were critical to the success of treatment of the wounded in the Korean War.[17] During the Vietnam War, rapidity and accessibility of transportation, as well as definitive medical therapy, were further refined. A critical factor was the development and deployment of reliable, rapid, and durable air transport equipment (particularly the UH-ID or "Huey" helicopter). The success of delivery of medical care to severely injured patients is exemplified by two facts. First, mortality decreased to one per cent for all patients who reached medical therapy. Second, and equally important, no soldier in Vietnam was more than 35 minutes away from a medical facility capable of delivering definitive, life-saving care.[18] Unfortunately, that statement cannot be made concerning victims of traffic accidents in the United States today.

Another significant development with regard to transportation of patients developed in the 1960s in another part of the world. In 1967, Pantridge and associates[19] demonstrated in Belfast that ventricular fibrillation could be successfully treated outside the hospital and proposed the use of "mobile coronary care units" for this purpose. Until that time, virtually any vehicle that could carry an ill or injured patient in the recumbent position could legitimately claim to be an ambulance. However, Pantridge's work, coupled with the success of medical evacuation in Vietnam, led to the development of the concept of delivering resuscitative medical care at the scene of an accident or injury, with the ultimate goal of providing accessibility to definitive medical care. Both rapidity of transportation and delivery of expert medical care at the scene were necessary to accomplish this. In some cases these facets were combined to startling degrees. For instance, in the initial "Medicopter" system, developed at Ohio State University, medical teams actually patrolled the highways in helicopters for 3- to 4-hour periods, in order to avoid the 3 to 6 minutes it took to warm the aircraft's engines.[20]

Emergency medical services (EMS) systems, including well-equipped ambulances, rapidly mushroomed throughout the country during the late 1960s, aided in part by the National Highway Traffic Safety Act of 1966 and the Emergency Medical Services System Act of 1973 (Public Law 93–154). Some systems followed the Belfast example and utilized physicians and nurses in the ambulance. However, the more common practice was that pioneered by Nagel and coworkers[21] in Florida, which utilized general purpose mobile intensive care unit ambulances staffed by EMTs and paramedics in radio and telemetry contact with a physician at a control hospital. By 1978, there were over 250 paramedic or EMT training sites throughout the country to prepare personnel for transportation of the ill and injured.[22] During the 1970s, the development of emergency medicine as a specialty and the staffing of numerous emergency departments with career emergency physicians contributed to prehospital care of the critically ill and injured.

The earliest use of civilian air transportation in this country developed as a result of the need for transport of critically ill neonates. In the 1960s, these air transport systems were developed at several centers throughout the country. In addition, in Baltimore, Cowley and associates developed the use of state police helicopters to transport patients from the scene of accidents. Since that time air transport has developed rapidly, and there are now over 35 hospital-based air transport helicopters in this country. In addition there are numerous air ambulance services that provide fixed-wing transportation.

GOALS OF TRANSPORTATION OF INJURED PATIENTS

The primary goal of transporting the ill or injured child is optimizing the patient's access to appropriate medical care. This access must be safe and yet rapid, since delays in delivery of medical care may adversely affect outcome, particularly in critically ill children.[24, 25] However, the transportation process must also be safe, both as transportation itself and as a means of extricating the patient from the site of the accident. For example, a patient with a cervical spine injury requires rapid transportation to definitive medical care; however, protection of the cervical spine while the patient is moved from the site of the accident is equally important.

Medical care may be classified either as resuscitative or definitive. These are separate yet closely related areas. Resuscitative care includes assuring that the patient has a patent airway, supporting the circulation, and placing an intravenous (IV) line with appropriate fluids. Definitive care includes operative, nonoperative, and, in some cases, intensive care management of the patient at the hospital. In cases in which the accident occurs a great distance from the hospital, there may be a delay in delivering definitive medical care, yet communication between physicians at the site of medical control and trained paramedical personnel can result in immediate delivery of resuscitative care for the patient's specific injuries.

The goals of care for the injured patient are (1) to provide an effective airway with adequate ventilation; (2) to treat shock; (3) to prevent further damage or deterioration, and (4) to maximize efficiency and rapidity in delivery of the preceding goals.

Airway and Ventilation

The goal of providing respiratory support to an injured child during transport includes providing a patent airway with adequate ventilation, preventing vomiting and aspiration, and delivering humidified oxygen to patients in shock. Providing a patent airway with adequate ventilation requires a systematic assessment of the airway with provision of the appropriate means of therapy. In some cases, either endotracheal intubation or (more rarely) needle cricothyroidotomy may be necessary. In the prehospital phase of care, the degree of invasiveness utilized in providing an airway depends upon both the patient's condition and the level of training of the personnel staffing the system. For example, if the system utilizes well-trained paramedics, endotracheal intubation or cricothyroidotomy may be used to provide an airway, provided that there are appropriate indications for these procedures. *However, in most pediatric patients, bag and mask ventilation can be easily provided in the field, unless there has been direct laryngeal or tracheal injury or massive aspiration.*

A potentially useful adjunct in the prehospital phase of care has been the development of pediatric esophageal obdurator airways (EOA) and esophageal gastric tube airways (EGTA). These airways should be used only in patients over 120 cm in length who are unconscious and in whom bag and mask ventilation is unsuccessful. Particular caution should be exercised in maintaining neutral, in-line cervical traction while placing these devices, since cervical spine injury cannot be excluded in the unconscious patient without x-rays. Regardless of the means used to provide airway and ventilation, patency of the airway and adequacy of ventilation should be reassessed throughout the transport, since clinical deterioration may occur. Details of airway management are presented in Chapters 1 and 3.

Preventing vomiting and aspiration always requires consideration, since gastric distention occurs much more commonly in children. A functioning nasogastric tube should be placed in all children who require ventilatory assistance as well as those with a distended abdomen. After the stomach has been emptied, the tube should be aspirated frequently during transport to remove accumulated air, secretions, and blood. These provisions are particularly important in the semiconscious or obtunded patient.

Although oxygen is not a cure for any traumatic disease, one of the goals of therapy for shock is increased oxygen delivery. Therefore, any patients requiring ventilatory assistance and those with signs of shock should have humidified oxygen delivered until they can be evaluated definitively.

Treatment of Shock

Field stabilization and treatment of shock involves several components. The first of these is control of bleeding, either by direct pressure, elevation of the affected area, or use of military anti-shock trousers (MAST). MAST are external counterpressure devices that serve to control bleeding, to increase effective circulatory blood volume, and to increase total peripheral resistance. When appropriate indications are present (Table 33–1), these trousers may be utilized in the field treatment of shock but only when ordered by the medical control physician. Second, virtually all pediatric patients with serious injuries, including those involved in high-energy trauma (motor vehicle accident, auto-pedestrian collisions, and falls from greater than 10 ft, and those with penetrating

Table 33–1. INDICATIONS FOR MAST*

General	
	Blood pressure ≥ 60 mm Hg
	Blood pressure < ⅔ normal and symptoms of shock
Specific	
	Pelvic fractures
	Multiple leg fractures
	Abdominal or retroperitoneal bleeding
	Lower extremity soft tissue bleeding
Contraindications	
	Pulmonary edema
	Pregnancy (use leg sections only)

*MAST = military anti-shock trousers.

injuries) should have an IV line placed to *restore effective circulatory volume,* since clinical deterioration may occur rapidly in these patients.

Percutaneous IV lines can usually be placed in the antecubital fossa, the greater saphenous vein at the ankle, or the fifth interdigital vein on the dorsum of the hand (see Chapter 1, pp. 9–12). Third, as mentioned previously, one of the goals of shock therapy is *increased oxygen delivery to the tissues.* In any patient with serious injuries or significant blood loss or in whom respiratory support is instituted, supplemental humidified oxygen should be provided until the child can be further assessed.

Perhaps the most common error in caring for injured children is inadequate volume replacement for hypovolemic shock. Familiarity with the normal blood pressure and blood volume of children can prevent this. Minimum normal blood pressure in children is 80 mm Hg plus twice the age in years; normal blood volume is 85 ml/kg regardless of the age of the child. Remembering these simple figures as well as the subtle signs and symptoms of shock listed in Chapter 1 (pp. 12–18) will prevent many errors in treating injured children.

Lactated Ringer's or normal saline solution is usually the fluid of choice for resuscitation of patients in shock during the prehospital phase of care, inasmuch as they restore effective circulatory volume, are more cost effective than colloids, and are rarely associated with significant complications.

In children without hypotension who have other signs of shock (impaired capillary refill, increased diastolic blood pressure, tachycardia, tachypnea), one fourth of the total blood volume should be infused in 5 minutes or less.[28] When hypotension or massive bleeding is present, one half of the total blood volume should be rapidly infused. If a child has no signs of shock but has evidence of internal or external bleeding, the blood loss should be estimated and replaced, up to one fourth to one half of the child's blood volume. After fluid infusion has begun, the injured child should be constantly reassessed, since additional fluid bolus therapy may be required.

All physicians, nurses, and paramedical personnel should be familiar with the principles of control of bleeding, use of MAST, fluid infusion therapy, and supplemental oxygen therapy in children. These elements form the basis of rational prehospital stabilization of the patient in shock.

Preventing Further Damage or Deterioration

This ancient concept dates from Hiprocrates's dictum *"primum non nocere"* (First, do not harm). Its importance has not diminished since that time, and it should guide all resuscitative and definitive care efforts in the injured child. Prehospital first aid measures for specific injuries can be life saving, and examples are listed below by body area.

Chest Injury

Penetrating injuries to the chest should be covered with a Vaseline gauze or other occlusive dressing to ensure that air will not enter the chest. Patients with flail chest should be placed with the flail segment down or have the flail area stabilized with sandbags. If tension pneumothorax is suspected, needle aspiration of the chest can be easily performed, either in the field or during transport by those trained in the techniques. In cases of long transport times, the use of Heimlich valves may be necessary to ensure that tension pneumothorax does not redevelop.

Cervical Spine

Although cervical spine injuries are relatively less common in children than in adults, prehospital care should be predicted on its possibility, since the sequelae from a spinal cord injury can be devastating. Extrication and initial first aid measures can almost always be performed while assuring stability of the cervical spine. On rare occasions, provision of a patent airway with adequate ventilation conflicts with optimal spine stabilization. In those cases, judicious application of the necessary measures to relieve airway obstruction and provide ventilation should be utilized. Clearly, preventing spine injury will be of little value if the patient is anoxic for prolonged periods.

In-line cervical traction, backboards, and rigid cervical collars are the mainstays of spine protection, and field personnel should be well-trained in their use. Emergency department personnel, including physicians, nurses, and x-ray technicians, should be equally conversant with these devices. Many patients have had the spine adequately protected by paramedics in the field only to have these measures ignored in the emergency department.[29] A normal neurologic examination does not preclude an unstable spine fracture; only adequate x-rays can assess the integrity of the spinal column. Occasionally, even when physical examination and x-rays are normal, but the history is highly suggestive of injury, precautions should still be taken to stabilize the spine until tomograms can be performed.

For example, up to 67 per cent of children with spinal cord injury have complete or severe partial spinal cord lesions, even though there is no radiographically demonstrable fracture.[30] In patients with this syndrome of spinal cord injury without radiographic abnormality (SCIWORA), there is usually a history of transient paresthesia, numbness, or subjective paralysis. In any child with such history, cervical spine immobilization should be continued even after radiographs have been performed until a neurosurgeon can evaluate the patient.

Head Injury

There is an understandable tendency for prehospital care personnel to assume that a child with a severe head injury requires immediate transport. In fact, very few children require immediate neurosurgical intervention, and only 20 to 30 per cent of all children with severe head injuries have intracranial mass lesions.[31, 32] Immediate therapy *is* required for severe head injury, but the basic elements of this care can be provided in the field.

A complete discussion of the evaluation of the head-injured patient is given in Chapter 16. However, it is critical to note that prehospital care personnel should be well-trained in performing a basic *field* mini-neurologic examination, since clinical deterioration is highly significant in head injuries. Field evaluation of head-injured patients can be completed in less than a minute and consists of three parts: determination of level of consciousness (as judged by the Glasgow Coma Scale); measurement of pupillary light response, and examination for lateralized extremity weakness or abnormal posturing.

Review of radio communications between paramedics and medical control physicians frequently reveals communications such as "the patient is comatose." However, this statement has very little meaning and the patient is better served if the paramedic can communicate the essentials of the level of consciousness as specified by the Glasgow Coma Scale (see Table 1–4, p. 25). Use of this system requires a minimal amount of training, and virtually all nurses and emergency medical technicians (EMTs) can be taught to use it. Even if the specific elements of the scale are not computed in the field, the concepts of this system can clearly communicate the patient's level of consciousness. For example, the statement that "the patient is unable to speak or open the eyes and responds to pain with decerebration" clearly communicates the essentials of the Glasgow Coma Scale score. Clinical deterioration can be clearly documented, since this scale is precise enough that changes of 2 points are significant, and changes of 3 points require urgent neurosurgical intervention.[33] In hypotensive patients, decreasing levels of consciousness may be due to shock instead of head injury. Further, the use of neurologic depressants (e.g., alcohol or drugs) must also be considered.

The pupils should be assessed with regard to size, asymmetry, and reactivity to light. A unilaterally dilated pupil may be secondary to increased intracranial pressure due to an intracranial mass lesion. Alteration of pupillary reactivity can also indicate the severity of initial impact injury, even in the absence of an intracranial mass lesion. One caution is necessary in this regard. Patients with direct trauma to the eye may have a unilaterally dilated pupil secondary to ocular injury, without a severe head injury.

Movement of the extremities, including spontaneous movement and movement on commands, should be evaluated in all patients. Mass lesions may cause unilateral extremity weakness or hemiparesis secondary to increased intracranial pressure. If the patient's level of consciousness is depressed, assessment of movement may be more difficult but can usually be carried out by carefully evaluating spontaneous movements. In addition to evaluating lateralized extremity weakness, the presence of abnormal posturing (decerebrate, decorticate, or flaccid) should be noted.

By evaluating the patient's level of consciousness and pupillary light response and the presence of lateralized extremity weakness, prehospital personnel can effectively communicate the condition of the head-injured patient in the field. Patients should be considered to have a severe head injury if the Glasgow Coma Scale (GCS) score is 10 or lower; if a decrease in the GCS of 2 points is documented; or if pupillary asymmetry, lateralized extremity weakness, depressed skull fractures, or open skull fractures are present and associated with depressed level of consciousness (GCS $\leq$ 10). In patients with a rapidly decreasing level of consciousness (GCS decreased by 3 points) or in those with all three signs of depressed level of consciousness (pupil asymmetry, lateralized extremity weakness, or abnormal posturing), the possibility is great that there is a rapidly expanding intracranial mass lesion.

Children with head injury can benefit greatly from provision of basic measures in the prehospital phase of care. It is most important by far to provide an adequate airway and treat shock. Hypoxia, hypercarbia, and hypotension greatly compound the problem of head injury. Provision of an airway with adequate ventilation (usually with mild hyperventilation) can greatly benefit the head-injured patient. Shock is rarely due to isolated head injuries, so other injuries can usually be found in the head-injured patient who presents with hypotension. Adequate volume restoration with Ringer's lactate solution should be provided.

Properly positioning the head increases venous return and can greatly decrease intracranial pressure. The head should be kept in a midline position relative to the body and elevated 30 to 40 degrees from the waist, unless thoracic or lumbar spine injury is suspected. Bleeding from the head should be covered with pressure dressings prior to elevation, which prevents air embolism in cases of dural sinus tears. Steroids should be administered only under orders from the medical control physician.[34, 35]

Hypothermia

Children, and infants in particular, are much more susceptible to heat loss. This is partly due to their large body surface area as well as to their less effective homeostatic thermoregulatory mechanisms. This problem should be anticipated and planned for during the prehospital phase of care, since hypothermia greatly increases oxygen consumption and adversely affects the child's other injuries, especially shock. In burned children, great care should be taken to maintain a neutral thermal environment, since massive losses of fluid couple with hypothermia to significantly affect outcome. During interhospital transfers of infants, special transport isolettes may be used; however, for prehospital use, warming blankets are usually sufficient. The need to prevent hypothermia should not keep prehospital personnel from reassessing stability of cardiorespiratory function or other injuries. Constant reassessment of blood pressure, for example, should be undertaken in patients with hypovolemia. This can always be done while maintaining the essentials of a neutral thermal environment. Once the patient is inside the ambulance, heat can usually be regulated to ensure that minimal heat loss occurs while reassessment takes place.

Fractures

The presence of pain, swelling, or deformity should alert prehospital personnel to the possibility of a fracture in children. Ambulance personnel may assume that children with extremity pain may have sprains. However, young children have a relative degree of bony weakness at the epiphyseal plate, and epiphyseal injuries are at least as common as sprains in children.[36] Any child with pain, swelling, or deformity of an extremity should have the extremity splinted and distal pulse and neurologic status should be assessed. There are relatively few indications for field reduction of fractures in children, except when distal neurovascular compromise is present or bony fragments are causing possible skin necrosis.

Maximum Efficiency and Rapidity

Respiratory support, shock treatment, and measures to prevent deterioration must all be delivered both rapidly and effectively. Ideally, there should be minimal delays between resuscitative care and definitive care of the patient's injuries. As indicated previously, definitive care is nearly always delivered in the hospital setting. However, the basic elements of resuscitative care can be delivered either in the field or at the hospital. There are conflicting opinions, even among experienced surgeons, as to whether resuscitative care should be delivered in the field or at the hospital. The controversy between proponents of field stabilization and "scoop and run" philosophies exemplifies this conflict.

The "scoop and run" philosophy dictates that the central factor of importance in prehospital care of the injured patient is to deliver the patient to definitive medical care as quickly as possible. Field stabilization proponents argue that the delivery of resuscitative medical care at the scene of the injury can be equally as important to outcome as the time required for delivery of definitive care. Stated simply, "scoop and run" advocates note that the patient needs to be delivered to medical care as soon as possible, whereas field stabilization proponents argue that certain specific aspects of resuscitative care need to be delivered to the patient at the scene of the accident. Although both groups agree that time is of the essence to efficient care of the injured patient, they disagree on the location where resuscitative care should be delivered.

The clearest argument for field stabilization of the trauma patient arises from data from the Seattle Fire Department and Harborview Medical Center. Oreskovich[37] noted that a carefully planned prehospital care system, meticulous training and preparation of prehospital personnel, and strict medical control by the trauma surgeon resulted in startling results with field stabilization of seriously injured patients. The Seattle system clearly emphasizes the goals of provision of a patent airway, shock treatment, and prevention of further damage. The efficiency of this system is attested to by its response time. The average time from arrival of the paramedic unit at the scene of the accident to arrival at the hospital emergency room door was 22 minutes. Of 100 trauma patients who required cardiopulmonary resuscitation at the scene of accident or immediately upon arrival at the hospital, 20 per cent survived to be discharged from the hospital. This experience underlines the fact that judicious field stabilization may be delivered rapidly, efficiently, and with good outcomes.

Additional support for the concept of field stabilization of the injured patient is implicit in data from the head injury study in San Diego County.[38] In that system, head-injured patients are treated rapidly and aggressively in the field with regard to provision of an airway and circulatory support. These efforts, coupled with early diagnosis and intensive management in the hospital, have resulted in favorable outcomes for their series of severe head-injured patients.

However, significant planning, training, education, and effective medical control are necessary in any prehospital care system in which field stabilization is emphasized. Furthermore, "scoop and run" transports are indicated in certain specific instances. For example, patients with penetrating cardiac injuries may need to be rushed to the nearest site for definitive care without prior stabilization.[39] The final decision on field stabilization or "scoop and run" is left to the medical control physician.

COMPONENTS

Medical Control

The foundation upon which all transportation systems rest is the concept of medical control. The increasing sophistication of these systems indicates that quality medical care can be delivered in the initial phase after injury to trauma victims. However, this can occur only if there is careful prospective planning, adequate medical input, and continued monitoring of the transportation system. Virtually every aspect of the system, including financing, training, communication, and equipment, requires significant physician input to assure that timely, appropriate care is delivered. Medical control refers to the concept that trained physician input guides the overall function of the transportation system. This input is *prospective* (in establishing protocols, standing orders, and training for emergency personnel), *immediate* (in communicating specific orders to paramedical personnel in the field), and *retrospective* (inasmuch as monitoring the accountability of the system is necessary).[40] Further, prehospital care, including transportation of the patient, is best delivered when it is an extension of hospital emergency care to the field. Since medical care delivery is involved to significant degrees in even the simplest of transportation systems, it is virtually impossible for such a system to function without genuine medical control.

The responsibility for medical control may fall to any of a number of groups of physicians. Classically, surgeons, cardiologists, and, to an increasing degree, emergency physicians have been called upon to assume administrative and medical responsibilities for planning and implementing prehospital care. Planning should begin with the EMS Council and should be carefully coordinated within existing systems. The medical control physician should be responsible for planning and implementing prospective, immediate, and retrospective components of prehospital care. A significant amount of time, energy, and expertise are necessary for effective medical control.

Medical control may also be construed in the more narrow sense of responsibility for the immediate phase of patient care. The clearest example of this is in evaluating communications from paramedics and issuing orders for the care of the patient in the field. Clearly, medical control in this sense requires that the physician be in the emergency department to respond to calls. Emergency physicians have generally been responsible for this aspect of medical control in recent years. In well-staffed regional centers, trauma surgeons may be available to handle medical control duties for seriously injured patients.[41] Regardless of the type of physician responsible for medical control, this position requires significant expertise in the field of emergency care as well as immediate availability.

An additional point that deserves emphasis relates to transportation systems in which more than one hospital desires to serve as the medical control facility for the system. In many metropolitan areas, this has provoked significant controversy. In these areas, the base-station hospital may be responsible for triaging patients either to the medical control hospital or to other (perhaps nearer, but also perhaps less well-equipped) hospitals. This may create significant problems, since the decision regarding the hospital to which the patient is transported may result in perceived inequities among hospital emergency departments and hospital administrators. In most instances, the state or regional EMS Council is responsible for evaluating and assigning medical control to a given hospital. These councils should also monitor medical control to ensure that patients receive optimal medical care and that inequities in assigning patients do not occur.

Financial Aspects

Perhaps the most neglected aspect of transportation of ill and injured patients is financial management. Flashing lights and the possibility of life-saving intervention draw the curiosity and attention of lay, paramedical, and medical personnel. However, the fact remains that this care must be paid for in one form or another. Federal budget cuts in EMS grants have focused an increasing amount of attention on the question of who bears the financial burden for transportation of emergency patients.

In a general sense, the answer to that question depends upon whether transportation is considered a private or a public service. In system in which transportation is considered a private service, the financial burden of the service falls upon the users of the service. Specifically, individual charges are billed to those patients who are transported. When transportation is considered to be a public service, the taxpayer subsidizes the system to substantial degrees. In most systems, some combination of these two viewpoints is utilized. Even in systems in which individual patient billing is utilized, public payments effectively serve to subsidize the system.

To a large extent, the assignment of transportation costs also depends upon the existing system upon which transportation is based. EMS transportation services may be designed to function under a number of systems: fire department, police department, health department, hospital, volunteer services, or commercial ambulance providers. There are advantages and disadvantages to each of these systems. Both fire department and police department services have the advantage that they are already linked to communication systems for emergency services; personnel are trained to deal with emergency situations; vehicle maintenance provisions are operational; and, particularly in fire department, facilities are located strategically to respond in a timely fashion to emergencies. In the case of fire department services, an additional advantage may be that the fire fighter's time is more optimally utilized when medical care is one of his duties. Problems associated with these systems are that neither have expertise in billing for their services; career development is geared toward fire or law enforcement goals (not medical care); and, in certain situations, the medical and fire or law enforcement roles may overlap or conflict.

Health department or hospital-based systems have the advantages of optimizing coordination of prehospital and hospital care, utilizing personnel effectively between emergency calls, and expertise in billing. Disadvantages of these systems are that large vehicle maintenance facilities and communication systems are usually not readily available. Volunteer services benefit from decreased costs and increased enthusiasm but may suffer from lack of availability of personnel, cost of linking with communication systems, and maintenance of vehicles and facilities. Commercial ambulance agencies share these problems, but offset the costs through billing. Successful systems may be based on any of these models, provided sufficient financial planning and management are utilized.

The expenses of patient transportation may be divided into transportation, communication, and administrative costs. Regardless of how and where a transportation system is based, these costs must be considered in instituting the maintaining the system. Failure to provide adequate financial management may force some EMS transportation systems to close, particularly at a time when federal funds for these purposes are declining. Although federal, state, county, and local, or private, funds may be available, particularly during the development or start-up phase, once the system is operational, the balance between grants and collections must be maintained if the system is to survive. In situations in which individual billings are utilized, third-party payers have recognized that transportation costs can be a legitimately reimbursable health care expense. However, up to 20 per cent of patients who are covered by private medical insurers are not covered for emergency transportation costs.

Training

With the existing number and location of prehospital care systems in this country, the vast majority of seriously injured patients have their initial medical care delivered by field personnel. The initial 20 minutes to 1 hour following a patient's injury may be spent with ambulance personnel or paramedics, depending upon the distance to the nearest appropriate medical facility. For this reason, ambulance and rescue personnel require rigorous training to ensure that the patient's initial triage and treatment are optimal. This is particularly true with regard to pediatric patients, and each member of the prehospital care system should be well-trained in pediatric resuscitative measures.

However, the amount, type, and degree of medical care delivered in the field depends upon the local system responsible for delivering such care. In some areas, EMS councils and medical control officers have elected to develop a system using basic life support and extrication procedures alone. By contrast, other systems provide a high degree of medical control coupled with extremely well-trained paramedics, who perform endotracheal intubation, cricothyroidotomy, and central venous cannulation in the field, when appropriate indications are present.[37, 41] Each EMS system should be developed on a logical basis at the local level, integrating a number of factors, including equipment, finances, medical control, personnel, and EMS council input. The degree and intensity of training logically depend on the level of prehospital care to be delivered in any given system. Regardless of the degree of prehospital care delivered, training is equally important in any system. Advanced life support (ALS) requires a longer, more intense period of training than less sophisticated systems. However, emergency medical personnel in rural systems with basic life support (BLS) capability still require careful training in those procedures and techniques for which they are approved.

At the present time, nomenclature for prehospital providers is not well standardized, although efforts to correct this have been undertaken. In 1972, the Department of Transportation published standards of training for emergency medical technicians (EMT). These standards were revised in 1977, with expansion to the 15-module Caroline curriculum for paramedics. Despite the overlapping nomenclature and the lack of widely accepted standardization of training, the following terms generally describe the basic categories of field providers.

Emergency Medical Technicians–Ambulance (EMT–A)

Also known as EMT–1 or EMT–Basic, these field providers receive between 81 and 150 hours of didactic clinical training. This training is intended to allow the student to deliver three general goals of care: (1) recognition of life-threatening illnesses or injuries, (2) provision of advanced first aid, and (3) provision of basic life support. Depending upon the system, EMT–As may also be responsible for extrication of the patient. In systems providing BLS alone, the EMT–A is the sole provider of prehospital care, whereas ALS systems most often use EMT–As as first responders, who are backed up by more advanced paramedics as second responders.

Emergency Medical Technicians–Paramedics (EMT–P)

EMT–Ps represent a higher level of care to the patient and thus require additional training. In general, paramedics may be trained to provide advanced life support, including extrication, IV therapy, drug infusion, placement of MAST, provision of an airway, defibrillation, and other advanced procedures. However, the specific procedures and the training required to perform such procedures, vary widely according to the requirements of the prehospital care training system. Most paramedic training programs utilize the elements of the Caroline curriculum, although the length of training varies from 500 to 2000 hours.

Instructors responsible for training EMT–As and EMT–Ps may come from a number of fields. Certified paramedics, emergency physicians, cardiologists, surgeons, respiratory therapists, and emergency nurses have all been successfully used in such training. The critical factor is identifying instructors committed to quality prehospital care, who are willing to dedicate themselves to the task of training prehospital personnel.

Communications

There are four basic categories of prehospital communication in any EMS system, inlcuding public access, dispatch of emergency personnel, medical communications, and interagency communication. These categories are linked by a threefold communication system. The first element of this system is a communications center responsible for receiving incoming calls, coordinating location of ambulance vehicles, and dispatching appropriate emergency personnel to the scene. The second element is mobile equipment capable of allowing field personnel to communicate with medical control physicians and of sending appropriate telemetry. The final element is appropriate hospital equipment allowing hospital to field, hospital to dispatch, and interhospital communications. All such equipment and the communications over them are subject to Federal Communications Commission Regulations, which are detailed in FCC regulations part 90.

In many areas of the country, public access to the EMS system for all emergencies occurs through the use of the 911 telephone number. In areas in which the 911 number is not used, police, fire, and hospital emergency services telephone numbers should be prominently displayed.

Once a call has been placed to activate the EMS system, the dispatcher is responsible for assessing the type of accident that has occurred, as well as the type and number of vehicles and personnel that are needed to respond to the emergency. The dispatcher must be constantly aware of the location of all ambulance units in his area in order to be sure that the closest appropriate vehicle is dispatched. Furthermore, he must alert other agencies to coordinate traffic, law enforcement, and fire department efforts. Because the dispatcher must assess the possibility of injuries and assume responsibility for mobilizing appropriate personnel rapidly, it is usually advisable to ensure that dispatchers have had significant experience in field provision of emergency care.

When the team of EMTs has been dispatched, they must initially assess the situation at the scene of the accident and, in some cases, call for additional paramedical personnel or support units from the police or fire department. As individual patients are assessed, one of two things may happen, depending upon the individual EMS system, the level of training of the initial responders, and the degree of the patient's injuries. First, many modern EMS systems have provided basic, initial treatment protocols for patients who fall into specific treatment categories. Second, in some areas prehospital protocols have not been established, in which case immediate radio communication with medical control is necessary. In either case, the EMTs are responsible for informing the medical control hospital of their assessment at the site of illness or injury. This serves to alert the hospital to the possibility of patients being transported to their center and, when injuries are of sufficient severity, medical control physicians may order treatment to be delivered in the field. In other cases, it may be necessary to provide immediate transportation of the patient to medical care. EMT units should continually update the medical control facility on the patient's condition during transportation.

Interagency communication refers to the necessity for planning a response to emergencies as well as to the ability to coordinate delivery of appropriate resources to the site of accident or injury. Police, fire department, ambulance agency, EMS council, and medical control representatives must develop open lines of communications between their respective agencies. This can be accomplished only through appropriate planning, and regular meetings between these agencies assist in the delivery of quality prehospital medical care. In many urban areas, this degree of cooperation has been extensively developed. For example, some cities utilize police cruisers to rush blood samples from the site of injury to the receiving hospital. This enables the hospital to have type-specific blood available for patients with massive injuries at the time they arrive at the hospital emergency department.

Equipment

Prior to the development in the 1960s of the concept of prehospital care, virtually any vehicle that could carry a patient in the supine position could be considered an ambulance. A crouched-over ambulance attendant, a stretcher, a cramped patient, and possibly a portable oxygen bottle was a familiar picture in the "hearse-type" ambulance. The present-day ambulance, with its sophisticated equipment and capabilities, stands in sharp contrast to the hearse-type ambulance of the 1950s. In addition to transporting patients to medical care, ambulances now offer the possibility of providing medical care to the patient while en route to definitive treatment facilities. The American College of Surgeons, the Department of Transportation, and others[3–6] have contributed to the development of standards for ambulance services. In addition to rigorous training of ambulance personnel, provision of appropriate equipment is necessary for the delivery of effective prehospital care. The American College of Surgeons publication "Essential Equipment for Ambulances"[3] details specific equipment needs for ambulances, but basic categories will be addressed here.

Although ambulances may vary in size, shape, and configuration, all should be capable of carrying one or more patients in a recumbent position on a stretcher capable of being secured to the floor of the vehicle. In addition, there must be sufficient room for ambulance attendants to provide basic care to the patient while en route to the hospital. Adequate illumination and facilities to control the temperature of the patient compartment must be furnished.

Equipment for securing the airway should be included, with the type of equipment dependent on the level of sophistication of prehospital care. Suction devices, humidified oxygen, and oropharyngeal airways are basic requisites, but esophageal, endotracheal, or surgical airways may also be included if paramedics or physicians are available to provide this level of care. Bag and mask devices (including adult, child, and infant sizes) should be available and must have valves capable of use in cold weather conditions.

Equipment for spinal immobilization is a necessity, including short and long rigid backboards and rigid cervical collars. Rigid splints should be provided for splinting extremity fractures, although some systems continue to use the somewhat outdated air splints. Hare or Thomas splints should be available for use when femoral fractures are present. For systems in which the EMTs are trained in their use, MAST in adult and pediatric sizes should be available.

IV solutions should include 5 per cent dextrose and water, lactated Ringer's, solution, and 5 per cent dextrose in 0.45 per cent normal saline, all in soft, plastic containers. Glass bottles containing IV solutions are likely to shatter and their use should be avoided in the field. An overhead mechanism for securing and stabilizing IV solutions must be available. Specific needs for IV therapy in the pediatric age group include small indwelling catheters (20- and 22-gauge plastic catheters, and 19, 22, and 25-gauge "butterfly" catheters), T-connectors (see Chapter 34,

p. 527), short arm and foot boards, and tape to secure the catheters.

The type and number of medications carried on any ambulance depend on local law and medical control input. Significant cooperation between medical control physicians and field personnel is necessary to establish and update appropriate medications. All medications should be given with physician's orders, either verbally over the radio or via established prehospital protocols.

General equipment, including extrication equipment, clean sheets for burn victims, obstetric kits, blood pressure manometers of appropriate sizes (5 mm, 7 mm, and 9.5 mm), a two-way radio with telemetry capabilities, poison kits (with ipecac and activated charcoal), aluminum foil or survival blankets (to control heat loss in infants and young children), mouth gags, tape, sterile dressings, and 4-inch and 6-inch soft rubber bandages. A cardioscope with pediatric leads and defibrillator (with pediatric paddles) should be available if advanced EMTs staff the system.

The reader is encouraged to consult other references[3, 42–44] as well as with existing prehospital care systems to establish appropriate equipment needs for local circumstances. Equipment should be assessed and restocked after each ambulance run. Occasionally, continued experience within any given system results in changes in equipment, medications, or prehospital protocols. An ongoing dialogue between medical control and ambulance units is necessary for these changes.

Evaluation

According to numerous studies, in order for emergency medical personnel to maintain proficiency in the skills necessary for prehospital care, they must take periodic courses to update their knowledge.[45–47] Evaluation of the prehospital system is necessary to ensure that the goals of the system are being met as well as to assess the technical aspects of the provision of care. Evaluation of prehospital services should include regular monthly audits of ambulance runs (particularly ALS runs); skill updates for ambulance attendants, EMT–As, EMT–Ps, nurses, and physicians; and assessment of response times. Effective dialogue between emergency physicians and prehospital personnel is key to continued evaluation and often improves the quality of care delivered to the patient. In areas in which prehospital personnel may not be exposed to large volumes of patients with any given injury, clinical skills may decay more rapidly. Training facilities with large-volume emergency departments may elect to provide clinical rotations for these personnel on a regular basis in order to update their training and skills.

Records

As in any aspect of medical care, meticulous attention to detail in providing adequate records of the patient's care is an absolute necessity.[6] Although the legal ramifications of detailed record keeping are important, by far the most overriding concern is appropriate care of the patient. Unless patient data are observed and recorded in an orderly fashion, serious errors in diagnosis and management may result. A well-organized prehospital care form for recording patient data should include patient identification data, time of initial call, arrival at the scene of accident or injury, arrival at the hospital, past history, vital signs, and physical assessment. Additional space should be available for updated vital signs, verbal orders, radio communications, therapy utilized in the field, and so on. In cases in which radio communication is utilized, both field and hospital personnel should record these communications. In most cases, hospitals should tape record all ALS communications.

Well-kept records benefit the patient and help protect the providers of prehospital care and the medical control physicians who are responsible for such care. In addition, these records may be used for ongoing evaluation of the prehospital care system.

INTERHOSPITAL TRANSFER

With the increasing availability of trauma centers and other specialized regional centers (including children's hospitals, head and spinal cord injury centers, burn units, and replantation facilities), interhospital transportation of injured patients has increased in frequency and importance. There are three stringent requirements in any interhospital transfer: (1) correction of major physiologic derangements (airway, circulation, other injuries); (2) communication with the hospital and physician to which the patient is being referred prior to and during transport, and including transmission of records; (3) adequate monitoring of vital signs, blood pressure, nasogastric tube, and so on during transport, with anticipation of possible clinical deterioration.

Every patient who is transferred to another hospital for definitive care should be judiciously stabilized prior to undergoing interhospital transportation. In some patients with critical injuries, only a relative degree of stabilization may be assured. In other cases, such as a patient with acute subdural hematoma who requires neurosurgical intervention, the amount of time taken for stabilization may adversely affect outcome. However, it is particularly important in children to provide the maximum stabilization possible. This includes providing an adequate airway, supporting the circulation, controlling hemorrhage, splinting fractures, placing a nasogastric tube and IV line, and providing basic therapy for head injuries (when indicated). The details of these measures have been outlined elsewhere in this chapter and are elaborated on in the individual chapters that concern each body area.

Communication is a critical factor in interhospital transportation, particularly in pediatric patients. In the past, many patients were transferred to other hospitals without any communication among physicians, nurses, and other hospital staff. This not only results in inadequate care for the patient during transport but also does not allow the receiving facility to adequately prepare for the patient. Furthermore, in some cases, patients have been transferred to referral centers at which no beds were available. Every interhospital transfer must have clear communication established between the referring physician and the facility to which the patient is being transferred. Physician-to-physician communication is an absolute requirement.[48, 49]

This communication must convey appropriate information on the patient's history, diagnostic work-up, and current status and must establish a clear plan of therapy for the patient undergoing transportation. This latter aspect is particularly important in children, since many pediatric interhospital transfers are undertaken specifically because the referring hospital lacks either the facilities or expertise for care of the injured child. Specific treatment plans should be established, including type and rate of IV fluid infusion, medications, and other indicated therapy. In addition to verbal communication, copies of the patient's chart and diagnostic work-up (including x-rays) should also accompany the patient. Courtesy, as well as adequate follow-up care, dictates that the receiving hospital update the referring hospital and physician on the patient's progress and final disposition.

Once the patient has been initially stabilized and appropriate communication has been established, the patient requires adequate monitoring in anticipation of possible deterioration. The amount of monitoring required varies according to the patient's injuries. All patients undergoing transportation should have frequent (every 15 minutes) monitoring of the vital signs. Blood pressure may drop precipitously in critically ill children, so an appropriately sized blood pressure cuff or Doppler ultrasound should be available. Patients who are receiving ventilatory assistance should be evaluated frequently to assure that chest wall rise and breath sounds reflect adequate ventilation. Patients receiving ventilatory assistance and those with abdominal trauma should have a nasogastric tube placed. The tube should be aspirated frequently during transportation to empty the stomach of air and solid matter. When severe head injury is present, the neurologic status, including level of consciousness, pupillary size and reactivity, and presence or absence of lateralized extremity weakness should be frequently assessed. If clinical deterioration in any body area does occur during the interhospital transportation, the receiving hospital should be contacted immediately for further orders.

AIR TRANSPORTATION

Although it may seem incongruous that lessons gleaned from combat in two wars should lead to saving civilians' lives, aeromedical transportation owes a great debt to the experience gained in military transport of injured patients. Without the massive air transport experience in the Korean and Vietnam wars, it is unlikely that our present understanding of rotary and fixed-wing transportation of ill and injured patients would have developed to its present level of sophistication. As indicated in the historical review in this chapter, successful extension of air transportation to both neonates and patients injured in motor vehicle accidents occurred as early as the 1960s.[23–26, 50] Since that time, air transportation of injured patients has undergone extensive growth.

Air transportation may be effected using either rotary-wing (helicopters) or fixed-wing aircraft. In general, rotary-wing aircraft are utilized on short flights, whereas fixed-wing aircraft is utilized on transports of 100 miles or longer. Some states have followed the model utilized in Maryland by Cowley and associates,[7, 23] in which state police helicopters transport patients. Far more common is the concept of hospital-based helicopters, which are usually leased from air transportation companies. Details of the lease and maintenance arrangements are available from these companies.* Use of hospital-based leased helicopters has the advantage of decreased response time. In addition, most companies are able to provide fixed-wing transportation when appropriate indications are present.

The clearest advantages of air transportation of injured patients are time, geographic considerations, and the need for regionalization of specialized care. Most helicopters used for medical transportation have speeds in excess of 100 miles/hour, enabling much faster transportation than ground vehicles could offer. Fixed-wing medical aircraft travel at speeds over 200 miles/per hour, offering a significant time advantage in situations in which flights exceed 100 miles. In addition, with flights over 100 miles, fixed-wing aircraft are much lower in cost, largely owing to the fact that they are much more fuel efficient than helicopters.

Geographic advantages are perhaps most pronounced in urban areas, where heavy traffic may significantly delay ground transportation. In the Houston experience, air transportation of patients from the scene of the accident has been life-saving in some cases.[52] In rural areas or in mountainous terrain, air transport may also represent a significant benefit.

An additional advantage of air transportation involves the concept of regionalization of specialized care. Early reports indicate that regionalization of some facets of critical care may result in lower morbidity and mortality.[11, 23, 53–55] When transportation to these regionalized centers is indicated, the development of 24-hour availability of a specially trained transport teams offers a significant advantage to the patient. This is particularly true in the case of pediatric patients, many of whom are referred to regional pediatric centers specifically because of the expertise available. Transportation teams at regional centers focus on delivery of expert medical care at the earliest possible time. In this regard, the critical issue is not how long it takes the patient to arrive at the regional center, but rather how long it takes the centers expert care to be delivered to the child. In addition to dispatching the transport team rapidly and efficiently, an even faster means of delivery of expert care is via immediate consultation over radio and telephone systems, since this care can be instituted even while the transport aircraft and personnel are being mobilized.

There are several possible disadvantages to the use of air transportation, including the increased cost and noise, space limitations, and dangers posed by flight and/or weather. Although very few detailed cost analyses have been prepared with regard to air transport,[55] cost can be within 1 per cent of similar ground transportation, particularly when transport distances exceed 25 miles.[56] Nonetheless, an adequate number of air transports per year is necessary to justify a hospital-based system.[27] Although noise presents only minor problems in fixed-wing aircraft, the roar of rotary-wing aircraft may prevent hearing blood pressure, heart or breath sounds, or even verbal communications. Doppler ultrasound equipment should be carried on all air transport to assist in detecting blood pressure. The transport team should be prepared to care for the patient under the noisiest of conditions. In some aircraft (UH-ID, for example), the transport team may need to utilize either hand signals or written communications.

Although very few aircraft have as much space as ground ambulances, most patients (particularly children) can be adequately cared for in both rotary and fixed-wing aircraft. Dangers posed by flight and/or weather are very real, but accidents involving medical aircraft have been exceedingly rare. Data from numerous centers[7, 11, 23, 51, 55] indicate that air transport is very safe, providing pilots are judicious in assessing the capability of flight.

*Rocky Mountain Helicopters, Box 1337, Provo, Utah, Attn: Russ Spray, Director, Medical Group; Aerospatiale Helicopter Corporation, 2701 Forum Drive, Grand Prairie, Texas; Evergreen Air Services, Medical Transport Group, Denver Colorado.

When air transportation is considered, several aspects are of importance. First, appropriate indications should be present, including considerations of time, geography, referral to specialized regional centers, and the specifics of the patient's diagnosis. In general, patients with myocardial infarctions are better transported by ground, since the stress and turbulence may predispose to increased cardiac irritability or arrhythmias. Patients with unstable spinal cord injury should be considered carefully prior to attempting air transportation, since turbulence may worsen the injury, unless great caution is taken to stabilize the spine.[57]

Consideration of the effects of altitude on the patient are essential. Rotary-wing aircraft may ascent to 12,000 ft or more without pressurization. Although many fixed-wing medical aircraft are pressurized, altitude is still a consideration, since most aircraft maintain an ambient pressure of only approximately 6000 ft above sea level.[58] The most important altitude-related effects are hypoxia and gas expansion. Patients whose cardiorespiratory status is well compensated on room air at sea level may undergo decompensation at 10,000 ft. Examples include children with multiple trauma, congenital heart disease, chronic pulmonary disease, or sickle cell disease. For this reason, all pediatric patients undergoing air transport should receive humidified oxygen during transportation.

Gas expansion may present significant problems either by distending a hollow viscus or through expansion of intrapleural air. Nasogastric and chest tubes must be carefully assessed and reassessed throughout flight to assure proper function. Many air transport systems prefer the use of Heimlich flutter valves for tube thoracostomy lines.[58] In addition, altitude may affect MAST trouser or endotracheal tube cuff pressure, which should be re-evaluated during flight.

Some patients experience an exaggerated vestibular response to either altitude or turbulence, which may produce nausea and vomiting. A nasogastric tube to empty the stomach and prevent aspiration may be necessary. When nausea and vomiting occur, sedation or antiemetics may be necessary, particularly in patients with spinal cord injury or elevated intracranial pressure.

When securing the patient in the aircraft, appropriate access to the patient should be maintained. IV lines, endotracheal tubes, chest tubes, and so on should all be in a position to be observed and serviced when necessary. IV fluid infusion rates may vary radically with altitude or turbulence. Constant infusion pumps are advantageous for maintaining proper IV flow rates.

An additional consideration relates to the concept of field stabilization versus "scoop and run" for injured children. Occasional transportation from the scene of accidents or injuries requires a "scoop and run" approach. However, when the pediatric transport team is involved in interhospital transfers, it is usually preferable to stabilize the patient (to whatever degree possible) before entering the aircraft. Although major resuscitative procedures can be performed in most aircraft, noise and space limitations make it preferable to perform these procedures prior to air transport whenever possible.[56]

A final element necessary for all air transportation systems is planning. Careful assessments of the need for the system; well-marked, well-lighted helipads; public relations; interface with various phases of medical care; assessment of equipment and personnel needs; and training must all be provided.

REFERENCES

1. Boyd DR: Emergency medical services systems. *In* Pascarelli EP (ed.): Hospital-Based Ambulatory Care. Norwalk, Appleton-Century-Crofts, 1982.
2. Eisenberg MS, Hallstrom A, Bergner L: Long-term survival after out-of-hospital cardiac arrest. N Engl J Med 306:1340, 1982.
3. Committee on Trauma, American College of Surgeons: Essential equipment for ambulances. Bull Am Coll Surg 66:17, 1981.
4. Committee on Trauma, American College of Surgeons: Standards for emergency ambulance services. Bull Am Coll Surg 52:131, 1967.
5. Committee on Trauma, American College of Surgeons: Treatment protocol for pre-hospital management of the trauma patient. Bull Am Coll Surg 65:23, 1980.
6. Committee on Trauma, American College of Surgeons: Advanced trauma life support course. 1984.
7. Cowley RA, Hudson F, Scanlan E, et al.: An economical and proved helicopter program for transporting the emergency critically ill and injured patient in Maryland. J Trauma 13:1029, 1973.
8. Steedman J: The History and Statutes of the Royal Infirmary of Edinburgh. Edinburgh, 1778.
9. The Dundee Advertiser, March 27, 1835.
10. Hort H: The conveyance of patients to and from the hospital. 1720–1850. Med His. 22:397, 1978.
11. Dobrin RS, Black B, Gilman JI, Massaro TA: The development of a pediatric emergency transport system. Pediatr Clin North Am 27:633, 1980.
12. Johnson A Jr: Treatise on aeromedical evacuation: I. Administration and some medical considerations. Aviat Space Environ Med 48:546, 1977.

13. Guilford FR, Soboroff BJ: Air evacuation: A historical review. J Aviat Med 18:601, 1947.
14. Forsee JH: Forward surgery of the severely wounded. Am Surg. 17:508, 1951.
15. Funsch HF, Wareff MJ, Watkins PB: Wings for wounded warriors. JAMA 200:391, 1967.
16. Neel S: Army aeromedical evacuation procedures in Vietnam. JAMA 204:99, 1968.
17. Artz CP: Battle Casualties in Korea. Studies of the Surgical Research Team. Washington, D.C., Army Medical Service Graduate School, 1955.
18. Hardoway RM III: Viet Nam wound analysis. J Trauma 18:635, 1978.
19. Pantridge JF, Geddes JS: Mobile intensive care unit in the management of myocardial infarction. Lancet 2:271, 1967.
20. Roberts S, Bailey C, Vandermade JR, Marable SA; Medicopter: An airborne intensive care unit. Ann Surg 172:325, 1970.
21. Nagel EL, Hirshman JC, Nussenfeld SR et al.: Telemetry-medical command to coronary and other mobile emergency care systems. JAMA 214:332, 1970.
22. Eisenberg M, Bergner L, Hollstrom A: Paramedic programs and out-of-hospital cardiac arrest. Am J Pub Health 69:30, 1979.
23. Mackenzie CF, Shin B, Fisher R, Crowley RA: Two-year mortality in 760 patients transported by helicopter direct from the road accident scene. Am Surg 45:101, 1979.
24. Cunningham MD, Smith FR: Stabilization and transport of severely ill infants. Pediatr Clin North Am 20:359, 1973.
25. Pettett G, Meronstein GB, Battaglia FC et al.: An analysis of air transport results in the sick newborn infant. Part I. The transport team. Pediatrics 55:774, 1975.
26. Harris BH, Orr RE, Boles ET Jr: Aeromedical transport for infants and children J Pediatr Surg 10:719, 1975.
27. Cooper MA, Klippel AP, Seymour JA: A hospital-based helicopter service: Will it fly? Am Emerg Med 9:451, 1980.
28. Morse TS: Evaluation and initial management. *In* Touloukian RJ (ed.): Pediatric Trauma. New York, John Wiley and Sons, 1978, pp. 21–42.
29. George J: Emergency Care and the Law. Rockville, Md., Aspen Publications, 1978.
30. Pang D, Wilberger JE: Spinal cord injury without radiographic abnormalities in children. J Neurosurg 57:114, 1982.
31. Mayer T, Walker ML, Shasha I et al.: Effect of multiple trauma on outcome of pediatric patients with neurologic injuries. Child's Brain 8:189, 1981.
32. Bruce DA, Raphaely RC, Goldberg AI, et al.: Pathophysiology, treatment and outcome following severe head injury in children. Child's Brain 5:174, 1979.
33. Langfitt TW, Genarelli TA: Can the outcome from head injury be improved? J Neurosurg 56:19, 1982.
34. Saul TG, Ducker TB, Soloman M, Carro M: Steroids in severe head injury: A prospective randomized trial. J Neurosurg 54:596, 1981.
35. Cooper PR, Moody S, Clark WK, et al.: Dexamethasone and severe head injury: J Neurosurg 51:307, 1979.
36. Salter RB: Birth and pediatric fractures. *In* Heppenstall RB: Fracture Treatment and Healing. Philadelphia, W. B. Saunders Company, 1980, pp. 189–234.
37. Oreskovich M: Prehospital surgical care. Presented to the 67th Annual Clinical Congress, American College of Surgeons, San Francisco, California, 1981.
38. Bowers SA, Marshall LF: Outcome in 200 consecutive cases of severe head injury treated in San Diego County: A prospective analysis. Neurosurgery 6:237, 1980.
39. Gervin AS, Fischer RP: The importance of prompt transport in salvage of patients with penetrating heart wounds. J Trauma 22:443, 1982.
40. McSwain NE Jr: Medical control-What is it? JACEP 7:114, 1978.
41. Harner TJ, Oreskovich MR, Copass MK, et al.: Role of emergency thoracotomy in the resuscitation of moribund trauma victims. Am J Surg 142:96, 1981.
42. Caroline N: Emergency Care in the Field: A Manual for Paramedics. Pittsburgh, ADV Agency, 1975.
43. Harless KW, Morris AH, Cengiz M, et al.: Civilian ground and air transport of adults with acute respiratory failure. JAMA 240:361, 1978.
44. Safar P, Esposito G, Benson DM: Ambulance design and equipment for mobile intensive care. Arch Surg 102:163, 1971.
45. Strate RG, Fischer RP: Midesophageal perforation by esophageal obdurator airways. J Trauma 16:503, 1976.
46. Pilcher DB: Ambulance critique review. JACEP 3:383, 1974.
47. Pilcher DB, Gettinger CE, Seligson D: Recurrent themes in ambulance critique review sessions over eight years. J Trauma 19:324, 1979.
48. Committee on Trauma, American College of Surgeons: Interhospital transfer of patients. Bull Am Coll Surg 69:29, 1984.
49. American College of Emergency Physicians: Emergency care guidelines. Ann Emerg Med 11:222, 1982.
50. Arp LJ, Dillon RE, Long MT, et al.: An emergency air-ground transport system for newborn infants with respiratory distress syndrome. Pa Med 72:74, 1969.
51. Evergreen Air Services, Medical Transport Group, Denver, Colorado.
52. Duke JH, Clarke WP: A university-staffed, private hospital-based air transport service. Arch Surg 116:703, 1981.
53. West JG, Trunkey DD, Lim RC: Systems of trauma care: A study of two countries. Arch Surg 116:703, 1981.
54. Marless KW, Morris AH, Cenzig M, et al.: Civilian ground and air transport of adults with acute respiratory failure. JAMA 240:361, 1976.
55. Gill W, Champion HR, Long WB, et al.: A clinical experience of major trauma in Maryland. Md State Med J 25:55, 1976.
56. Black RE, Mayer T, Walker ML, et al.: Air transport of pediatric emergency cases. N Engl J Med 307:1465, 1982.
57. Holdsworth FW: Fracture, dislocation and fracture-dislocation of the spine. J Bone Joint Surg 52:153, 1970.
58. Cooper MA: Critical Care Air Transport. *In* Kravis TC, Warner CG (eds.): Emergency Medicine: A Comprehensive Review. Rockville, Md., Aspen Publications, 1983.

CHAPTER

34 Care of the Injured Child in the General Emergency Department

THOM A. MAYER

Pediatric emergencies account for at least 16 million emergency department visits per year.[1] Further, 60 per cent of all deaths in children aged 1 to 14 years are due to emergency medical service (EMS) diseases, of which trauma is the number-one killer.[2] The episodic nature of trauma and the fact that most physicians' offices are not well equipped to care for even minor injuries, dictate that most trauma care will be delivered in emergency facilities.

Over 90 per cent of the 16 million pediatric emergency visits are to emergency departments of general hospitals. In fact, of the 126 member hospitals of the National Association of Children's Hospitals and Related Institutions, only 36 have active emergency departments. In 1979, a total of 1.2 million patients were seen at these emergency departments.[3] Therefore, the vast majority of cases of pediatric trauma are evaluated in general emergency rooms, which treat ten times as many adults as pediatric patients, with 40 times as many adult EMS deaths.[2]

Because general emergency departments evaluate and treat a larger number of adult patients, the relative rarity of pediatric emergency visits make allocation of resources a critical problem. Commitment to care of pediatric patients is necessary for each emergency medical system if the death and disability from pediatric trauma are to be decreased. Committing resources for treatment of emergency medical system diseases, however, does not ensure that pediatric emergency care will be appropriately encompassed, for several reasons.

Children are not simply small adults; they are both qualitatively and quantitatively different. Care of the pediatric patient involves recognition of the developmental stages through which children progress. Appropriate treatment for a given problem differs according to a child's age. These differences are both anatomic and pathophysiologic in nature. For example, the rates of chest compressions and breaths for cardiopulmonary resuscitation differ significantly according to age.[4, 5]

Further, the child's response to disease, and to trauma in particular, differs from that of adults. Although the physiologic response to hemorrhage in children is similar to that of adults, there is a smaller margin for error and shock progresses more rapidly in the child.[6] A 5-cm scalp laceration bleeds just as briskly in a child as in an adult, but the amount of blood lost represents a relatively larger percentage of the total blood volume. Thus, injuries that would be considered minor or moderate in an adult may be more severe in a child. As a further example, hypothermia may represent a significant threat to life in injured infants or young children because their homeostatic mechanisms are not as effective as those of adults and their body surface areas are proportionately greater.[7]

In addition, children are at risk for certain specific injuries that are less common in adults. Fifty per cent of duodenal hematomas, for example, occur in children under age 12, and 80 per cent are in patients less than 20 years of age.[8, 9] Abdominal trauma producing mild to moderate pain with obstructive symptoms developing over the following 24 to 72 hours is a classic history for this entity. In a child, this history should raise the suspicion of duodenal hematoma; that diagnosis would be much less likely in an adult.

Pediatric head injury represents another area in which the child's response to trauma differs significantly from that of adults. Classically, a history of head injury with loss of consciousness followed by a lucid interval indicates the strong possibility of an epidural hematoma. However, in children, diffuse cerebral edema is the most common cause of this clinical picture.[10, 11] These observations are of extreme importance to the clinician because of their implications for prognosis and treatment.

Children are not simply "adults in miniature," and their response to trauma differs in significant aspects from that of adults. Thus, all physicians who care for injured children should be prepared to recognize these differences, since the majority of injured pediatric patients are initially cared for in the general emergency department. In one sense, the entire purpose of this book is to address those differences and the therapeutic implications that arise from them. The purpose of this chapter in particular is to highlight certain aspects of the care of the injured child with regard to training, equipment needs, evaluation, and therapy.

TRAINING

The greatest problem in training medical personnel to care for the injured child relates to the relatively small number of cases of pediatric trauma that are seen in any given emergency room. The majority of emergency physicians have had little formal training in the recognition and management of pediatric emergencies.[12, 13] The small percentage of total visits by injured children makes it unlikely that expertise in this field can be gained by personal experience alone.

Training must be designed to maximize efficiency and proficiency in caring for an event that occurs with relatively low frequency. This training should address professionals at all levels of medical care, including physicians, nurses, and emergency medical technicians (EMTs). The need for training physicians is obvious, since they are ultimately responsible for the care of the child. However, it is equally important to ensure that other members of the medical team are well-prepared in caring for children. EMTs are particularly important in this regard, since they are responsible for implementing the physician's initial orders in all children transported by ambulance. (For specific information on training personnel for prehospital care, see Chapter 33.)

Training for pediatric emergencies requires preparation and effective dialogue to assure appropriate education, consultation, and referral. Preparation and dialogue are inseparable in effecting the goal of improved training, inasmuch as the appropriate sources of education are also the sources for consultation and referral.[14, 15] The nearest and best sources of information on the care of injured children are the community's pediatricians. Many of these pediatricians are quite active in evaluating and treating their private patients in the emergency department, but pediatricians are rarely in the emergency department when a pediatric victim of serious trauma initially arrives. However, their input to the care of pediatric emergencies should be sought in every EMS system. Further, a child's private pediatrician should generally be informed whenever the child is evaluated at the emergency department, regardless of the severity of the injury.

Other sources of education, consultation, and referral should also be actively sought. These include local EMS councils, state and local chapters of the American College of Emergency Physicians and American Academy of Pediatrics, and nearby referral centers. These referral centers may include children's hospitals, burn centers, centers for the care of head and spinal cord injuries, microvascular replantation teams, and so on. It is ultimately the responsibility of emergency physicians to seek information from these sources. This provides education (since representatives from these centers are usually available for in-service lectures) and also establishes clear lines of referral and consultation when specific injuries are encountered. Information on referral agreements should be written into the policies and procedures manual and clearly communicated to all staff emergency physicians to ensure that delays in consultation and referral are minimized.

EQUIPMENT

Once appropriate training has been established for members of the emergency system, implementation of care requires appropriate equipment for pediatric patients. The emergency department director, with the assistance of the head nurse or supervisor, should be responsible for assuring that this equipment is available. Table 34–1 lists equipment for pediatric emergencies, but essential items are discussed here.

Resuscitative Equipment

Pediatric resuscitative equipment is absolutely essential in any emergency depart-

Table 34–1. EQUIPMENT FOR PEDIATRIC EMERGENCIES

Resuscitative Equipment
EKG machine with: pediatric leads (adhesive or needle leads)
pediatric paddles
low defibrillation current (10 watt/second minimum)
Small and large laryngoscope handles
Spare bulbs for laryngoscope (small and large)
Laryngoscope blades
Miller 0 (newborn)
Miller 1 (1 month to 1 year)
Miller 2 (2 to 10 years)
Wis-Foregger 3
Macentosh 3
Wis-Hipple 1½ (1 to 2 years)
Masks
Rendell Baker 0 (newborn)
Rendell Baker 1 (1 month to 1 year)
Rendell Baker 2 (1 to 2 years)
Rendell Baker 3 (2 to 10 years)
Adult (adolescent)
Stylets
Airways (size 000-3)
Endotracheal tubes (size 3.0 Foregger to 6.5 Foregger in 0.5 mm increments)
Pediatric Magill or ENT forceps
Anesthesia bags (0.5l to 20l)
Pediatric esophageal airway
Pediatric MAST trousers (David Clark Co., Inc., Worcester, Mass.)
Nasogastric tubes Nos. 5, 8, 10, 14, and 16 French (Argyle Co., Chicago, Ill.) or Nos. 10 and 11 Andersen (Andersen Company, Cincinnati, Ohio)
Suction catheters (Nos. 5, 8, 10, and 14)

IV Equipment
IV infusion pump
Mini-Drip buretrols
IV catheters-Butterfly (Abbott Labs, North Chicago, Ill.)
19-, 21-, 23-, and 25-gauge
IV catheters, plastic
20- and 22-gauge
T-Connector (Abbott Labs, Chicago, Ill.)
Steristrips (3-M Surgical Products, St. Paul, Minn.)
Pediatric arm and foot boards

Examination Equipment
Pediatric stethoscope
Blood pressure cuffs (5 mm, 7.5 mm, and 9.0 mm)
Doppler ultrasound equipment
Tape measure
Pediatric visual acuity chart (with animals, objects, or directional Es)
Pediatric otoscope specula (disposable)
Ear curettes

Other Equipment
Papoose board (Olympus Products)
Pediatric rigid cervical collars
Pediatric Thomas or Hare splints
Pediatric growth charts (to plot age versus height and weight)
Foley or French urinary catheters (Nos. 5, 8, 10, and 12)
Urine collection bags (U-Bags; Hallister Co., Chicago, Ill.)
Chest tubes Nos. 8, 12, and 16 French (Argyle Company, North Chicago, Ill.)
Infant warmer

ment. Necessary items include infant and preschool-sized ventilation masks and bags, endotracheal tubes, laryngoscope blades, and small stylets. Small Magill forceps or ENT forceps may be of value in assisting with intubation. Pediatric esophageal obdurator airways are available and may be of use in the prehospital phase of care, although airway management is usually more appropriately delivered by bag and mask or endotracheal intubation.[16] Any child who receives respiratory support should have the stomach decompressed; therefore appropriately sized soft nasogastric tubes should be available for this purpose. Andersen tubes (No. 10 or 11)* are preferred, but a No. 5, 8, 12, or 16 French nasogastric tube can be used. Additional equipment that may be necessary during resuscitation includes small chest tubes (No. 8 through No. 16 Fr)† pediatric rigid cervical collars, pediatric MAST, and small urinary catheters (No. 5 to No. 8 Fr). Electrocardiographic monitoring equipment should include pediatric leads, pediatric paddles, and a defibrillator with a lower limit of 10 watt/second.

*Anderson Company, Cincinnati, Ohio.
†Argyle Company.

Blood Pressure Equipment

Accurate determination of blood pressure in children requires an appropriately sized cuff, since inaccurate readings occur if the cuff is too large or too small. In general the blood pressure cuff should cover approximately two thirds of the child's upper arm in order to obtain an accurate reading. Proper cuff sizes by age, are the following: 14 years and older, 12 cm; 8 to 14 years, 9.5 cm; 5 to 8 years, 7 cm, and 5 years and younger, 5 cm. Occasionally blood pressure cannot be auscultated accurately even with appropriately sized cuffs, particularly in the infant. Doppler ultrasound equipment is useful in determining arterial pressure in these circumstances, and this equipment should be readily available, if not physically present, in the emergency room.

Intravenous Line Equipment

Obtaining venous access in children is discussed in detail in Chapter 1 (pp. 9–12). Specific equipment needs include small intravenous (IV) cannulas (25-, 23-, and 21-gauge "butterflies" and 22- and 20-gauge plastic cannulas), T-connectors,* pediatric armboards, sterilized cutdown trays, and minidrip buretrols. An infusion pump and pressure bag should be readily available. Central venous cannulation is not the preferred method of obtaining emergency venous access in children but may be utilized once initial stabilization has been provided. Once access to the circulation has been obtained, protecting the IV line is critical, since precious time is lost in replacing it. One means of preventing dislodgment of pediatric IVs is the use of T-connectors. Because of the relatively shorter length of the IV cannula in children, the weight of the IV tubing may dislodge the catheter, resulting in infiltration of the IV. The use of an appropriately taped T-connector allows the tubing to be taped more securely and with less weight on the catheter itself (Fig. 34–1).

All IV lines should be securely taped, but this does not require massive amounts of tape or restraint. Instead, carefully applied arm or foot boards and tape or Steristrips† effectively secure most IVs (Figs. 34–2 and 34–3). A medicine cup can be taped over the catheter site itself to prevent dislodgment. It is particularly important that the nurse and physician be able to see the IV line clearly to be sure that infiltration has not occurred or that the tubing has not become disconnected. Resuscitations may be unsuccessful because medications are being infused either into the tissue or the patient's bed instead of into the vein.

*Abbott Laboratories, North Chicago, Illinois.
†3-M Surgical Products, St. Paul, Minnesota.

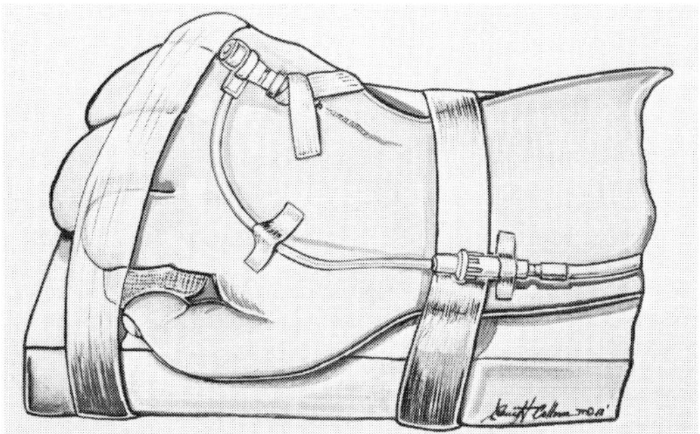

Figure 34–1. The use of a T-connector in pediatric patients allows the intravenous tubing to be taped more securely and prevents dislodgment of the catheter.

EXAMINATION AND TREATMENT

Evaluation

The approach to the examination and treatment of children is somewhat a matter of personal style, but several points deserve emphasis. First, the overall approach to the pediatric patient must be as nonthreatening as possible. The strange surroundings of the emergency department, noise from other patients, the pain from the injury itself, anticipation of pain from treatment of the injury, as well as the possibility of previous unpleasant encounters with physicians all combine to put the child in a state of anxiety, confusion, and fear. Introducing yourself to the parents and talking briefly with the child often save a great deal of time and result as well in a more thorough and pleasant examination. Second, the elements of the physical examination and any procedures to be performed should be explained to the child and to the parents. Some physicians prefer that parents and grandparents be excluded from the examination and treatment area. Others feel that the presence of the parents may be helpful during the examination. However, family members are usually asked to leave if any invasive procedures are performed (laceration repair, lumbar puncture, chest tube insertion, and so on). On some occasions, both the physician and parents may feel more comfortable when a family member remains with the child during these procedures.

Third, the child must always be approached with gentleness. Sudden movements and probing fingers are frightening even if they are not painful. All devices, including the stethoscope, otoscope, and opthalmoscope are potentially threatening to the child. The use of finger puppets during the examination is frequently quite helpful. Placing the puppet on the stethoscope, otoscope, or other equipment can change fright to interest or even laughter in many children (Fig. 34–4).

This small investment of time and effort in the initial phase usually calms the child and the parents and often makes physical restraint unnecessary, even when lacerations are repaired. When restraint is needed, several means are available. Commercial restraints with Velcro closures (see Fig. 19–3) effectively restrain all but the most combative

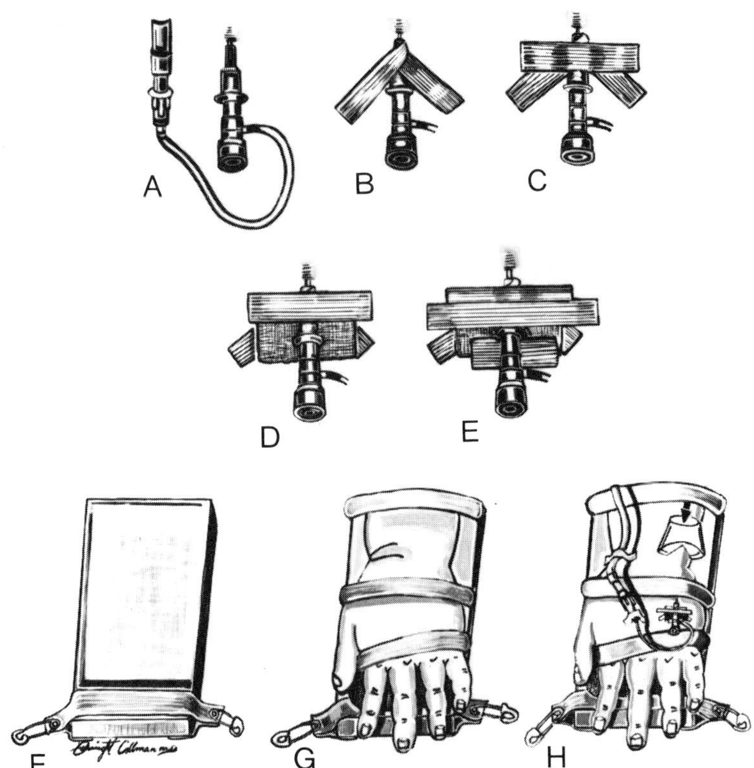

Figure 34–2. Appropriate technique for securing a peripheral angiocatheter. *A,* A T-connector is attached to the catheter and then to the intravenous tubing. *B,* The hub of the angiocatheter is taped to the skin. *C,* An additional piece of tape is placed over the hub of the catheter. *D,* A two-by-two or piece of cotton is placed underneath the catheter, keeping it at approximately the same angle as it was when it entered the vein. *E,* The two-by-two is then secured to the skin with tape. *F,* An arm or foot board should always be used to secure the extremity, and the board should be taped or pinned to the patient's bed. In older children it may not be necessary to secure the board to the bed. *G,* The arm should be taped securely to the board to prevent unnecessary movement. *H,* A medicine cup can be taped over the catheter to prevent dislodgment.

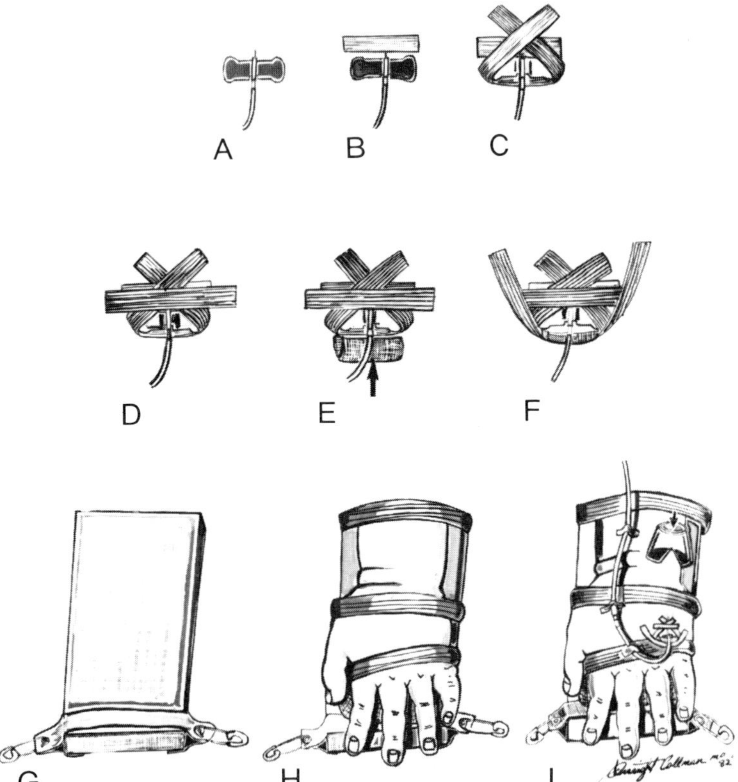

Figure 34–3. Appropriate technique for securing a "butterfly" catheter. *A,* The catheter should be advanced into the vein, as evidenced by entry of blood into the proximal portion of the tubing. *B,* The line should be flushed with intravenous solution, and the catheter taped to the skin at the point of entry. *C,* The butterfly portion of the catheter should be taped to the skin as well. *D,* Following this, an additional piece of tape should be placed under the butterfly portion of the catheter. *E,* A two-by-two or piece of cotton should be placed under the butterfly portion of the catheter and *(F)* taped to the skin. *G,* An arm board should be utilized to prevent movement. *H,* The arm should be securely taped to the board and padded, wherever necessary. *I,* Once the catheter has been placed and taped, a medicine cup may be used to prevent dislodgment.

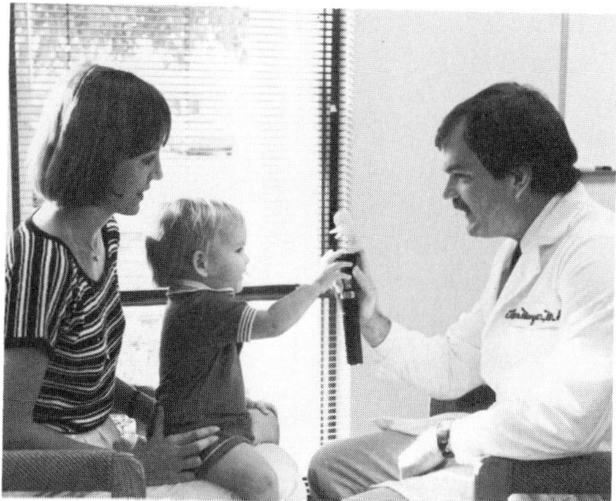

Figure 34–4. Use of finger puppets during the initial examination of the pediatric patient can often change the patient's initial fright to laughter. The puppets can be used on virtually any piece of diagnostic equipment and can greatly ease children's anxieties.

children. A simple bed sheet can serve the same purpose if an attendent is available to assist (Fig. 34–5). Finally, physical restraint with an adequate number of assistants is sometimes attempted but is seldom effective, since the child's ability to wriggle and thrash usually exceeds the number of hands and arms available for restraint. Once a child is effectively restrained, the majority will usually submit to the procedure. Many physicians find it helpful to talk with the patient throughout the procedure, since this frequently has a soothing effect. Others have used stereo headphones and music for the same purpose.

Therapy

Most physicians are aware that drug dosages in infants and children are different from those in adults. Much less well-known, however, are the specific dosages for children and the fact that metabolism and excretion of drugs are also often different in children. Assuming that a child is one-half the size of an adult and therefore should take one-half of the drug dosage may result in disastrous consequences. Up to 50 per cent of pediatric emergency patients evaluated in general emergency rooms have been found to be undermedicated when seen on referral.[17, 18]

Whenever there is a question regarding proper medication dosage, the physician or nurse should always consult a drug reference. A list of emergency medications can be found in Table 34–2 of this chapter, and most pediatric textbooks contain such a reference.[19, 20] Such a source should always be readily available in every emergency department. Extremely urgent problems, such as cardiac arrest, do not allow time to check the drug dosage. Every physician who cares for injured children should be well acquainted with the dosage of medications required in these cases (see Table 1–3).

Because children's previous experiences with physicians and medical care may preclude the ability to calm them sufficiently, several medications have been used to induce drowsiness, cooperation, and mild analgesia. The physician is well-served by familiarity with the following medications, since they may be used as aids for diagnostic examination or treatment purposes.

Sedation and Anesthesia

Nitrous Oxide

Nitrous oxide inhalational anesthesia is rapid and effective and induces a euphoric state in the majority of children. It requires the child's cooperation, and great care must be taken to ensure that oxygen is administered simultaneously, since 100 per cent nitrous oxide can produce hypotension and cardiac arrest.[21] Although some centers use this method with good results, it has not gained wide acceptance.[22, 23]

Seconal

In a 2 mg/kg dose, given intramuscularly (IM) or orally, Seconal induces mild sedation. It is frequently used in crying children in whom examination of the abdomen is difficult. Since oral Seconal requires 20 to 60 minutes to take effect, the IM route is usually preferred.

Cardiac Cocktail

Originally used as a sedative prior to cardiac catheterization, this mixture of meperidine (Demerol), promethazine (Phenergan), and chlorpromazine (Thorazine) is quite effective in safely producing moderate sedation. The dose must be carefully checked to avoid overmedication (Table 34–3), and the drugs should be given by deep IM injection, since meperidine is extremely irritating to soft tissue. The injection begins to take effect in 20 to 30 minutes, with the maximum

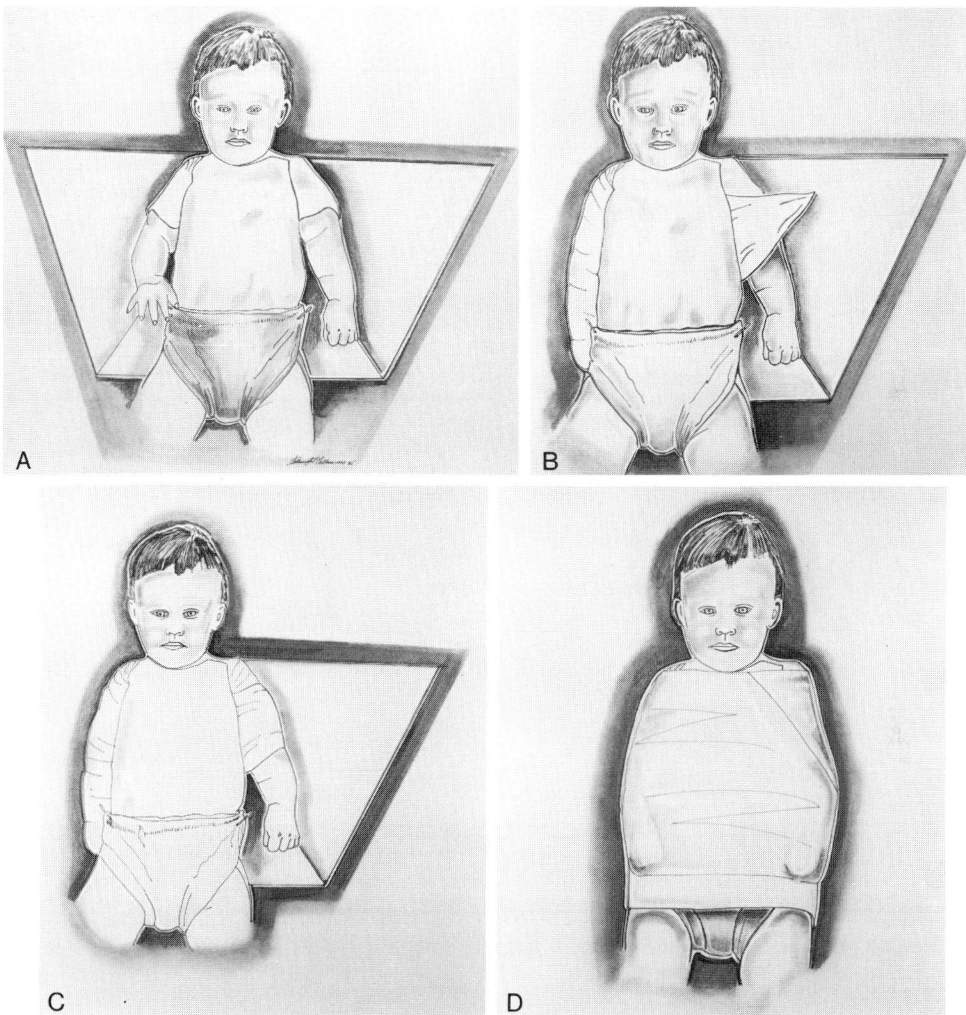

Figure 34–5. A bed sheet can be used for restraining small children. *A*, The sheet should be folded into a triangle, and the infant placed upon it. *B*, The sheet should be placed over the right arm, under the back, and over the left arm of the patient. *C*, The portion of the sheet over the left arm is then tucked under the back. *D*, The left side of the sheet is then placed over the body and tucked under the back. This system effectively restrains all but the most active children.

Table 34–2. PEDIATRIC RESUSCITATION MEDICATIONS

Drug	Dose	How Supplied	Remarks
Atropine sulfate	0.01 mg/kg	0.4 mg/ml	Dose may be doubled in asystole
Bretylium tosylate	5–30 mg/kg	50 mg/ml, 10 ml ampule	Start at 5 mg/kg and increase in 5 mg/kg increments
Calcium chloride 10 per cent	20 mg/kg/dose	100 mg/ml	Dilute 1:1 with sterile water; give slowly; asystole, electromechanical dissociation
Dopamine HCL	5–20 μg/kg/min	40 mg/ml	See "Rule of Six," p. 8
Epinephrine HCL (1:10,000)	0.01 mg/kg/dose	0.1 mg/cc	Asystole; ventricular fibrillation
Furosemide	1 mg/kg/dose	10 mg/ml	Dose may be doubled
Isoproterenol HCL	0.1–0.5 μg/kg/dose	1 mg/5 ml	See "Rule of Six," p. 8
Lidocaine (bolus)	1 mg/kg	20 mg/ml	Ventricular arrhythmias
Lidocaine (infusion)	30 μg/kg/min	20 mg/ml	
Sodium bicarbonate	1–2 mg/kg/dose	1 mEq/ml	Additional doses on basis of blood gases; dilute 1:1 with sterile water in infants
Naloxone	0.01 mg/kg/dose	0.4 mg/ml	May repeat every 2 to 3 minutes
Mannitol (bolus)	1 g/kg/dose	1 g/ml	Use only with neurosurgical consultation
Mannitol (infusion)	300 mg/kg g 3 h	Use only with neurosurgical consultation	
Sodium nitroprusside	0.5 μg/kg/min	10 mg/ml	Usual effect at 1–10 μg/kg/min
Dextrose 50 per cent	500 mg-1 gm/kg max = 25 gm	500 mg/ml, 50 ml syringe	Dilute 1:1 in infants
Diazepam	0.3 mg/kg/dose		Give slowly
Diphenylhydantoin	10–15 mg/kg/dose for seizures		Dilute in normal saline
Dexamethasone	1.5 mg/kg initially, then 1.5 mg/kg/day	4 mg/ml	
Diazoxide	5–10 mg/kg	4 mg/ml	
Aminophylline	5–7 mg/kg loading 0.9 mg/kg/hr infusion		
Morphine	0.1 mg/kg		Observe closely for respiratory depression
Phenobarbital	5–10 mg/kg		May repeat every 10 minutes for status epilepticus up to 25 mg/kg
Propranolol	0.01–0.15 mg/kg up to 10 mg		Hypotension, hypoglyceia, and bradycardia are side-effects
Methylprednisone	5 mg/kg 1–2 mg/kg		For sepsis or shock; for bronchospasm
Acetaminophen	10–15 mg/kg	Pediatric tablets 80 mg; elixir 120 mg/5 ml; Tempra Drops 60 mg/0.6 ml; Liquiprin 120 mg/2.5 ml	Toxic dose 140 mg/kg
N-Acetylcysteine 10%	Loading: 140 mg/kg/po Maintenance: 70 mg/kg g 4 hr × 17	Acetaminophen overdose	Dilute to 5%
Ampicillin	50–400 mg/kg/day		Dosage varies with severity of disease
Activated charcoal	1 g/kg		Mix with water

Table 34–3. PEDIATRIC COCKTAILS

		Dosage	Maximum Dose
I	Demerol (meperidine)	2 mg/kg	50 mg
	Thorazine (chlorpromazine)	0.5 mg/kg	12.5 mg
	Phenergan (promethazines)	0.5 mg/kg	12.5 mg
II	Demerol (meperidine)	2 mg/kg	50 mg
	Phenergan (promethazine)	2 mg/kg	50 mg

response at 45 minutes. This combination of medications can be quite effective in children who require repair of facial lacerations, in whom movement and crying would prevent optimal surgical technique.

LIDOCAINE

Even when mild sedation is used, most children with lacerations require local or field block anesthesia for repair. Either 0.5 or 1 per cent epinephrine (1:100,000) may be used, but higher concentrations should be avoided in the child to prevent side effects. Up to 3 to 4 mg/kg of lidocaine may be safely used for local or field blocks in children. To decrease the amount of pain when lidocaine is injected, two points deserve emphasis. First, the lidocaine should be as near body temperature as possible, and it may be kept in a controlled warmer for this purpose. Second, the injection should always be undertaken with as small a needle as possible (usually 27-gauge but never larger than 25-gauge). A slightly longer time is required for injection, but it is much less painful.

Additional areas in which therapy in children differs in approach or content from adults are addressed in the chapters that deal with each specific body area. Recognition of the fact that children *are* different and preparation for the diagnostic and therapeutic implications that these differences entail will make a significant difference in outcome. There is certainly no greater thrill in medicine than effectively resuscitating a critically ill child. This is possible only through appropriate preparation and education.

REFERENCES

1. Meier EM: The pediatric emergency patient. Emer Med 13:29, 1981.
2. Holbrook PR: Prehospital care of critically ill children Crit Care Med 8:537, 1980.
3. Annual Report, National Association of children's Hospitals and Related Institutions, 1979.
4. Chameides L, Melker R, Raye JR, et al.: Resuscitation of children. *In* McIntyre KM, Lewis AJ (eds.): Textbook of Advanced Cardiac Life Support. Dallas, American Heart Association, 1981.
5. Ehrlich R, Emmett SM, Rodriguez-Torres R: Pediatric cardiac resuscitation trauma: A six-year study. J Pediatr 84:152, 1974.
6. Rowe MI: Shock and resuscitation. *In* Welch KJ (ed.): Complications of Pediatric Surgery. Philadelphia, W. B. Saunders Co., 1982, pp. 14–38.
7. Smith RM: Anesthesia for Infants and Children. 4th ed. St. Louis, C. V. Mosby Co., 1980.
8. Margolis IB, Cornazzo AJ, Finn MD: Intramural duodenal hematoma. Am J Surg 132:779, 1976.
9. Janson KL, Stockinger F: Duodenal hematoma. Critical analysis of recent treatment techniques. Am J Surg 129:304, 1975.
10. Bruce DA, Alavi A, Bilaniuk L, et al.: Diffuse cerebral swelling following head injury in children: The syndrome of "malignant brain edema." J Neurosurg 170, 1981.
11. Bruce DA, Raphaely RC, Goldberg AI, et al.: Pathophysiology, treatment and outcome following severe head injury in children. Child's Brain 5:174, 1979.
12. Ludwig S, Fleisher G, Henretig F: Pediatric training in emergency medicine residency programs. Ann Emerg Med 11:170, 1982.
13. Halperin R, Meyer AR, Alpert JJ: Utilization of pediatric emergency services. Pediatr Clin North Am 26:747, 1979.
14. Wingert WA: Delivery of emergency care to children: Who is responsible? (letter). Pediatrics 62:124, 1978.
15. Haller JA: An overview of pediatric trauma. *In* Toularkian RJ (ed.): Pediatric Trauma. New York, John Wiley & Sons, 1978, 88:3–20.
16. Melker R: CPR in neonates, infants, and children. *In* Auerbach PS, Budassi SA (eds.): Cardiac Arrest and CPR. Rockville, Aspen Systems, 1983, pp. 165–178.
17. Wingert WA, Friedman DB, Larson WR: Pediatric emergency room patients: A comparison of patients seen during the day and the night. Am J Dis Child 115:48, 1968.
18. Alpert JJ, Feinbloom R: Advances in hospital ambulatory care for children. Pediatr Clin North Am 21:263, 1974.
19. Vaughan VC, McKay RJ (eds.): Textbook of Pediatrics. 11th ed. Philadelphia, W. B. Saunders Co., 1981.
20. Rudolph A (ed.): Pediatrics. Norwalk, Ct., Appleton-Century-Crofts, 1983.
21. Dripps RD, Eckendorff JE, Vandam LD (eds.): Introduction to Anesthesia: The Principles of Safe Practice. Philadelphia, W. B. Saunders, 1977.
22. Gregory GA; Pediatric anesthesia. *In* Miller RD (ed.): Anesthesia. New York, Churchill Livingstone, 1981.
23. Smith RM: Fundamental Differences in Anesthesia for Infants and Children. St. Louis, C. V. Mosby, 1980.

INDEX

Note: Page numbers in italics refer to illustrations; page numbers followed by t refer to tables.

Abdominal bleeding, celiotomy for, 336
Abdominal distention, 330–331
Abdominal girth, *330*, 330–331
Abdominal injuries, 328–338
  assessment of, 27–29, 328–335
  auscultation and, 331
  blunt, 328–329, 329t
    surgical treatment of, 337–338
  conservative therapy for, 338
  diagnostic studies of, 332–335, 332t, *333–334*, 333t
  examination of pelvis, perineum and rectum in, 331, 332t
  girth measurement in, *330*, 330–331
  hemorrhage in, 335–336, 336t
  history of, 328
  indications for surgery in, 335–338, 335t
  inspection of, 329–330
  management of, 335–338
  mechanism of, 328–329
  palpation and, 331
  penetrating, 329
    surgical treatment of, 336–337
  peritoneal lavage and, *333–334*, 333–335, 333t
  physical diagnosis of, 329–335
  radiographic evaluation of, 192–194, *193*
  vascular, 409
Abdominal thrust, 4
Acetaminophen, antidote to, 452t
  for resuscitation, 532t
  in emergency room poisoning episodes, 445t
N-Acetylcysteine, for resuscitation, 532t
Acidosis, fluid and electrolyte management in, 107–108
  in poisoning cases, 456
  metabolic, 145–146
Acids, antidote to, 452t
Acquired coagulopathies, 222–223
Acquired heart disease, 205
Activated charcoal, for resuscitation, 532t
Acute renal failure (ARF), 140–157
  dialysis and, 150–151, 154–156
  differential diagnosis of, 141–142
  drug use in, 150, 152t–153t
  enteral alimentation in, 149t
  fluid and electrolyte management in, 111
  laboratory features of, 141t
  management problems in, 143–148
  medications and, 238
  natural history of, 157
  nutritional management in, 148–150, 149t
Acute renal failure (ARF) (*Continued*)
  parenchymal involvement in, 140–141
  postrenal, 141
  post-traumatic, 139–159
  pre-renal (functional), 140
  therapeutic considerations in, 142–143
  volume overload in, 146
Acute renal parenchymal failure (ARPF), 140–141
  causes of, 140
  diagnosis of, 141–142, 141t
  laboratory features of, 141t
  therapy for, 142–143
Acute tubular necrosis (ATN), 140
Adolescent, minimum daily protein requirements for, 148
  nasal intubation in, *60*, 60–62
Adolescent poisoning, common drugs in, 445t
Adrenal disease, 231–232
Adult poisoning, common drugs in, 445t
Aggravated rape, definition of, 435
Air transportation, 520–522
Airway, and breathing, 2–5
  esophageal obturator, 4
  patent, maintenance of, *56–57*, 56–62, 58t, *59–61*, 59t
      during transportation, 510
  positioning of, 3, *3*
  surgical opening of, 5, *6*, 62
Airway control, 3–5
  flow sheet for, *2*
Airway obstruction, 20
  complete, *489–490*, 489–492, 491t, *492*
  partial, *488*, 488–489
Airway obstructive disease, 485–494
  infectious, 485–487
  types of, 486t
Albumin, for shock resuscitation, 14
Albuterol, for asthma, 244t
Alcohol/drug combination, in emergency room poisoning episodes, 445t
Alkali, antidote to, 452t
Alkaloids, antidote to, 452t
Alkalosis, fluid and electrolyte management in, 108–109
Aluminum pop-tops, ingestion of, 495, *496*
Alveolar bone, intruded tooth in, *321*, 321–322
Alveolar fractures, 326, *326*
Ambu bags, 54
Amikacin, and ARF, 152t

Amin-aid, and enteral alimentation in ARF, 149t
Aminess tablets, and enteral alimentation in ARF, 149t
Aminoacidopathies, 232
Amino acids, essential, 125
 nonessential, 125–126
ϵ-Aminocaproic acid (Amicar), for mucous membrane bleeding, 221
Aminoglycosides, and ARF, 152t
Aminophylline, for asthma, 243–244, 244t
 for resuscitation, 532t
Amitriptyline, in emergency room poisoning episodes, 445t
Amoxicillin, and ARF, 153t
Amphetamine, antidote to, 452t
 in emergency room poisoning episodes, 445t
Ampicillin, for cystic fibrosis, 247t
 for head injury, 283
 for neurologic injury, 26t, 27
 for resuscitation, 532t
Amputation, for hand injuries, 403–404, *404*
 traumatic, treatment of, 34
Analgesics, for burns, 417
Anemia, 223
 medullary compensation of, *224*
Anesthesia, and acute spinal cord lesions, 87
 and burn patients, 87
 drugs used in, 74–83, 76t
 fluid and blood replacement during, 84–87
 for minor trauma, 87–89
 humidification during, 84
 in pediatric emergencies, 530, 533, 533t
 increase in IOP during, 87
 induction of, 58t, 59t, 72–74
 maintenance of, 74
 maintenance of respiration during, 83–84
 rapid sequence intubation for, 72–73
 special considerations during, 87
Anesthetic airway, rapid sequence technique for, 72–73
Anesthetized patient, extensive monitoring of, 69–72, 70t, 71t
 intraoperative management of, 68–89
 routine monitoring of, 68–69, 69t
Angulation, spontaneous correction of, 354, *355*
Animal bites, 466–483
 of hand, 393
Anion gap, 99
Ankle fractures, 378–380
 radiographic evaluation of, 175–176
Ankle blocks, 88–89
Antacids, use of, prior to surgery, 67–68
Antibiotics, for cystic fibrosis, 247t
 for head injury, 283
Anticholinergics, antidote to, 452t
Anticholinesterases, antidote to, 452t
 for clinical anesthesia, 83
Anticonvulsants, and ARF, 152t
Antidiuretic hormone (ADH), hyponatremia and, 103
 inappropriate secretion of, 103, 247
Antidotal therapy, for poisoning, 451, 451t, 452t–454t, 454
 for pre-hospital phase of care, 451t
 local and systemic, 452t–454t
Antihistamine, antidote to, 452t
Antimicrobials, and ARF, 152t
Antivenin therapy, 480–481
 for latrodectism, 471
Aorta, coarctation of, 212
Aortic laceration, radiographic evaluation of, 191–192
Apnea, 277
Aquatic animal bites, 473
Arrhythmias. See *Cardiac arrhythmias*
Arsenic, antidote to, 452t
Arterial blood pressure monitoring, of ICU patient, 116–117, *118*
Arterial cannulation, 70
Arterial oxygen content, 208–209
Arterial oxygen tension, 72
Arthropod stings and bites, 470–473
Ascorbic acid, daily requirements of, 126t
Asphyxia, traumatic, 259
Aspiration, needle, 20
Aspirin, and platelet function, 220
 in emergency room poisoning episodes, 445t
Asthma, 243–244
 drug therapy for, 244t
Asystole, 8
Atelectasis, radiographic evaluation of, 191
Atrial filling pressure, cardiac lesions and, 209–211
Atropine, 74
 antidote to, 452t
 for asthma, 244t
 for cardiac arrest, 7t, 8
 use of, prior to anesthesia, 73
  prior to surgery, 67
Atropine sulfate, for resuscitation, 64t, 532t
 for scorpion stings, 472
Auscultation, of abdomen, 331
Automobile accidents, dental injuries caused by, 317
Azotemia, prerenal, 140–141, 141t

Bacterial endocarditis, 214
Bacterial tracheitis, 487
 pathophysiology of, *488*
Bag and mask ventilation, 4, 54
Balloon-tipped catheter, 495–496, *496*
Barbiturate coma, in near drowning victims, 463
Barbiturates, for clinical anesthesia, 79
Barium salts, antidote to, 452t
Basilar pneumothorax, 186, *186*
Battered child syndrome. See *Child abuse*
Beck's triad, 22
Belladonna alkaloids, antodote to, 452t
"Belly-breathing," 330
Belt marks, 425
Benzodiazepines, for clinical anesthesia, 79–80
Berlin's edema, 312, *312–313*
Betamethasone dipropionate (Diprosone), for hymenoptera stings, 472
 for scorpion stings, 472
Bier's block, 88
Bilateral rib fractures, 430
Biochemical parameters, in nutritional support, 137, 137t
Biotin, daily requirements of, 126t
Birth fractures, 361–363, *362–363*
Bite marks, 427, *427*
Bites, 293–294, 294t, 393, 466–483

Black widow spider (Latrodectus) bites, *470*, 470–471
Bladder, injuries to, 30, 338, 349–350, *349–350*
  radiographic evaluation of, 198–199, *199*
Bladder decompression, by catheterization, 29–30, *30*
  purpose of, 29
Blalock-Taussig shunt, 209
Bleeding. See also *Hemorrhage*
  abnormal. See also *Hemostatic disorders*
    common causes of, 218
    evaluation of, 217–218, 218t
  as complication of peritoneal dialysis, 154
  external, 17
  internal, 17–18, *18*
Blood flow distribution, cardiac lesions and, 212
Blood gas determinations, for ICU patients, 119–120
Blood gases, intra-arterial, monitoring of, 72
Blood loss, estimating degree of, 13–14
  following shock, 17–18, *18*
  hypotension and, 13
  shock and, 13
Blood pressure, following head injury, 277
Blood pressure equipment, 526
Blood replacement, during anesthesia, 84–87
Blood transfusion, whole, vs. component therapy, 46–48, 46t
Blood volume, 12
Blowout fractures, *304–305*, 304–306
Blows and thrusts, 4
Blunt trauma, and abdominal injuries, 328–329, 329t
  to bladder, 338
Body fluid compartments, 98, *98*
Body fluid electrolyte composition, 98, *98*
Body volume, and composition, 98–100, *98–99*
Boehler's angle, for calcaneal fracture, 175, *175*
Bolus feeding, 130
Bone, alveolar, intruded tooth in, *321*, 321–322
  long, plastic bowing of, 166, *166*
  teeth-supporting, injuries to, 326, *326*
Bone shortening, spontaneous correction of, 356, *356*
Bony injuries, to hand, 401
Boxer's fracture, *164*, 169
Brachial plexus block, 88
Brachial vein cutdown, 10
Branding, burns inflicted by, 426–427
Breathing, airway and, 2–5
Bretylium, for cardiac arrest, 7t, 9
  for resuscitation, 532t
Bromides, antidote to, 452t
Bronchopulmonary dysplasia, 242–243
Brown recluse spider (Loxosceles) bites, *471*, 471–472
Bruises, 424–425, *425*
  child abuse and, 424–426, 424t, *425*
  circumferential, 425
  estimating ages of, 424t
  lung, 190, *190*
Bryant's skin traction, 383, *383*
  for birth fractures, 362
"Bucket-handle" fracture, 388
Buckle fracture, cortical, incomplete, *164*
  of radius and ulna, 364, *364*
Burns, 413–420
  analgesics for, 417
Burns (*Continued*)
  anesthesia for, 87
  chemical, 418–419
    of eye, *306*, 306–307, 306t
  child abuse and, *426*, 426–427
  classification of, 414, 414t
  electrical injury and, 418
  fluid and electrolyte management in, 111
  fluid resuscitation for, after 48 hrs, 415t, 416
    during first 24 hrs, 415–416, 415t
    during second 24 hrs, 415t, 416
    problems during, 416
  fluid therapy for, 414–416, 415t
  inhalation injury and, 417–418
  initial evaluation of, 413–414
  minor, 417
  outcome of, 419–420
  peripheral vascular compromise and, 416–417
  reconstruction following, 397–398
  third degree, from gasoline, *396*
  to hand, 394–398, *396–397*
    emergency care of, 396
Burr holes, 26, 284
"Butterfly" catheter, *529*
Butyrophenones, for clinical anesthesia, 80

Cadmium, antidote to, 452t
Caffey's disease, 432
Calcaneal fracture, Boehler's angle for, 175, *175*
Calcium, daily requirements of, 126t
  TPN infusion of, 132t
Calcium balance, in ARF, 146–147
Calcium chloride, for cardiac arrest, 7t, 8
  for resuscitation, 64t, 532t
Calcium gluconate, for hyperkalemia, 145, 145t
  for Latrodectus bites, 470
  for resuscitation, 64t
  for scorpion stings, 472
Caloric balance, effect of trauma on, 127t
Calorie count, 128
Calories, for injured children, 127
  in TPN infusate composition, 132t
Canalicular lacerations, 303–304, *304*
Canalicular trauma, 302
Candida precipitans, in TPN infection, 135
Capillary hydrostatic pressure, edema and, 106
Capillary permeability, edema and, 105
Car seat burns, 432
Carbamates, antidote to, 452t
Carbenicillin, and ARF, 153t
  for cystic fibrosis, 247t
Carbon monoxide, antidote to, 452t
Cardiac arrest, 6–9, 7t, *8*
Cardiac arrhythmias, head injuries and, 207
  in poisoning cases, 456
Cardiac cocktails, 530, 533, 533t
Cardiac compressions, 63
Cardiac drugs, pathophysiologic changes induced by, 213
Cardiac lesions, and afterload, 211
  and atrial filling pressure, 209–211
  and blood flow distribution, 212
  and contractility, 211–212
Cardiac pathophysiologic abnormalities, 208–213
Cardiac rate and rhythm, 212–213

Cardiac rupture, 268
Cardiac system, preanesthetic treatment and stabilization of, 62–65, *63*, 64t
Cardiac tamponade, 268–269
hemopericardium with, 206
Cardiac valvar injury, 268
Cardiogenic shock, 39t
Cardiopulmonary resuscitation (CPR), 63, *63*
Cardiorespiratory injury, diagnosis of, 254–255
initial resuscitation following, 255
reassessment following, 255
Cardiorespiratory values, baseline, 4t
Cardiotoxicity, hyperkalemia and, 109
Cardiovascular problems, in near drowning victims, 464
Cardiovascular system, arterial blood pressure monitoring of, 116–117, *118*
central venous pressure monitoring of, 117, 119, 119t
effects of chest trauma on, 205–206
effects of CNS trauma on, 206–207
effects of trauma on, 205–208
EKG of, 116
examination and monitoring of, 65
intensive care monitoring of, 116–119
near drowning affecting, 461
pulmonary artery catheterization in evaluation of, 119
vital signs in evaluation of, 116
Carotid artery injury, 408–409
Cat bites, 469
Catharsis, of ingested poisons, 451
Catheter-related hazards, of TPN, 134–135, 134t
Caudal anesthesia, 88
Cefamandole (Mandol), and ARF, 152t
Cefazolin (Ancef, Kefzol), and ARF, 152t
Cefoperazone (Cefobid), and ARF, 152t
Cefotaxime (Claforan), and ARF, 152t
Celiotomy, to control bleeding, 336
Central nervous system (CNS), near drowning and, 459–461
preanesthetic treatment and stabilization of, 65–66
Central nervous system trauma, child abuse and, 428
effects of, on cardiovascular system, 206–207
Central venous pressure (CVP) monitoring, catheter for, 14
indications for, 71t
of ICU patient, 117, 119, 119t
Centruroides species, sting of, 472, *472*
Cephalexin (Keflex), for Loxosceles bites, 472
Cephalic vein cutdown, 10
Cephalosporins, and ARF, 152t–153t
Cephalothin (Keflin), and ARF, 153t
Cerebral edema, 282
following head injury, 282
in poisoning cases, 456
Cerebral hyperemia, 282
Cerebral support, for near drowning victims, 462–463
Cervical spine, injury to, 27, *27*
preventing damage to, 511–512
radiographic evaluation of, *178–179*, 178–180, 251–252
Cervicomediastinal injuries, 409
Cheeks, lacerations of, 295–296
Chemical burns, 418–419
of eye, *306*, 306–307, 306t
Chemosis, 307, *308*
Chest trauma. See *Thoracic trauma*
Chest tube, in tension pneumothorax, 20–21, *21*
Cheyne-Stokes respirations, 277
Child(ren), baseline cardiorespiratory values in, 4t
battered. See *Child abuse*
blood volume in, 12
cardiac compressions for, 63
causes of death in, *502*
DC countershock in, 7t, 9
incidence of fractures in, 353
indications for thoracotomy in, 255–256
injured, evaluation and management of, 1–36
nasal intubation in, 60
normal, nutritional requirements of, 125–127, 125t
respiratory rates in, 273, 276t
on hemodialysis, 238–239
on medications, 237–238
on peritoneal dialysis, 239–240
periosteum in, 353, *353*
small, cannulation in, 9
urine output in, 13
vascular injuries in, 406
Weech mnemonics for, 64t
Child abuse, 421–434
age distribution of, *422*
and other inflicted injuries, 431
bite marks and, 427, *427*
bruising in, 424–426, 424t, *425*
burns in, *426*, 426–427
clinical history in, 422–424, 424t
areas of emphasis in, 423–424
CNS trauma and, 428
common and characteristic findings in, 424–431
considerations for physician in suspected cases of, 432–434
fractures indicating, 429–430, *430*
head trauma and, 427–428
intra-abdominal injuries and, 431
magnitude of problem of, 421
national study on, 421t
ocular manifestations of, 314–315
pancreatic trauma and, 431
physical findings mimicking, 431–432, *432*
physician's responsibilities in, 421–422
radiographic evaluation in, 200–201, *201*
sexual. See *Sexual abuse*
skeletal injuries and, 428–431
skeletal surveys for, 430–431
skin trauma and, 424–427, 424t, *425–427*
supporting parents in cases of, 434
victims of, interdisciplinary approach to, 436–443
Child protection, in abuse cases, 432–433
Child protective services, 433
Chloral hydrate, and ARF, 152t
Chloramphenicol, and ARF, 153t
Chlorates, antidote to, 453t
Chlordiazepoxide, in emergency room poisoning episodes, 445t
Chlorpromazine (Thorazine), pediatric cocktail, 533t
Choking child, back blows to, *489*
chest thrusts to, *490*
conscious, 489–490, *489–490*, 491t

Choking child (*Continued*)
Heimlich maneuver in, 489–490, *490*
unconscious, 491–492, 491t, *492*
Cholinergic compounds, antidote to, 452t
Chorioretinal rupture, 313, *313*
Christmas disease, 221–222
treatment of, 219t
Chronic anemia, 223
Chronic cardiac disease, injuries to children with, 205–215
Chronic lung disease, injuries to children with, 241–248
Chronic renal disease, clinical characteristics of, 234t
effect of, on tolerance limits, 233–234, *234*, 234t
electrolyte therapy in, 237
estimating magnitude of, 235
identifying and assessing, 234–235
injuries to children with, 233–240
laboratory features of, 235
maintenance fluid therapy in, 237
medications for, 237–238
physical characteristics of, 234–235
resuscitation fluid therapy in, 236–237
Chylothorax, following chest trauma, 262
radiographic evaluation of, 188, *189*
Cigarette burns, 427
Cimetidine, use of, prior to surgery, 67
Circulation, assessment of, 5–12
Circulatory volume, restoration of, 14–16, *15*, 43–45
Clavicle, birth fractures of, 362
fractures of, 256–257, 376–377, *377*
radiographic evaluation of, 173, *174*
retrosternal dislocation of, 185, *185*
Clindamycin, for cystic fibrosis, 247t
Clonidine, for hypertension, 148t
Closed pneumothorax, following chest trauma, 260, *260*
Coagulation, in ICU patients, 121–122
Coagulation factor cascade, schema of, *217*
Coagulopathies, acquired, 222–223
in near drowning victims, 461–462, 464
management of, 221–223
Coarctation, of aorta, 212
Cocaine, administration of, before nasal intubation, 60
in emergency room poisoning episodes, 445t
Codeine, and ARF, 152t
Codeine combinations, in emergency room poisoning episodes, 445t
Coin rubbing (CiaGio), 432, *432*
Coins, ingestion of, 495
Colloid solutions, for shock resuscitation, 14
vs. crystalloids, 44–45
Coma, barbiturate, in near drowning victims, 463
Comb marks, 425, *425*
Commotio retinae, 312, *312–313*
Communication system, of pediatric trauma center, 504
of transportation system, 517–518
Complete airway obstruction, *489–490*, 489–492, 491t, *492*
Complete fracture, *162*, 165
Component therapy, vs. whole blood, 46–48, 46t
Computerized tomography (CT), for severe head injury, 280
Computerized tomography (CT) (*Continued*)
renal injury and, 344
Condylar neck, fractures through, 299–300
Congenital heart disease, 205
cyanotic, oxygen content in, 208–209
Conjunctival crepitus, 307–308
Conjunctival edema, 307, *308*
Conjunctival hemorrhage, 307, *307*
Conjunctival injuries, 307
Conscious choking child, 489–490, *489–490*, 491t
Consciousness, level of, following head injury, 276
Continuous positive airway pressure (CPAP), 89–90
Contractility, cardiac, lesions affecting, 207–212
Controlyte, and enteral alimentation in ARF, 149t
Controlyte formula, 130t
Contusion. See specific types
Copper, antidote to, 452t
Corn oil, and enteral alimentation in ARF, 149t
Corneal abrasion, foreign bodies and, 308–309, *309*
Corneal lacerations, 310, *310*
Coronary artery rupture, 268
Cottonmouth snake, 474
Court testimony, in abuse cases, 433–434
Creatinine excretion, 128
Crepitus, conjunctival, 307–308
Cricothyroidotomy, needle, 5, *6*, 491
surgical, 491–492, *492*
Criticare NH formula, 130t
Crotalid envenomation, classification and treatment of, 476t
field treatment of, 477–478
hospital care for, 478–479
Crotalidae family, 474
Croup, 486–487
clinical scoring of, 486t
Crown-root fractures, 320
Cryoprecipitate, for shock therapy, 47–48
Crystalloid solutions, for shock resuscitation, 14–16, *15*
vs. colloids, 44–45
Cubitus valgus, 371
Cubitus varus, 371, *371*, 374, *374*
Cyanide, antidote to, 452t
Cyanocobalamin, daily requirements of, 126t
Cyclopentolate hydrochloride (Cyclogyl), for corneal abrasion, 309
Cystic fibrosis (CF), 244–248
antibiotics and, 247t
electrolyte disturbance and, 247
fluid disturbance and, 247
gastrointestinal disease and, 246–247
infections and, 247, 247t
problems and considerations of trauma and, 245t
pulmonary disease in, 245–246

Dental injuries, 317–327. See also *Tooth*
causes of, 317
clinical examination of, 318
diagnosis of, 317–318, 318t
infection and, 326–327
Dentin, tooth, fractures of, 318–319, *319–320*
Depolarizing muscle relaxants, 81–82

Depressed skull fracture, 183, *183*
Dermal exposure, to poisons, 449–450
Detoxification, of ingested poisons, 451
Dexamethasone, for controlling ICP, 65
for neck injury, 27
for neurologic injury, 26t
for resuscitation, 64t, 532t
Dextran, for resuscitation, 14
Dextrose, for resuscitation, 532t
Diabetes mellitus, 226–229, 227t, 228t
management of trauma in patient with, 226–227, 227t
treatment of, 219t
Dialysis, after trauma, 150–151, 154–156
indications for, 150
selecting type of, 150–151, 154–156
to eliminate absorbed poison, 455
Diaphragmatic injury, radiographic evaluation of, 192
Diaphragmatic rupture, 264–266, *265*
Diastatic suture fracture, 182, *182*
Diazepam (Valium), for hymenoptera stings, 473
for Latrodectus bites, 470
for resuscitation, 64, 532t
for scorpion stings, 472
for status epilepticus, 283
in emergency room poisoning episodes, 445t
Diazoxide, for hypertension, 148t
for resuscitation, 532t
Dietary history, 127–128
Diethylstilbesterol (DES), for pregnancy prophylaxis, 442
Diphenylhydantoin, for neurologic injury, 27
for resuscitation, 532t
in emergency room poisoning episodes, 445t
Direct current (DC) countershock, for ventricular fibrillation, 7t, 9
Disequilibrium syndrome, 156
Dislocations, 353–357, 363–368
Displaced fractures, of clavicle, 377, *377*
of radius and ulna, 364–365, *364–365*
Disseminated intravascular coagulation (DIC), 222–223
treatment of, 219t
Distributive shock, 39t
Diuretics, for head injury, 284
to eliminate absorbed poison, *454*, 454–455
Division of emergency medical services (DEMS), components of, *503*
Dobhoff tube, 129
Dog bites, 294, 466, *467*
Dopamine, for cardiac arrest, 7t, 8, *8*
for resuscitation, 64t, 532t
Droperidol, for clinical anesthesia, 80
Drowning, near, 459–465
and coagulation disorders, 461–462, 464
and fluid and electrolyte disturbances, 461
pathophysiology of, 459–462
prognosis for, 464–465
treatment of, 462–464
Drug reaction, psychedelic, in poisoning cases, 457
Drug therapy, for asthma, 244t
for head injury, 284
Drug use, effect of ARF on, 150, 152t–153t
Drug withdrawal states, acute, in poisoning cases, 457
Drugs, cardiac, pathophysiologic changes induced by, 213
use of, for resuscitation, 63–65, 64t
Duck embryo vaccine (DEV), 468
Dunking burn, 426
Duodenal hematoma, intramural, 431
Dysplasia, bronchopulmonary, 242–243

Ear, foreign bodies in, 484
lacerations of, 296
Eastern coral snake, 474
Edema, cerebral, following head injury, 282
in poisoning cases, 456
conjunctival, 307, *308*
definition of, 105
fluid and electrolyte management in, 105–107
pathogenesis of, 105t
primary (initiating) factors in, 105–106
secondary (amplifying) factors in, 106
treatment of, 106–107
Edrophonium, for clinical anesthesia, 83
Ehlers-Danlos syndrome, 220
Elapid envenomation, 476t, 479
Elapidae family, 474
Elbow, fractures and dislocations of, 367–376
radiographic evaluation of, 170–173, *171–172*
Electrical injury, 418
Electrocardiogram, of ICU patient, 116
Electrocardiographic abnormalities, head injuries and, 207
Electrolyte balance, in ICU patients, 122
Electrolyte disturbances, cystic fibrosis and, 247
near drowing and, 461
Electrolyte imbalance, in TPN, 135t, 136
Electrolyte management, 98–112
special problems in, 102–111
Electrolyte reqiurements, daily, 100t
Electrolyte therapy, in ARF, 143–144
in chronic renal disease, 237
Electrolyte tolerance limits, effect of renal disease on, 233–234, *234*, 234t
normal, 233
Electrolytes, TPN infusion of, 132t, 133
Emergency custody, in abuse cases, 433
Emergency department, care of injured child in, 524–533
equipment of, 525–527, 526t
training of personnel for, 525
Emergency medical technicians–ambulance (EMT-A), 517
Emergency medical technicians–paramedics (EMT-P), 517
Emphysema, subcutaneous, 256, *257*
Enamel, tooth, fractures of, 318–319, *319–320*
Encephalopathy, hyponatremia and, 103
hypoxic ischemic, 459–460
in hemodialysis patients, 156
End-expiratory carbon dioxide partial pressure (Eco_2), 120
Endocarditis, bacterial, 214
Endocrine disease, injuries to children with, 226–232
Endotracheal intubation, 4–5, 7t, 58–60, 58t, *59*, 59t

Endotracheal intubation (*Continued*)
indications for, 58
Endotracheal tube dimensions, 59t
Enflurane, 75–77, 76t
Ensure formula, 130t
Enteral alimentation, 129–131, 130t
in ARF, 149t
Envenomation, antivenin for, 454t, 480–482
clinical classification of, 475–476, 476t
crotalid, classification and treatment of, 476t
field treatment of, 477–478
hospital care of, 478–479
elapid, classification of, 476t
subacute phase of, 482–483
Epicondyle, medial. See *Medial epicondyle*
Epiglottitis, 487
Epinephrine, for asthma, 243, 244t
for brachial plexus block, 88
for cardiac arrest, 7, 7t
for hymenoptera stings, 473
for resuscitation, 64t, 532t
Epiphyseal plate, anatomy of, 357–358
fractures of, 166–168, *166–169*, 357–361, *358–360*
histology of, 357–358
injuries of, and growth disturbance, 360–361, *360–361*
diagnosis of, 358
healing of, 360
treatment of, 361
physiology of, 357–358
Epistaxis, factor replacement therapy for, 221
Equine bites, 469, *469*
Esophageal foreign bodies, balloon tipped catheter technique for removal of, 495–496, *496*
Esophageal gastric tube airway (EGTA), *57*
use of, during transportation, 510
Esophageal injury, radiographic evaluation of, 191
Esophageal obturator airway (EOA), 4, 54–58, *55–57*
placement of, *56*
use of, during transportation, 510
Esophagus, corrosive injury to, 266
evaluation of, following chest trauma, 266, *267*
foreign bodies in, 494–496, *496*
perforation of, 266, *267*
Ethylene glycol, antidote to, 452t
Exsanguinating hemorrhage, fluid therapy for, 14
Extensor tendon injuries, 398–399
External jugular vein cutdown, 10
Extracellular fluid (ECF), 98, *98*
Extradural hematoma, *280*, 280–281
Extraocular muscles, trauma to, 308
Extremities, movement of, following head injury, 277
of ICU patient, 123
Extremity injury, 31
evaluation of, 66
Eye injuries, 301–315
anterior segment involvement in, 310, *311–312*, 312
chemical burns and, *306*, 306–307, 306t
child abuse and, 314–315
examination of, 301–302, *302*, 302t
Eye injuries (*Continued*)
posterior segment involvement in, *312–314*, 312–315
sports-related, 314
Eyeball, injuries to, 308–309
Eyebrows, lacerations of, 295, *295*
Eyelid, lacerations of, 294–295, 303, *303*
loss of, 303

Facial fractures, 297–300, *299*
examination and diagnosis of, 297–298
treatment of, 298
Facial nerve branches, injuries to, 295–296
Facial scars, secondary repair of, 296–297
Facial slap marks, *425*
Facial trauma, 287–300
anesthesia for, 289
animal bites and, *467*, *469*
initial assessment of, 288–289, 288t
radiographic evaluation of, 183–184, *184*
Factor replacement therapy, for hemophilia, 221
Factor VIII, for hemophilia, 221
inhibitor to, 222
Falls, dental injuries caused by, 317
Fat, TPN infusion of, 132t, 133
Fat stores, 128
Fat-soluble vitamins, daily requirements of, 126t
Feeding, enteral. See *Enteral alimentation*
Femoral diaphysis, radiographic evaluation of, 177
Femoral epiphysis, injury of, 381, *381*, 386, *386*
Femoral neck, fractures of, 384–386
complications of, 385–386, *386*
treatment of, 385, *385*
Femoral shaft, fractures of, 382–384
complications of, 384, *384*
diagnosis of, *382*, 382–383
treatment of, 383–384, *383–384*
Femoral vein cannulation, 10
Femur, fractures of, 382–386, *382–386*
birth trauma and, 362–363, *363*
injuries to epiphysis of, 381, *381*, 386, *386*
Fentanyl, 78–79
Fibrillation, ventricular, 7t, 9
Fibula, radiographic evaluation of, 176
Fibular epiphysis, injury of, 378
separation of, *357*
Fick equation, 43
"Fiddler" spider bites, *471*, 471–472
Fights, dental injuries caused by, 317
Figure of eight bandage, for fractured clavicle, 377, *377*
Fingertip injuries, *402*, 403
First aid treatment, for poisonings, 448–451, 449t
Flail chest, 21–22
following chest trauma, 257–258, *258*
therapy for, 258
Flexor tendon injuries, *399*, 399–400
Fluid disturbances, cystic fibrosis and, 247
near drowning and, 461
Fluid imbalance, in TPN, 136
Fluid management, 98–112
Fluid replacement, during anesthesia, 84–87

Fluid resuscitation, post-burn, after 48 hrs, 415t, 416
during first 24 hrs, 415–416, 415t
during second 24 hrs, 415t, 416
problems during, 416
Fluid therapy, 100–102
for head injury, *274*, 275
in ARF, 143–144
in poisoning cases, 457
pathophysiologic basis for, 414–416, 415t
Fluoride, antidote to, 452t
Flurazepam, in emergency room poisoning episodes, 445t
Fly bites, 473
Folic acid, daily requirements of, 126t
Fontan operation, 210
Foot, fractures of, 377–378
radiographic evaluation of, 173–175, *174–175*
Forearm, radiographic evaluation of, 170, *170*
Foreign bodies, 484–497
corneal abrasion and, 308–309, *309*
protruding from brain, 282, *282*
Formulas, enteral hyperalimentation, 130t
Fractures. See also specific types
complications of, differences in, 356
diagnostic problems in, 354
estimating age of, 428–429, *429–430*
healing of, 354
incidence of, 353
indicating child abuse, 429–430, *430*
preventing damage to, 513
radiographic appearance of, 164–165, *165–167*
site-specific, 363–388
special features of, 353–357
special types of, 357–363
treatment of, 33–34, 356–357
types of, *161–162*, *164–169*, 165–168
Fresh frozen plasma, 47
Frog leg position, for genital examination, *440*
Fructosemia, 230
Fundus examination, following head injury, 276–277
Furosemide, for ARPF, 142–143
for edema, 106–107
for neurologic injury, 26, 26t
for resuscitation, 64t, 532t

Galactosemia, 230
Gallamine, for clinical anesthesia, 82
Gardner-Wells tongs, *27*
Gas flow rates, 54, 55t
Gasoline burns, of hand, *396*
Gastric evacuation, of ingested poisons, 450
Gastric intubation, 5
Gastric lavage, of ingested poisons, 450–451
Gastric pH, prior to surgery, 67–68
Gastrointestinal disease, cystic fibrosis and, 246–247
Gastrointestinal system, of ICU patients, 122
presence of foreign bodies in, 494–497
radiographic evaluation of, 193–194
General anesthesia, for facial injury, 289
General emergency department, care of injured child in, 524–533
Genital examination, of sexually abused child, *440*, 440–442
Genitalia, male, injury to, 351
Genitourinary injuries, 341–351
assessment of, 29–31, *30*
physical signs of, 329t, 343t
radiographic evaluation of, 194, *195–200*, 196–200
Gentamicin, and ARF, 152t
for cystic fibrosis, 247t
Gerota's fascia, 345, 348
Gibson's sign, 265
Glasgow Coma Scale (GCS), 25, 25t, 121, 284, *284*, 512–513
Glass, ingestion of, 495
Globe, injuries to, 308–310
Glomerular disease, 233, 234t
clinical findings of, 234t
laboratory features of, 235
resuscitation fluid therapy in, 236
Glomerular filtration rate (GFR), 139
decline in, 140
Glucose, TPN infusion of, 132, 132t
with insulin, for hyperkalemia, 145, 145t
Glucose abnormalities, in TPN, 135t, 136
Glycopyrrolate, prior to anesthesia, 73
prior to surgery, 67
Gold, antidote to, 453t
Gonorrhea, test for, 441
Grab marks, 424
Great vessels, chest trauma involving, 269–270
non-penetrating injuries to, 269, *269*
penetrating injuries to, 269–270
Greenstick fractures, of clavicle, 376–377
of radius and ulna, 364–365, *364–365*
Gunshot wounds, to abdomen, 336

Haemophilus influenzae, bacterial tracheitis caused by, 487
epiglottitis caused by, 487
Hair brush injuries, 425, *425*
Halothane, 74, 75–77, 76t
Hand, anatomy of, 391
radiographic evaluation of, *164*, 169
Hand injuries, 390–404
amputations for, 403–404, *404*
bony, 401
burns and, 394–398, *396–397*
care of, 391–393
compound, 392
dressings for, 394
evaluation of, 390–391
prosthesis for, 404
sling for, 394
vascular, 392, 403
Head injuries, 272–284
absence of respiratory effort after, 24
adult vs. pediatric patient with, 272
assessment of, 23–27, 25t, 26t
burr holes in treatment of, 284
child abuse and, 427–428
diuretics for, 284
effects of, on cardiovascular system, 206–207
fixed, dilated pupils in, 24
fluid therapy for, *274*, 275
hemorrhage in, 24
history of, 23–24
initial approach to, 273, *274*, 275
initial treatment of, 282–283, 283t
mild, evaluation of, 278, 278t
mini-neurologic examination in, 275–277

Head injuries (*Continued*)
moderate to severe, CT scans for, 280
evaluation of, 278–280
laboratory tests for, 278–279
skull radiographs for, 279–280
oxygenation, ventilation and perfusion in, 24
phases of, 272
preventing deterioration of, 512–513
severe, antibiotic therapy for, 283
treatment of, 282–284, 283t, 284t
steroids for, 284
trauma scoring in, 284, *284*
treatment of, 25–27, 26t, 282–284
Heart, chest trauma affecting, 266, 268
non-penetrating injuries to, 266, 268
penetrating injuries to, 268
Heart murmur, unexplained, 213–214
Heavy metals, antidote to, 453t
Heimlich manuever, 4
in choking child, 489–490, *490*
Hematocrit values, following shock, 14
Hematoma, duodenal, intramural, 431
intracranial, 280–281, *280–281*
pulmonary, 190–191, 263
Hemodialysis, 238–239
complications of, 156
general principles of, 155
procedure for, 155–156
Hemoperfusion, to eliminate absorbed poison, 455
Hemopericardium, with tamponade, 206
Hemophilia, 221–222
factor replacement therapy for, 221
treatment of, 219t
Hemopneumothorax, *187*
Hemoptysis, cystic fibrosis and, 246
Hemorrhage. See also *Bleeding*
abdominal, 335–336, 336t
and head injury, 24
conjunctival, 307, *307*
effect of, on cardiovascular system, 207–208
exsanguinating, fluid therapy for, 14
vitreous, 312
Hemorrhagic shock, hemostatic response to, 40–42
effects of, 207–208
Hemostasis, decreasing blood loss through, 48–49
effect of trauma on, 235–236, 236t
in hemorrhagic shock, 40–42
liver function and, 222
normal, 216–217, *216–217*
Hemostatic disorders. See also *Bleeding, abnormal*
emergency treatment of, 219t
injuries to children with, 216–225
laboratory evaluation of, 218t
Hemothorax, 21
following chest trauma, 261
radiographic evaluation of, 187–188, *188*
Henoch-Schönlein purpura, 220
Heparin, TPN infusion of, 132t
Heroin/morphine, in emergency room poisoning episodes, 445t
Hetastarch, for shock resuscitation, 14
High-frequency positive pressure ventilation (HFPPV), 62
Hip, dislocation of, 386–387
complications of, 387
diagnosis of, 386, *387*
Hip (*Continued*)
dislocation of, treatment of, 386–387
fractures of, 384–387
radiographic evaluation of, *177*, 177–178
Horse bites, 469, *469*
Horse serum allergies, skin testing for, 481–482
Hospital care, for near drowning victims, 462–464
Hot water immersion burns, 426, *426*
Household agents, causing eye burns, 306t
Human bites, 293–294
to hand, 393
Human diploid cell rabies vaccine (HDCV), 468–469
Human rabies immune globulin (HRIG), 468–469
Humeral diaphysis, radiographic evaluation of, 173
Humeral epiphysis, proximal, fracture-separation of, 376, *376*
Humerus, birth fractures of, 362, *362*
lateral condylar fractures of, 370–371, *371*
supracondylar fracture of, 371–374
complications of, 374, *374*
diagnosis of, 372, *372*
pathologic anatomy of, 371–372, *372*
treatment of, 372–374, *373*
Humidification, during anesthesia, and surgery, 84
Hydralazine, for hypertension, 148t
Hydrocortisone, for asthma, 244, 244t
for bronchopulmonary dysplasia, 242
for renal disease, 238
Hydrocortisone sodium succinate (Solu-Cortef), for adrenal disease, 231
Hymenoptera stings, 472–473, *473*
Hyperemia, cerebral, 282
Hyperkalemia, 144–145
causes of, 109t
drug treatment of, 145t
electrocardiographic changes seen in, *144*
fluid and electrolyte management in, 109–110
therapy for, 109–110, 110t
Hypernatremia, causes of, 104t
fluid and electrolyte management in, 104–105
Hyperphosphatemia, in ARF, 146
Hypertension, 147
head injuries and, 206–207
medications for, 148t
Hyperthyroidism, 231
Hyperuricemia, 147
Hyperventilation, neurogenic, central, 277
Hyphema, traumatic, 310, *311*
Hypocalcemia, in ARF, 146–147
Hypochlorites, antidote to, 453t
Hypoglycemia, 229–230
Hypokalemia, causes of, 110t
fluid and electrolyte management in, 110–111
potassium for, 237
Hyponatremia, ADH and, 103
causes of, 103t
encephalopathy and, 103
fluid and electrolyte management in, 102–104
sodium concentration and, 103–104
treatment of, 103

Hypotension, blood loss and, 13
  in poisoning cases, 456
Hypothermia, in near drowning victims, 463
  prevention of, during transportation, 513
Hypothyroidism, 230–231
Hypovolemic shock, causes of, 39t
  development of, 40–42
  management of, 39–49
Hypoxemia, pathophysiology of, 241–242
Hypoxia, in trauma victims, 40
Hypoxic ischemic encephalopathy, 459–460

Iatrogenic injuries, 411–412
Idiopathic thrombocytopenic purpura, 219t
Immersion burns, hot water, 426, *426*
Immersion hypothermia, 460–461
Immune system, malnutrition and, 128–129
Implosion effect, of pulmonary contusion, 262
Incest, definition of, 435
Incomplete apposition, spontaneous correction of, 354, *355*
Incomplete fracture, *161*, *164–165*, 165–166, *172*
Increased intracranial pressure, in near drowning victims, 463–464
Indecent liberties, definition of, 435
Inertial effect, of pulmonary contusion, 262
Infant, cardiac compressions for, 63, *63*
  DC countershock in, 7t, 9
  gross motor development in, 424t
  indications for thoracotomy in, 255–256
  minimum daily protein requirements for, 148
  respiratory system of, 53
  urine output in, 13
  vascular injuries in, 406
  Weech mnemonics for, 64t
Infantile cortical hyperostosis, 432
Infection, cystic fibrosis and susceptibility to, 247, 247t
  dental injuries and, 326–327
  in ICU patient, 122–123
  in TPN catheter-related hazards, 134–135, 134t
Infectious airway obstructive disease, 485–487
Infusate composition, for TPN, 132–133, 132t
Infusion feeding, 130
Ingestion exposure, to poisons, 450–451
Inhalation agents, 74–77, 76t
  comparison of, 76t
Inhalation exposure, to poisons, 450
Inhalation injury, 417–418
Inherited clotting factor deficiencies, 221–222
Injury. See *Trauma* and *Trauma patient*
Inspired oxygen concentration monitoring, 69
Insulin therapy, protocol for, 228t
Intensive care monitoring, 113–123
  invasive, and therapy, 123
  medications and, 123
  systems approach to, 113–115, *114–115*
  team concept of, 115–116
Interhospital transfer, 519–520
Intermittent positive pressure breathing (IPPB), following surgery, 90
Internal pneumatic stabilization, for flail chest, 258
Intestines, blunt injury to, 338
  foreign bodies in, 496–497
Intra-abdominal injuries, child abuse and, 431
Intra-arterial blood gases, 72
Intracardiac injection, 8
Intracardiac septal rupture, 268
Intracellular fluid (ICF), 98, *98*
Intracerebral hematoma, 281, *281*
Intracranial hematoma, 280–281, *280–281*
Intracranial injuries, child abuse and, 428
  types of, 280–282
Intracranial pressure (ICP), control of, 65–66
  increased, in near drowning victims, 463–464
Intramural duodenal hematoma, 431
Intraocular foreign bodies, 313–314, *314*
Intraocular pressure (IOP), during anesthesia, 87
Intraorbital foreign bodies, 314
Intraosseous fluid infusion, 11–12
  advantages of, 11–12
Intrathoracic foreign bodies, 262
Intravenous access, in TPN, 131, *131*
Intravenous agents, 77–81
Intravenous line(s), failure to secure, 74
  placement of, 63
Intravenous line equipment, 527, *527*, *528–529*
Intubation equipment, 58t
Invasive hemodynamic monitoring, of anesthetized patient, 70–71
Invasive monitoring, and therapy, for ICU patients, 123
Iodine, daily requirements of, 126t
Iron, antidote to, 453t
  daily requirements of, 126t
  TPN infusion of, 132t
Isocal formula, 130t
Isoetharine, for asthma, 244t
Isoflurane, 75–77, 76t
Isoniazid, antidote to, 453t
Isoproterenol, for asthma, 244t
  for cardiac arrest, 7t, 8, *8*
  for resuscitation, 64t, 532t

Juvenile diabetes. See *Diabetes mellitus*

Kanamycin, and ARF, 152t
Kayexalate, for hyperkalemia, 109–110, 110t, 144–145, 145t
Ketamine, 73
  for clinical anesthesia, 80–81
Ketotic hypoglycemia, 229
Kidney, autoregulation of, 139
  effect of morphine on, 78
  injuries to. See *Renal injuries*
  radiographic evaluation of, 194, *195–198*, 196–197
Kidney disease. See *Acute renal failure; Chronic renal disease*
Kirschner wires, for extensor tendon injuries, 398
Knee. See also *Patella*
  injuries to, 380–384
  internal derangements of, 382
  radiographic evaluation of, 176–177
Knee-chest position, for genital examination, *440*

Laboratory monitoring, of anesthetized patient, 72
Laboratory tests, for head injury, 278–279

Lacerations, pulmonary, *263*, 263–264
renal, 345, *347*, 348
surgical care of, 289–296
Large-bore intravenous catheterization, 62
Laryngeal axes, schematic drawing of, *59*
Laryngeal foreign bodies, 488–492
Laryngeal obstruction, 491t
Laryngotracheitis (croup), 486–487
clinical scoring of, 486t
Lateral condyle, of humerus, fractures of, 370-371, *371*
Latrodectus bites, *470*, 470–471
Law enforcement protocols, in abuse cases, 433, 435–437
Lazarus-Nelson technique, for peritoneal lavage, *334*
Lead, antidote to, 453t
Lens, trauma to, 310, 312, *312*
Lidocaine, for brachial plexus block, 88
for cardiac arrest, 7t, 9
for Loxosceles bites, 472
for resuscitation, 64t, 532t
for skin injury, 393
for ventricular tachycardia, 212
in pediatric emergencies, 533
Life support, in poisoning cases, 455
Ligament injuries, to hand, 392, 402
Ligaments, torn, incidence of, 357, *357*
Linear skull fracture, *182*, 182–183
Lipid abnormalities, in TPN patients, 135t, 136–137
Lipids, TPN infusion of, 132t, 133
Lips, lacerations of, 295
Liver, of ICU patient, 122
radiographic evaluation of, 192, *193*
Liver disease, treatment of, 219t
Liver dysfunction, in TPN patients, 135t, 137
Liver function, hemostasis and, 222
Local anesthesia, for facial injury, 289
Loop marks, 425, *425*
Loxosceles bites, *471*, 471–472
Loxosceles reclusa, 471
Lung disease, chronic, injuries to children with, 241–248
Lungs, bruised, 190, *190*
chest trauma and, 262–264
Lye, and esophageal corrosive injury, 266

Magnesium, daily requirements of, 126t
TPN infusion of, 132t
Maintenance fluids, 100–101, 100t, 101t
administration of, 102
daily requirements of, 100t
in chronic renal disease, 237
selection of, 102
Male external genitalia, injury to, 351
Malignant brain edema, 272–273
syndrome of, 272, 282
Malnutrition, and immune system, 128–129
Malunion, in supracondylar fracture of humerus, 374
spontaneous correction of, 354, *354–356*
Mandibular fractures, *299*, 299–300
Mannitol, for ARPF, 142
for intracranial pressure, 464
for neurologic injury, 26, 26t
for poison treatment, 454
for resuscitation, 64t, 532t
Marcus-Gunn pupil, 301
Marijuana, in emergency room poisoning episodes, 445t
Masks, 58t
oxygen administration by, 73
Maxilla, fractures of, 299, *299*
MCT oil, 130t
and enteral alimentation in ARF, 149t
Medial epicondyle, avulsion of, 369–370, *370*
complications of, 369–370
treatment of, 369, *370*
Medical control, of transportation system, 514–515
Medical facility care, for sexually abused child, 437–443
Medical records, in abuse cases, 433
Medications, emergency, for cardiac arrest, 7t
for ICU patients, 123
for renal disease, 237–238
preoperative, 66–68
renal failure and, 238
Menke's syndrome, 201
Meperidine (Demerol), 70
and ARF, 152t
for Latrodectus bites, 470–471
pediatric cocktail, 533t
Mercury, antidote to, 453t
Metabolic acidosis, 145–146
causes of, 107t
fluid and electrolyte management in, 107–108
Metabolic alkalosis, causes of, 109t
fluid and electrolyte management in, 108–109
Metabolic complications, of peritoneal dialysis, 154–155
of TPN, 135–137, 135t
Metabolic disease, injuries to children with, 226–232
Metabolic-nutritional system, 122
Metaphyseal avulsion fractures, 200, *201*
Metaphyseal corner fractures, 200, *201*
Metaphyseal fractures, of long bones, 429–430, *430*
Metaproterenol, for asthma, 244t
Metatarsals, fractures of, 377–378
Methadone, in emergency room poisoning episodes, 445t
Methanol, antidote to, 453t
Methaqualone, in emergency room poisoning episodes, 445t
Methemoglobinemic agents, antidote to, 453t
Methicillin, and ARF, 153t
for head injury, 283
for neurologic injury, 26t, 27
Methyldopa, for hypertension, 148t
Methylprednisolone (Solu-Medrol), for hemorrhagic shock, 208
for hymenoptera stings, 473
for Loxosceles bites, 471
for resuscitation, 532t
Metoclopramide, for enteral feeding, 129
Metocurine, for clinical anesthesia, 82
Micrurus fulvius, 474
Military anti-shock trousers (MAST), 9
during transportation, 510
for restoring circulatory volume, 45
for shock resuscitation, 16
indications for, 511t
Mineral imbalance, in TPN, 135t, 136
Mineral requirements, daily, 126–127, 126t
TPN infusion of, 132t, 133

Mini-heurologic examination, 24–25, 25t
Minimal alveolar concentration (MAC), 75
Minor trauma, anesthesia for, 87–89
Minoxidil, for hypertension, 148t
Modified Injury Severity Scale (MISS), 284, *284*
Mongolian spots, 431–432
Monitoring, of surgical patient, 68–72, 69t, 70t, 71t
Monteggia's fracture-dislocation, 170, *170*, 367, *367*
Morphine, 77–78
  and ARF, 152t
  for Latrodectus bites, 471
  for resuscitation, 532t
  hemodynamic effects of, 78
  preoperative use of, 67
  renal effects of, 78
Motor development, in infants and toddlers, 424t
Mouth-to-mouth ventilation, 4
Moxalactum (Moxam), and ARF, 153t
Mucous membrane bleeding, factor replacement therapy for, 221
Multiple fractures, of different ages, 429
Multisystem trauma, evaluation and treatment of, 52–53
Muscle relaxants, 81–83
Musculoskeletal injuries, 353–388
  evaluation of, 31–33
    radiographic, *162*, *164–167*
Myocardial contusion, 205–206, 268
  management of, 206
Myocardial rupture, 268

Nafcillin, and ARF, 153t
  for cystic fibrosis, 247t
Nail injuries, 392, 402–403
Naloxone, for resuscitation, 64t, 532t
Narcotics, 77–79
  and ARF, 152t
  antidote to, 453t
  in anesthetics, 77–79
Nasal fractures, *298*, 298–299
Nasal intubation, *60*, 60–62
  supplemental oxygen during, *60–61*
Nasal septal injury, 298
Nasal tube insertion, 4
Naso-orbital-ethmoid region, fractures of, 299, *299*
Nasogastric (NG) tube, stomach evacuation with, 73–74
Nasotracheal intubation, 60–61
"Natriuretic factor," 99
Neck injury, assessment of, 27, *27*
Needle aspiration, in tension pneumothorax, 20
Needle cricothyroidotomy, 5, *6*, 491
Needle pericardiocentesis, 22–23, *23*
Neonate, respiratory system of, 53
Neoplastic disorders, injury and, 223–225, *224*
Neostigmine, antidote to, 452t
  for clinical anesthesia, 83
Neurogenic hyperventilation, central, 277
Neurogenic pulmonary edema, head injuries and, 207
Neurologic injury, assessment of, 23–27
  history of, 23–24
  to hand, 400–401
  treatment of, 25–27, 26t
Neurologic-psychologic system, intensive care monitoring of, 121
Neutral protamine Hagedorn (NPH) insulin, 226–227
Newborn, birth fractures in, 361–363
  respiratory system of, 53
Niacin, daily requirements of, 126t
Nitrites, antidote to, 453t
Nitrobenzene, antidote to, 453t
Nitrogen balance, effect of trauma on, 127t
Nitrous oxide (N_2O), 75
  in pediatric emergencies, 530
Non-narcotics, for clinical anesthesia, 79–81
"Nonrebreathing systems," 54
Nondepolarizing muscle relaxants, 82–83
Nonketotic hypoglycemia, 229
Nontoxic ingestion, 448
Norcuron, for clinical anesthesia, 83
Nose, foreign bodies in, 484–485
  fractures of, *298*, 298–299
  lacerations of, 295
Nutrition, total parenteral. See *Total parenteral nutrition (TPN)*
Nutritional assessment, 127–129
  in monitoring therapy, 137
Nutritional management, in ARF, 148–150, 149t
Nutritional requirements, normal, 125–127, 125t
  of injured children, 127
Nutritional support, 125–138
  biochemical parameters in, 137, 137t
  necessity for, 129

Obstructive shock, 39t
Occipital fracture, Towne's view of, *182*
Ocular exposure, to poisons, 448–449, 449t
Ocular trauma. See *Eye injuries*
Odontoid fractures, 180
Olecranon fossa, 371
Opaque foreign bodies, removal of, 175
Open pneumothorax, 22
  following chest trauma, 259, *259*
Operating room, transport to, 68
Oral axes, schematic drawing of, *59*
Oral bleeding, factor replacement therapy for, 221
Oral intubation, 4–5, 61–62
Orbit, injuries to, 304
Organic acidemias, 232
Organophosphates, antidote to, 452t
Os calcis, fractures of, 378
Osmolar monitoring, 102
Osmolite formula, 130t
Otorrhea, following head injury, 277
Oxacillin, and ARF, 153t
Oxalate, antidote to, 453t
Oxygen, supplemental, during nasal intubation, *60–61*
Oxygen delivery, by mask, 75
  flow rates for, 54, 55t
  following shock, 16–17, 45–48
  for asthma, 244t
Oxygen-powered resuscitator, 55, *56*
Oxygenation, in cyanotic congenital heart disease, 208–209
  in head injury, 24
  of trauma patient, 54–56, *55–56*, 55t

Palpation, of abdomen, 331
Pancreas, of ICU patient, 122
radiographic evaluation of, 194
Pancreatic trauma, 338
child abuse and, 431
Pancuronium bromide (Pavulon), 74
as muscle relaxant, 73
for clinical anesthesia, 82
for controlling ICP, 66
Pantothenic acid, daily requirements of, 126t
Paracentesis, findings of, 334–335
site for, *333*
technique of, 333, *334*
Paraldehyde, and ARF, 152t
Parents, in child abuse cases, reaction of, 423
supporting, 434
Partial airway obstruction, *488*, 488–489
Partial breathing systems, 54, *55*
Partial thromboplastin time (PPT), 217
Patella. See also *Knee*
dislocation of, 381–382, *382*
complications of, 382, *382*
diagnosis of, 381–382
treatment of, 382
fractures of, 177
Patent airway, maintenance of, *56–57*, 56–62, 58t, *59–61*, 59t
Pathologic fracture, 168
PCP/PCP combinations, in emergency room poisoning episodes, 445t
Pediatric cocktails, 533t
Pediatric emergencies, equipment for, 525–527, 526t
examination and treatment of, 527, 530, *530*
sedation and anesthesia in, 530, 533, 533t
therapy in, 530, 532t
training for, 525
Pediatric endotracheal tube dimensions, 59t
Pediatric genital examination, frog leg position for, *440*
knee-chest position for, *440*
Pediatric intensive care unit, 505
Pediatric resuscitation medications, 532t
Pediatric surgical operating room, 505
Pediatric trauma center, 501–506
Pelvic trauma, evaluation of, 332t
Pelvis, "bucket-handle" fracture of, 388
examination of, 331
fractures of, 387–388
diagnosis of, 387
treatment of, 388
vascular injury associated with, 409–410
radiographic evaluation of, *177*, 177–178
stable fractures of, 388
straddle injury of, 388
unstable fractures of, 388
Penetrating trauma, and abdominal injuries, 329
Penetrating wounds, 293
Penicillin, and ARF, 153t
Penis, injury to, 351
Pentazocine, in emergency room poisoning episodes, 445t
Percutaneous central venous cannulation, 9–10
Percutaneous peripheral vein cannulation, 9
alternatives to, 9–10
Percutaneous suprapubic catheterization, bladder decompression by, 30, *30*
Perfusion, and head injury, 24
Pericardial tamponade, 22–23
needle pericardiocentesis for, 22–23, *23*
Perineum, examination of, 331
Periosteum, 353, *353*
Peripheral angiocatheter, *528*
Peripheral nerve injury, in supracondylar fracture of humerus, 374
Peripheral vascular compromise, burns and, 416–417
Peripheral vascular injuries, 410
Peripheral venous cutdown, 10, *11*
Peritoneal dialysis, 151, 154–155, 239–240
complications of, 154–155
general principles of, 151
procedure for, 151, 154
Peritoneal lavage, 29
and abdominal injuries, *333–334*, 333–335, 333t
complications of, 335
findings of, 334–335
indications for, 333t
Lazarus-Nelson technique for, 333, *334*
site for, *333*
Peritonitis, 155
pH, elevated, alkalosis and, 108–109
gastric, prior to surgery, 67–68
low, acidosis and, 107–108
Pharyngeal axes, schematic drawing of, *59*
Phenobarbital, and ARF, 152t
for resuscitation, 532t
in emergency room poisoning episodes, 445t
Phenothiazines, antidote to, 453t
Phenylephrine, use of, before nasal intubation, 60
Phenytoin (Dilantin), and ARF, 152t
for resuscitation, 532t
for seizures, 283
Phosgene, antidote to, 453t
Phosphorus, daily requirements of, 126t
TPN infusion of, 132t
Phosphorus balance, in ARF, 146
Photography, in abuse cases, 433
Physical examination, following injury, 18–34
Physostigmine, antidote to, 452t
Pinch marks, 424
"Ping-pong" fracture, 183
Piperacillin, and ARF, 153t
Pit vipers, 474
Plantar responses, following head injury, 277
Plasma, fresh frozen, 47
Plasma coagulation factors, biologic half-lives of, 222t
Plasma colloid concentration, edema and, 105–106
Plasma colloid osmotic pressure (PCOP), pulmonary edema and, 44
Plastic bowing, of long bones, 166, *166*
Platelet disorders, management of, 218–221, 219t
Platelets, for shock therapy, 47
Pleural space, thoracic trauma and, 260–262
Pneumocephalus, *281*, 281–282
Pneumomediastinum, radiographic evaluation of, 186–187, *187*
Pneumothorax, 21
cystic fibrosis and, 245–246
radiographic evaluation of, 186, *186*
Poison(s), 444, 446–448, *446*, 447t, 448t
absorbed, elimination of, *454*, 454–455
Poisoned patients, referral of, 457
Poisoning, 444–458
adolescent and adult, common drugs in, 445t

Poisoning (*Continued*)
age predisposition to, 444t
antidotal therapy for, 451, 451t, 452t–454t, 454
classification of, by mode of exposure, 446t
evaluation of, 444, 446–448
first aid procedures in, 448–451, 449t
general management of, 448–457
in children under 5, 445t
rating scales for severity of symptoms in, 447t
Poisoning history, key questions in obtaining, *446*
Polycose formula, 130t
Polycose liquid, and enteral alimentation in ARF, 149t
Positive end expiratory pressure (PEEP), 89–91
Post-traumatic renal failure, 139–159
Postrenal failure, 141
Postrenal transplant patient, 240
Potassium, for hypokalemia, 110–111, 237
TPN infusion of, 132t
Potassium tolerance limits, 233
Prazosin, for hypertension, 148t
Pre-renal (functional) failure, 140
Prealbumin levels, 128
Preanesthetic treatment, and stabilization, 53–66
Prednisone, for asthma, 244t
for serum sickness, 482
for thrombocytopenia, 219t, 220
Pregnancy, prophylaxis against, 442
Preload, cardiac disease and, 207
cardiac lesions requiring, 209–211
Preoperative medications, 66–68
Prerenal azotemia, 140–141, 141t
Primary survey, and resuscitative measures, 2–18
Primary tooth, replanting of, 325–326
Probenecid, for venereal disease, 442
Procaine penicillin, for venereal disease, 442
Promethazine (Phenergan), 533t
Propoxyphene, in emergency room poisoning episodes, 445t
Propranolol, for resuscitation, 532t
Prosthesis, for hand injuries, 404
Protein, 125–126
requirements of, in infants and adolescents, 148
in injured children, 127
normal, 125–126
TPN infusion of, 132, 132t
problems associated with, 135t, 136
Protein malnutrition, and immune system, 128–129
Protein stores, 128
Prothrombin time (PT), 217
Pseudomonas aeruginosa, cystic fibrosis and, 247
Psychedelic drug reaction, in poisoning cases, 457
Psychiatric evaluation, of suicidal patients, 458
Psychosocial history, in abuse cases, 423
Pulled elbow, clinical features of, 367–368
diagnosis of, 388
pathologic anatomy of, *368*,
treatment of, 368
Pulmonary artery catheterization, 14, 119, 119t
Pulmonary contusion, following chest trauma, *262*, 262–263
radiographic evaluation of, 190, *190*
Pulmonary disease, cystic fibrosis and, 245–246
Pulmonary edema, neurogenic, head injuries and, 207
PCOP and, 44
Pulmonary hematoma, 190–191, 263
Pulmonary hemorrhage, cystic fibrosis and, 246
Pulmonary injury, radiographic evaluation of, 186–191, *186–191*
Pulmonary laceration, *263*, 263–264
radiographic evaluation of, 190–191, *190–191*
Pulmonary shunt, for ICU patients, 120–121
Pulmonary support, for near drowning victims, 462
Pulmonary system, in freshwater or saltwater submersion, 459
Pulp, tooth, fractures of, 318–319, *319–320*
Pulse, following head injury, 277
Pupils, asymmetry of, 302t
examination of, after head injury, 276
fixed, dilated, 24
Pyridostigmine, antidote to, 452t
for clinical anesthesia, 83

Quaternary ammonium compounds, antidote to, 453t

Rabid wound, treatment of, 294t
Rabies, diagnosis of, 467–468
epidemiology of, 466–467
treatment for, 468–469
"Raccoon eye," 279
Racemic epinephrine, for croup, 486
Radial epiphysis, fracture-separation of, *363*, 363–364, 368–369, *369*
Radial head, subluxation of, 432
Radiographic evaluation, of abdominal trauma, 192–194, *193*
of ankle, 175–176
of aortic laceration, 191–192
of atelectasis, 191
of battered child syndrome, 200–201, *201*
of bladder, 198–199, *199*
of chylothorax, 188, *189*
of clavicle, 173, *174*
of diaphragmatic injury, 192
of elbow, 170–173, *171–172*
of esophageal injury, 191
of facial trauma, 183–184, *184*
of femoral diaphysis, 177
of fibula, 176
of foot, 173–175, *174–175*
of gastrointestinal tract, 193–194
of genitourinary trauma, 194, *195–200*, 196–200
of hand, *164*, 169
of hemothorax, 187–188, *188*
of hips, *177*, 177–178
of humeral diaphysis, 173
of injured child, 160–202
of kidney, 194, *195–198*, 196–197
for injury, 343–344
of knee, 176–177
of liver, 192, *193*
of mid forearm, 170, *170*
of musculoskeletal trauma, *162*, *164–167*
of pancreas, 194

Radiographic evaluation (*Continued*)
of pelvis, *177*, 177–178
of pneumomediastinum, 186–187, *187*
of pneumothorax, 186, *186*
of pulmonary injuries, 186–191, *186–191*
of shoulder, 173
of skull, 180–182, *182*
of spine, *178–179*, 178–180
of spleen, 192–193, *193*
of thoracic trauma, 184–185, *185*
of tibia, 176, *176*
of tracheobronchial injury, 188, 190
of ureter, 197–198, *198*
of urethra, 199–200, *200*
of wrist and distal forearm, 170
site-specific, 160–161, *160–161*, 169–182, *170–172, 174–179, 182*
Radius, fractures of, 364–365, *364*, *365*, 367, *367*
Rape, definition of, 435
Rape kit, 439
Rapid-sequence intubation, of anesthesia, 72–73
Rattlesnakes, 474
Records, of transportation systems, 519
Rectum, examination of, 331, 332t
Red blood cells, 47
disorders of, 223
Refractory shock, 336t
Regional anesthesia, 87–89
Regional evaluation, in secondary survey, 18–34
Regional pediatric trauma centers, 501–506
Renal abnormalities, in near drowning victims, 464
Renal contusion, 345, *347*
radiographic evaluation of, 194, *195*
Renal disease, chronic. See *Chronic renal disease*
Renal failure, acute. See *Acute renal failure*
Renal function, effects of trauma on, 235, 236t
evaluation of, 66
normal, 139
Renal injuries, 30, 341–345
cause of, 341–345
classification of, 345–351
conservative vs. surgical therapy for, 344–345
CT evaluation of, 344
diagnosis of, *342*, 342–344, 343t
history of, *342*, 342–343
management of, 343t
physical examination for, 343, 343t
radiographic studies for, 343–344
urinalysis for, 343
Renal laceration, 345, *347*, 348
burst or shattered type of, *346*, 348
CT scanning of, *196–197*
radiographic evaluation of, 194, *195*
Renal response, to shock, 139
Renal system, near drowing and, 461
Renal system fluid intake and output, and electrolyte balance, in ICU patients, 122
Renal vascular injury, 348–349, *349*
Reptile bites, 470
Respiration, following head injury, 277
maintenance of, during surgery, 83–84
Respiratory acidosis, causes of, 107t
fluid and electrolyte management in, 107
Respiratory alkalosis, causes of, 108t
fluid and electrolyte management in, 108
Respiratory effort, absence of, head injury and, 24
Respiratory failure, in poisoning cases, 456
Respiratory pathophysiology, 241–242
Respiratory rates, normal, 273, 276t
Respiratory system, intensive care monitoring of, 119–121
preanesthetic treatment and stabilization of, 53–62, 55t, *55–57*, 58t, 59t, *59–61*
Resuscitation, use of drugs and fluids for, 63–65, 64t
Resuscitation fluid therapy, in chronic renal disease, 236–237
Resuscitative measures, primary survey and, 2–18
Resuscitive equipment, pediatric, 525–526, 526t
Retina, contusion edema of, 312, *312–313*
traumatic detachment of, 313
Retinitis sclopetaria, 313, *313*
Retroperitoneal trauma, diagnostic studies for evaluation of, 332t
Reversal agents, 83
Rhinorrhea, following head injury, 277
Rib fractures, 185, 257, *257*
Riboflavin, daily requirements of, 126t
Ringer's solution, for cardiac arrest, 6
for head injury, 275
for hemorrhage, 335
for peritoneal lavage, 333
for shock resuscitation, 14–16, *15*
Root fractures, 320, *320*
Routine monitoring, of anesthetized patient, 68–69, 69t
Rule of six method, for dopamine and isoproterenol infusions, 8, *8*

S-29, and enteral alimentation in ARF, 149t
Safety pins, ingestion of, 495
Salt solution, for head injury, 275
Salter-Harris classification, of epiphyseal growth plate injuries, 166–168, *166–168*
Saphenous vein cutdown, 10, *11*
Scalp injuries, child abuse and, 427
Scalp lacerations, 296
Scar maturation, 292
Schönlein-Henoch purpura, 220
Scleral lacerations, 310, *310*, *311*
use of protective shield following, *311*
Scorpion stings, 472, *472*
Scrotum, injury to, 351
Seconal, in pediatric emergencies, 530
Sedation, for facial injury, 289
in pediatric emergencies, 530, 533, 533t
Sedatives, and ARF, 152t
Seizures, 283
in poisoning cases, 456
Sellick maneuver, 73
Serum albumin levels, 128
Serum creatinine concentration, renal disease and, 235
Serum glucose monitoring, 122
Serum potassium concentration, elevated, 109
measurement of, 109
Serum sickness, 482
Serum sodium concentration abnormalities, 146
Sexual abuse, 435–443
definition of, 435
psychologic effects of, 442–443

Shock, 12–18, *15*, *18*. See also specific types
blood loss and, 13, 40–42, 207–208
classification and causes of, 39t
definition of, 12, 39
effect of, on cardiovascular surgery, 207–208
in pediatric patient, 42–43
laboratory indicators of, 14
pathophysiology of, 39–40
progressing, clinical indicators of, 13
recognition of, 12–13
renal response to, 139
treatment of, 14–18, *15*, *18*, 43–49
during transportation, 510–511, 511t
urine output and, 13
Shoulder, fractures of, 376–377, *376–377*
radiographic evaluation of, 173
Silver, antidote to, 453t
Similac, and enteral alimentation in ARF, 149t
Sinus bradycardia, head injuries and, 206
Sinus tachycardia, head injuries and, 207
Skeletal injuries, child abuse and, 428–431
evaluation of, 31–33
Skeletal surveys, 430–431
Skin, of ICU patient, 123
Skin injury, 31, 393–394, *394*
child abuse and, 424–427, 424t, *425–427*
Skin testing, for horse serum allergies, 481–482
Skull, radiographic evaluation of, 180–182, *182*
for severe head injury, 279–280
indications for, 278t
Skull fractures, classification of, 279–280
location of, 279
types of, 182–183, *182–183*
Skull injuries, child abuse and, 427–428
Slap marks, 424–425, *425*
SMA, and enteral alimentation in ARF, 149t
Snake venom, 474–475
Snakebites, 473–476
clinical symptoms of, 475
management of, 476–483
"Sniffing" position, 3, *3*
Sodium, TPN infusion of, 132t
Sodium bicarbonate, for cardiac arrest, 7, 7t
for hyperkalemia, 145, 145t
for resuscitation, 64t, 532t
for shock, 16
for urine alkalization, 454
Sodium nitroprusside, for hypertension, 148t
for resuscitation, 64t, 532t
Sodium tolerance limits, 233
Soft tissue trauma, 287–300
thoracic, 185
treatment of, *32–33*, 34
Spalling effect, of pulmonary contusion, 262
Speed (amphetamine) overdose, in emergency room poisoning episodes, 445t
Spinal cord injury, 249–252
diagnosis of, 249–250
emergency management of, 249
evaluation of, 249
radiological examination of, *250–251*, 250–252
rehabilitation following, 252
resuscitation in, 249
therapy for, 252
Spinal cord lesions, anesthesia in patients with, 87
Spine, birth fractures of, 363
radiographic evaluation of, *178–179*, 178–180, *250–251*, 251
Spiral fractures, 430, *430*
Splash burns, 426, *426*
Spleen, blunt injuries to, 337–338
CT scanning of, 192–193, *193*
Splinting procedures, for evulsed teeth, *324*, 325
Sports, dental injuries caused by, 317
ocular trauma in, 314
Stab wounds, to abdomen, 336–337
Staphylococcus aureus infection, and endocarditis, 214
and peritonitis, 155
and tracheitis, 485
susceptibility to, in cystic fibrosis, 247
Staphylococcus epidermidis infection, and peritonitis, 155
in TPN patients, 134
Starling's law, 207
Status epilepticus, 283
Sternal compressions, for cardiac arrest, 7, *7t*
Sternal fractures, 185, 259
Steroid therapy, for head injury, 284
Still's murmur, 213
Stomach, foreign bodies in, 496–497, *497*
Stomach evacuation, with NG tube, 73–74
"Straddle" injury, of pelvis, 388
Subclavian vein cannulation, hazards of, 10
Subcutaneous emphysema, 256, *257*
Subdural hematoma, 281, *281*
Sublimaze, use of, prior to surgery, 67
Submersion. See also *Drowning, near*
factors determining survival time in cases of, 460–461
Succinylcholine, 73, 74
for clinical anesthesia, 81–82
"Sucking chest wound," 22
Suicidal patients, evaluation and referral of, 458
Suicide attempts, 444, 444t
Sumacal, and enteral alimentation in ARF, 149t
Supracondylar fracture, of humerus, 371–374, *371–374*
spontaneous correction of, *355*
Surgery, abdominal injuries requiring, 335t
postoperative considerations, 89–91
premedication, 66–68
preparation for, 66–68
transport to, 68
Surgical cricothyroidotomy, 491–492, *492*
Sustacal formula, 130t
Syndrome of inappropriate antidiuretic hormone (SIADH), 103, 247
Systemic lupus erythematosus, treatment of, 219t

T-connectors, pediatric, 527, *527*
"Tear drop" configuration, to bladder, 199, *199*
Temperature, following head injury, 277
Temperature alteration, in poisoning cases, 457
Temperature monitoring, of ICU patient, 116
of surgical patient, 69
Tendon injuries, 398–400, *399*
Tension pneumothorax, 20–21, 186
following chest trauma, 260–261, *261*
Tetanus immunization, *32–33*
Tetralogy of Fallot, 209, 212
Thalassemia major, medullary compensation in, *224*
Thallium, antidote to, 453t

THAM, respiratory acidosis and, 107
Thermal trauma. See *Burns*
Thiamine, daily requirements of, 126t
Thigh, injuries to, 380–384
Thiopental, 73
  for clinical anesthesia, 79
  for controlling ICP, 66
Thomas splint, 383, *383*
Thoracic cage, soft tissue injury to, 256
Thoracic trauma, 254–270
  evaluation of, 19–23, 254–256
    radiographic, 184–185, *185*
  local, effects of, 205–206
  major, examination following, 206
  mortality in, 270
  pathophysiology of, 254
  prevention of deterioration of, 511
  soft tissue injury in, 185
  specific injuries in, 256–270
  treatment of, 254–256
  unique features of, 256
Thoracolumbar spine, radiographic evaluation of, 180
Thoracotomy, early, indications for, 255–256
Throat, foreign bodies in, 485
Thrombocytopenia, 218, 219t, 220
Thromboembolic problems, in TPN catheter-related hazards, 134, 134t
Thyroid disease, 230–231
Thyroid storm, 231
Tibia, fracture of, 379–380, *380*
  radiographic evaluation of, 176, *176*
Tibial epiphysis, injury of, 378–380, *378–380*
Ticarcillin, and ARF, 153t
  for cystic fibrosis, 247t
Tissue loss, wounds with, 292–293, *293*
Tissue oxygenation, 208
  following shock, 16–17
Tobramycin, and ARF, 152t
  for cystic fibrosis, 247t
Toddler, gross motor development of, 424t
Tooth, and supporting bone, classification of injury to, 318t
  crack or crazing (infarction) of, 318, *319*
  displacement or loosening of, 321–325
  evulsed, 322–323, *324–325*, 325
    follow-up treatment of, 325, *325*
    splinting procedures for, *324*, 325
  fractures of, 318–319, *319–320*
  injuries to, 318–326. See also *Dental injuries*
  intruded, *321*, 321–322
  mobility (subluxation) of, 321
  partial extrusion of, from socket, 322, *322–323*
  primary, replanting of, 325–326
  sensitivity of, 321
Tooth socket, displacement within, 322, *323*
Topical exposure, to poisons, 449–450
Total body water (TBW), 98, *98*
Total parenteral nutrition (TPN), 131–137
  catheter-related hazards of, 134–135, 134t
  complications of, 134–137, 135t
  infusate composition for, 132–133, 132t
  initiation of, 133–134
  intravenous access in, central, 131, *131*
    peripheral, 131
  metabolic complications of, 135–137, 135t
Towne's view, of occipital fracture, *182*
Toxidromes, characteristics of, 448, 448t
Tracheitis, bacterial, 487, *488*
Tracheobronchial foreign bodies, 492–494, *493*
Tracheobronchial injury, 264
  radiographic evaluation of, 188, 190
Tracheostomy. See *Cricothyroidotomy*
Traction epiphyses, avulsion of, 361
Training, of field personnel, 516–517
Transfer considerations, burn patients and, 419
Transcapillary refill phenomenon, 40
Transcutaneous oxygen monitoring, 120
Transferrin levels, 128
Transfusion, of blood and blood components, 45
Transillumination, 293
Transport system, emergency medical technicians and, 504
Transportation, of injured child, 508–522
    by air, 520–522
    components of, 514–519
    efficiency and rapidity of, 513–514
    goals of, 509–514
    historical aspects of, 508–509
    preventing deterioration during, 511–513
Transtracheal catheter ventilation, 62
Trauma. See also specific types
  effect of, on caloric and nitrogen balance, 127t
    on cardiovascular system, 205–208
    on hemostasis, 235–236, 236t
    on renal function, 235, 236t
  history of, 18
  major, cardiac pathophysiologic abnormalities affecting, 208–213
  minor, anesthesia for, 87–89
  physical examination following, 18–34
  prior, in child abuse cases, 423
  psychologic impact of, 34–36
  regional evaluation of, 18–34
  resuscitative measures following, 2–18
  site of, radiographic evaluation of, 160–161, *160–161*
Trauma patient, 1–36
  intraoperative management of, 68–89
  postoperative considerations involving, 89–91
  preanesthetic treatment and stabilization of, 53–66
  preparation of, for surgery, 66–68
  primary survey of, 1, 2–18
  radiographic evaluation of, 160–202
  secondary survey of, 1–2, 18–34
  transportation of, 508–522
Trauma scoring, in head injury, 284, *284*
Trenchkoff catheter, 154
Tricuspid obstruction, 210
Tricyclic antidepressants, antidote to, 454t
Trocath catheter, 154
Tropicamide (Mydriacyl), for corneal abrasion, 309
d-Tubocurarine, as muscle relaxant, 73
  for clinical anesthesia, 82
Tubulointerstitial disease, 233, 234t
  clinical findings of, 234t
  laboratory features of, 235
  resuscitation fluid therapy in, 236

Ulna, fractures of, 364–365, *364*, *365*, 367, *367*
Ulnar nerve, traction injury of, 369–370
Unconscious choking child, 491–492, 491t, *492*

Unstable fractures, of radius and ulna, 365, *365*
pitfalls in treatment of, 365, *365–366*
Uremia, 148–149
treatment of, 219t
Ureter, radiographic evaluation of, 197–198, *198*
Ureteral injuries, 31, 349
Urethra, radiographic evaluation of, 199–200, *200*
Urethral injuries, 30–31, 350, *350*
Urinalysis, in renal injury, 343
Urine alkalization, sodium bicarbonate for, 454
Urine output, following shock, 13
measurement of, 71–72

Vaginal foreign bodies, 497
Vaginal injuries, 351
Vancomycin, and ARF, 153t
Vascular abnormalities, 220–221
Vascular disorders, management of, 218–221, 219t
Vascular injuries, 406–412
diagnosis of, 407–408
emergency treatment of, 408
etiology of, 407
special considerations in, 406–407
to hand, 403
Vasoconstriction, peripheral, cardiac disease and, 207
Vasomotor nephropathy, 140
Venereal disease, treatment for, 442
Venom, snake, 474–475
Venous access, 9–12, *11*
Vented esophageal tube airway (VETA), *57*, 58
Ventilation, and treatment of head injury, 24
assessment of, 3–4, 4t
bag and mask, 4
maintaining, during transportation, 510
mouth-to-mouth, 4
of trauma patient, 54
Ventilation therapy, 52–91
Ventilatory assistance, 120
Ventricular fibrillation, 7t, 9
"Vibratory" systolic murmur, 213
Vital signs, examination of, following head injury, 277
of ICU patient, 116
Vitamin(s), requirements of, daily, 126(t)
in injured children, 127
TPN infusion of, 132t, 133
Vitamin K deficiency, coagulopathies due to, 222
treatment of, 219t
Vitreous hemorrhage, 312
Vivonex formula, 130t
Volkmann's ischemia, clinical manifestations of, 384, *384*
in supracondylar fracture of humerus, 374
Volume monitoring, 101–102
Volume overload, in ARF, 146
von Willebrand's disease, 220
treatment of, 219t
Vulvar injuries, 351

Warfarin, antidote to, 454t
Water, TPN infusion of, 132t, 133
Water intake and output, representative values for, 101t
Water moccasin snake, 474
Water requirements, in ARF, 143–144
modification of, 101t
Water tolerance limits, effect of renal disease on, 233–234, *234*, 234t
normal, 233
Water-soluble vitamins, daily requirements of, 126t
Weech mnemonics, 64t
Whiplash-shaken-infant-syndrome, 428
Whole blood transfusion, for shock therapy, 47
vs. component therapy, 46–48, 46t
Wounds, closure of, 290–292, *291–292*
debridement of, 290, *290*
penetrating, 293
rabies-infected, treatment of, 294t
with tissue loss, 292–293, *293*
Wrist, fracture-separation of, 363–367
radiographic evaluation of, 170

X-rays. See *Radiographic evaluation*
Xylometazoline, use of, before nasal intubation, 60